Cajal's Neuronal Forest

Cajal's Neuronal Forest

SCIENCE AND ART

JAVIER DEFELIPE, PhD

RESEARCH PROFESSOR
CONSEJO SUPERIOR DE INVESTIGACIONES CIENTÍFICAS
INSTITUTO CAJAL
AND
LABORATORIO CAJAL DE CIRCUITOS CORTICALES
CENTRO DE TECNOLOGÍA BIOMÉDICA
UNIVERSIDAD POLITÉCNICA DE MADRID
MADRID, SPAIN

OXFORD
UNIVERSITY PRESS

OXFORD
UNIVERSITY PRESS

Oxford University Press is a department of the University of Oxford. It furthers the University's objective of excellence in research, scholarship, and education by publishing worldwide. Oxford is a registered trade mark of Oxford University Press in the UK and certain other countries.

Published in the United States of America by Oxford University Press
198 Madison Avenue, New York, NY 10016, United States of America.

Library of Congress Cataloging-in-Publication Data
Names: DeFelipe, Javier, author.
Title: Cajal's neuronal forest: science and art / by Javier DeFelipe.
Description: New York, NY: Oxford University Press, [2018] |
Includes bibliographical references and index.
Identifiers: LCCN 2017015627 | ISBN 9780190842833 (alk. paper)
Subjects: | MESH: Nervous System | Medical Illustration | Neurology—history | Pictorial Works
Classification: LCC QM451 | NLM WL 17 | DDC 611.8—dc23
LC record available at https://lccn.loc.gov/2017015627

9 8 7 6 5 4 3 2
Printed by Sheridan Books, Inc.

GOBIERNO DE ESPAÑA | MINISTERIO DE ECONOMÍA, INDUSTRIA Y COMPETITIVIDAD
FECYT FUNDACIÓN ESPAÑOLA PARA LA CIENCIA Y LA TECNOLOGÍA
FUNDACIÓN RAMÓN ARECES
GOBIERNO DE ESPAÑA | MINISTERIO DE ECONOMÍA, INDUSTRIA Y COMPETITIVIDAD
CSIC CONSEJO SUPERIOR DE INVESTIGACIONES CIENTÍFICAS
FUNDACIÓN TATIANA PÉREZ DE GUZMÁN EL BUENO

To my wife, Alicia, and my daughter, Alicia, with all my love

CONTENTS

FOREWORD: PASKO RAKIC

When I was approached to write a Foreword for *Cajal's Neuronal Forest: Science and Art*, I was very busy writing my own research papers and grant applications, as well as traveling and lecturing abroad. So, I really did not look forward to additional writing obligations. However, when I examined the invitation in more detail and looked at the book transcript online, I recognized that it was an offer I could not refuse for at least three reasons.

First, the invitation to write the Foreword came from my colleague and friend Javier DeFelipe. He is a highly accomplished neuroscientist and no one else is more appropriate, more knowledgeable, and more deserving to write this book. He has devoted his life to help in our understanding of the uniqueness of the human brain, particularly the human cerebral cortex (e.g., DeFelipe, 1993; DeFelipe et al., 2002; DeFelipe, 2011). He resisted the temptation of the sophisticated and complex experimental methods that can be used only in simple animal models of the brain in order to focus on what is possible to do in humans. I was sympathetic to this cause because, in response to the question posed by Alan Alda at the 2014 Science Forum in New York City to a distinguished group of scientists including several Nobel laureates in disciplines that range from cancer research and neuroscience to nanotechnology and astrophysics—"What is the single most important question in science?—I argued that it is "understanding the brain." I met with some resistance.

"What do you mean? How about the origin of the universe?" argued one astrophysicist, citing new theories of the Big Bang and cosmic inflation.

I then asked, "Which organ did [scientists] use to make these theories?" And by the audience's reaction and the panel's subsequent responses, it seemed to me that I won that argument. And this Foreword is for a book about the brain.

My second reason for writing this Foreword is that the book about Santiago Ramón y Cajal reminded me of a New Year's Eve dinner in Long Island about one decade ago that was also attended by Nobel Laureate Marshal Nirenberg, who received the prize for breaking the genetic code. He liked to lighten such evenings with intellectual conversations and social games that involve some challenging questions. One, posed just before midnight, was: "If we learn that our planet will be inevitably and totally destroyed by a huge incoming meteor and we have only one rocket ready and capable of sending a two-pound (one-kilogram) object to a parallel universe to inform some possibly existing, and quite different, but intelligent creatures about the human beings who populated the now-extinguished planet Earth, what would you send in this rocket?" As expected, people had quite diverse ideas, such as "How about the Bible?" or "How about the painting of Mona Lisa or a transcript of Beethoven's Eighth Symphony?" Marshal, as a scientist, suggested that we should send "a DNA sequence library from the human genome resources." I commented that this would not enable these creatures to reconstruct our brain, the organ that created our civilization. They also could not read and understand the Bible regardless of the language in which it is printed. Therefore, I suggested we send Cajal's book with his drawings of the neurons. I argued that, even if they could not understand Spanish, his drawings, by themselves, would give them an idea of the complexity and possible extraordinary capacity of our brain better than any other single object. Because we had already had some drinks, most people agreed.

My third reason is more private and personal. I probably would not be in science if I had not seen Cajal's book, which was available in the Belgrade Medical Library in French (*Histologie du système nerveux de l'homme & des vertébrés*). I had entered medical school on the advice of my father and was, at the time, being trained to become a physician—more specifically, a neurosurgeon. However, deep in my heart I always dreamed of becoming an artist. After seeing the drawings in Cajal's book, I recognized that it still might be possible to do both. Thus, after obtaining my MD degree, I started to work on my graduate thesis dissertation, which was illustrated by my India ink drawings (see some sixty-two of them reproduced in the chapter "Development of the Human Central Nervous System" published years later in the Haymaker and Adams reference book on *Histology and Histopathology of the Nervous System* [Sidman and Rakic, 1982]). Although I subsequently entered the field of cellular and molecular developmental neurobiology and neurogenetics (e.g., reviewed in Rakic [2007]), I always tried to illustrate my ideas with drawings. In an interview in *Nature*, I stated my opinion that "both science and art want to find some meaning or order in the larger picture of chaos" (Dove, 2005). Thus, by suggesting to send a book with Cajal's drawings into space, I thought we would inform these imaginary creatures of something about the organization of the brain that has enabled us to be both rational and artistic beings. Later, I learned there were some parallelisms, because Cajal also grew up with artistic inclinations and wanted to become an artist. We were both guided by our fathers to choose to study medicine, but we both found a way to incorporate art into our research work. I am honored and privileged to write this Foreword to a book that celebrates Cajal's unparalleled artistic achievements within the field of science.

Cajal is considered to be one of our greatest scientists, and among his numerous recognitions is the 1906 Nobel Prize for Physiology or Medicine. He was truly a Renaissance Man—not just a scientist, but also a painter, photographer, physician, bodybuilder, chess player, writer, and publisher. He is a household name among scientists in all disciplines, and most of them know him also as an artist. However, he is less well known by the general population as an artist such as Leonardo da Vinci. To remedy this void, Dr. DeFelipe has brought to life a book that contains an exquisite selection of drawings, many of them unknown even to most scientists. For those unfamiliar with the fine structure of the nervous system, a quick look at the images might seem the work of a contemporary artist with a live imagination to create intricate, whimsical patterns populated with creatures with twisted branches in a winter landscape. A beautiful selection is included with evocative images that transcend their scientific purpose and reach an artistic status. They belong on the walls of a contemporary art gallery.

Javier DeFelipe is not new to this endeavor; he has already written several popular books that connect Cajal's scientific and artistic talents. Most notably, *Cajal's Butterflies of the Soul*, published by Oxford University Press a few years ago (DeFelipe, 2009), was intended to showcase the artistic value of the drawings of pioneering neuroscientists, including Cajal, Golgi, and Nissl, to name a few. The selection of images was based not only on the scientific information they provide, but also and especially based on their beauty, proving how science can intersect with art. It is not surprising that *Butterflies of the Soul* has been the best seller at meetings of the Society for Neuroscience every year since its publication in 2009.

This current book, *Cajal's Neuronal Forest*, continues and expands the path started with *Butterflies of the Soul*, and is also divided into two parts. The first part is devoted to contextualize the work of Cajal and other early neuroscientists. It contains ample information about the techniques, scientific ideas, and controversies in neuroscience at the turn of the nineteenth century, and it is illustrated profusely with beautiful scientific drawings and pictures from the time. These early works show how different scientists had different ideas and interpretations about the structure of our most appreciated organ, and how the most prominent figures, such as Cajal, created a school of thought, and developed personal styles in drawing that make their work recognizable, sometimes unmistakably. In the same way we can pinpoint a Monet or a Van Gogh, these drawings can be recognized as a Cajal or as a Golgi. And attributing the merit to the authors is much easier than in the world of art, because there are no known forgeries in this field! The influence of the master could be such that not only the school of thought, but also the drawing style, was transmitted to disciples all over the world, including three of the prominent disciples of Cajal: Rafael Lorente de Nó, Pío del Río-Hortega, and Fernando de Castro.

Dr.DeFelipe demonstrates his expertise well in the first part of the book when he explains the techniques used to generate samples and stainings, as well as their advantages and limitations. Thus, he describes not only technical details about the stainings used at the time to expose the shape of the neurons and their connections, but also gives a firsthand explanation of their possible functional significance and possible role in neuropsychiatric disease in the proper historical context. But more notably, what transpires in this first part is his attraction to the scientific drawings that reflect the beauty of the nervous system and also his love for the history of neuroscience, trying to understand how some stubborn scientists were able to start deciphering the intricacies of the nervous system through persistent observation.

Javier DeFelipe incorporates many beautiful images in this section to illustrate how ideas and hypotheses emerged from those same drawings, and how different interpretations arose from them, leading to controversy and discussions that are at the core of any scientific advancement. It is a very scholarly and richly illustrated journey through the birth and early steps of neuroscience that is accessible and entertaining for experts and laypeople. One can also feel Dr. Felipe's admiration of Cajal, how he shined with a different light, able to see what others could not see, and make the correct interpretations that were confirmed with more advanced methods time and time again.

In Part I you will receive an expert explanation about one of the biggest and most famous disagreements in the history of science, which occurred at the occasion of granting the 1906 Nobel Prize in Stockholm, which Cajal shared with Italian scientist Camillo Golgi. The controversy is known as the Reticular Theory Versus the Neuron Doctrine. Both Nobel laureates used the very same method developed originally by Golgi, and later adopted and used so successfully by Cajal. However, they had a very different interpretation of the nature and function of neuronal shapes and the network of their connections; ultimately, Cajal won the battle. This controversy also shows the importance of the use of common sense in both science and art. Dr. DeFelipe provides many more details of the atmosphere in the scientific community at the time of Cajal, from which we can learn even in these days. It is also interesting that Cajal made his famous drawings before a time when sophisticated photomicroscopes were available, using only the camera lucida to contour the shapes, and his sharp vision and skilled hand to complete detailed drawings. Despite this, Cajal's drawings are remarkably precise and reproducible when compared with contemporary "objective'" images obtained by modern methods and equipment. DeFelipe also provides some examples comparing, side by side, Cajal's drawings with images obtained using sophisticated modern microscopes. It is highly instructive that despite using the rather crude methods available at the time, Cajal's interpretations and conclusions have endured. Cajal always resisted the temptation as an artist to exaggerate or slightly elaborate images beyond reality. Many novelty-driven contemporary scientists could learn from his accuracy and modesty in interpretation.

One of the last sections in Part I is dedicated to the artistic inclinations of Cajal, how he wanted to become an artist when he was young, and how this passion is reflected not only in his virtuosity of drawing what he saw in the microscopic but also in his photographic work. Cajal developed specific techniques for color photography that were cutting edge at that time, some of which are also shown in this book.

The second part of the book is dedicated to the scientific drawings of Cajal—a collection of 275 original figures, selected for their beauty and scientific relevance, but also favoring relatively unknown drawings, to give them more exposure. Part II is the core of the book, where science and history slip though the pages, and art and sensations blend. It is truly a visit to an enchanted forest populated by extraordinary neuronal trees, long branching of axons and twisted dendrites intermingled to create interesting, almost surreal patterns. In this part, one almost does not need much verbal explanation, similar to how one does not need to read detailed descriptions of paintings while enjoying them in a museum.

Javier DeFelipe has a very original, productive, and successful career of his own, but he has always been interested and surrounded by Cajal's figures. Javier started his scientific career at the Instituto Cajal (the Neurobiology Research Institute created in 1922 and whose first managing director was Cajal). I can imagine the fascination that Javier felt when looking at the original preparations and drawings by Cajal preserved at the Institute.

After defending his PhD dissertation, Javier landed in the lab of Ted Jones, where he focused his work on the microstructure and connectivity of the cerebral cortex. He also found the time—teaming with his mentor, Jones—to translate and edit the works of Cajal on the cerebral cortex (DeFelipe and Jones, 1988) and on degeneration and regeneration of the nervous system (DeFelipe and Jones, 1991). When DeFelipe later returned to Spain, he went back to the Cajal Institute and, in addition to his prolific and outstanding scientific contributions, he continued to explore, study, and publicize the works of Cajal, writing articles about his work, his opinions, and how his legacy has influenced and still survives in modern neuroscience. Starting in 2006, to commemorate the 100th anniversary of Cajal's 1906 Nobel Prize in Physiology or Medicine, he organized the exhibition Neuroscapes, the inauguration of which I had the privilege to attend, joined by Ted Jones, Torsten Wiesel, and Peter Somogyi in Barcelona. The goal of the exhibition was to link science and art, and it consisted of more than 400 scientific images about the brain submitted by scientific groups and private individuals that were selected based on aesthetic merits. The exhibit was a great success and was attended by more than 35,000 people in its first three weeks. Later, the exhibition toured 17 other cities in Spain and 16 cities in the United States, Europe and Asia.

In the words of my deceased friend and DeFelipe's mentor, Ted Jones, "Cajal has found a modern embodiment in the author whose eye for the beauty revealed by the microscope and gift for romantic language provide a vision of the nervous system that matches that of the master himself."

Cajal is not the only or even rare example of a person with the ability to combine science and art. In Leonardo da Vinci's drawings, there is no border between artistic skills and his ability to convey evidence and scientific information. Galileo Galilei, who also wanted to be a painter but was urged by his father to study medicine, later used considerable artistic talent to convey the essence of the moon's surface in impressive watercolors. Likewise, Charles Darwin was both an exceptional writer and an artist. However, their contributions to science were often separate from their contribution to art. In contrast, Cajal used both art and science in this work—for him they were the same.

I am quite familiar with many of the Cajal publications and actually have in my library several of his books, including the original two comprehensive volumes in French, which induced me to become a scientist. So I thought that, in this book, I would probably recognize most of the figures. I was wrong (this time). Just going from drawing to drawing, I was astonished by the beauty of unexpected and stunning shapes, some which look like abstract paintings. However, they are "true"; they secretly expose and explain to us visually the miracle of the brain architecture. Thus, there is no doubt in my mind that this book will be a lasting monument to

Cajal's scientific legacy as well as convincing evidence that art and science are part of the same humanity enabled by our brain.

So, the least I can do is write a Foreword to the book about Cajal's drawings of the cells in the cosmos of the brain. However, when faced with an empty sheet of paper, I recognized it is not an easy task to say something appropriate, good, and *new*! Shall I say less than that? How to give justice to this wonderful book, except to recommend that you buy it, place it in your library, look at it once in a while, and spend time enjoying each page. When I say you should buy it, I do not mean you should do so only if you are a neuroscientist, neurologist, or psychiatrist. I mean you should have it no matter who you are—even if you do not have a background in biology or medicine. Enjoy these drawings and admire the complexity of myriads of forms that seem to be deceivably random, yet are so precise and repeatable from generation to generation in a way that makes it possible to celebrate the beauty of life and think about who we are and where we came from.

Pasko Rakic
Yale University School of Medicine
New Haven, Connecticut

References

DeFelipe, J. (1993) Neocortical neuronal diversity: Chemical heterogeneity revealed by colocalization studies of classic neurotransmitters, neuropeptides, calcium-binding proteins, and cell surface molecules. *Cereb. Cortex* 3, 273–289.

DeFelipe, J. (2009) *Cajal's butterflies of the soul: Science and art*. New York: Oxford University Press.

DeFelipe, J. (2011) The evolution of the human nature of cortical circuits, and intellectual creativity. *Front. Neuroanat.* 5, 1–29.

DeFelipe, J., Alonso-Nanclares, L., and Arellano, J. I. (2002) Microstructure of neocortex: Comparative aspects. *J. Neurocytol.* 31 (3–5), 299–316.

DeFelipe, J., and Jones, E. G. (1988) *Cajal and the cerebral cortex: An annotated translation of the complete writings*. New York: Oxford University Press.

DeFelipe, J., and Jones, E. G. (1991) *Cajal's degeneration and regeneration of the nervous system*. New York: Oxford University Press.

Dove, A. (2005) Profile: Pasko Rakic. *Nat. Med.* 11, 362.

Rakic, P. (2007) The radial edifice of cortical architecture: From neuronal silhouettes to genetic engineering. Special Issue on: Centenary of neuroscience discovery: Reflecting on the Nobel Prize to Golgi and Cajal in 1906. *Brain Res. Rev.* 55, 204–219.

Sidman, R. L., and Rakic, P. (1982) Development of the human central nervous system. In *Histology and histopathology of the nervous system*, ed. W. Haymaker and R. D. Adams, 3–145. Springfield, IL: C.C. Thomas.

FOREWORD: CONSEJO SUPERIOR DE INVESTIGACIONES CIENTÍFICAS

The Spanish National Research Council (Consejo Superior de Investigaciones Científicas, or CSIC) is the largest public institution dedicated to multidisciplinary research in Spain and the third largest in Europe aiming to promote Spain's competitiveness and to foster scientific, educational, and economic development. CSIC research is driven by its 125 centers and institutes, which are spread across the country, with more than 12,000 staff members, including more than 3000 staff researchers and a similar figure of contracted PhDs and researchers under formation programs. The CSIC also manages a large number of strategic national and international research facilities and has very strong ties with universities, technology centers, hospitals, and nonprofit organizations focused on research and development (R&D) throughout joint research groups. The CSIC is strongly connected to the productive sector through R&D contracts and technology transfer activities, and it remains the reference institution among Latin American universities in collaborative projects and joint publications. Regarding the origin of the CSIC in 1939, one cannot help but be aware of the fact that the alma mater of this national organization is Santiago Ramón y Cajal (1852–1934). Following the award of the Nobel Prize in Physiology or Medicine to Cajal in 1906, he was appointed chair of the board of the Junta para Ampliación de Estudios e Investigaciones Biológicas (JAE, 1907–1939) of the Spanish Ministry of Public Instruction and Fine Arts. Cajal's strategy as JAE president (1907–1932) effected the largest renovation process and scientific modernization in Spain during the early twentieth century. Cajal encouraged critical changes in the educational structures of the Spanish society during his very long presidency of JAE, germ of the CSIC. Cajal was appointed director of the Laboratorio de Investigaciones Biológicas in 1920, a research center founded in 1902 by order of HM the King Alfonso XIII that later gave rise to the Cajal Institute in 1922. The Cajal Institute was incorporated in the CSIC November 24, 1939. For its more than 100 years of existence, renowned CSIC scientists and professionals have spread worldwide their contributions to the remarkable advancement of neurobiology. Today, the Cajal Institute is prepared to confront future challenges and to maintain the leading role in neurobiological research in Spain, always keeping in mind that the final destination of knowledge is the well-being of society.

Cajal is considered one of the founders of modern neuroscience. To this day, his work is mentioned constantly in all forms of scientific publications. Although his contributions to current concepts of brain function and organization are widely publicized, his carefully rendered drawings—a rare mix of artistic skill and scientific insight—are much less known. It is therefore a great pleasure to contribute to the publication of his outstanding work by editing a representative sample of his drawings kept at the Cajal Institute. It is also with great pleasure that we participate in the production of this marvelous book, not only because its represents an excellent opportunity to commemorate Cajal, but also because *Cajal's Neuronal Forest: Science and Art* contains a fantastic new compilation of a vast collection of beautiful figures produced throughout the nineteenth century and the beginning of the twentieth century. Javier DeFelipe, the author of this book, is a full professor at the CSIC and is considered an international expert on the microanatomy of the cerebral cortex. From a biographical perspective, he is one of the greatest authorities in historical studies to have tackled Cajal's science. Indeed, he has written several excellent articles, chapters, and books regarding the influence of Cajal in modern neuroscience and on the link between the study of the brain and art. Thus, we consider Prof. DeFelipe to be the perfect author for this type of book.

We are confident that *Cajal's Neuronal Forest: Science and Art* will serve as both an inexhaustible source for artistic inspiration in general and as a way to divulge and increase interest in the nervous system. Together with the highly motivated organization of this well planned editorial initiative, we are sure that this sample of the Cajal Legacy will be seen as an aesthetic experience, as well, for those who approach it for the first time. It might be that science and art often travel together.

Ricardo Martínez Murillo
Director, Instituto Cajal
Consejo Superior de Investigaciones Científicas, CSIC
Madrid, Spain

FOREWORD: RAMÓN ARECES FOUNDATION

It is with great pride that the Ramón Areces Foundation has collaborated in *Cajal's Neuronal Forest: Science and Art*. This is a singular book because of its beauty and its meaning. It makes the work and talent of Santiago Ramón y Cajal, one of the most important personalities to grace the world of science, even more valuable. I sincerely congratulate Oxford University Press and the author of the work, Javier DeFelipe, on this initiative because it projects the work of Santiago Ramón y Cajal beyond the scientific community.

One of the main missions of our institution is to contribute to strengthening the science system in Spain. We have been doing so for four decades now. However, this strengthening is only possible with the support of Spanish scientists. This is a priority task for us—even more so our current environment, in which science no longer has borders. Santiago Ramón y Cajal demonstrated this almost a century ago with his contributions to neuroscience. His findings are still in force today and have contributed significantly to a greater knowledge of the brain. Cajal put his talent, his abilities, and his creativity at the service of humanity.

The pages of *Cajal's Neuronal Forest* show the originality of the scientific approaches of Santiago Ramón y Cajal. His drawings, of great beauty and quality, are filled with brilliance despite the scarce resources of his time, when the imaging techniques of today did not exist. The value of these works of art describe, with great detail, the structure of one of the most perfect and unknown machines of the human body. Cajal had the virtue of seeing and understanding the forest, the trees, and the leaves of the brain. This is why his work endures.

Raimundo Pérez-Hernández y Torra
Director, Ramón Areces Foundation
Madrid, Spain

FOREWORD: SPANISH FOUNDATION FOR SCIENCE AND TECHNOLOGY

It is a pleasure and a source of pride to have collaborated in an initiative that shines light on the figure of Santiago Ramón y Cajal, one of Spain's most distinguished scientists and the one who has made the greatest contribution to science at the international level.

Cajal is considered the father of neurobiology, and many of his observations are at the frontier of human knowledge even today. But, Cajal was also passionate about art. His talent as a draftsman allowed him to give his ideas visual form, allowing even inexpert viewers to immerse themselves in his research. I thank and congratulate Oxford University Press and Javier DeFelipe for making possible *Cajal's Neuronal Forest: Science and Art*.

Among other objectives, the Spanish Foundation for Science and Technology (FECYT) aims to bring science closer to society through initiatives that rouse the public's curiosity, interest, and participation. FECYT's Art and Science Programme includes activities to connect these two areas of knowledge that so often seem distant from one another, combining artistic vision and creation with scientific research and curiosity. So it should come as no surprise that FECYT would participate in the production of this book, an indispensable collection of illustrations that are magnificent not only for their outstanding beauty, but also for the greatness of the scientific impulse they describe.

In his *Recuerdos de mi vida* (*Recollections of My Life*; 1917), Santiago Ramón y Cajal wrote:

> Those who are bewitched by the investigation of the infinitely small will continue to find in the bosom of the living, millions of palpitating cells that, if they are to surrender their secrets and give the halo of fame to the investigator, demand a clear and persistent intelligence to contemplate, admire and understand them.

Cajal's Neuronal Forest brings together many of these "palpitating cells": small works of art that—without a doubt—invite us to contemplate, to admire, to surprise ourselves, and (why not?) to yearn for understanding, to embark on adventures to uncharted territories of knowledge that only science is able to conquer.

José Ignacio Fernández Vera,
General Director
Spanish Foundation for Science and Technology
Madrid, Spain

FOREWORD: TATIANA PÉREZ DE GUZMÁN EL BUENO FOUNDATION

The Tatiana Pérez de Guzmán el Bueno Foundation, which funds research into neuroscience and the environment, endorses the publication of this book with the utmost interest and satisfaction. *Cajal's Neuronal Forest: Science and Art* harmonizes both worlds through the lively artistic imagination of its author, Javier DeFelipe.

Our Foundation made the decision to support neuroscience and the environment to reflect the personal interests of its founder, Tatiana Pérez de Guzmán el Bueno. Doña Tatiana, as she was called by those closest to her, was a noble lady whose family has long roots in the history of Spain, dating back to the thirteenth century. Together with her husband, Don Julio Peláez Avendaño, a physicist, she decided to leave her belongings to the Foundation in her name to benefit the people and to preserve their historical heritage. Doña Tatiana delighted in nature and in tending her greenhouse. She also had a deep respect for science—a respect shared by her husband. They declared that the Foundation should support scientific research. Thus, when the Foundation Council had to settle on which fields to endow, the environment and neuroscience were natural choices. Certainly, knowledge from environmental and neuroscientific research are keys to helping people, which is the ultimate goal of the Foundation.

In the field of neuroscience, our Foundation contributes through its "Plan in Support of Neuroscience in Spain," which includes yearly calls for predoctoral fellowships, biennial calls for research projects, a chair in neuroscience at the Medical School of the Autonomous University of Madrid, and funding for courses and conferences, such as those held during Cajal week at the Royal National Academy of Medicine of Spain.

Neuroscience is certainly grounded solidly in Spain. Santiago Ramón y Cajal, the central figure in this book, is the founder of modern neuroscience. Cajal himself was an artist too. His drawings of the structure of the nervous system and its cells are true works of art. *Cajal's Neuronal Forest* gives us the opportunity to experience great pleasure in contemplating the beauty of the brain, which is, in a final analysis, a sample of the beauty of nature itself.

Teodoro Sánchez-Ávila Sánchez-Migallón,
President Fundación Tatiana Pérez de Guzmán el Bueno
Madrid, Spain

PREFACE

During the nineteenth century, when the detailed analysis of the nervous system began, most scientific figures presented by the neuroanatomists were their own drawings because microphotography was not yet a well-developed technique. Therefore, a successful neuroanatomist required a combination of artistic talent and an ability to interpret microscopic images effectively. The problem was that these illustrations were not necessarily free of technical errors and they may have been subject to the scientists' own interpretations. Indeed, in some cases, these drawings were considered to be basically artistic interpretations rather than accurate copies of the histological preparations. Furthermore, there are many examples showing that even using the same microscopes and the same techniques, scientists "see" differently through the microscope. As a result, this period of scientific "art" and skepticism represents a fascinating page in the history of neuroscience because it provided the basis of our current understanding of the anatomy of the nervous system.

Importantly, during the decades after the introduction of light microscopy, little progress was made in understanding the structure and function of the nervous system. The main reason for this lack of information was due to the fact that, with the histological techniques available, the visualization of nerve cells was incomplete, because it was often only feasible to observe the cell body and the proximal portions of the dendrites and axon. Thus, it was not possible to follow the trajectory of the thin axons or to visualize the terminal axonal arbors. Hence, it was still not technically feasible to address one of the key requirements for studying the organization of the nervous system—namely, the tracing of the connections between neurons. In 1873, a giant step for neuroscience occurred with the introduction of the staining method of the *reazione nera* (black reaction) of Camillo Golgi (1843–1926). With this new method, the observation of neurons and glia with all their parts became feasible, and all of a sudden it was possible to begin studying the tracing of the connections between neurons. Nevertheless, this method was not fully exploited until Santiago Ramón y Cajal (1852–1934) arrived on the scene in 1888.

As illustrated by his marvelous drawings, the studies of Cajal no doubt contributed, more than those of any other researcher at the time, to the growth of modern neuroscience. Cajal was captivated by the beautiful shapes of the cells of the nervous system, which he saw through an artist's eye. He and other scientists saw some neurons as trees, such as the pyramidal cells of the cerebral cortex and the Purkinje cells of the cerebellar cortex, and likened glial cells to bushes. Given their high density and arrangement, neurons and glial cells seemed to constitute a thick forest, a seemingly impenetrable terrain of interacting cells mediating cognition and behavior. The great challenge was, and still is, to uncover its mysteries that, from a structural point of view, were beautifully described in the writings of Cajal in *Recuerdos de mi vida* (Cajal, 1917b, Madrid, pages 100–101):

The great enigma in the organization of the brain revolves around our need to ascertain how the nervous ramifications end and how neurons are mutually connected. Referring to the previously mentioned simile, the idea was to inquire how the roots and branches of the trees in the gray matter terminate, so that in such a dense jungle, in which there are no gaps thanks to its refined complexity, the trunks, branches, and leaves touch everywhere.

It may seem incredible that a simple histological staining technique such as the Golgi method and the microscopes available at the time of Cajal represented the principal tools that changed the course of the history of neuroscience. In their quest to unravel the mysteries of the brain, the researchers of the day encountered an almost infinite number of cellular forms with an extraordinary beauty, allowing the discovery of a new artistic world—the neuronal forest, giving free rein to their imagination and a new way to view the brain. Nevertheless, it is important to highlight that, despite the common misconception—especially among the general public—that the drawings of Cajal (and other authors of the time) are pieces of art, these drawings are in fact copies of histological preparations. It is true that early scientists needed artistic capabilities because they had to draw what they saw when they looked through a microscope (similar to what artists do when they draw from nature) and, indeed, these drawings are of course beautiful and look like pieces of art. However, those scientists were, in fact, merely illustrating the microscopic world with no license for artistic interpretation.

This book is divided into two parts. Part I is based mainly on previous publications by myself (some of them in Spanish) or prepared in collaboration with other authors, particularly with the great neuroanatomist Ted Jones, with whom I had the great honor and pleasure of working for many years until he passed away unexpectedly in 2011. Part I is divided into sections A and B. Section A focuses on the scientific atmosphere in Cajal's times and, in particular, on the history of the neuron and the anatomical challenge of the study of neuronal connections. This section also contains a discussion of the methods used and a reflection on why, in that period, there were many examples of differing interpretations of the microscopic world by scientists, even though they were using the same staining and microscope techniques. I focus on two of the most critical differences in the interpretation of the microscopic images at that time, both of which have had a profound impact on the history of neuroscience—namely, the different interpretations of the connections between neurons (the Reticular Theory versus the Neuron Doctrine), and the discovery of dendritic spines and the debate on their significance.

Section B examines the artistic skills and emotions of Cajal and other important pioneers in neuroscience, using their own words to describe the artistic emotions they experienced when visualizing the neural elements. This section also deals with the verification in recent years of many of the descriptions and illustrations of the early neuroanatomists, particularly those of Cajal. This has been achieved through the examination of Cajal's own histological preparations, currently housed in the Legado Cajal at the Instituto Cajal in Madrid. Similarly, many of the descriptions and illustrations of Cajal and other scientists have been confirmed in recent years using modern techniques. Thus, I have included some examples that illustrate the similarities between the old drawings and the modern images obtained using such techniques. The last part of this section deals with how the neuronal forests have served as an unlimited source of artistic and poetic inspiration to many scientists, not only in the early days of the research of the brain, but also during modern times.

It is true that the discovery of the Golgi method represented a major innovation in analyzing the nervous system. However, many other methods yield not only very important results, but also beautiful multicolor images of the brain. This world of color and shape represents an aesthetic stimulus for the eyes of both scientists and artists, and at the same time provides a source of great inspiration. As a result, numerous art exhibitions across the globe have been organized, which indicates the increasing interest in the link between the study of the brain and art. Here I highlight one of these exhibitions—*Paisajes Neuronales*, or Neuroscapes, which took place in 2006. This exhibition was first presented in Barcelona as a special event to celebrate the 100th anniversary of the Nobel Prize for Physiology or Medicine (1906) awarded jointly to Cajal and Golgi for their contributions in the field of neuroscience. More than 35,000 people visited this exhibition in the first three weeks alone. Many of the visitors (including famous writers and artists) participated in the event by briefly describing what they "saw" in the images.

The last part of Section B emphasizes how these initiatives—and others like them—not only serve to bring the world of neuroscience a step closer to the general public, but also represent a very interesting bridge between science and art. As you will see, many images of the brain look like paintings by artists belonging to a large variety of artistic movements, including paintings by Pierre-Auguste Renoir or Joan Miró. Finally, to help guide you through the text of Part I, it is illustrated with 114 figures that include old drawings as well as images of the brain using modern techniques. Many of these figures are composite images, containing drawings by Golgi and Cajal as well as other great pioneers of neuroscience, such as the well-known disciples of Cajal, Pío del Río-Hortega and Fernando de Castro, and other scientists such as Alzheimer, Deiters, Dogiel Golgi, Kölliker, Meynert, Ranvier, and Retzius. In many cases, these drawings have been retouched and restored to remove stains, wrinkles, or other artifacts, and some of them are reproduced from the original drawings.

Part II represents the main body of the book and consists of 275 additional original drawings by Cajal, which he published throughout the course of his scientific career, covering virtually all his research fields of interest. The vast majority of these illustrations were drawn by Cajal; the remaining figures were produced by his disciples, as indicated in the figures legends. When I chose these drawings, I took into account three factors. First, the beauty of the image; second, the scientific importance of the illustration; and third, its "originality" in terms of how frequently the drawing had been published previously, if at all.

Each image is accompanied by a title based on the description given by Cajal, the original legend, and its source to enable those of you interested in a particular figure to satisfy your curiosity regarding its significance within the context of the time in which it was created. Nevertheless, because most of the legends of these figures are in Spanish and some are in French, I translated them into English to make them accessible to all readers. The original labeling of the drawings used to describe the illustrations and the indications of Cajal to the printer to reproduce the figures have been preserved as well. Thus, the figures in Part II have been reproduced as they are today, without removing stains or other artifacts, except for the "Museo Cajal" stamps and the corresponding numbers that were used to mark and catalog the drawings after the death of Cajal. Unfortunately, many of these stamps were on top of the drawing and it was necessary to remove them to restore the original drawing. Thus, Part II of the book is not only of great scientific relevance, as it contains a large collection of Cajal's drawings, but also you will find detailed technical information, such as the types of drawing tools (e.g., pencils or ink) and papers that Cajal used, how he rectified some of the illustrations, his indications to the printer about the final size of the drawing that should be in the printed copy, or other instructions. These drawings are currently housed in the Legado Cajal at the Instituto Cajal, and permission for their use in this book was kindly granted.

In preparing *Cajal's Neuronal Forest*, I feel very grateful and indebted to all current members of my laboratory for their technical and scientific support; and for their companionship, friendship, and encouragement: Lidia Alonso-Nanclares, Mª del Carmen Álvarez, Alejandro Antón, Guillermo Aparicio, Lidia Blázquez-Llorca, Ruth Benavides-Piccione Débora Cano, Marta Domínguez, Isabel Fernaud, Montserrat Fernández, Pilar Flores-Romero, Diana Furcila, Ana García, Juncal González, Asta

Kastanauskaite, Gonzalo León-Espinosa, Miriam Marín, Ángel Merchán, Miguel Miguens, Marta Montero, Alberto Muñoz, Sandra Ostos, Mª Carmen Regalado, José Rodrigo-Rodríguez, Yago Rodríguez, Concepción Rojo, Andrea Santuy, Silvia Tapia, Marta Turégano, and Lorena Valdés.

The retouching and preparation of the images were largely done by myself, with much assistance from Ana García, particularly for many of the drawings of Cajal. I also express my gratitude to María de los Ángeles Langa, a librarian at the Instituto Cajal, for her help in obtaining some of the books and articles from which I extracted some of the figures and quotes included here. I am also grateful to Nick Guthrie for his excellent editorial assistance and Ángel Acebes for his help translating the legends of the figures of the insect brain into English. I am indebted to the grandson, granddaughter, and great-grandson of Cajal—Santiago Ramón y Cajal Junquera, María de los Ángeles Ramón y Cajal Junquera, and Santiago Ramón y Cajal Asensio, respectively—for their continuous support and for granting us permission to use Cajal's original drawings. I also thank all colleagues and friends, whose names appear in the figure legends, for kindly supplying or preparing some of the figures included in the book. I extend my gratitude to Craig Allen Panner (Associate Editorial Director, Medicine Books of Oxford University Press) for his enthusiastic support, encouragement, and help in this project. Finally, I thank my friends and colleagues at the Instituto Cajal, as well as Emilio Lora-Tamayo (President, Consejo Superior de Investigaciones Científicas) and Ramón Rodríguez (Chief Editor, Department of Publications, Consejo Superior de Investigaciones Científicas), for their encouragement and assistance in this project. I also thank the Fundación Española para la Ciencia y la Tecnología (FCYT), the Fundación Tatiana Pérez de Guzmán el Bueno, and the Fundación Ramón Areces (Spain) for sponsoring the book. This work was supported by grants from the Spanish Ministerio de Economía y Competitividad (grant SAF 2015-66603-P and thc Cajal Bluc Brain Projcct, Spanish partner of the Blue Brain Project initiative from école polytechnique fédérale de Lausanne), and the European Union's Horizon 2020 research and innovation program under grant agreement no. 720270 (Human Brain Project).

Javier DeFelipe
Madrid, Spain
March 1, 2017

PART I

INTRODUCTION

Introductory Remarks

Almost everything that humankind creates has a touch of art, despite the fact that we do not need beauty or an aesthetic perception to survive. Rather, we simply derive intellectual pleasure, which is also true of other mental activities, such as reading a book or listening to music. For centuries, many philosophers and scientists have tried to define, explain, and locate various aspects of human cognition, including artistic talent. As we will see in Section B, "Artistic skills and emotions of Cajal," it is somewhat surprising that during the early days of the study of the brain, artistic talent was a necessary ability to be a successful neuroanatomist; the majority of the scientific illustrations were drawings done directly with the naked eye or using a microscope. Much has changed in neuroscience over the years, not only the tools we use to study the brain, but also the way in which we go about our investigations. A good example of this development is shown in Figure 1. The drawing by Leonardo da Vinci (1452–1519) on the left of this figure shows the central nervous system and cranial nerves, which were believed to be hollow and capable of transmitting the so-called "animal or generating forces," a vital fluid contained within the ventricles and nerves. Da Vinci was one of the pioneers in trying to explain in detail by physical laws how the brain processes visual information and other sensory stimuli, and integrates this information "through the soul." Da Vinci believed that the anatomical visual system played an essential role in artistic perception and he developed a mechanistic model based on the ventricular or cellular doctrine of brain functions (see Pevsner, 2002). This doctrine represents a medieval view of the localization of mental faculties in the ventricular system, according to the anatomic and functional concepts described by the great Greek physician Galen of Pergamon (129–ca. 215 AD). In general, different attributes of the mind were located in different ventricles; the two lateral ventricles together constituted the first "cell" (small room) that receives input from all the sense organs and was the site of the sensus communis (common sense), integrating information across the different sensory modalities. This integration gives rise to images, and therefore fantasy and imagination were also located here. The second or middle cell was the site of cognitive processes: reasoning, judgment, and thought. The third cell or ventricle was the site of memory (see Pevsner, 2002). On the right of Figure 1, a schematic drawing of the human central nervous system by Lewellys F. Barker (1867–1943) is shown. This illustration was published in his book *The Nervous System and Its Constituent Neurons*, and I have chosen to include it here because it is a wonderful example of "modern" neurological anatomy that demonstrates to the students of medicine and psychology that the central nervous system works as a whole. It is amazing

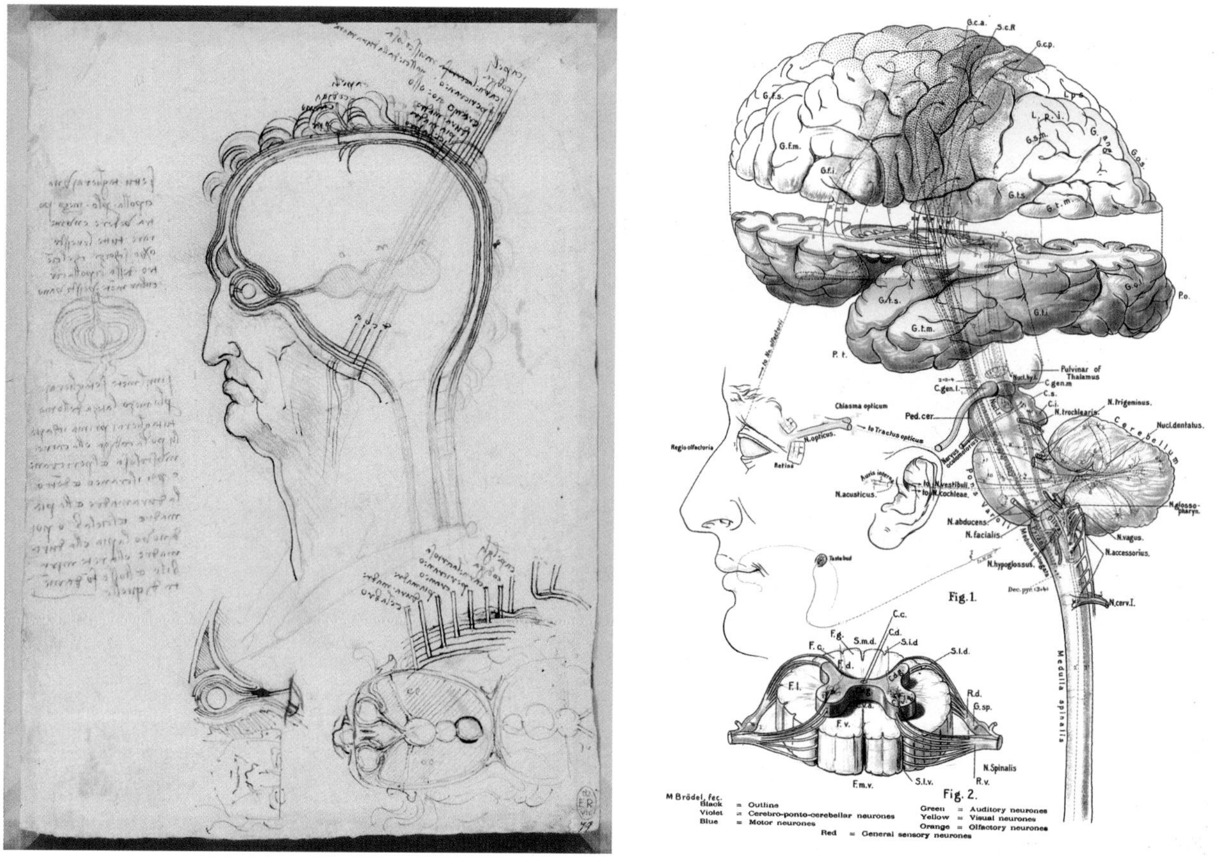

FIGURE 1. *Left*, Leonardo da Vinci, *Quaderni d'anatomia* (1490 [Keele and Pedretti, 1979]). The central nervous system and cranial nerves. This is a schematic representation of the ventricles and their relationship to the central nervous system and cranial nerves. The main drawing shows the layers covering the brain compared with the layers of an onion cut in half (on the left of the image). At the bottom of the drawing, the ventricles viewed from above are illustrated, including the optic and auditory nerves entering the anterior ventricle. Royal Collection Trust/© Her Majesty Queen Elizabeth II, 2017. *Right*, Lewellys F. Barker (1899), "The nervous system and its constituent neurones"; schematic drawing to illustrate some of the multiple relationships between different parts of the human central nervous system.

to observe the decidedly modern appearance of this "connectomic" illustration of the central nervous system, despite the fact that it was published as far back as 1899.

In the nervous system, there are billions of neurons and glial cells, the discovery of which has a long, fascinating history in which many researchers have participated up to the present day. The great challenge is to find out how the neurons and glia are structured in the different regions of the brain, and how neuronal circuits (local and long distance) contribute to the functional organization of the brain, giving rise to cognition and behavior. From a biological standpoint, perhaps the cardinal question is: What neural substrates make a human being human? Thanks to the remarkable development and evolution of the brain, we are able to perform extremely complicated, extraordinary tasks such as writing a book, composing a symphony, or inventing the computer. So, the question is: Who am I (Figure 2)? Answering this question is extremely difficult—not only because of brain complexity and the technical difficulties involved, but also because ethical limitations do not allow all the necessary data sets to be acquired directly from human brains (DeFelipe, 2015a).

In general, neurons can be divided into distinct morphological and functional regions: a receptor apparatus (formed by the dendrites and cell body or soma), the emission apparatus (the axon), and the distribution apparatus (terminal axonal arborization).

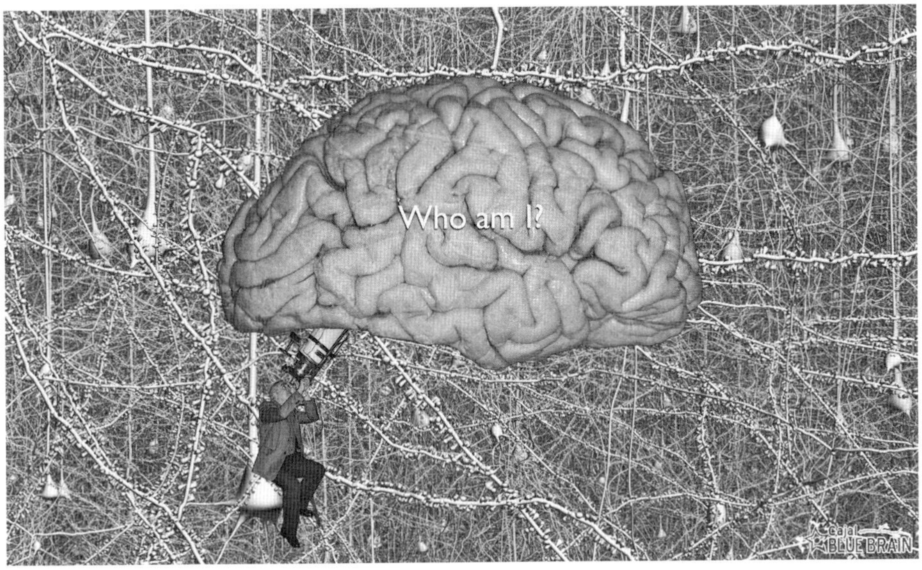

FIGURE 2. Artistic composition illustrating the lack of knowledge about the human nature of our brain and the interest in its study.

The exchange of information between neurons mainly takes place through two types of highly specialized structures: chemical synapses (the majority) and electrical synapses. The space between the cell bodies of the neurons, glia, and blood vessels—the neuropil—is occupied by a very dense network of axonal, dendritic, and glial processes. In the neuropil there is a high density of synapses; for example, in the human temporal cortex, there are approximately 1000×10^6 synapses/mm^3 of neuropil. Indeed, the neuropil represents between 90% and 98% of the volume of the cerebral cortex (Alonso et al., 2008). Thus, the main problem when analyzing the structure of the nervous system is its extreme complexity, particularly in higher vertebrates (Figure 3).

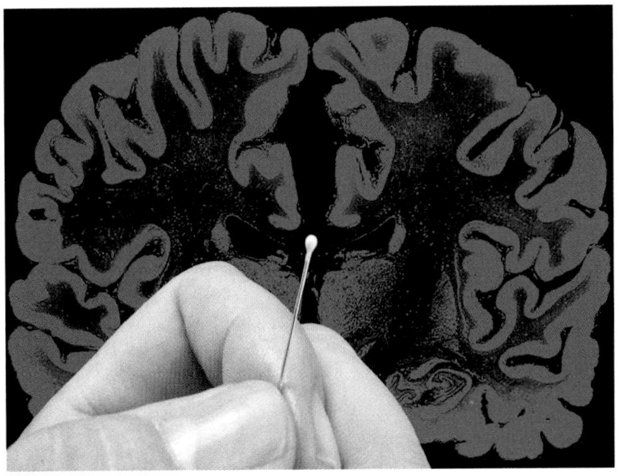

FIGURE 3. The complexity of the brain. Artistic composition showing a coronal histological section of the human brain and a hand holding a pin with a pinhead (approximately 1 mm^3) to illustrate graphically the complexity of the brain. In a volume of human cerebral cortex similar to the pinhead in this figure, there are about 27,000 neurons and 1000 million synapses (Alonso-Nanclares et al., 2008). The diameter of the pin (0.5 mm) is equivalent to the thickness of a cortical column. Because a human pyramidal neuron typically has a dendritic tree with a minimum total length of several millimeters, in this volume there would be several hundred meters of dendrites. For example, considering a medium-size pyramidal neuron with a dendritic length of 10 mm, there would be approximately 270 m of dendrites in this 1 mm^3. Furthermore, the brain is one of the organs of the body with the highest metabolic demands and, thus, there is a very dense network of blood vessels in association with the neurons and glia. Figure and text taken from DeFelipe (2015a).

Throughout the history of neuroscience, scientists have sought to develop appropriate methods to analyze different aspects of the structure and function of the nervous system. Back in the nineteenth century, a giant step for neuroscience occurred in 1873 with the introduction of the *reazione nera* (black reaction) staining method of Camillo Golgi (1843–1926) (Figure 4, *left*). With this new method, the observation of neurons and glia with all their parts became feasible and, all of a sudden, it was possible to begin tracing the connections between neurons. Nevertheless,

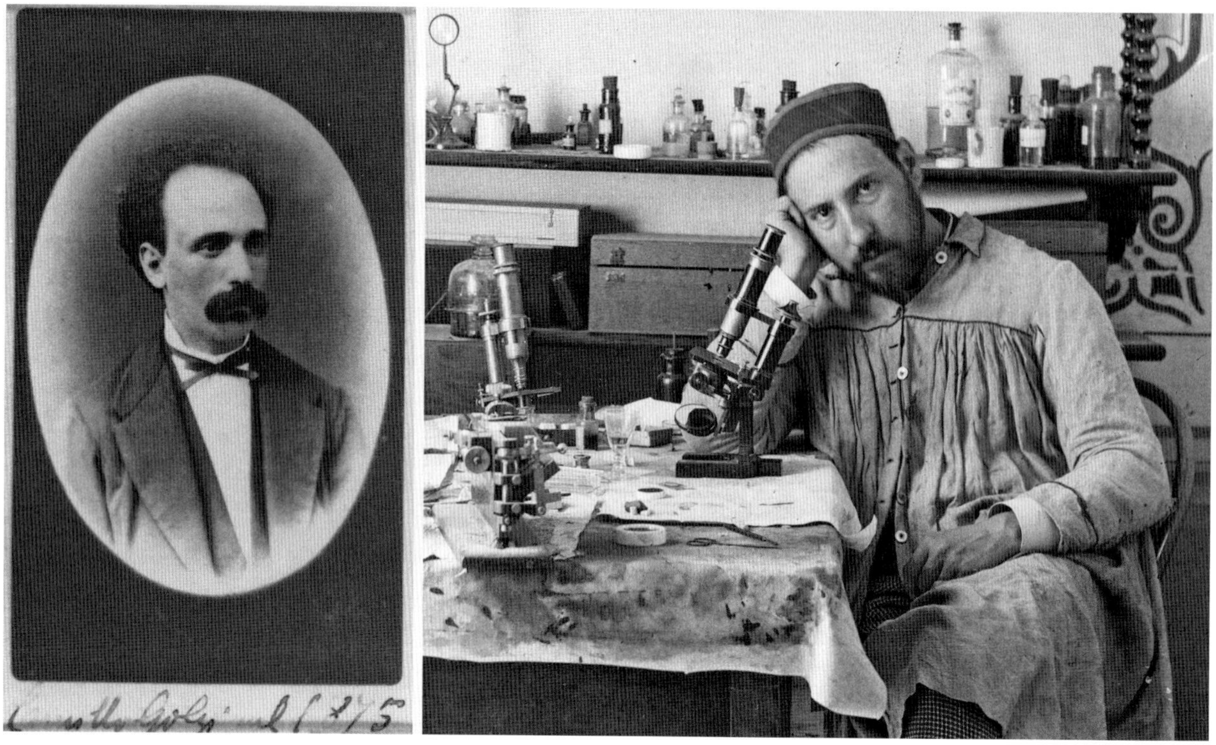

FIGURE 4. *Left*, Golgi in 1875, at the time when he discovered the black reaction. Courtesy of Paolo Mazzarello, Golgi Museum, University of Pavia, Italy. *Right*, Cajal in his laboratory in Valencia (1885), before he "discovered" the Golgi method. See Section A, "The discovery of the Golgi method," for further details.

as we will see in Section A, "The discovery of the Golgi method," this method was not fully exploited until Santiago Ramón y Cajal (1852–1934) arrived on the scene several years later, in 1888 (Figure 4, *right*). It may seem incredible that this simple histological staining technique and the microscopes available at the time of Golgi and Cajal (Figure 5) represented the principal tools that were to change the course of the history of neuroscience. This fact could be taken as a lesson to demonstrate that the development of science does not only depend on the methods available, but also on the way they are exploited. As we will see, the Golgi method represents a good example of a technique that was available to scientists but was not fully exploited until an individual made an important discovery or an astute interpretation that generated new concepts.

Indeed, the studies of Cajal no doubt contributed more than those of any other researcher at the time to the growth of modern neuroscience and, therefore, he is considered the father of modern neuroscience (DeFelipe, 2002b). He published almost 300 articles and several books of great importance, such as the classics *Textura del Sistema Nervioso del Hombre y de los Vertebrados* (Cajal, 1899–1904) and *Estudios sobre la degeneración y regeneración del sistema nervioso* (Cajal, 1913–1914). He also received numerous awards and distinctions (Figure 6, *left* and *center*), including some of the most prestigious awards of his time: the Moscow Award (1900); the Helmholt gold medal (1905); and the Nobel Prize for Physiology or Medicine (1906), which he shared with Golgi. Over the years, Cajal has also received many tributes, such as the homage during the US National Aeronautics and Space Administration "Neurolab" space flight mission in 1998 (Figure 6, *right*). One of the most remarkable international meetings held in his honor was in 2005, in Petilla de Aragón, a small village in Navarra (northern Spain), where Cajal was born (Figure 7). Despite hundreds of studies since the time of Cajal, there are still no criteria accepted by the scientific community to determine the fundamental

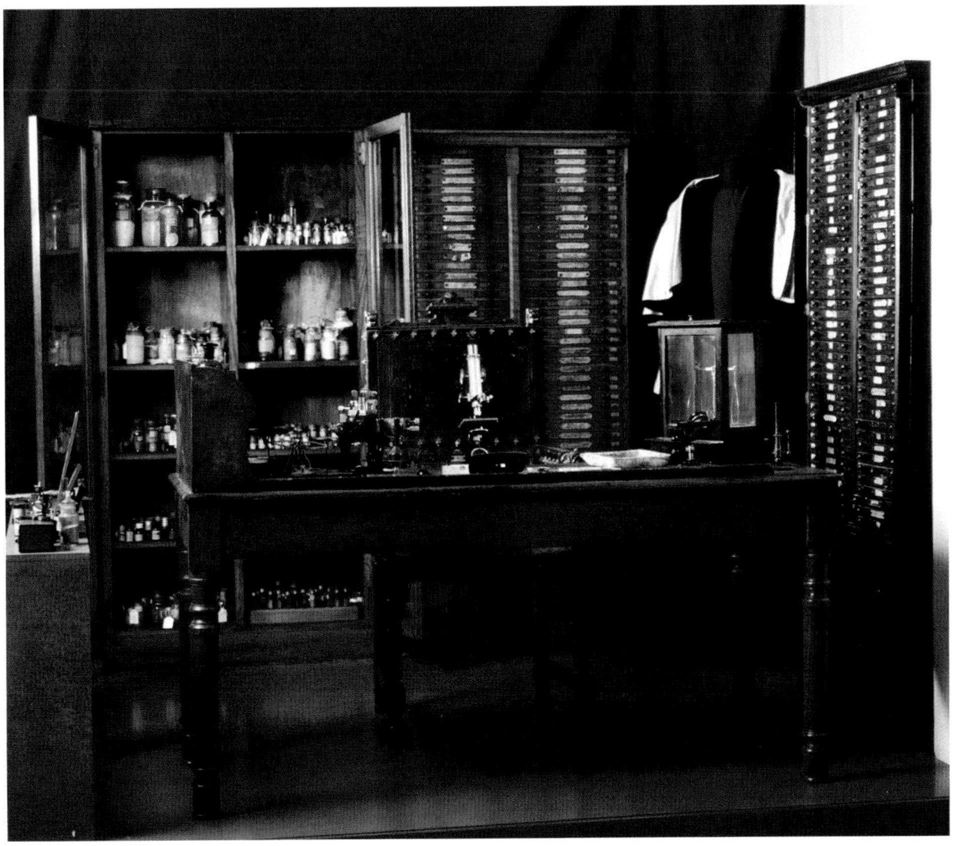

FIGURE 5. Part of the laboratory of Cajal exhibited in the Cajal Institute library (Consejo Superior de Investigaciones Científicas, Madrid). Worktable with some laboratory equipment including a light microscope, one microtome, and two weighing scales. Also shown are two wardrobes for histological preparations (*center / right* and *right*), one wardrobe for histological reagents (*center / left*), a chair, and Cajal's academic gown.

morphological, molecular, and physiological characteristics that distinguish between the various types of cortical neurons. However, this meeting did allow us to reach a series of basic agreements that currently provide guidance to the scientific community on the nomenclature of cortical interneurons, known as *Petilla terminology* (Ascoli et al., 2008).

A Note on Microphotography and Illustrations of Histological Preparations

At the beginning of the nineteenth century and for several decades afterward, microphotography was not a well-established technique to study histology. Certainly, several types of microphotographic accessories were available for light microscopy at that time, some of which were very sophisticated (Figure 8), but good techniques of microphotography had not yet been developed. Interestingly, Cajal was a great photographer and a pioneer in the development of color photography (Figure 9). He published an excellent book in 1912 titled *Fotografía de los Colores: Fundamentos Científicos y Reglas Prácticas* and produced beautiful color pictures (Figures 10 and 11). One of Cajal's photographs is shown on the right of Figure 11—a still life in color with flowers and fruit, which is aesthetically similar to the typical paintings of still lifes at the time, such as the one that appears on the left of Figure 11. It seems clear that Cajal used color photography as an artistic tool to satisfy his aesthetic feelings. However, in the case of scientific illustrations, the problem was that obtaining high-quality microscopic images, particularly high-power microphotographs, was a difficult task.

Moreover, the structure of the nervous system is very complex and the selective staining methods used, such as the Golgi method, do not define all

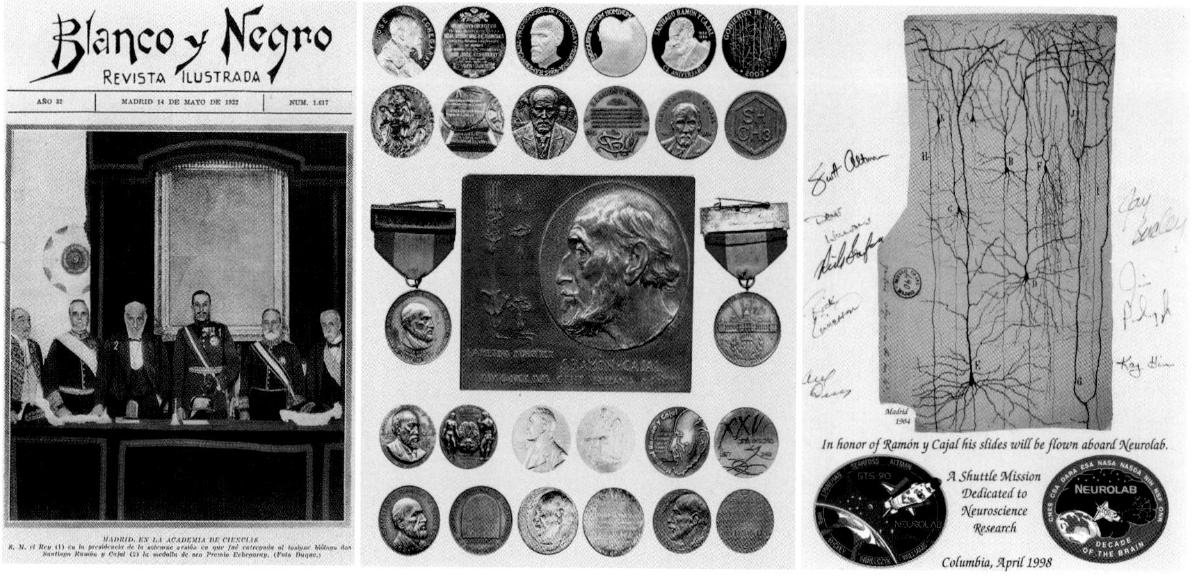
Blanco y Negro
Revista Ilustrada
Año 32
Madrid 14 de Mayo de 1922
Núm. 1.617
In honor of Ramón y Cajal his slides will be flown aboard Neurolab.
A Shuttle Mission Dedicated to Neuroscience Research
NEUROLAB
DECADE OF THE BRAIN
Columbia, April 1998

FIGURE 6. *Left*, Cover of the magazine *Blanco y Negro* (1922) to illustrate the award of the Echegaray Medal to Cajal at the Academia de Ciencias Exactas, Físicas y Naturales (Madrid), in the presence of His Majesty the King of Spain Alfonso XIII (1886–1941). *Center*, Photograph showing a plaque and some medals that Cajal received in recognition of his studies. The images of the medals were kindly supplied by Pere Berbel (Instituto de Neurociencias, Alicante). *Right*, Copy of one of the nine Cajal drawings that traveled aboard the Space Shuttle Columbia as a tribute to him during the US National Aeronautics and Space Administration Neurolab mission. The signatures are those of the crew members: Scott D. Altman, Jay C. Buckey, Richard M. Linnehan, Kathryn P. Hire, James A. Pawelczyk, Richard A. Searfoss, and Dafydd Rhys Williams. See Note 1.

the elements labeled in a given region in the same preparation or in the same focal plane. As previously discussed in DeFelipe and Jones (1992), very little of a neuron is in view at any one time and its examination requires continual movements of the fine focus and of the microscope slide. Therefore, as we will see in Section A, "Drawing as a tool," most of the scientific figures presented during this early period were drawn by the neuroanatomists themselves, which provided them with an outlet to express and build on their own artistic talents.

As with the painters of landscapes, when the scientists drew the images observed in a histological preparation, it was clearly not possible for them to reproduce the whole microscopic field of the histological samples observed. Therefore, they limited themselves to illustrating only those elements they considered most relevant to whatever they were describing (Figure 12). It is not surprising, then, that these illustrations sometimes contained technical errors and relied on the subjective interpretations of the individual scientists themselves, which often impeded the acceptance of the drawings by their peers in the scientific community. That said, one important reason for the difficulties in the exchange of information between scientists at the time was that often the drawings were not considered to be true copies of the histological preparations, but rather they were deemed to be artistic representations of them—an issue that continues to make the interpretation of these figures problematic to this day. As we will see in Section A, "Differences in the interpretation," a clear consequence of the creativity, subjectivity, ambiguity, and skepticism that abounded during this early period was to make it one of great fascination in the history of neuroscience.

The Anatomical Challenge of the Study of Neuronal Connections

It is important to keep in mind that for decades after the introduction of light microscopy, little progress was made in understanding the structure and function of the nervous system. As mentioned earlier, this lack of information was mainly a result of the fact that with the histological techniques

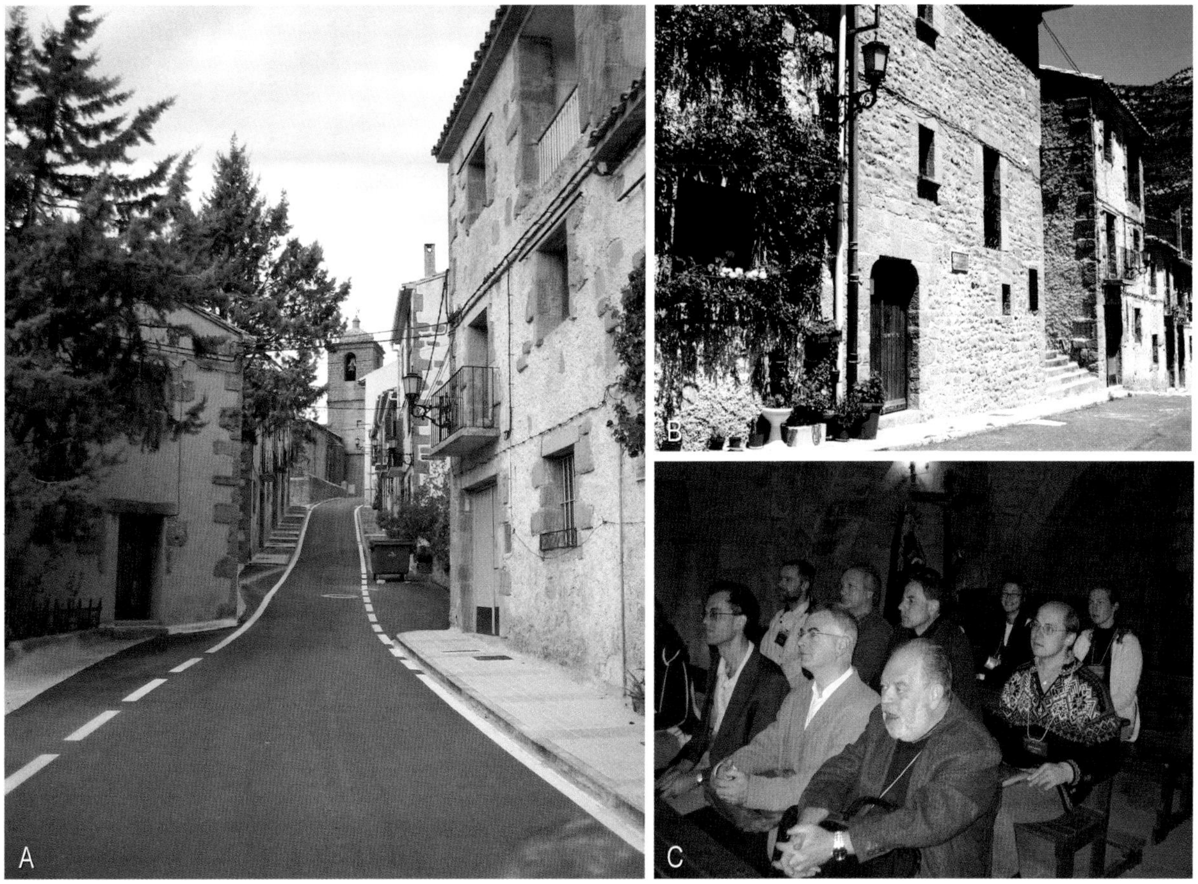

FIGURE 7. Petilla de Aragón (Navarra), birthplace of Cajal. **A**, Photograph of Main Street. The church of San Millán (XII-XIII century) can be seen in the background. **B**, The house where Cajal was born, located on Main Street. **C**, Image taken from inside the Church of San Millán during one of the scientific sessions of the international meeting on classification of cortical neurons "Petilla terminology" (Ascoli et al., 2008). First row: Bernardo Rudy, György Buzsáki, and Giorgio Ascoli. Second row: Carl Petersen, Andreas Burkhalter, Tamás Freund, and Gábor Tamás. Third row: Ruth Benavides-Piccione and Lidia Alonso-Nanclares.

available before the discovery of the black reaction of Golgi, the visualization of nerve cells was incomplete; often, it was only feasible to observe the cell body and the proximal portions of the dendrites and axon. For example, in the classic book of Rudolf Albert von Kölliker (1817–1905) published in 1852, the year Cajal was born, the structure of the nervous system was described in a very simple manner (Figure 13). Another interesting example is the illustration of the hippocampal formation by Kupffer (1859) (Figure 14), where all fields can be recognized but without details about the possible connections and scant anatomical information.

For a long time the relationship between nerve cells and nerve fibers remained unclear. Indeed, in the mid nineteenth century there were two hypotheses: one suggested that a nerve fiber is an outgrowth from a single cell (e.g., Bidder and Kupffer, 1857; His, 1886), whereas the alternative maintained that nerve cells and fibers were two independent elements in the nervous system. In this latter case, it was proposed that the nerve fibers differentiate within a continuous protoplasmic meshwork during very early stages of development (the "protoplasmic bridge" theory by Hensen [1864]). An essential step in the microanatomical analysis of the nervous system was the initial introduction of methods to dissociate this tissue manually and mechanically with dissection needles, with or without the use of chemical agents to harden the tissue and facilitate the dissection of

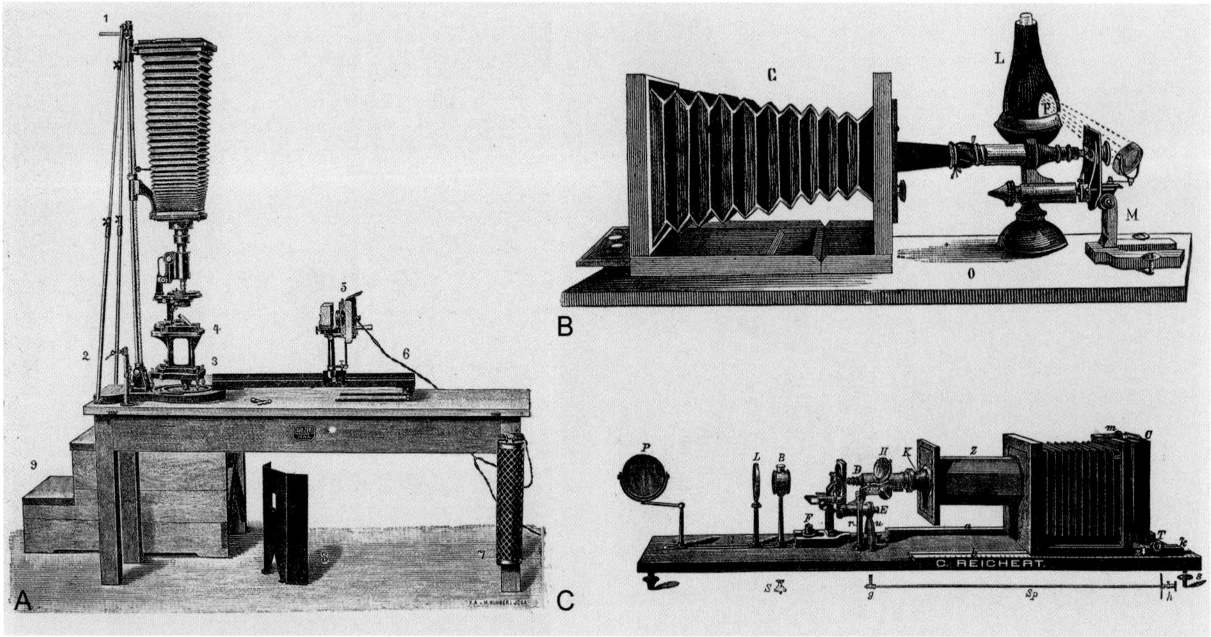

FIGURE 8. Illustrations of photomicrography devices (**A**, **B**, **C**) published by Cajal in various editions of the *Manual de histología normal y de técnica micrográfica* (A, 1889b; B, 1893c; C, 1914).

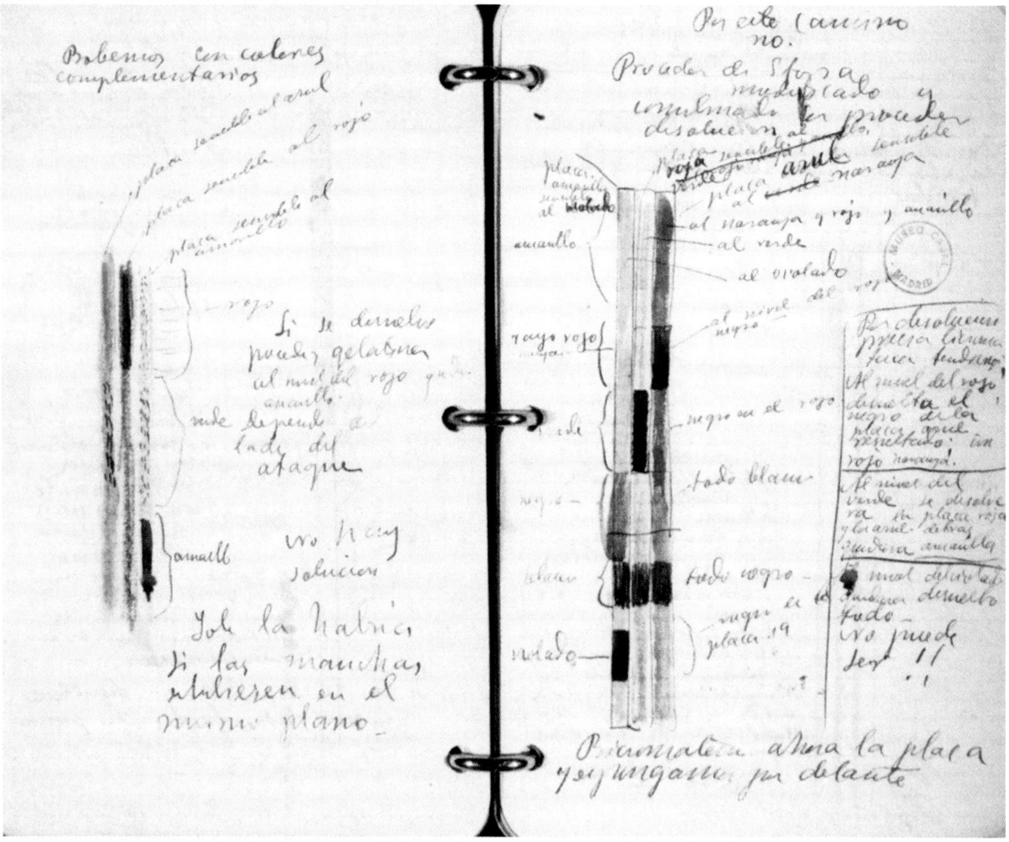

FIGURE 9. Notebook and protocols of Cajal with notes on color photography.

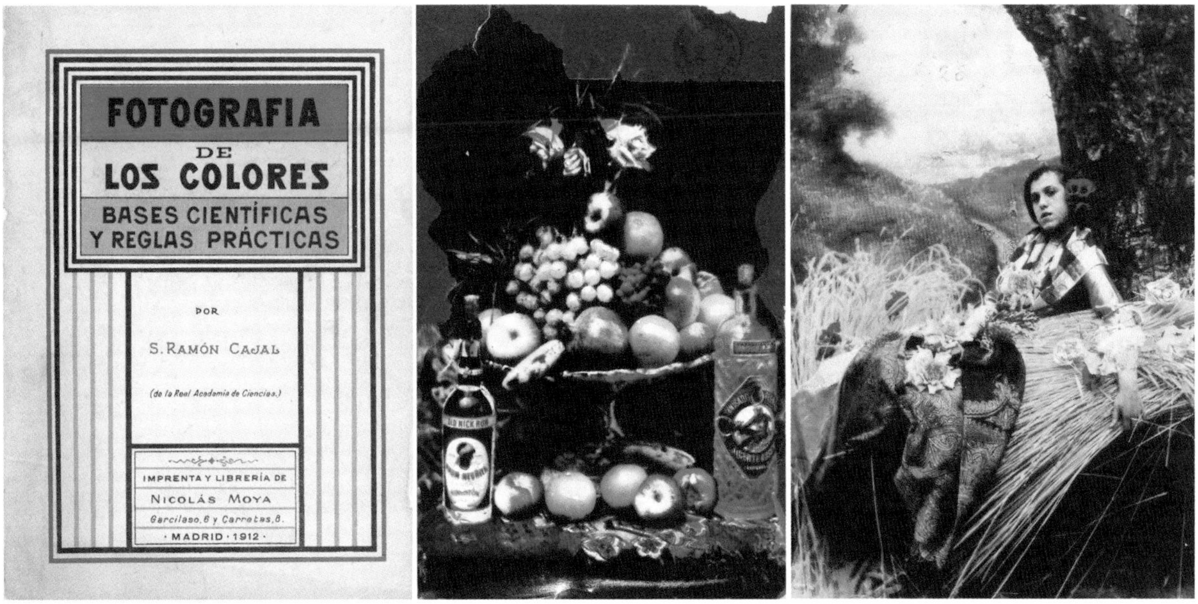

FIGURE 10. *Left*, Cover of Cajal's book *Fotografía de los Colores*, 1912. *Center*, Cajal's photograph, a still life in color with flowers, fruit, and bottles (trichrome procedure on paper), 1907. *Right*, Composition in color with a young girl (trichrome procedure on paper), 1907. Taken from DeFelipe et al. (2007).

nerves, ganglia, and nerve cells. Using this method, in 1833 and 1836, Christian Gottfried Ehrenberg (1795–1876) described "granules" (nerve cells) in the gray matter of the brain and ganglia, noting that these elements were often multipolar with several processes. However, Ehrenberg did not attribute any special significance to the granules, but rather these findings simply served to demonstrate that the gray matter of the nervous system was not a homogeneous amorphous mass, as assumed by several authors at that time (Clarke and Jacyna, 1987). These observations were confirmed by several researchers who initially proposed that all these processes were similar in nature. However, several authors soon indicated that only one of the processes had the characteristics of a nerve fiber (Barker, 1899).

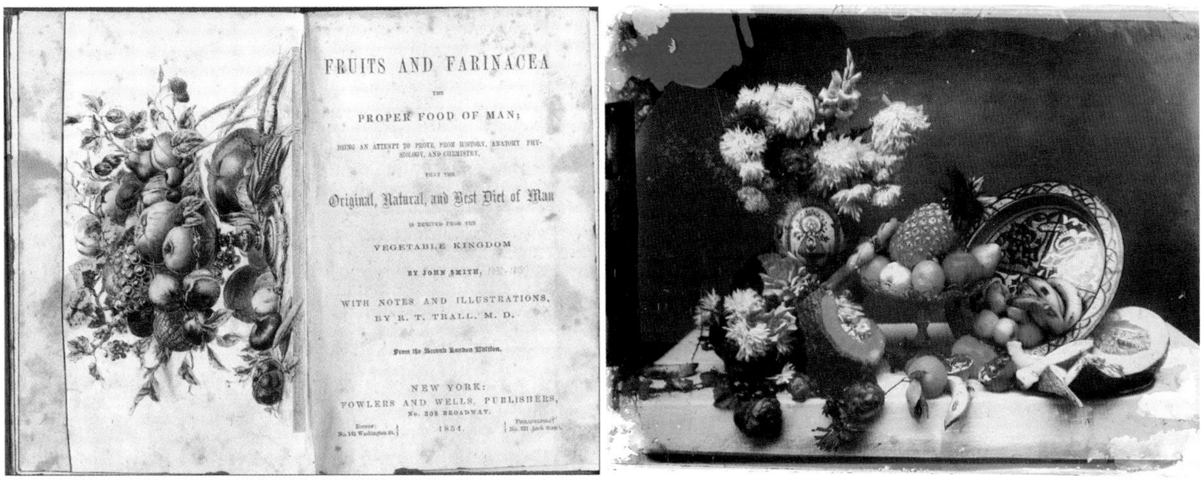

FIGURE 11. *Left,* Image taken from John Smith's book, *Fruits and Farinacea: The Proper Food of Man* (1854). *Right,* Still life by Cajal (see Figure 10 for technical details). Note the aesthetic resemblance between the drawing in the book and the photograph by Cajal.

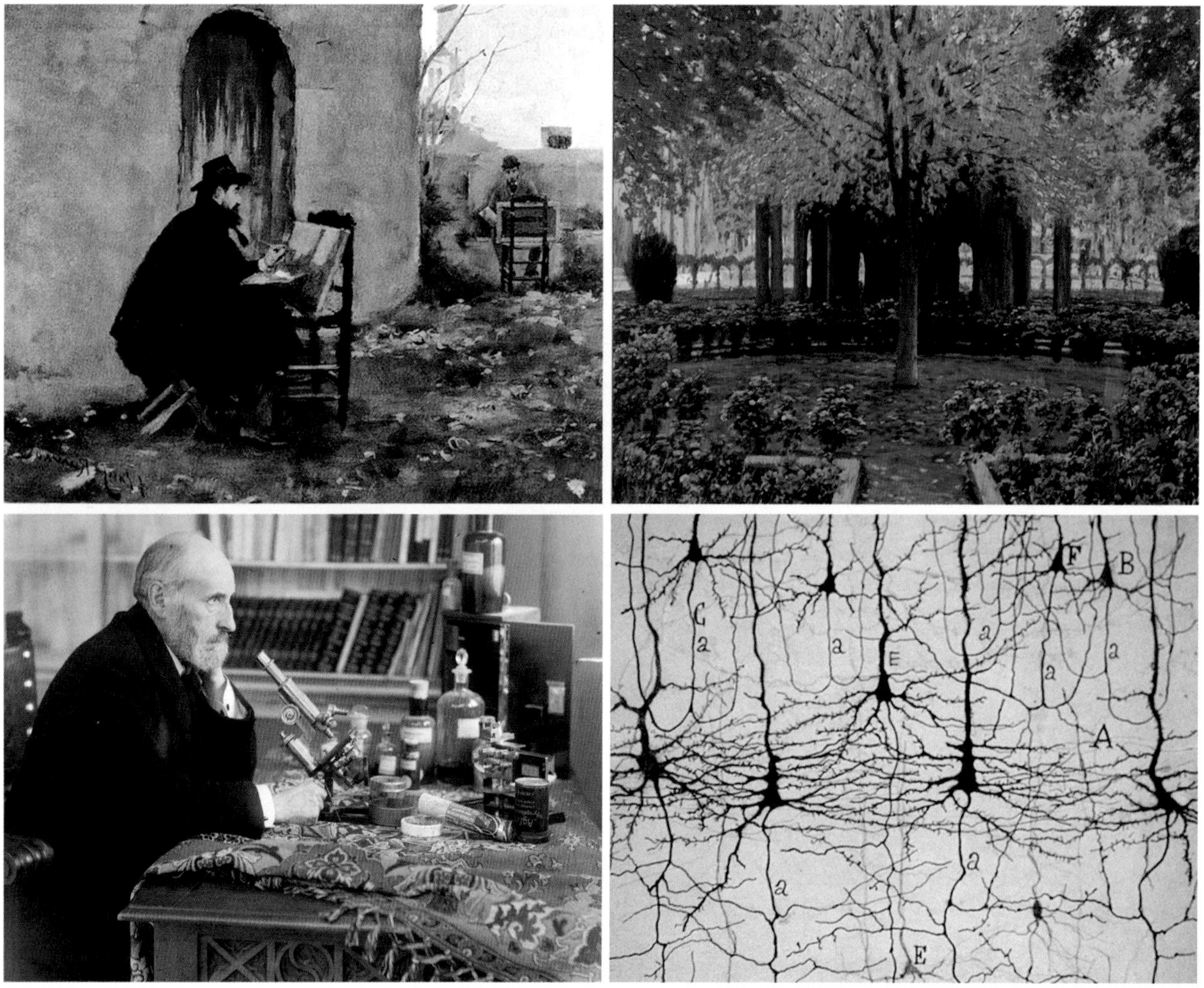

FIGURE 12. Art and science. *First row*: paintings by artists Santiago Rusiñol (1861–1931) and Ramón Casas (1866–1932). *Left*, "Ramón Casas y Santiago Rusiñol, retratándose" (1890). This image has been flipped horizontally to facilitate the composition of the figure. *Right*, "Glorieta de Cipreses-Jardines Aranjuez" (Rusiñol, 1919). *Second row, Left*, self-portrait photograph of Cajal. *Right*, original drawing by Cajal to illustrate neurons impregnated with the Golgi method in the cat visual cortex (Cajal, 1921).

Among these scientists, Robert Remak (1815–1865) is considered to be the first to have clearly illustrated the continuity between the axon and cell body, and to have distinguished the two main types of fibers that we recognize today: myelinated and unmyelinated fibers, described in 1838 by Remak as a "primitive band within a very thin-walled tube and organic fiber" (as cited in Van der Loos, 1967; Brazier, 1988). Otto Friedrich Karl Deiters (1834–1863) improved the dissociation method by introducing the treatment of the tissue with potassium dichromate. In 1865, two years after he died, the important generalization that all multipolar ganglion cells of vertebrates have two morphological and functional types of processes was published (Deiters, 1865). The first type was an axon that became myelinated, then called an *Achsencylinderfortsatz* (cylinderaxil prolongation), a term introduced in 1839 by J. F. Rosenthal (a student of Purkinje [Shepherd, 1991]); the second was several short, branching processes (dendrites) that he called *Protoplasmafortsätze* (protoplasmic prolongations). Furthermore, he distinguished a principal axon, (a) in Figure 15, originating from the soma and several thin axons emerging from the

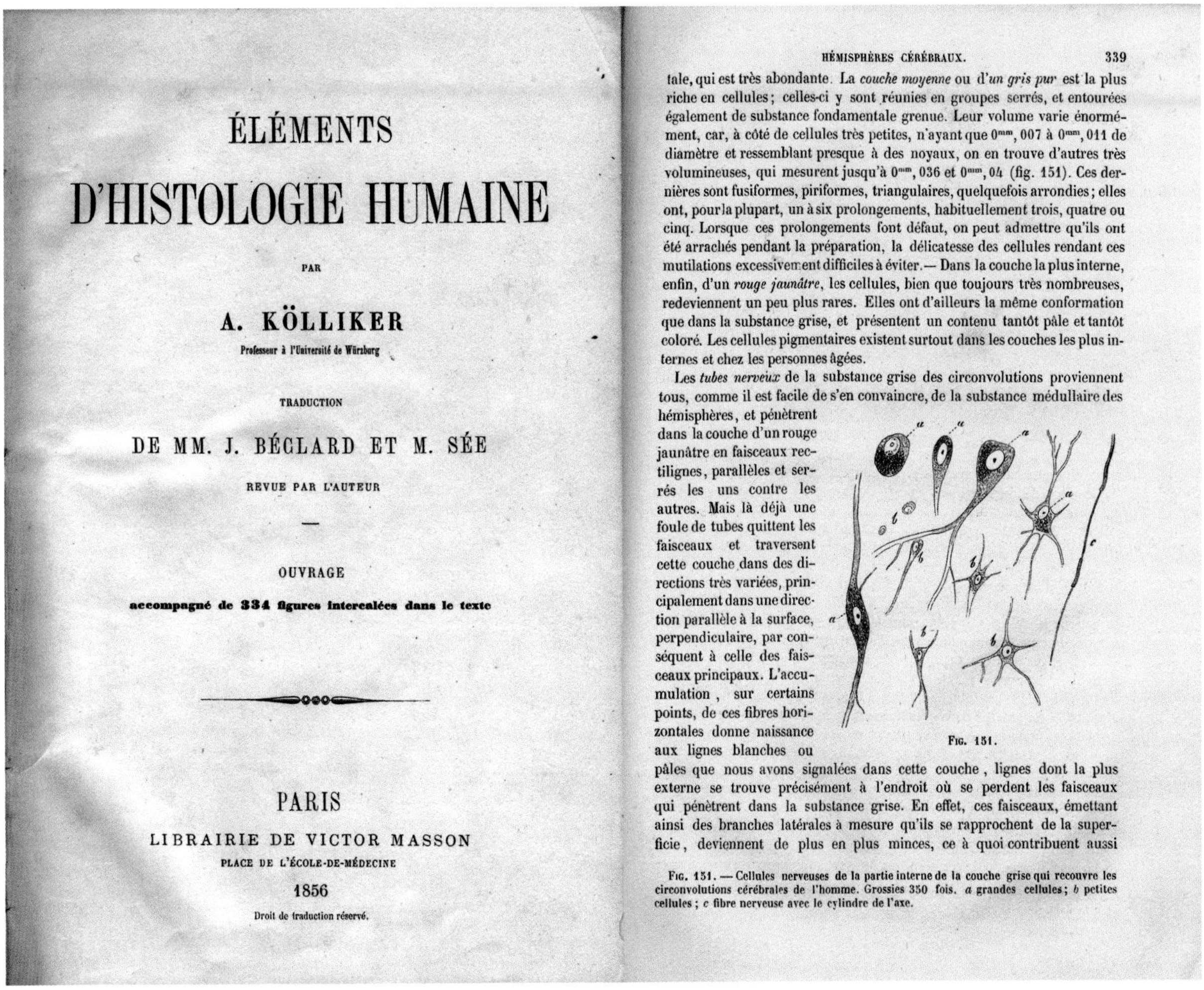

ÉLÉMENTS

D'HISTOLOGIE HUMAINE

PAR

A. KÖLLIKER

Professeur à l'Université de Würzburg

TRADUCTION

DE MM. J. BÉCLARD ET M. SÉE

REVUE PAR L'AUTEUR

OUVRAGE

accompagné de 334 figures intercalées dans le texte

PARIS

LIBRAIRIE DE VICTOR MASSON

PLACE DE L'ÉCOLE-DE-MÉDECINE

1856

Droit de traduction réservé.

HÉMISPHÈRES CÉRÉBRAUX. 339

tale, qui est très abondante. La *couche moyenne* ou d'*un gris pur* est la plus riche en cellules; celles-ci y sont réunies en groupes serrés, et entourées également de substance fondamentale grenue. Leur volume varie énormément, car, à côté de cellules très petites, n'ayant que 0mm,007 à 0mm,011 de diamètre et ressemblant presque à des noyaux, on en trouve d'autres très volumineuses, qui mesurent jusqu'à 0mm,036 et 0mm,04 (fig. 151). Ces dernières sont fusiformes, piriformes, triangulaires, quelquefois arrondies; elles ont, pour la plupart, un à six prolongements, habituellement trois, quatre ou cinq. Lorsque ces prolongements font défaut, on peut admettre qu'ils ont été arrachés pendant la préparation, la délicatesse des cellules rendant ces mutilations excessivement difficiles à éviter.— Dans la couche la plus interne, enfin, d'un *rouge jaunâtre*, les cellules, bien que toujours très nombreuses, redeviennent un peu plus rares. Elles ont d'ailleurs la même conformation que dans la substance grise, et présentent un contenu tantôt pâle et tantôt coloré. Les cellules pigmentaires existent surtout dans les couches les plus internes et chez les personnes âgées.

Les *tubes nerveux* de la substance grise des circonvolutions proviennent tous, comme il est facile de s'en convaincre, de la substance médullaire des hémisphères, et pénètrent dans la couche d'un rouge jaunâtre en faisceaux rectilignes, parallèles et serrés les uns contre les autres. Mais là déjà une foule de tubes quittent les faisceaux et traversent cette couche dans des directions très variées, principalement dans une direction parallèle à la surface, perpendiculaire, par conséquent à celle des faisceaux principaux. L'accumulation, sur certains points, de ces fibres horizontales donne naissance aux lignes blanches ou pâles que nous avons signalées dans cette couche, lignes dont la plus externe se trouve précisément à l'endroit où se perdent les faisceaux qui pénètrent dans la substance grise. En effet, ces faisceaux, émettant ainsi des branches latérales à mesure qu'ils se rapprochent de la superficie, deviennent de plus en plus minces, ce à quoi contribuent aussi

Fig. 151.

Fig. 151. — Cellules nerveuses de la partie interne de la couche grise qui recouvre les circonvolutions cérébrales de l'homme. Grossies 350 fois. *a* grandes cellules; *b* petites cellules; *c* fibre nerveuse avec le cylindre de l'axe.

FIGURE 13. *Left*, cover of the French edition (1856) of Kölliker's classic book *Handbuch der Gewebelehre des Menschen* (1852). *Right*, Figure 151 of the book where various morphological types of nerve cells in the human cerebral cortex are illustrated.

dendrites, giving rise to a second axonic system. According to Cajal (1899–1904), the discovery of this "second axonic system" was the starting point that led to the reticular theory (*vid.* Section A, "The Reticular Theory and Precursors of the Neuron Theory"). It is true that Deiters' method of mechanical dissociation (1865) enabled the morphology of a neuron to be completely visualized (Figure 15), but it was a technique that was very difficult to perform. Moreover, other disadvantages were that the cells were not observed in situ and the dissociation might have introduced artifacts affecting, for example, the shape of the dissociated cells. Cajal, in his autobiography *Recuerdos de mi vida: Historia de mi labor científica* (*Recollections of My Life: The Story of My Scientific Work*; 1917b, page 71) wrote:

> The procedure of mechanical dissociation . . . , applied to the analysis of the ganglia, of the retina, of the spinal cord or of the brain, the delicate operation of detaching the cells from their matrix of cement and of unraveling and extending their branched processes with needles, constituted a task for a Benedictine. What a delight it was when, by dint of much patience, we could completely isolate a neuroglial element, with its typical spider-like form, or a colossal motor neuron from the spinal cord, free and well separated with its robust axis

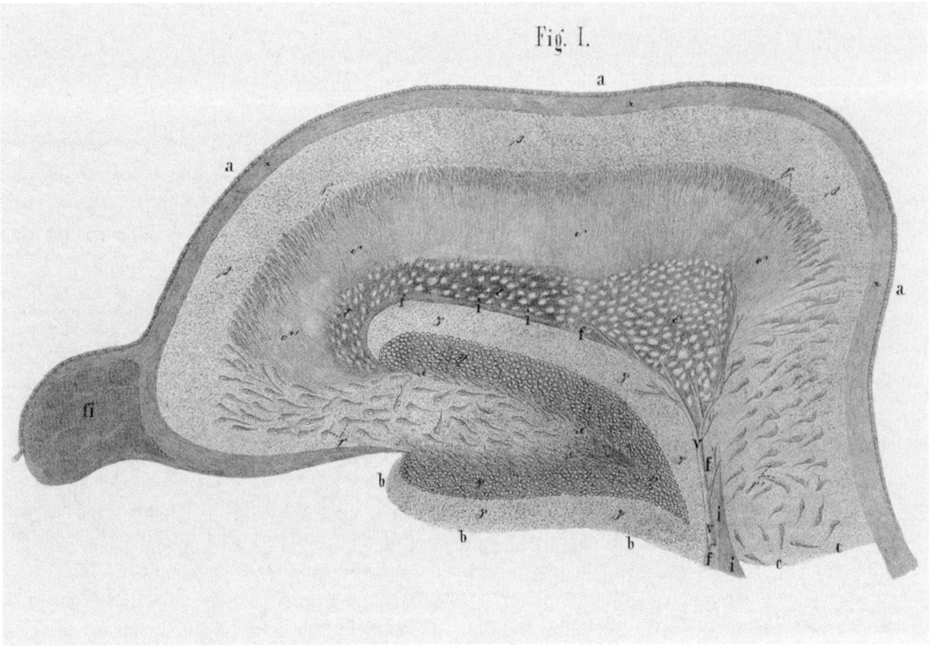

FIGURE 14. Illustration of the hippocampal formation taken from Kupffer (1859). The same hippocampal regions can be distinguished as in the drawings of Golgi (Figure 19) and Cajal (Figure 39), but with a rather rudimentary structure. See Note 2 for the transcription of the legend.

cylinder and dendrites! What a triumph to capture the bifurcation of the single process [axon] from a dissociated spinal ganglia, or to clear a pyramidal cell from its neuroglial bramble thicket, that is, the noble and enigmatic cell of thought!

Thus, it was not possible to follow the trajectory of the thin axons or to visualize the terminal axonal arbors. Hence, it was still not technically feasible to address one of the key needs to study the organization of the nervous system—the tracing of the

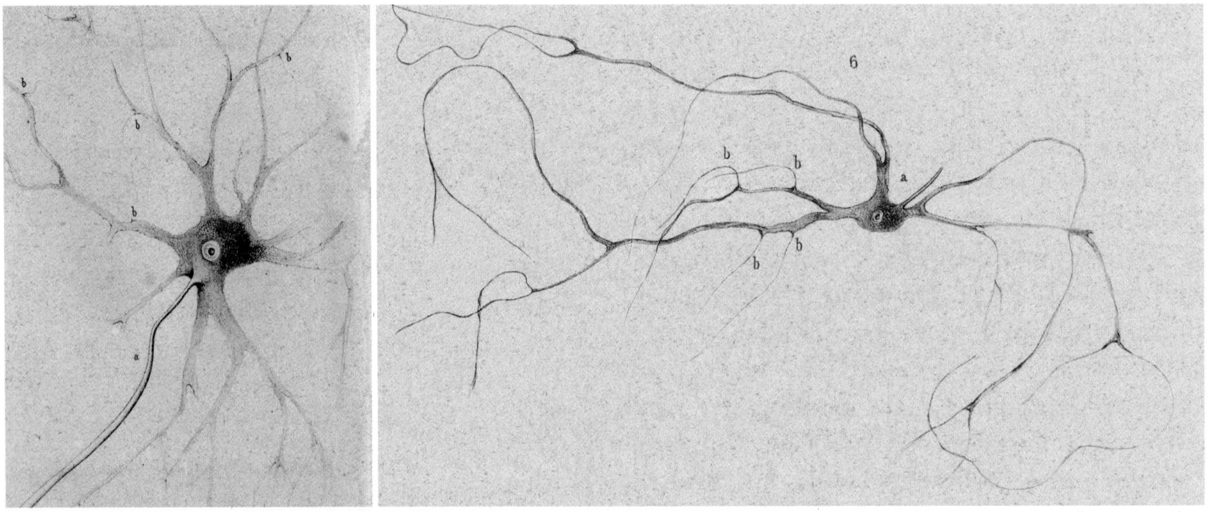

FIGURE 15. Drawings by Deiters (1865) to illustrate nerve cells (spinal cord of the ox). Method of mechanical dissociation. Deiters distinguished a principal axon (a) originating from the soma and several thin axons arising from the dendrites (b, "second axonic system"). According to Cajal, the erroneous interpretation of this second axonic plexus was the starting point of the reticular theory. See Section A, "Neuron doctrine versus the reticular theory," for further details.

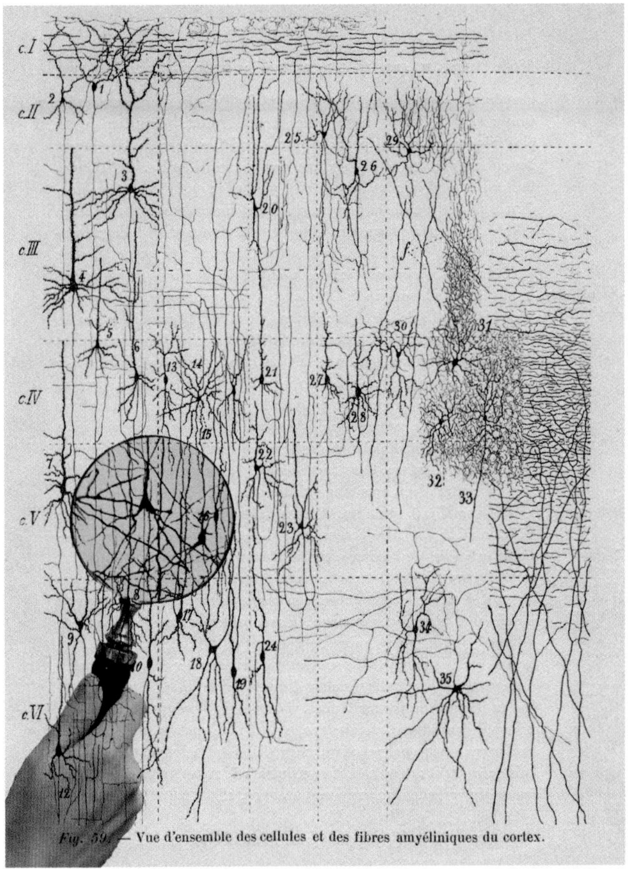

FIGURE 16. *Exploradores de la mente*, artistic composition to illustrate that progress in the study of the structure of the brain, at an intermediate resolution as can be achieved by optical microscopy, is based on the development of optical instruments and staining techniques (which at the beginning were rudimentary), as well as subjective interpretation of the microscopic world. Taken from DeFelipe (2014).

connections between neurons. This was again beautifully described by Cajal in *Recuerdos de mi vida* (1917b, pages 100–101):

> The great enigma in the organization of the brain revolves around our need to ascertain how the nervous ramifications end and how neurons are mutually connected. Referring to a simile already mentioned, the idea was to inquire how the roots and branches of the trees in the grey matter terminate, so that in such a dense jungle, in which there are no gaps thanks to its refined complexity, the trunks, branches and leaves touch everywhere.

As we will see in detail in Section A, "The Discovery of the *Reazione Nera:* Commencing the Detailed Study of the Structure of the Nervous System," this methodological void was resolved primarily with the discovery of the black reaction of Golgi. At last, the study of the microscopic world of the brain with the black reaction attracted many scientists to try to unravel the mysteries of its organization (Figure 16). In this search, scientists encountered an almost infinite number of cellular forms with an extraordinary beauty, allowing the discovery of a new artistic world, the "neuronal forest," giving free rein to their imagination and a new way of viewing the brain.

SECTION A

The Scientific Atmosphere in Cajal's Times

The Discovery of the *Reazione Nera*: Commencing the Detailed Study of the Structure of the Nervous System

On February 16, 1873, a revolution began in the world of neuroscience. On this date, Golgi sent the following letter to his friend Niccolò Manfredi (Mazzarello, 1999, page 63):

> I spend long hours at the microscope. I am delighted that I have found a new reaction to demonstrate even to the blind the structure of the interstitial stroma of the cerebral cortex. I let the silver nitrate react with pieces of brain hardened in potassium dichromate. I have obtained magnificent results and hope to do even better in the future.

In this letter, Golgi was referring to a new technique to stain the nervous system, allowing neurons and glia to be visualized, labeling them black (*reazione nera*). This method, named the *Golgi method* after its discoverer, was published in the *Gazzeta Medica Italiani* on August 2, 1873 (Golgi, 1873): *Sulla struttura della sostanza grigia del cervello* (On the Structure of the Gray Substance of the Cerebrum). In this article he said (page 244), "Taking advantage of the method, found by me, to stain black the elements of the brain . . . I happened to discover some facts concerning the structure of the cerebral grey matter that I believe merit immediate communication."

Thanks to a very simple staining protocol, requiring a "prolonged immersion of the tissue, previously hardened with potassium or ammonium dichromate, in a 0.50 or 1.0% solution of silver nitrate" (Golgi, 1873, page 244), for the first time it was possible to observe neurons and glia in a histological preparation (Figure 17) with all their parts (cell body, dendrites, and axon, in the case of neurons; cell body and processes in the case of glia which were described later). Furthermore, thanks to the Golgi method, it was possible to observe many cells at once in a given section and in situ, "in their natural position and shape," as Cajal said in *Textura del sistema nervioso del hombre y de los vertebrados* (Cajal [1899–1904]; Vol.1, 1899, page 24), without any possible artifacts that might be produced by dissociation methods. Figure 18 shows an example of the power of the Golgi method and its potential for studying the microanatomy of the nervous system when compared with the early days of the study of the nervous system.

Golgi used this method to examine many regions of the nervous system, providing new insights into the neuroanatomy of these structures, and he illustrated his findings with beautiful drawings, as shown in Figure 17 and Figures 19 through 22. Figures 20 and 22A show different types of neurons and glial cells in the hippocampal formation and cerebellar cortex, in great morphological detail, albeit with

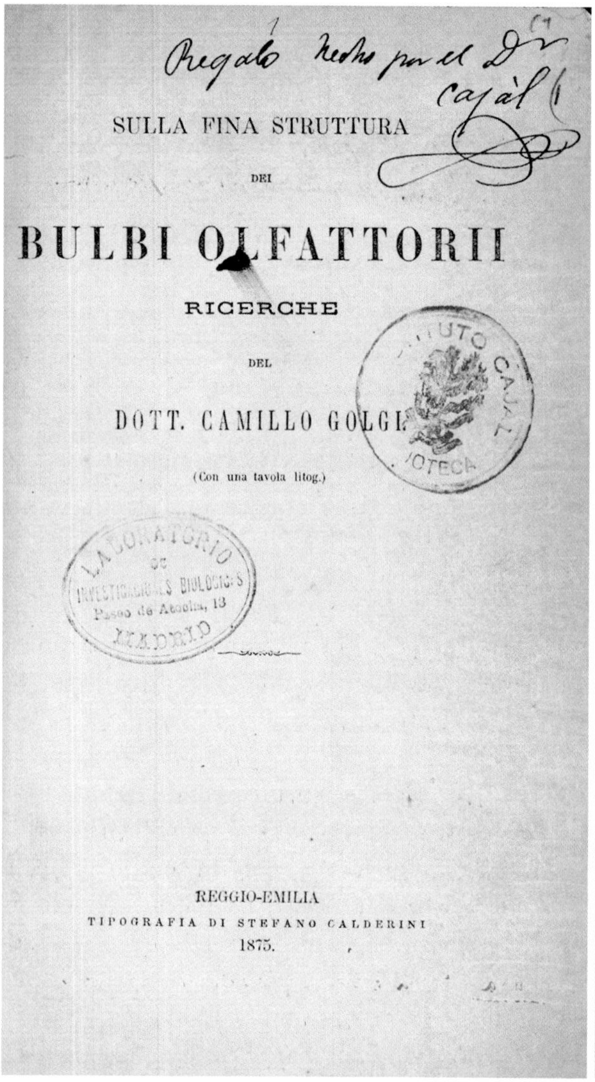

SULLA FINA STRUTTURA

DEI

BULBI OLFATTORII

RICERCHE

DEL

DOTT. CAMILLO GOLGI

(Con una tavola litog.)

REGGIO-EMILIA

TIPOGRAFIA DI STEFANO CALDERINI

1875.

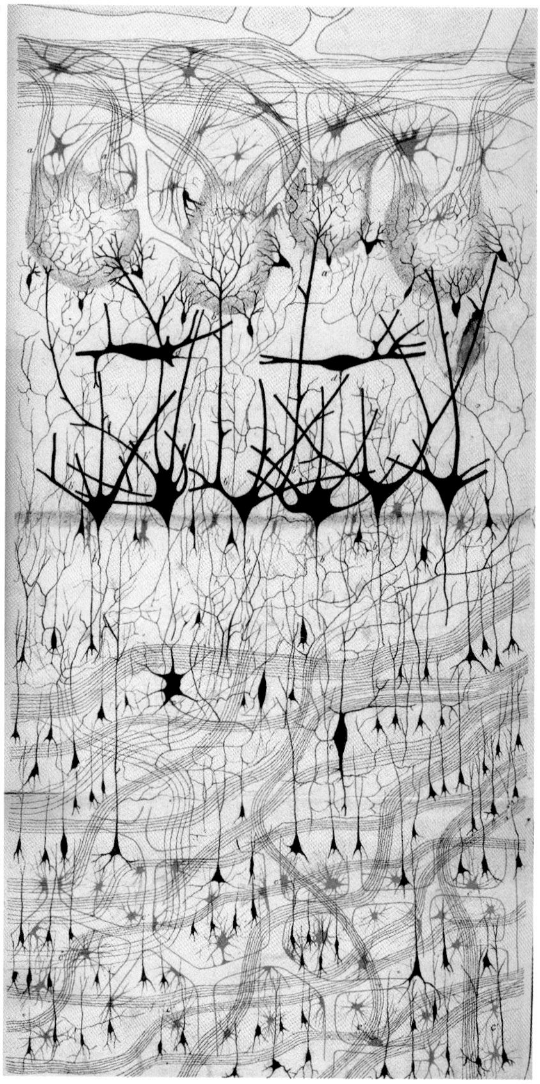

FIGURE 17. The first illustration by Golgi of a Golgi–impregnated preparation of the nervous system. "Semi-schematic drawing of a fragment of a vertical section of the olfactory bulb of a dog" (page 22). Taken from Golgi (1875). See Note 3 for a transcription of the legend.

some important exceptions, such as the dendritic arborizations of the hippocampal pyramidal cells and of Purkinje cells that appear free of dendritic spines (Figure 22B, C; see Section A, "Differences in the interpretation," for further discussion on this).

Another important advantage of the Golgi method was that only a small portion of the neurons in a given preparation were stained (Figure 23), permitting individual neurons to be examined in great morphological detail, which, for instance, allowed dendritic spines to be discovered (see Section A, "Dendritic spines"). Thus, it was at last possible to characterize and classify neurons, and potentially to study their connections. These characteristics of the Golgi method gave rise to another great advance—namely, that of tracing the first accurate circuit diagrams of the nervous system (DeFelipe, 2002a, 2002b) (see Section A, "Neuron doctrine").

The Discovery of the Golgi Method by Cajal and the Influence of Maestre de San Juan and Simarro

Cajal would probably not have achieved such eminence in science without the Golgi method, but it is intriguing to consider why such a long time passed

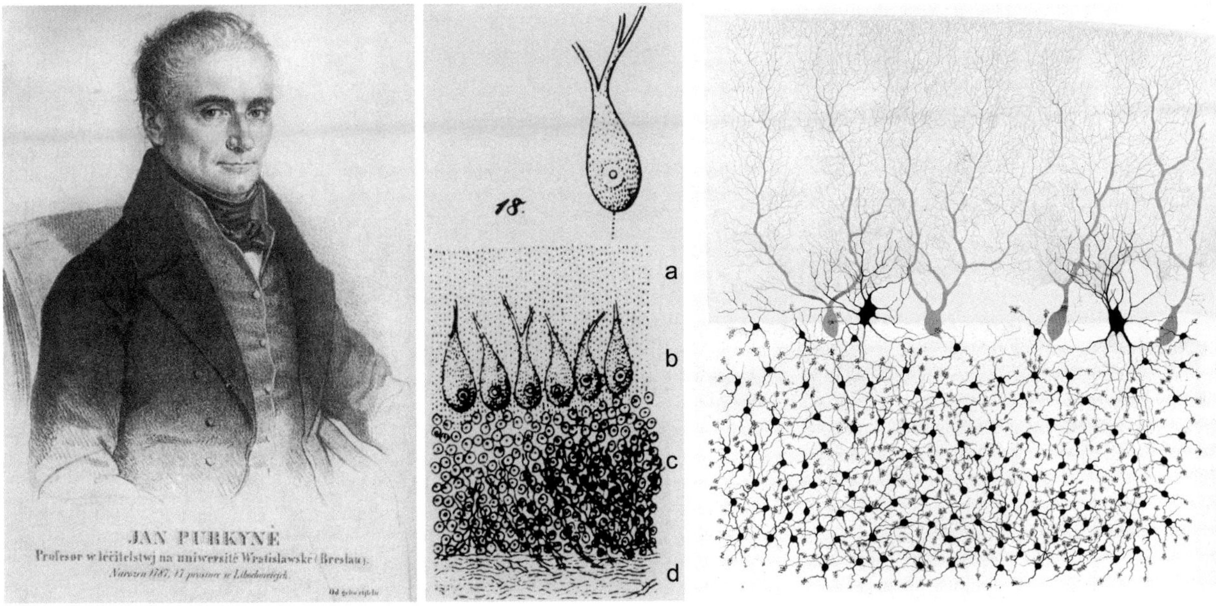

FIGURE 18. *Left*, Photograph of Jan Evangelista Purkinje (1787–1869). *Center*, Illustration of the first nerve cell identified (Purkinje, 1838), the large corpuscles of the cerebellum that were later called *Purkinje cells*. This illustration is also important because it was the first to show the cytoarchitecture of a region of the nervous system (Shepherd, 1991): a, molecular layer; b, large corpuscles; c, granules; d, fibers. *Right*, Illustration taken from Golgi showing the cytoarchitecture of the cerebellum visualized with the Golgi method. Note the great improvement in the visualization of the microanatomy of the Purkinje cells and granule cells. This drawing by Golgi was taken from Golgi (1882–1883). See Note 4 for a transcription of the legend.

between the method of Golgi being discovered in 1873 and it becoming popular among the scientific community during the 1890s when its potential was finally exploited. With few exceptions, the method of Golgi went virtually unnoticed. One of the most interesting examples is provided by the studies of Fridtjof Nansen (1861–1930), a Norwegian explorer, scientist, and diplomat who received the Nobel Peace Prize in 1922. In his publication on ganglion cells of invertebrates and the spinal cord of fish, *The Structure and Combination of the Histological Elements of the Central Nervous System* (Nansen, 1887) (Figure 24), Nansen not only attached great importance to the Golgi method, but also emphasized that there were no anastomoses between the processes of the ganglion cells (pages 75, 145 and 146):

> I shall now mention a method whose importance for our future knowledge of the nervous system can scarcely be overestimated, as it affords really quite marvelous preparations and far surpasses every method hitherto known. This is the black *chromo-silver method* of Prof. Golgi (at Pavia). By modifications of this method I have obtained excellent preparations, even from the spinal nerve-cord of Fishes, in which nobody before has succeeded . . . . *A direct combination between the ganglion cells is*, as we have seen, *not acceptable*. In spite of the most persevering investigations I have not been able to find any direct anastomosis of indubitable nature between the processes of the ganglion cells. Where I thought to have found an anastomosis it always on application of the strongest lenses resolved itself into an optical illusion. . . . If a direct combination is the common mode of combination between the cells, as most authors suppose, direct anastomoses between their processes ought, of course, to be quite common. When one has examined so many preparations (stained by the most perfect methods) as I have, without finding one anastomosis of indubitable nature, I think one must be entitled to say, that *direct anastomosis between the processes of the ganglion cells does not exist, as a rule.*

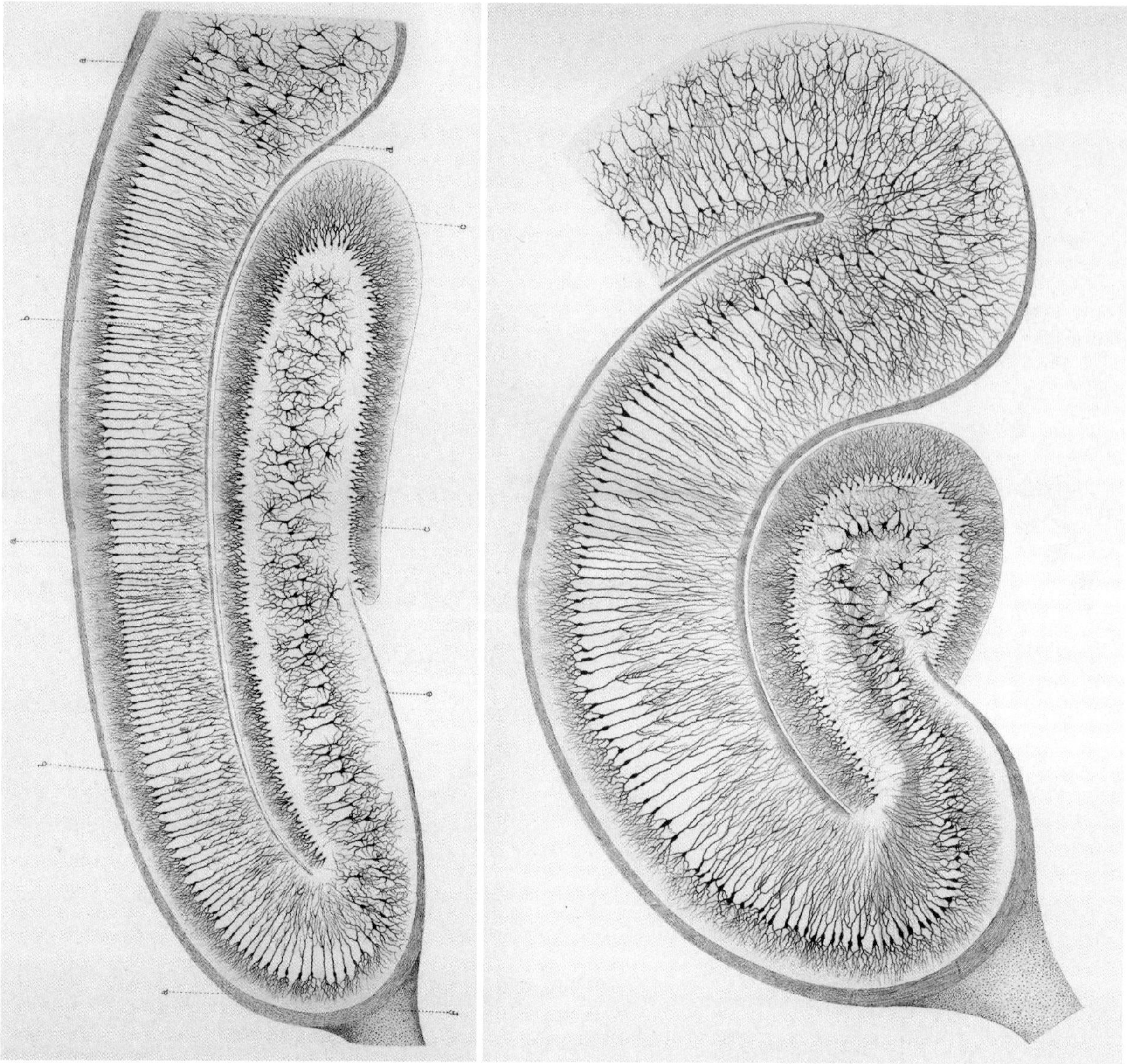

FIGURE 19. Drawings of the hippocampal formation by Golgi (1883). See Note 5 for a transcription of the legend.

It may be that the reasons why this publication went virtually unnoticed were that Nansen did not generalize his findings to the rest of the nervous system and that he did not confirm his observations in higher vertebrates. In addition, he did not have a distinguished scientist supporting his findings, unlike Cajal who was supported by Kölliker (see Section B, "Artistic skills and emotions").

In this regard, in *Recuerdos de mi vida* (Cajal, 1917b, page 76), Cajal wondered why the method of Golgi had not led to an explosion of excitement in the scientific community:

I expressed in former paragraphs the surprise which I experienced upon seeing with my own eyes the wonderful revelatory powers of the chrome-silver reaction and the absence of any excitement aroused in the scientific world by its discovery. How can one explain such strange indifference? Today, when I am better acquainted with the psychology of scientific men, I find it very natural . . . . Out of respect for the master, no pupil is wont to use methods of investigation which he has not learned from him. As for the great investigators, they would consider

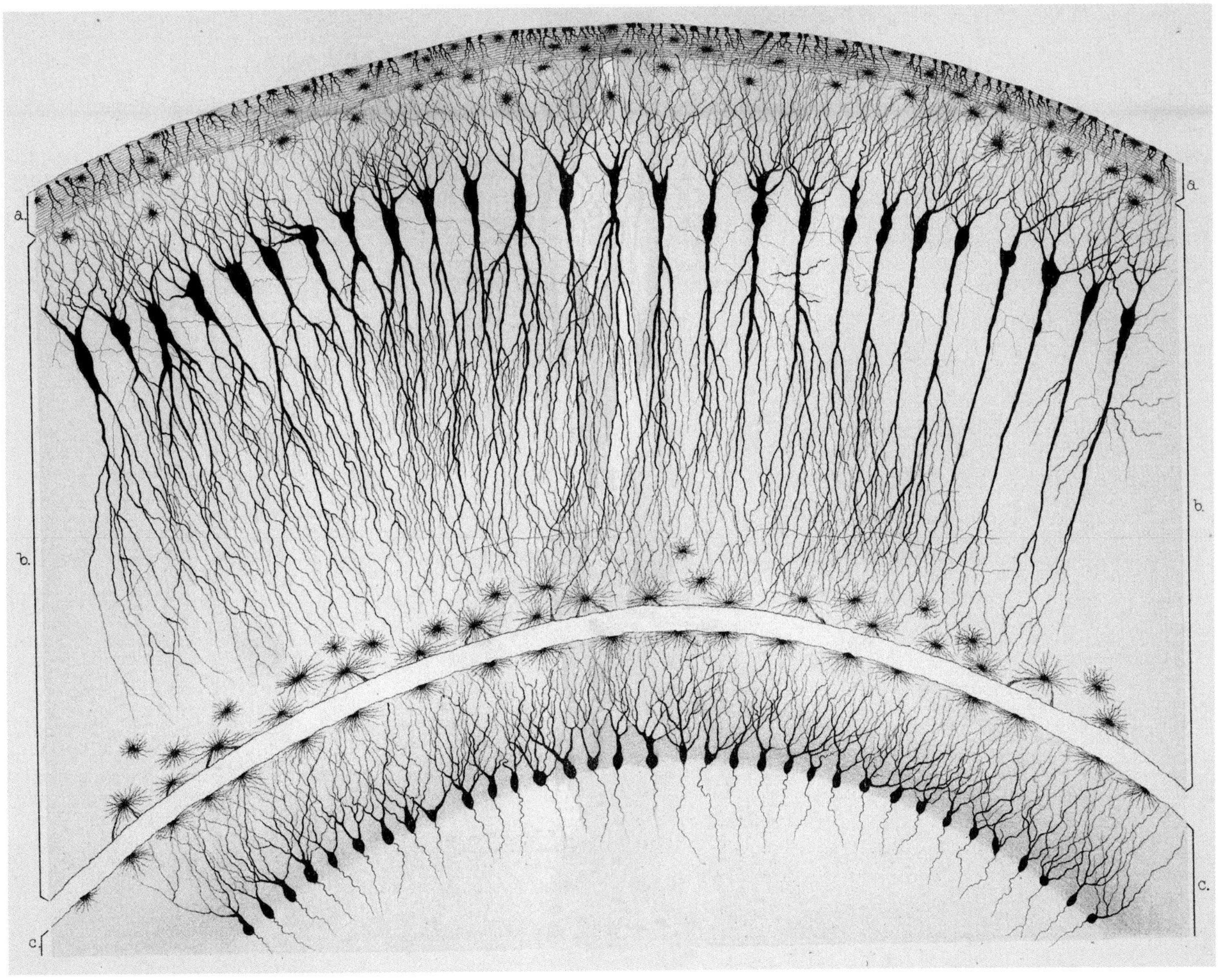

FIGURE 20. Drawing by Golgi (1883) to illustrate the cellular components in different hippocampal layers. See Note 6 for a transcription of the legend.

themselves dishonored if they worked with the methods of others.

These words of Cajal reflect the scientific atmosphere at the time, which can be seen in the very training that Cajal himself received (DeFelipe 2002b) (Figures 25 and 26). When Cajal was studying for his doctorate (*Patogenia de la inflamación* [see Merchán-Pérez, 2001]) and attending the doctoral course of normal and pathological histology in 1877, one of the principal texts used was the *Tratado de Histología Normal y Patológica* by Aureliano Maestre de San Juan (1828–1890), professor of histology at the Faculty of Medicine in Madrid (Figure 26, *upper right*). Indeed, it was this professor who first introduced Cajal to the field of microscopy. According to Cajal, he was so impressed by some of the beautiful histological preparations that Maestre de San Juan showed him that he decided to set up a laboratory of microscopy "as an indispensable complement of descriptive anatomy." In *Recuerdos de mi vida* (Cajal, 1917b, page 6), Cajal says,

> During the honeymoon of the microscope, I did nothing but satisfy my curiosity without method, merely scratching the surface of matters. I was offered a wonderful field of explorations, full of very agreeable surprises. With this spirit of spellbound spectator, I examined the blood corpuscles, epithelial cells, muscle fibers, nerve fibers, etc., pausing here and there to draw or photograph the most captivating scenes in the life of the infinitely small.

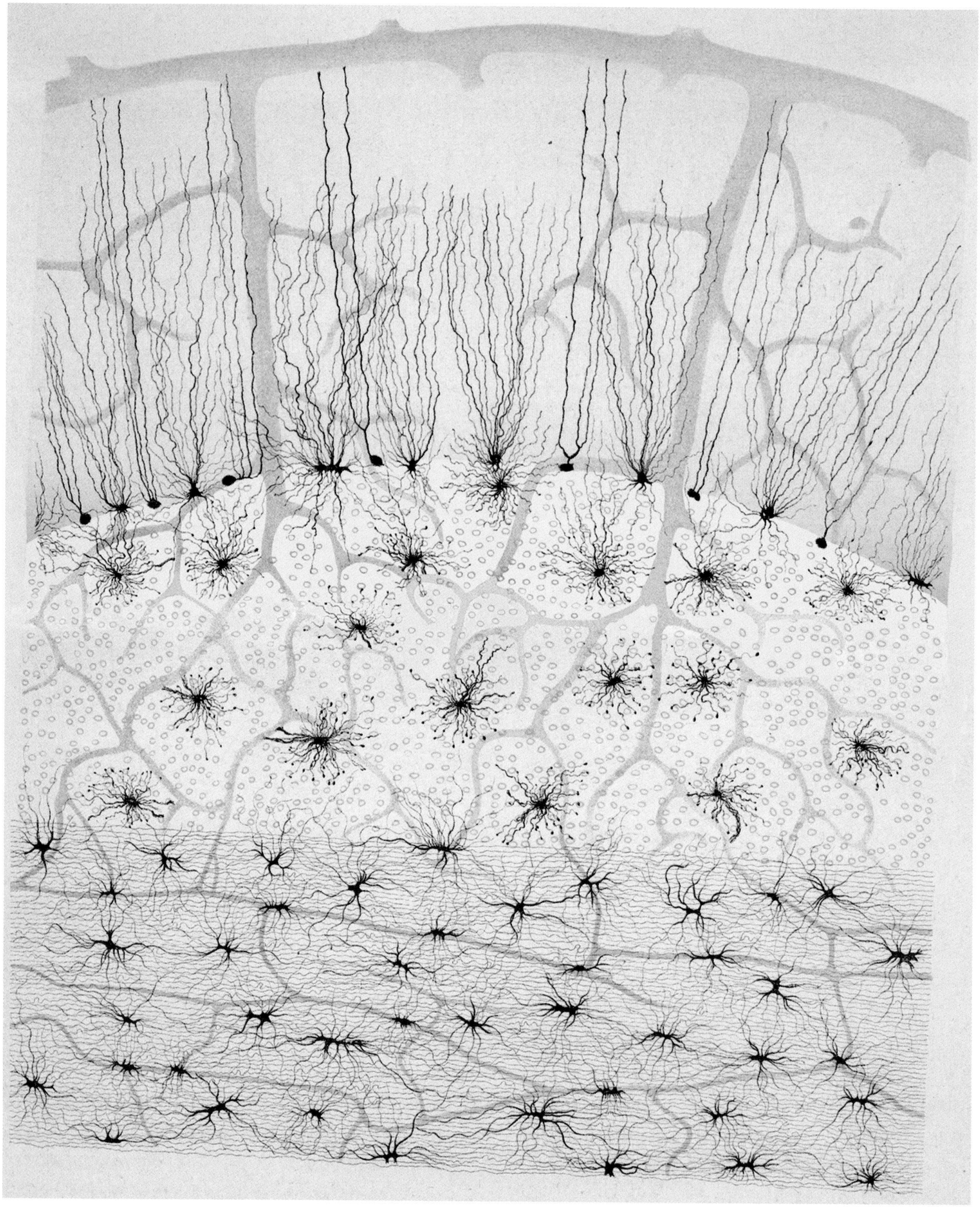

FIGURE 21. Drawing by Golgi (1882–1883) to illustrate glial cells in the cerebellum. See Note 7 for a transcription of the legend.

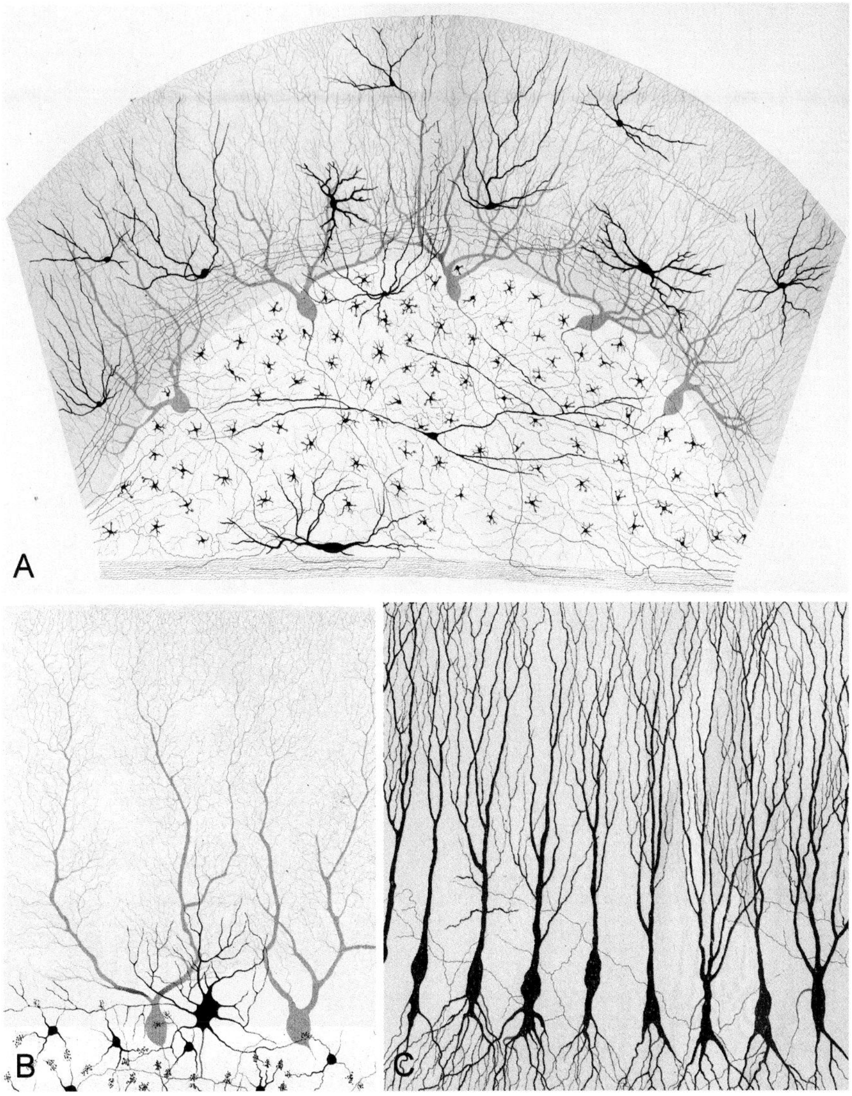

FIGURE 22. Drawings by Golgi of neurons stained with the method of Golgi. **A**, Different types of neurons in the cerebellum. Taken from Golgi (1882–1883). **B, C**, Details at higher magnification of Figure 18, *right*, and Figure 20 (this image has been rotated 180°), to illustrate the lack of spines in the dendrites of Purkinje cells of the cerebellum and in the pyramidal cells of the hippocampus, respectively. See Note 8 for a transcription of **A**.

However, in Maestre de San Juan's book, published in 1879 (Figure 27), and even in the second edition printed in 1885, there was no mention of the Golgi method. This was also true of another interesting book that Cajal used: *Tratado Elemental de Anatomía y Fisiología Normal y Patológica del Sistema Nervioso*, published by José Crous (1846–1887), Professor of Medical Pathology, in 1878. Crous' book neatly reflects just how rudimentary the knowledge of the organization of the brain was at that time (Figure 28). Thus, despite the years that had passed since its publication, the Golgi method was not commonly referred to in most of the contemporary texts available at the time.

Nevertheless, Cajal was aware of the existence of the Golgi method, even though he had not tested it, because he considered it to be of little use (Cajal, 1917b, page 73):

> But, as I mentioned, the admirable method of Golgi was then (1887–1888) unknown to the immense majority of neurologists or was underestimated

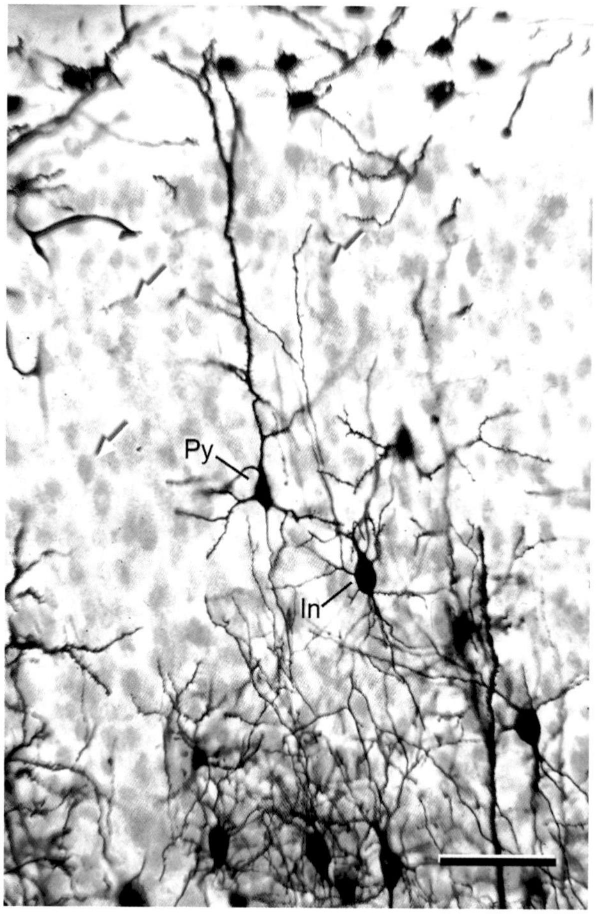

FIGURE 23. Preparation of mouse cerebral cortex stained with the Golgi method and counterstained with the method of Nissl (prepared in my laboratory). With the method of Golgi, only the cell body and its processes are stained in black, whereas when using the method of Nissl, only the cell bodies are stained in blue (white arrows indicate some stained cells). Note that with the method of Golgi, only a small proportion of the cells are stained. In, interneuron; Py; pyramidal cell. Scale bar: 100 μm.

> by the few who had precise information about it. Ranvier's book, my technical bible of those days, devoted only a few descriptive lines to it, written in an indifferent style. It was evident that the French savant had not tried it. Naturally, the readers of Ranvier, like myself, thought this method to be unworthy to be used.

If we compare Figure 13 of Kölliker (1852) with Figure 27 of Maestre de San Juan, we can see that although 27 years had elapsed since the publication of Kölliker's book, both drawings are very similar. This represents a good example of the slow progress in microanatomy resulting from the lack of appropriate methods and/or the incapacity to exploit the methods available. It was in this scientific setting that Cajal was interested in using this silver chromate method, thanks to Luis Simarro (1851–1921), a psychiatrist and neurologist who was also an enthusiast of histology (Figures 29 and 30). Interestingly, Simarro learned this method from Louis Antoine Ranvier (1835–1922) and introduced some modifications (Fernandez and Breathnach, 2001). It was in 1887, during a visit to Madrid, that Cajal—who was living in Valencia at the time—was invited into Simarro's own house, where he first saw a Golgi-impregnated preparation (Cajal, 1917b, pages 34–35) (Figure 31):

> I owe to Luis Simarro the unforgettable favour of having been shown the first good preparations made by the method of silver chromate which I ever saw, and of his having called my attention to the exceptional importance of the book of the Italian savant devoted to the examination of the fine structure of the gray matter [Golgi, 1885a] . . . . In fact, in 1887, it was in the house of Dr. Simarro at 41 Arco de Santa María Street [now called Augusto Figueroa, Madrid], that for the first time I had the privilege of viewing sections of the brain stained with the method of Weigert-Pal, and particularly . . . the sections impregnated by the silver method of the sage of Pavia. (See Note 9.)

Cajal was captivated by this marvelous staining method. The historical moment when he discovered the properties of the Golgi method is beautifully described in several of his writings, especially in the French translation (Cajal [1909–1911]; Vol. 1, 1909, pages 28–29) of the *Textura* (Cajal, 1899–1904), which represents an excellent example of his typical vivid writing style and enthusiasm (Figure 32):

> In summary, a method was necessary to selectively stain an element, or at most a small number of elements, that would appear to be isolated among the remaining invisible elements. Could the dream of such a technique truly become reality, in which the microscope becomes a scalpel and histology a fine

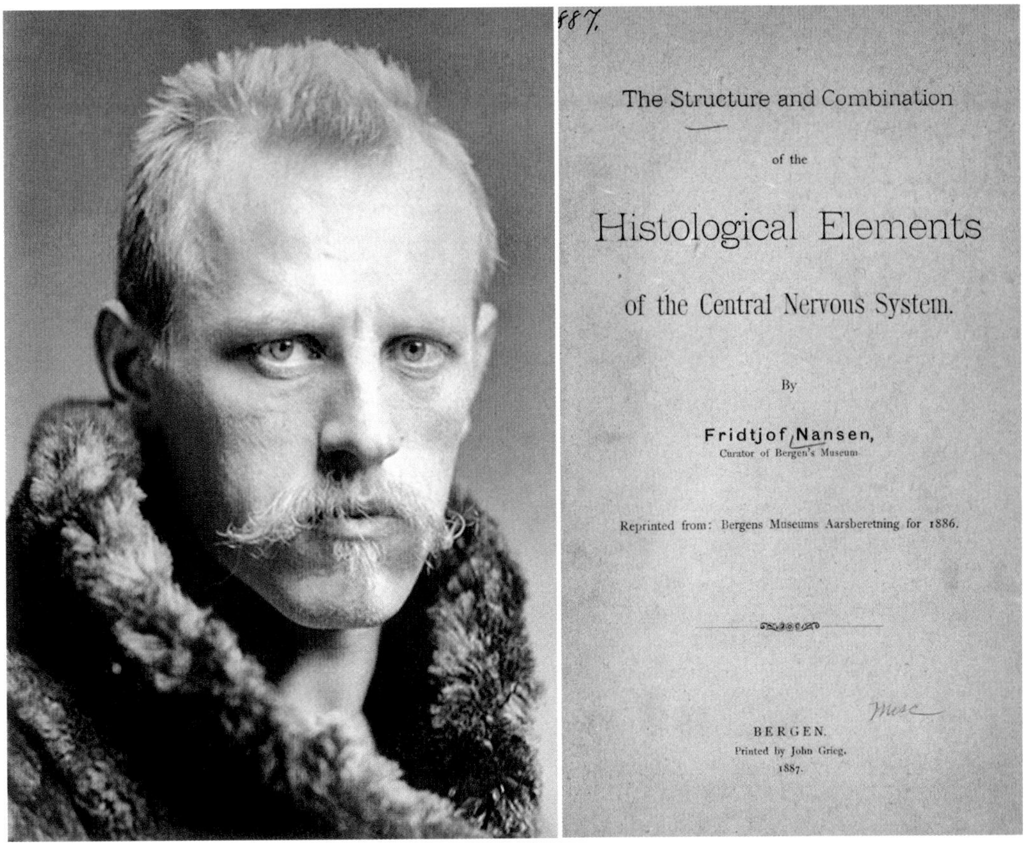
887.

The Structure and Combination

of the

Histological Elements

of the Central Nervous System.

By

Fridtjof Nansen,
Curator of Bergen's Museum.

Reprinted from: Bergens Museums Aarsberetning for 1886.

BERGEN.
Printed by John Grieg.
1887.

FIGURE 24. Portrait of Fridtjof Nansen and the first page of his book *The Structure and Combination of the Histological Elements of the Central Nervous System* (1887).

[tool for] anatomical dissection? A piece of nervous tissue was left hardening for several days in Müller's pure liquid [potassium dichromate] or in a mixture of this [fixative] with osmic acid. Whether it was the distraction of the histologist or the curiosity of the scientist, the tissue was then immersed in a bath of silver nitrate. The appearance of gleaming needles with shimmering gold reflections soon attracted the attention. The tissue was cut, and the sections were dehydrated, cleared, and then examined [with the microscope]. What an unexpected spectacle! On the perfectly translucent yellow background sparse black filaments appeared that were smooth and thin or thorny and thick, as well as black triangular, stellate or fusiform bodies! One would have thought that they were designs in Chinese ink on transparent Japanese paper. The eye was disconcerted, accustomed as it was to the inextricable network [observed] in the sections stained with carmine and hematoxylin where the indecision of the mind has to be reinforced by its capacity to criticize and interpret. Here everything was simple, clear and unconfused. It was no longer necessary to interpret [microscopically] the findings to verify that the cell has multiple branches covered with "frost," embracing an amazingly large space with their undulations. A slender fiber that originated from the cell elongated over enormous distances and suddenly opened out in a spray of innumerable sprouting fibers. A corpuscle confined to the surface of a ventricle where it sends out a shaft, which is branched at the surface of the [brain], and other cells [appeared] like comatulids or phalangidas. [See Note 10.] The amazed eye could not be torn away from this contemplation. The technique that had been dreamed of is a reality! The metallic impregnation has unexpectedly achieved this fine dissection. This is the Golgi method! . . . whose clear and decisive images

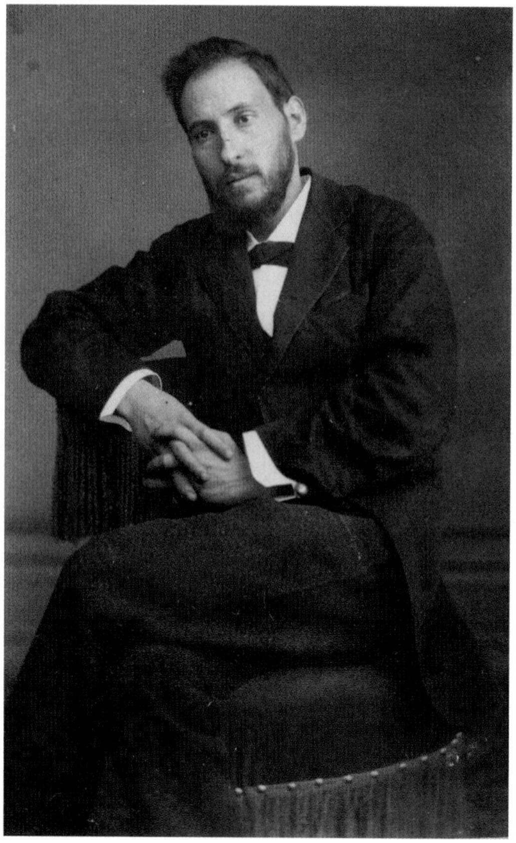

FIGURE 25. Santiago Ramón y Cajal, 1877.

enable us to cast off the famous net of Gerlach, the [dendritic] arms of Valentin and Wagner, as well as many another fanciful hypothesis.

After the meeting with Simarro, Cajal immediately started to use the Golgi method and set about examining practically the whole nervous system. One year later, he had published his first important study titled *Estructura de los Centros Nerviosos de las Aves* (Structure of the Avian Nerve Centers) (Cajal, 1888), based on results obtained with this method in the avian cerebellum (Figure 33). In this study, Cajal made two great contributions. First, he described for the first time the existence of dendritic spines (which he also named), structures that currently generate particular interest (see Section A, "Dendritic spines"). Second, Cajal confirmed Golgi's conclusion that dendrites end freely; but, in contrast to Golgi, Cajal added the critical conclusion that this also applies to axons and their branches (see Section A, "Neuron doctrine").

The observations, concepts, and theories of Cajal published during the next few years were soon to have a profound impact on the researchers of the era. As a result, distinguished institutions and researchers invited Cajal to expound on his findings. One of his most important early conferences was the Croonian Lecture (Cajal, 1894a,b) delivered on March 8th at the Royal Society of London (Burlington House) in 1894. In this lecture, Cajal presented his microanatomical results obtained in small mammals. He presented data regarding the morphological aspects of his studies and also, importantly, emphasized the implications relating to neuronal circuitry by suggesting the routes followed by the impulses in complex regions, including the cerebral cortex (Figure 34). In several of these illustrations, he traced how the axons originating in different functional regions of the brain contact with neurons in particular regions (multifunctional integration of inputs from different sources) and how these neurons distribute the "processed" information within that particular region and to other brain regions (Figures 35 and 36). In addition, Cajal proposed mechanisms for brain plasticity, and presented the histological hypothesis of *trabajo mental o gimnasia cerebral* (mental work or mental gymnastics), which surprisingly gives the impression that it might have been taken from a current publication reporting on findings that had used highly sophisticated methods (DeFelipe, 2006).

During this period, Cajal skillfully described the microorganization of almost every region of the central nervous system (Figure 37), and the results were summarized in his classic book *Textura del sistema nervioso del hombre y de los vertebrados* (Cajal, 1899–1904). This text was more widely disseminated through a French translation "*Histologie du système nerveux de l'homme et des vertébrés*" (Cajal, 1909–1911) and subsequently received even greater exposure through the two English translations, one by Neely Swanson and Larry W. Swanson and the other by Pedro Pasik and Tauba Pasik. It is still widely used as a reference book. Furthermore, from the very onset of his studies with the Golgi method, Cajal made important discoveries and formulated fundamental

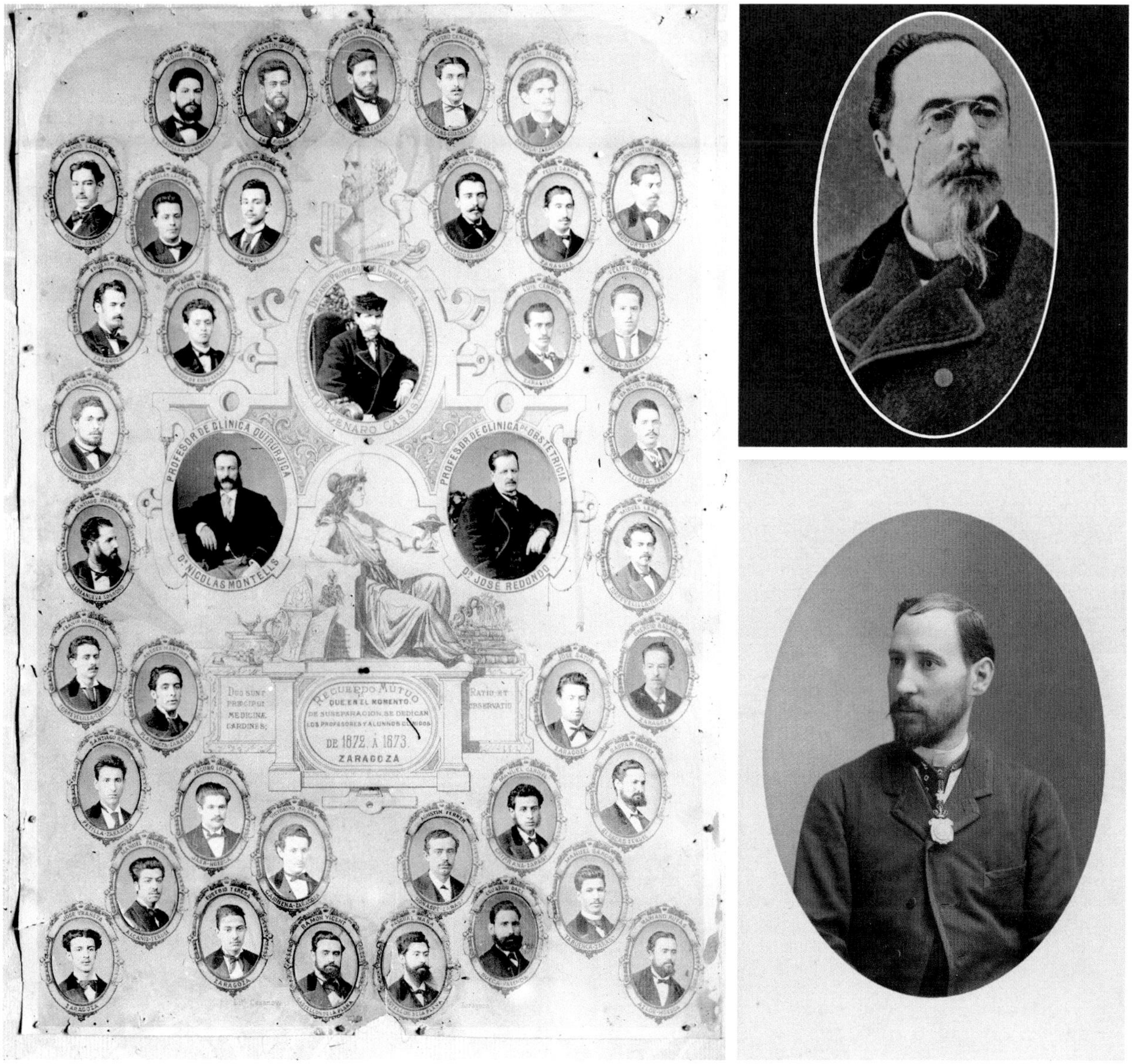

FIGURE 26. *Left*, Class graduation photograph of when Cajal obtained his medicine degree in 1873. *Upper right*, Portrait of Maestre de San Juan. *Lower right*, Photograph of Cajal in 1884, when he had recently transferred to the chair of Anatomy in Valencia.

theories regarding the development of the nervous system. For example, Cajal discovered and named the axonal growth cone (*cono de crecimiento*) (Cajal, 1890a), and he also devised the hypothesis of chemotaxis or chemotactism (Cajal, 1893b), later to be called *neurotropism*. Currently, these early contributions represent two of the most exciting fields of research in neuronal development. Finally, it is impressive that, by 1894, which was only a few years after Cajal had started using the Golgi method, he was able to devise accurate circuit diagrams of the nervous system, including complex structures such as the cerebral cortex (e.g., Cajal, 1891a, 1894b, 1903a) (Figures 34–36).

Drawing as a Tool to Illustrate Microscopic Images

When considering the history of neuroscience, it is fascinating to think that the description of microscopic images relied mainly on drawings because, unlike in modern laboratories, imaging techniques such as highly developed microphotography were

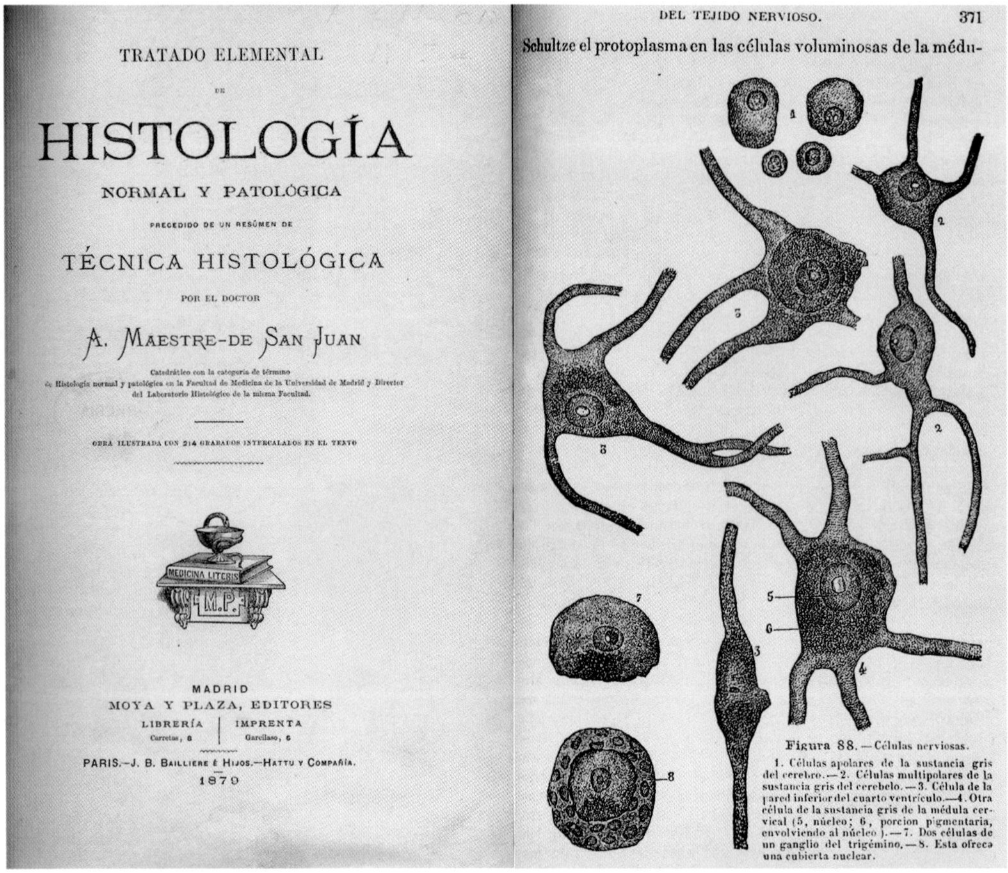
TRATADO ELEMENTAL

DE

HISTOLOGÍA

NORMAL Y PATOLÓGICA

PRECEDIDO DE UN RESÚMEN DE

TÉCNICA HISTOLÓGICA

POR EL DOCTOR

A. MAESTRE-DE SAN JUAN

Catedrático con la categoría de término de Histología normal y patológica en la Facultad de Medicina de la Universidad de Madrid y Director del Laboratorio Histológico de la misma Facultad.

OBRA ILUSTRADA CON 214 GRABADOS INTERCALADOS EN EL TEXTO

MEDICINA LITERIS

M.P.

MADRID

MOYA Y PLAZA, EDITORES

LIBRERÍA Carretas, 8 | IMPRENTA Garcilaso, 6

PARIS.—J. B. BAILLIERE É HIJOS.—HATTU Y COMPAÑÍA.

1879

DEL TEJIDO NERVIOSO. 371

Schultze el protoplasma en las células voluminosas de la médu-

Figura 88.—Células nerviosas.

1. Células apolares de la sustancia gris del cerebro.—2. Células multipolares de la sustancia gris del cerebelo.—3. Célula de la pared inferior del cuarto ventrículo.—4. Otra célula de la sustancia gris de la médula cervical (5, núcleo; 6, porcion pigmentaria, envolviendo al núcleo).—7. Dos células de un ganglio del trigémino.—8. Esta ofreca una cubierta nuclear.

FIGURE 27. Morphological types of nerve cells (taken from Maestre de San Juan, 1879, page 371). Cajal would have read the following regarding the morphological types of nerve cells in this book: "The nerve cell may or may not present prolongations of its protoplasm, and from that comes their division into: 1st, apolar, that is to say, without any protoplasmic prolongation . . . ; and 2nd, others [nerve cells] that show a variable number of prolongations."

not yet available. Several types of paper or cardboard (see Note 11) were used and the scientists would generally draw freehand on these, using a range of common media such as Indian ink, watercolor dyes, pencils, and pens (either separately or in different combinations). Scientists would draw either directly or with the help of a camera lucida—a plotting device that attaches to the microscope and projects the optical microscope image onto a drawing table. This makes it possible for the observer to trace the image and achieve an accurate drawing of the structures in question, aided by the fact that the paper, pencil, and histological preparation can all be visualized simultaneously (Figure 38). Anyone who has tried to draw a Golgi-impregnated neuron (or indeed one that has been filled using a different method) in detail at high magnification knows how difficult it is to achieve a complete impression of the neuron and its possible connections with other neurons without the aid of a camera lucida or some newer form of plotting device. Further detail regarding the different types of microscopic image reproduction methods and the material used for the illustrations can be found in the publications of Cajal, especially in his *Manual de histología normal y de técnica micrográfica* (*Handbook of Normal Histology and Micrographic Technique*), first published in 1889 (Cajal, 1889b) and re-edited over the years to include additional and corrected content. An English version was also published with the help of his disciple, Jorge Francisco Tello (1880–1958) (Cajal and Tello, 1933).

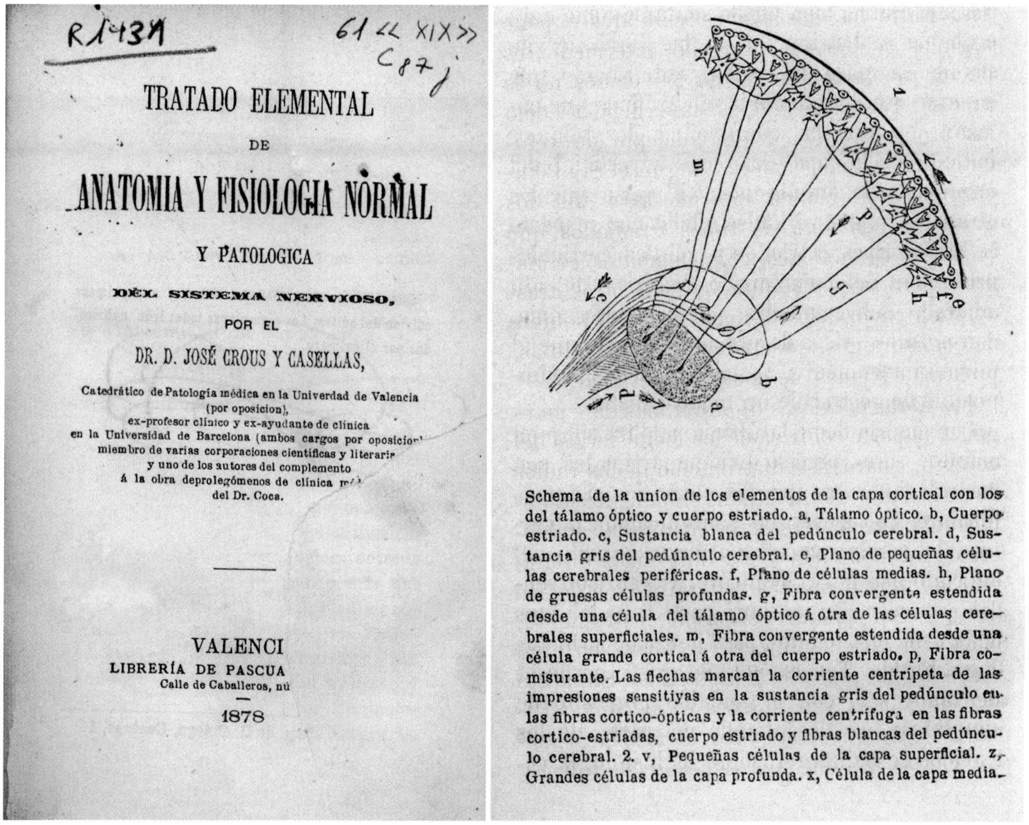

TRATADO ELEMENTAL
DE
ANATOMIA Y FISIOLOGIA NORMAL
Y PATOLOGICA
DEL SISTEMA NERVIOSO,
POR EL
DR. D. JOSÉ CROUS Y CASELLAS,
Catedrático de Patología médica en la Univerdad de Valencia
(por oposicion),
ex-profesor clínico y ex-ayudante de clínica
en la Universidad de Barcelona (ambos cargos por oposicion)
miembro de varias corporaciones científicas y literarias
y uno de los autores del complemento
á la obra deprolegómenos de clínica médica
del Dr. Coca.

VALENCI
LIBRERÍA DE PASCUA
Calle de Caballeros, nú
1878

Schema de la union de los elementos de la capa cortical con los del tálamo óptico y cuerpo estriado. a, Tálamo óptico. b, Cuerpo estriado. c, Sustancia blanca del pedúnculo cerebral. d, Sustancia gris del pedúnculo cerebral. e, Plano de pequeñas células cerebrales periféricas. f, Plano de células medias. h, Plano de gruesas células profundas. g, Fibra convergente estendida desde una célula del tálamo óptico á otra de las células cerebrales superficiales. m, Fibra convergente estendida desde una célula grande cortical á otra del cuerpo estriado. p, Fibra comisurante. Las flechas marcan la corriente centrípeta de las impresiones sensitiyas en la sustancia gris del pedúnculo en las fibras cortico-ópticas y la corriente centrífuga en las fibras cortico-estriadas, cuerpo estriado y fibras blancas del pedúnculo cerebral. 2. v, Pequeñas células de la capa superficial. z, Grandes células de la capa profunda. x, Célula de la capa media.

FIGURE 28. Taken from Crous (1878, page 47): "Scheme of the union of the elements of the cortical layer with those of the optic thalamus and corpus striatum. *a*, optic thalamus. *b*, corpus striatum. *c*, white matter of the cerebral peduncle . . . . Arrows indicate the centripetal and centrifugal currents."

However, it should be noted that in the majority of his publications, Cajal did not include a section with a detailed description of the methods used, and only on a rare occasion did he mention that a camera lucida had been used. For example, in the "Explanation of the plates" section in his 1891 paper *Sur la structure de l'écorce cérébrale de quelques mammifères* (On the Structure of the Cerebral Cortex of Certain Mammals) (Cajal, 1891b, page 173), Cajal wrote:

> The majority of our figures have been made using the Zeiss camera lucida, with the objective C of that manufacturer, and employing sometimes ocular 4, sometimes ocular 2. Figures 4 and 5 have been made with the very powerful E and Zeiss 1.30 apochromatic objectives.

However, Cajal appeared to prefer drawing directly, and used the camera lucida only when absolutely necessary, according to several accounts from those who knew him. On the first centenary of the birth of Cajal, one of his former students, Julian de la Villa wrote (de La Villa, 1952, page 24):

> The drawing was generated directly from the preparation; with the microscope on his left and the paper on his right, exact reproductions of [the preparations] began to appear. Although the camera lucida was known to him, because it was cumbersome to use, he preferred to avoid it.

It is also important to note that many of the illustrations by Cajal were composite drawings, especially those in which several cells were represented. Observation of Cajal's own histological preparations (now stored at the Instituto Cajal) clearly shows that this is the case and, indeed, Cajal mentioned this point in some of his publications, including *La rétine des vertébrés* (The Retina of Vertebrates) published in 1893 (Cajal, 1893b). In the "Explanation

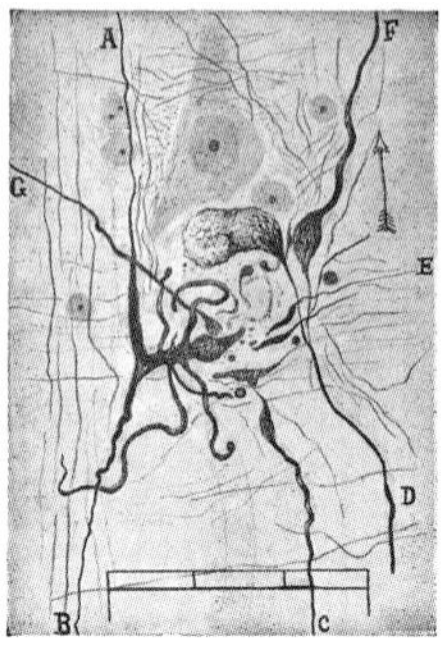

— 375 —

y monstruosas, en continuación con fibras de paso. Diríase que los retoños han sido atraídos hacia el territorio de la placa, á

Fig. 310.—Detalles de una placa de Fischer en vías de formación.—A, axon de proyección hipertrofiado junto á la placa, á la que envía recia colateral acabada en bulbo y numerosas ramas terminales; D, G, F, fibras terminadas en la región de la placa mediante botones ó bolas. (De un dibujo de Simarro).

influjo de alguna substancia especial neurotrópica. Ciertas mazas colosales, de retículo semidisgregado (D), parecen representar cilindros-ejes centrípetos bruscamente terminados (1).

(1) Por desgracia, el trabajo del Dr. Simarro, que data ya de cuatro años, permanece inédito todavía, no obstante el interés biológico de los datos que contiene.

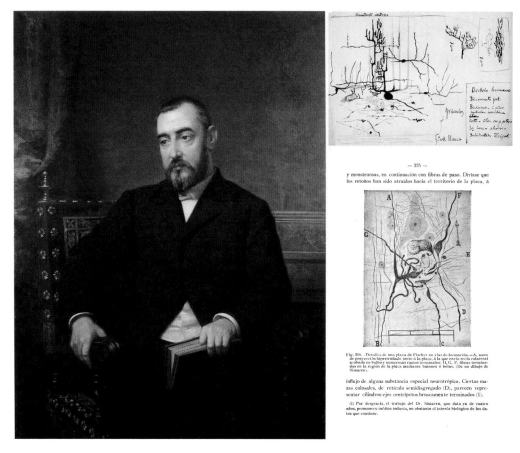

FIGURE 29. *Left*, Luis Simarro (Legado Cajal, Instituto Cajal). *Upper right*, Drawing from Simarro showing cells of the human cerebellum stained with the Golgi method (Legado Simarro, Universidad Complutense, Madrid. See Figure 31: Courtesy of Iñigo Azcoitia and Alberto Muñoz, Universidad Complutense). *Lower right*, Simarro's drawing of a senile plaque ("plaque of Fischer" [Fischer, 1912]) that was reproduced by Cajal in Figure 310 of the book *Estudios sobre la degeneración y regeneración del sistema nervioso* (Moya, Madrid, 1913–1914, page 375 [Vol. 2]): "Details of a plaque of Fischer in formation. *A*, hypertrophied projection axon, next to the plaque, to which it sends a thick collateral ending in a bulb and numerous terminal branches; *D, G, F*, fibers ending in buds or balls in the region of the plaque. (From a drawing by Simarro.) . . . It appears as if the sprouts had been attracted towards the region of the plaque under the influence of some special neurotropic substance" (see DeFelipe and Jones, 1991). The original drawing is held in the *Archivo Fernando de Castro*.

of the Plates" section of this article (page 247), he wrote:

> The majority of our figures have been made using the camera lucida of Abbe with a Zeiss C objective. We have reproduced, in the figures of large size, cells found in different sections of the retina of the same animal. However, they are represented as if they were seen in a single plane.

It is clear, then, that the complexities of particular regions of the nervous system were represented synthetically through the use of composite drawings in many of Cajal's illustrations. Although it is true that adopting this approach for illustrating microscopic observations was the source of a certain amount of skepticism, this was, in fact, also one of his most important contributions, because copying accurately the most relevant elements of the image to highlight the most important features of the structure being studied required both interpretative skills and artistic talent (Figure 39). As a consequence, the drawing of neural elements became an art. As we see in the next section, this provided an outlet for early neuroanatomists to express and develop their artistic talent.

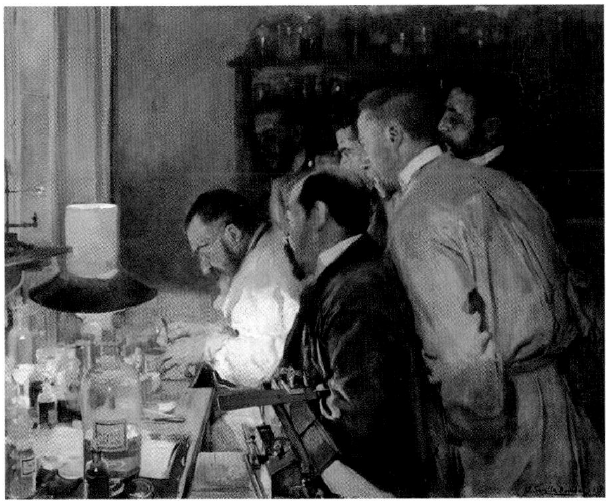

FIGURE 30. *Una investigación o el Dr. Simarro en el laboratorio* (1897) (An investigation or Dr. Simarro in the laboratory), by the painter Joaquin Sorolla Bastida (1863–1923), showing Luis Simarro (white coat) working in his laboratory. The large glass jar that appears in the foreground contains potassium dichromate, which—together with silver nitrate—make up the two main ingredients of the Golgi method (see the letter that Golgi sent to his friend Niccolò Manfredi, page 17). Madrid, Museo Sorolla (Inv. 417).

Differences in the Interpretation of the Microscopic World

Although it may seem reasonable to assume that what set Cajal apart from other scientists was an advantage in terms of the microscopes used or the histological preparations themselves, this was not the case. The microscopes used by all scientists at the time were, in fact, the same and the tissue preparations were similar. The key difference between Cajal and others was how he sought out detail relentlessly, noticing and interpreting it in ways that others did not. There are many examples that reveal differences in the interpretation of the microscopic world, such as the differences that can be seen between the drawings of the hippocampus by Golgi (Figure 19) and Cajal (Figure 39A). However, perhaps two of the most significant examples of such differing interpretations concern the connections between neurons (the neuron doctrine versus the reticular theory), and the debate about the existence of dendritic

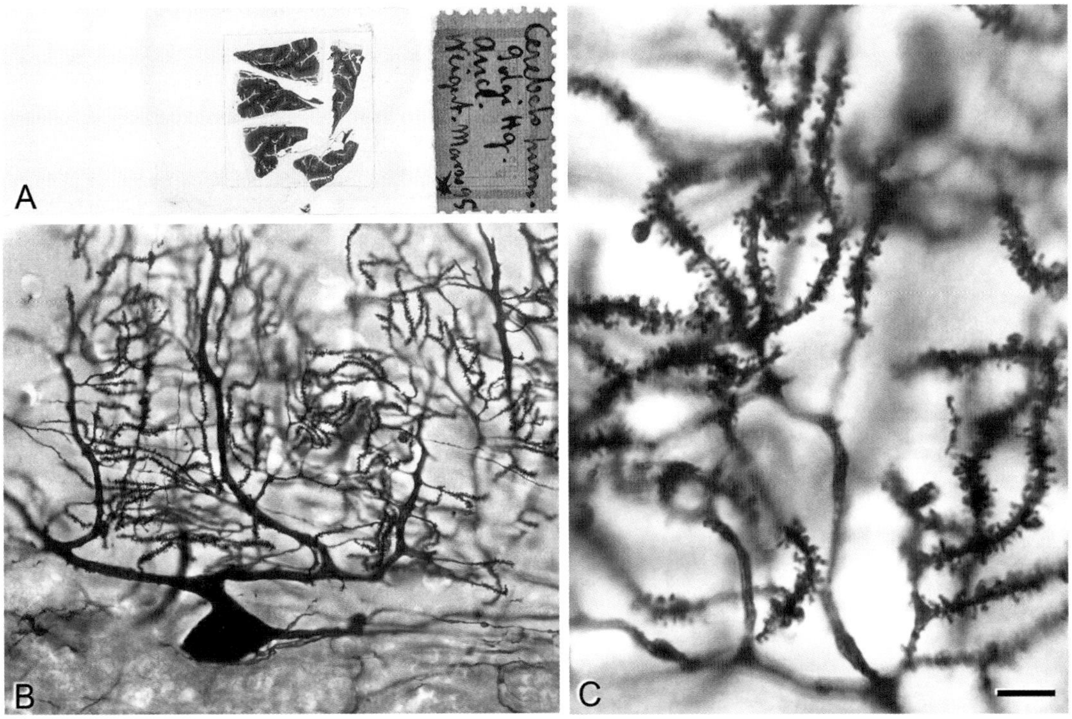

FIGURE 31. **A**, Photograph of a preparation from Simarro of the human cerebellum stained with the Golgi method in combination with the Weigert method. **B**, Low-power photomicrograph showing a typical Purkinje cell. **C**, Higher magnification of **B** showing dendritic spines. Scale bar (in C): 30 μm in **B**; 4.5 μm in **C**. The histological images (Legado Simarro, Universidad Complutense, Madrid) were taken by Iñigo Azcoitia and Alberto Muñoz (Universidad Complutense). Dendritic spines were discovered by Cajal in 1888 (see Section A, "Dendritic spines," for details).

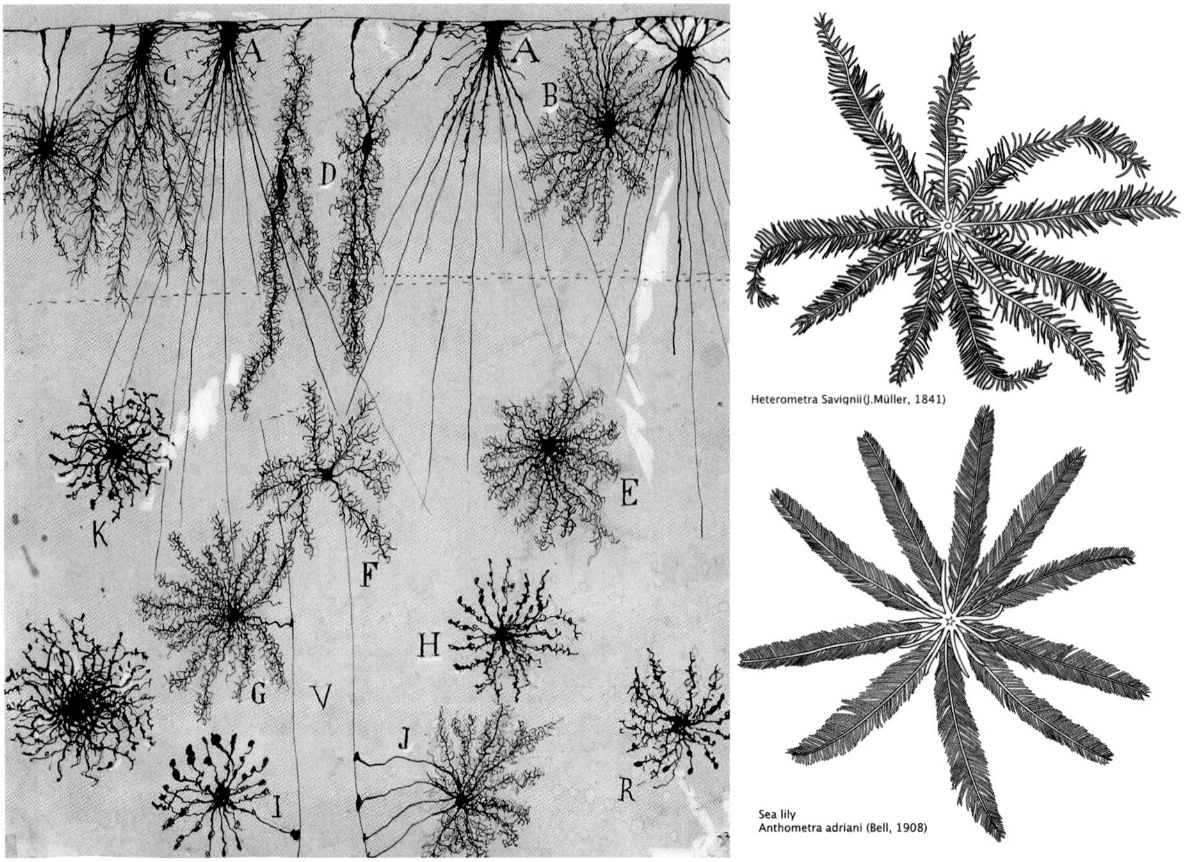

FIGURE 32. *Left,* Cajal's drawing of Golgi-impregnated neuroglia. The figure legend states: "Neuroglia of the superficial layers of the cerebrum: child of two months. Golgi Method. *A, B, [C], D,* neuroglial cells of the plexiform layer; *E, F, [G, H, K], R,* neuroglial cells of the second and third layers; *V,* blood vessel; *I, J,* neuroglial cells with vascular [pedicles]" (Cajal [1899–1904]; Vol. 2, 1904, page 853). The astrocyte vascular end-feet on blood vessels confirmed the observation made by Golgi (1885b), who often noticed that Golgi-impregnated processes from neuroglial cells were frequently in contact with both blood vessels (vascular end-feet or "sucker processes") and neurons. This finding prompted Golgi to suggest that the main function of glial cells was to supply nutrients to the nerve cells. *Right,* Two representative examples of sea lilies (class: Crinoidea, order: Comatulida): Top, *Alecto savignii = Heterometra savignii* (Müller, 1841) and bottom, *Anthometra adriani* (Bell, 1908). Original drawings from photographs of natural specimens by Ruth Morona (Departamento de Biología Celular, Facultad de Biología, Universidad Complutense de Madrid). Taken from DeFelipe (2014).

spines and their significance. These two subjects are discussed next.

NEURON DOCTRINE VERSUS THE RETICULAR THEORY

These two conflicting ideas about how neurons were connected suggested quite different functional consequences. The reticular theory maintained that nerve currents flow through a continuous network of neuronal processes. However, according to the neuron theory, these currents went from cell to cell via a point of contact "in much the same way that electric current crosses a splice between two wires" (Cajal [1909–1911]; Vol. 1, 1909, page 92). These new ideas about the connections between neurons therefore led to novel theories about the relationship between neuronal circuits and brain function (DeFelipe, 2010b).

The Reticular Theory and Precursors of the Neuron Theory

During this early period, the most common view regarding the organization of the nervous system was the reticular theory. According to Cajal (1899–1904),

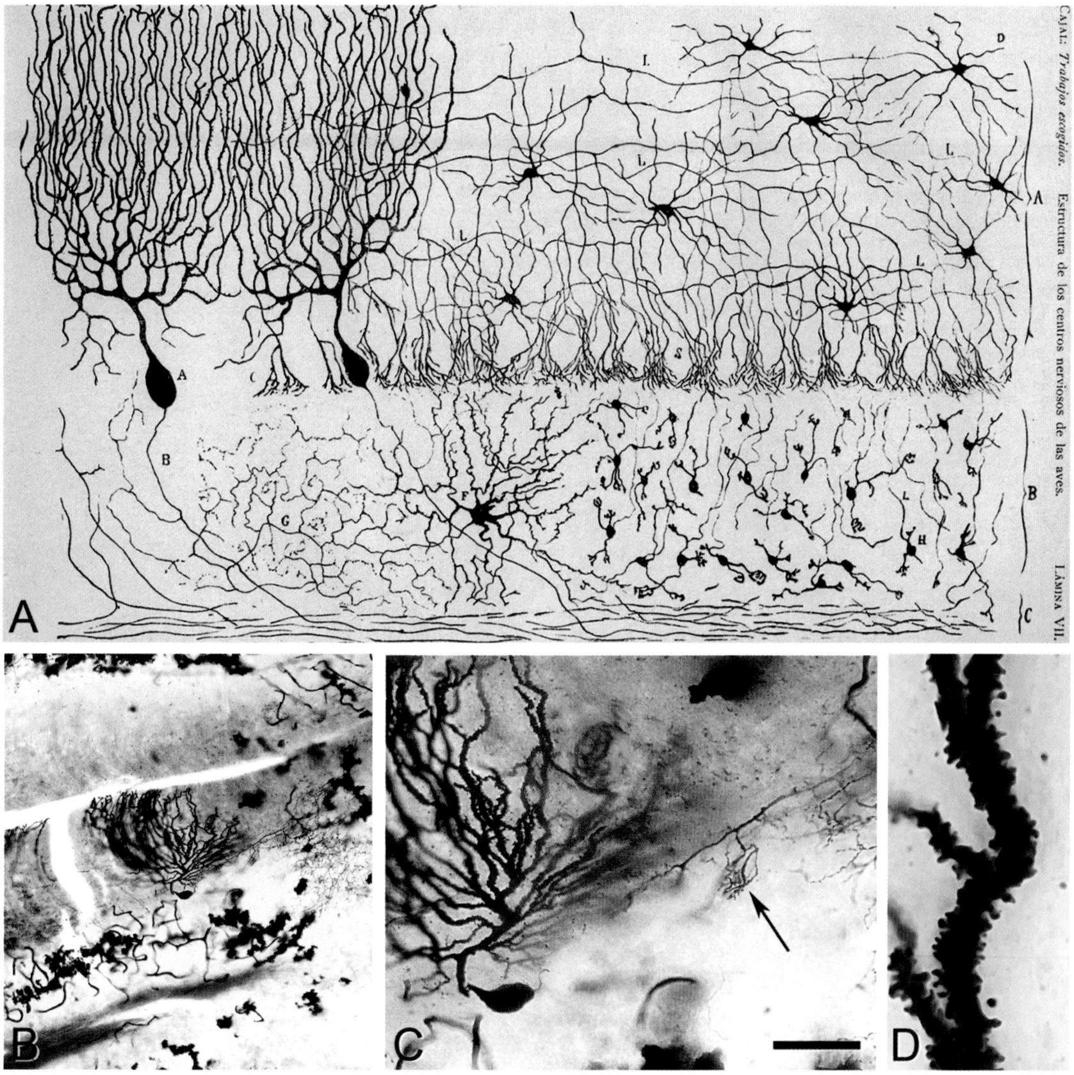

FIGURE 33. First illustration by Cajal of a Golgi-impregnated preparation of the nervous system (Cajal, 1888, page 10). **A**, Illustration with the legend: "Vertical section of a cerebellar convolution of a hen. Impregnation by the Golgi method. A, represents the molecular zone, B, designates the granular layer and C the white matter." **B**, Photomicrograph from one of Cajal's preparations of the cerebellum of an adult bird stained with the Golgi method. **C**, Higher magnification of **B** to illustrate a Purkinje cell and a basket formation (arrow). **D**, Dendrite of the Purkinje cell, which is covered by spines. In the text, Cajal wrote: "The surface of [the dendrites of Purkinje cells] appears to be covered with thorns or short spines . . . (At the beginning, we thought that these eminences were the result of a tumultuous precipitation of the silver but the constancy of its existence and its presence, even in preparations in which the reaction appears to be very delicate in the remaining elements, incline us to believe this to be a normal condition)" (pages 4–5). Scale bar (in **C**): 200 μm in **B**; 60 μm in **C**; 8.4 μm in **D**. The histological images were obtained by Pablo García-López, Virginia García-Marín, and Miguel Freire (Legado Cajal, Instituto Cajal).

the origin of the reticular theory was the result of a misinterpretation of Deiters (1865) that from the surface of the dendritic processes arose fine fibrils that continued as myelinated fibers, giving rise to a second axonic system (Figure 15). This observation was extremely influential. In the words of Cajal (1899–1904; Vol. 1, 1899, page 20):

Unfortunately, Deiters, trusting too much in the deceptive appearance of the protoplasmic expansions that were incompletely dissociated or examined in [histological] sections, admitted the possibility that fine fibrils could arise from their surfaces, and that perhaps these fibrils were continuous with real medullated tubes [myelinated fibers]. Such conjecture

444 Prof. Santiago Ramón y Cajal.

THE CROONIAN LECTURE.—"La fine Structure des Centres Nerveux." By SANTIAGO RAMÓN Y CAJAL, Professor ot Histology, University of Madrid. Received March 1,—Read March 8, 1894.

A l'invitation gracieuse que m'ont faite les honorables membres de cette société savante de venir dans cette séance rendre compte de mes travaux sur la structure des centres nerveux, mon premier dessein, je ne le cacherai pas, a été de renoncer à un honneur que je jugeais par trop disproportionné avec mes mérites; mais je songeai ensuite que votre bienveillance à m'écouter ne saurait être moindre que la générosité de votre invitation, et je me suis résigné au rôle, peu flatteur du reste, d'interrompre un moment l'harmonieux concert de vos beaux travaux. J'ai d'autant plus besoin de toute votre indulgence que je vais vous entretenir d'un sujet qui vous est parfaitement connu. Tout ce que je vais vous dire, des maîtres aussi éminents que His, Kölliker, Waldeyer, von Lenhossék, van Gehuchten, l'ont déjà publié et résumé d'une manière presque irréprochable. Je vais essayer cependant de vous donner, moi aussi, un aperçu de la structure du système nerveux central, et pour cela je m'inspirerai surtout, comme on m'en a prié, de mes propres recherches.

Les centres nerveux des mammifères, spécialement ceux de l'homme, représentent le véritable chef-d'œuvre de la nature, la machine la plus subtilement compliquée que la vie puisse nous offrir. En dépit de cette complication, capable de décourager les esprits les plus hardis, il n'a pourtant jamais manqué de patients anatomistes qui, utilisant la technique de leur époque, ont tenté de débrouiller la trame délicate de l'axe encéphalo-spinal. Ils étaient guidés, cela ne fait point de doute, par l'espoir que la découverte de la clef structurale des centres nerveux jetterait une vive lumière sur les importantes activités de ces organes. Les premières données positives, quoique incomplètes, relatives à la fine anatomie des substances grise et blanche, nous les devons à Ehrenberg, qui en 1833 découvrit les fibres nerveuses, à Rémak, à Hannover, à Helmholtz, à Wagner, qui, à la même époque, ou quelques années plus tard, trouvèrent les corpuscules multipolaires et crurent que ces expansions ramifiées des cellules étaient en continuation avec les fibres nerveuses. En 1865 Deiters, un des plus sagaces observateurs que l'anatomie ait jamais eus, nous fit faire un grand pas dans la connaissance de la morphologie de la cellule nerveuse; il démontra que dans toute cellule nerveuse il y avait toujours des expansions de deux sortes, c'est-à-dire que, outre les expansions ramifiées ou protoplasmiques, il s'en trouve une autre non ramifiée, ou cylindre-axe, se continuant directement avec un tube

462 Prof. Santiago Ramón y Cajal.

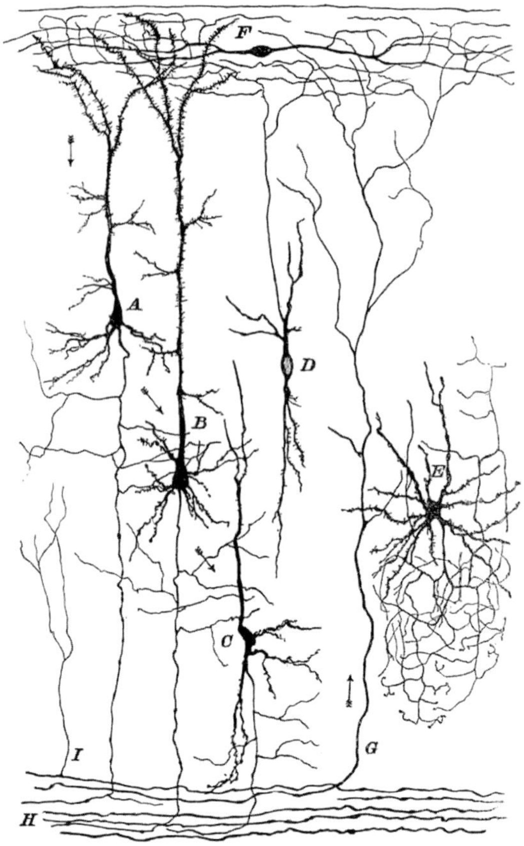

FIG. 6. Les principaux types cellulaires de l'écorce cérébrale des mammifères. A, cellule pyramidale à taille moyenne; B, cellule pyramidale géante; C, cellule polymorphe; D, cellule dont le cylindre-axe est ascendant; E, cellule de Golgi; F, cellule, spéciale de la couche moléculaire; G, fibre se terminant librement dans l'épaisseur de l'écorce; H, substance blanche; I, collatérale de la substance blanche.

FIGURE 34. Cajal's schematic representation of the major types of neurons in the cerebral cortex of small mammals. The arrows indicate the possible routes followed by nerve impulses. Taken from Cajal (1894b).

was the origin of an erroneous theory formulated by Gerlach, which has exerted a dismal influence on the direction of neurological research for more than twenty years.

After these studies, several scientists supported the reticular theory, proposing different types of networks (Figure 40). However, it was Joseph von Gerlach (1820–1896) who really developed the reticular theory and, thus, he is considered the father of this theory (Gerlach, 1872). Gerlach confirmed the observations of Deiters that nerve cells had a principal cylinder-axis (axon) and that the protoplasmic processes (dendrites) gave rise to another axonal plexus, but he added the observation that the protoplasmic processes formed a network (dendritic network). Thus, Gerlach proposed that the conduction of nervous activity takes place through a network of neural elements formed by dendrites (dendritic network) and axons (axonal network) (Figure 40B). That is, the axons have two origins—the direct (cell body) and indirect (dendritic network)—such that the connections between nerve cells was double, because it was both through the main axon and through the dendritic network, which in turn was part of the axonal network. Part of the success of this theory was a result of the idea that if the nervous system consisted of a continuous

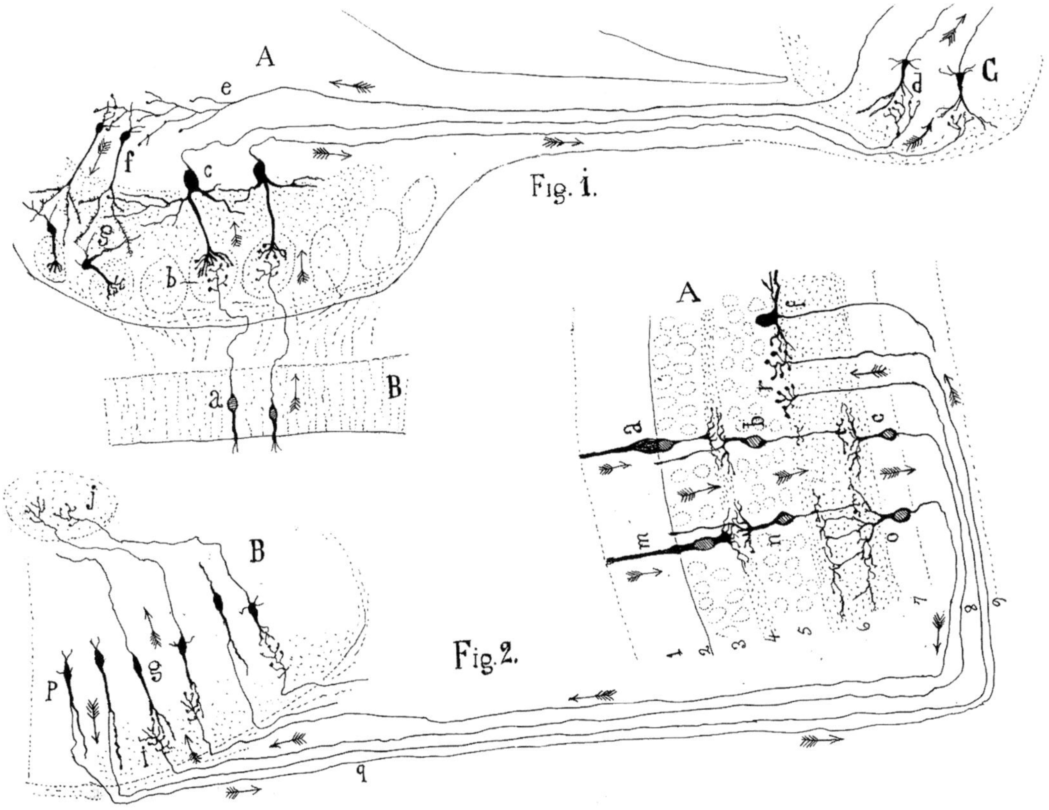

FIGURE 35. Cajal's scheme showing the current flow in the visual and olfactory systems. This drawing was reproduced in his article "*Significación fisiológica de las expansiones protoplásmicas y nerviosas de las células de la substancia gris*" (Cajal, 1891a). The legend states: "Figure 1. Scheme of cellular connections in the olfactory mucosa, olfactory bulb, tractus, and olfactory lobe of the cerebrum. The arrows indicate the direction of the currents. *A*, olfactory bulb; *B*, mucosa; *C*, olfactory lobe. *a, b, c, d,* one-way or centripetal pathway through which sensory or olfactory excitation passes. *e, f, g,* centrifugal pathway through which the [nervous] centers can act on the elements of the bulb, granules and nerve cells, whose protoplasmic processes penetrate the glomeruli" (pages 673–679). "Figure 2. Scheme of the visual excitation pathway through the retina, optic nerve and optic lobe of the birds. *A*, retina; *B*, optic lobe. *a, b, c,* represent a cone, a bipolar cell and a ganglion cell of the retina, respectively, the order through which visual excitation travels. *m, n, o,* parallel current emanating from the rod also involves bipolar and ganglion cells. *g,* cells of the optic lobe that receive the visual excitation and transfer it to *j,* the central ganglion. *p, q, r,* centrifugal currents that start in certain fusiform cells of the optic lobe and terminate in *r,* in the retina at the level of the spongioblasts; *f,* a spongioblast" (pages 715–723). Arrows indicate the direction of current flow.

network of processes, without interruptions, it could be relatively easy to explain how the nervous currents in the brain could pass from one nerve cell to another. That is, the passing of information from one nerve cell to another would be the result of the continuity of their processes. Figure 40C and D show drawings by Aleksander Dogiel (1852–1922), supporting the reticular theory. Figure 40C illustrates two neurons connected through a thick common dendrite ("interprotoplasmic bridges") rather than existing as independent elements. This is a particularly interesting figure because it was produced with the aid of a camera lucida—a good example indicating that the use of this device did not preclude the observer from making incorrect observations. Indeed, there were two major opponents of the reticular theory, Wilhelm His (1831–1904) and August-Henri Forel (1848–1931) (Figure 41). Referring to these two researchers, Cajal wrote (1899–1904; Vol. 1, 1899, page 59):

> They struggle against the doctrine of the networks, and they prepared our minds to accept the theory of contacts and of the free ending of the nervous processes.

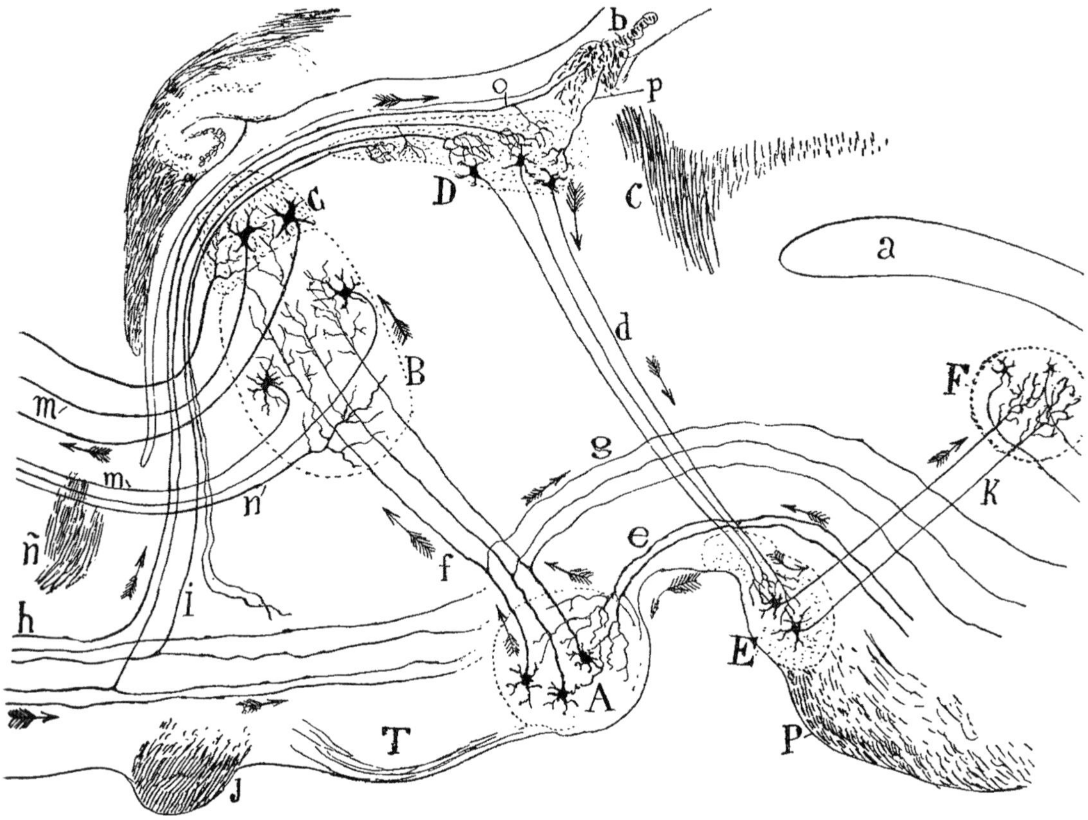

FIGURE 36. "Diagram of the pathways [afferent and efferent] of the mammillary body, habenular nuclei, and anterior and medial thalamic nuclei. *A*, medial mammillary nucleus; *B*, anterior medial nucleus of the thalamus; *C*, [anterior ventral nucleus]; *D*, habenular nuclei; *E*, interpeduncular nucleus; *F*, dorsal tegmental nucleus; *J*, optic chiasm; *a*, cerebral aqueduct of Sylvius; *b*, habenular commissure; *c*, posterior commissure; *d*, fasciculus retroflexus of Meyner; *e*, peduncle of the mammillary body; *f*, tract of Vicq d'Azyr [mammillo-thalamic tract]; *g*, mammillo-tegmental bundle of Gudden; *h, stria terminalis; i, stria medullaris; m*, thalamo-cortical fibers; *n*, cortico-thalamic fibers; *o*, fiber of the *stria medullaris* going into the habenular commissure to arborize within the habenular nuclei of the contralateral side; *p*, fiber coming from the opposite side. [Arrows indicate the direction of impulses]." Taken from Cajal (1903a, page 14).

Both of these scientists reached the same conclusion separately, based on different observations. Wilhelm His found that the surface of the nerve cells did not anastomose with other nerve cells, and he proposed that the nerve cell was the embryological or genetic unit of the nervous system (His, 1886, 1889). Forel began to work in the laboratory of Bernard von Gudden (1824–1886), where he learned the experimental methods to study von Gudden degeneration and the connections in the nervous system. This method was devised by August Waller (1816–1870) to study spinal nerve degeneration, through which secondary degeneration was discovered (better known as *Wallerian degeneration*, in honor of its discoverer). Waller (1850, 1852) found that when an axon is sectioned, the portion that was separated from the cell body ("trophic center") degenerated and disappeared whereas the portion joined to the cell of origin maintained its structure. The method of von Gudden consisted of inducing secondary atrophy in central structures of the nervous system after extirping the sense organs or the cranial nerves of young animals. As a consequence, atrophy of the nerve cells from which the damaged axons originated would occur first and, later, these cells would disappear completely (von Gudden, 1870). Forel (1887, 1890–1891) rejected the reticular theory, based on the pathological and physiological evidence obtained with the method of von Gudden. Forel argued that after a lesion in a given region of

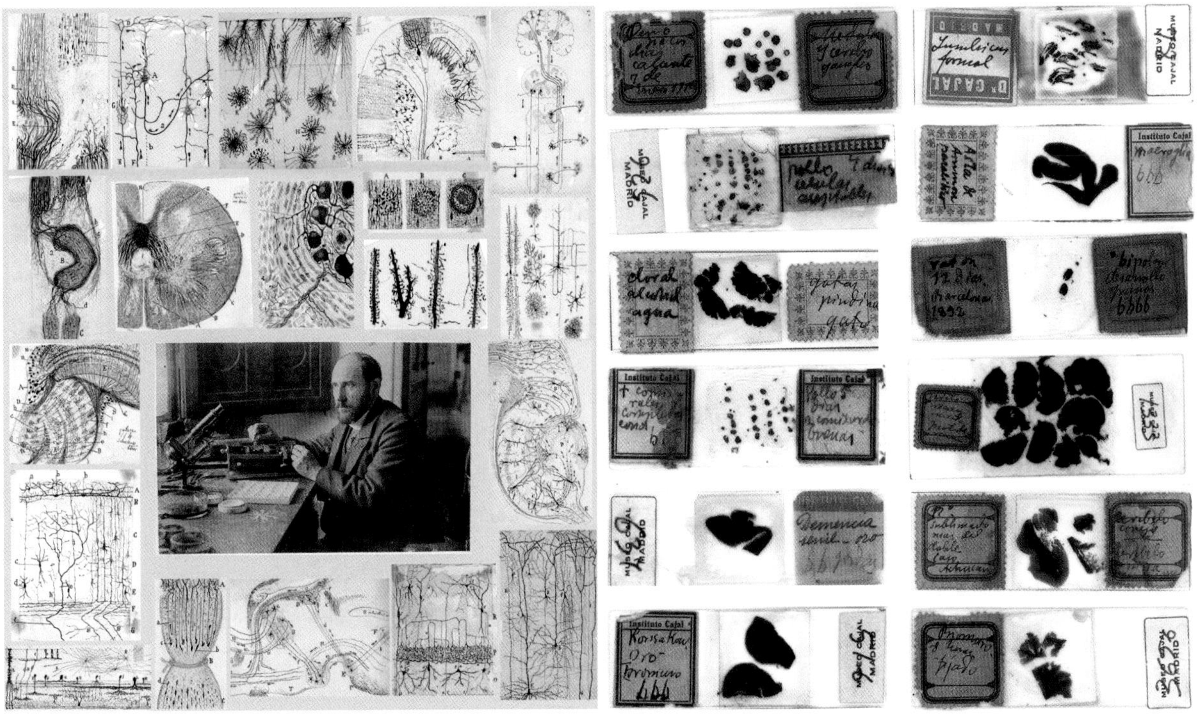

FIGURE 37. *Left,* Photograph of Cajal and some of his drawings to illustrate the diversity of his studies on the structure of the nervous system. Cajal took this photograph himself in 1888 in his laboratory in Barcelona, and it shows him cutting a piece of brain tissue with a microtome. *Right,* Photographs of typical Cajal preparations, labeled in Cajal's own handwriting—currently housed in the Legado Cajal at the Instituto Cajal. These slides contain sections from blocks of various regions of the brain from several species, stained with different techniques.

the nervous system, cell atrophy was restricted to a particular group of cells, without extending to another group of cells, as would be expected if they formed a mesh.

According to Cajal (1899–1904;Vol.1, 1899, page 90), the ideas of His and Forel were not accepted by the reticularists for mainly methodological reasons, and also because their studies were performed in embryonic or young animals:

> It was necessary to demonstrate *de visu*, and in the adult, that nervous ramifications terminated freely, and in conditions in which it were not possible to question this fact, neither due to the embryonic nature of the material presented, nor because of the incomplete staining of the fibers.

For example, Hans Held (1866–1942) described a separation in the trapezoid nucleus of the embryo or in newborn animals: a line of demarcation (*Grenxlinie*) between the giant basket terminals (*Endkörb*)—later called *chalices of Held*—and the cell body of the neurons with which they contacted. However, he proposed that during development, these terminal axons were fused to the cell bodies (Figure 42 [Held, 1897a, 1897b]). This idea was generalized to other parts of the nervous system (Held, 1902, 1904, 1905, 1929), indicating that axon terminals were not only fused with the cell bodies, but also with the dendrites. As a result, the reticular theory represented the main concept regarding the organization of the nervous system.

Golgi, Cajal, and the Nobel Prize Lectures in 1906

A remarkable moment in the history of the neuron was when Golgi examined the silver-impregnated preparations using the method of the *reazione nera* and concluded that the reticular theory put forward by Gerlach was wrong, because Golgi thought dendrites ended freely, and only the axons and their collaterals were seen to anastomose (Golgi,

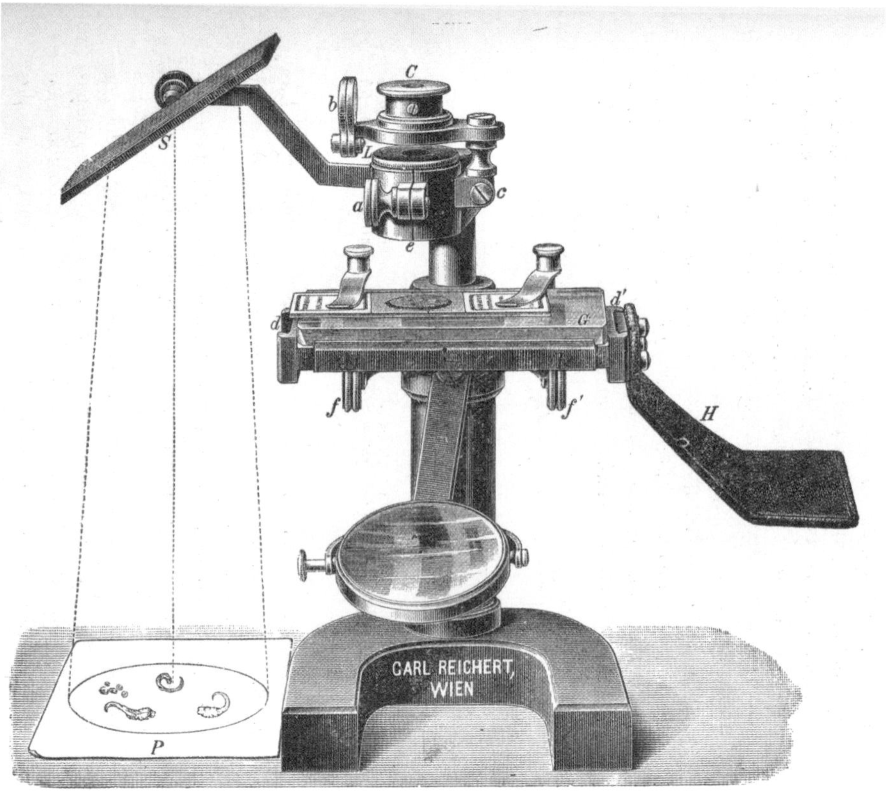

FIGURE 38. Reichert microscope, with a camera lucida of the Abbe type, published by Cajal in his book *Manual de histología normal y de técnica micrográfica* (Cajal, 1914).

1882–1883, 1883, 1885b). Therefore, he suggested that the nervous system consisted of a *rete nervosa diffusa* (diffuse nervous network)—an idea that he even supported during his Nobel Prize lecture in 1906 (Golgi, 1929) (Figure 43). When they jointly received the Nobel Prize for Physiology or Medicine in 1906, the lectures of Cajal and Golgi provided a good reflection of the state of scientific thought at the time (DeFelipe, 2002b). Golgi started his lecture *La dottrina del neurone: teoria e fati* (The Neuron Doctrine: Theory and Facts) (Golgi, 1929, page 1) by saying (kindly translated by Fiorenzo Conti, University of Ancona, Italy):

> It might appear odd that, having always opposed the neuron doctrine—though its point of departure is undoubtedly to be found in my own studies—I should choose this very problem as the subject of my lecture, particularly at a time when this doctrine is considered by many to be on the wane.

In contrast, Cajal's Nobel lecture *Structure et connexions des neurones* (The Structure and Connections of Neurons) expounded his most fundamental results and vigorously opposed Golgi's stance (Cajal, 1907a). Regarding Golgi's Nobel lecture, Cajal later said in his autobiography, *Recuerdos de mi vida* (Cajal, 1917b, page 489):

> Contrary to what we all expected, instead of pointing out the valuable facts which he [Golgi] had discovered, he tried to refloat his almost forgotten theory of the interstitial nervous nets.

As discussed previously (see DeFelipe, 2002b), Cajal is well known for his vivid discussions in support of the neuron doctrine and he is recognized as one of the scientists who contributed significantly to the victory of the neuron doctrine in its battle against the reticular theory. A good example is when Cajal was annoyed because Golgi—in his Nobel

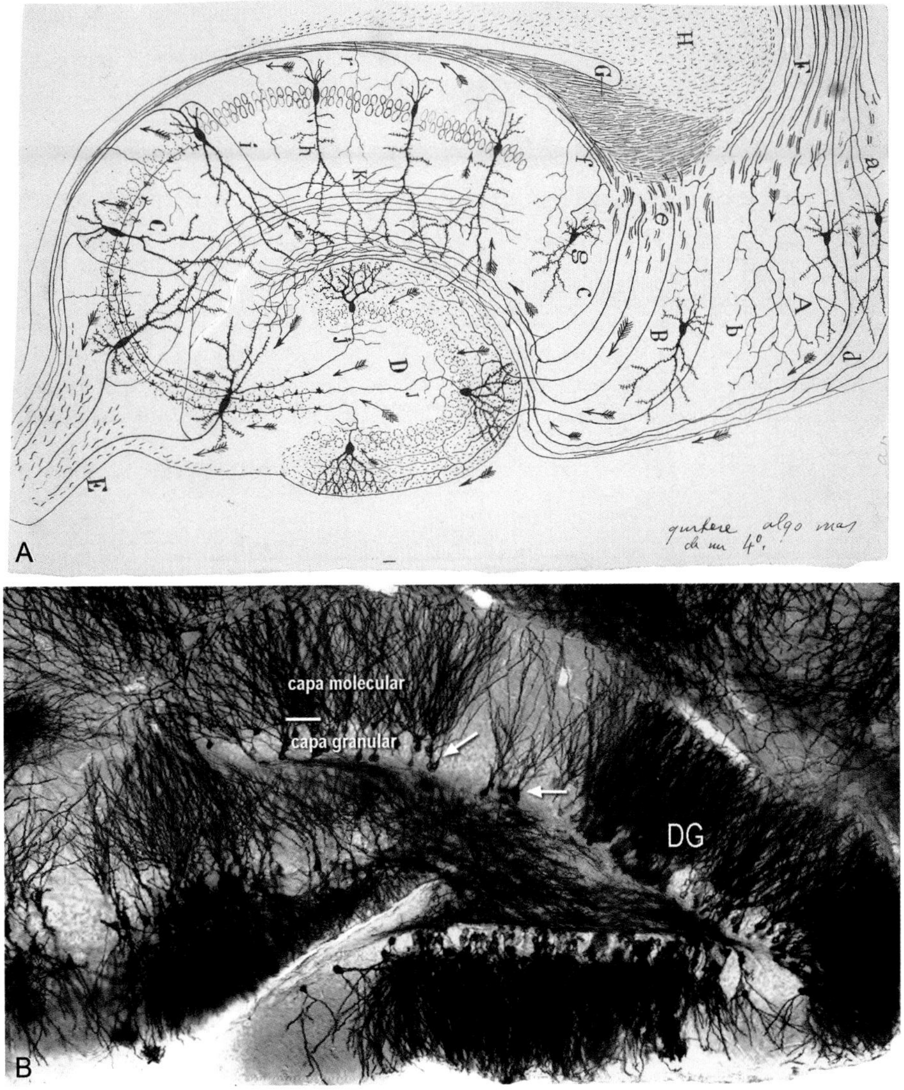

FIGURE 39. **A**, Drawing taken from Cajal (1901–1902, page 88) showing the structure and connections of the hippocampus from small mammals based on the Golgi method. The translation of the legend is as follows: "Scheme of the structure and connections of Ammon's horn. *A*, ganglion of the occipital pole; *B*, subiculum; *C*, Ammon's horn; *D*, fascia dentata; *E*, fimbria; *F*, cingulum; *G*, crossed angular bundle; *H*, corpus callosum; *a*, axons penetrating the cingulum; *b*, cingular fibers terminating in the focus of the occipital pole; *c*, perforant spheno-ammonic fibers; *d*, perforant cingular fibers; *e*, plane of the superior spheno-ammonic fibers; *g*, cell of the subiculum; [*h*, pyramidal cells of the superior region of Ammon's horn; *i*, ascending collaterals of the large pyramidal cells; *j*, axon of a granule cell; *r*, collaterals of the fibers of the alveus]." **B**, Photomicrograph from the dentate gyrus (DG; see *D* in **A**) stained with the method of Golgi. The figure shows many labeled granule cells, the predominant cell type in the DG. These neurons are densely packed, with their cell bodies located in the granular layer ("capa granular"). They give rise to a V-shaped dendritic arbor extending throughout the molecular layer ("capa molecular"). The axons of these neurons invade the hilar region (arrows in *D* in **A**). This image, together with its text, was presented by Michael Frotscher (Albert-Ludwigs-Universitat Freiburg, Germany) in the exhibition Neuroscapes 2006 (DeFelipe et al., 2007).

lecture—did not even allude to the works of Cajal or mention the studies of other relevant researchers, such as Forel, His, Retzius, Waldeyer, Kölliker, van Gehuchten, von Lenhossék, and Edinger among others. He said (Cajal, 1917b, page 489):

For the anatomist of Pavia [see Note 9], nothing of interest had been added to his early studies by Forel, His, myself, Retzius, Waldeyer, Kölliker, van Gehuchten, v. Lenhossék, Edinger, my brother [Pedro], Tello, Athias, or even by his compatriot Lugaro . . . .

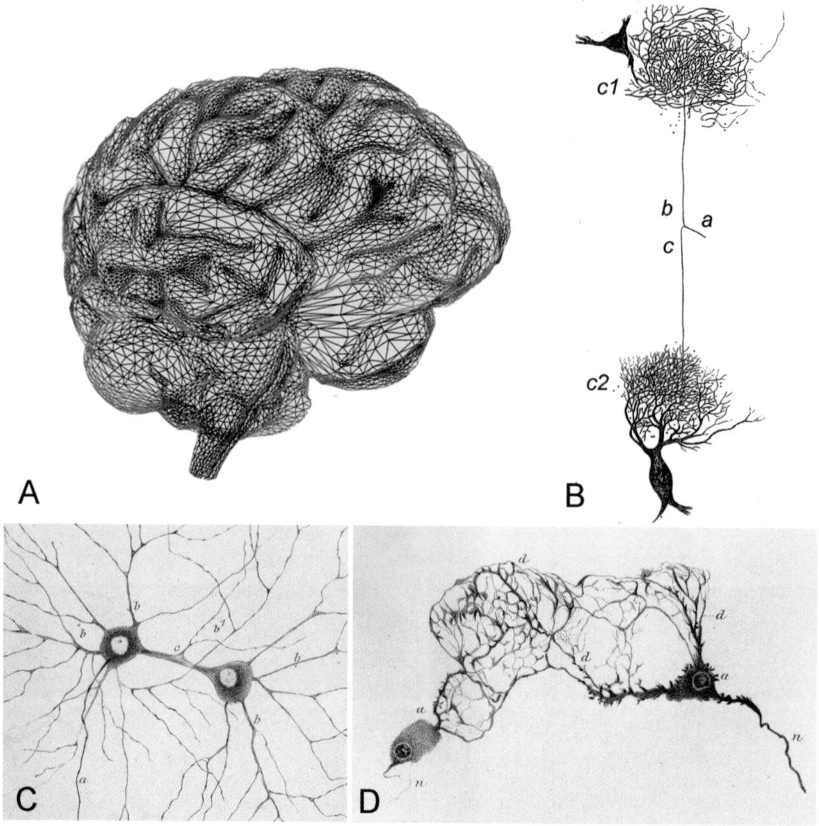

FIGURE 40. Reticular theory. **A**, Schematic illustration to show the brain as made up of a mesh of neuronal processes. This drawing of the brain was kindly provided by Juan Sanz (computer animation specialist). **B**, Drawing by Gerlach (1872) showing two nerve cells from the spinal cord of the ox (prepared with carmine and ammonia). According to Gerlach, the conduction of nervous activity takes place through a network of neural elements formed by dendrites (dendritic network) and axons (axonal network). **C**, **D**, Drawings of ganglion cells of the human retina and cells of the dog gallbladder ganglia by Dogiel in 1893 and 1899, respectively.

> The noble and most discrete Retzius was in consternation; Holmgren, Henschen, and all the Swedish neurologists and histologists contemplated the speaker with stupefaction. And I was trembling with impatience as I saw that the most elementary respect for the conventions prevented me from giving an opportune and categorical correction to so many odious errors and so many deliberate omissions.

Importantly, Cajal confirmed Golgi's conclusion that dendrites end freely in studies in which Cajal also used the method of Golgi. However, in contrast to Golgi, Cajal came to the critical conclusion that this also applied to axons and their branches (Cajal, 1888, page 9):

> We have carried out detailed studies to investigate the course and connections of the nerve fibers in the cerebral and cerebellar convolutions of the human, monkey, dog, etc. We have not been able to see an anastomosis between the ramifications of two different nervous prolongations, nor between the filaments emanating from the same expansion of Deiters [axons]. While the fibers are interlaced in a very complicated manner, engendering an intricate and dense plexus, they never form a net . . . it could be said that each [nerve cell] is an absolutely autonomous physiological canton [unit].

Indeed, from the outset of Cajal's studies with the Golgi method in 1887, he provided many examples from throughout the nervous system to support his observation that dendrites and axons end freely. However, the path leading up to this point was not an easy one, and the differences between researchers

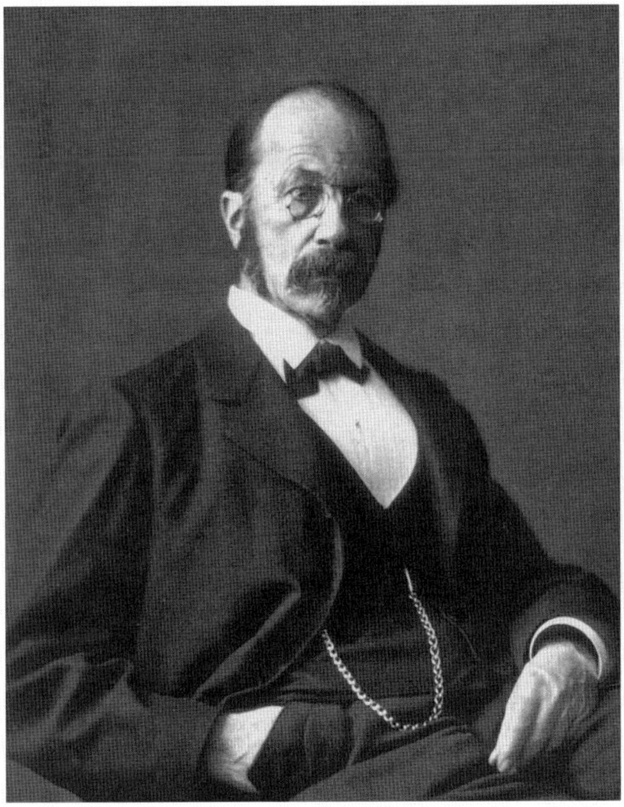

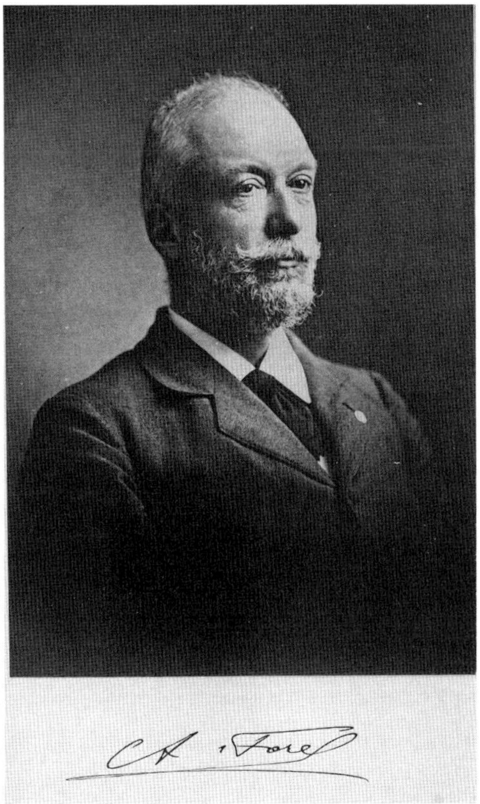

FIGURE 41. Precursors of the neuronal theory: Wilhelm His and August-Henri Forel.

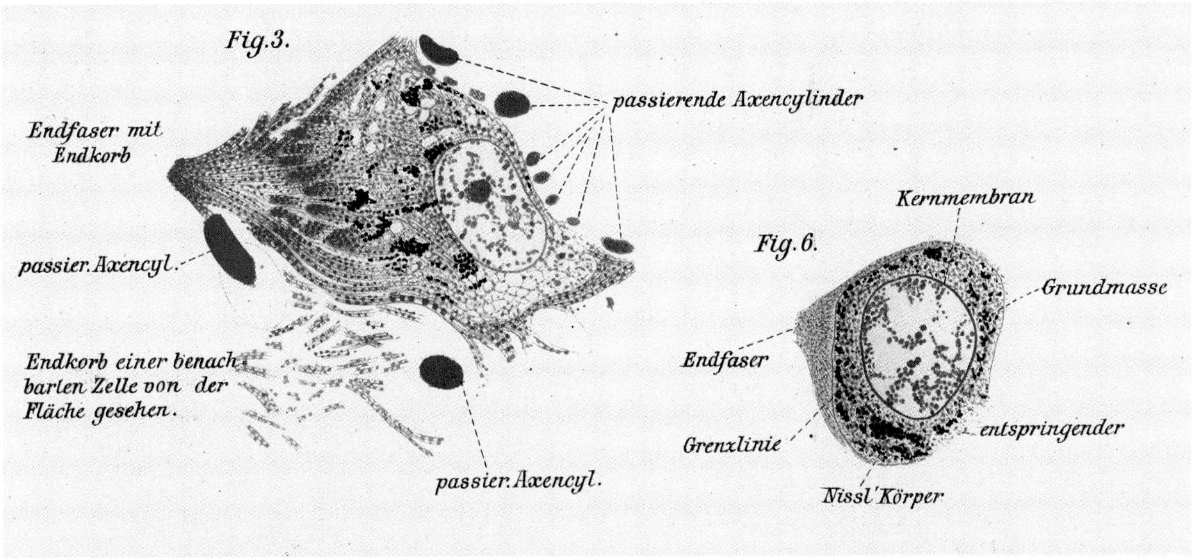

FIGURE 42. Drawings by Held (1897a) to show the development of the giant basket terminals in the trapezoid nucleus stained with erythrosine/methylene blue. According to Held, in the newborn animal (*fig. 6*; nine-day-old dog, paraffin section 3 μm thick), there is a demarcation line (*Grenzlinie*) between the terminal fiber (*Endfaser*) and the cell body. However, in the adult (*fig. 3*; rabbit paraffin section, 1.5 μm thick), Held thought the terminal axons were fused to the cell body.

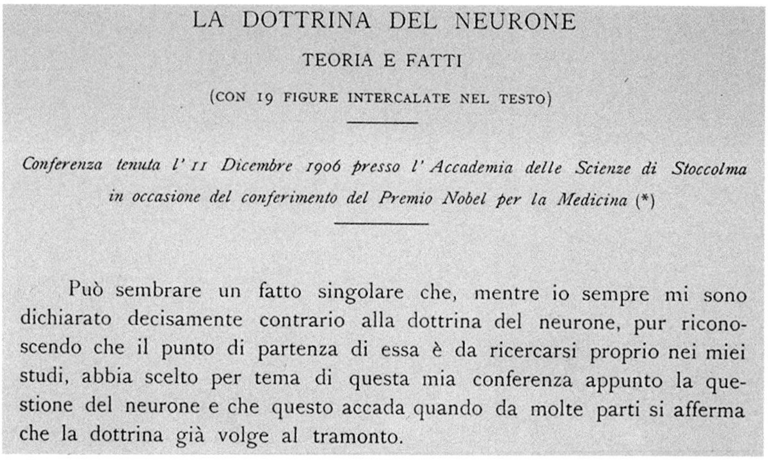

LA DOTTRINA DEL NEURONE

TEORIA E FATTI

(CON 19 FIGURE INTERCALATE NEL TESTO)

Conferenza tenuta l' 11 Dicembre 1906 presso l' Accademia delle Scienze di Stoccolma in occasione del conferimento del Premio Nobel per la Medicina (*)

Può sembrare un fatto singolare che, mentre io sempre mi sono dichiarato decisamente contrario alla dottrina del neurone, pur riconoscendo che il punto di partenza di essa è da ricercarsi proprio nei miei studi, abbia scelto per tema di questa mia conferenza appunto la questione del neurone e che questo accada quando da molte parti si afferma che la dottrina già volge al tramonto.

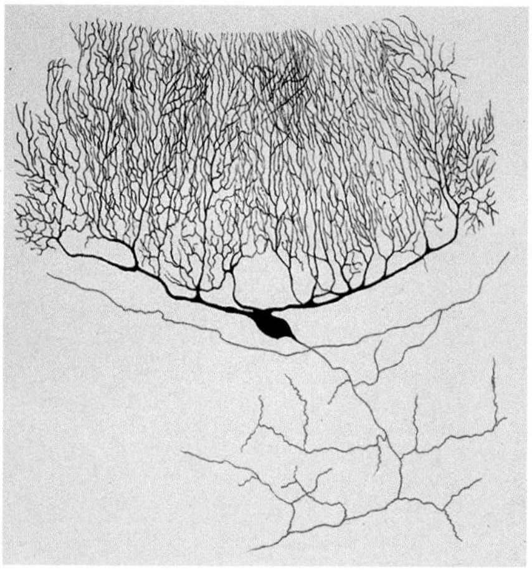

FIGURE 43. *Left*, Introductory paragraph of the Nobel Prize lecture given by Golgi in 1906 (Golgi, 1929). *Right*, Drawing by Golgi illustrating a Purkinje cell of the cerebellum (Figure 4 of his lecture). The axon is shown in red.

in favor or against the neuron doctrine were based mainly on the interpretation of the microscopic images and on the results obtained with the different experimental approaches they used, or based on

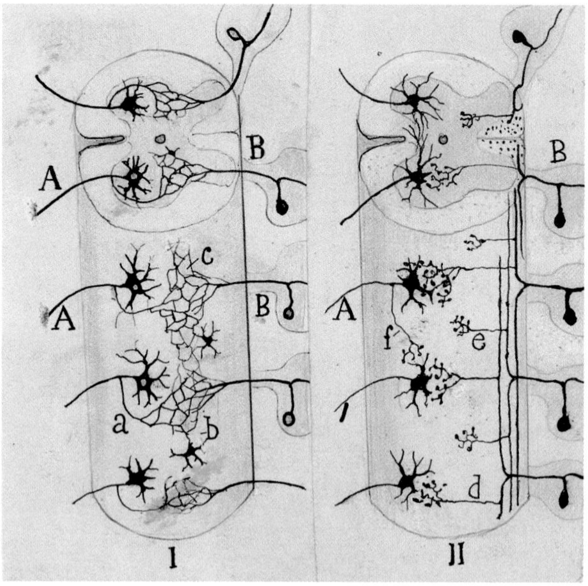

FIGURE 44. Cajal's drawing to explain the differences between the neuron and the reticular theories. The figure legend states: "Scheme to compare the concept of Golgi regarding the sensory-motor connections of the spinal cord (I) with the results of my investigations (II). *A*, anterior roots; *B*, posterior roots; *a*, collateral of a motor root; *b*, cells with a short axon which, according to Golgi, would intervene in the formation of the network; *c*, diffuse interstitial network; *d*, our long collaterals in contact with the motor cells; *e*, short collaterals." This figure was reproduced as Figure 9 in *Recuerdos de mi vida* (Cajal, 1917b, page 125).

logical intuition. For example, Cajal considered that the free arborization of neurons would explain more easily plastic changes in the brain through the formation of new connections (Cajal, 1894b, page 467):

> As opposed to the reticular theory, the theory that cellular processes could develop free arborizations seems not only the most likely, but also the most encouraging. A continuous pre-established net—like a lattice of telegraphic wires in which no new stations or new lines can be created—somehow rigid, immutable, incapable of being modified, goes against the concept that all we hold of the organ of thought, which within certain limits, is malleable and capable of being perfected by means of well-directed mental gymnastics.

Therefore, the way in which connections between neurons were established was another important issue that had to be addressed by scientists. This was summarized by Cajal in *Recuerdos de mi vida* (1917b) in the following poetic and characteristic anthropomorphic prose that he often used to describe various aspects of the nervous system (pages 167–168):

> What mysterious forces preside the appearance of the processes [dendrites and axon], promoting their growth and ramification, provoking the coherent migration of the cells and fibers in predetermined directions, as if obeying a wise architectonic plan, and finally establishing those protoplasmic kisses,

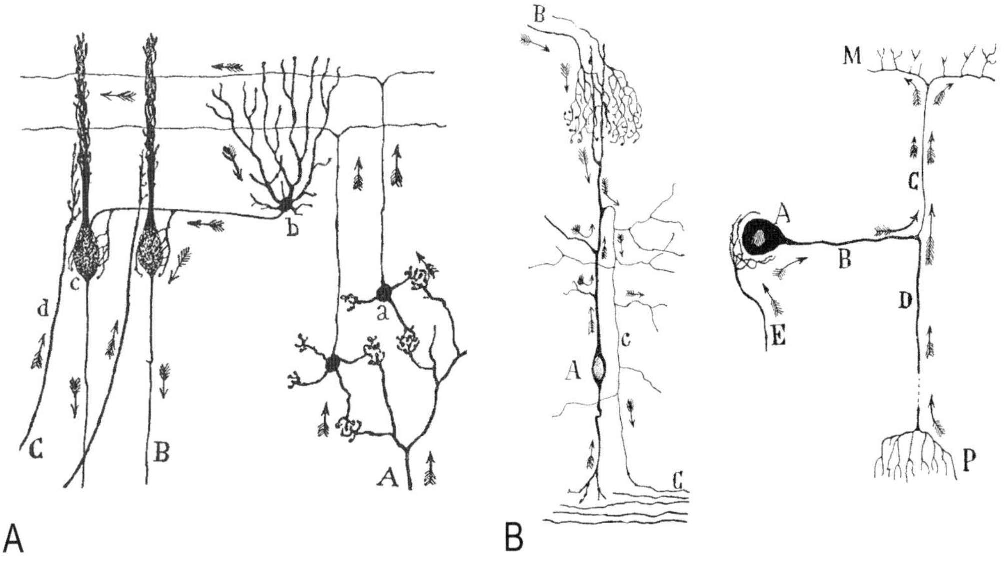

FIGURE 45. **A**, Cajal's drawing to illustrate the participation of basket cells in the transmission of afferent impulses in the cerebellum based on the theory of dynamic polarization. The legend states: "*A*, mossy fiber; *B*, Purkinje cell axons; *C*, climbing fiber; a, granule cell; b, basket cell; c, Purkinje cell [side view]." Taken from Cajal (1899–1904; Vol. 2, 1904, page 446). **B**, Cajal's drawing reproduced in his article "*Leyes de la morfología y dinamismo de las células nerviosas*" (1897b, pages 3 [left] and 7 [right]). The legend states: *Left*, "Crosier cell of the optic lobe of the sparrow. *A*, soma; *B*, fibers arriving from the retina; *c*, central white matter; *C*, axon. Arrows indicate the direction of the current [flow]." *Right*, "Scheme showing the current flows in a sensory ganglion cell of mammals. *A*, soma; *B*, shaft; *D*, axipetal or peripheral process that provides currents; *C*, axon that carries the impulses to the spinal cord; *E*, fiber constituent of the pericellular arborization; *M*, spinal cord; [*P*, skin]."

the *intercellular articulations* [synapses] that appear to constitute the final ecstasy of an epic love story?

The Law of Dynamic Polarization of Nerve Cells

Important implications stemmed from believing that nerve currents flow through a continuous rather than a discontinuous network of neuronal processes (Figure 44). Thus, the new ideas about the connections between neurons led to novel theories about the relationship between neuronal circuits and brain function. Cajal wrote (Cajal [1909–1911]; Vol. 1, 1909, page 92):

> The cell bodies [dendrites and axons] terminate freely but nevertheless, the flow of currents is not impeded in such an infinitely interrupted, fragmented nervous system. How can such currents flow? There can be only one answer, by contact, in much the same way that electric current crosses a splice between two wires.

It was commonly thought that dendrites played a nourishing role whereas axons transmitted nervous impulses in a cellulifugal direction (a generalization based mostly on the cellulifugal conduction in the axons of the spinal motor neurons). However, there was no general consensus or definite ideas about the role of dendrites in the processing of information. In 1889, Cajal thought it was clear that the dendrites played a role in receiving currents (Cajal, 1889a), at least in certain cases, and two years later he tried to generalize this idea in the Law of Dynamic Polarization (Cajal, 1891a). This law was based on the direction followed by the impulses in regions of the nervous system where, through their activity, it was apparently clear which anatomical routes the impulse followed, such as in the visual and olfactory systems (Figure 35). In the words of Cajal (1891a, page 675):

> If in such inquiry, the [dendritic] arborization is always shown as a receptor apparatus and the [axonal arborization] as an apparatus for the *application* of the [impulses], then by analogy we would have attained a rule to judge the direction of the currents in the [nerve cells within the central nervous system].

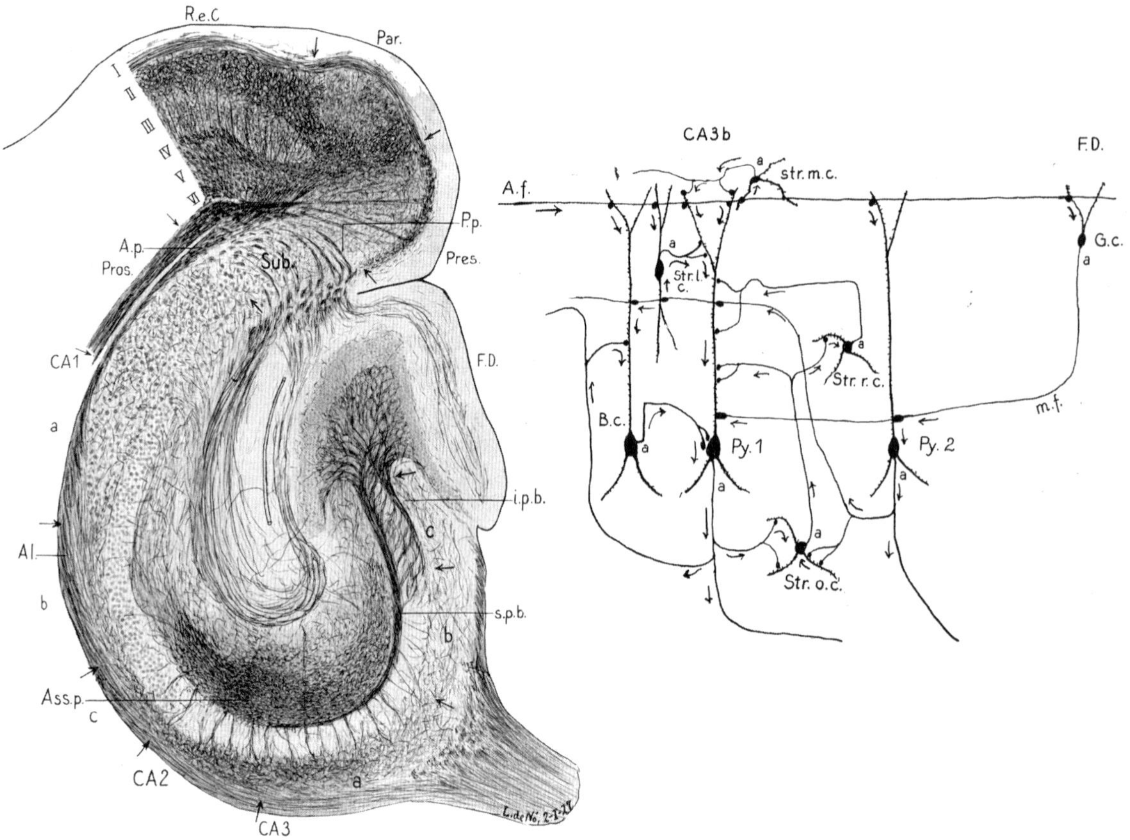

FIGURE 46. Drawing taken from Lorente de Nó (1934) to illustrate the hippocampal formation (*left*) and synaptic circuits in CA3 (*right*). *Left,* The legend states: "Horizontal section through the brain of an adult mouse. Cajal's reduced silver method; fixation in pyridine 50%. The lettering is as in Figure 2 [*R.e.* Regio entorhinalis; *Aa, lib, B, C* its fields; *Par.* Parasubiculum; *Sub.* Subiculum with its two fields (*a, b*); *Pres.* Presubiculum; *Pros.* Prosubiculum with its three fields (*a, b, c*); *CA2* field CA2; *CA3* field CA3 with its three subfields (*a, b, c*); *CA4* field CA4; *F.d.* Fascia dentata; *Fi.* Fimbria]; besides, *s. p. b.* and *i. p. b.* supra and infrapyramidal bundles of mossy fibres from the Fascia dentata. *A.p.* alvear path from the Area entorhinalis; *P. p.* perforant path from the Area entorhinalis; *AI.* Alveus or white substance; *Ass. p.* Association (axial) path in front of *CA2*. The layers of the Area entorhinalis have been marked with roman numerals (I–VI). Note the presence between III and IV of an association path, which ends in the parasubiculum (*Par.*)" (page 117). *Right,* The legend states: "Several of the many possible paths between the afferent fibres of the perforant path and the effector pyramid, *Py.* 1; field *CA 3b.* The afferent fibre *A.f.* establishes contacts with the pyramids *Py.* 1 and *Py.* 2, with the cells with short axis cylinder of the Stratum moleculare *(str. m. c.),* lacunosum *(str. l. c.)* and pyramidale (basket cell, *B. c.)* and with the granules of the Fascia dentata (g. *c.).* When these cells discharge, their impulses are transmitted to cell *Py.* 1. Besides, when cells *Py* discharge, other cells with short axis cylinder, of the Stratum radiatum *(Str. r. c.)* and oriens *(Str. o. c.)* which were not affected by the afferent impulse are brought into activity; their impulses are again transmitted to cell *Py.* 1. The axons are marked with *a*" (page 169).

Cajal proposed that neurons could be divided into three functionally distinct regions: a receptor apparatus (formed by the dendrites and soma), an emission apparatus (the axon), and a distribution apparatus (terminal axonal arborization) (Figure 45A). He later realized that the soma does not always intervene in the conduction of the impulses and that sometimes impulse activity goes directly from the dendrites to the axon (Cajal, 1897b) (Figure 45B). Thus, the law of dynamic polarization became the theory of axipetal polarization:

> The soma and dendrites display axipetal conduction, whereby they transmit the nervous waves towards the axon. Conversely, the axon or cylinder-axis has somatofugal or dendrifugal conduction, propagating the impulses received by the soma or dendrites towards the terminal axonal arborizations . . . . This

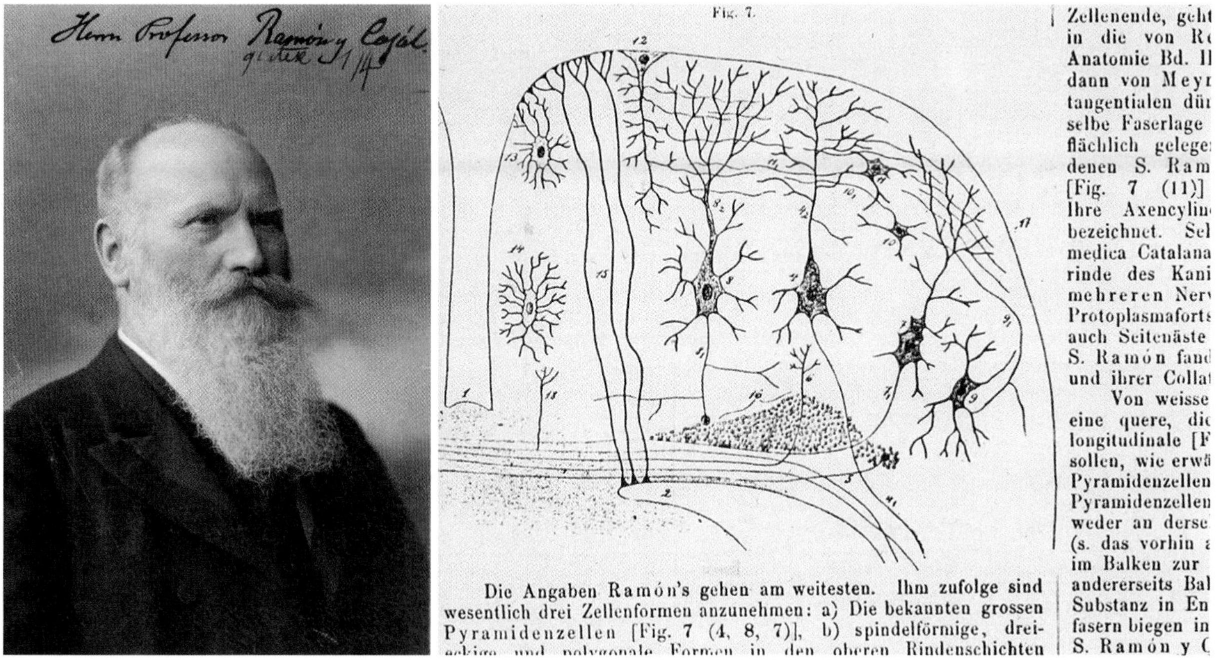

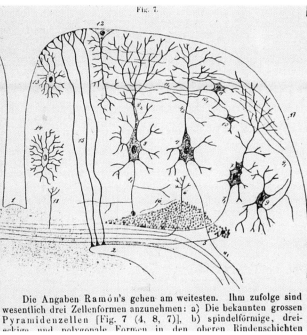

FIGURE 47. *Left*, Portrait of Wilhelm von Waldeyer-Hartz dedicated to Cajal (Legado Cajal, Instituto Cajal). *Right*, Drawing taken from von Waldeyer-Hartz's work published in the journal *Deutsche Medizinische Wochenschrift* in 1891, describing some of the findings of Cajal.

> formula can be applied universally without exception, both in vertebrates and invertebrates. (Cajal, 1897b, page 2)

Thanks to the theory of dynamic polarization, it was possible for Cajal and other scientists to trace and interpret the flow of information in complex microcircuits of the nervous system. For example, when Rafael Lorente de Nó (1934) described the complex connectivity of CA3 in Figure 46, he made the following comment: "Arrows indicate the direction of transmission of the impulses according to Cajal's law of axonal polarisation. If this law is not accomplished, i.e., if the synapse is not irreversible, the interpretation of the diagram would be quite different from that proposed in the text" (page 169). Therefore, this theory was very important because it served to theorize about the functional organization of neural connections.

Nevertheless, in the decades following Cajal's early histological investigations, the introduction of new methods for the study of the electrophysiology of neurons led to changes in key aspects of the theory of dynamic polarization. This was summarized masterfully in the highly influential review by Theodore Bullock titled "Neuron Doctrine and Electrophysiology" (1959). In this article, Bullock wrote the famous phrase "these changes in viewpoint add up to a quiet but sweeping revolution" (page 998) and made the following important points (page 1002):

> Physiologically, however, we have a new appreciation of the complexity-within-unity of the neuron. Like a person, it is truly a functional unit, but it is composed of parts of very different function not only with respect to metabolism and maintenance but also in the realms of processing diverse input and determining output—that is, of integration. The impulse is not the only form of nerve cell activity; excitation of one part of the neuron does not necessarily involve the whole neuron; many dendrites may not propagate impulses at all; and the synapse is not the only locus of selection, evaluation, fatigue, and persistent change. Several forms of graded activity—for example, pace-maker, synaptic, and local potentials— each confined to a circumscribed region or repeating regions of the neuron, can separately or sequentially integrate

0354239001001

DIE

NEURONENLEHRE

UND IHRE ANHÄNGER.

EIN BEITRAG
ZUR LÖSUNG DES PROBLEMS DER BEZIEHUNGEN
ZWISCHEN NERVENZELLE, FASER UND GRAU.

VON

DR. FRANZ NISSL,
A.O. PROFESSOR IN HEIDELBERG.

MIT 2 TAFELN.

JENA
VERLAG VON GUSTAV FISCHER
1903.

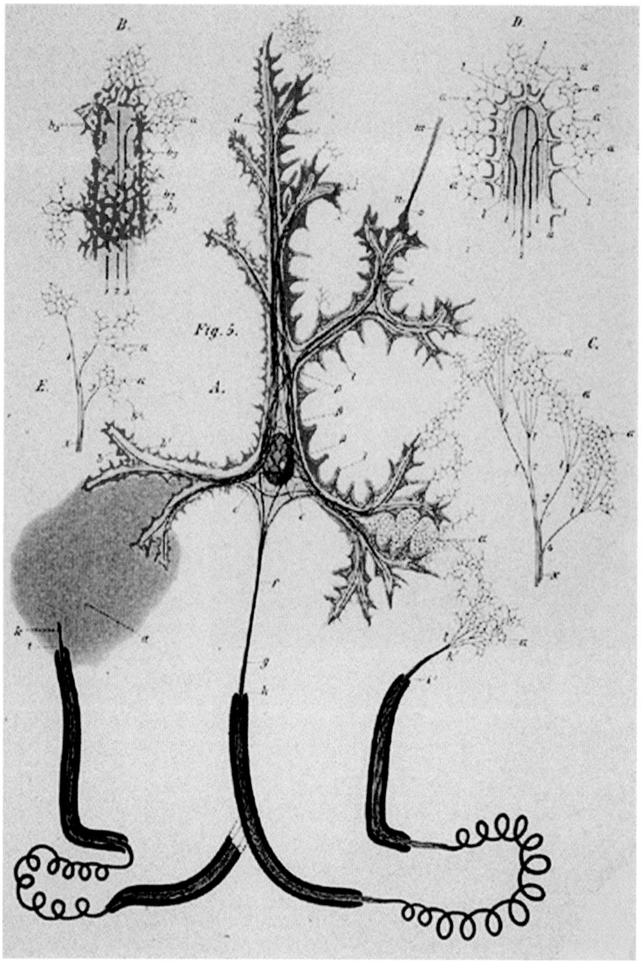

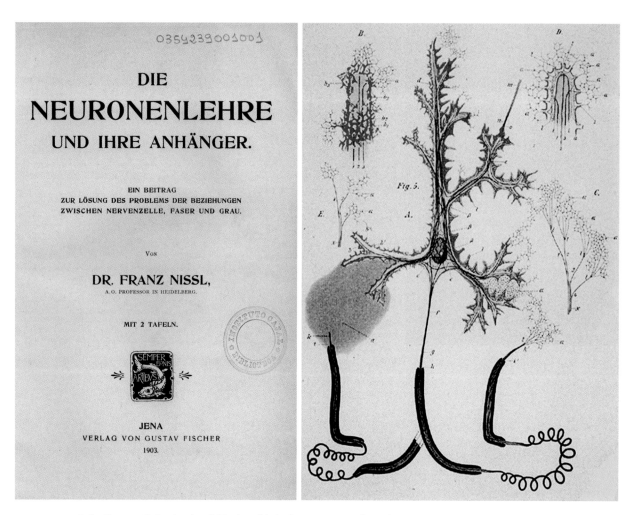

FIGURE 48. *Left*, Cover of the book of Nissl published in 1903. *Right*, Schematic drawing by Nissl supporting reticularism: "Schematic drawings that show, on one hand, what we know about the elemental structure of the nervous system of vertebrates (left half of neuron *A*) and, on the other, how one can imagine the elemental structure of the nervous system (right half of neuron *A*) . . . if we imagine the gray substance in the sense of Apathy as a reticulum of elemental [neuro] fibrils" (page 475). Taken from Nissl (1903).

arriving events, with the history and milieu to determine output in the restricted region where spikes are initiated. The size, number, and distribution over the neuron of these functionally differentiated regions and the labile coupling functions between the successive processes that eventually determine what information is transferred to the next neuron provide an enormous range of possible complexity within this single cellular unit. In the face of this gradual but sweeping change in functional concepts, any statement but the most diffuse about expectations for the future must be very dangerous. Nevertheless I will venture to suggest that in the near future we will gain significant new insight at this unitary level of neurophysiology with respect to the functions and differentiations among dendrites, the chemical and perhaps ultramicroscopic specification of different kinds of surface membrane, additional labile processes, sites of possible persistent change, and the normal functional significance of intercellular reactions mediated by graded activity without the intervention of all-or-none impulses.

Introduction of the Term *Neuron* and the Renascence of Reticularism

Cajal's early studies with the Golgi method were so decisive that they represented the main core of the review published by Wilhelm von Waldeyer-Hartz

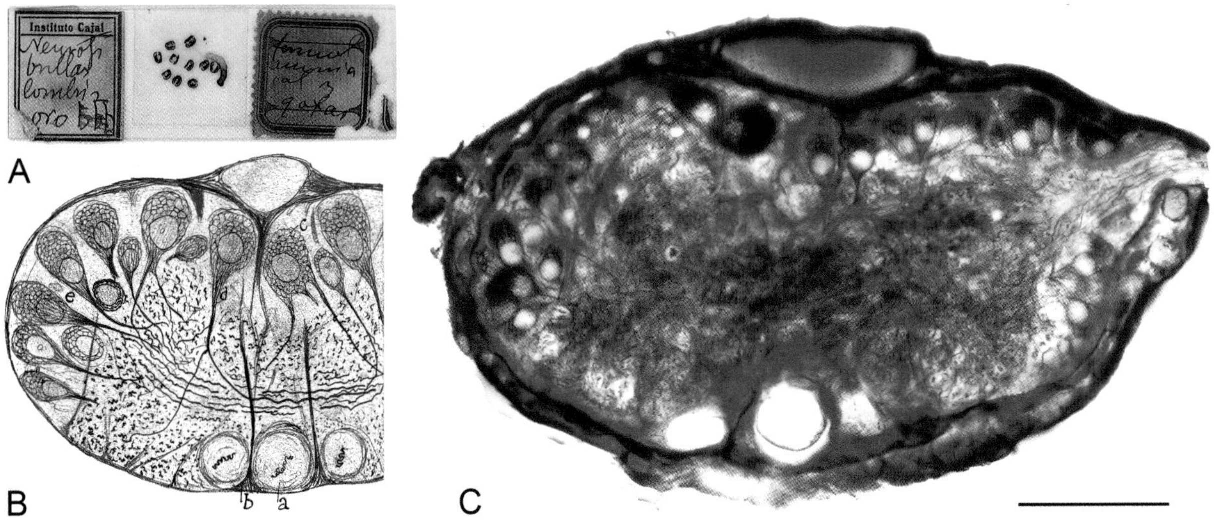

FIGURE 49. **A**, Photograph of Cajal's preparation of an earthworm stained with his reduced silver nitrate/gold-toning method. **B**, Cajal's drawing (1904) of a transverse section of a ganglion of the earthworm's (*Lumbricus agricola*) ventral chain. The legend states: "*a*, colossal tube [axon]; *b*, neuroglial column; *c*, multipolar corpuscle [neuron]; *d*, commissural cell; *e*, unipolar elements [cells]" (page 282). **C**, Photomicrograph taken from a section in *a* to illustrate the same structures as those observed in Cajal's drawing. Scale bar: 500 μm. The histological images were obtained by Virginia García-Marín, Pablo García-López and Miguel Freire (Legado Cajal, Instituto Cajal).

(1836–1921) in the journal *Deutsche Medizinische Wochenschrift* in 1891 (Figure 47). In this article, the term *neuron* was introduced to denominate the nerve cells and, at last, the so-called neuron doctrine became popular. By the end of the nineteenth century, this theory was the one that was most widely accepted by researchers in the field as an explanation for the organization of the nervous system (Shepherd, 1991; Jones, 1994), although several prestigious researchers were detractors. In addition to Golgi, distinguished reticularists included Franz Nissl (1860–1919) (Figure 48), Stephen von Apáthy (1863–1922), and, somewhat surprisingly, also Held, the great specialist in the study of axonal terminations.

One of the most important experiments that challenged the neuron doctrine was performed by Albrecht Bethe (DeFelipe, 2002b), who in 1901 started to publish several influential experimental papers on the regeneration of nerve fibers, claiming that axons regenerated from the anastomosis of multiple cells (Bethe, 1901). In mammals that were a few days of age, Bethe cut the sciatic nerve and covered the stumps in such a way that their union was apparently not possible. According to Bethe, the microscopic examination of the scar in these preparations showed the discontinuity between the two segments, but regeneration of the peripheral stump occurred as indicated by the reestablishment of physiological excitability. Thus, he concluded that nerves that were separated from their trophic centers were capable of autoregeneration (Bethe, 1903a, 1903b), as had been claimed by earlier physiologists and pathologists who supported the polygenetic theory of axon growth and regeneration. This theory states that the regenerated axons could result from the fusion of numerous axon segments produced by the differentiation and transformation of the ensheathing cells of the old nerve fibers.

These new experiments and their conclusions supporting the reticular theory were pivotal in prompting Cajal to set out on another big project in 1905: to study degeneration and regeneration in the nervous system, using mainly the reduced silver nitrate method, a new technique that he had improved himself (Cajal, 1903b, 1904) (Figure 49). In the words of Cajal (1917b, page 456):

> So fulminant and widespread did the contagion of reticularism become in 1903, due mainly to the

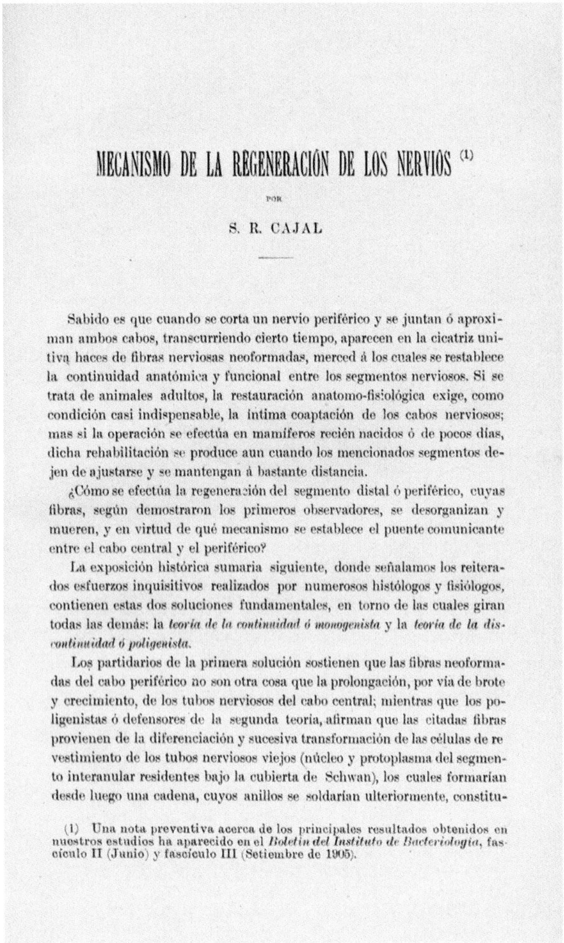

MECANISMO DE LA REGENERACIÓN DE LOS NERVIOS (1)

POR

S. R. CAJAL

Sabido es que cuando se corta un nervio periférico y se juntan ó aproximan ambos cabos, transcurriendo cierto tiempo, aparecen en la cicatriz unitiva haces de fibras nerviosas neoformadas, merced á los cuales se restablece la continuidad anatómica y funcional entre los segmentos nerviosos. Si se trata de animales adultos, la restauración anatomo-fisiológica exige, como condición casi indispensable, la íntima coaptación de los cabos nerviosos; mas si la operación se efectúa en mamíferos recién nacidos ó de pocos días, dicha rehabilitación se produce aun cuando los mencionados segmentos dejen de ajustarse y se mantengan á bastante distancia.

¿Cómo se efectúa la regeneración del segmento distal ó periférico, cuyas fibras, según demostraron los primeros observadores, se desorganizan y mueren, y en virtud de qué mecanismo se establece el puente comunicante entre el cabo central y el periférico?

La exposición histórica sumaria siguiente, donde señalamos los reiterados esfuerzos inquisitivos realizados por numerosos histólogos y fisiólogos, contienen estas dos soluciones fundamentales, en torno de las cuales giran todas las demás: la *teoría de la continuidad ó monogenista* y la *teoría de la discontinuidad ó poligenista*.

Los partidarios de la primera solución sostienen que las fibras neoformadas del cabo periférico no son otra cosa que la prolongación, por vía de brote y crecimiento, de los tubos nerviosos del cabo central; mientras que los poligenistas ó defensores de la segunda teoría, afirman que las citadas fibras provienen de la diferenciación y sucesiva transformación de las células de revestimiento de los tubos nerviosos viejos (núcleo y protoplasma del segmento interanular residentes bajo la cubierta de Schwan), los cuales formarían desde luego una cadena, cuyos anillos se soldarían ulteriormente, constitu-

(1) Una nota preventiva acerca de los principales resultados obtenidos en nuestros estudios ha aparecido en el *Boletín del Instituto de Bacteriología*, fascículo II (Junio) y fascículo III (Setiembre de 1905).

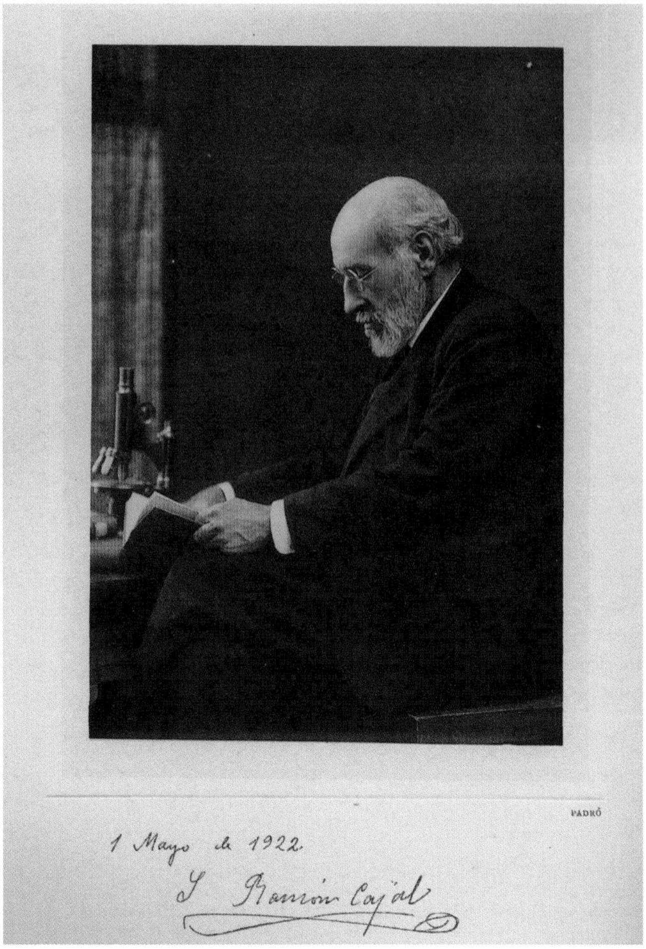

FIGURE 50. *Left,* First page of the article "*Mecanismo de la regeneración de los nervios*" (Cajal, 1906). This article is a more complete study of the results he published as a preliminary note titled "*Sobre la degeneración y regeneración de los nervios*" (Cajal, 1905). *Right,* Cajal in 1922, reading a book.

attractive statements of A. Bethe, that the illustrious Waldeyer wavered in his neuronist faith . . . , and even the illustrious Van Gehuchten, who was one of the pillars of neuronism weakened (who would have thought it!); he without renouncing the orthodox doctrine completely, made the following humiliating concession to the dissidents: The adult nerve cell possesses a perfect individuality, and is the product of a single neuroblast; but in the pathological state, for example, during the process of nervous regeneration, the new axons result from the fusion and differentiation of a chain of peripheral neuroblasts . . . . The details given demonstrate to the reader the truly dangerous situation that had been reached . . . the reticular chimera is so invasive and inconsistent in its objections, so arrogant and misplaced that the patience of the neuronists reached its limits. It was necessary to correct the general aberration. Some scholars wrote to me in a reproaching tone, puzzled by my silence and perhaps considering me as the most compelled to take up arms in favor of the truth: What are you doing? Why don't you defend yourself?

Cajal published numerous articles about this subject, which were summarized in another classic book, *Estudios sobre la degeneración y regeneración del sistema nervioso* (Cajal, 1913–1914). From the beginning of these studies using the reduced silver nitrate method (Cajal, 1905) (Figure 50), it was clear that

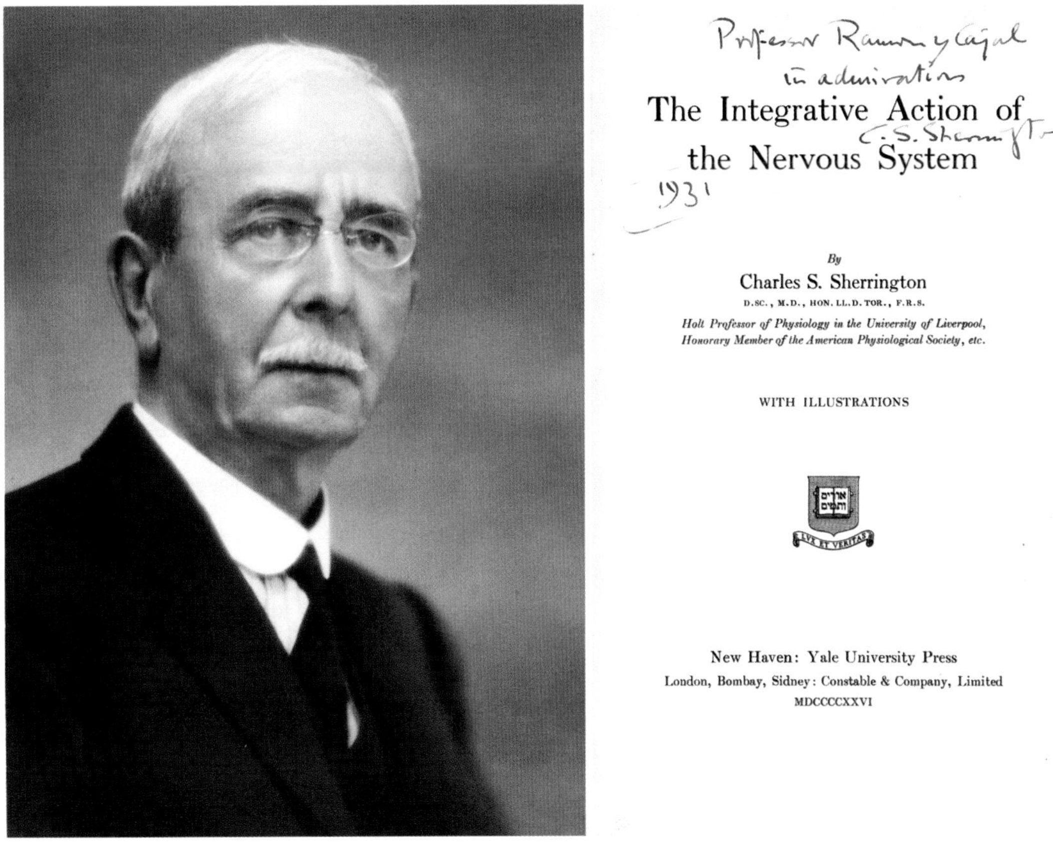
Professor Ramon y Cajal
in admiration
C. S. Sherrington
1931
The Integrative Action of
the Nervous System
By
Charles S. Sherrington
D.SC., M.D., HON. LL.D. TOR., F.R.S.
Holt Professor of Physiology in the University of Liverpool,
Honorary Member of the American Physiological Society, etc.
WITH ILLUSTRATIONS
LUX ET VERITAS
New Haven: Yale University Press
London, Bombay, Sidney: Constable & Company, Limited
MDCCCCXXVI

FIGURE 51. Portrait of Charles Sherrington included in the 1947 edition of his book *The Integrative Action of the Nervous System.*

the new fibers that appeared in the peripheral stump of a cut nerve originated from the sprouting of axons of the central stump and, as a result, the neuron doctrine once again became widely accepted. The differences in interpretation and the many, fundamental contributions of Cajal to the neuron doctrine were summarized in several of his own articles and books, especially in *¿Neuronismo o reticularismo?* published in 1933.

Nevertheless, despite the wealth of experimental data (from physiological and Wallerian secondary degeneration studies) and histological observations supporting the neuron doctrine, the crucial observation that there was a physical separation between the neurons took a long time to appear because the light microscope was not powerful enough to address this issue. As a result of the optical limitations of light microscopy, the contact areas between the axon terminals and soma and/or dendrites were, at best, displayed only as a single membrane. For those researchers in favor of the neuron doctrine, this was presumably because the limiting membranes of the presynaptic and postsynaptic element were so close that only one membrane could be distinguished. Thus, the neuron doctrine was generally accepted, but with certain doubts, and exceptions were proposed up to the middle of the twentieth century. This situation was summarized beautifully by Charles Sherrington (1857–1952) in his classic book *The Integrative Action of the Nervous System* (Figure 51). Sherrington, who in 1897 introduced the term *synapse*, for the hypothetical one-way contact between axon terminals and somata or dendrites, wrote the following with regard to this subject (Sherrington, 1947, page 17):

> As to the existence or non-existence of a surface of separation or membrane between neurone and

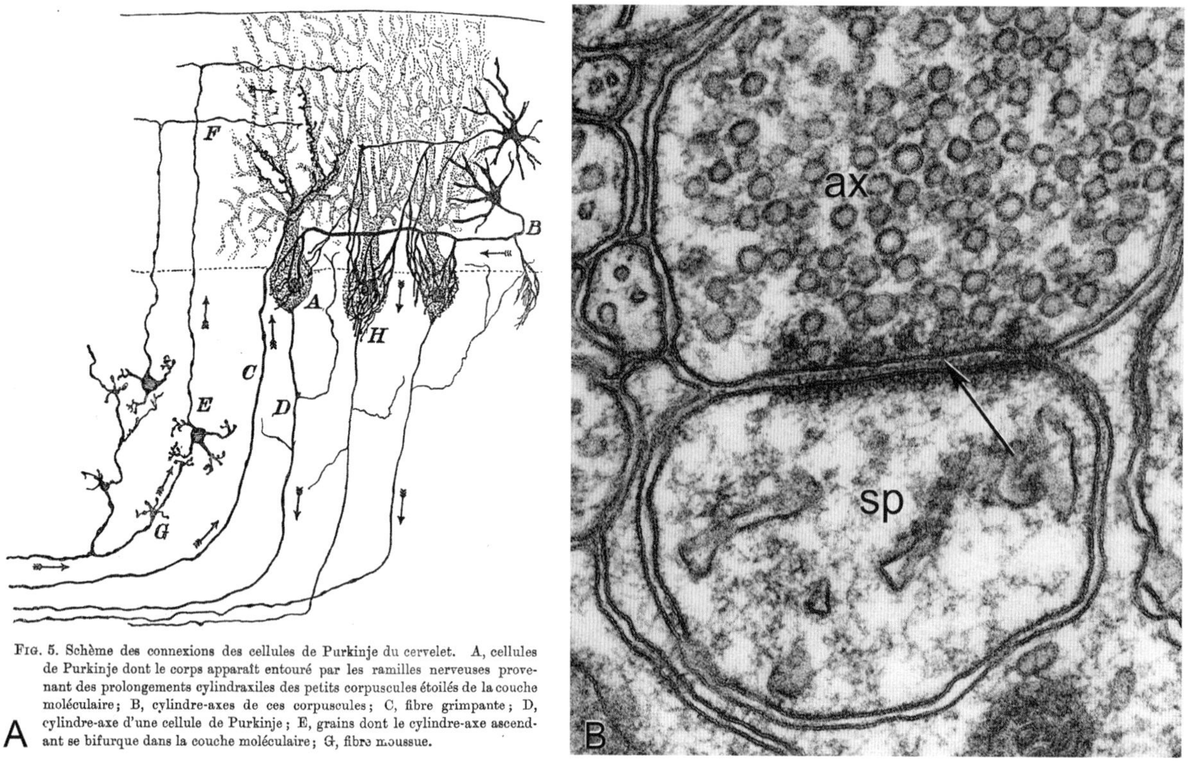
F
B
C
E
D
A
H
G
Fig. 5. Schème des connexions des cellules de Purkinje du cervelet. A, cellules de Purkinje dont le corps apparaît entouré par les ramilles nerveuses provenant des prolongements cylindraxiles des petits corpuscules étoilés de la couche moléculaire; B, cylindre-axes de ces corpuscules; C, fibre grimpante; D, cylindre-axe d'une cellule de Purkinje; E, grains dont le cylindre-axe ascendant se bifurque dans la couche moléculaire; G, fibre moussue.
A
ax
sp
B

FIGURE 52. **A**, Schematic drawing by Cajal to show connections of Purkinje cells in the cerebellum and the possible flow of information (arrows) (Cajal, 1894b). The legend states: "*A*, Purkinje cells whose bodies appear surrounded by the nervous branchlets coming from the axis cylinder prolongations of the small stellate corpuscles of the molecular layer; *B*, axis cylinders of these corpuscles; *C*, climbing fibers; *D*, axis cylinder of a Purkinje cell; *E*, granules whose ascending axis cylinder *F* bifurcates in the molecular layer; G, mossy fiber" (page 459). "Axis cylinder" is equivalent to "axon." **B**, Electron micrograph of a typical synapse. In this figure a synapse established between a parallel fiber varicosity (ax) and a dendritic spine of a Purkinje cell dendrite (sp) in the molecular layer of the rat cerebellum is shown. The presynaptic varicosity is filled with spherical synaptic vesicles that contain the neurotransmitter (glutamate). The synaptic cleft (between the pre- and postsynaptic membranes) is indicated by an arrow. (Courtesy of Constantino Sotelo, Instituto de Neurociencias, Alicante, Spain.)

neurone, that is a structural question on which histology might be competent to give valuable information. In certain cases, especially in Invertebrata, observation (Apáthy, Bethe, etc.) indicates that many nerve-cells are actually continuous one with another. It is noteworthy that in several of these cases the irreversibility of direction of conduction which is characteristic of spinal reflex-arcs is not demonstrable . . . . But in the neurone-chains on the gray-centred system of vertebrates, histology on the whole furnishes evidence that a surface of separation does exist between neurone and neurone . . . . It seems therefore likely that the nexus between neurone and neurone in the reflex-arc, at least in the spinal arc of the vertebrate, involves a surface of separation between neurone and neurone; and this as a transverse membrane across the conductor must be an important element in intercellular conduction . . . . In view, therefore, of the probable importance physiologically of this mode of nexus between neurone and neurone it is convenient to have a term for it. The term introduced has been *synapse* (Foster and Sherrington, 1897).

Confirmation of the Free Ending of the Nervous Processes: The Discovery of the Synaptic Cleft

It was not until the introduction of electron microscopy during the 1950s that the structural issues raised by Sherrington could be resolved. Along with the development of new methods to prepare nervous tissue for fine structural analysis (for example, fixation in osmium tetroxide and/or aldehydes, epoxy embedding, and so on [Robertson, 1953; Palade and Palay, 1954; De Robertis and Bennett, 1955; Palay, 1956; De Robertis, 1959; Gray, 1959a, 1959b), this novel microscopy technique allowed the examination of the ultrastructure of the synapse. This made it possible to confirm one of the main tenets of the neural doctrine—namely, that presynaptic and postsynaptic elements are separated physically by a space about 10 to 20 nm wide, known as the *synaptic cleft* (reviewed in Peters et al., 1991). Figure 52A shows a schematic drawing by Cajal demonstrating the connections of Purkinje cells in the cerebellum (Cajal, 1894b). When referring to the connections between the granule cells and the Purkinje cells of the cerebellum in the text, Cajal (1894b, page 460) described "a very intimate contact" of the granule cell axons with the dendritic spines of Purkinje:

> The granules of the cerebellum . . . possess an axis cylinder [axon] of extraordinary fineness. This ascends to the molecular zone, where it bifurcates at various heights, thus producing a longitudinal fibril that runs in a parallel manner along the whole cerebellar lamella. These interesting fibrils that we have called parallel [fibers] because they are arranged in parallel in relation to the cerebellar lamellae, become positioned in very intimate contact, during their trajectory, with the spinous contours of the protoplasmic [dendritic] branches of Purkinje cells.

Figure 52B shows—at the structural level—one of these "intimate contacts" in which a synapse established between a parallel fiber varicosity (ax) and a dendritic spine of a Purkinje cell dendrite (sp) is observed, including the synaptic cleft. Thus, Cajal proposed that dendritic spines established synapses, but it was necessary to wait several decades until the advent of electron microscopy to visualize the space that exists between the axon terminals and the dendrites.

Neoreticularism and the Neuron Doctrine in the Present Day

Although the neuron doctrine was largely supported by the appearance of new techniques to study the nervous system at the anatomical, physiological, and molecular levels, these very same techniques have revealed many exceptions that challenge the neuron doctrine and the law of dynamic (or axipetal) polarization. As discussed recently in DeFelipe (2015a and references contained therein; see also Bullock et al., 2005), a large variety of synaptic relationships have been observed, including dendrodendritic, somatosomatic, somatodendritic, dendrosomatic, dendroaxonic and somatoaxonic synapses. Cells may also be coupled electrically, and the direction of transmission may be bidirectional through small channels known as *gap junctions*. These junctions connect the cytoplasm of the adjoining neurons, permitting the diffusion of small molecules and the flow of electric current. Moreover, the transmitter released at synaptic or nonsynaptic sites may diffuse and act on other synaptic contacts, or on extrasynaptic receptors. A further example of the diversity of these interactions is the ephatic coupling that takes place between closely apposed neuronal elements without obvious membrane specializations. Yet another is the proposal that glial cells are involved in information processing through their bidirectional signaling with neurons. We also now know that the activity of neuronal circuits is strongly influenced by neuromodulators (such as dopamine, serotonin, and acetylcholine), which are secreted by a small group of neurons and diffuse through large regions of the nervous system. Neurohormones, released by neurosecretory cells, also have an effect on many brain regions via the circulatory system.

Despite this ever-increasing complexity, it is important to keep in mind that there are general principles or rules for the design of brain circuits, the discovery of which is fundamental to understanding more fully brain organization and function. For instance, chemical axodendritic synapses are by far the most common type of synapse (followed by axosomatic synapses), at least in mammals. Other types of synapses are not found in all regions of the nervous system, and when they are present, they are usually only established between certain types of neurons. A further point to consider is the functional significance of the various

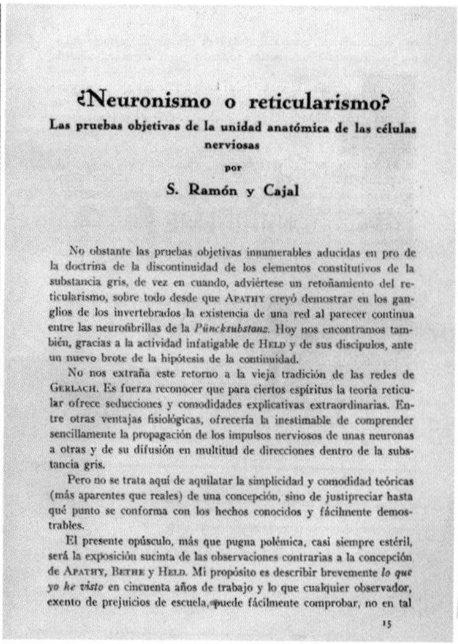

¿Neuronismo o reticularismo?

Las pruebas objetivas de la unidad anatómica de las células nerviosas

por

S. Ramón y Cajal

No obstante las pruebas objetivas innumerables aducidas en pro de la doctrina de la discontinuidad de los elementos constitutivos de la substancia gris, de vez en cuando, adviértese un retoñamiento del reticularismo, sobre todo desde que APATHY creyó demostrar en los ganglios de los invertebrados la existencia de una red al parecer continua entre las neurofibrillas de la *Püncksubstanz*. Hoy nos encontramos también, gracias a la actividad infatigable de HELD y de sus discípulos, ante un nuevo brote de la hipótesis de la continuidad.

No nos extraña este retorno a la vieja tradición de las redes de GERLACH. Es fuerza reconocer que para ciertos espíritus la teoría reticular ofrece seducciones y comodidades explicativas extraordinarias. Entre otras ventajas fisiológicas, ofrecería la inestimable de comprender sencillamente la propagación de los impulsos nerviosos de unas neuronas a otras y de su difusión en multitud de direcciones dentro de la substancia gris.

Pero no se trata aquí de aquilatar la simplicidad y comodidad teóricas (más aparentes que reales) de una concepción, sino de justipreciar hasta qué punto se conforma con los hechos conocidos y fácilmente demostrables.

El presente opúsculo, más que pugna polémica, casi siempre estéril, será la exposición sucinta de las observaciones contrarias a la concepción de APATHY, BETHE y HELD. Mi propósito es describir brevemente *lo que yo he visto* en cincuenta años de trabajo y lo que cualquier observador, exento de prejuicios de escuela, puede fácilmente comprobar, no en tal

15

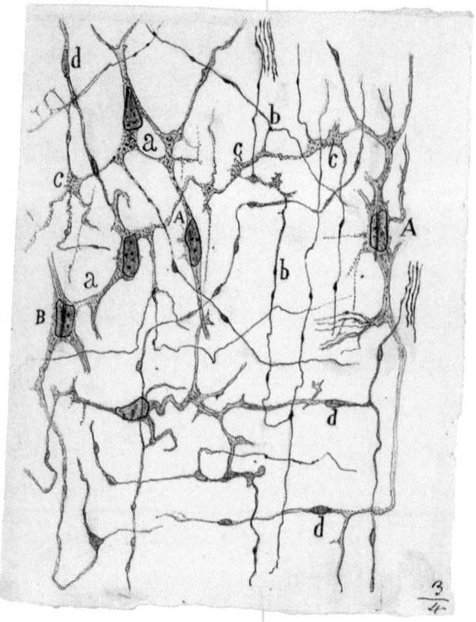

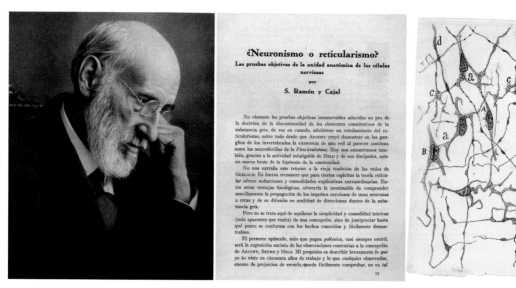

FIGURE 53. *Left,* Photograph of Cajal with his face resting on one hand as if deep in thought. *Center,* First page of the article of by Cajal "*¿Neuronismo o reticularismo?*" (1933), in which he summarized the main observations opposing the reticular theory. *Right,* Cell of the Auerbach's plexus (or myenteric plexus) stained with methyl blue. Taken from Cajal (1892a). The legend states: "*A,* Elongated cells; *B,* stellate cell; *a,* intercellular anastomoses" (page 26).

forms of overall brain connectivity. For example, the brain's wiring—its "synaptome" (DeFelipe 2010b)—is the anatomical basis for a large variety of functions that require information to be communicated rapidly from one point to another. The neuronal circuits involved in reflexes are a typical example of this because they involve relatively simple, fast, automatic actions that occur at a subconscious level. Other, much more complex functions related to the synaptome include information processing in large but discrete circuits in the sensory and motor systems, and in the brain regions associated with language, calculation, writing, and reasoning. The modulatory systems, however, act on multiple neuronal circuits and brain areas. This diffuse action is related to the overall moods and states of the brain (for example, attentiveness, sleep, and anxiety).

Finally, returning to Cajal and the subject of the anastomosis, there is a common misinterpretation that Cajal denied its existence, although this was not the case. In fact, on occasion, Cajal described the existence of anastomoses, sometimes called *puentes inter-protoplásmicos o inter-nerviosos* (interprotoplasmic or internervous bridges; Figure 53, right) (Cajal 1889c; Cajal, 1892a; Cajal and Sala, 1891), but he was convinced that most of the connections between neurons were by contact or contiguity, not continuity. Thus, once again ahead of his time, Cajal in his article "*¿Neuronismo or reticularismo?*" (1933, page 142 (Figure 53), commented:

> We are neither exclusive nor dogmatic. We are proud of retaining a mental flexibility that is not embarrassed by the need to rectify. Exceptions may arise to the neuronal discontinuity that is so evident in innumerable examples. We ourselves have reported some, for example, those that are probably present in the glands, vessels and intestine . . . . For this reason, we have previously pointed out, and we insist on this, that when dealing with the morphology and connections of neurons, we must abide by the law of large numbers, that is, we must adhere to a rigorously statistical criterion.

In conclusion, although there are notable exceptions and important additions to our knowledge about how neurons function and interchange information with other neural elements, currently the neuron doctrine continues to be one of the foundations on which our concept of the anatomical and functional organization of the nervous system is based (Shepherd, 1991, 2016).

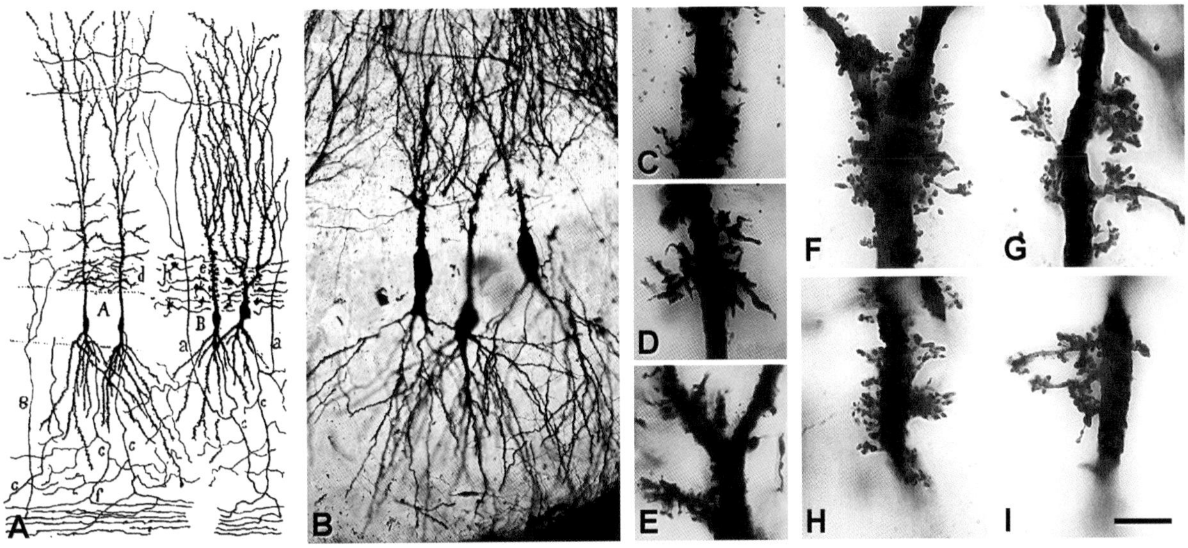

FIGURE 54. Complex dendritic spines (thorny excrescences) of CA3 pyramidal neurons. **A**, Cajal's drawing showing pyramidal cells with thorny excrescences in the CA3 (taken from Cajal, 1893a, page 70). **B–I**, Photomicrographs of Cajal's original histological preparations. **B**, CA3 pyramidal cells of the rabbit stained by the Golgi method. **C–I**, Examples of thorny excrescences on CA3 pyramidal neurons. **C–E**, Dendrites from a newborn child's CA3 pyramidal neurons stained by the Golgi method. **F–I**, Dendrites of rabbit CA3 pyramidal neurons stained by Kenyon's variant of the Golgi method (preparations housed in the Legado Cajal at the Instituto Cajal). Scale bar (in I): **B**, 55 μm; **C–I**, 11 μm. Taken from Blazquez-Llorca et al. (2011).

DENDRITIC SPINES: TRUE ANATOMICAL STRUCTURES VERSUS ARTIFACTS

What follows is a discussion on the discovery of dendritic spines and their interpretation based on a recent publication by me (DeFelipe, 2015b). As we have seen, dendritic spines were discovered and named by Cajal in 1888 in his first important article based on results obtained with the Golgi method (Figure 33). In this article, Cajal (1888, pages 4–5) said:

> The surface of [the dendrites of Purkinje cells] appears to be covered with thorns or short spines . . . . At the beginning, we thought that these eminences were the result of a tumultuous precipitation of the silver but the constancy of its existence and its presence, even in preparations in which the reaction appears to be very delicate in the remaining elements, inclines us to believe this to be a normal condition.

However, in this article he did not discuss the possible function of dendritic spines. Two years later, Cajal described the existence of these structures in the pyramidal cells of the cerebral cortex and interpreted them as possible targets of axons (Cajal, 1890b, page 25):

> Layer of the small pyramids—We will only add two details to the description given by Golgi: first, the peripheral arborizations of the ascending shaft bristles with short spines ending in a small swelling. The gulfs that are between such collateral spines receive the impression of innumerable small fibers of the superficial layer. Exactly the same disposition is possessed by the terminal peripheral arborizations of the large pyramids.

It was not until 1892 that he more specifically referred to the dendritic spines as key elements for transmission by contact in both the cerebellar and cerebral cortices (Cajal, 1892b). In this article, when referring to the connections between the axonal plexus of layer I and the ascending dendritic tufts of pyramidal cells ending in this layer, he wrote (page 462):

> It is impossible not to consider this singular arrangement, which, by the way, is found with the same

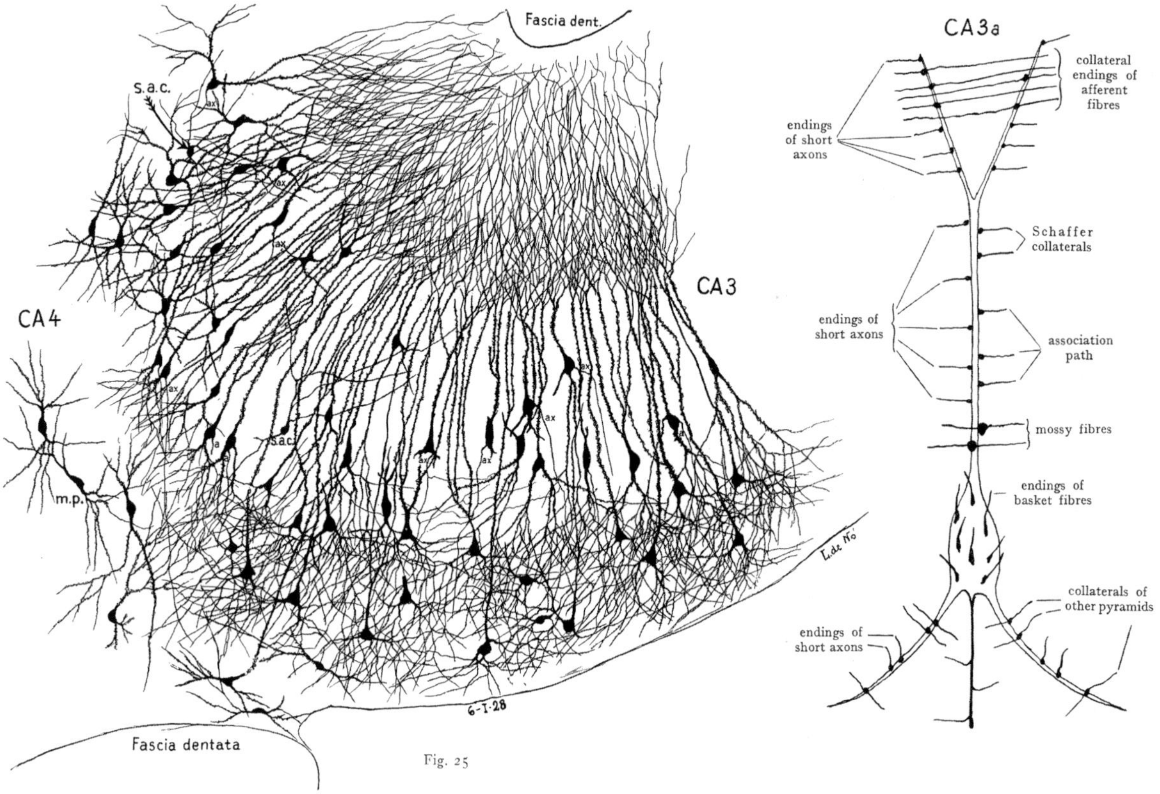

FIGURE 55. Drawings taken from Lorente de Nó (1934) to illustrate part of the CA3 field at the border with CA4 (*left* [page 149]) and a diagram showing the different types of synapses established on a CA3 pyramid cell, including the synapses formed by mossy fibers [page 168].(see also Figure 46).

> characteristics in all vertebrates, as an important example of neural transmission by contact, comparable to that occurring in the cerebellum between the tiny parallel fibers and the [dendritic] arborizations of the Purkinje cells. This contact would be transverse or oblique, on account of which the terminal [dendritic] branches of the pyramidal cells possess short collateral spines, in the gaps between which the thinnest small axonal fibers bereft of myelin seem to be tightly caught.

Furthermore, in 1893, he also discovered and named the typical thorny excrescences of hippocampal pyramidal cells of CA3 (Cajal, 1893a). He proposed that these large and often branched structures served as points of contact with the mossy fibers from the dentate gyrus (Figure 54). This observation was confirmed by various authors, although some doubts remained. Lorente de Nó (1934) was among those who believed that this issue was still debatable. He made the following interesting comment regarding the pyramidal cells of CA3 (Figure 55) and the thorny excrescences: "The initial part of the shaft has very thick thorns destined to come in contact with the mossy thickenings of the axons from the Fascia dentata" (page 131). This sentence was accompanied by the following footnote:

> Kölliker, who in general considered all thorns in the pyramids as an artefact, expressed his belief that the mentioned thorns are also an artefact. Possibly Kölliker saw giant pyramids of CA2 without thorns and thought that the thorns of CA3 were not preexistent. Whether the thorns are a part of the pyramid, or the endings of mossy fibres stained without the fibre, I would not dare to decide. The fact that Cajal stained thorns of the pyramids of the common cortex with Erlich's methylene blue method is a very

> powerful argument in favor of the assumption that they are a part of the pyramid itself. However, one sometimes sees pictures in Golgi preparations which seem to indicate that the thorns are endings of fibres stained alone, i.e., without the fibre. At any rate, there is no doubt that each thorn is a synapse. In the actual case of the big thorns of CA3 pyramids, it is interesting to note that they appear in every pyramid of CA3, and never in a pyramid of CA2, although many cells of both fields may be stained at the same time. That an artefact should appear always in a cell, and always in the same manner, never in another cell lying almost in immediate contact with it is impossible.

Currently, it is well established that thorny excrescences are postsynaptic specializations of CA3 pyramidal neurons that establish excitatory synapses with mossy fibers (Andersen et al., 2007). In addition, in the immature nervous system, Cajal observed the presence of short dendritic protrusions that were different to dendritic spines. He described these protrusions as "irregular projections very seldom ending as bulbs" and proposed that they were most likely transitory (Cajal, 1933). Later, these transitory protrusions were called *filopodia*. After these studies, numerous researchers confirmed the existence of dendritic spines (e.g., Retzius, 1891a; Schaffer, 1892; Edinger, 1893; Demoor, 1896; Stefanowska, 1897, 1901; Hatai, 1903). Among the later researchers, it is interesting to highlight the studies of Micheline Stefanowska—one of the very few female neuroscientists of that time. Her work was based on the 1890s hypothesis of amoeboid movement of neurons to possible changes in brain circuits as plastic responses of the normal brain or after experimental manipulation. For example, it was proposed that inactivity during sleep could be explained by a retraction of dendritic processes (theory of the histophysiology of sleep). This retraction would reduce considerably the number of contacts and thus "the association of the individual cellular activities" (DeFelipe, 2006). Stefanowska focused on the "pyriform appendages"—the name she used to refer to the dendritic spines. She proposed that these pyriform appendages could change temporarily both their shape and number in the brain during normal activity, and that similar changes may occur in the brain of experimental animals under certain experimental conditions, such as electrical stimulation of the cerebral cortex or after the administration of sedatives (morphine, chloral hydrate, and chloroform). As we will see, in general, the conclusions regarding the activity-dependent changes in dendritic spines have received particular attention again in recent times because many of these ideas have been confirmed with modern techniques.

Dendritic Spines and the Methylene Blue Method

It is important to note that a number of other authors believed the dendritic spines were artifacts, including distinguished scientists such as Kölliker (1896)—see Lorente de Nó's comment earlier—and even Golgi himself did not believe that the dendritic spines were actual neuronal structures. The structures were considered to be needle-shaped crystallizations of silver chromate on the neuron surface, and so they were left out of early drawings in which the dendrites were represented as being smooth in appearance (Figure 22B, C and Figure 56A). Although differing interpretations of the microscope images played a part in this skepticism (Figure 56), it was also because the dendritic spines were not visible with methods other than either the Golgi method or an adapted version of it called the *Golgi-Cox method* (Cox, 1891) that involved submerging the tissue samples in a potassium dichromate–mercuric chloride mixture. Moreover, Semi Meyer (1895, 1896, 1897) reported he could find no evidence these structures existed when using a variant of the methylene blue technique. This technique started out as a bacterial stain and was introduced by Paul Ehrlich (1881), although a few years later (in 1886), this same scientist discovered that injecting the stain directly into the blood vessels of living animals led to peripheral nerve fiber staining (Ehrlich, 1886). The resulting images were comparable with the Golgi method images, which contributed to the popularity of Ehrlich's approach. Several scientists went on to adapt this methylene

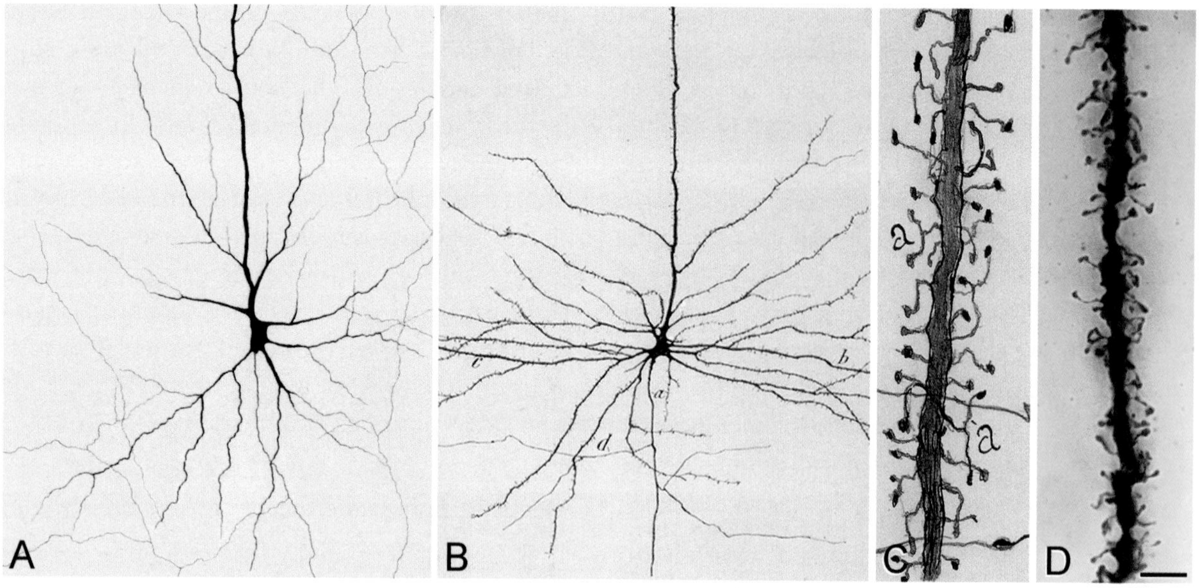

FIGURE 56. Pyramidal cells of the human cerebral cortex. **A**, Drawing by Golgi (1882–1883) to illustrate a pyramidal cell of the human motor cortex stained with the Golgi method. The axon appears in red. **B**, Drawing by Cajal (1899) to illustrate a pyramidal cell of the human motor cortex. *a*, initial part of the axon; *b*, dendrites; *d*, axonal collaterals. **C**, Drawing by Cajal to illustrate the dendritic spines of pyramidal cells (cerebral cortex of a 2-month-old child). Taken from Cajal (1933). Note that Golgi does not draw dendritic spines. However, in the drawing of Cajal shown in **B**, it can be seen that the surface of the dendrites are covered with dendrites spines. **D**, Photomicrograph of a preparation by Cajal of the human motor cortex (15-day-old child) stained using the Golgi method. The image illustrates an apical dendrite of a layer V pyramidal cell covered with spines. Scale bar in **D**: 8 μm. The histological image was obtained by Pablo García-López, Virginia García-Marín, and Miguel Freire (Legado Cajal, Instituto Cajal). Figure and legend taken from DeFelipe (2014).

blue method, including Bethe and Dogiel, who deserve a special mention here. Bethe (1895) achieved better staining preservation throughout the various steps involved in the histological processing of the sections by introducing ammonium molybdate fixation. Modifications that were included by Dogiel (1896) made it possible to use the technique with thin, freshly cut slices of central nervous tissue.

The Golgi method and the adapted Cox method both stained dendritic spines consistently, and this staining occurred in particular neuronal regions. Cajal saw this as strong evidence that dendritic spines did, indeed, exist, and came to the conclusion that they must be extremely important for the structure and function of neurons. Cajal (1896, page 124) stated:

> Dendritic spines are constantly present at the same regions of the [dendritic] arborizations, no matter what animal is studied, and are always lacking at certain sites, such as the [axon initial segment], cell body and origin of the thick [dendritic] processes.

Nevertheless, Cajal revisited this matter (using the methylene blue method this time), partly in response to the contrasting findings of Meyer and partly because of the skepticism of Kölliker, who Cajal held in high regard. Using the same method as Meyer, Cajal observed the dendrites were stained so pale that it would not be surprising if their dendritic spines were stained much paler—to the point of being invisible—given that dendritic spines would clearly hold much less stain than dendrites, which are much larger. Thus, Cajal concluded that the method used by Meyer was not suitable for demonstrating the presence of dendritic spines. Cajal went on to adapt the methylene blue method, adopting aspects of the procedures used by Bethe and Dogiel, which resulted in the staining of the dendritic spines (Cajal, 1896) (Figure 57). Others also confirmed that dendritic spines were visible with the methylene blue method (e.g., Turner and Aber, 1900; Soukhanoff et al., 1904), which ruled out the possibility of them

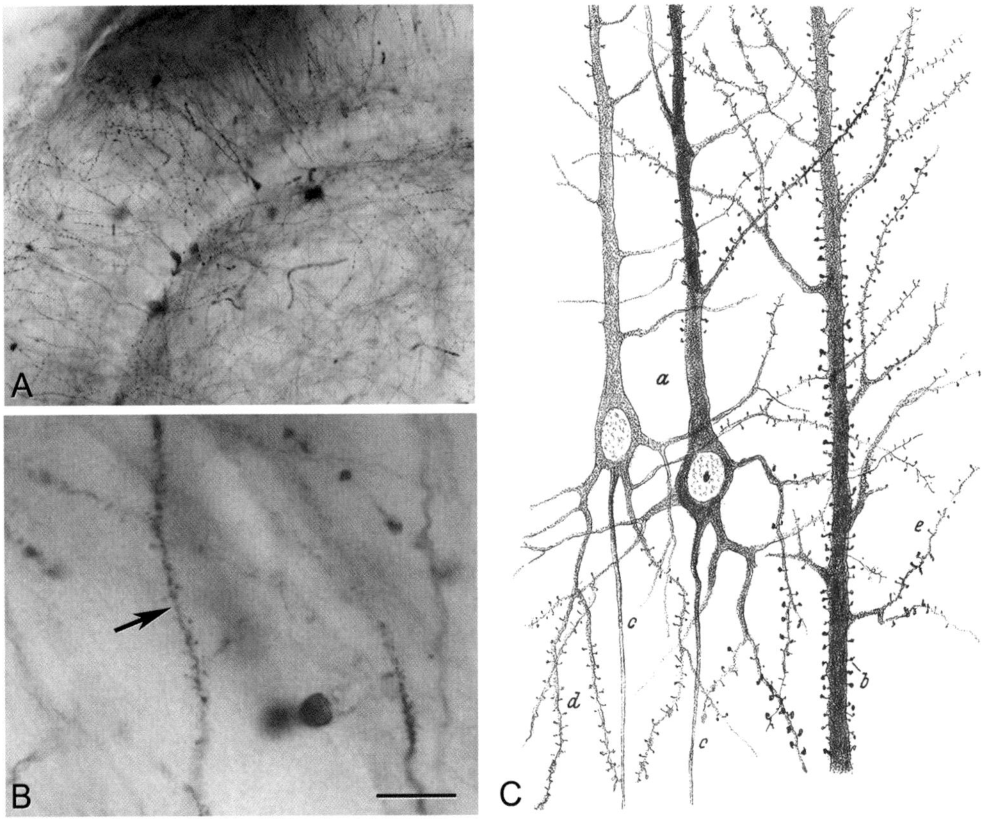

FIGURE 57. Dendritic spines stained with the methylene blue method. **A**, **B**, Low- and high-magnification photomicrographs, respectively, of a preparation by Cajal of the hippocampus stained with the methylene blue method (preparation housed in the Legado Cajal at the Instituto Cajal). These photomicrographs are from unpublished material from DeFelipe and Jones (1988). Scale bar (in B): **A**, 120 µm; **B**, 10 µm. **C**, Drawing used by Cajal (1896, page 127) to show the existence of dendritic spines on pyramidal cells using the methylene blue method. Figure and legend taken from DeFelipe (2015b).

being artifacts, leading to the conclusion they were, indeed, anatomical structures.

Interestingly, some years later Golgi recognized the existence of dendritic spines (Golgi, 1901), as we can see from the fact that he included them in several of his drawings (e.g., Figure 58). However, in the text he did not mention these structures. This change in his interpretation of the microscopic images was probably a result of emergence of new evidence obtained with the methylene blue method used by Cajal and others scientists, but Golgi did not seem to attribute any functional relevance to these structures. This is a good example of the way in which the observer might change how they interpret and illustrate what they are seeing, influenced by the mental image or predisposition they have about the structure being analyzed. This also clearly demonstrates why it is sometimes so difficult to interpret the figures of the early neuroanatomists, because we cannot be sure how accurate these illustrations are. Thus, it was (and continues to be) important for researchers to check the veracity of Cajal's drawings by analyzing their own histological preparations (Figure 49; Figure 56C, D; Figure 57; Figure 59) (e.g., see DeFelipe and Jones, 1988, 1991) or by using more modern methods to analyze the nervous system to determine whether his interpretations were indeed accurate (see the section "Confirmation That Dendritic Spines Are Postsynaptic Structures").

Other Interpretations of the Dendritic Spines

It is also interesting to note that it was not only the *existence* of the dendritic spines that was controversial among scientists; their *function* was an equally

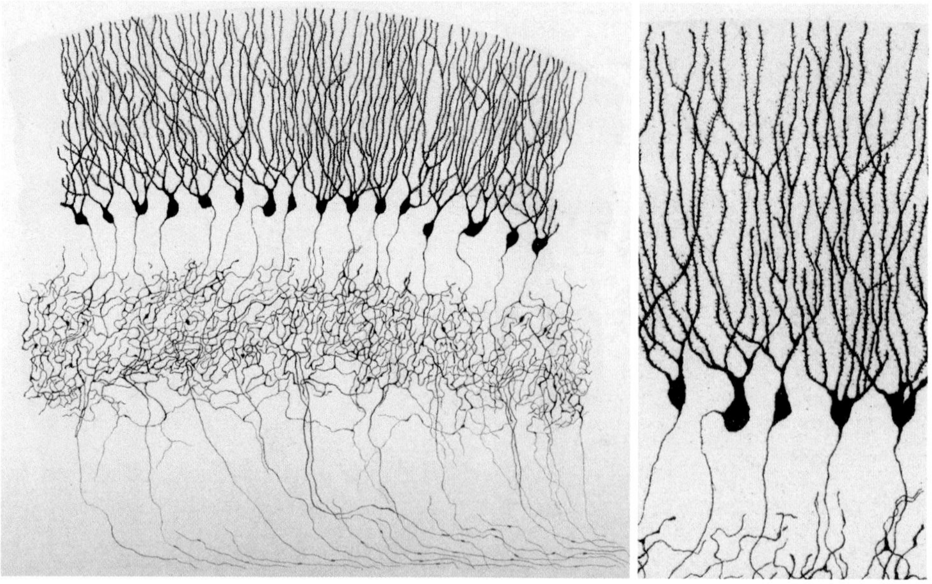

FIGURE 58. Illustration by Golgi (1901) of a Golgi-impregnated preparation of the dentate gyrus. "*Fascia dentata del grande piede di Hippocampo.*" *Left*, Panoramic view. Golgi used this drawing to illustrate that the axons of granule cells formed a very complex nervous network ("*rete nervosa*"). See Note 12 for the transcription of the legend. *Right*, High magnification of the drawing illustrating that Golgi recognized the presence of dendritic spines. Figure and legend taken from DeFelipe (2015b).

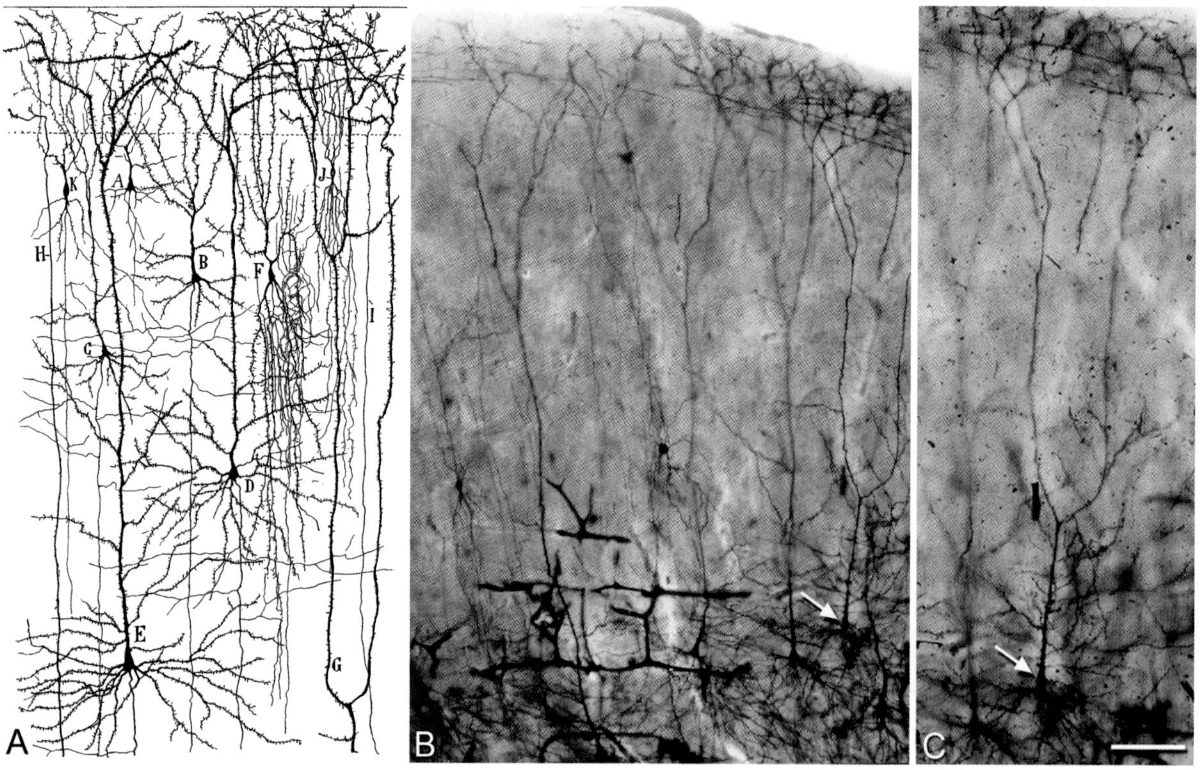

FIGURE 59. **A**, Cajal's drawing (1899) from a Golgi stained preparation to illustrate some of the neuronal components of supragranular layers of the human cerebral cortex. The translation of the legend is as follows: "First, second, and third layers of the precentral gyrus of a child of one month. *A, B, C*, small pyramids; *D, E*, medium pyramids; *F*, bitufted cell, whose axon formed terminal nests; *G*, dendritic shaft emanating from a large pyramid of the fourth layer; *H, I*, thin dendritic shafts of cells of the sixth and seven layers: *J*, small bitufted cell; *K*, fusiform cell with long axon" (page 139). **B**, **C**, Low- and high-magnification photomicrographs, respectively, from one of Cajal's preparations of the postcentral gyrus of a newborn child, showing a layer V pyramidal cell (arrows)—impregnated by the Golgi method—with an apical dendrite that forms a tuft in layer I. Notice the similar morphological appearance of this cell and the one shown in **A** in Figure 68A.

contentious issue in these early days. Some accepted that dendritic spines existed, but offered very different interpretations from Cajal regarding their role. The two very different functions proposed by Bethe and Held illustrate this point well (Figure 60). The drawings by Bethe (1903a) presented the dendritic spines in the same way as Cajal had, but Bethe postulated that these were, in fact, the initial points of an interstitial network of the gray matter that Nissl called *nervöses Grau* (Figure 60A) (quoted in Cajal, 1909, 1911: Vol.1, 1909, page 69). Held accepted that dendritic spines existed, but interpreted them as being the end-feet (axons ended in distinct terminals), or *Endfüsse*, which had either been split or were not completely stained (Figure 60B) by the neurofibrillar methods. He believed these axon terminals joined together with the dendrites, in the same way as end-feet do on cell bodies (Held, 1897a, 1897b, 1902, 1904, 1905, 1929). Held also proposed the possibility of an interstitial network, which would make communication between pyramidal cells possible via anastomoses between these "dendritic spines" and the nerve fibers (Held, 1929).

Cajal focused on this article by Held (1929), setting out to disprove his hypothesis. He was motivated to do so not only because he disagreed with the ideas put forward by Held, but also because the German anatomist had wrongly credited Golgi with having discovered dendritic spines. In "*¿Neuronismo o reticularismo?*" (Cajal, 1933), Cajal made a compelling case that countered the interpretation of Held, in which Cajal argued that even the thinnest of axons were visible, whereas the dendritic spines of pyramidal cells or Purkinje cells were never stained by the neurofibrillar methods. To illustrate this point, Cajal included an exquisite schematic drawing (see

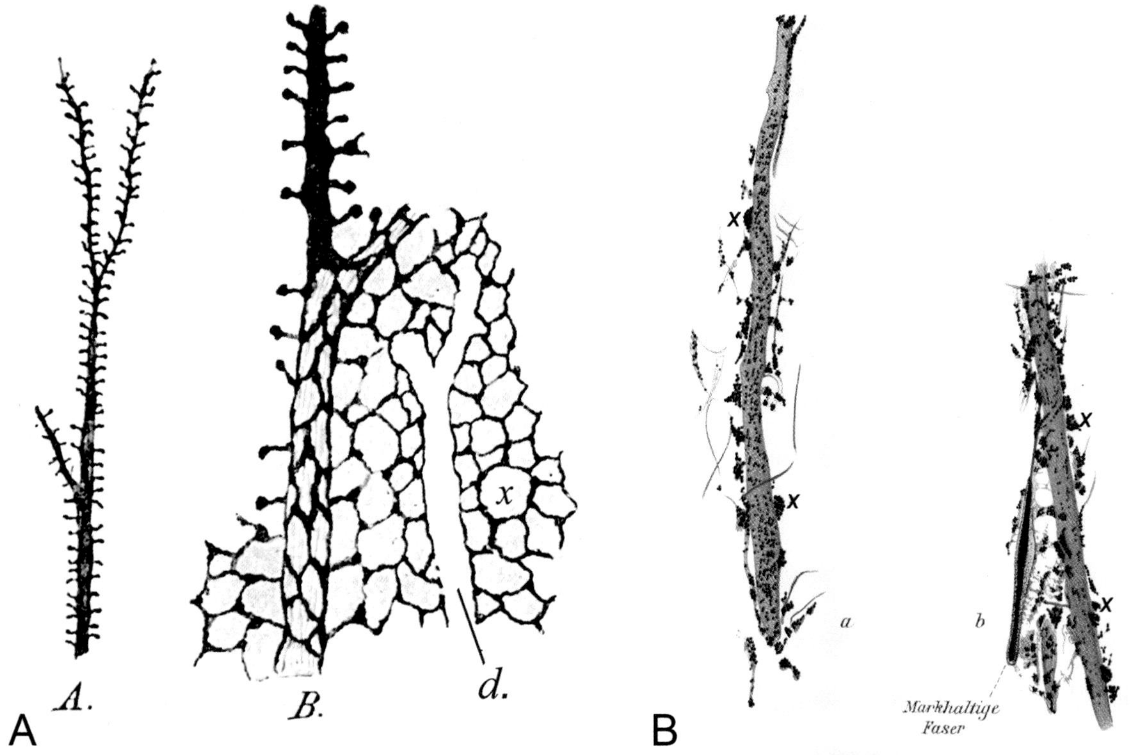

FIGURE 60. Different interpretation of dendritic spines. **A**, Drawings by Bethe (1903a) to illustrate dendritic spines stained with the ammonium molybdate method. *A*, An apical dendrite of a pyramidal cell covered with dendritic spines. *B*, Schematic representation to illustrate his hypothesis that dendritic spines were the starting points of an interstitial network of the gray matter. *d*, Unstained apical dendrite. **B**, Drawings by Held (1897b) to show dendrites innervated by end-feet or axon terminals (some of them are marked with an x). See text for further details. Figure and legend taken from DeFelipe (2015b).

panel A in Figure 63), showing the collateral axonal branches of the pyramidal cells making contact with the dendritic spines, following his analysis of the "extremely complex, diffuse nerve plexuses" of the cerebral cortex (Cajal, 1933, pages 94 and 98):

> I referred particularly to this intricate plexus when I lamented the insurmountable difficulties facing the analysis of the cortical synapses . . . . Note how these collaterals cross and enter into transversal or oblique contact with a great number of the dendritic shafts. It is probable that collaterals rest on the spines which cover the protoplasmic surfaces [dendrites] like down . . . . I have never seen anastomoses between the spines and the nerve fibers, despite having devoted particular attention to them since 1888.

Following his discovery of dendritic spines, Cajal postulated that they formed connections with axon terminals, and in his final publications he referred to such connections as *synapses* at times (e.g., Cajal, 1933).

Dendritic Spines and Cajal's "Final Lesson"

In the correspondence of Cajal, there is a letter that he wrote to his disciple Lorente de Nó (Figure 61A, C), which is particularly interesting for the subject of dendritic spines and could be considered his final lesson, because this letter is dated October 15, 1934, two days before he died in his home in Madrid (Figure 62). In this letter he writes:

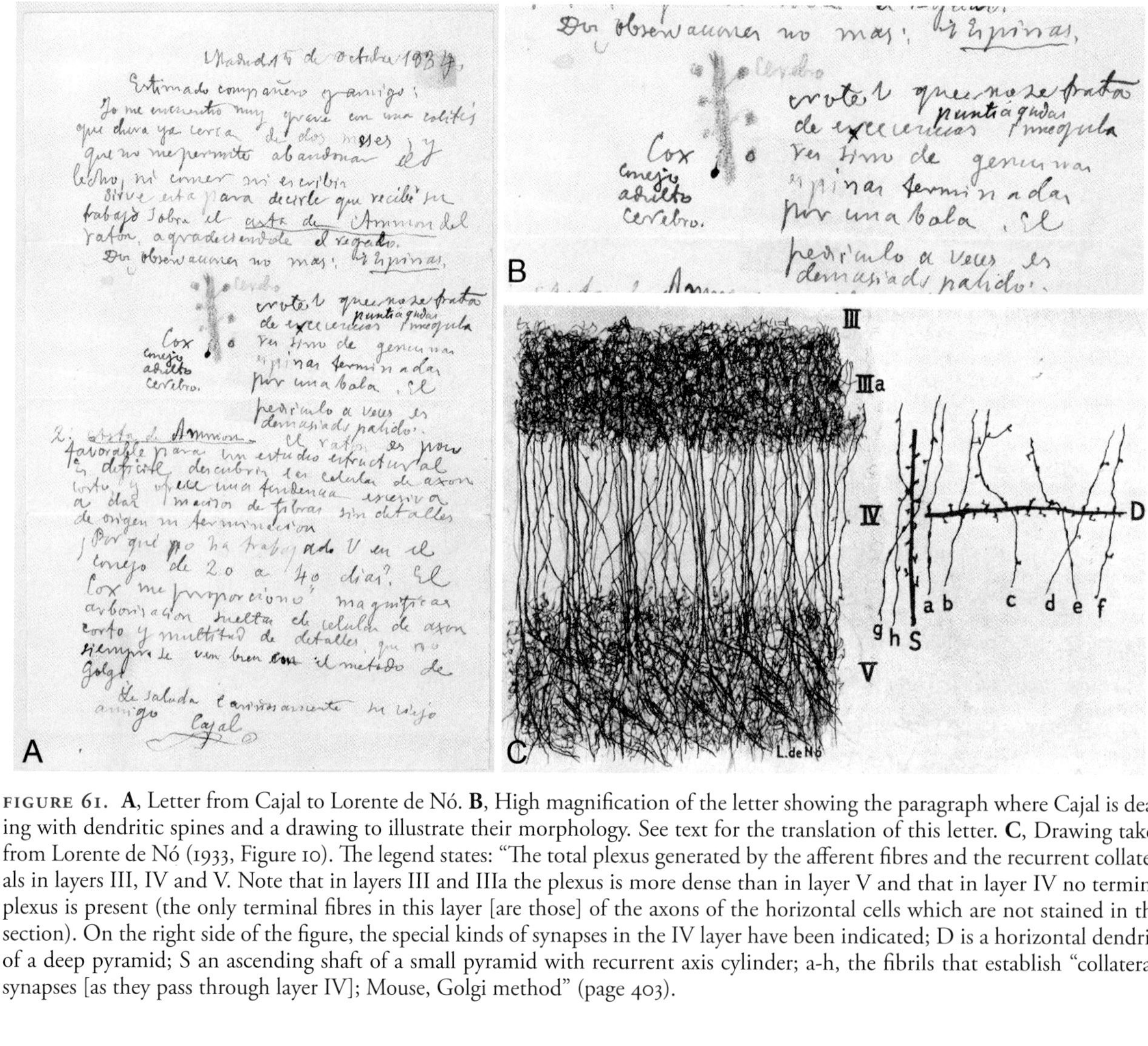

FIGURE 61. **A**, Letter from Cajal to Lorente de Nó. **B**, High magnification of the letter showing the paragraph where Cajal is dealing with dendritic spines and a drawing to illustrate their morphology. See text for the translation of this letter. **C**, Drawing taken from Lorente de Nó (1933, Figure 10). The legend states: "The total plexus generated by the afferent fibres and the recurrent collaterals in layers III, IV and V. Note that in layers III and IIIa the plexus is more dense than in layer V and that in layer IV no terminal plexus is present (the only terminal fibres in this layer [are those] of the axons of the horizontal cells which are not stained in this section). On the right side of the figure, the special kinds of synapses in the IV layer have been indicated; D is a horizontal dendrite of a deep pyramid; S an ascending shaft of a small pyramid with recurrent axis cylinder; a-h, the fibrils that establish "collateral" synapses [as they pass through layer IV]; Mouse, Golgi method" (page 403).

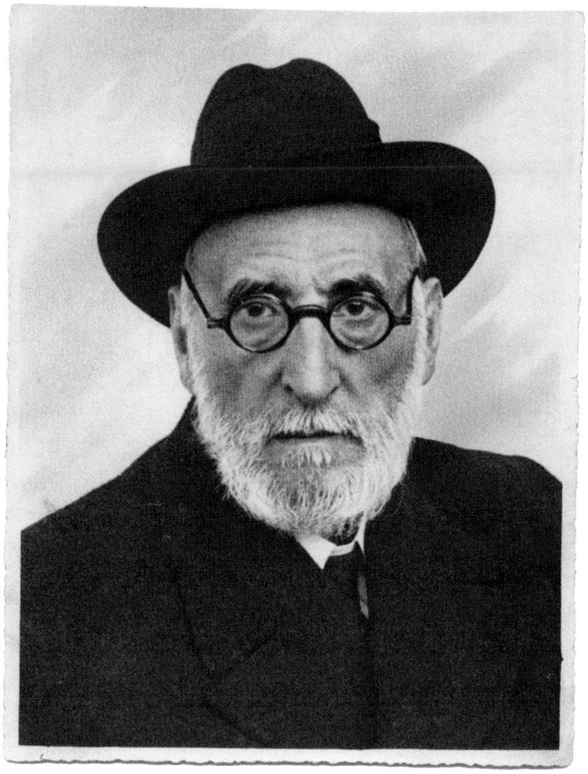

FIGURE 62. Photograph of Cajal taken in Valencia in 1933. From the private collection of his son Luis Ramón y Cajal Fañanás, kindly provided by his daughter María Ángeles Ramón y Cajal Junquera.

Dear colleague and friend,

I am very seriously sick with a colitis that has lasted nearly two months and does not allow me to leave the bed, eat or write. This letter serves to tell you that I received your work on the Ammon's horn of the mouse, and I am thankful for the gift.

Only two observations:

1 spines, note that they are not sharp irregular excrescences, but genuine spines terminating with a ball. The pedicle [neck] is sometimes too pale.

2 Ammon's horn, the mouse is not very favorable for a structural study. It is difficult to find short axon cells and there is an excessive tendency to [stain] clumps of fibers without details of their origin or termination.

Why have not you worked with 20- to 40-day-old rabbits? The [method of] Cox gave me magnificent isolated [axonal] arborizations of short-axon cells and multitude of details that can not always be seen with the method of Golgi.

Warm greetings from your old friend,
Cajal

In this letter, Cajal drew typical dendritic spines to point out that they are not sharp, irregular excrescences but small protrusions with a bulbous head (the spine head), and that the neck that connects the head of the spine to the shaft of the dendrite is often too lightly stained (Figure 61A, B). Interestingly, in the first study of Lorente de Nó on the cerebral cortex (Lorente de Nó, 1922), when he was only 20 years old and working in the laboratory of Cajal, the young researcher used the term *espina*, as Cajal did. However, in his classic studies of the entorhinal cortex and hippocampal formation (Lorente de Nó, 1933, 1934), which were written in English, he used the term "thorn" instead of "spine," which is probably what Cajal was referring to when he used "spine" in his letter (note that "espina" in Spanish translates to both "spine" and "thorn" in English). For example, Lorente de Nó described some of the connections made by the recurrent axonal collaterals of neurons of layers III, IV, V, and VI in layer IV of the entorhinal cortex of the mouse (Lorente de Nó, 1933, page 403) as follows: "*D* is a horizontal dendrite of a deep pyramid and *a-f* are recurrent collaterals, which [pass over and] establish synapses with the thorns of the dendrite. *S* is an ascending shaft of a pyramid with recurrent axon (layer V) [that has] similar "collateral" contacts (*g, h*)" (Figure 61C). In de Nó's 1934 article, for example, he described CA4 neurons as follows (page 132):

> The body has smooth contours, but the main dendrites and even their branches are covered with big thorns which are characteristic of contacts with the mossy fibres of the fascia dentata. However, the whole length of the dendrites does not have such thick thorns; the terminal part has only fine thorns and establishes contacts with other fibres.

Therefore, by the 1930s, it was assumed that dendritic spines were postsynaptic elements, although the term *spine* had not yet replaced other terms definitively. However, according to Shepherd (2010), the first physiological studies were performed some years later by Hsiang-Tung Chang, who in 1952 published a highly influential article on the functional analysis of the characteristics of dendritic spines and their contributions to the integrative actions of dendrites. In this article, titled "Cortical Neurons with Particular Reference to the Apical Dendrites," Chang made the following interesting observations about dendritic spines, which he named "gemmules" (page 196):

> If the end bulbs of the gemmules are the receptive apparatus for presynaptic impulses, the process of postsynaptic excitation initiated there must be greatly attenuated during its passage through the stems of the gemmules, which probably offer considerable ohmic resistance because of their extreme slenderness. As another consequence of this morphological arrangement, the bulb-headed gemmules around the dendritic process will constitute a sort of mechanical barrier preventing the synaptic knobs from touching the dendritic surface directly.

Confirmation that Dendritic Spines are Postsynaptic Structures

The final confirmation that dendritic spines are postsynaptic structures came several years later, when electron microscopy was introduced to study the nervous system (Figure 63). The first electron microscope study of dendritic spines showing they establish synaptic connections was published by George Gray (1959a, 1959b), and these observations were confirmed and extended by several authors (e.g., Jones and Powell, 1969; Peters and Kaiserman-Abramof, 1969, 1970).

Combination of the Golgi Method and Electron Microscopy Direct demonstration that the dendritic spines of Golgi-impregnated neurons established synapses came with the introduction of the combination of the Golgi method and electron

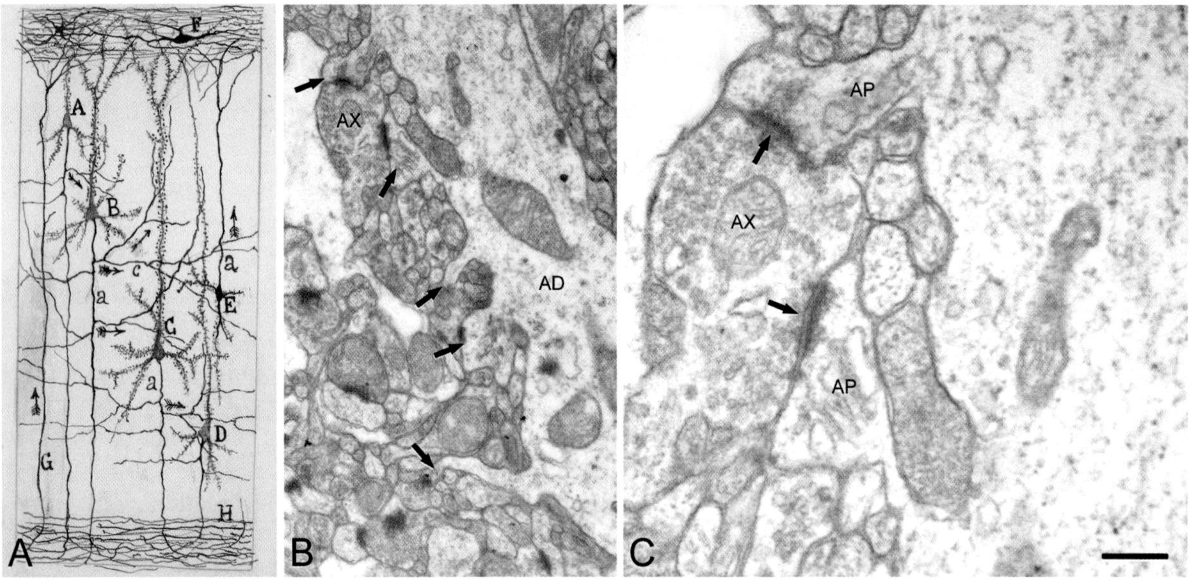

FIGURE 63. Drawing and images showing dendritic spines as postsynaptic structures. **A**, Schematic drawing by Cajal (1933) to show synaptic connections and the possible flow of information through neural circuits in the cerebral cortex. The legend states: "*A,* small pyramid; *B* and *C,* medium and giant pyramids, respectively; a, axon; [c], nervous collaterals that appear to cross and touch the dendrites and the trunks [apical dendrites] of the pyramids; H, white matter; [E, Martinotti cell with ascending axon]; F, special cells of the first layer of cerebral cortex; G, fiber coming from the white matter. The arrows mark the supposed direction of the nervous current" (page 95). **B**, Electron micrograph of a typical apical dendrite (AD) of the human cerebral cortex, showing dendritic spines with different shapes (arrows). **C**, High magnification of **A** to illustrate an axon terminal (AX) that establishes synaptic contacts (arrows) simultaneously with two dendritic spines. AP, spine apparatus. Scale bar (in C): **B**, 0.60 μm; **C**, 0.15 μm. Taken from unpublished material (Alonso-Nanclares et al., 2008). Figure and legend taken from DeFelipe (2015b).

microscopy, particularly the gold-toning technique of Alfonso Fairén and colleagues (1977). This method involves deimpregnation of previously Golgi-impregnated neurons, followed by the study of their fine structure by electron microscope. The original impregnation deposit of silver chromate (which produces an intense, homogeneous intracellular labeling that masks postsynaptic densities) is replaced by a deposit of gold particles. At the electron microscope level, this deposit is visible as fine particles that mark the profiles of the deimpregnated neurons while allowing the visualization of the cytological details of the labeled neuron. Thus, this technique enables the accurate study of the ultrastructural characteristics and synaptic connections of Golgi-impregnated neurons, including dendritic spines, because the postsynaptic densities can be clearly distinguished (Figure 64).

Further development of combinations of a variety of techniques (degeneration methods,

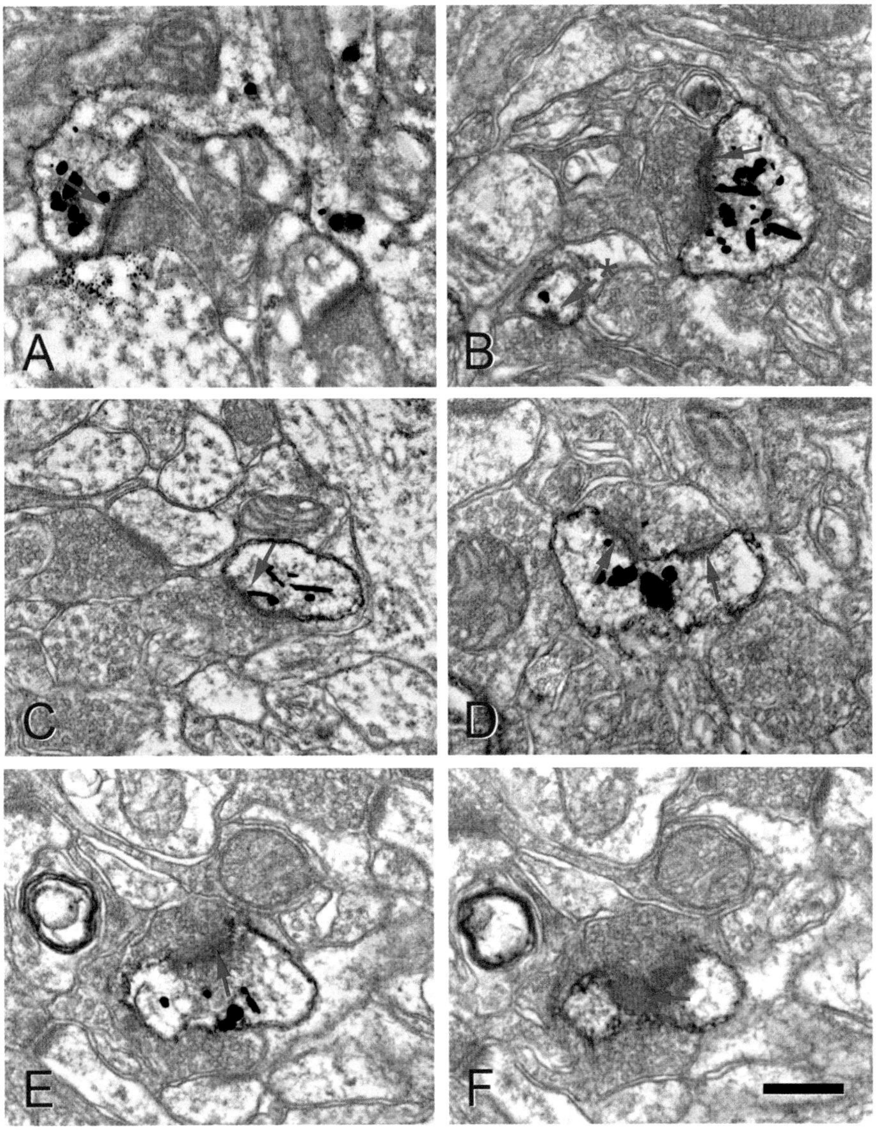

FIGURE 64. Examples of dendritic spines of Golgi-impregnated neurons forming synapses (**A–F**) in the adult mouse neocortex (gold-toning technique). The gold particles allow the postsynaptic densities (PSDs; red arrows) to be clearly distinguished when present. Note the small size of the postsynaptic density (60 nm) in the head of a small spine in **B** (asterisk). **E** and **F** are consecutive sections of a spine head to illustrate a PSD cut tangentially. Scale bar (in F): **A**, 560 nm; **B, C**, 350 nm; **D**, 300 nm; **E**, **F**, 280 nm. Taken from Arellano et al. (2007).

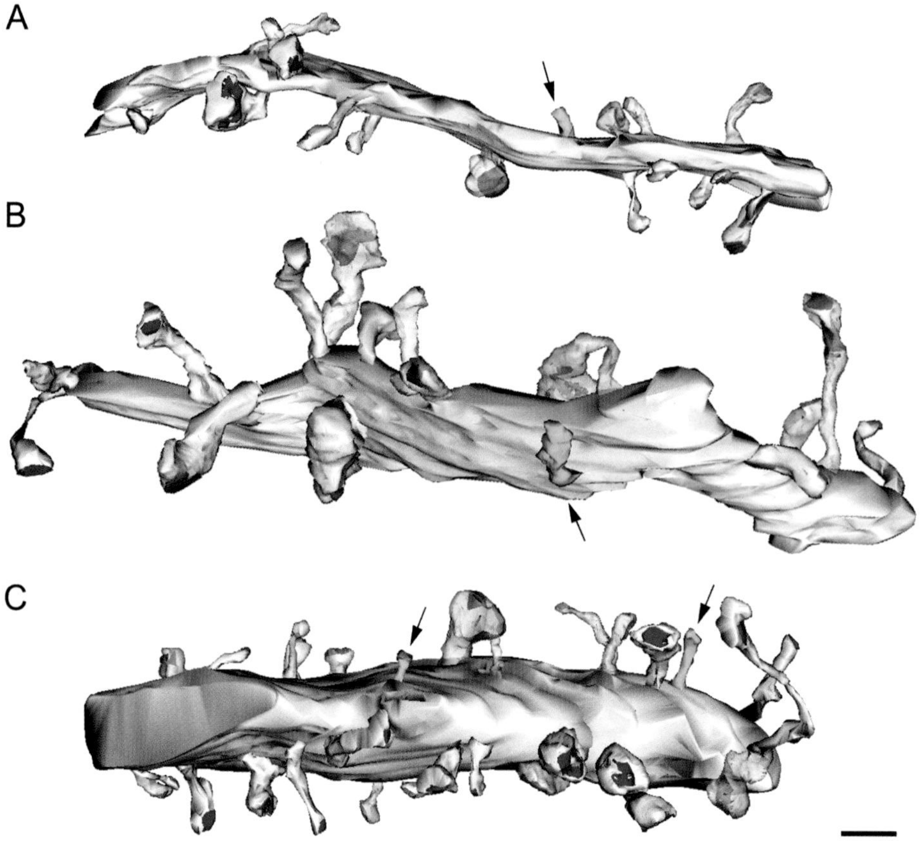

FIGURE 65. Reconstructions of electron micrographs from serial sections of dendritic segments in the adult mouse neocortex to illustrate the distribution of some nonsynaptic spines (blue) indicated by arrows. The remaining spines establish synaptic contacts (red, PSD). (**A**, **B**) Basal dendrites. (**C**) Apical dendrite. Scale bar: 2000 nm. Taken from Arellano et al. (2007).

immunocytochemistry, and so forth) for correlative light and electron microscopy soon followed. The application of these methods allowed the detailed examination of the afferent and efferent connections and chemical characteristics of Golgi-impregnated neurons (e.g., Frotscher and Léránth, 1986). As a result of all these advances, currently it is well established that almost all dendritic spines establish at least one excitatory glutamatergic synapse; only a small portion of dendritic spines have been found to be nonsynaptic (Figure 65) (Arellano et al., 2007; Bosch et al., 2015).

Dendritic Spines: Their Features and Role as a Key Component in Microcircuits Finally, the collective work of many authors has shown that dendritic spines are very numerous on many kinds of dendrites and they constitute the majority of postsynaptic targets of excitatory axons in the vertebrate brain. Dendritic spines are particularly abundant in the cerebral cortex, cerebellar cortex, and basal ganglia. Thus, they represent a key component in many different types of microcircuits. Moreover, the studies on visual deprivation and mental retardation carried out during the 1960s and 1970s (e.g., Globus and Scheibel, 1967; Valverde, 1971; Marín-Padilla, 1972; Purpura, 1974) also generated considerable interest in dendritic spines. The visual deprivation studies indicated that the formation and maintenance of spines depends on synaptic activity, and they can be modulated by sensory experience. In contrast, the studies of mental retardation identified changes in the morphology and density of spines (Figure 66), suggesting dendritic spines might alter synaptic inputs to pyramidal neurons.

More recent studies have confirmed and extended these early observations, showing alterations of dendritic spines in many different brain pathologies

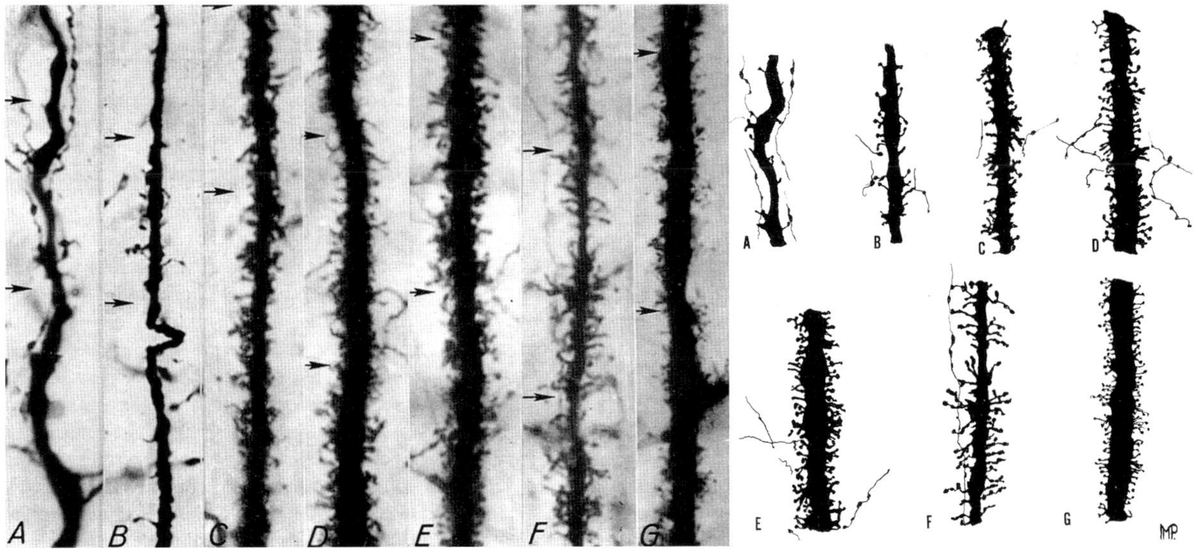

FIGURE 66. *Left*, Detail of the apical dendrites of the giant pyramidal neurons (layer V) of the human cerebral cortex in a variety of normal and abnormal cases. They are all reproduced at the same magnification to facilitate their comparative analysis. Each one represents a section of the apical dendrite of layer V pyramidal neuron crossing the territory of layer III of the cerebral cortex. The apical dendritic segments illustrated here belong to the following cases: **A**, A five-month fetus. **B**, A seven-month fetus. **C**, A newborn. **D**, A two-month-old infant. **E**, An eight-month-old infant. **F**, A newborn girl with D1 (13–15) trisomy (Patau syndrome). **G**, An 18-month-old mentally retarded girl with 21 trisomy (Down syndrome, mongolism). They illustrate the morphological characteristics of the human dendritic spine of the pyramidal neurons of the motor cortex during the course of prenatal and early postnatal cortical development, and those of two infants with proven chromosomal trisomies. Rapid Golgi method. *Right*, Camera lucida drawings made from the Golgi preparations of each one of the apical dendrites shown in Figure 1 *[Left]* to illustrate perhaps [more] clearly and with more detail the morphological characteristics of the apical dendritic spines of normal and abnormal human cerebral cortices. The dendritic segments reproduced in these drawings are those marked by arrows in the apical dendrites shown in Figure 1 [*Left*]. The drawing of each dendritic segment is identified by the same capital letter used in the identification of the different apical dendrites of Figure 1 [*Left*]. Figure and legend taken from Marín-Padilla (1972).

and after different experimental conditions. Also, it is clear at present that dendritic spines are highly plastic structures and that they are key elements in learning, memory, and cognition (for recent reviews see Russo et al., 2010; Yuste, 2010; Penzes et al., 2011; Rochefort and Konnerth, 2012; Spires-Jones and Knafo, 2012; Kuwajima et al., 2013; Rácz and Weinberg, 2013; Segal, 2016; Heck and Benavides-Piccione, 2016). All these features make the study of dendritic spines a major goal in neuroscience.

SECTION B

The Golden Era for Artistic Creativity in Neuroscience

Artistic Skills and Emotions of Cajal and Other Early Neuroanatomists

Cajal was captivated by the beautiful shapes of the cells of the nervous system, which he saw through an artist's eye. In Figure 67, we can see two interesting photographs taken by Cajal himself. On the left of the figure, Cajal is looking through a microscope while his daughter Paula is posing in a colorful dress with a basket of flowers. My interpretation of this photograph is that Cajal wants to convey that science and art can coexist. The picture on the right seems to me as if Paula was like an angel or a muse of scientific inspiration (DeFelipe, 2010a).

He and other scientists saw some neurons as trees or other plants, such as the pyramidal cells of the cerebral cortex and the Purkinje cells of the cerebellar cortex, and likened glial cells to bushes (Figure 68). Figure 68C has been taken from a re-edition of the first-century book *De Materia Medica* by Pedacio Dioscorides (third book)—the main manual of pharmacopoeia during the Middle Ages and the Renaissance. The re-edition dates back to 1568 and it was doctor and naturalist Pietro Andrea Gregorio Mattioli (1501–1577) who was responsible for its publication. It is interesting to note how closely the drawing on the left resembles Purkinje cells (Figure 68B) and illustrates the plant known as cleavers, sticky willy, Velcro weed, or grip grass (*Galium aparine*) of the family Rubiaceae.

Given their high density and arrangement, neurons and glial cells seemed to constitute a thick forest (Figure 69). In the words of Cajal (1894a, pages 159–160):

> The cerebral cortex is similar to a garden filled with innumerable trees, the pyramidal cells, which can multiply their branches thanks to intelligent cultivation, send their roots deeper and produce more exquisite flowers and fruits every day.

As pointed out previously in DeFelipe (2013) and DeFelipe et al. (2014), the similarities between the neuronal forest and an actual forest in nature were so obvious to him that he applied the vocabulary of nature to his histological findings: "ivy," "creeper," "mossy," "tuft," "nest," "glade," "vegetation," "bud," "pyriform," "elegant and leafy tree," "spines," "garden plants," "series of hyacinths," "field spikes," "climbing vines," "pinkish efflorescences," and so on. These terms have become commonplace in scientific texts nowadays, which is interesting to note given that they stem from such a romantic approach to studying the brain—a form of romanticism that is not normally reflected in modern-day scientific writing styles that are purely technical in nature. It is difficult to imagine a publication nowadays describing our interest in the study of the microanatomy of the brain with, for example, the following beautiful romantic prose used by Cajal in *Recuerdos de mi vida* (1917b, page 345):

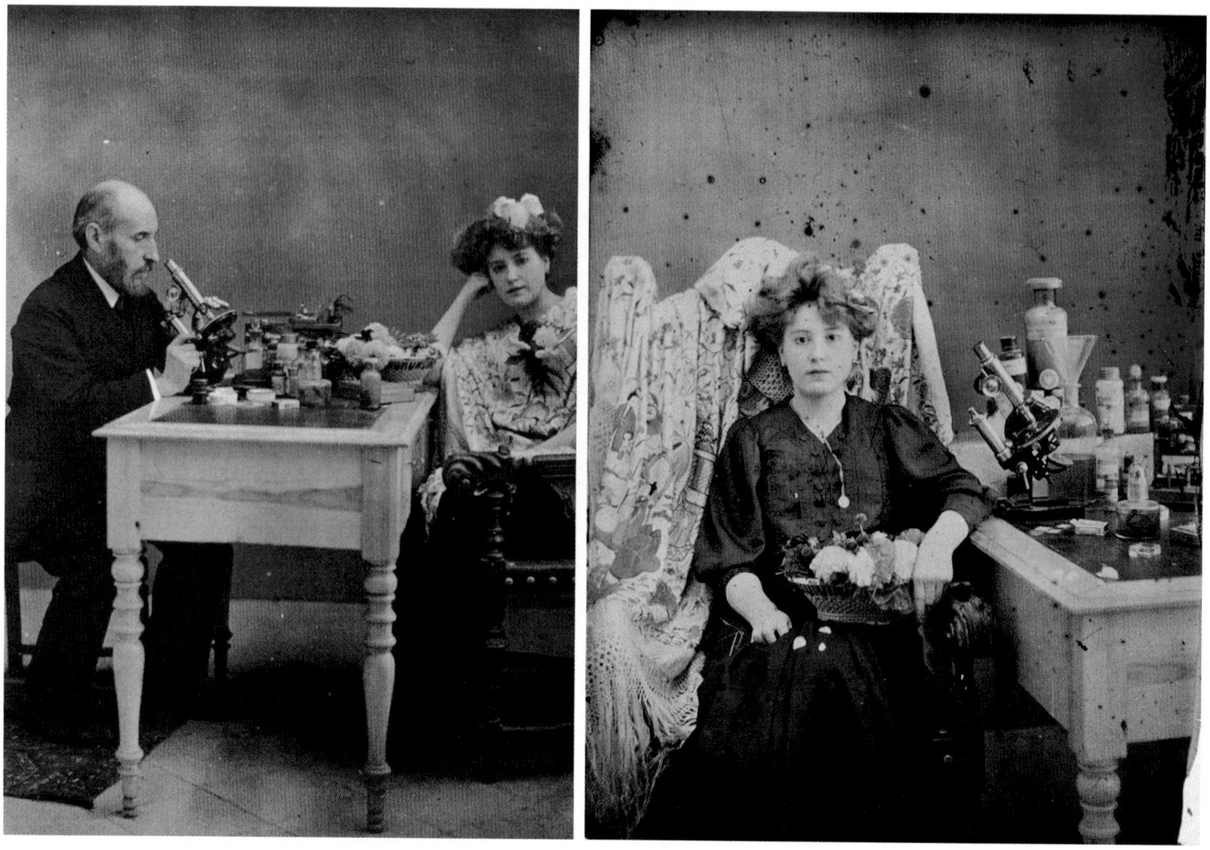

FIGURE 67. Photographs taken by Cajal of himself and his daughter, Paula. From the private collection of Silvia Cañadas, daughter of Paula Ramón y Cajal. Taken from DeFelipe (2010a).

I felt at that time the most lively curiosity—somehow romantic—for the enigmatic organization of the organ of the soul. Humans—I said to myself—reign over Nature through the architectural perfection of their brains . . . . To know the brain—we said to ourselves in our idealistic enthusiasm—is equivalent to discovering the material course of thought and will . . . . Like the entomologist hunting for brightly colored butterflies, my attention was drawn to the flower garden of the grey matter, which contained cells with delicate and elegant forms, the mysterious butterflies of the soul, the beating of whose wings may some day (who knows?) clarify the secret of mental life . . . . Even from the aesthetic point of view, the nervous tissue contains the most charming attractions. In our parks are there any trees more elegant and luxurious than the Purkinje cells from the cerebellum or the psychic cell that is the famous cerebral pyramid?

One amusing anecdote reveals how Cajal's boyhood dreams of becoming an artist (Figure 70) were thwarted by his father's misgivings. He spoke about this in an interview in 1900 (Ramón y Cajal-Junquera, 2007):

> Undoubtedly, only artists devote themselves to science . . . I realized that if I wanted to make a name for myself as a painter, my hands needed to become precision instruments. I owe what I am today to my boyhood artistic hobbies, which my father opposed fiercely. To date, I must have done over 12,000 drawings. To the layman, they look like strange drawings, with details that measure thousandths of a millimeter, but they reveal the mysterious worlds of the architecture of the brain . . . . Look [Cajal said to the journalist, showing one of his drawings], here I am pursuing a goal of great interest to painters: appreciating line and color in the brain.

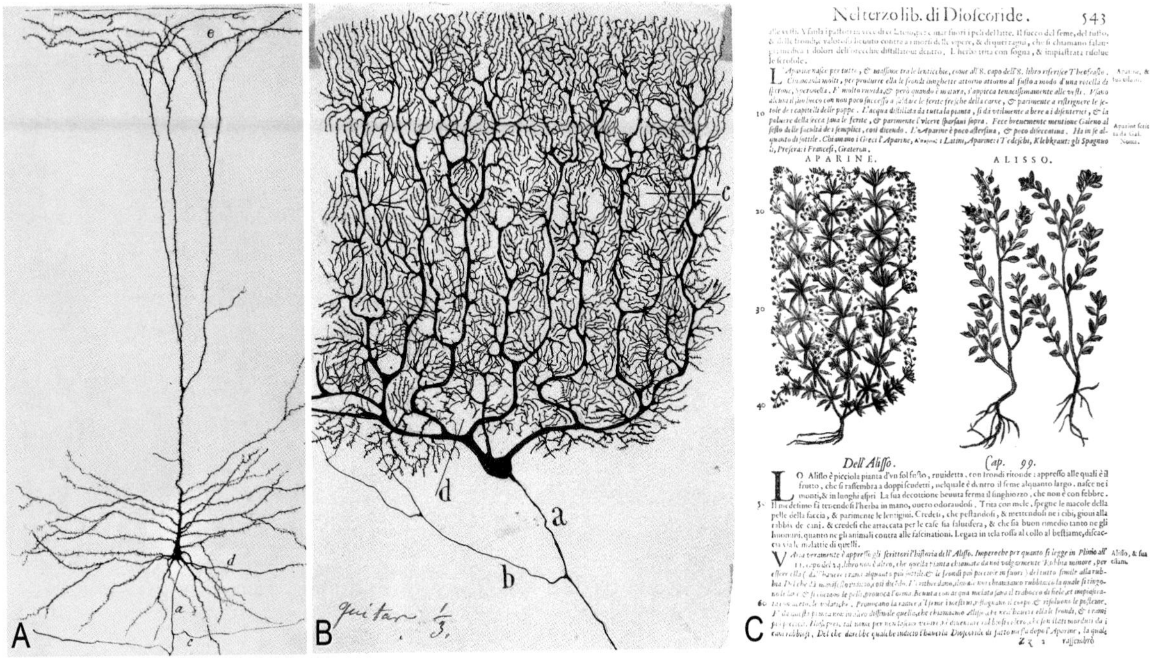

FIGURE 68. **A**, **B**, Cajal's drawings from Golgi-stained preparations to illustrate the pyramidal (*a*) and Purkinje (*b*) cells in the human cerebral cortex and cerebellum, respectively. In **A**: "*a*," "*c*," "*d*" and "*e*" indicate axon, collaterals, long basal dendrites, and terminal (dendritic) tuft, respectively. In **B**: "*a*," "*b*," "*c*," and "*d*" indicate axon, recurrent collaterals, holes occupied by capillaries, and holes occupied by basket cells, respectively. These figures were reproduced in *Textura del sistema nervioso del hombre y de los vertebrados* (Cajal 1899–1904, figures 689 [*left*], and 10 and 365 [*right*]). **C**, Illustrations of plants from the book *De Materia Medica* (see text for details). Note the similarity between the plant on the left (cleavers) and the Purkinje cell shown in **B**. The infusion of the flowers of this plant is used as a diuretic, and its ground seeds are a coffee substitute. According to neurologist Ivan Iniesta (The Walton Centre for Neurology and Neurosurgery, Liverpool) "Another curiosity about this plant in relation to the neurons is that it is covered with small spurs, which make it adhere like Velcro (or as a synapse, by contiguity) to clothing or body hair." Courtesy of Ivan Iniesta.

Later, in his autographical *Recuerdos de mi vida: Mi infancia y juventud* (*Recollections of My Life: My Childhood and Youth*) (Cajal, 1901a, pages 52 and 84–86), Cajal wrote:

> And translating my dreams on to paper, with a pencil as my magic wand, I forged a world as I pleased, populated with all the things that fueled my dreams. Dantesque landscapes, bright and pleasant valleys, desolating wars, Greek and Roman heroes, the great events of history . . . all paraded through my restless pencil . . . my father, who was already averse to all kinds of aesthetic tendencies . . . and wearied, no doubt, of depriving me of pencils and taking away my drawings, and seeing the ardent vocation towards painting which I exhibited, he decided to determine whether those scrawls had any merit promising their author the glories of a Velázquez . . . . As there was no one in the town sufficiently qualified in the art of drawing, the author of my days turned to a plasterer and decorator from afar, who had arrived in Ayerbe around that time . . . to paint the walls of the church, damaged and scorched by a recent fire . . . . I timidly displayed my picture . . . the house painter looked at it and looked at it again, and after moving his head significantly and adopting a solemn and judicial attitude he exclaimed:
>
> "What a daub! Neither is this an Apostle, nor has the figure proportions, nor are the draperies right . . . this child will never be an artist." In fact, the opinion of this dauber of walls was received in my family like the pronouncement of an Academy of Fine Arts. It was decided, therefore, that I should renounce my madness for drawing and prepare myself to follow a medical career.

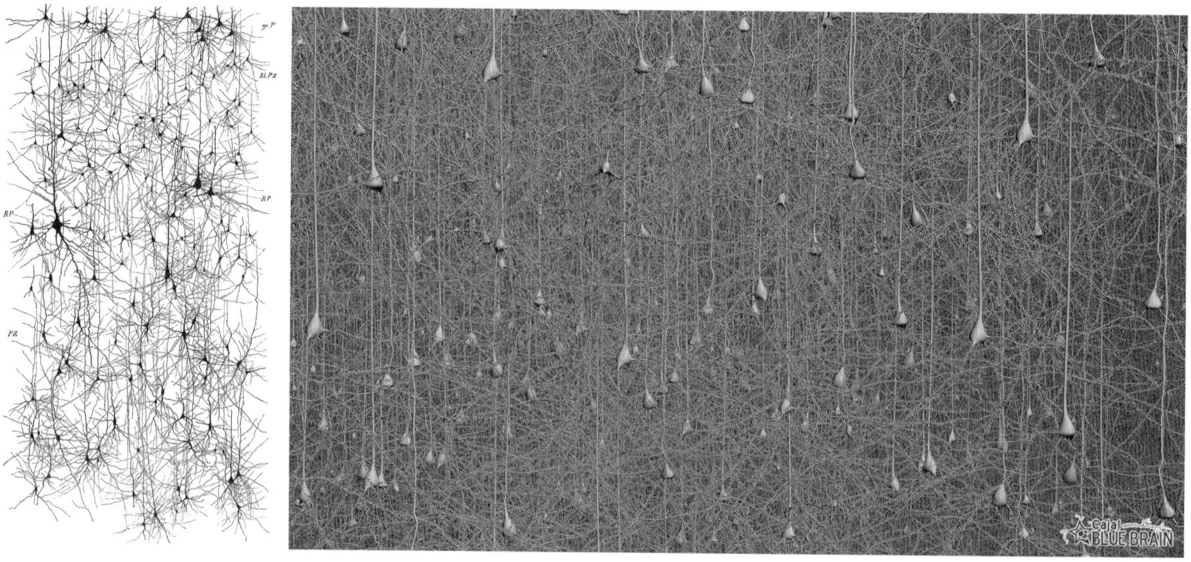

FIGURE 69. **A**, Drawings of the human cerebral cortex (Golgi method) taken from Kölliker (1893), illustrating a forest-like appearance. **B**, Computer-generated image to illustrate the complexity of the cerebral cortex, which resembles a neuronal forest. This image was taken from the video *Bosque Neuronal* (Cajal Blue Brain Project) created (in alphabetical order) by Sofía Bayona, Ruth Benavides-Piccione, Juan Pedro Brito, Eva Cortés, Javier DeFelipe, José Miguel Espadero, Susana Mata, Luis Pastor, Ángel Rodríguez, and Luis Miguel Serrano.

The bridge between science and art was also well expressed by Cajal in *Recuerdos de mi vida* (1917b, pages 155–156), when referring to the intellectual pleasure he felt when observing and drawing from his histological preparations:

> My work began at nine o'clock in the morning and usually lasted until around midnight. Most curiously, my work caused me pleasure, a delightful intoxication, an irresistible enchantment. Indeed, leaving aside the egocentric flattery, the garden of neurology offers the investigator captivating spectacles and incomparable artistic emotions. In it, my aesthetic instincts were at last fully satisfied.

Cajal was not alone in possessing these skills and experiencing such emotions. His well-known disciples Pío del Río-Hortega (1882–1945) and Fernando

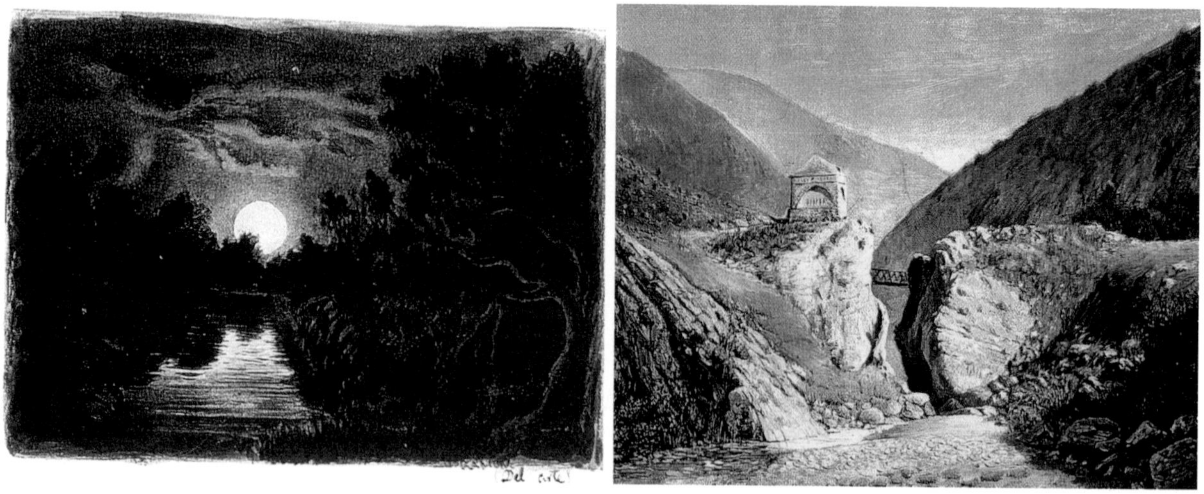

FIGURE 70. *Left*, Watercolor by Cajal in 1865. *Right*, Oil painting on canvas by Cajal in 1878. Landscape between Biescas and Panticosa (Huesca, Spain). Taken from DeFelipe et al. (2007).

de Castro (1896–1967) did too (Figure 71). Many of the great pioneers of neuroscience were also of like mind, such as Alzheimer, Deiters, Dogiel, Golgi, Kölliker, Meynert, Ranvier, and Retzius (Figure 72). Figures 73 through 84 show some examples of drawings by these and other scientists.

Figure 85 shows another beautiful drawing representing the visual system of the fly that Cajal published in 1915 with Domingo Sánchez y Sánchez (1860–1947), who was his main collaborator in the histological study of the nervous system of invertebrates. In Part II of the book, there is a large collection of illustrations, drawn by Cajal and Sánchez, that highlights the relative simplicity and extraordinary beauty of the nervous system of these tiny organisms (Cajal and Sánchez, 1915).

It should be noted that Cajal had staining techniques other than the Golgi method at his disposal, and many others have emerged since the times of his work. This has greatly facilitated the analysis of particular architectonic aspects of the nervous system, and the morphology and cytology of neurons and glia, through the use of different fixation and staining protocols. These techniques not only served to unravel the complex organization of the nervous system, but also revealed a beautiful microscopic world, with an almost infinite variety of forms and colors. The coming together of art and science was brilliantly described by Del Río-Hortega in his article on art and science "*Arte y artificio de la ciencia histológica*" (Del Río-Hortega, 1933, page 200):

> After using one of those technical processes that requires the careful combination of several complementary colors: red and green, yellow and blue, the histologist finally got a true picture from which

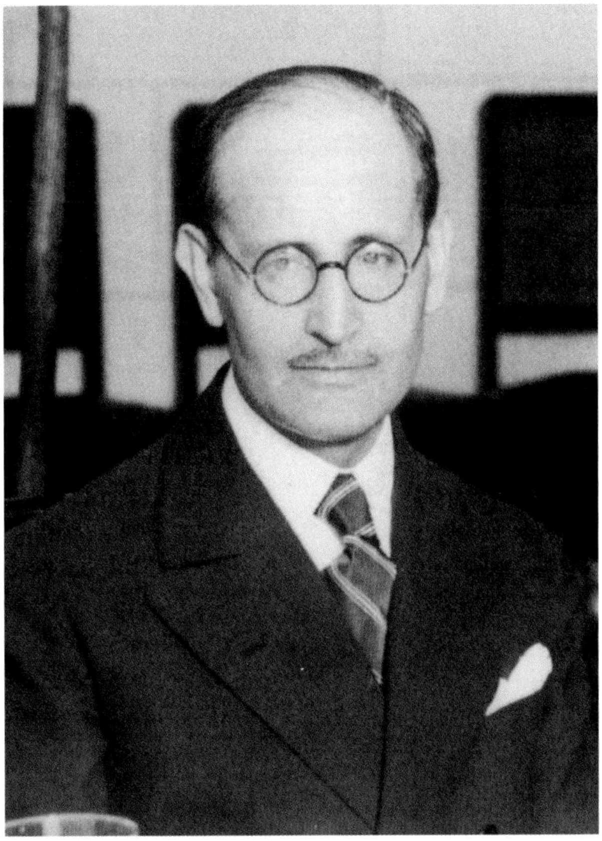

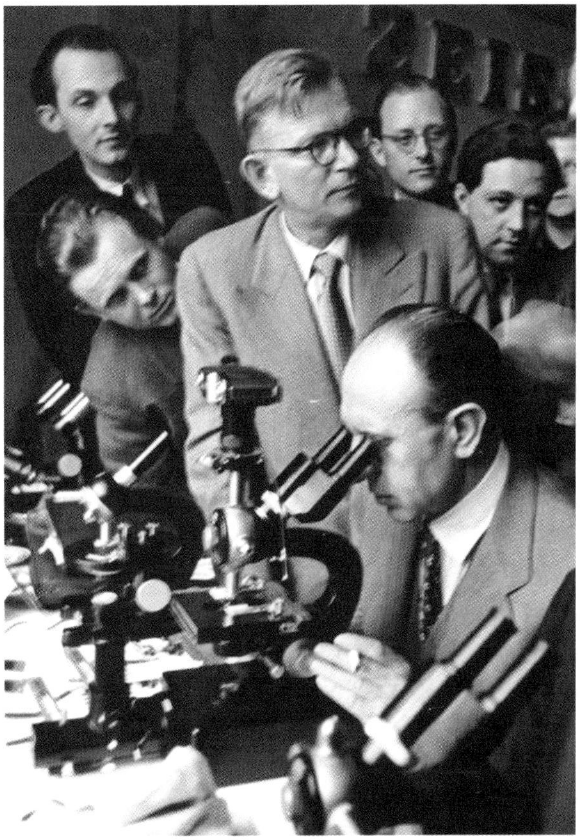

FIGURE 71. *Left*, Pío del Río-Hortega (1882–1945). *Right*, Fernando de Castro (1896–1967), looking through the microscope at the Congress of Wiesbaden held in 1950 (*Archivo Fernando de Castro*). Taken from DeFelipe (2010a).

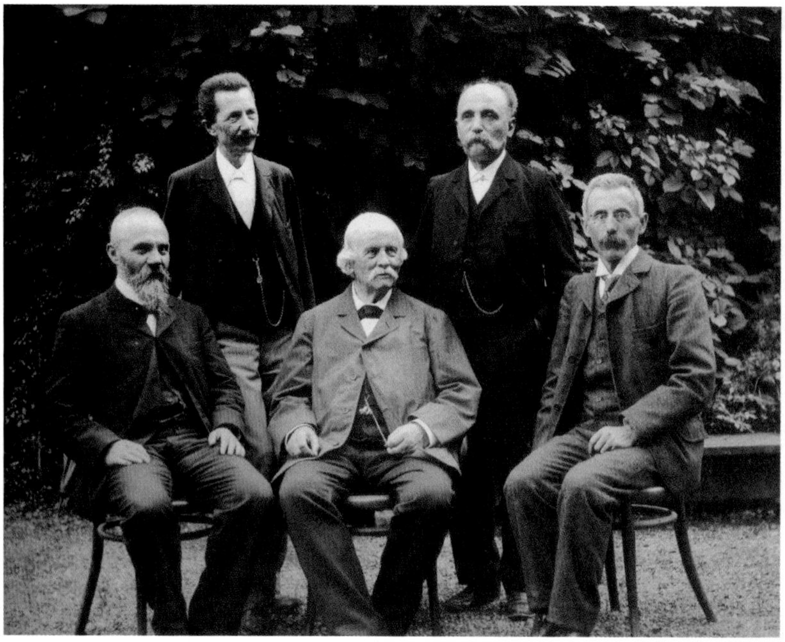

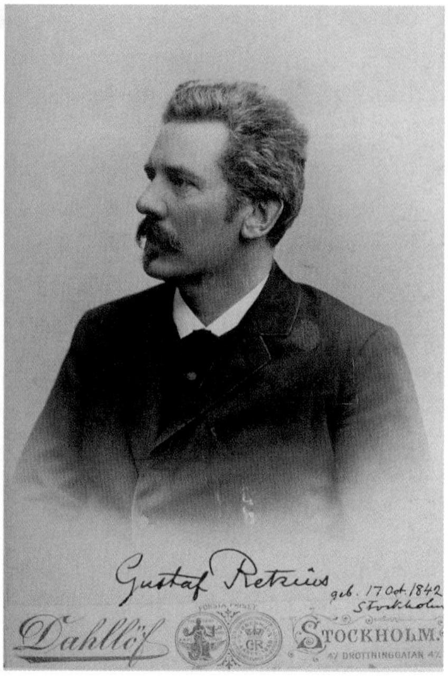

FIGURE 72. *Left*, From left to right, back row: Giulio Bizzozero (1846–1901) and Camillo Golgi (1843–1926); front row, Edoardo Perroncito (1847–1936), Rudolf Albert von Kölliker (1817–1905), and Romeo Fusari (1857–1919). *Right*, Gustav Magnus Retzius (1842–1919). Courtesy of Paolo Mazzarello, University Pavia. Taken from DeFelipe (2010a).

> three sources of pure emotion could be derived: that which stems from the beauty of the landscape itself, with its polychromatic nature, its tones and [depth]; that which emanates from the observer himself, who feels the hidden satisfaction of achieving his purpose; and that which emerges from the novelty of the details resolved, [that is,] the discovery of unknown truths.

Another example of romantic prose is the description of the relationships between neurons, glia, and blood vessels by Del Río-Hortega also in "*Arte y artificio de la ciencia histológica.*" He used the drawing shown in Figure 86 as an example of artistic inspiration that may emerge from a histological preparation. This figure was accompanied by the following legend (Del Río-Hortega, 1933, page 193):

> In the landscape of the brain there are endless irrigation canals—blood vessels—, and on their banks the bush-like cells—glia—collaborate in nerve function.

Such captivating and emotive observations would not have been possible without chemicals such as pyridine, methylene blue, mercuric chloride, osmic acid, and silver solutions, which made "selective" visualization of specific elements possible. For example, these chemicals form the basis of methods that allow different glial cell types—but not neurons—to be visualized, whereas other procedures permit the labeling of mainly neurons, including their dendritic and axonal processes. The development of other selective staining methods permitted investigation of the different organelle types found in the perikaryon, including Nissl bodies, mitochondria, neurofibrils, and the Golgi apparatus, as well as pigments, fat, and lipids, among others. The staining procedures not only included a large number of reagents and methods, but also numerous modifications introduced by several scientists, such as Weigert staining for glia, Cajal's gold chloride sublimate method, the method of Mann–Alzheimer, the method of Alzheimer–Mallory, the method of Bielschowsky, and so on.

It is interesting to note that the drawings of spinal ganglion cells of the pigeon by Edmund Vincent Cowdry (1888–1975) have great aesthetic appeal (Figure 87). As shown in Figures 88 through 90, the senile plaque drawings by Alois Alzheimer (1864–1915), Oskar Fischer (1876–1942), and Georges Marinesco (1863–1938) are also very aesthetically

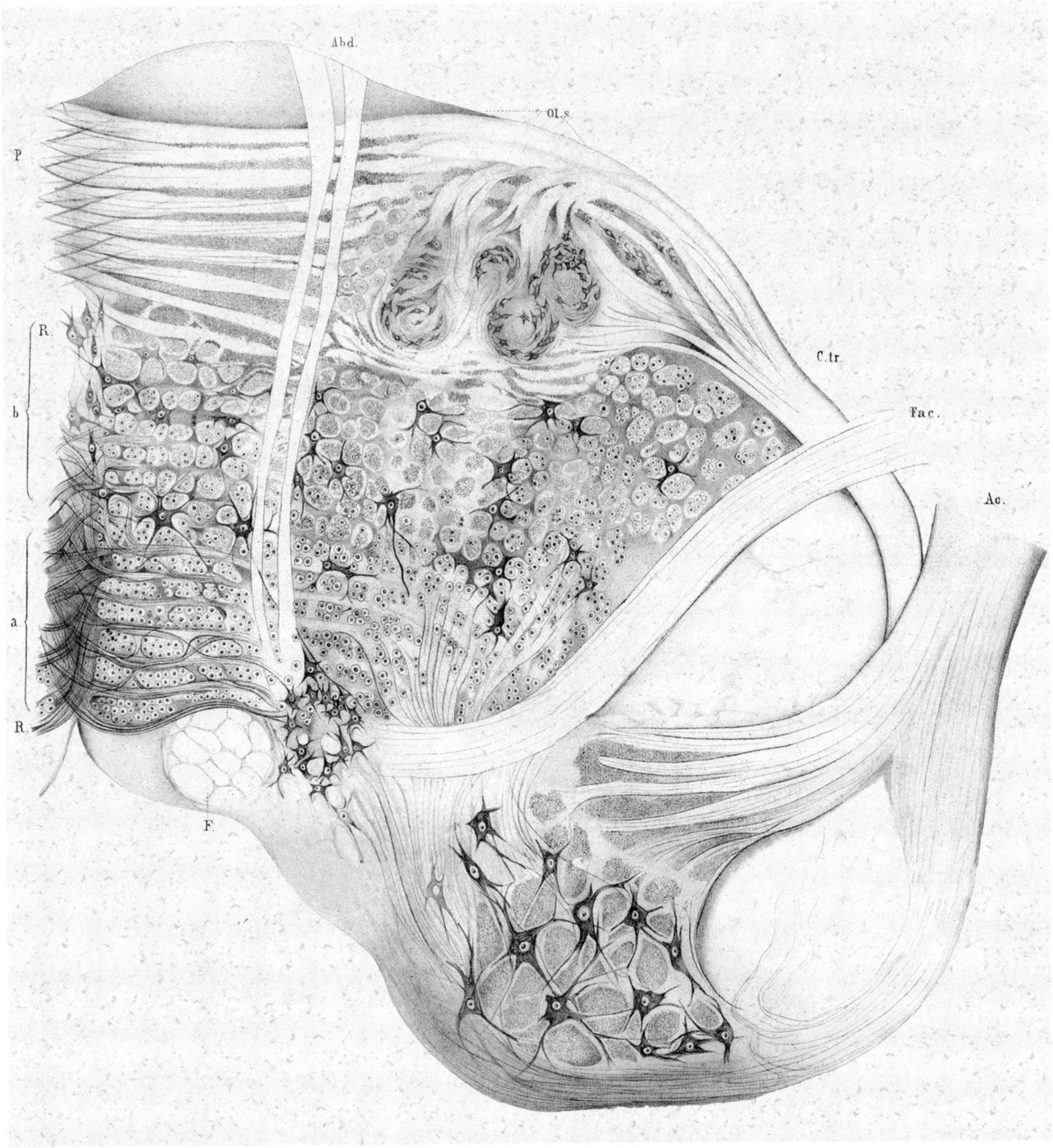

FIGURE 73. Human medulla oblongata by Otto Friedrich Karl Deiters (1834–1863). See Note 13 for the transcription of the legend. Taken from Deiters (1865).

pleasing, as are the illustrations by other scientists showing changes in neurons in cases of dementia precox, aging, or Alzheimer's disease (Figure 91).

Further examples of the remarkable drawings produced at that time are shown in Figures 92 through 94, in which various aspects of the normal and altered nervous system are shown in a wealth of detail and color.

As outlined in the introduction, a consequence of the creativity, subjectivity, ambiguity, and skepticism that abounded during Cajal's times was that fellow scientists were reluctant to accept their findings at times.

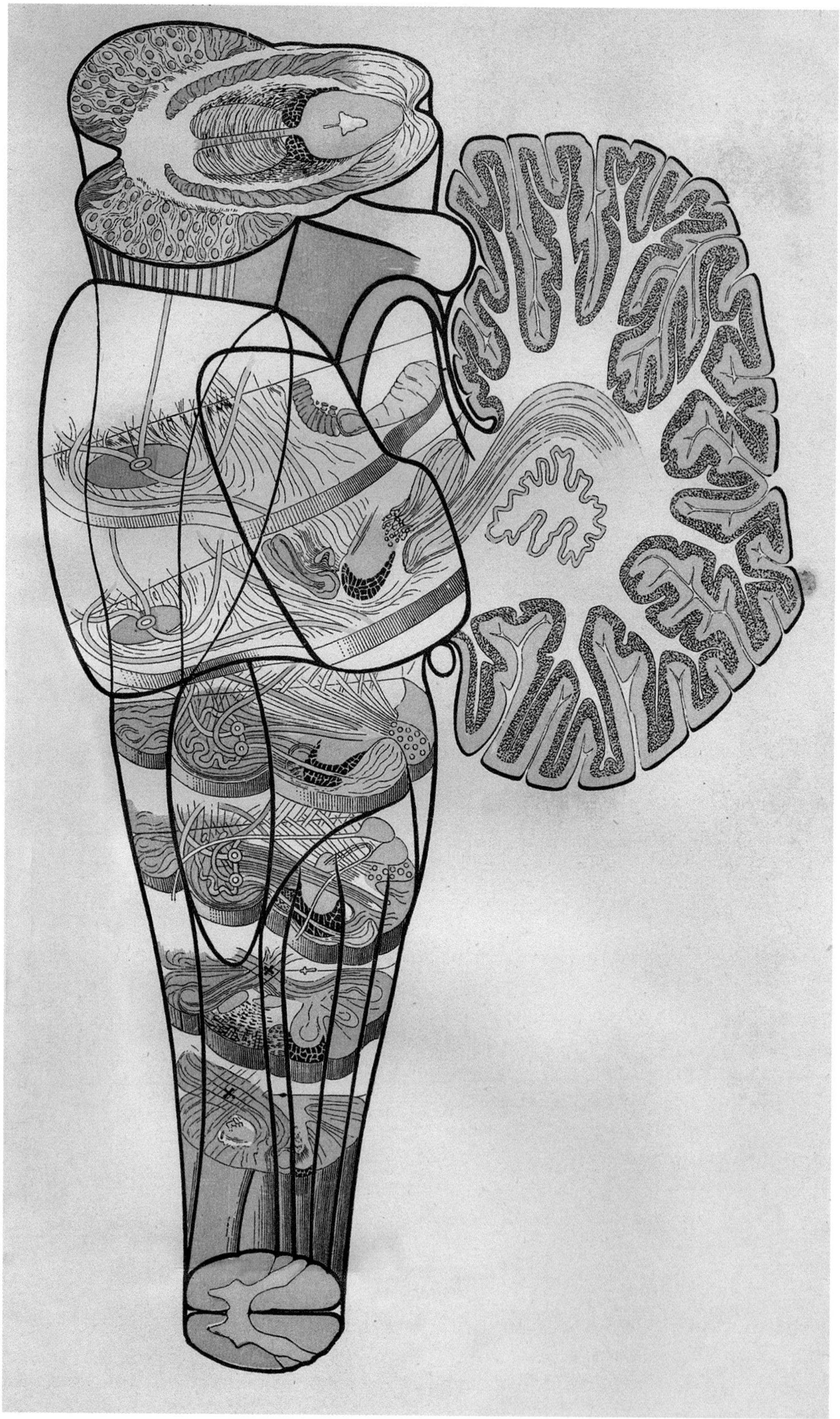

FIGURE 74. Brainstem and cerebellum by Theodor Meynert (1833–1892). See Note 14 for the transcription of the legend. Taken from Meynert (1874).

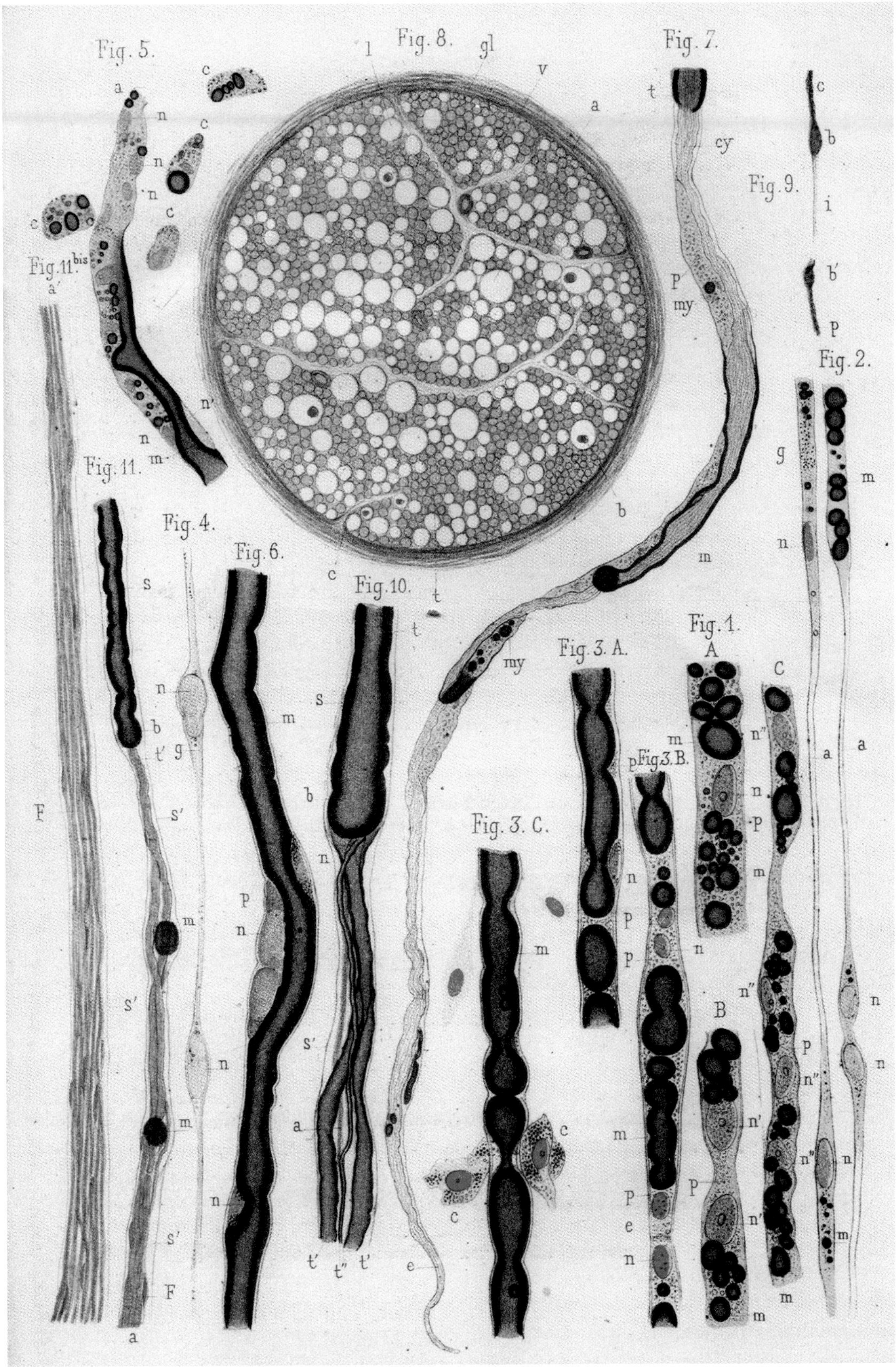

FIGURE 75. Nerve fibers by Louis Antoine Ranvier (1835–1922). See Note 15 for the transcription of the legend. Taken from Ranvier (1878).

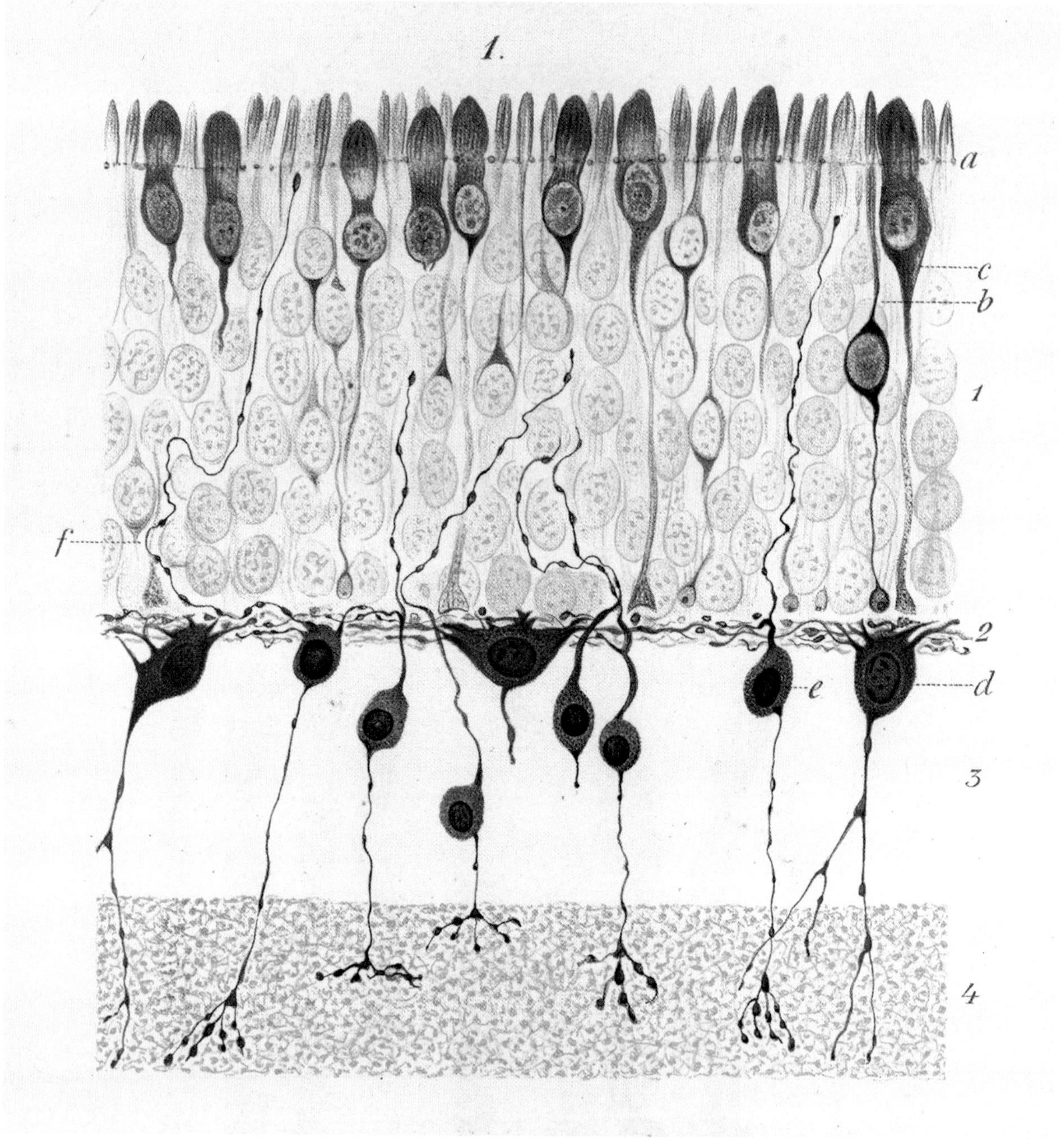

FIGURE 76. Diagram of the structure of the retina by Aleksander Dogiel (1852–1922). See Note 16 for the transcription of the legend. Taken from Dogiel (1891).

Cajal's disciple Del Río-Hortega made the following interesting observation in his article "*Arte y artificio de la ciencia histológica*" (Del Río-Hortega, 1933, page 198):

> In each country, preference is usually given to a technical procedure that leads to discoveries with a particular characteristic. From this derives the fact that scientific truth is not the same in all countries and even that there are truths for all tastes. That which is the most sublime expression of a perfect technique here, is despised with the insult of being an artifact that distorts and disfigures reality there. And so it happens that what many consider to be the absolute truth, others regard as a relative truth, and some as pure fiction.

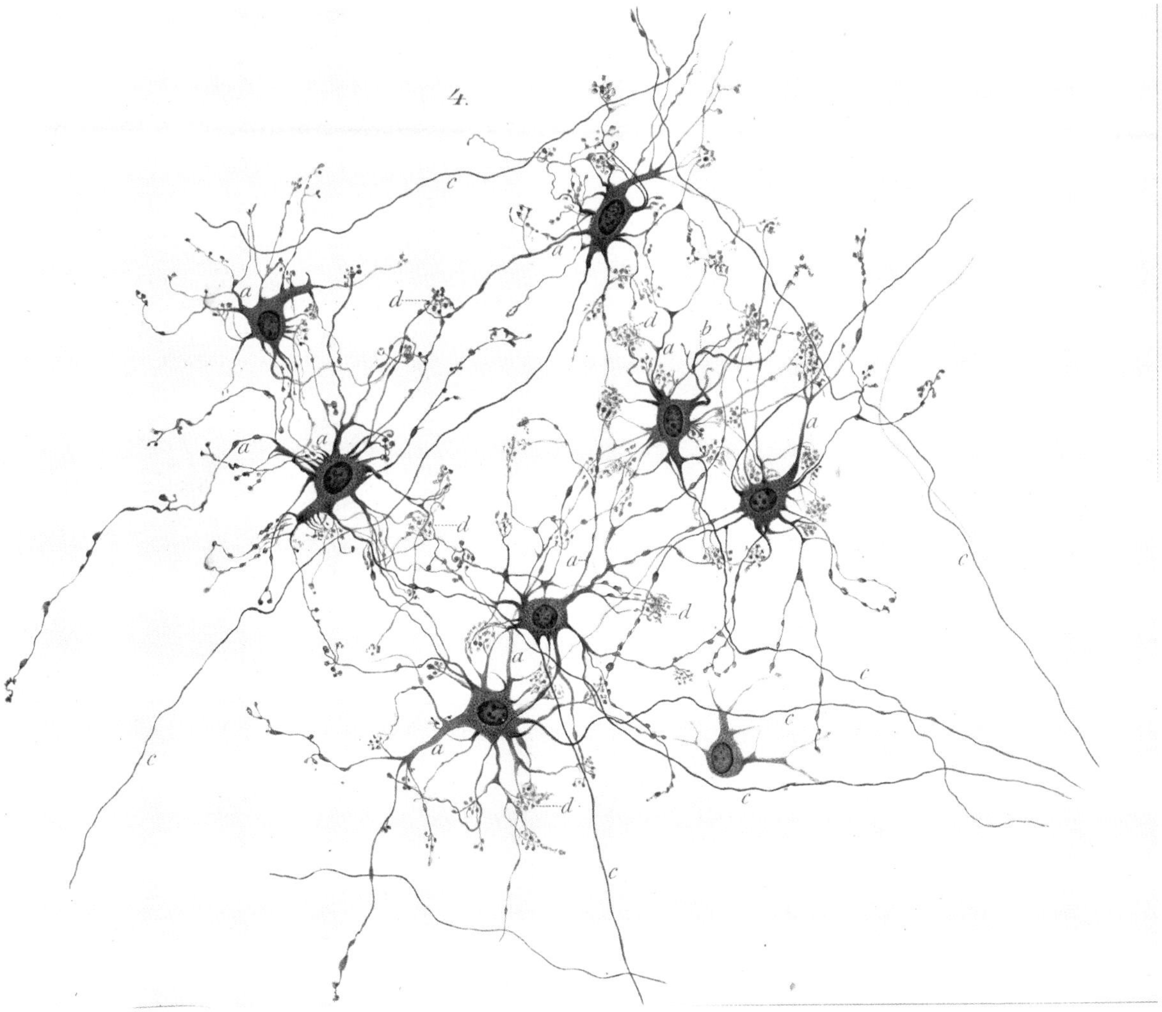

FIGURE 77. Large stellate cells in the retina by Aleksander Dogiel (1852–1922). See Note 17 for the transcription of the legend. Taken from Dogiel (1891).

Returning to Cajal, in his *Recuerdos de mi vida* (1917b, page 6) there is a passage in which he wonders why light microscopy was not introduced during the teaching of medicine, because the microscope opened up a marvelous field of exploration and greatly facilitated a better understanding of the normal anatomy and pathology of the body in general. This was probably partly a result of the fact that the introduction of achromatic lenses, coupled with other improvements in optical microscopy, during the late 1820s and early 1830s, led to the demonstration that the "globules" described by the earlier microscopists were artifacts produced by the chromatic and spherical aberrations of the optical lens used in old microscopes (Hughes, 1959). Perhaps this led some of the professors at that time to believe that observations with optical microscopy should be considered with caution.

> The preparations being so easy to make, I was completely surprised by the almost total absence of any curiosity on the part of our professors, who spent their time talking to us at great length about healthy and diseased cells without making the slightest effort to become acquainted visually with those transcendental and mysterious protagonists of life and suffering. What am I saying!—Many, perhaps the majority of professors in those days, underestimated the microscope, even considering it prejudicial to the progress of Biology! In the opinion of these academic reactionaries, the marvelous published descriptions

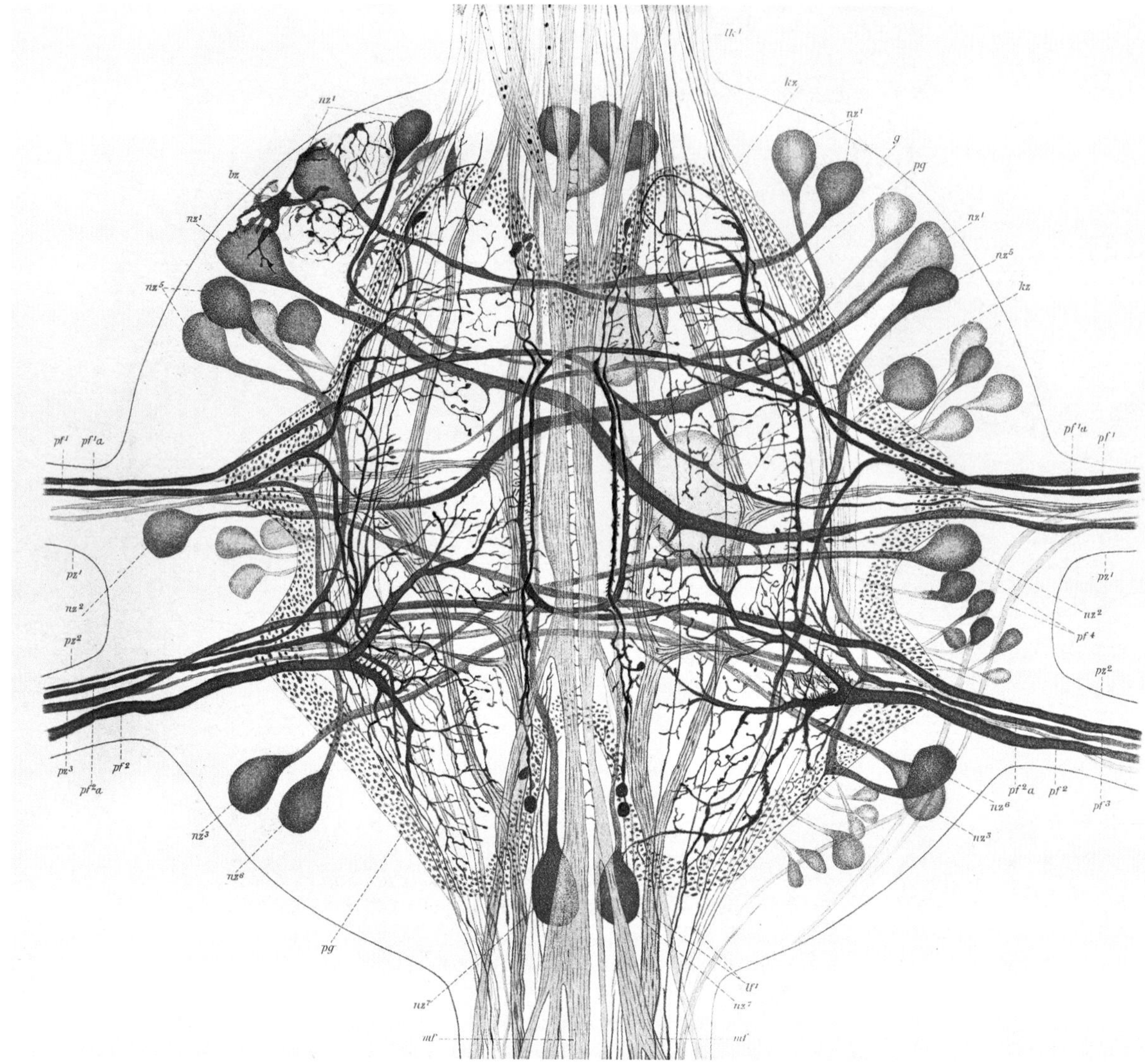

FIGURE 78. Central nervous system of the leech by Gustav Magnus Retzius (1842–1919). See Note 18 for the transcription of the legend. Taken from Retzius (1891b).

of cells and of invisible parasites were pure fantasy. I remember a certain professor in Madrid who was never willing to look though the eyepiece of a magnifying instrument [ocular of a microscope], and who referred to microscopic Anatomy as *Celestial Anatomy* [ironically useless anatomy]. This phrase, which became popular, is a good reflection of the attitude of that generation of professors.

Another clear example of this skepticism is revealed by the words of Prof. Arthur van Gehuchten (1861–1914) in a speech that he gave during an event at the University of Louvrain, which was celebrating him having spent 25 years teaching there. van Gehuchten described the momentous day at the renowned Congress of the German Society of Anatomy (October 1889, University of Berlin) when Cajal was discovered by Kölliker who, as mentioned previously, was one of the leading neuroscientists of the day. In an excerpt from his speech, van Gehuchten (1913, pages 32–33) recounts that pivotal moment, underlining the scale of the problems encountered by Cajal and others scientists at the time:

The facts described [by Cajal] in his first publications were so strange that the histologists of the

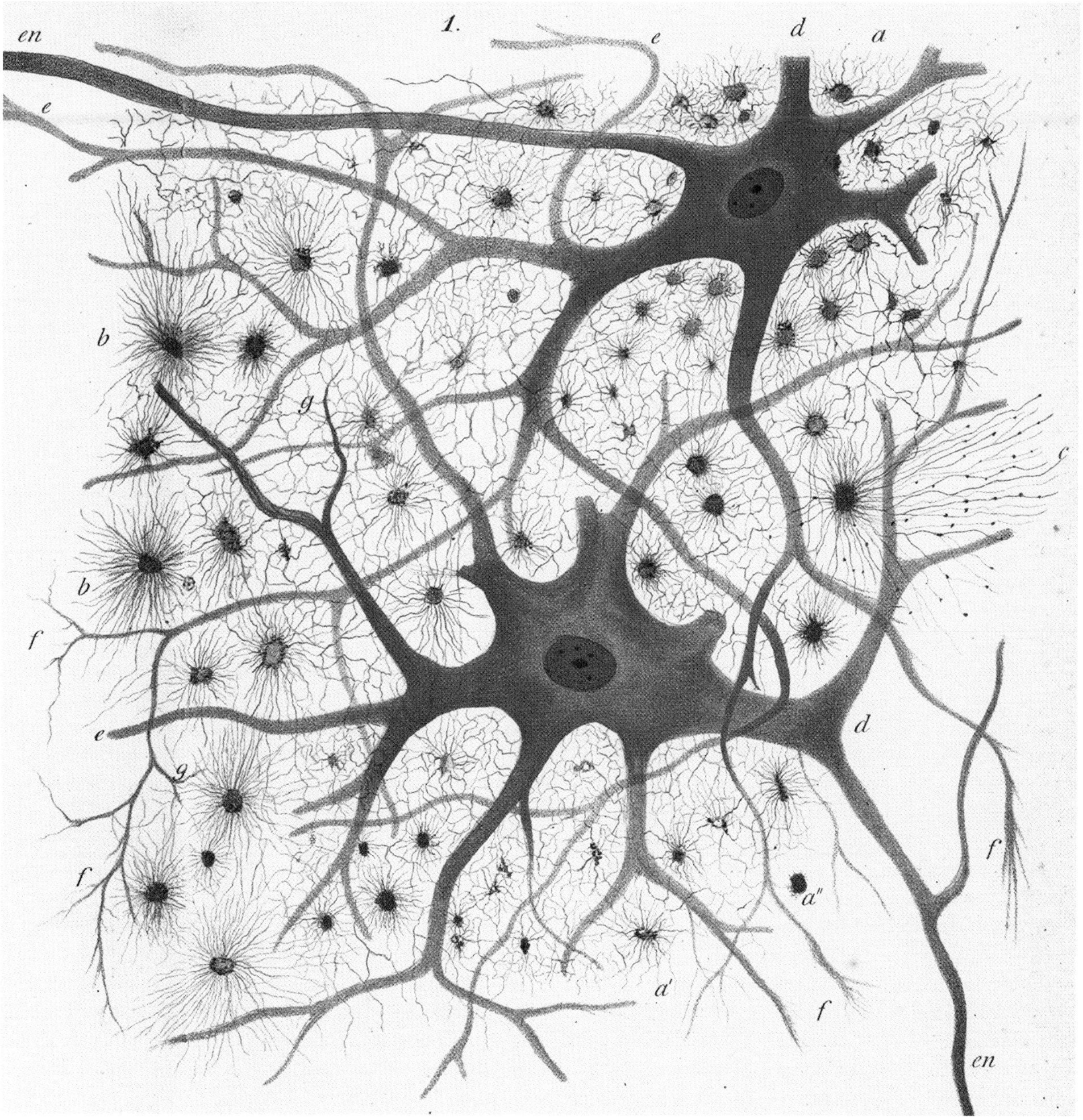

FIGURE 79. Drawings of different cellular elements of the spinal cord by Michail Lavdowsky (1846–1902). See Note 19 for the transcription of the legend. Taken from Lavdowsky (1891).

time . . . received them with the greatest skepticism. The distrust was such that, at the anatomical congress held in Berlin in 1889, Cajal, who afterwards became the great histologist of Madrid, found himself alone, provoking around him only smiles of incredulity . . . . I can still see him taking aside Kölliker, who was then the unquestioned master of German histology, and dragging him into a corner of the demonstration hall to show him under the microscope his admirable preparations, and to convince him at the same time of the reality of the facts which he claimed to have discovered. This demonstration was so decisive that a few months later the Würzbourg histologist [Kölliker] confirmed all the facts stated by Cajal.

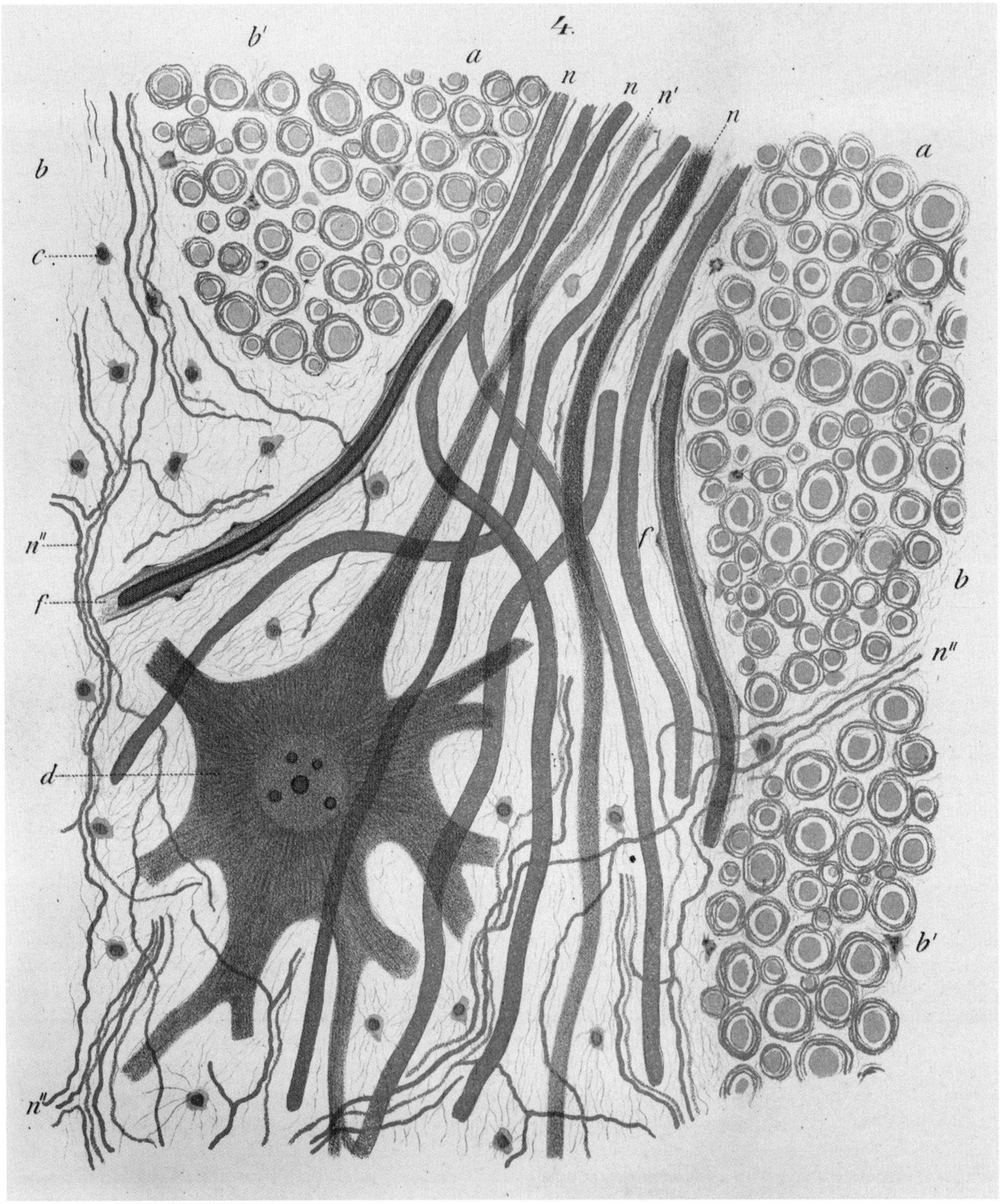

FIGURE 80. Drawing to illustrate some aspects of the histological organization of the spinal cord, I, by Michail Lavdowsky (1846–1902). See Note 20 for the transcription of the legend. Taken from Lavdowsky (1891).

Cajal's findings had such an impact on Kölliker that the German neuroscientist declared (Cajal, 1917b, page 147):

The results that you have obtained are so beautiful that I am planning to immediately undertake a series of confirmatory studies by adopting your

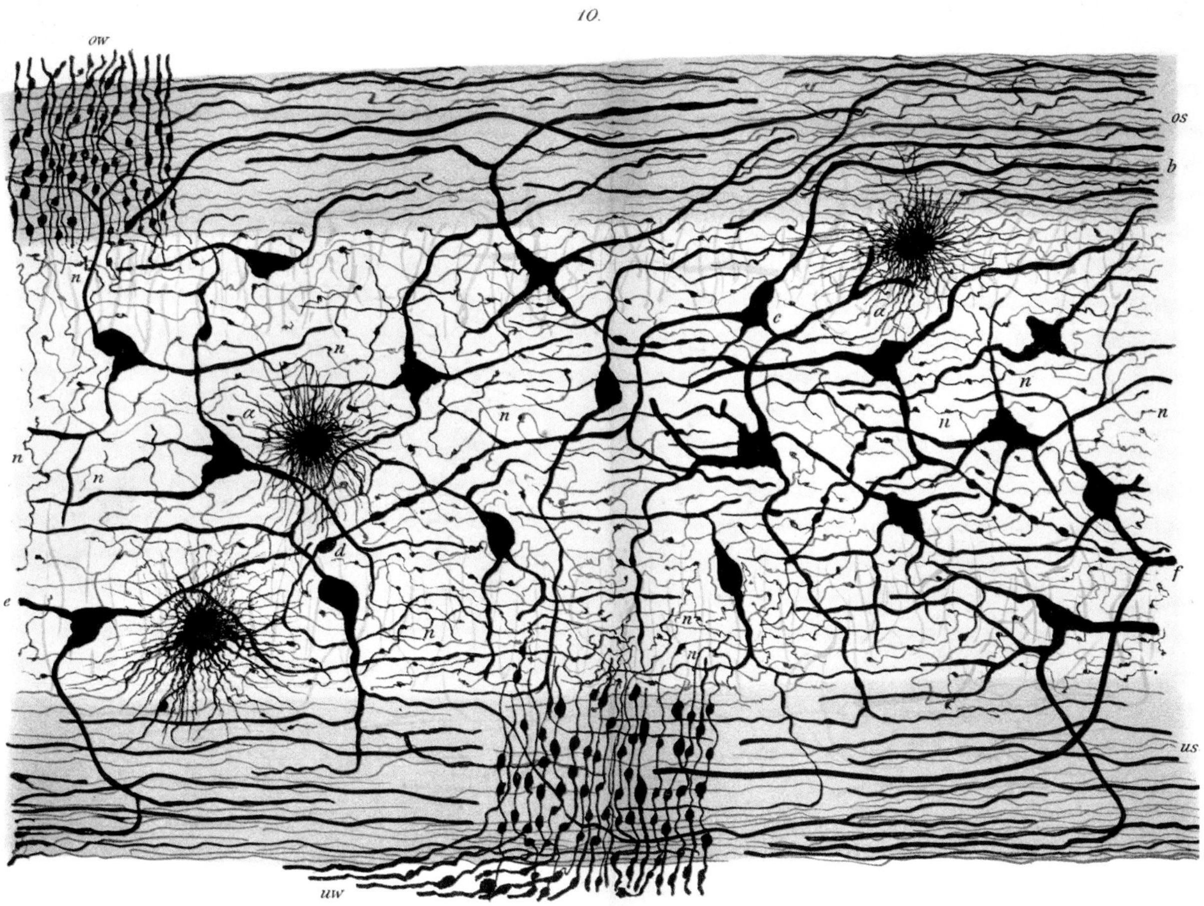

FIGURE 81. Drawing to illustrate some aspects of the histological organization of the spinal cord, II, by Michail Lavdowsky (1846–1902). See Note 21 for the transcription of the legend. Taken from Lavdowsky (1891).

> methodology. I have discovered you, and I wish to make my discovery known in Germany.

Cajal was emboldened by the outcome of his visit to the Congress of Anatomy and this, together with his captivation of the sheer beauty of the histological preparations, meant that he would maintain his focus on the intriguing mysteries of the nervous system for the rest of his days.

VERIFICATION OF THE DRAWINGS OF CAJAL AND OTHER SCIENTISTS

The phrase "exact representations" used by Cajal to define his drawings has commonly been misinterpreted. It does not mean the copying of everything that could be seen in a given microscopic field, but rather the exact reproduction of details extracted from it. This was duly verified several decades later by means of the examination of Cajal's own histological preparations, currently housed in the *Legado Cajal* at the Instituto Cajal in Madrid (e.g., DeFelipe and Jones, 1988, 1992; Garcia-Lopez et al., 2010). For example, it has been demonstrated that his drawings of cells are very similar to cells found in his extant preparations as seen in Figures 33, 49, 54, 56, 57, and 59. Figures 95 and 96 show other examples from the original preparations of de Castro.

Similarly, many of the descriptions and illustrations of Cajal and other scientists have been confirmed in recent years using modern techniques. Some examples are shown in Figures 97 through 101.

As discussed in DeFelipe (2010a), you should keep in mind that, in many cases, the chemical reaction that labels the cellular and subcellular elements

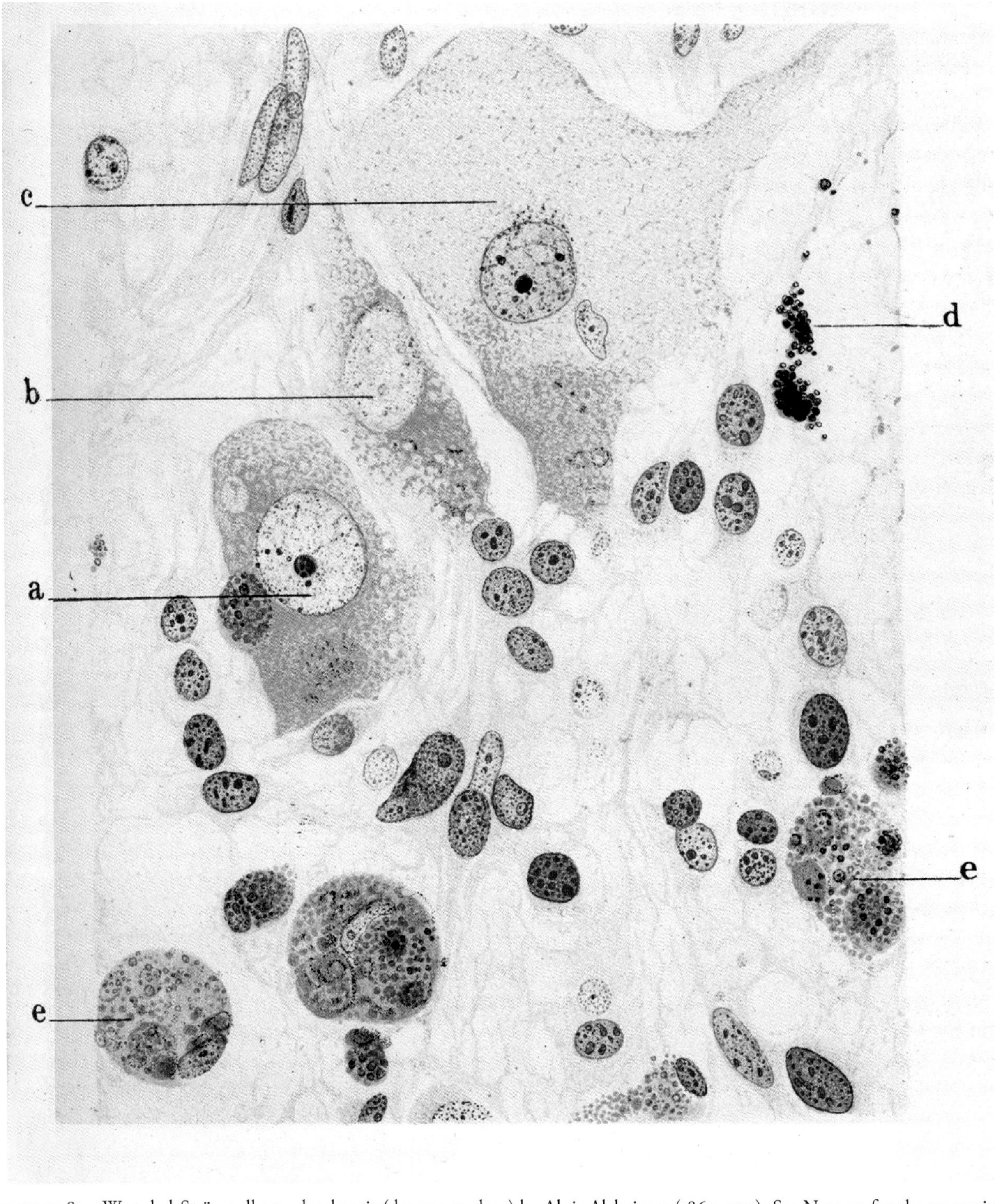

FIGURE 82. Westphal-Strümpell pseudosclerosis (dentate nucleus) by Alois Alzheimer (1864–1915). See Note 22 for the transcription of the legend. Taken from von Hoesslin and Alzheimer (1912).

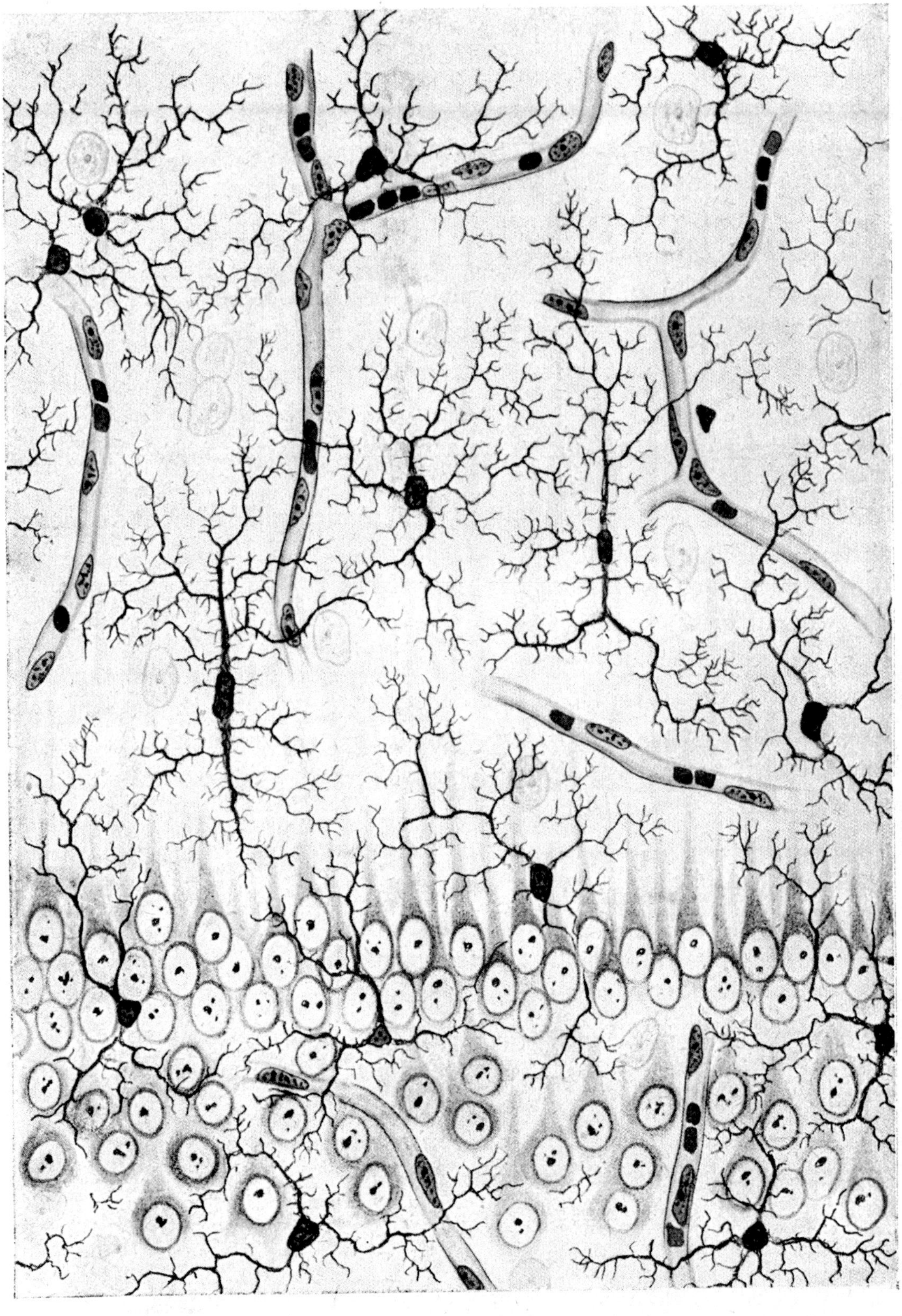

FIGURE 83. Microglial cells in the Ammon's horn (*stratum radiatum*) of the rabbit by Pío del Río-Hortega (1882–1945). See Note 23 for the transcription of the legend. Taken from Del Río-Hortega (1920).

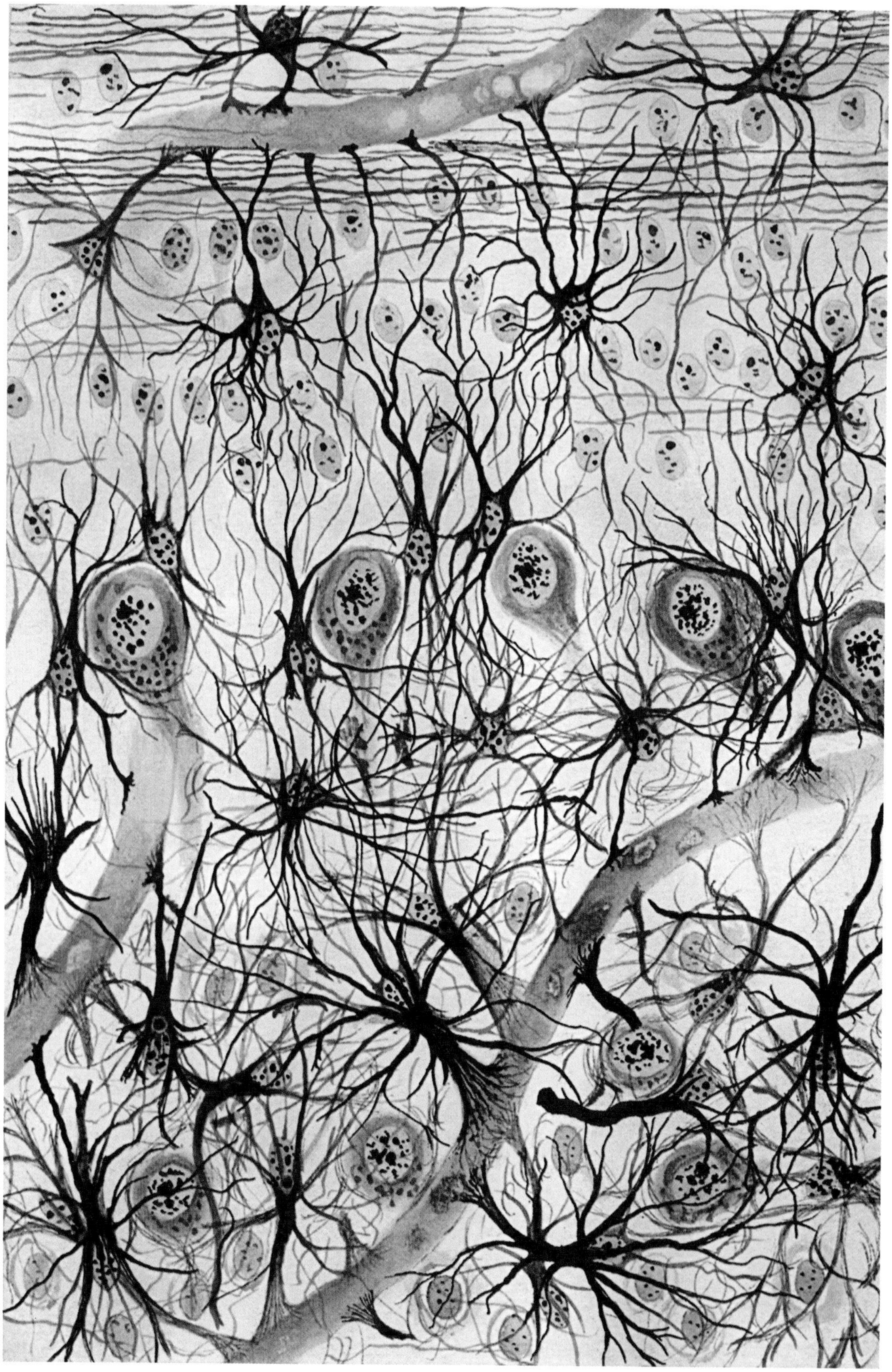

FIGURE 84. Human olfactory bulb by Fernando de Castro (1896–1967). See Note 24 for the transcription of the legend. Taken from de Castro (1920).

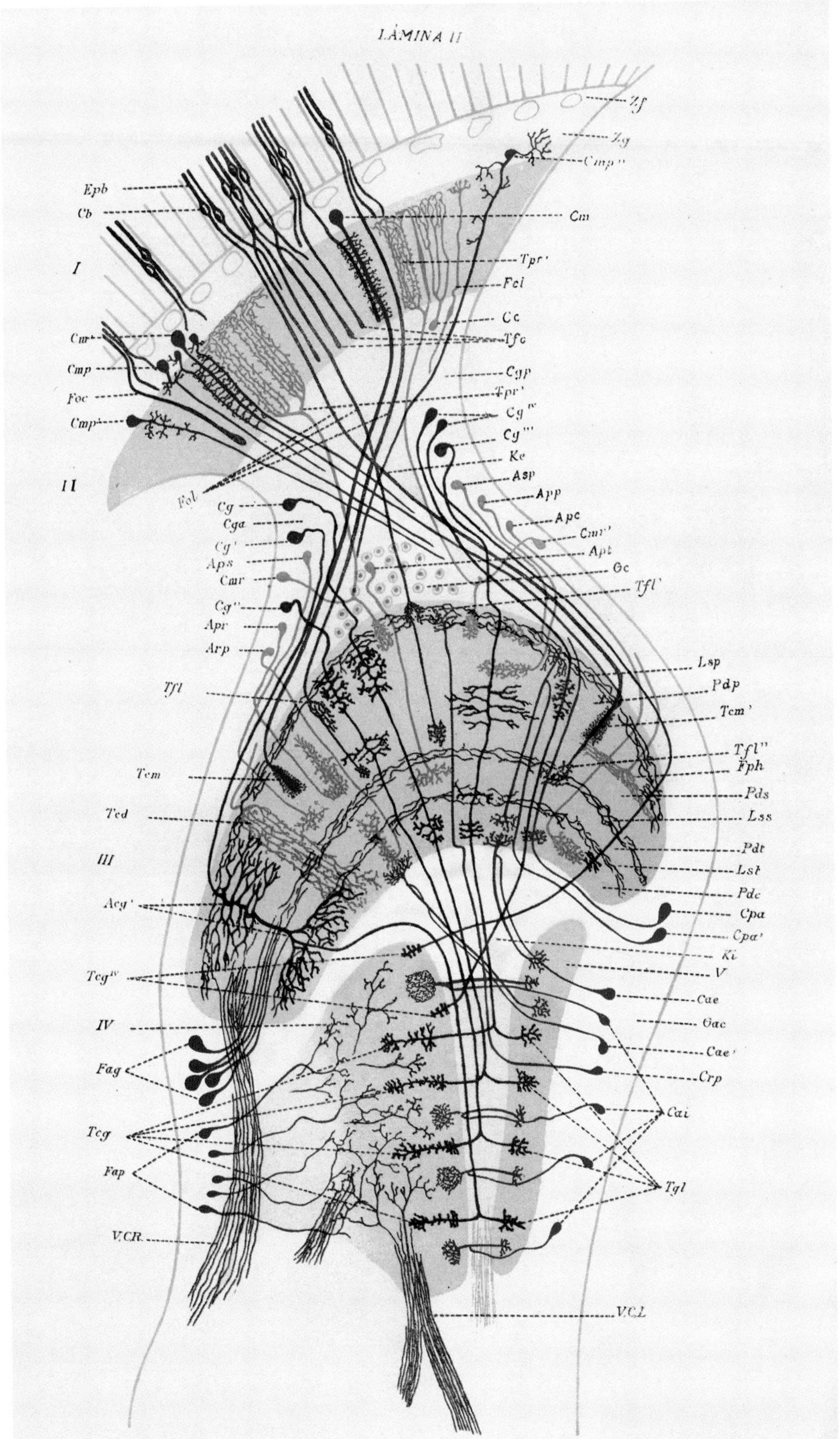

FIGURE 85. Schema of the retina and visual centers of the fly. See Note 25 for the transcription of the legend. Taken from Cajal and Sánchez (1915).

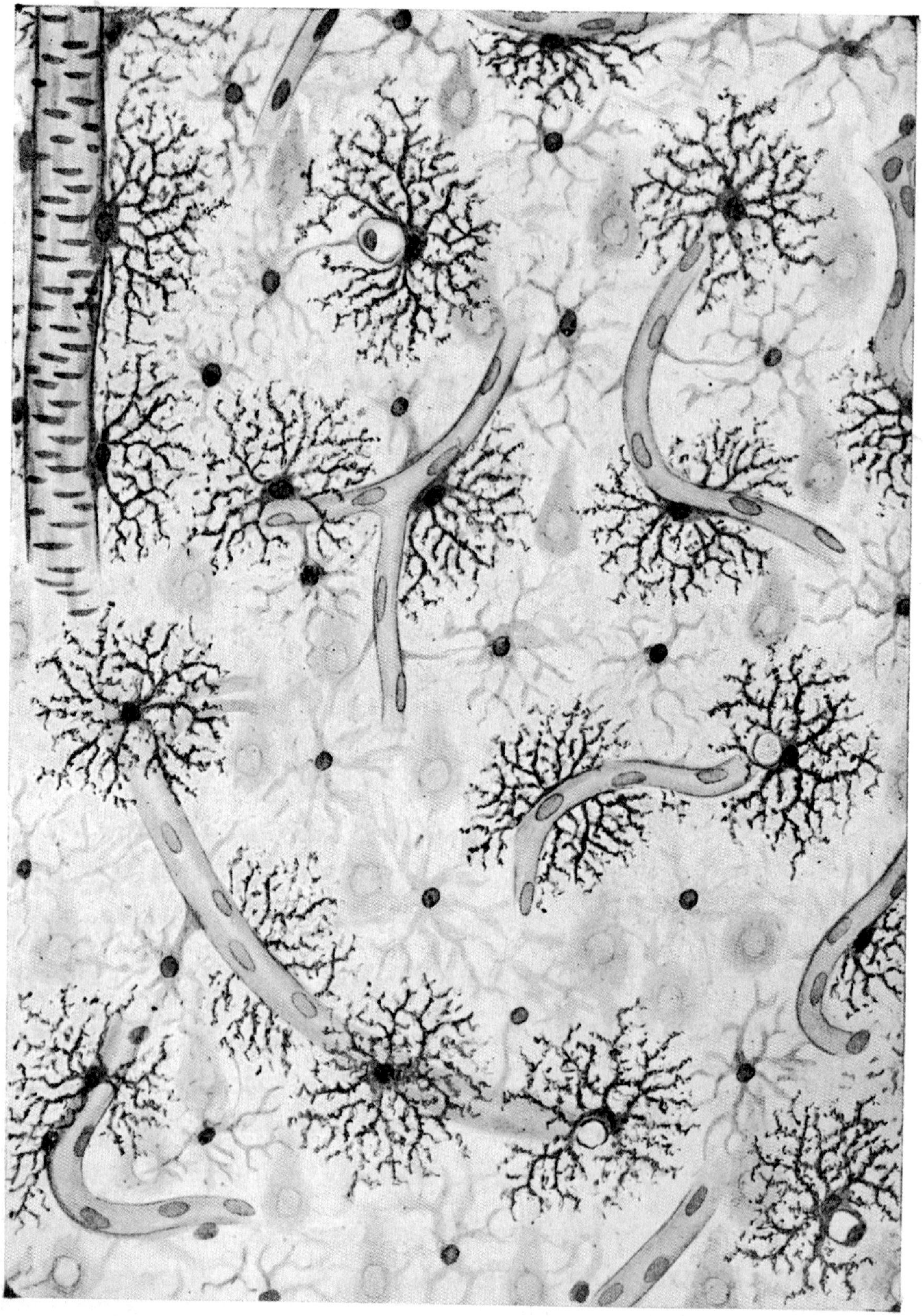

FIGURE 86. Drawings by Del Río-Hortega illustrating the distribution of perivascular glia in the cerebral cortex. Taken from Del Río-Hortega (1933).

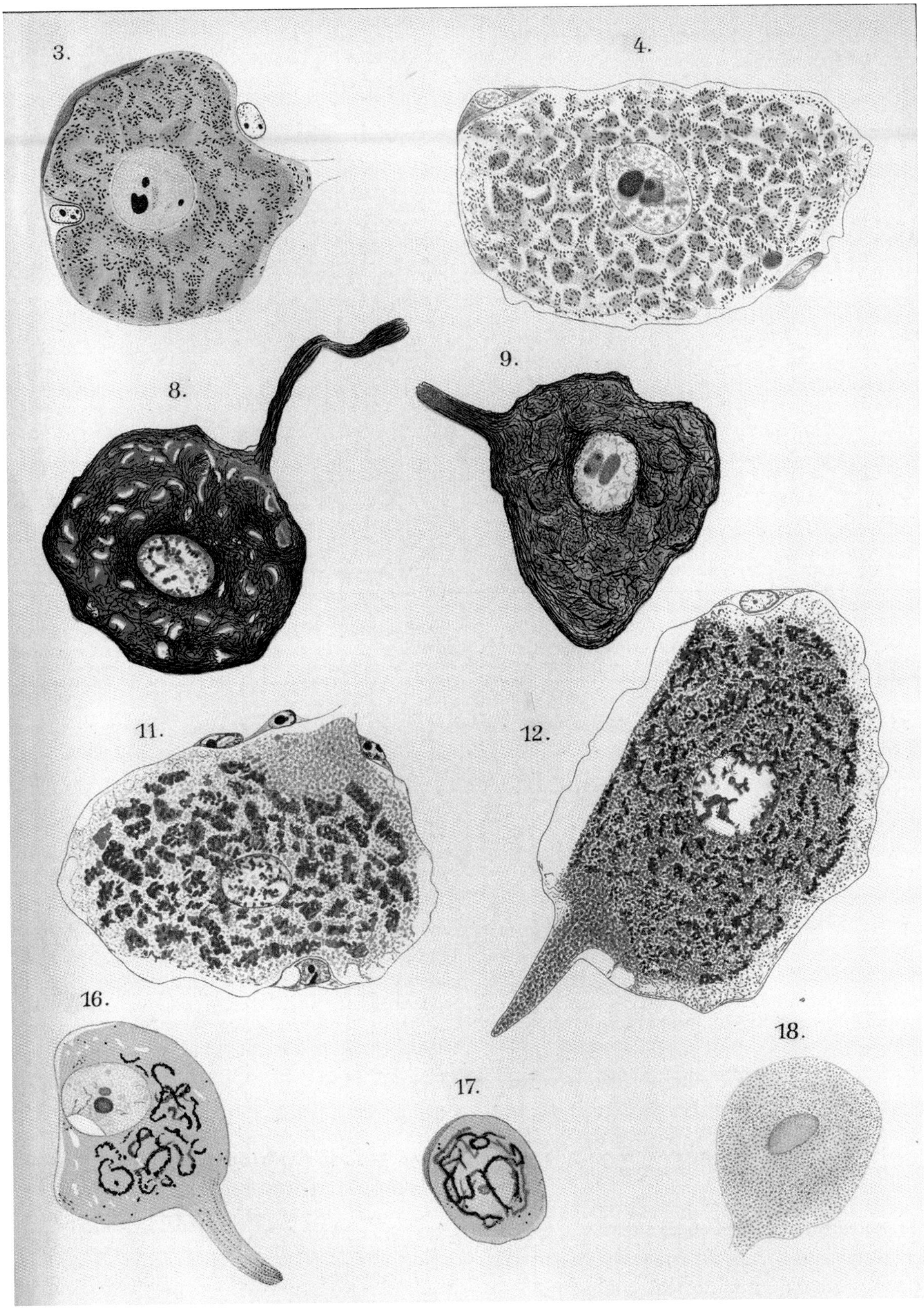

FIGURE 87. Drawings from preparations of spinal ganglion cells of the pigeon showing the relations of mitochondria and other cytoplasmic constituents. See Note 26 for the transcription of the legend. Taken from Cowdry (1913).

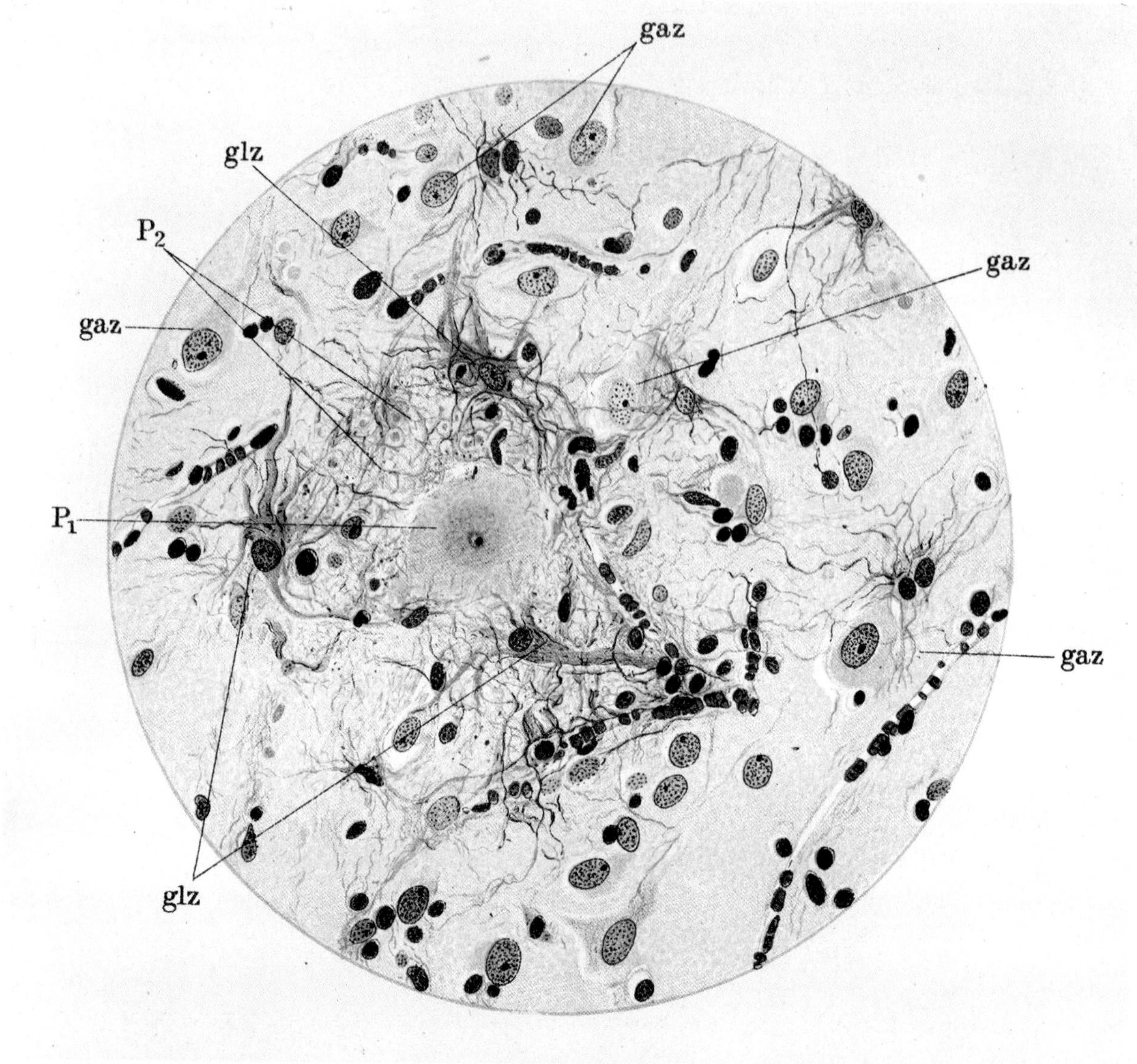

FIGURE 88. Drawing of a senile plaque from Alzheimer (1911) using the Weigert method to stain glia. See Note 27 for the transcription of the legend.

in the nervous system is unknown. Furthermore, in some cases the labeling has proved to be an artifact of the techniques, or the authors' incorrect interpretation. However, in general, these methods represent the roots of our knowledge of the cytology, histology, and connectivity of the nervous system. Indeed, these techniques and the methods derived from them were used for decades after being discovered and continue to be used extensively to this day. Ted Jones—one of the most distinguished modern neuroanatomists and with whom I had the great honor and pleasure of working for many years until he passed away unexpectedly in 2011—summarized this well (Jones, 2007):

> It is salutary for us to recognize that the years subsequent to Cajal's last major papers in the early 1920s were years in which the techniques at the disposal of neuroanatomists remained those that Cajal himself had used or that had been in existence even before he commenced his research. Not that these were years of impoverished discovery . . . the post-Cajal years were those of active research on the long tract connections in the nervous system, an area in which the

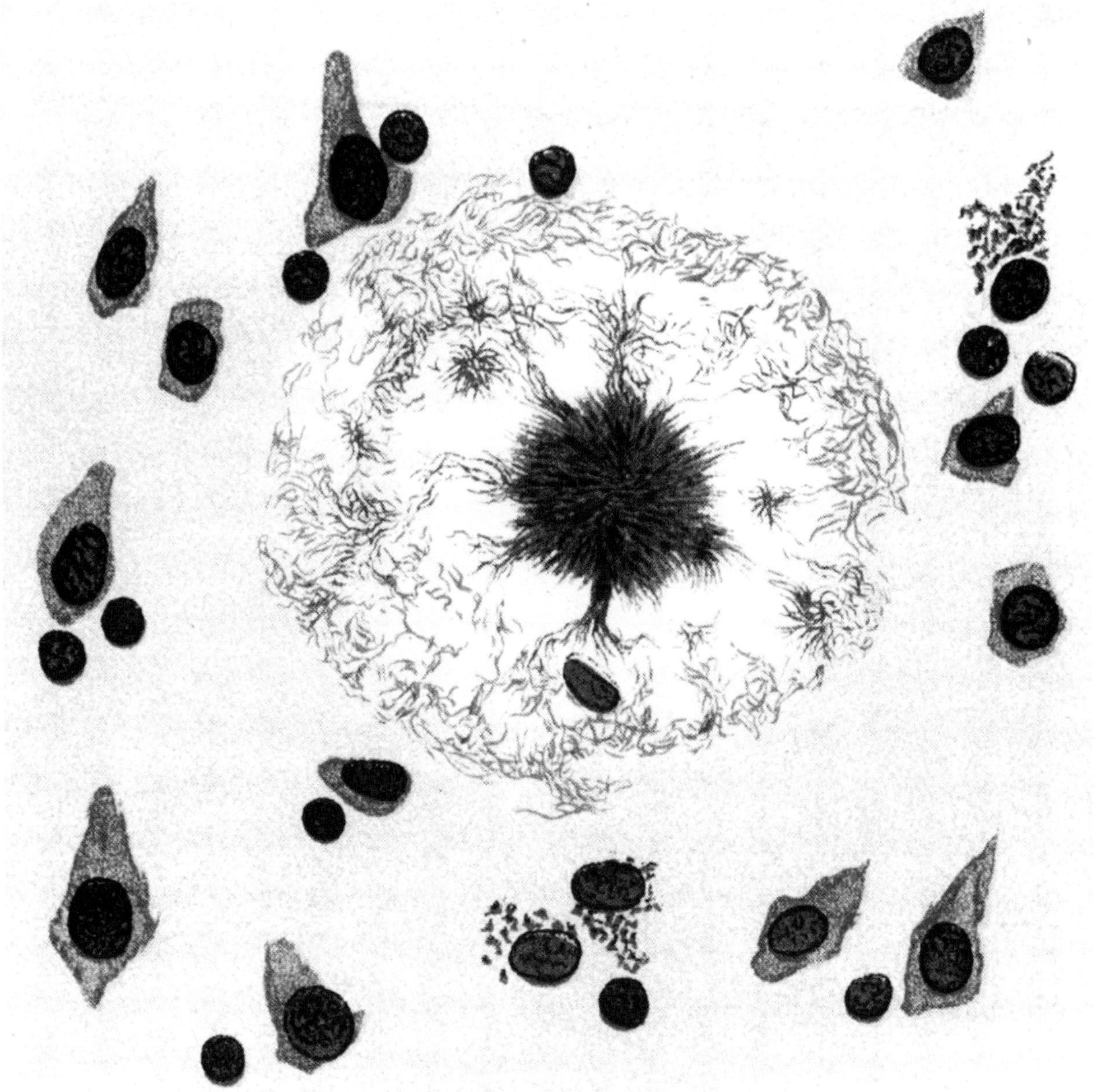

FIGURE 89. Drawing of a senile plaque from Fischer (1912) stained with carbol methylene blue/methylene violet. See Note 28 for the transcription of the legend.

Golgi technique could yield little. But it is also true to say that these important investigations on the spinal, brainstem and thalamocortical pathways were conducted with techniques that predated Cajal's perfection of the Golgi technique.

THE NEURONAL FOREST AS A SOURCE OF ARTISTIC INSPIRATION

As described in *El Jardín de la Neurología: Sobre lo bello, el arte y el cerebro* (DeFelipe, 2014), the surgical removal of the "the stone of madness" in people considered insane or with epilepsy served as a subject for several painters during the sixteenth century. One of the most famous paintings is the *Extracción de la piedra de la locura* (*Extracting the Stone of Madness*) (Museo del Prado, Madrid) by Jeroen van Anthoniszoon Aeken, known as El Bosco (1450–1516), in which he mocks the deception and ignorance of those affected (Figure 102). However, it turns out that what is extracted from the patient's

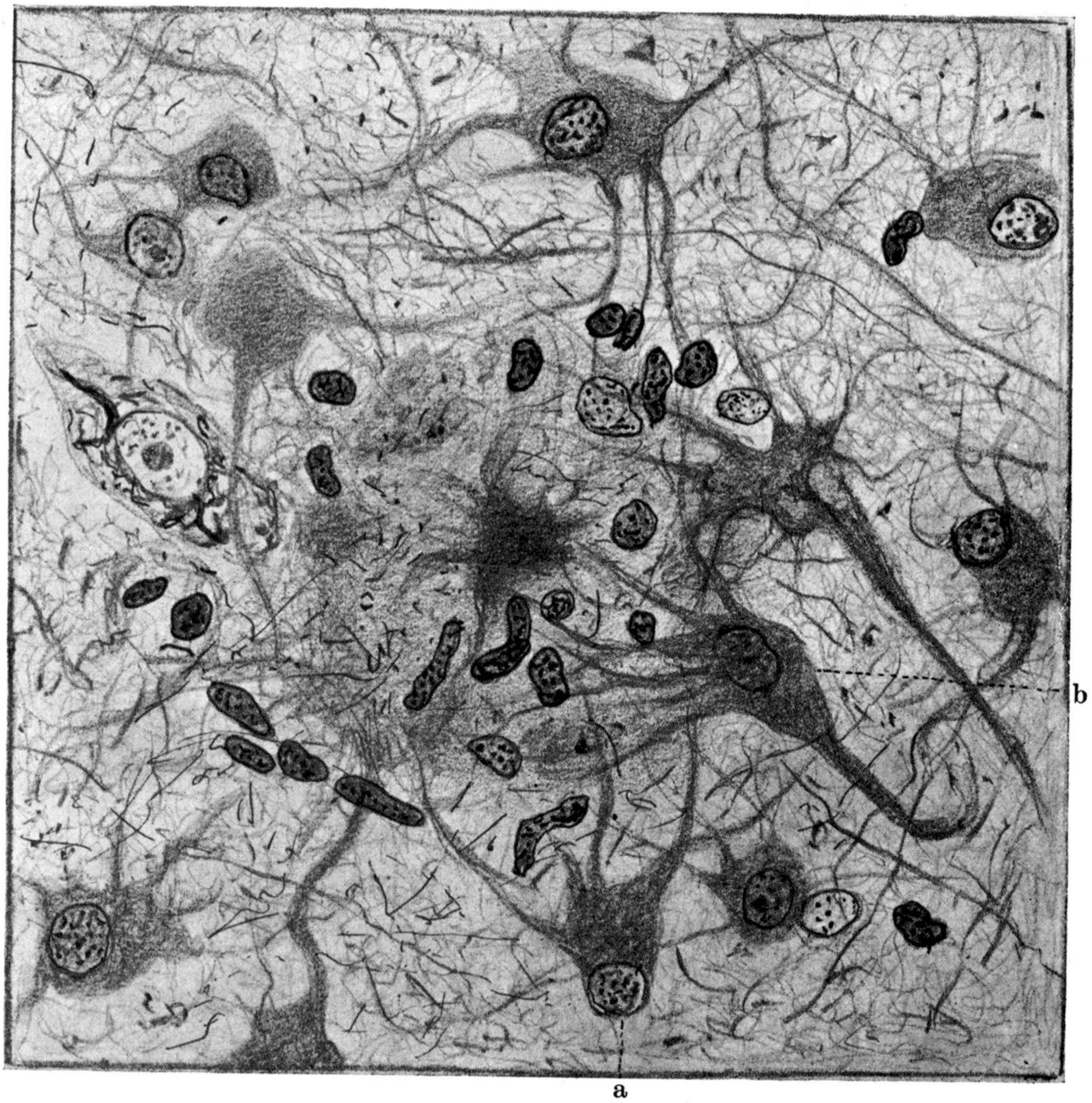

FIGURE 90. Drawing of a senile plaque from Marinesco and Minea (1912). See Note 29 for the transcription of the legend.

head is not a stone but a flower—a type of tulip like the one that can be seen on the table. Thus, we could fantasize that this painting was a forerunner to the work of El Bosco, and was suggesting that neurons are comparable with plants. Who could have imagined that the forest that Cajal painted when he was only 13 years old, shown in Figure 70, would later lead to drawings illustrating the neuronal forest that constitutes the brain?

These neuronal forests have served as an unlimited source of artistic and poetic inspiration to many scientists. Indeed, Figure 103 is an artistic illustration showing a mysterious object, the brain, arising through the mist and emerging from the entangled branches of the trees that constitute the enchanting neuronal forest. The panel on the right of this figure shows a garden where the sculpture ("the scientist"), which is seen in the foreground, is looking toward

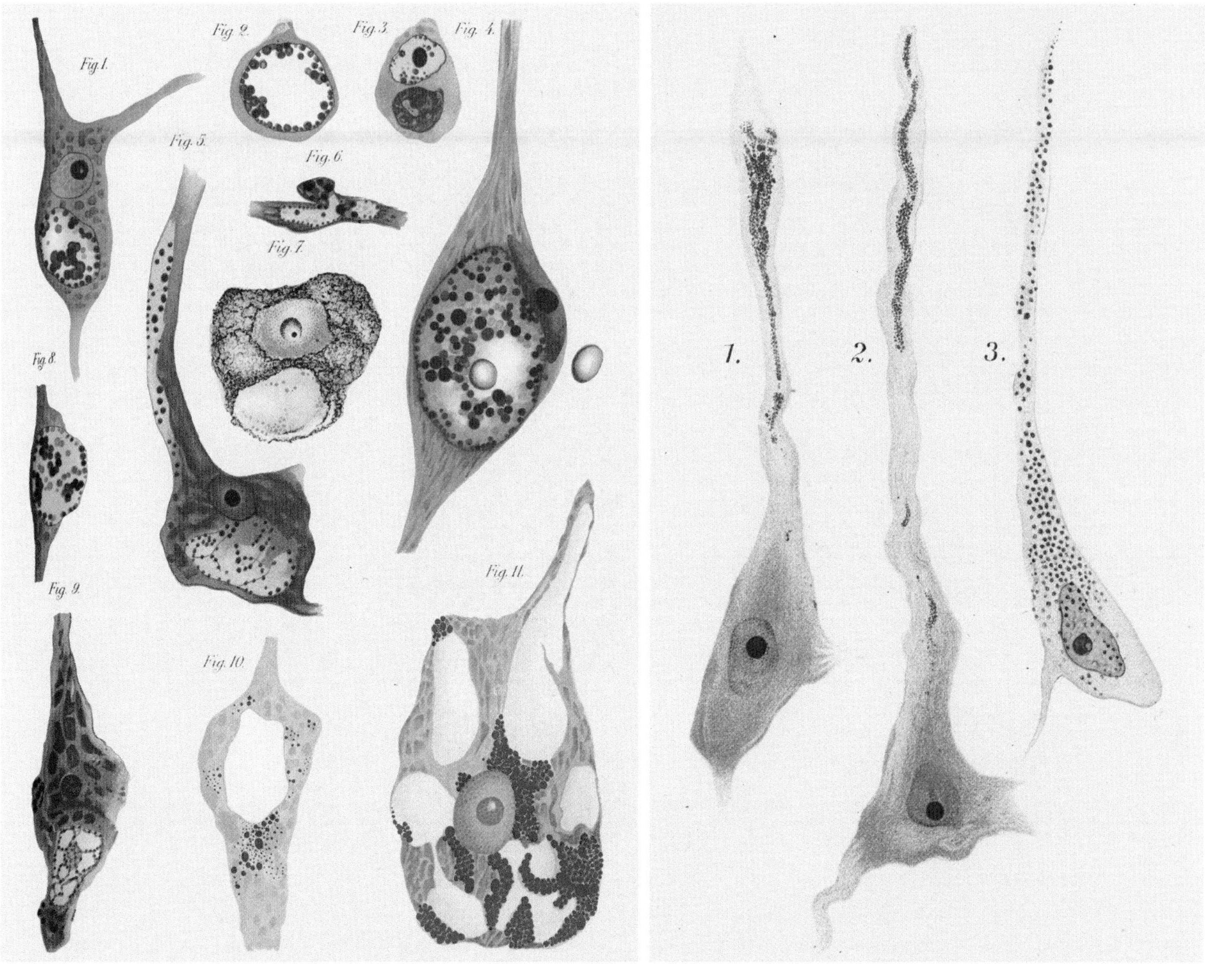

FIGURE 91. Changes in neurons in cases of dementia precox, aging, or Alzheimer's disease. *Left*, Drawings showing the changes in neurons of the medulla oblongata associated with dementia precox, using different methods: *Figures 1–4*, Mann-Alzheimer method; *Figures 5 and 6*, Alzheimer-Mallory method; *Figure 7*, Bielschowscky method; *Figures 8 and 9*, Weigert method to stain neuroglia; and *Figures 10 and 11*, Daddi-Herxheimer method. See Note 30 for the transcription of the legend. Taken from Rezza (1913). *Right, Figures 1 and 2*, neurons from the hippocampus of a twenty-two-year-old horse; *Figure 3*, ganglion cell from the hippocampus of a case of senile dementia. See Note 31 for the transcription of the legend. Taken from Simchowicz (1911).

the end of the pathway, where the fog obscures the view, making it difficult to distinguish the details of the trees in the background. In this case, the fog represents the technical difficulties scientists have to face when studying the elements that make up the neuronal forest.

Without a doubt, the discovery of the Golgi method represented a major innovation that facilitated the study of the nervous system. However, many other methods yielded not only very important results, but also beautiful, multicolor images of the brain. As previously discussed in Cajal's *Butterflies of the Soul* (DeFelipe, 2010a), the methods to analyze the nervous system have evolved dramatically over the years from the era of Cajal to the present day. Three main stages—or "explosions of colors"—can be distinguished. The first explosion started with the study of the normal and altered cytology of neural cells, the second involved the introduction of fluorescence microscopy and confocal laser scanning microscopy, and the third was the introduction of green fluorescent protein (GFP) and the Brainbow. What follows is a modified extract of the text published in Cajal's *Butterflies of the Soul* (DeFelipe, 2010a, pages 39–50):

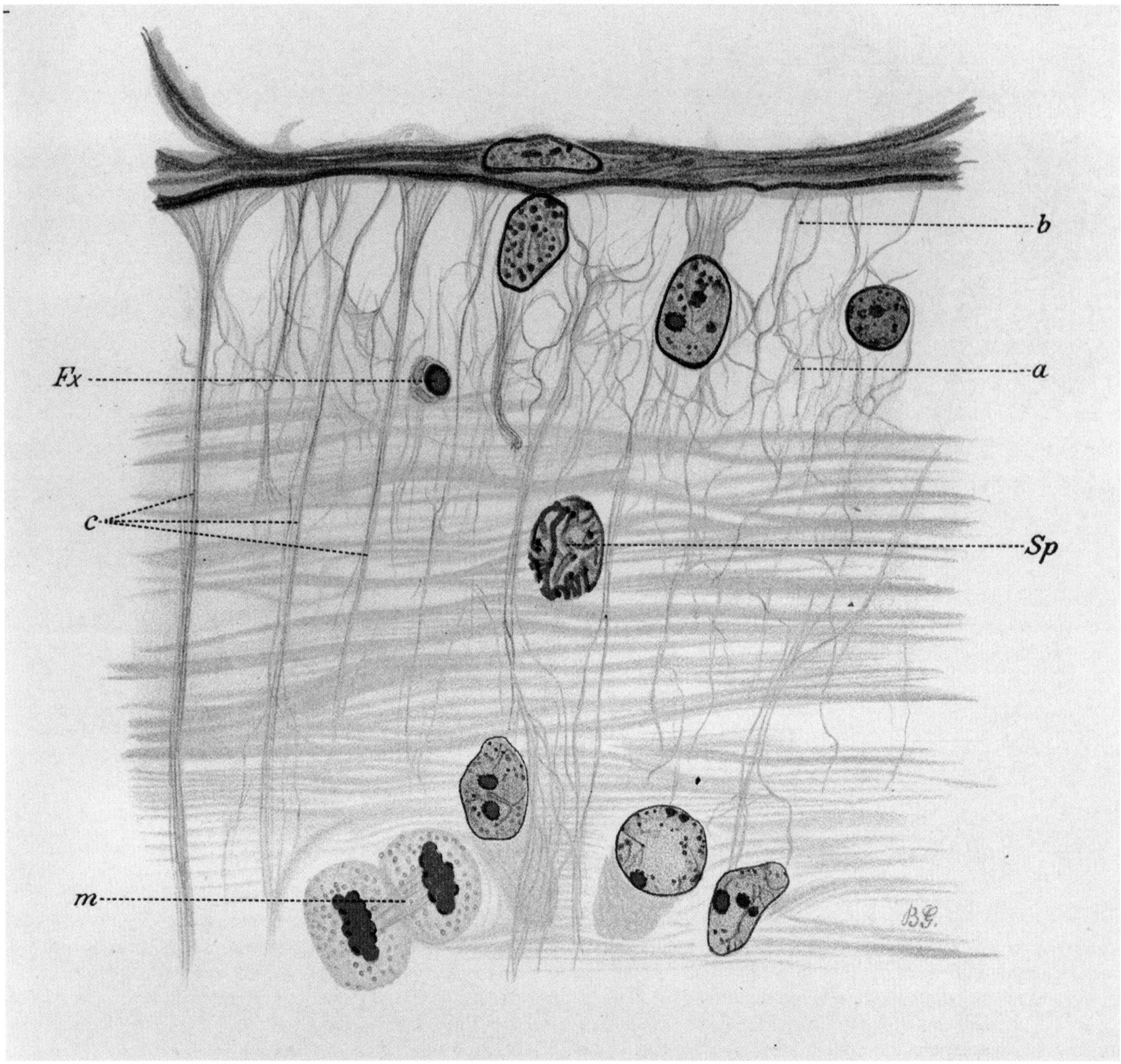

FIGURE 92. Normal histology of the spinal cord of the newborn rabbit. Taken from Spatz (1918). See Note 32 for the transcription of the legend.

The first explosion came mainly when scientists at the time of Cajal began to examine cytoplasmic organelles in detail to address the possible changes associated with the functional state of nerve cells. One of the questions was whether the activity of neurons produces chemical or morphological changes in their constitution. For this purpose, a variety of methods were developed that involved the use of different dyes. Through these colorants, researchers could analyze cytological characteristics and infer the chemical composition in both normal and altered states. During the first three decades of 1900, marvelous drawings were produced to illustrate different characteristics of the normal and altered cytology and histology of the nervous system in general. The staining procedures included a large number of reagents and methods, such as eosin, toluidine blue, reduced silver nitrate, silver carbonate, methylene blue, erythrosine, carmine, hematoxylin, and so on, as well as numerous modifications introduced by different scientists, such as Weigert staining for glia, Cajal's gold chloride

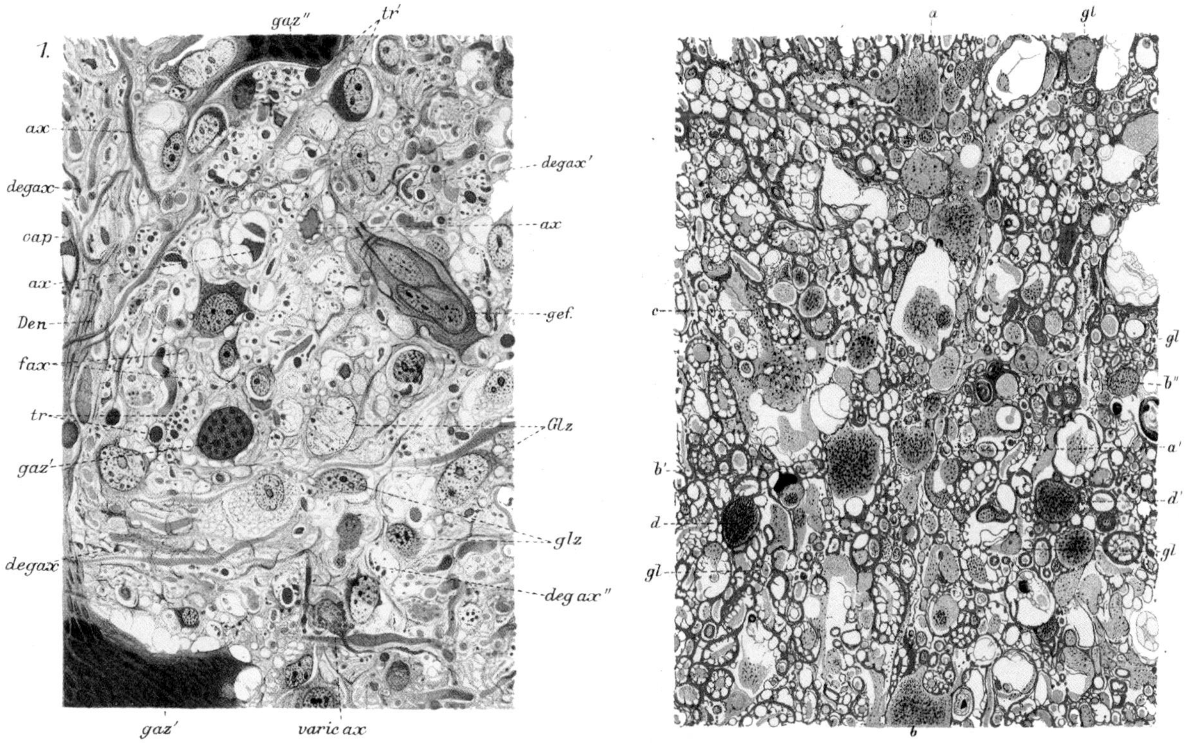

FIGURE 93. Drawings showing histological alterations in acute myelitis and encephalitis. Taken from Lotmar (1918). The legend states: *Left*, "Degeneration of fine nervous structures (axis cylinder, eventually thin dendrites) in the marginal region of the anterior horn. Method of Mann" (page 426). See Note 33 for the transcription of the legend. *Right*, "General view of a transverse section through the marginal region of a focus in the white matter of the spinal cord showing axon swelling. Fuchsin staining" (page 430). See Note 34 for the transcription of the legend.

sublimate method, and the three different methods conceived by Mann-Alzheimer, Alzheimer-Mallory, and Bielschowsky. As shown in Figures 87 through 94, the images obtained with these methods were often particularly beautiful and it is important to point out that many of these techniques remain widely used in many areas of neuroscience. Those of you interested in the description of the protocols of these methods should refer to the book *Elementos de Técnica Micrográfica del Sistema Nervioso* (*Principles of Micrographical Technique for the Nervous System*) by Cajal and de Castro (1933), which has been recently translated to English (Merchán et al., 2016).

The second explosion occurred during the late 1970s, when fluorescence microscopy and the use of fluorescent dyes or fluorochrome stains to visualize a molecule of interest in specimens became a commonly used technique in neuroscience. For instance, Kuypers and his colleagues studied long-range connections using Bisbenzimide and Nuclear Yellow to produce green and golden-yellow retrograde labeling of the neuronal nuclei, and True Blue and Fast Blue was used to produce blue retrograde labeling of the neuron's cytoplasm (Kuypers et al., 1980). At the same time, the availability of a variety of neural-specific antibodies and secondary antibodies conjugated to different fluorescent tags (e.g., rhodamine-conjugated [red] and fluorescein-conjugated [green] secondary antisera) facilitated colocalization studies in which two or more substances could be identified in a given neuron (e.g., Hendry et al., 1984). Combinations of various techniques served to examine other aspects of the organization of the nervous system. For example, combining retrograde tracing and fluorescent dye injection with indirect immunofluorescence histochemistry permitted the neurochemical characterization of neurons that could be identified by

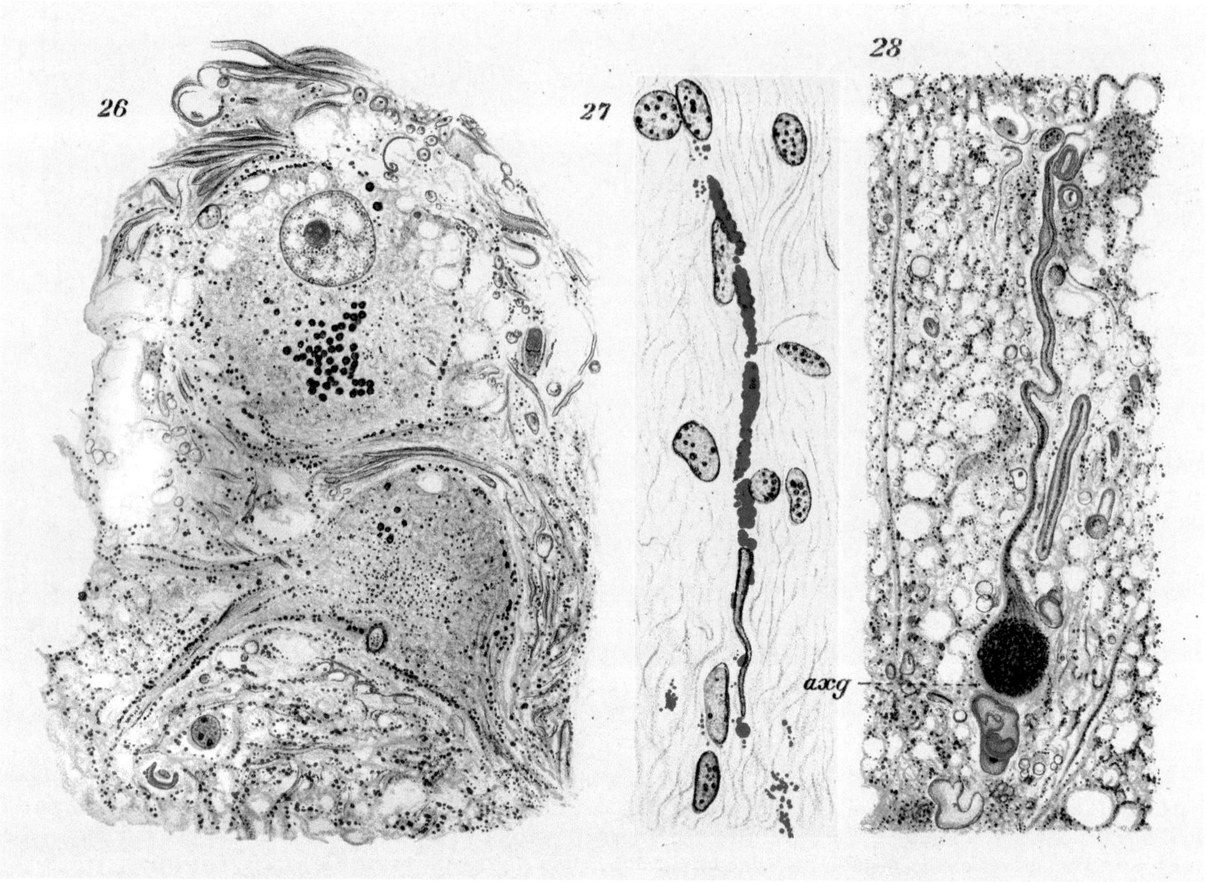

FIGURE 94. Pathological changes in the brain. Taken from Creutzfeldt (1921). See Note 35 for the transcription of the legend.

their projection site and their labeling in different colors (e.g., Skirboll et al., 1984). Thus, multicolor images using several fluorophores could be obtained by combining several single-color images. However, one of the limitations of fluorescent microscopy is that interference of the fluorescent emissions occurs above and below the focal plane and, therefore, it is not possible to obtain high-resolution optical images of thick specimens. This problem was resolved with the introduction of confocal laser scanning microscopy, which became a standard technique toward the end of the 1980s. Because confocal microscopy images are acquired point by point (optical sectioning), and these images can be computer reconstructed in three dimensions, it is possible—and indeed relatively easy—to analyze complex spatial relationships between neural elements visualized with different colors in thick sections.

The third explosion has come in recent years from the identification of the green fluorescent protein, or GFP, originally isolated from the jellyfish *Aequorea victoria*. The GFP gene can be introduced into intact cells and organisms in such a way that when the gene for GFP is fused to the gene encoding a given protein, the expressed protein preserves its normal activity whereas GFP maintains its fluorescence, providing us with a very useful marker for gene expression (Tsien, 1998). Engineering of GFP has permitted brighter and more stable variants to be generated, with various excitation and emission spectra, marking a new era for imaging in cell biology (Giepmans et al., 2006). The impact of GFP and its variants has been extraordinary. Indeed, Martin Chalfie, Osamu Shimomura, and Roger Y. Tsien were awarded the 2008 Nobel Prize in Chemistry "for their discovery and development of

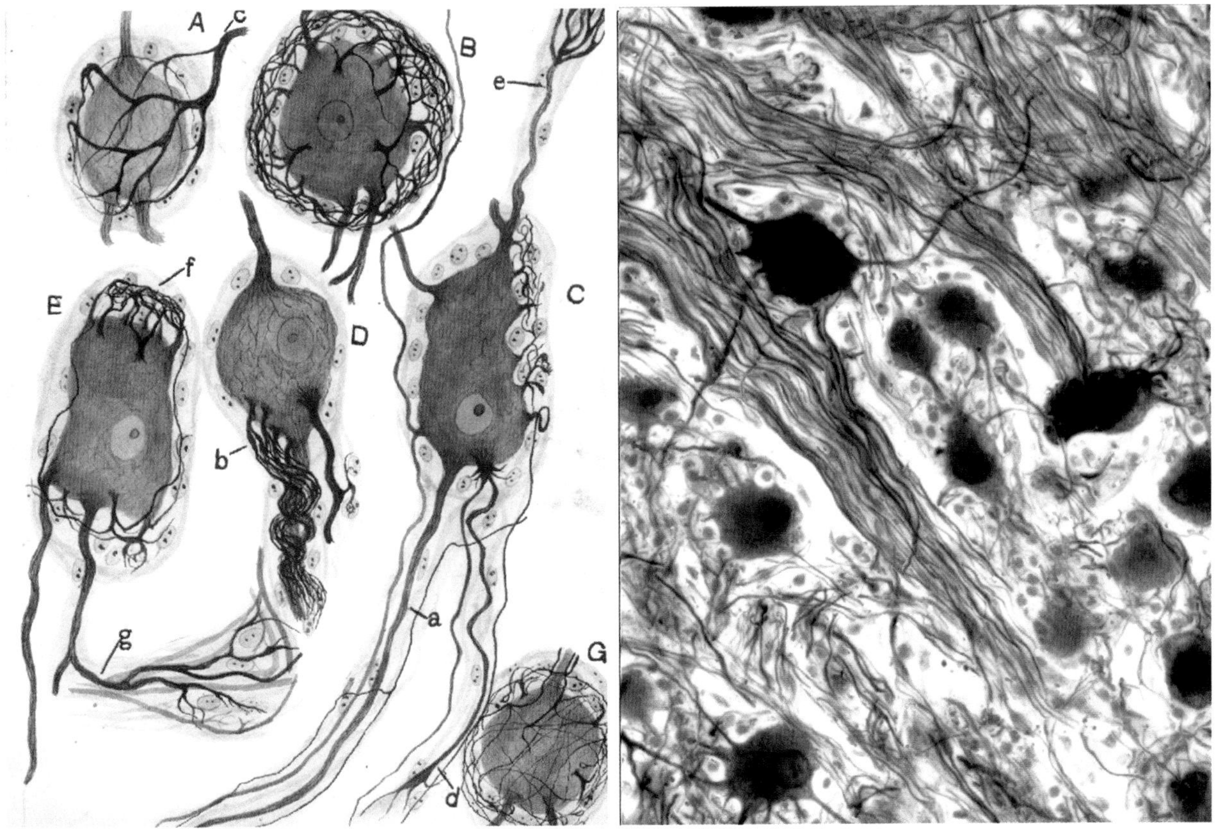

FIGURE 95. *Left*, An original sketch by de Castro showing the special features of the dendrites of the cervical sympathetic neurons published in "*Sobre la fina anatomía de los ganglios simpáticos, vertebrales y prevertebrales de los simios*" (de Castro, 1926). *Right*, Upper cervical ganglion from a cat (autonomic nervous system)—histological preparation using Cajal–Castro's reduced silver impregnation (mosaic × 10). Photomicrograph obtained from an original slide from Prof. Fernando de Castro (*Archivo Fernando De Castro*), to whom the original drawing also belongs. The histological image was taken by Miguel A. Merchán. Figure and legend taken from *Cajal and de Castro's Neurohistological Methods* (Merchán et al., 2016).

the green fluorescent protein." The application of this technology to the study of brain circuits yields very visually appealing results and now represents one of the most exciting and promising areas in neuroanatomy. For example, transgenic mice have been generated in which red, green, yellow, or cyan fluorescent proteins (called *XFPs*) are selectively expressed in neurons, such that the labeling is similar to Golgi staining but with bright colors. Mice expressing spectrally distinct XFPs can be crossed to generate "bi-" or "tricolor" animals in which the possible connections between the labeled neurons can be visualized (Feng et al., 2000).

One of the most fascinating new tools is the combinatorial color method, called *Brainbow*, in which, rather than labeling neurons in one of two or three colors, they can be labeled in one of more than one hundred colors (Livet et al., 2007). The combinatorial expression of red, green, and blue XFPs at various levels can generate a large spectrum of colors. Lichtman and colleagues (2008, page 419) drew a useful analogy between the Brainbow and an RGB video monitor "which combines different intensities of three channels (red, green and blue) to generate almost the entire color spectrum that the human visual system can perceive."

In summary, the analysis of the cells and regions of the nervous system has been aided by the work of many scientists carried out over a long period, leading to an improvement in these methods, which has provided scientists with the means to approach their research from many different angles. Thus, it has been the cumulative work of these scientists that

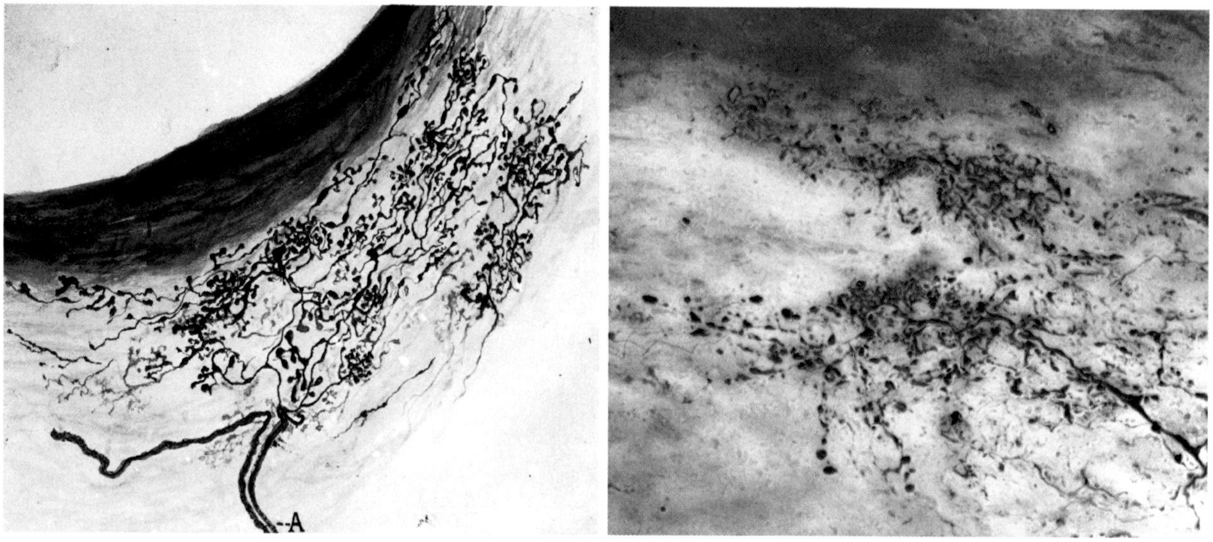

FIGURE 96. Methods for the demonstration of neuronal morphology, Ehrlich's method and variants using methyl blue. Intravital staining with methyl blue carried out by Prof. Fernando de Castro to study the fibers of the carotid sinus. (Modification of Cajal's method. Fixed in ammonium molybdate. Adult cat carotid). *Left*, Original pen-and-ink wash drawing by de Castro published in "*Sur la structure et l'innervation du sinus carotidien de l'homme et des mammifères: Nouveaux faits sur l'innervation et la fonction du glomus caroticum*" (de Castro, 1928). *Right*, Photomicrograph to illustrate a terminal field of fibers in the aortic wall. The background blue staining is due to the intravital diffusion of the stain (×20). Photomicrograph obtained from an original slide from Professor Fernando De Castro (*Archivo Fernando de Castro*), to whom the original drawing also belongs. The histological image was taken by Miguel A. Merchán. Figure and legend taken from *Cajal and de Castro's Neurohistological Methods* (Merchán et al., 2016).

has been crucial in revealing the knowledge that we currently have regarding the structure of the nervous system—or as Peters and colleagues (1991, page 14) so succinctly stated in the classic book *The Fine Structure of the Nervous System*:

> Our image of the nerve cell at the light microscope level is like a collage of many overlapping views, patiently accrued during a century of study.

The collage in Figure 104 could be considered an attempt to illustrate this observation by Peters and colleagues. This figure is the cover of the book *Paisajes Neuronales: Homenaje a Santiago Ramón y Cajal* (DeFelipe et al., 2007) that was published as a result of the international exhibition held in Barcelona in 2006 titled *Paisajes Neuronales* 2006 (Neuroscapes 2006). This exhibition is an example of the increasing interest in the link between the study of the brain and art, which has given rise to numerous other exhibitions around the world. Neuroscapes 2006 was first presented in Barcelona as a special event to celebrate the one-hundredth anniversary of the Nobel Prize for Physiology or Medicine (1906) awarded jointly to Cajal and Golgi for their contributions in the field of the neurosciences. The Neuroscapes 2006 exhibition was inaugurated in the city of Barcelona on April 6, 2006, before its international launch during the Cajal Centenary Conference on the Cerebral Cortex, held at the CosmoCaixa Science Museum in Barcelona, April 25–29. A total of 433 images from sixty-two laboratories around the world were submitted to Neuroscapes for consideration. Each piece of work submitted was reviewed independently by a panel of artists and by the directors of the Neuroscapes exhibition (Javier DeFelipe, Instituto Cajal , Madrid; Henry Markram, Brain Mind Institute, Lausanne; and Jorge Wagensberg, Director of the Area of Environment and Science of La Caixa Foundation, Barcelona). Under the presidency of Torsten Wiesel (Figure 105, *right*) (who together with David H. Hubel received the 1981 Nobel Prize in Physiology or Medicine for their discoveries concerning information processing in the visual system), the organizing committee of Neuroscapes presented the Neuroscapes 2006 Award to Tamily Weissman

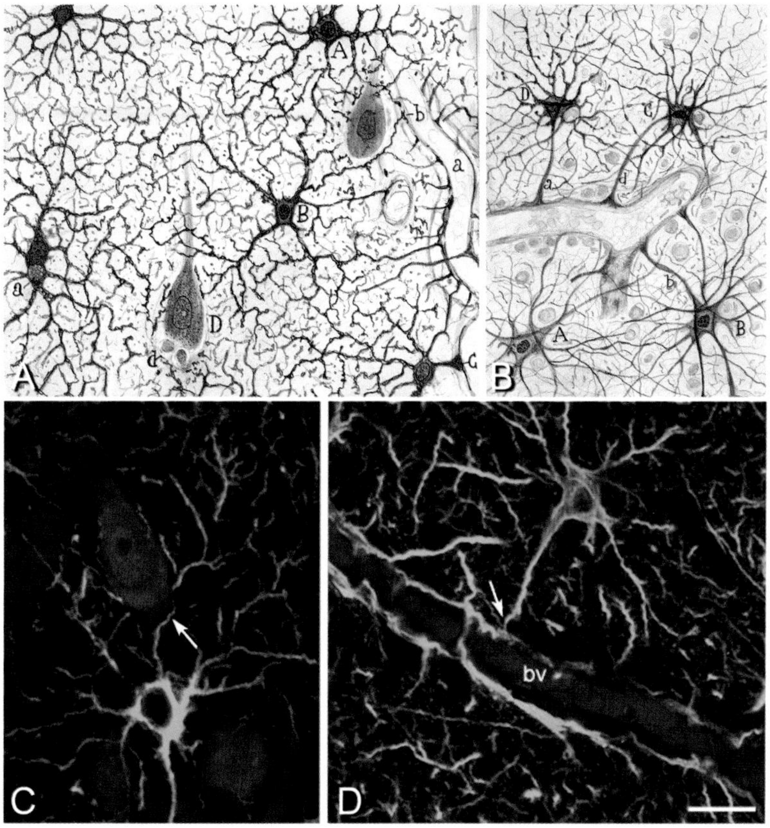

FIGURE 97. **A**, **B**, Drawings by Cajal illustrating astrocytes of the gray matter and white matter, respectively, of the human cerebral cortex. Taken from Cajal (1913). **C**, **D**, Images obtained with a laser confocal microscope to illustrate the relationship of astrocytes with neurons and blood vessels by immunocytochemical techniques of double staining, using anti-NeuN and anti- glial fibrillary acidic protein (GFAP) antibodies, which marks neurons (red) and astrocytes (green), respectively. **C**, Image showing the presence of GFAP-positive astrocytic processes in the neuropil and adjacent to NeuN-positive neurons (arrow). **D**, GFAP-positive astrocytic perivascular end-feet (arrow) located around a capillary (Bv). These capillaries are identified by nonspecific staining of red blood cells. Note the similarity between panels **C** and **D**, and the drawings of Cajal shown in **A** and **B**. Calibration bar (in **D**): 15 μm in **C** and **D**. Figure taken from DeFelipe (2014).

and Jeff Lichtman (Harvard University, United States). The piece by these authors (Figure 105, *left*) received the most votes from the scientists attending the Cajal Centenary Conference meeting, based on its aesthetic appeal. During the first three weeks alone, more than 35,000 people visited the exhibition. Many of the visitors (including famous writers and artists) participated in the event by briefly describing what they "saw" in the images. Thus, this event not only served to bring the world of neuroscience a step closer to the general public, but was also a very interesting bridge between science and art. Since its inauguration in Barcelona, the exhibition has been presented in seventeen cities in Spain and sixteen cities in various countries of America, Europe, and Asia.

Figures 106 and 107 show several other beautiful examples of the study of the brain acting as a source of artistic inspiration today (also presented in Neuroscapes 2006). Figure 106 looks like a painting by Pierre-Auguste Renoir (1841–1919) and Figure 107 resembles a painting by Joan Miró (1893–1983). Many other examples of images of the nervous system look like paintings from a wide variety of artistic movements.

As indicated in Cajal's *Butterflies of the Soul*, while reflecting on the Brainbow mouse, the comment of Russian writer Vladimir Nabokov (1899–1977)

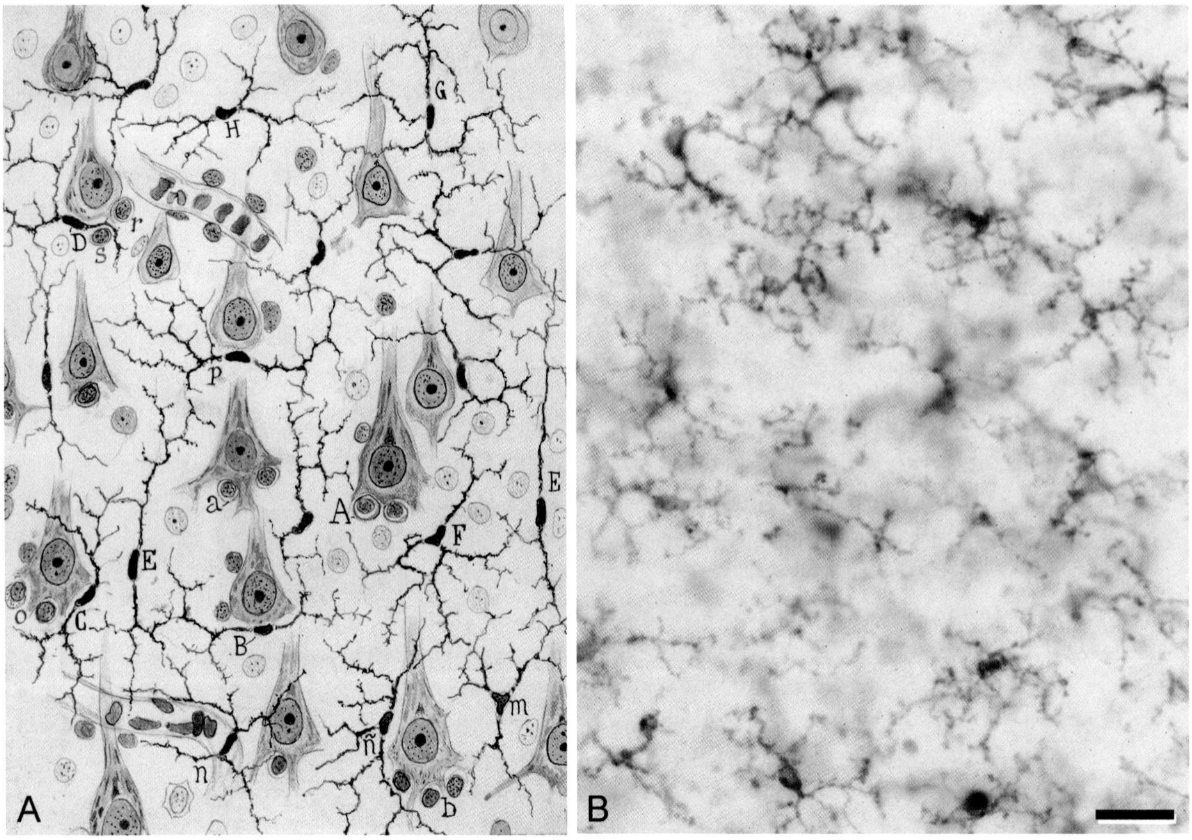

FIGURE 98. **A**, Drawing by Cajal to illustrate microglial cells of the human cerebral cortex. Taken from Cajal (1920). **B**, Photomicrograph of the human cerebral cortex stained immunocytochemically with anti-LN3 antibody to visualize microglial cells. Note the similarity between this image and the drawing in panel **A**. Calibration bar: 25 µm. Figure taken from DeFelipe (2014).

comes to mind when he said it was "as if genes were painting in aquarelle." Vladimir Nabokov, mainly known for his novel *Lolita* (Nabokov, 1955), was a grapheme-color synesthete—meaning, he was an individual with synesthesia, a phenomenon in which stimulation of one sensory or cognitive pathway leads to associated experiences in a second, unstimulated stream (e.g., Hubbard, 2007, and references contain therein). He made this comment in a television interview in 1962 (Smith, 1962) on his life and work. After saying, "I have this rather freakish gift of seeing letters in colour," the interviewer asked him, "What colours are your own initials, VN?" Nabokov answered:

> V is a kind of pale, transparent pink . . . : this is one of the closest colours that I can connect with the V. And the N, on the other hand, is a greyish-yellowish oatmeal colour. But a funny thing happens: my wife has this gift of seeing letters in colour, too, but her colours are completely different. There are, perhaps, two or three letters where we coincide, but otherwise the colours are quite different. It turned out, we discovered one day, that my son . . . sees letters in colours, too . . . . Then we asked him to list his colours and we discovered that in one case, one letter which he sees as purple, or perhaps mauve, is pink to me and blue to my wife. This is the letter M. So the combination of pink and blue makes lilac in his case. Which is as if his genes were painting in aquarelle.

It is amazing that this metaphor of Nabokov has been, in a sense, "brought to life" by the generation of transgenic animals in which subsets of neurons are genetically labeled with multiple, distinct colors, such as the Brainbow mice, in which rather than in aquarelle, genes are painted with fluorescent

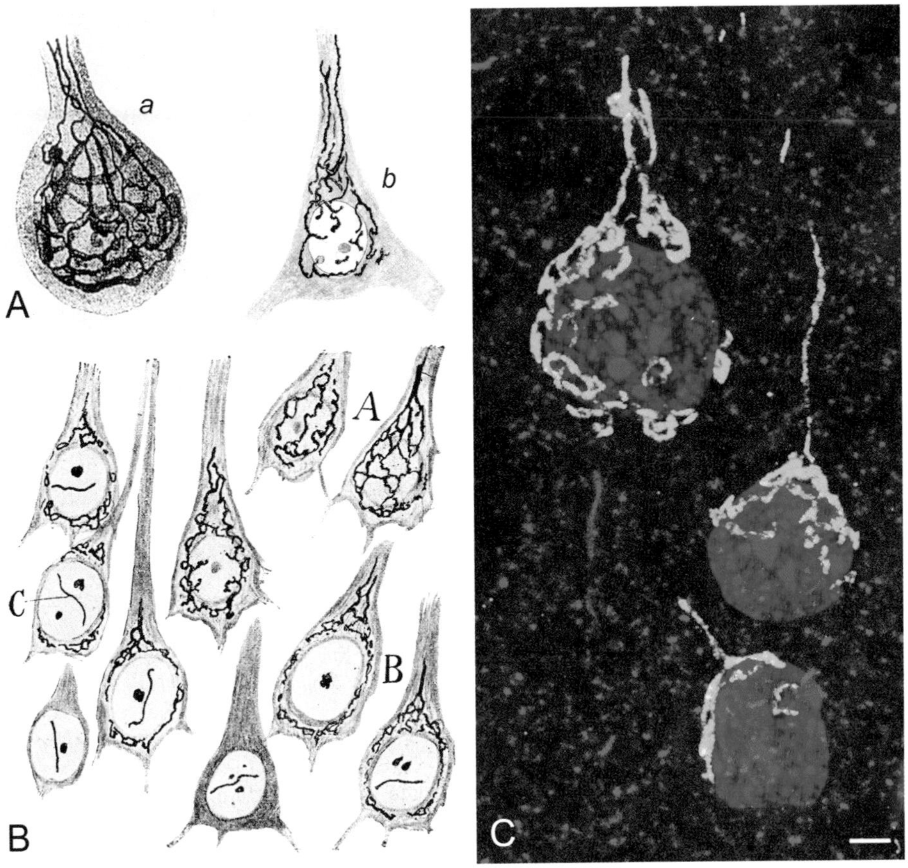

FIGURE 99. **A**, Drawings by Golgi to illustrate the *apparato reticolare interno* (internal reticular apparatus; Golgi apparatus). A first illustration of the Golgi apparatus published in 1898. Taken from Golgi (1889). Courtesy of *Sistema Museale di Ateneo - Museo per la Storia dell'Università di Pavia*. **B**, Drawing by Cajal to illustrate the Golgi apparatus of pyramidal cells in deep layers of the rabbit cerebral cortex. Taken from the book *Histologie du système nerveux de l'homme et des vertébrés* (Cajal 1909–1911). **C**, Photomicrograph obtained with a confocal microscope of a section of the rat somatosensory cortex (layer V) stained with DAPI (blue) and, in addition, double-stained using antibodies directed against the protein synaptopodin (red) and the Golgi complex using the antibody GM130 (green). Calibration bar: 3 μm. Taken from Anton-Fernández et al. (2015). Figure taken from DeFelipe (2014).

proteins—a great revelation for literary and artistic inspiration for a grapheme-color synesthete like Nabokov and also an insight, for those without synethesia, into what it feels like to see bright colors where such colors would usually be lacking.

This world of colors and shapes clearly represents an aesthetic stimulus for the eyes of both scientists and artists, and at the same time a source of inspiration. For example, as mentioned in the book *El Jardín de la Neurología* (DeFelipe, 2014), I do not know why Cajal used the word *mariposa* (butterfly), but during the presentation of my book Cajal's *Butterflies of the Soul* at the congress of the Society for Neuroscience held in Chicago, Illinois, United States, in 2009, one of the attendees, Alan Kay (professor of biology at the University of Iowa, United States) told me that in ancient Greek, *butterfly* is also "psyche" and symbolizes the soul. Because Cajal had a great interest in art and there are many artistic representations of psyche, perhaps he was aware of the relationship between the psyche and the butterfly. Thus, pyramidal cells—that is, the butterflies of the soul of Cajal—would be the main elements responsible for mental activity. Reflecting on this relationship, the painting by François Gérard (1770–1837) *Cupid and Psyche* (Figure 108, *left*) is truly inspiring because, in addition to representing a metaphysical allegory (the union of the human

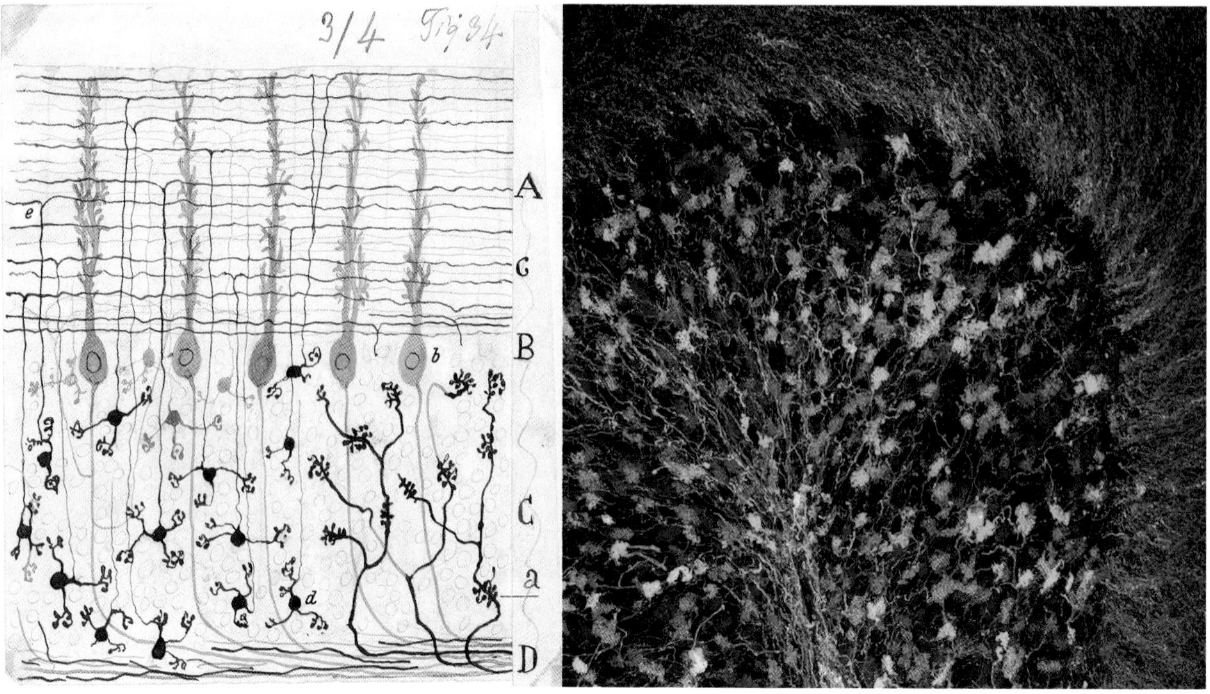

FIGURE 100. *Left*, Drawing by Cajal of the cerebellar cortex stained with the Golgi method. Taken from *Recuerdos de mi vida* (Cajal, 1917b). *Right, Mossy Fiber Cascade*, image presented by Tamily Weissman and Jeff Lichtman (Harvard University, United States) to the exhibition Neuroscapes 2006 (DeFelipe et al., 2007). This color image of the cerebellum was taken from a mouse that was genetically modified to express fluorescent proteins in subsets of cells throughout the nervous system. Note that it looks like a painting by Claude Monet (1840–1926). See Note 36 for the description of this image by the authors. Figure modified from DeFelipe (2014).

soul with divine love), it is also a love story. Thus, the kiss of Cupid that prompts Psyche to fall in love could be likened to the formation of the synaptic kisses that Cajal speaks of in *Recuerdos de mi vida* (1917b) "that appear to constitute the final ecstasy of an epic love story" (pages 42–43), allowing mental activity (the "beating of wings of butterflies"; page 68). As a perfect ending to this connection between butterflies and pyramidal cells, it turns out that Nabokov had a passion for the study of butterflies. In fact, during the 1940s he was responsible for organizing the butterfly collection of the Museum of Comparative Zoology at Harvard University, and his contributions in the field of entomology were such that one genus was named in his honor: *Nabokovia*. The last novel by Nabokov, *Look at the Harlequins!* (1974) includes a drawing of an imaginary butterfly with multiple colors (Figure 108, *center*), which he dedicated to his wife, Véra. This butterfly makes the case for the poetic relationship between the multicolored Brainbow mouse and the previously mentioned synesthesia that Nabokov had. I imagine that he might have envisaged a pyramidal cell of a Brainbow mouse as having an appearance not unlike this butterfly if Nabokov had had the opportunity to learn of the Brainbow mouse. Finally, on the bottom right of Figure 108, a drawing of a "neuronal butterfly" can be seen, inspired by the butterflies of the soul of Cajal and his drawings.

Visual artistic creativity is clearly a product of the brain, which interprets the external world by processing the information it receives through its neuronal circuits, beginning with the eyes and traveling into the brain (retina, optic nerve, thalamus, cerebral cortex, and so on). Thus, in the retina—where different markers with different colors are used to show up different types of cells and their connections (Figure 109A)—a "journey" begins into the interior of the brain through routes (nerve fibers) that connect the different parts of

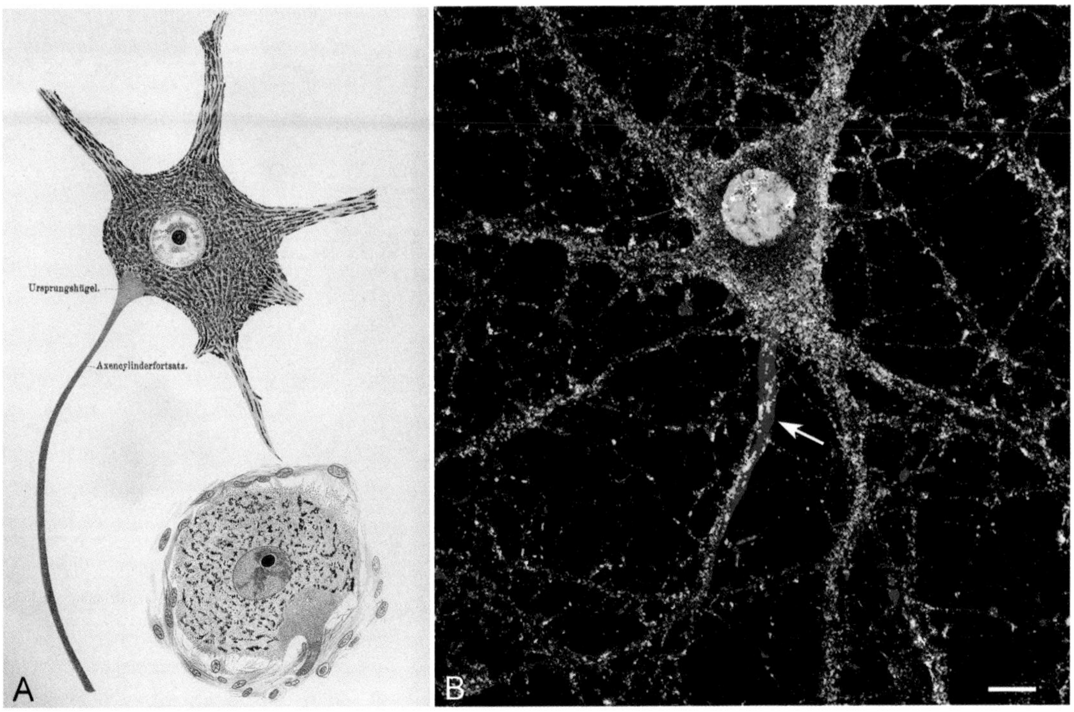

FIGURE 101. **A**, Neurons of the spinal cord stained with erythrosine/methylene blue. The axon initial segment (*Axencylinderfortsatz*; prolongation of the cylinder-axis) of the cell in the upper part of the figure appears reddish. Taken from Held (1895). **B**, Photomicrograph obtained with a confocal microscope of a neuron in the hippocampus of the mouse that had grown in culture for 18 days. The cell has been stained in red with a marker for actin (phalloidin) and immunostained for α-actinin-2 (green) and antiphospho-IκBα to mark the axon initial segment (blue) (arrow). The preparation was counterstained with DAPI to visualize the neuronal nucleus (cyan). This study was conducted to examine the morphological and molecular characteristics of the axon initial segment. Note that in both cases (**A** and **B**) the axon initial segment (*Axencylinderfortsatz* in **A**; arrow in **B**) can be distinguished easily from other neuronal processes. Calibration bar: 15 μm. Taken from Sánchez-Ponce et al. (2011).

the brain. The trajectories of these fibers can be visualized in vivo as a color map that is obtained by diffusion tensor imaging (Figure 109B). It is interesting to contemplate whether this image is in some way indicative of the mental flow involved in the creative process of abstract painters or artists such as van Gogh during the creation of their paintings (Figure 109C).

As mentioned in *Butterflies of the Soul* (DeFelipe, 2010a), the similarities between scientific illustrations and some paintings created by artists make me wonder whether the artist was unconsciously painting not only what his brain was interpreting, but—to some extent—what his own brain contains. Indeed, the photomicrographic images of crystallized neurotransmitters, when visualized using polarized light microscopy, resemble the cubist paintings or abstract art of Franz Marc (1880–1916) or Juan Gris (1887–1927) (Figure 110). Figure 111 shows an artistic composite illustration comprising a collage of digital images of the major neurotransmitters in the brain (glutamate, γ-aminobutyric acid, norepinephrine, serotonin, acetylcholine, and dopamine) superimposed on a picture of a human brain. This cocktail of "colorful" neurotransmitters is intended to show that the inexhaustible artistic creativity of the human mind seems to have a parallel multicolor world within the microscopic universe of the brain.

The more art I see, the more I am amazed and the more interested I become in the striking resemblance between art that is created by our brain and the natural beauty of its neural landscapes, especially when the artist produces such art inadvertently. In addition to the examples described previously, the

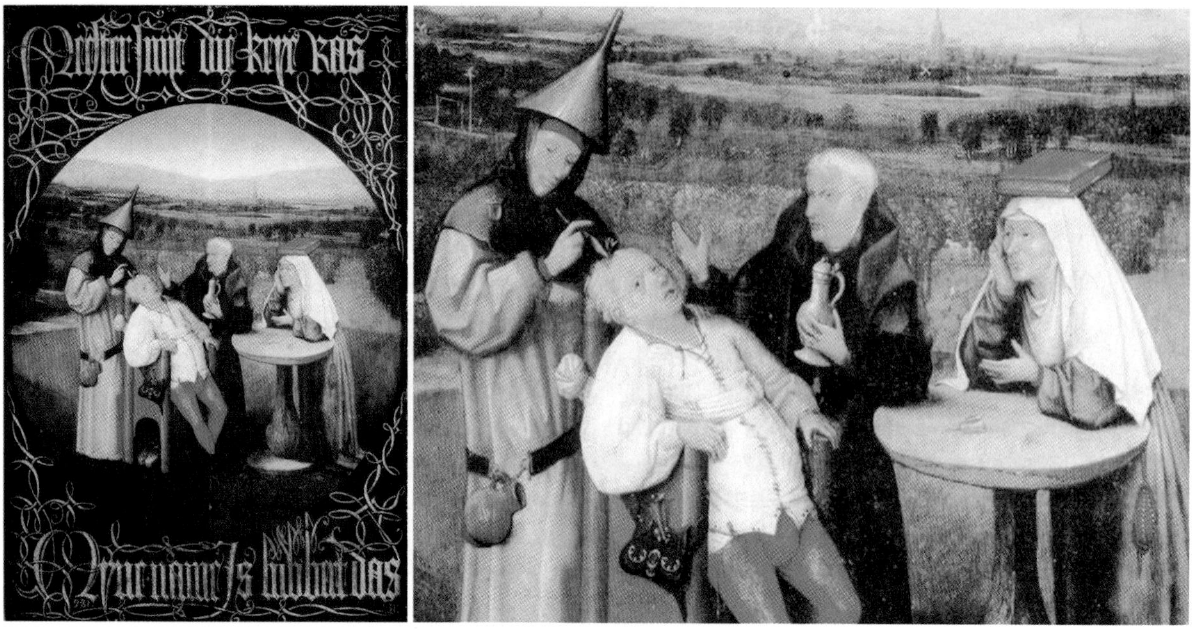

FIGURE 102. *Extracting the Stone of Madness* by El Bosco (1490). *Right*: Detail showing the central theme of the work. In the painting, a supposed healer appears with an upside-down funnel on his head (figurative representation of madness that appears in many medieval representations of individuals who have lost their mind). This seems to suggest that it is in fact him who is crazy rather than the patient. The supposed surgeon removes the "stone of madness" from the head of an individual facing the viewer of the painting. However, it is noteworthy that what is extracted is a flower, a tulip (similar to the one that is on the table). A dagger can be seen passing through his purse, which is a symbol of his scam. A monk and a nun also appear; the cleric, holding a pitcher, seems to bless the surgery, whereas the nun has a closed book on her head, which could represent an allegory to superstition and ignorance that was often attributed to the clergy. According to some scholars of this work, the circular central theme of the painting could represent a mirror reflecting those who believe they are in possession of knowledge, but that, ultimately, are more ignorant than those who intended to have their illness cured. The legend that is written on the painting says on the top *Meester snijt die keye ras* (Master, rid me of this stone soon) and, at the bottom, *Myne name is lubbert das* (My name is Lubbert Das). Lubber Das was a satirical character of Dutch literature representing stupidity, so the character of the picture might be saying "my name is fool." Taken from DeFelipe (2014).

theme of the grapevines by Cristóbal Guerra, illustrated at the top of Figure 112, are particularly interesting. These paintings are remarkably similar to images obtained today with the confocal microscope when studying the microanatomical alterations in Alzheimer's disease of the most typical and abundant neurons of the cerebral cortex: the pyramidal cells. The dendrites of these neurons have dendritic spines (bottom of Figure 112), which are key in the processes of memory, learning, and cognition (see Section A, "Dendritic spines"). This figure shows the contact between the amyloid plaques (red), typical of the disease, and dendritic spines (green), causing the alteration of the dendritic spines, which has been related to cognitive decline (e.g., Merino-Serrais et al., 2013). It is interesting to recall an unexpected, eye-opening moment that occurred during a talk I gave in Las Palmas de Gran Canaria. The artist Cristóbal Guerra, who was in the audience, was absolutely amazed by the similarity between his work and the amyloid plaques, and he told me that his mother was suffering from Alzheimer's disease!

Also, as can be seen in Figure 113, these amyloid plaques bear a striking resemblance to the nebulae and other objects observed in the universe. Indeed, the similarity between these celestial bodies and the plaques that appear in the brain of Alzheimer's patients is overwhelming, because it makes us think about the relationship between the macrocosm and microcosm. It is both strange and intriguing to think about this not only in terms of this clear similarity, but also in terms of the huge differences in scale. Although certain objects in the macrocosm, such as nebulae and black holes, have formidable

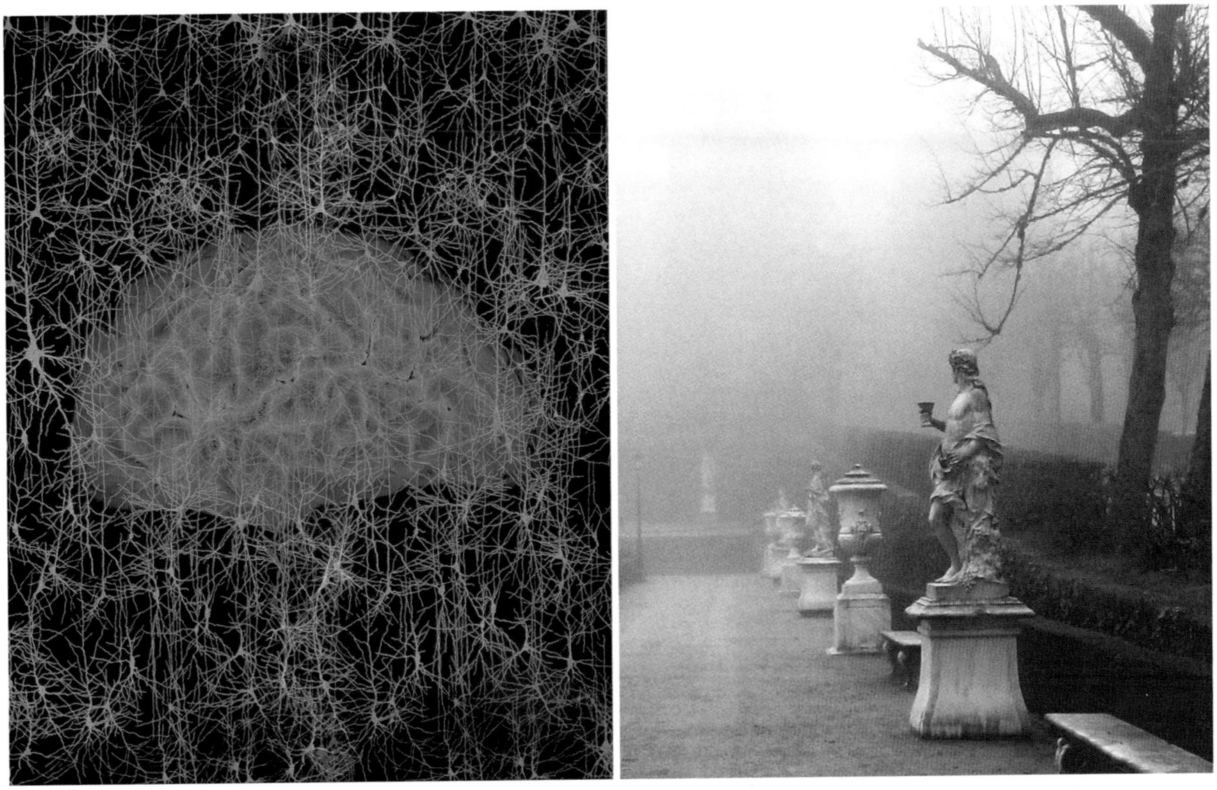

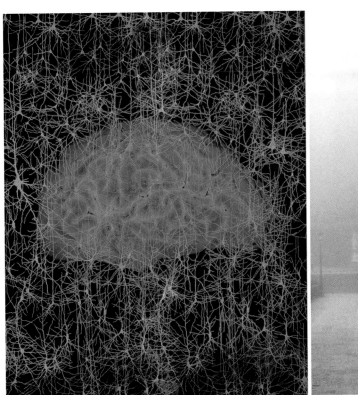

FIGURE 103. *Left*, Artistic composition showing a brain in the center that seems to emerge from the neurons in the image. *Right*, *Niebla* (2012) gardens of the *Granja de San Ildefonso* (Segovia, Spain). Taken from DeFelipe (2014).

dimensions (hundreds to billions of kilometers), in the microcosm of the brain, these plaques are only a few thousandths of a millimeter in diameter.

Finally, as shown in Figure 114, the similarities between the images obtained with the simulation of the universe and those visualized to study the nervous system are incredible. Panels A and B illustrate, at different scales, the morphology of the dark matter distribution in the universe, based on the Millennium-XXL Simulation (http://galformod.mpa-garching.mpg.de/portal/mxxl.html). Panels C and D show some examples of images from the nervous system. Panel A resembles the distribution of microglial cells in the cerebral cortex as viewed at a relatively low magnification (panel C). Panel B resembles the myenteric plexus of the gut as seen in panel D. Note that the scale bars are in parsecs in A and B, whereas in C and D they are in micrometers (see Note 40). To put this enormous difference in scale into perspective, it highlights that the conversion factor between a millimeter and a parsec is 3.24077929e-23. This is another astonishing similarity between the macro- and microcosm, and between certain aspects of the structure of the inert matter and the "intelligent matter" of the nervous system. We can only imagine what Cajal, who was fond of astronomy, might have made of these similarities. Metaphorically, it could be said that the similarity may reflect that, as the nervous system originates from the dust of stars, it in some way retains certain patterns of the organization of the universe.

It is perhaps fitting to finish with some words from Cajal, who once described the brain as being "rightly considered the masterpiece of creation." While reflecting on astronomy, death, and the human brain, he said (Cajal, 1917b, page 167):

> And what a distressing indifference of nature it is to abandon [in death] the masterpiece of creation, the sublime cerebral mirror, where it would appear that matter and [cosmic] force become aware of themselves!

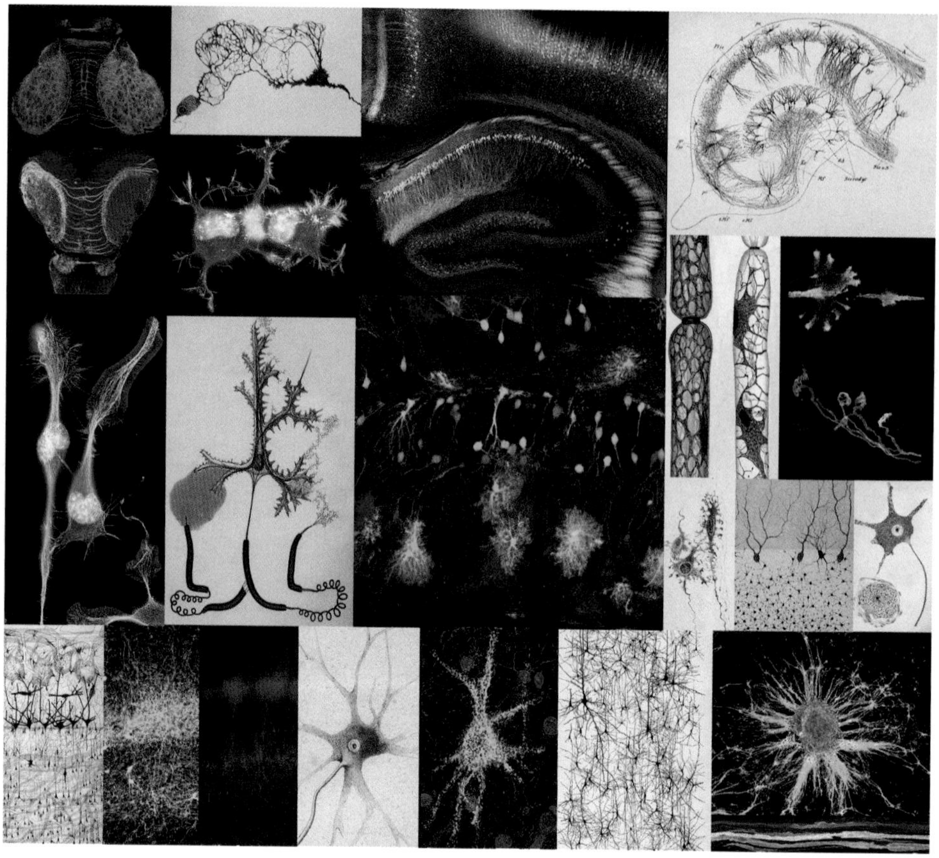

FIGURE 104. Combination of images of the nervous system composed of both drawings from early neuroscientists and modern images from several neuroscience laboratories around the world, illustrating current concepts and important discoveries in the field of neuroscience in an attractive and colorful way. Taken from DeFelipe et al. (2007).

Summary, Final Considerations, and Concluding Remarks

As described earlier in this book, the illustrations on which scientists to convey what they saw to the readers of their articles were often deemed to be artistic impressions that lacked accuracy, as opposed to exact copies of the histological image viewed—an issue that continues to hinder their interpretation to this very day. This early period in the history of neuroscience was as fascinating as it was controversial. It was a time that was associated with scientific "art" and skepticism, because these drawings required such artistic talent but also gave rise to such different interpretations. In *Textura* (Cajal, 1899–1904; Vol. 1, 1899, page X), Cajal emphasized just how important these drawings were and why:

> In an anatomical book the illustrations are almost more essential than the text: the [illustrations] represent the objective element, that is, nature, while the [text] represents the subjective element, in other words the author, whose intelligence constantly tends to distort and simplify the external reality due to the fatalism of brain organization. A good drawing, like a good microscope preparation, is a fragment of reality, scientific documents that indefinitely maintain their value and whose study will always be useful, whatever interpretation they might inspire.

Nowadays, microphotography and digital drawings are, of course, virtually the only methods used to illustrate microscopic observations. Certainly, microphotography allows a more reliable illustration of the microscopic world, is much less time-consuming compared with drawings, and has the added advantage that it is not necessary to have artistic skills. However, an important aspect of drawings,

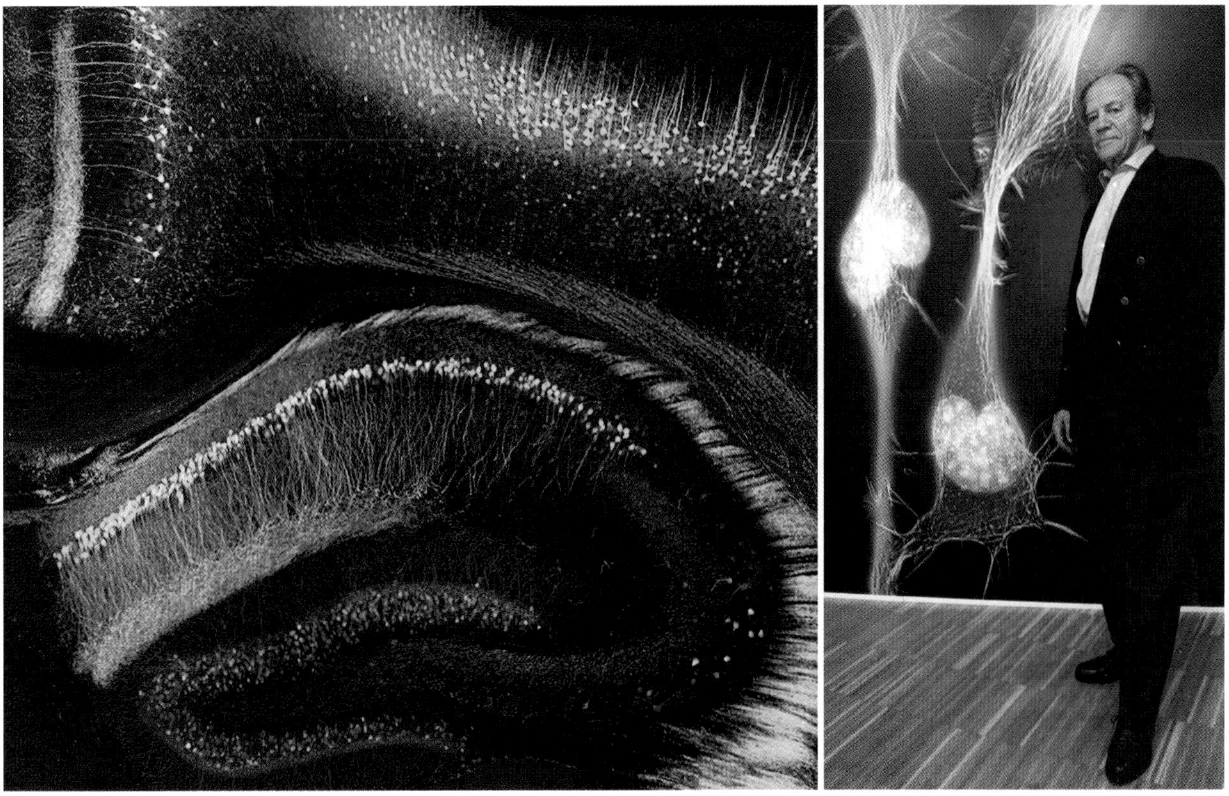

FIGURE 105. *Left,* Hippocampus with cortex of a mouse genetically modified to express fluorescent proteins (red, green, or yellow) in subsets of cells. Presented by Tamily Weissman and Jeff Lichtman (Harvard University, United States) to the exhibition Neuroscapes 2006 (DeFelipe et al., 2007). Note that the image looks like a painter's palette. See Note 37 for the description by the authors. *Right,* Photograph of Torsten Wiesel during the inauguration of Neuroscapes 2006 (kindly provided by *Diario Médico*; photograph taken by Rafa Marín). The image that is displayed in the background is a fluorescent light micrograph of in vitro differentiating mouse neuroblastoma cells. Torsten Wittmann (University of California, United States) presented this image in the exhibition Neuroscapes 2006 (DeFelipe et al., 2007).

which usually goes unnoticed, is that they provide the researcher with a more detailed observation of the microscopic world.

During his speech when joining the *Academia de Ciencias Exactas, Físicas y Naturales* (Academy of Exact, Physical and Natural Sciences) given on December 5, 1897, titled "*Fundamentos racionales y condiciones técnicas de la investigación biológica*" (which was also published in successive editions with additional and corrected content titled *Reglas y consejos sobre investigación científica*), Cajal wrote (Cajal, 1897a, page 19):

> If our study is concerned with an object related to Anatomy, Natural History, etc., observation will be accompanied by illustration because, in addition to other advantages, the act of copying something disciplines and strengthens attention. It forces us to examine the entire phenomenon, thus preventing the details that commonly go unnoticed in ordinary observation from escaping our attention.

As we have seen in this book and in Cajal's *Butterflies of the Soul* (DeFelipe, 2010a), many of the illustrations of these great scientists and artists can be considered to belong to artistic movements, such as modernism, surrealism, cubism, abstractionism, and impressionism. Therefore, although these early drawings are clearly of great value because of the fact that they form the basis of our current understanding of the microanatomy of the nervous system, they also represent an appealing bridge between art and neuroscience. Indeed, the neuronal forest that constitutes our brain has served as a never-ending source

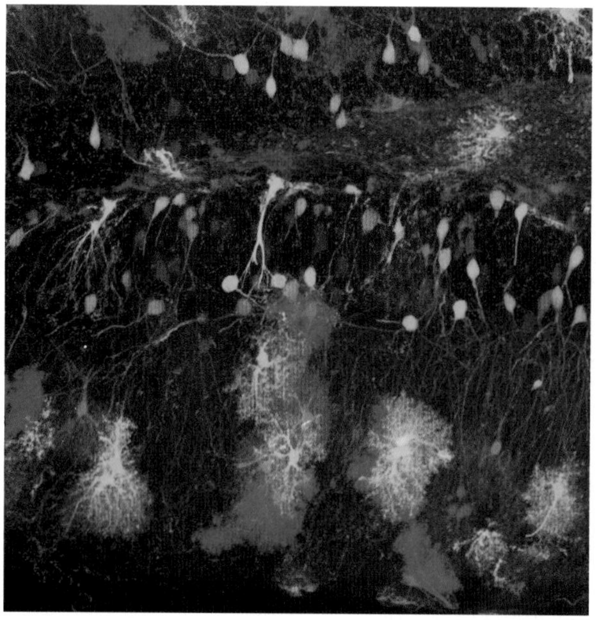

FIGURE 106. Hippocampus of a Brainbow mouse. This image was presented by Jean Livet, Joshua R. Sanes, and Jeff W. Lichtman (Harvard University, United States) to the exhibition Neuroscapes 2006 (DeFelipe et al., 2007) and resembles a painting by Renoir. See Note 38 for the description of this image by the authors.

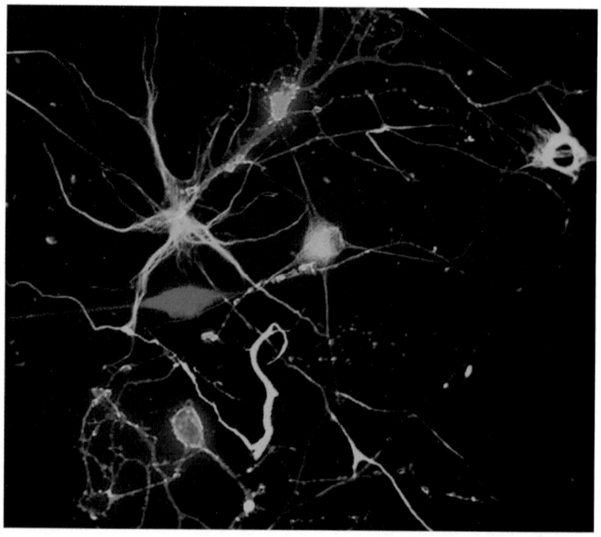

FIGURE 107. Neurosphere progeny from the adult human subventricular zone. This image was presented by Nader Sanai (University of California, United States), Alfredo Quiñones-Hinojosa (Johns Hopkins University, United States), Jose Manuel García-Verdugo (Universidad de Valencia, Spain), and Arturo Álvarez-Buylla (University of California, United States) to the exhibition Neuroscapes 2006 (DeFelipe et al., 2007). This figure looks like a painting by Miró. See Note 39 for the transcription of the legend.

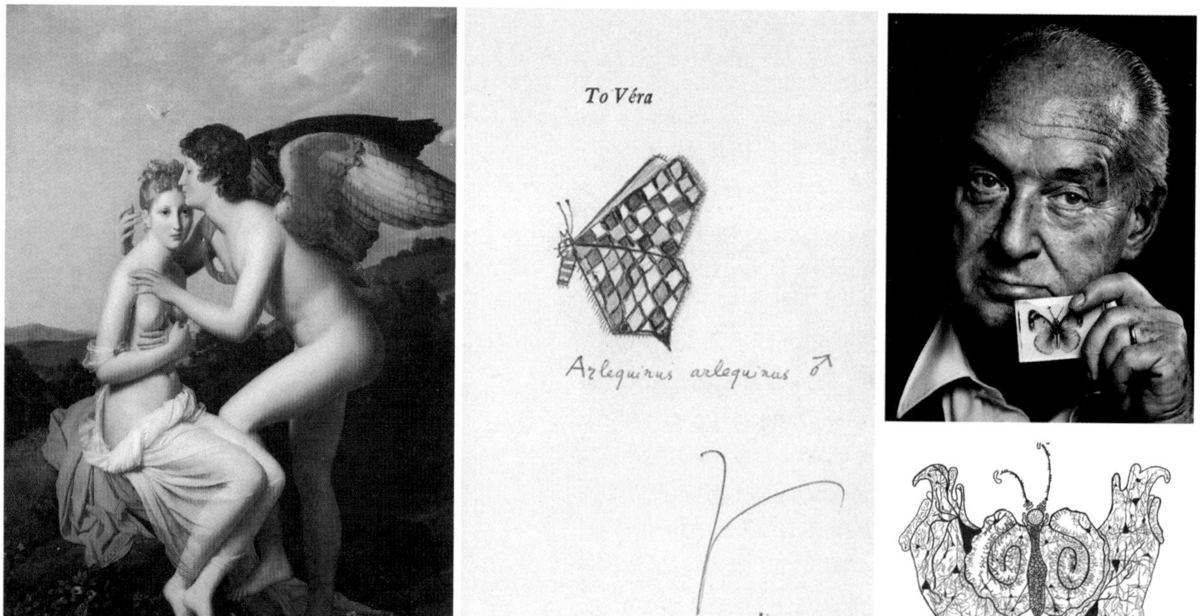

FIGURE 108. *Left, Cupid and Psyche,* also known as Psyche receiving Cupid's first kiss (1798), by François Gérard (1770–1837) (Louvre, Paris). The beautiful young princess Psyche is surprised by the first kiss of Cupid, son of the goddess Venus, who is invisible to her but awakens her love. A symbolic butterfly hovers over Psyche's head, which, besides symbolizing the soul, signifies the transformation from mortal to goddess that Psyche had to undergo to marry Cupid (the butterfly is also a symbol of transmutation). *Center*: drawing of an imaginary butterfly (with the fictitious name *Arlequinus arlequinus*) dedicated to Véra, wife of Nabokov, which appears in the book *Look at the Harlequins!* (Nabokov, 1974); Division of Rare and Manuscript Collections, Cornell University Library, United States. *Top right*, Photograph of Vladimir Nabokov holding a butterfly. *Bottom right, Mariposa Neuronal* (*Neuronal Butterfly*). Drawing by Débora Cano from the laboratory of Javier DeFelipe. Taken from DeFelipe (2014).

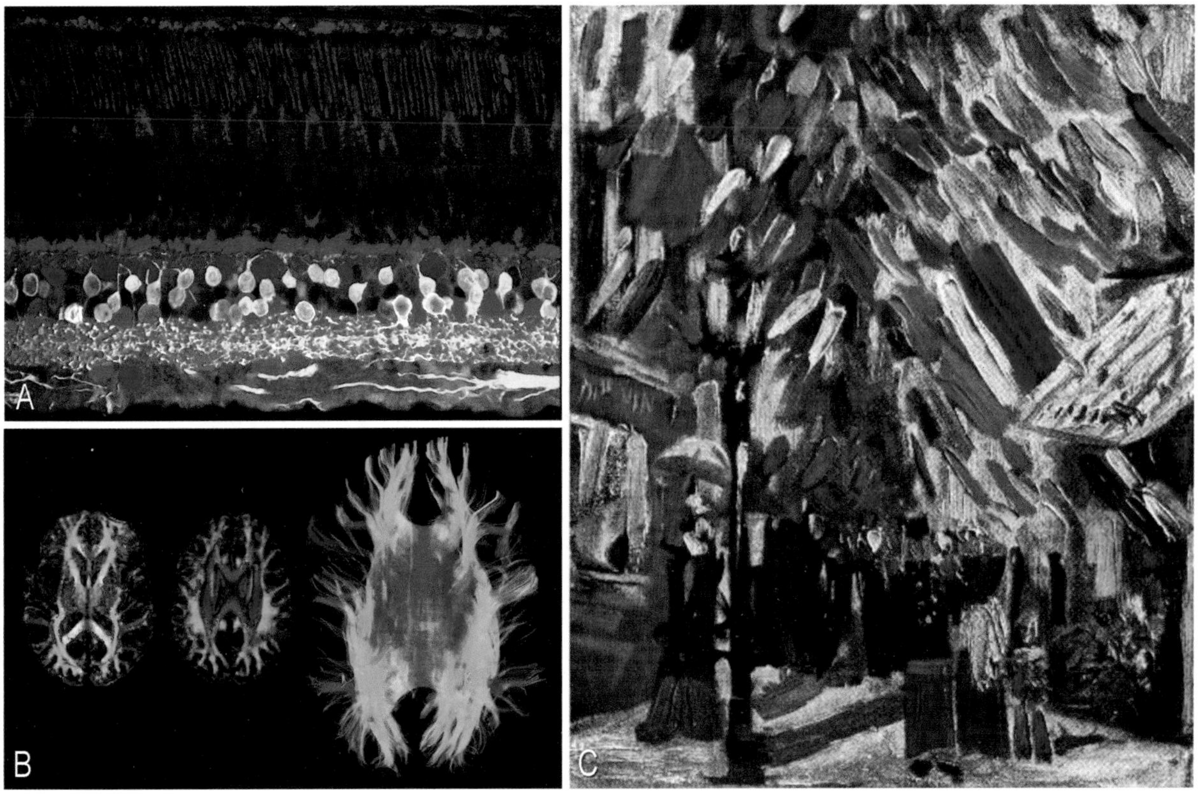

FIGURE 109. **A**, *Monkey Retina Cell Types* by Nicolás Cuenca and Gema Martínez-Navarrete (Universidad de Alicante, Spain), presented to the exhibition Neuroscapes 2006 (DeFelipe et al., 2007). This image is a confocal microscopy photograph of a monkey retinal section triply immunolabeled with antibodies against α-synuclein (red), calretinin (blue), and glycine (green) showing all retinal cell types and their connections. **B**, *Multicolored Brain*. Images showing bundles of fibers of human brain obtained with sequential diffusion tensor imaging on a 3-Tesla magnetic resonance (HDxt, GEHC), which is used extensively to map white matter tractography in the brain; *left* and *center*, panoramic images at different levels of the brain. *Right*, High-magnification image to illustrate the fibers of the corpus callosum and the superior longitudinal fasciculus. These techniques make it possible to determine the direction of the fiber tracts of the white matter. The color indicates the direction of the fibers (red, transversal; green, anteroposterior; blue, superior–inferior). Image courtesy of Juan Álvarez-Linera Prado, Fundación CIEN-Fundación Reina Sofía, Madrid. **C**, Multicolor painting by van Gogh, *The Fourteenth of July Celebration in Paris*. Taken from DeFelipe (2014).

of artistic and poetic inspiration to many scientists—not only at the time of Cajal, but also in the present day. No doubt the discovery of the method of Golgi represented a major innovation that facilitated the study of the nervous system. However, many other early methods—as well as modern techniques—of course yield very important results, while also providing us with beautiful, multicolor images of the brain. This world of colors and shapes represents an aesthetic visual stimulus for both scientists and artists and, at the same time, a rich source of inspiration. It is amazing to think that nature serves as a starting point for the aesthetic creativity in some artistic movements such as impressionism, in which it is transformed into an imaginary colorful world, and that—through our studies—a similar multicolor world with infinite shapes has been revealed in our own brain! It is as if the intangible, imaginary world of the artist comes true or is materialized in the very brain that has created it. As a consequence, in recent years there has been increasing interest in the link between the study of the brain and art, giving rise to numerous exhibitions around the world. These exhibitions not only serve to show the general public the sheer beauty of the brain, but also play a key role in disseminating neuroscience—with all of its charms and all of is challenges. The cells in our brain seem to constitute a thick forest, a seemingly

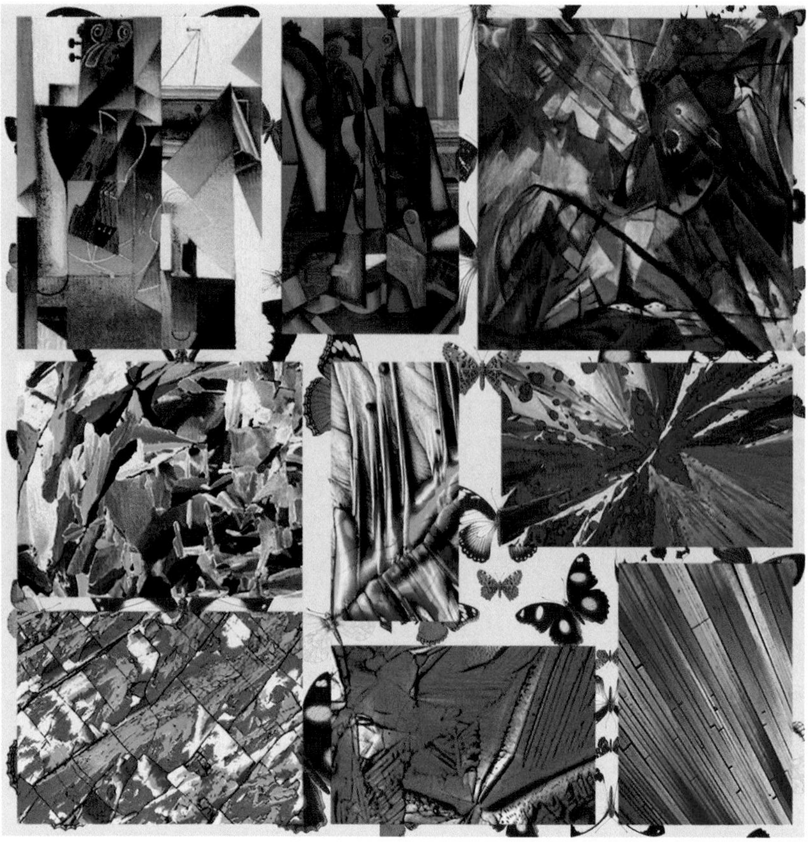

FIGURE 110. *From left to right, first row*: Paintings by artists Juan Gris (1887–1927; the first two pictures are *Violin and Engraving*, 1913, and *Violin and Guitar*, 1913, respectively) and Franz Marc (1880–1916; *Tyrol*, 1914). *Second row*, Polarized light photomicrographs showing glutamate, norepinephrine, and dopamine, respectively. *Third row*, Polarized light photomicrographs showing γ-aminobutyric acid, serotonin, and acetylcholine. Note the resemblance of the art and image of the neurotransmitters. Pictures of polarized light microscopy provided by Michael W. Davidson (Florida State University, United States). Modified from DeFelipe (2014).

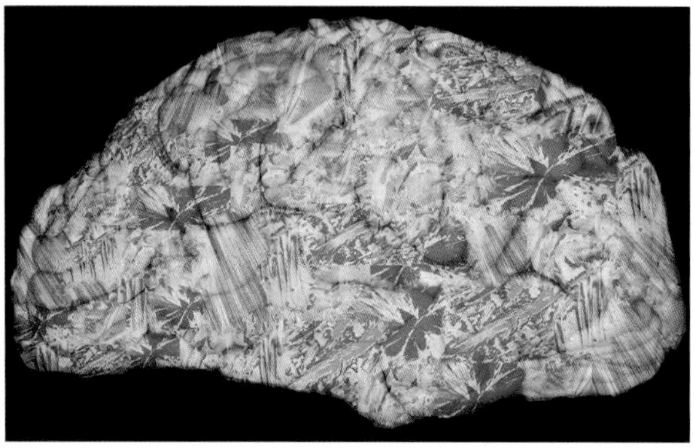

FIGURE 111. Artistic representation of the human brain in which the colors represent the major neurotransmitters found in the brain (see Figure 110). Taken from DeFelipe (2014).

impenetrable terrain of interacting cells that mediate cognition and behavior. However, thanks to the discovery and development of a variety of techniques from the times of Cajal up to the present day, the explorers of the brain are uncovering its mysteries little by little and discovering a wonderful new artistic world.

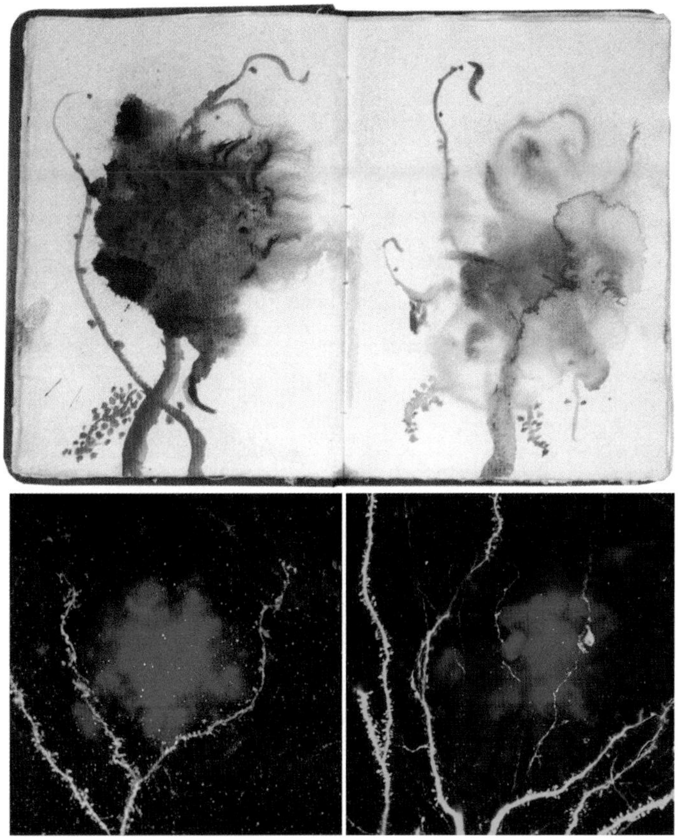

FIGURE 112. *Top panel*, Oil paintings of grapevines by Cristóbal Guerra (Guerra, 2009). *Lower panel*, Images taken with a confocal microscope to show the dendrites with spines (green) of pyramidal cells in the cerebral cortex of a double transgenic APP/PS1 mouse. In the brain of these mice, plaques develop that contain the peptide beta-amyloid (red; labeled with Congo Red), making these animals suitable for use as models for the study of Alzheimer's disease. Pyramidal cells were injected intracellularly with Lucifer Yellow (a fluorescent marker) that diffuses inside the neuron, allowing visualization of the complete cell morphology. These experiments are performed both in experimental animals and in autopsies from Alzheimer's patients to study how changes in the pyramidal cells are associated with cognitive impairment in this disease. The images were obtained in my laboratory by Ruth Benavides-Piccione. Taken from DeFelipe (2014).

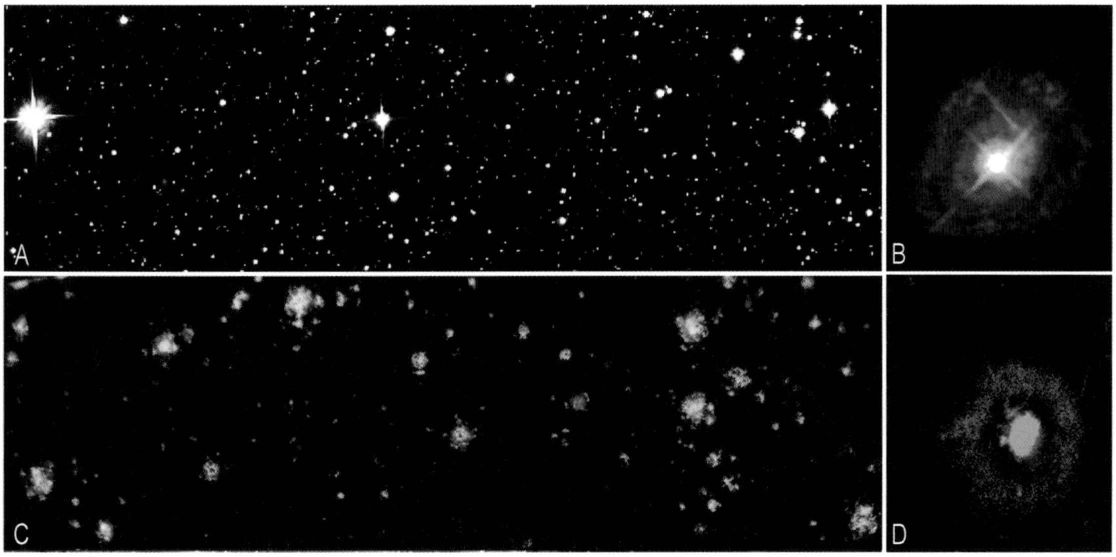

FIGURE 113. **A**, Image of space, from part of the photograph *Infant Stars in the Small Magellanic Cloud* (NASA, ESA, and A. Nota [STScI/ESA]). **B**, Image of a black hole titled *Anatomy of a Black Hole's Surroundings Revealed: Major Study Includes Observations with NASA's Hubble Space Telescope* (NASA, ESA, G. Kriss [STScI], and J. de Plaa [SRON Netherlands Institute for Space Research]). **C**, Panoramic photograph of amyloid plaques in the hippocampal formation of a patient with Alzheimer's disease. **D**, Detail of one of these plaques at higher magnification. Taken from DeFelipe (2014).

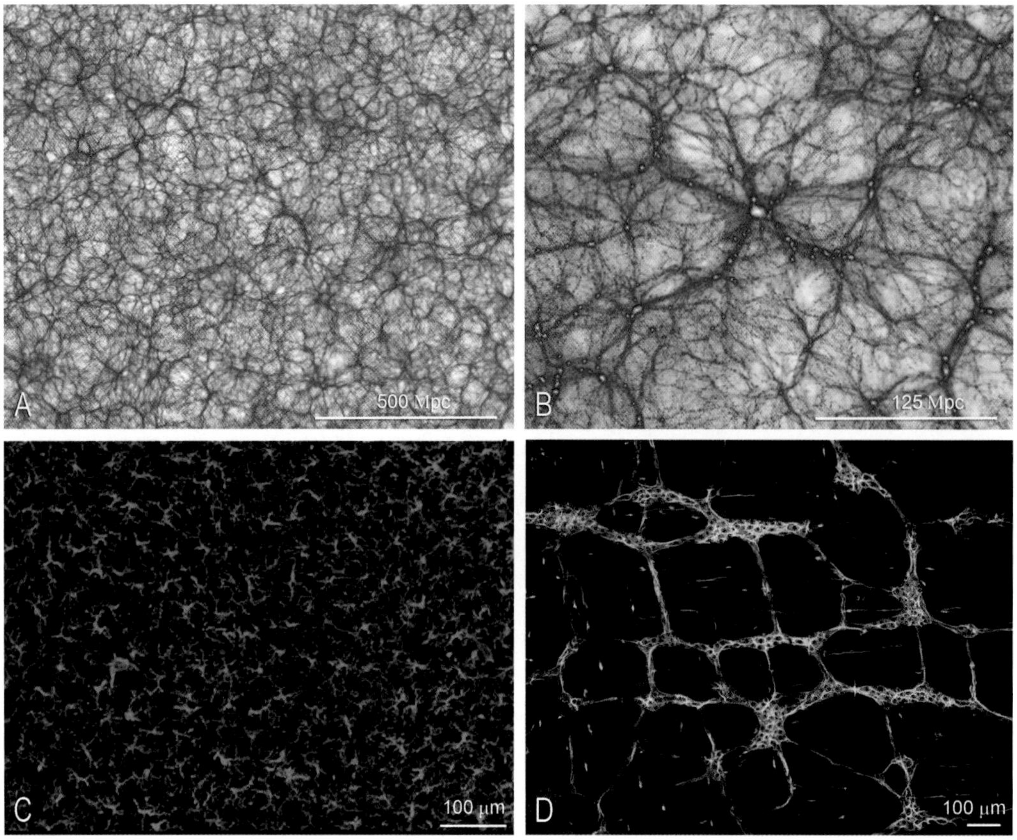

FIGURE 114. **A**, **B**, The dark matter distribution in the universe at the current time is shown, based on the *Millennium-XXL Simulation*, one of the largest N-body simulations carried out thus far (more than 10^{11} particles). The images highlight the morphology of the structure on different scales. Note that the filamentary structures that join high-density regions, which appear as yellow shading in **B**, look like neuronal connections. The high-density regions are predicted to host luminous galaxies. mpc, megaparsecs (10^6 parcecs; see Note 40). These images were kindly supplied by Raúl Angulo (Angulo et al., 2012). **C**, Photomicrograph, obtained with a confocal microscope, of a section of the mouse somatosensory cortex immunostained using the anti-antibody anti-Iba1 to label microglia cells (pseudocolored in blue). **D**, Photomicrograph showing a whole-mount preparation of the mouse distal colon myenteric plexus. Glia are labeled in blue by the fluorescent dipeptide derivative Ala-Lys-AMCA and in green by antiglial fibrillary acidic protein (conjugated with Cy2). Enteric neurons are labeled in red by the panneuronal marker anti-Hu. Note intracellular accumulation of Ala-Lys-AMCA in cells located between the meshes of ENS ganglia and nerve strands. Immunohistochemically, these cells are immunopositive for macrophage markers, and hence correspond to tissue-resident macrophages. The pattern of Ala-Lys-AMCA uptake provides evidence for the expression of functional PEPT2 transporters in enteric glial cells and tissue-resident macrophages in the ENS. Calibration bar is 100 μm. Figure and legend by Anne Rühl and Michael Schemann (Technical University of Munich, Germany).

1. Neurolab was a National Aeronautics and Space Administration (NASA) research mission to study how the nervous system responds in microgravity—a fundamental question for future long-duration space flights. Neurolab was born when the US president declared the 1990s the Decade of the Brain, and NASA proposed the Neurolab mission as its contribution. Other international space agencies also participated in the Neurolab mission. The seven-member crew was not only involved in various experiments with animals (rats, mice, fish, snails, and crickets) aboard the Space Shuttle *Columbia*, but also they were subjected to a number of sophisticated biomedical studies themselves. The shuttle was launched on April 17, 1998, and it landed on May 4, 1998, at Kennedy Space Center in Cape Canaveral, Florida. The shuttle reached an altitude of approximately 320 km above the planet's surface and traveled at a speed of approximately 7.5 km/s. Because the shuttle orbited Earth every ninety-two minutes, during the sixteen-day spaceflight there were sixteen sunsets and sixteen sunrises every twenty-four hours. Accordingly, the shuttle completed a total of 256 orbits around Earth.
2. Figure 1. Segmentum transversam e cornu Ammonis cuniculi petitum, circiter centies amplificatum. a.a.a. Hujus organi superficies lihera epithelio obtecta, quae in ventriculi lateralis cavum spectat. b.b.b. Gyrus in hemisphaerii superficie interna situs, qui fasciae dentatae apud hominem respondet. c.c.c. Transitus cornus Ammonis folii superioris in gyrum hippocampi; af. af. folium superius, bf.bf. folium inferius (cornus Ammonis.). f'. Introitus fissurae inter fasciam dentatam et gyrum hippocampi. f. Continuatio hujus flssurae inter ambo cornus Ammonis folia. fi. Fimbria. α. Stratum fibrarum nervearum. β. Stratum moleculare primum. γ. Stratum cellulosum. γ'γ'. Cellulae dispersae in cornus Ammonis folio inferiore et in eo loco ubi hujus organi folium superius in gyrum hippocampi transit. δδ. Stratum a peripheria ad cetrum striatum. δ'. Decussatio processuum cellularum. εε. Stratum reticulare. ζζζ. Stratum moleculare secundum. ηηη. Stratum granulosum. ϑϑϑ Fibrae e granis prodeuntes. ii. Fibrae e strato reticulari prodenntes, quae in gyri hippocampi superficiem tendunt. vv. Vas sanguiferum.
   Kupffer, G. (1859) *De cornus ammonis textura disquisitiones praecipue in cuniculis institutae. Dissertatio Inauguralis.* Universitate Literarum Caesarea Dorpatensi. Dorpati Livonorum: Typis Viduae (J.C. Schünmanni et C. Mattieseni).
3. *I singoli elementi riprodotti in questa tavola, vennero punto per punto con esattezza scrupolosa disegnati coll'aiuto della camera chiara di Oberhauser.* Il disegno rappresenta, semischematicamente, a 250 diametri circa di ingrandimento, un frammento di sezione verticale di un bulbo olfattorio di un cane. I tre diversi strati dell'organo sono indicati colle lettere *A B C* poste a lato. *A*, indica lo strato superficiale del bulbo, o strato delle fibre nervose periferiche. Esso vedesi essenzialmente costituito dai fasci di fibre nervose provenienti dalla mucosa olfattoria. Questi fasci, fra loro incrociandosi, si dirigono verso i glomeroli olfattori, entro i quali penetrano (in *a a a*), e si suddividono finamente. In mezzo agli stessi fasci si scorge anche un vaso sanguigno, che invia verticalmente verso l'interno dell'organo varie diramazioni. *B*, indica lo strato medio, o strato di sostanza grigia. Al confine periferico di questo stanno i glomeroli olfattori; al confine interno trovansi invece le grandi cellule nervose, disposte in regolare serie. Il prolungamento essenzialmente nervoso (*b b b*) (prolungamento-cillinder-axis) di queste ultime cellule, appare, con regola invariabile, verticalmente diretto verso gli strati interni del bulbo; i prolungamenti protoplasmatici (*b' b' b'*) si portano invece verso i glomeroli nei quali penetrano e si ramificano complicatamente. Quest'ultimo andamento nel disegno vedesi riprodotto soltanto per uno dei prolungamenti (*b''*). Verso il mezzo di questo medesimo strato *B* vennero disegnate anche due grandi cellule nervose solitarie fusiformi, il cui prolungamento nervoso, colorato in azzurro, scende,

ramificandosi, nello strato delle fibre nervose. All'ingiro dei glomeroli veggonsi alcune cellule nervose piccole. Di queste i prolungamenti rivolti verso i glomeroli hanno i caratteri dei protoplasmatici, mentre l'unico prolungamento che emana nell'opposta direzione (quello colorito in azzurro) ha i caratteri dei prolungamenti nervosi. *C*, finalmente indica lo strato interno o delle fibre nervose provenienti dal tractus. Nei vani lasciati dagli incrociantisi fasci stanno i piccoli elementi di forma prevalentemente piramidale, e di natura probabilmente nervosa. Nel mezzo dello strato veggonsi anche qui due cellule ben caratterizzate come nervose, sia per la forma e grandezza loro, sia per la presenza di un prolungamento appartenente evidentemente al tipo dei nervosi (quello colorito in azzurro). Le fibrille risultanti dalle suddivisioni di questo prolungamento s'uniscono ai fasci provenienti dal tractus. Le complicate ramificazioni delle fibre nervose vennero omesse nel disegno, perchè non risultasse troppo complicato; il modo di decorrere e di ramificarsi delle medesime fibre per altro, può essere con approssimazione rilevato verso la periferia dello strato *C*. Ivi alcune di tali fibre staccarsi dai fasci, e ramificandosi complicatamente oltrepassano con decorso tortuoso il confine della sostanza bianca, penetrano nello strato grigio, che parimenti attraversano, e molte di esse, ridotte a fibrille finissime, si ponno accompagnare fin entro i glomeroli. Lo stroma di cellule connettive venne riprodotto in modo possibilmente vicino al vero, per la quantità e pei suoi rapporti coi vasi, soltanto nelle parti profonde dello strato *C*, ove di fatto le cellule connettive raggiate sogliono essere assai numerose. Riguardo alle altre parti lo si vede soltanto accennato nella zona di confine tra la sostanza bianca e la grigia, nei glomeroli nello strato delle fibre nervose periferiche. (Veggansi le parti del disegno colorate in rosso). [I have added the letters *A, B, C*].

Golgi, C. (1875) *Sulla fina struttura del bulbi olfattorii*. Reggio-Emilia: Printer Stefano Calderini. [Reprinted from Golgi, C. (1875). Sulla fina struttura dei bulbi olfactorii. *Riv. Sper. Freniatr. Med. Leg.* 1, 405–425.]

4. Tavola XIX. *Frammento di sezione verticale di una circonvoluzione cerebellare del coniglio*. Disegno fatto a particolare illustrazione dello strato dei granuli.—Questi così detti granuli si presentano quali cellule nervose di forma globosa, piccolissime e fornite di 3, 4, 5 ed anche 6 prolungamenti, dei quali sempre uno solo offre i caratteri di prolungamento nervoso; siffatto prolungamento trova si appena accennato (filo rosso). I prolungamenti, che pare si possano chiamare protoplasmatici, sebbene si presentino in modo un po' diverso dai prolungamenti protoplasmatici delle altre cellule gangliari, finiscono con un piccolo ammasso granuloso, al quale spesso veggonsi confluire le estremità dei corrispondenti prolungamenti dei circostanti granuli. Nella zona di passaggio tra lo strato molecolare e lo strato dei granuli sono pur disegnate altre due cellule, che dalle cellule di Purkinje, a lato delle quali sono poste, si differenziano oltrechè per la forma del corpo cellulare e modo di ramificarsi dei prolungamenti protoplasmatici, anche, e sopratutto, pel contegno affatto diverso del prolungamento nervoso.—Queste due cellule appartengono al tipo che già trovasi illustrato nelle Tavole XIV e XVII.

   Golgi, C. (1882–1883) Sulla fina anatomia degli organi centrali del sistema nervoso: Rivista sperimentale di Freniatria, anni 1882–1883. In *Opera Omnia*, vol. I. *Istologia Normale* (1870–1883) 1903, 295–393. Milano: Ulrico Hoepli.

5. [*Left*] Tavola XXVIII. Figura specialmente destinata a far rilevare forma, disposizione e vicendevoli rapporti delle cellule nervose dei due strati grigi del grande piede di Hippocampo. In tutte le cellule gangliari il prolungamento nervoso venne soppresso. *a-a-a*, Strato midollare che riveste il grande piede di Hippocampo verso la superficie ventricolare. *b-b-b*, Strato grigio circonvoluto. *c-c-c*, Fascia dentata. *d-d*, Lamina midollare circonvoluta. *e*, Fascio di fibre nervose continuantesi colla fimbria e derivante dalle cellule appartenenti all'ultima porzione dello strato grigio circonvoluto. *f*, Fimbria. [*Right*] Tavola XXIX. *Sezione verticale-trasversale del grande piede di Hippocampo di gattino neonato*. Tutti i particolari come nella tavola precedente. In più qui trovasi disegnato in rosso il fascio di fibre nervose derivante dalle piccole cellule della fascia dentata e che, attraversando la zona occupata dai corpi delle cellule gangliari dello strato grigio circonvoluto, va ad unirsi alle fibre nervose della fimbria. Il contegno di questo fascio, e sopratutto il modo con cui le singole sue fibre si mettono in rapporto colle piccole cellule nervose della fascia dentata, apparirà in modo assai più chiaro nella tavola XXXI.

   Golgi, C. (1883) Sulla fina anatomia degli organi centrali del sistema nervoso: Rivista sperimentale di Freniatria, anni 1883. In *Opera Omnia*, vol. II. *Istologia Normale* (1883–1902) 1903, 397–536. Milano: Ulrico Hoepli.

6. Tavola XXX. *Frammento di sezione verticale del gran piede di Hippocampo del coniglio*. Le particolarità di struttura vi appariscono molto meno complicate che nel vero. *a–a*, Strato di fibre nervose limitante la superficie ventricolare del grande piede di *Hippocampo* (Alveus).—La superficie interna o ventricolare di tale strato, presenta un regolare rivestimento di cellule (epitelio ventricolare), il di cui corpo, che apparisce piatto verso la superficie libera, penetra più o meno profondamente nel tessuto, per suddividersi in una serie di processi, i quali, continuamente ramificandosi, si perdono a maggiore o minor distanza, in modo che non può essere con precisione

determinato.—Nel modo di comportarsi e nell'aspetto di questa singolare forma di epitelio, notasi una spiccata analogia coll'aspetto e contegno delle cellule della nevroglia. È superfluo il dire, che le fibre dell' *Alveus* invadono continuamente lo strato grigio, e che quindi fra i due strati, lungi dall'esistere il limite netto che si vede nel disegno, ha luogo invece un graduale passaggio dall'uno nell'altro. *b–b*, Strato grigio circonvoluto.—Disposizione, forma e rapporti delle cellule nervose che a tale strato appartengono.—Nello spessore del medesimo strato trovasi pure accennato, però con scarse fibrille, l'intreccio di complicata formazione, entro il quale vanno a perdersi le fibre della lamina midollare circonvoluta. *c–c*, Serie regolare di cellule nervose piccole della fascia dentata.—Il prolungamento nervoso di tali cellule è appena accennato, perchè le particolarità che lo riguardano, possono essere rilevate nelle tavole XXXI e XXXII. Degli elementi della nevroglia, che nei preparati spesso vedonsi riccamente distribuiti dapertutto, nella Tavola non ne venne disegnata che un'esigua rappresentanza.

Golgi, C. (1883). Sulla fina anatomia degli organi centrali del sistema nervoso: Rivista sperimentale di Freniatria, anni 1883. In *Opera Omnia*, vol. II. *Istologia Normale* (1883–1902) 1903, 397–536. Milano: Ulrico Hoepli.

7. Tavola XXI. *Frammento di sezione verticale di una circonvoluzione cerebellare dell'uomo*. Disegno fatto a particolare illustrazione dello stroma connettivo (*neuroglia*) dei tre diversi strati delle circonvoluzioni del cervelletto.—Lo strato molecolare vedesi attraversato da fasci di fibrille, derivanti da cellule connettive situate o al limite profondo dello strato medesimo, od anche più profondamente entro lo strato dei granuli.—Lo strato *limitante* di cellule connettive piatte della superficie libera non trovasi disegnato. Nello strato dei granuli le cellule connettive raggiate trovansi irregolarmente disseminate, per altro spiccano sempre i rapporti che tali elementi hanno colle pareti dei vasi; la connessione di quelli con questi o è diretta, essendo i corpi cellulari applicati sulle stesse pareti vasali, delle quali spesso direbbesi che fanno parte, oppure si effettua mediante più o meno robusti prolungamenti, i quali nel punto d'inserzione presentano una tenue espansione, ove più ove meno estesa. Eguali particolarità, anzi più evidenti, veggonsi nello stroma connettivo dello strato midollare. Qui per altro le cellule connettive hanno in prevalenza forma appiattita e presentansi più regolarmente disposte, in rapporto colla più o meno regolare disposizione in fasci delle fibre nervose. I vasi sanguigni che, ramificandosi, dalla superficie penetrano nell'interno della circonvoluzione, sono disegnati in tinta molto sbiadita, affinché più chiaramente appariscano gli elementi connettivi.

   Golgi, C. (1882–1883) Sulla fina anatomia degli organi centrali del sistema nervoso: Rivista sperimentale di Freniatria, anni 1883. In *Opera Omnia,* vol. I. *Istologia Normale* (1870–1883) 1903, 295–393. Milano: Ulrico Hoepli.

8. Tavola XX*. *Frammento di sezione verticale d'una circonvoluzione cerebellare dell'uomo*. Disegno specialmente dimostrante l'enorme complicazione di rapporti esistenti fra le fibre nervose e le cellule gangliari;—esso dev'essere qualificato come semischematico, perchè in certo modo rappresenta la sintesi di fatti dedotti dallo studio di parecchi preparati; per altro i singoli elementi disegnati, per situazione,—rapporti, forma e modo di ramificarsi delle fibre nervose e dei prolungamenti cellulari esattamente corrispondono al vero, almeno al loro modo di presentarsi nei pezzi trattati col metodo della colorazione nera. Ad onta della mancanza delle lettere indicative si possono ben distinguere i tre strati formanti le circonvoluzioni del cervelletto: *strato molecolare; strato dei granuli; strato delle fibre nervose*.

   Strato molecolare. Vi si vedono molto spiccate, per la tinta nera intensa, alcune fra le cellule nervose piccole proprie di tale strato.—Richiamo in modo speciale l'attenzione sulle molte differenze che, relativamente al punto di emanazione e contegno successivo, presenta il prolungamento nervoso (filo rosso), di cui tutte queste cellule son o provvedute. Riguardo a quelle che stanno nel terzo inferiore dello strato, deve essere notato che il medesimo prolungamento evidentemente si unisce al plesso di fibre nervose orizzontali ivi esistenti, esattamente uniformandosi, per andamento e modo di ramificarsi, alle singole fibre di cui il medesimo plesso è costituito. Nel terzo profondo dello strato è disegnata in rosso una parte del complicatissimo plesso accennato; alle fibre decorrenti parallelamente ai margini dello strato in questione s'inseriscono molte fibre che derivano dallo strato dei granuli: dalle medesime fibre emanano poi innumerevoli fibrille, che, ramificandosi con vicende svariate, si portano verso l'alto. Il plesso evidentemente non è cosi limitato come qui appare, ma s'estende a tutta la larghezza dello strato: il disegno corrisponde al suo più frequente modo di presentarsi ne'miei preparati. Lungo il margine profondo dello strato molecolare sono disegnate con tinta sbiadita alcune cellule di Purkinje. Il loro prolungamento nervoso, somministrante un certo numero di fibrille secondarie, può essere accompagnato fino allo strato delle fibre nervose.

   Strato dei granuli. Vi sono disegnati: 1.º I cosi detti granuli, però in quantità molto minore di quella che realmente esiste; il prolungamento nervoso, di cui ciascuno di questi elementi è provveduto, è appena accennato. Vuol essere notato che nell'uomo i medesimi elementi sono assai più piccoli che nel coniglio, gatto, vitello ecc. (Vedi Tav. XIX). 2.º Una cellula nervosa identica a quelle piccole dello strato molecolare è situata in alto, a livello del corpo delle cellule di Purkinje. 3.° Due cellule gangliari piuttosto grandi, l'una di forma triangolare situata verso il mezzo dello strato, l'altra di forma fusata, situata rasente allo strato midollare, Il prolungamento nervoso di queste cellule è appena accennato.—Siffatte cellule solitarie di forma svariata nel cervelletto dell'uomo sana abbastanza frequenti. *Strato delle fibre nervose.* Di tale strato non ne venne raffigurata che una sottile striscia. In mezzo alle fibre orizzontali schematicamente disegnate, se ne scorgono alcune esattamente riprodotte dal vero. Seguendo il loro decorso dal basso all'alto si vede che certunc conducono al corpo delle cellule di Purkinje, non essendo altro che altrettanti prolungamenti nervosi delle medesime, i quali conservano la loro individualità, sebbene diano origine ad alcune fibrille secondarie, e che certe altre invece, nel mentre attraversano lo strato dei granuli, si suddividono complicatamente, perdendosi in un plesso di cui è assai difficile, se non impossibile, scoprire il più fino contegno. Molte delle più spiccate ramificazioni di questa seconda categoria di fibre certamente penetrano nello strato molecolare, partecipando alla formazione del plesso ivi esistente; lo stesso accade di alcune ramificazioni delle fibrille emananti dal prolungamento nervoso delle cellule di Purkinje.

*La maggior parte delle particolarità, concernenti lo strato molecolare disegnato in questa tavola, sono riprodotte dalla tavola corredante una nota (*Sull'origine delle fibre nervose nel cervelletto*), che verrà quanto prima pubblicata dal distinto mio allievo sig. R. Fusari.

Golgi, C. (1882–1883) Sulla fina anatomia degli organi centrali del sistema nervoso: Rivista sperimentale di Freniatria, anni 1883. In *Opera Omnia,* vol. I. *Istologia Normale* (1870–1883) 1903, 295–393. Milano: Ulrico Hoepli.

9. Cajal commonly named Golgi "the sage of Pavia." The city of Pavia is where the university in which Golgi studied medicine can be found—the same university where he went on to become professor of histology and, later, rector.
10. Comatulids are marine crinoid invertebrates like sea lilies and feather stars. Phalangidas (or opiliones), also known as water harvestmen, are arachnids that superficially resemble true spiders but they have small, oval-shaped bodies and long legs. Cajal is probably referring to some neuroglial cells that when stained with the Golgi method, have a morphology that resembles these invertebrates (see Figure 32).
11. Nevertheless, Cajal was not particularly insistent on using artists' paper or another special type of paper, because many of his illustrations, including some used directly for half-tone reproduction, were drawn on notepaper and on the backs of letters or printed notices. Several examples showing these kind of papers can be seen in Part II of the book, in the gallery of original drawings by Cajal (for example, see Figure 120).
12. Tavola XLI. *Fascia dentata del grande piede di Hippocampo.* Il disegno particolarmente illustra il modo col quale un fascio di fibre nervose si mette in rapporto colle cellule gangliari della fascia dentata. Fra le fibre nervose ancora in istato di ben individualizzati elementi ed il prolungamento nervoso delle piccole cellule esiste un complicatissimo intreccio, rete nervosa.

Golgi, C. (1901) Sulla fina anatomia degli organi centrali del sistema nervoso. Lettera al Prof. Luigi Luciani [(1901) La lettera fu pubblicata in parte nel Trattato di fisiologia dell'uomo del Professore Luigi Luciani ordinario di Fisiologia nell'Universita di Roma. Milan: Societa editrice libraria.]. In *Opera Omnia.* Vol. II. *Istologia Normale* (1883–1902) 1903, 721–733. Milano: Ulrico Hoepli.

13. FIG. 14. Querschnitt durch eine Hälfte der medulla oblongata dicht vor ihrem Uebergang in den pons Varolii, mit Wurzelbündeln des nervus abducens, facialis und acusticus. *E* Fasern der Pyramiden; *R R* Raphe, rechts davon das Balkenwerk der formatio reticularis, innerhalb deren in der oberen Partie *b* schmalere, in der unteren *a* breitere Nervenprimitivfasern liegen; *Ol* (Ol. s.) Durchschnitt durch die obere Olive; *C.tr* Fasern des corpus trapezoides; *Cr.c* crura cerebelli ad medullam oblongatam mit den zahlreichen grossen Ganglienzellen, welche scheinbar zum Ursprung des Nervus acusticus *Ac* gehören; *Fac.* Nervus facialis; *F* derselbe Nerv im Querschnitt, Knie des facialis; *Abd.* Nervus abducens. Die Zeichnung ist nicht vollendet, so hätten *z.* B. bei *J* die Querschnitte der verschieden dicken Nervenfasern angegeben werden müssen, welche diese Stelle erfüllen. (Vergl. u. A. Seite 192, 231, 275.)

Deiters, O. F. K. (1865) *Untersuchungen über Gehirn und Rückenmark des Menschen und der Säugethiere*, ed. M. Schultze. Braunschweig: F. Vieweg und Sohn.

14. Tafel V. Der Grosshirnstamm.—Diese Tafel ist das Seitenstück zu der nach Buchstaben erläuterten schematischen Abbildung des Grosshirnstammes der Taf. III, daher die einleitendee Bemerkungen der bezüglichen Tafelerklärung auch hierfür nachzulesen sind. Die Bedeutung der Farben ist: Roth stellt die graue Substanz, blau die centrifugal leitenden Bahnen, hellbraun die centripetal leitenden Bahnen, gelb die aus dem Kleinhirn hervortretenden Arme und Bündel dar. Die Continuität der dargestellen Bündel und grauen Substanz tritt durch gleichfarbige Uebereinanderlagerung ihrer Querschnitte vor Augen. Der graue Boden der Rautengrube ist die Brücke hindurch nicht dargestellt, weil dadurch die Continuität des Processus cerebelli ad cerebellum unklar geworden wäre. Das in der Hirnschenkelebene Taf.

III mit vp bezeichnete Feld ist darum nicht blau gefärbt, weil gerade die fortlaufend durchgeführte Absetzung der Schleifenschichten, innerhalb der hintern Bahn des Stammes eine Grundlage der Orientirung abgibt. Auf folgende Unvollkommenheiten des Druckes mache ich aufmerksam: In der obersten, durch das verlängerte Mark gelegten Ebene, sollten die hellbraunen Fäden (Taf. III *fb fb*) gleichmässig bis an ihr hinteres Ende gefärbt sein, und ist das in derselben Ebene über den Quintusdurchschnitt nach vorn hinaus reichende Roth wegzudenken. Der äussere Contour des Vaguskernes in der zweiten Oblongatenebene (Taf. III *tr*) sollte gerade, nicht convex sein, weil hierdurch der innere Acusticuskern weggeschnitten wird. Das Vorderhorn in der untersten Oblongatenebene (entsprechend Taf. IV FIG. 6 *cra*) ist schlecht begränzt. Als Hauptobjekt der ganzen Darstellung bedarf diese Tafel hier keiner weiteren Erklärung.

Meynert, T. (1874) Skizze des menschlichen Grosshirnstammes nach seiner Aussenform und seinem inneren Bau. *Arch. Psychiatr. Nervenkr.* 4, 387–431.

15. FIG. 1. A, B, C. Trois tubes nerveux du segment périphérique du sciatique du pigeon, le troisième jour après la section.—Ces tubes, isolés après une heure de macération du nerf dans une solution d'acide osmique à 1 pour 100, ont été colorés au picrocarminate et conservés dans la glycérine substituée lentement au liquide colorant (*Voy*. p. 4). *A*, portion médiane d'un segment interannulaire, présentant un seul noyau hypertrophié *n*, entouré d'une masse de protoplasma *p*, et de gouttes de myéline teintes par l'osmium, *m*. *B*, partie centrale d´un segment interannulaire, présentant deux noyaux *n*′ *n*′, plongés dans une masse protoplasmique commune *p*. Entre les deux noyaux, le tube nerveux présente un léger rétrécissement. *C*, quatre noyaux n″ *n*″ *n*″ *n*″ se rencontrent dans un même segment interannulaire. Le protoplasma *p* qui les enveloppe n'est pas segmenté, et dans son intérieur sont également contenues des boules de myéline, *m*. FIG. 2. Deux tubes nerveux à myéline du segment périphérique du pneumogastrique du lapin, six jours après la section.—Dissociation après macération dans une solution d'acide osmique à l pour 100; coloration au moyen du picrocarminate; couservation dans la glycérine. Les portions *a a* de ces tubes, qui ne sont occupées ni par des gouttes de myéline ni par des noyaux, sont revenues sur elles-mêmes, et à leur niveau le tube nerveux est rétréci.—*n n*, noyaux proliférés des segments interannulaires; *m m*, gouttes de myéline; *g*, granulations graisseuses (*Voy*. p. 9). FIG. 3. *A, B, C.* Trois tubes nerveux du segment périphérique du sciatique du lapin, quatre jours après la section.—Même mode de préparation que pour les tubes représentés figure 2 (*Voy*. p. 9). *A*,—Le noyau *n* du segment, légèrement hypertrophié, comprime la myéline; autour de lui, le protoplasma *p*, s'étant accru, a refoulé en divers points la gaîne médullaire ou l'a complétement sectionnée. *B*, prolifération des noyaux *n* des segments interannulaires; *e*. étranglement annulaire, efacé en partie par le gonflement du protoplasma *p; m*, gaîne médullaire fragmentée. *C*, tube nerveux dont la gaîne médullaire est déprimée ou sectionnée par l'accroissement du protoplasma, et de chaque côté duquel se voient deux cellules du tissu connectif intrafasciculaire *c c* (*Voy*. p. 15). FIG. 4. Portion d'une fibre de Remak du segment périphérique du sciatique du lapin, cinq jours après la section. Mode de préparation indiqué à l'explication de la figure 2.—*n n*, noyaux hypertrophiés et légèrement étranglés; *g*, granulations graisseuses (*Voy*. p. 14). FIG. 5. Un tube nerveux de l'extrémité du segment supérieur du sciatique du rat, trois jours après la section. La figure est retournée; en *a* se trouve l'extrémité ouverte du tube sectionné, dont le calibre est occupé en grande partie par des cellules limphatiques, dans lesquelles on distingue les noyaux *n*, les granulations graisseuses et les gouttes de myéline qu'elles contiennent.—La gaîne médullaire *m* est déformée, rongée ou refoulée par les cellules lymphatiques.—*n*′ noyau du segment interannulaire.—*c c c c*. quatre cellules lymphatiques du tissu conjonctif intrafasciculaire, chargées de granulations graisseuses et de gouttes de myéline (*Voy*. p. 37). FIG. 6.—Tube nerveux du bourgeon central du nerf sciatique du lapin, quatre jours après la section. La portion qui a été dessinée a été prise un peu au-dessus de l'extrémité sectionnée. Même mode de préparation que pour les tubes représentés dans les figures précédentes.—*m*, gaîne médullaire refoulée en quelques points, mais non sectionnée par le protoplasma *p* et les noyaux proliférés *n n n* (*Voy*. p. 41). FIG. 7. Tube nerveux complétement isolé du bourgeon central du nerf sciatique du rat, trois jours après la section (*Voy*. p. 33).—*t*, terminaison de la gaîne médullaire normale; *cy*, cylindre axe strié; *p*, protoplasma granuleux qui l'entoure; *m*, portion de la gâine médullaire n'ayant subi qu'une résorption incomplète; *my*, boules de myéline; *e*, extrémité libre du cylindre axe au niveau de la section. FIG. 8.—Coupe transversale d'un des faisceaux du segmet périphérique du nerf sciatique du lapin, vingt-huit jours après la section.—Le durcissement du nerf a été obtenu par une macération d'une semaine dans une solution d'acide chromique à 2 pour 100, un séjour de vingt-quatre heures dans l'eau pour enlever l´excès du réactif et de vingt-quatre heures dans l'alcool pour donner au nerf une consistance convenable.—La coupe a été colorée au moyen du picrocarminate et elle a été montée dans le baume

du Canada après avoir été déshydratée par l'alcool et éclaircie par l'essence de girofle. (*Voy.* p. 10).—*gl*, gaîne lamelleuse; *v*, vaisseaux sanguins; *a*, gros tubes nerveux sans cylindre axe; *b*, tubes nerveux encore munis d'un cylindre axe; *t*, petits tubes nerveux sans cylindre axe; *c*, tissu conjonctif intrafasciculaire; *l*, lames intrafasciculaires. FIG. 9.—Nerf pneumogastrique du lapin enlevé soixante jours après la section, vu à l'œil nu et dessiné à sa grandeur naturelle après macération de vingt-quatre heures dans une solution d'acide osmique à 1 pour 100.—*c*, segment central; *b*, bourgeon central; *i*, segment intermédiaire on cicatriciel; *b'*, bourgeon périphérique; *p*, segment périphérique (*Voy.* p. 47). FIG. 10. Un gros tube nerveux à myéline du bourgeon central du nerf pneumogastrique du lapin, soixante-douze jours après la section, isolé après une macération de vingt-quatre heures dans une solution d'acide osmique à 1 pour 100. La gaîne médullaire du tube primitif *t* se termine par un bourgeon *b*, de l'extrémité duquel partent des tubes à myéline *t' t''* et des fibres sans myéline.—*s*, gaîne de Schwann du tube primitif formant aux tubes qui en émanent une gaîne secondaire, s' (*Voy.* p. 61). FIG. 11 et 11 *bis*. Tube nerveux du bourgeon central du nerf sciatique du lapin, quatre-vingt-dix jours après la section.—La figure 11 *bis* doit être reportée à la suite de la figure 11, de telle sorte que *a'* se continue avec *a* (*Voy*, p. 62).— Ce tube nerveux a été isolé après une macération de vingt-quatre heures dans l'acide osmique à 1 pour 100.— *t*, tube nerveux primitif entouré de sa gaîne de Schwann *s*, et se terminant par un bourgeon de sa gaîne médullaire *b*.—De l'extrémité de ce bourgeon part un tube secondaire *t'*, qui se divise et se subdivise pour donner un faisceau de tubes nerveux médullaires grêtes *F*, entouré d'une gaîne secondaire *s'*, émanation de la gaîne de Schwann; *m*, boules de myéline provenant de la gaîne médullaire de l'ancien tube.

Ranvier, L. (1878) *Leçons sur l'histologie du système nerveux*. Paris: Savy.

16. Tafel XIX. Die Abbildungen sind sämmtlich mit Hülfe der Camera lucida nach Präparaten der Retina gezeichnet, welche durch Methylenblau gefärbt und mit pikrinsaurem Ammoniak oder Ammonium-Pikrat-Osmiumsäure-Mischung fixirt worden waren. FIG. 1. Querschnitt durch die Retina. 1) Neuroepithelschicht; 2) äussere reticuläre Schicht; 3) Körnerschicht; 4) innere reticuläre Schicht; a) Membr. lim. externa; b) Stäbchen; c) Zapfen; d) grosse sternförmige Zellen mit äusseren und inneren Fortsätzen; e) bipolare Zellen mit den äusseren (horizontalen), dem intraepithelialen (f) und dem inneren Fortsatze; letzterer zerfällt in der inneren reticulären Schicht in ein Fibrillenbüschel. Reichert, Obj. 8a.

    Dogiel, A.S. (1891) Ueber die nervösen Elemente in der Retina des Menschen. *Arch. Mikrosk. Anat.* 38, 317–344.

17. Tafel XIX. Die Abbildungen sind sämmtlich mit Hülfe der Camera lucida nach Präparaten der Retina gezeichnet, welche durch Methylenblau gefärbt und mit pikrinsaurem Ammoniak oder Ammonium-Pikrat-Osmiumsäure-Mischung fixirt worden waren. Fig. 4 Fläcehenpräparat der Retina, nahe der Ora serrata. Grosse sternförmige Zellen mit den äusseren (a), den inneren (b) und den Axencylinderfortsätzen (c); d) terminale Netze, gebildet von den Verzweigungen der äusseren Fortsätze. Reichert, Obj. 8a.

    Dogiel, A.S. (1891) Ueber die nervösen Elemente in der Retina des Menschen. *Arch. Mikrosk. Anat.* 38, 317–344.

18. Tafel X. Das centrale Nervensystem von Hirudo medicinalis. FIG. 1 stellt das vierte Ganglion des Bauchstrangs, von der dorsalen Seite geseben, dar. Gez. bei Vér. Obj. 6 u. Ocul. 3 (eingeschob. Tubus). lk^1—vordere Längskommissur; lk^2—hintere Längskommissur; pz^1—vorderer lateraler peripherer Nervenzweig; pz^2—hinterer lateraler peripherer Nervenzweig; *g*—Grenzcontour des Ganglions; *pg*—Grenzcontour der Punktsubstanz; *mf*—Medianfasersystem; lf^1—longitudinale, einzeln durchziehende Nervenfasern; lf^2 ıongitudinale, durchziehende, gestreifte Bündelfasern, welche, im Ganglion in je zwei Bündel getheilt, von jedem Bündel zu den beiden peripheren Nervenzweigpaaren Aeste abgeben; nz^1—Ganglienzellen in der vorderen Partie des Ganglions, welche ihren Stammfortsatz unter Abgabe von Nebenfortsätzen durch die vordere Querkommissur in die entgegengesetzte Ganglionhälfte und weiter in den vorderen Nervenzweig hineinschicken; nz^2—Ganglienzellen in der mittleren Partie des Gangıions, welche den Stammfortsatz unter Abgabe von Nebenfortsätzen durch die hintere Querkommissur quer über das Ganglion in den hinteren Nervenzweig der entgegengesetzten Seite des Ganglions hinübersenden; nz^3—Ganglienzellen in der hinteren Partie des Ganglions, welche ihren Stammfortsatz unter Abgabe von Nebenfortsätzen durch die hintere Querkommissur in den hinteren Nervenzweig der entgegengesetzten Seite des Ganglions hinübersenden; nz^5, nz^6—Ganglienzellen, welche theils von vorn, theils von hinten her ihren Stammfortsatz in periphere Nervenzweige derselben Ganglionhälfte hineinsenden; nz^7—hinten im Ganglion und im Medianfelde belegene Ganglienzellen, welche ihren Stammfortsatz unter Abgabe von Nebenfortsätzen nach vorn hin durch das Ganglion hindurch in die vordere Längskommissur hineinsenden; *kz*—kolossale Ganglienzellen, deren Stammfortsätze nicht sichtbar sind; pf^1, pf^1a—zwei Paare von Nervenfasern, welche aus dem vorderen peripheren Nervenzweigpaare ins

Ganglion hineintreten, um sich in ihre Punktsubstanz zu verästeln und in dieser Weise zu endigen; das eine Paar (*pf*[1]) bleibt in derselben Hälfte des Ganglions, in welche es eingetreten ist, das andere Paar (*pf*[1]*a*) läuft in die andere Hälfte des Ganglions über, um gebogen in typischer Weise zu endigen; *pf*[2], *pf*[2]*a*, *pf*[3]—drei Paare von Nervenfasern, welche aus dem hinteren peripheren Nervenzweigpaare ins Ganglion hineintreten, um sich in ihre Punktsubstanz zu verästeln und in dieser Weise zu endigen; zwei Paare (*pf*[2], *pf*[2]*a*) bleiben in derselben Hälfte des Ganglions, in welche sie eingetreten sind, das dritte Paar (*pf*[3]) läuft in die andere Hälfte hinüber, um dort in typischer Weise zu endigen; *Pf*[4]—aus den peripheren Nervenzweigen kommende Fasern, welche den Typus des Medianfasersystems haben und im Ganglion verästelt endigen; *bz*—Bindegewebszellen in der Kapsel und im Inneren des Ganglions, wo sie Ganglienzellen umspinnen.
Retzius, G. (1891b) Zur Kenntniss des centralen Nervensystems der Würmer. *Biol. Untersuch. Neue Folge* 2, 1–28.

19. Tafel XIV, Fig. 1. Ein Zupfpräparat der grauen Substanz des Rückenmarkes vom Kalbe nach Maceration in Landois-Gierkescher Flüssigkeit und Färbung mit Methylblau und Fuschsin. Einschluss in Canadabalsam nach der Methode "Demidessiccation." a—das Neuroglianetz, bestehend aus kleinen a′ und grösseren b, c Gliazellen, von welchen zahlreiche Fasern ausgehen und als ein dicht gefilztes Netz oder Geflecht zusammenhägen. a″—scheinbare freie Kerne in demselben. d—zwei fast unversehrt isolirte Nervenzellen mit sogen. protoplasmatischen Fortsätzen—bei e und axencylindrischen—en, f—die feinen Verzweigungen der protoplasmatischen Fortsätze. g—scheinbarer Uebergang letzterer Fortsätze in das Neuroglianetz. Vergrösserung 1000.
Lavdowsky, M. (1891) Vom Aufbau des Rückenmarks. Histologisches über die Neuroglia und die Nervensubstanz. *Arch. Mikrosk. Anat.* 38, 264–301.

20. Tafel XIV, Fig. 4. Querschnitt des vorderen Hornes wom Rückenmark eines Hundes nach Erhärtung in Müller'scher Flüssigkeit und mehrjährigem Aufenthalt im Alkohol. Gefärbt mit Anilinblau (unlöslich in Alkohol) und Magdalaroth. Die Doppelfärbung ist etwas verschieden, wenn man die weisse Substanz mit der grauen vergleicht. In der weissen Substanz bei a sind die quergeschnittenen Axencylinder blau, umkreist durch die roth gefärbte Markscheide (Keratinscheide); in der grauen Substanz sind die Axencylinder theils blau oder violet (n′), grösstentheils aber schön rosa (n) tingirt. Einige von ihnen, f, behalten eine innerste Schicht der Keratinblätter bei und tragen also die sogenannte Axencylinderscheide (Axolemma). b—blau gefärbter Neurogliafilz der grauen Substanz mit Gliazellen c. b′—die Gliazellen der weissen Substanz. d—Nervenzelle, welche ihren Axencylinderfortsatz an die vordere Wurzel entsendet. n″—feinste Fasern des grauen "Nervengewirres," gefärbt durch Magdalaroth. Einige von den Fasern dringen in die Neurogliasepten, zwischen die Abtheilungen der vorderen weissen Stränge (n″, rechts). Vergr. 650.
Lavdowsky, M. (1891) Vom Aufbau des Rückenmarks. Histologisches über die Neuroglia und die Nervensubstanz. *Arch. Mikrosk. Anat.* 38, 264–301.

21. Tafel XVIII, Fig. 10. Sagittaler Längsschnitt des Rückenmarks von demselben Bufo, der sowohl die graue Substanz als auch den hinteren (oberen) os und vorderen (unteren) us Seitenstrang in sich fasst. a—drei Conglomerate von Neurogliazellen in Form grosser, mit zahlreichen Fortsätzen versehenen Körper. b, c, d—die Nervenzellen, deren Fortsätze theils in die hinteren Stränge eindringen, theils schräg durch die graue Substanz hinziehen und in ein Nervennetz übergehen. e, f—Nervenzellen, deren Fortsätze in die unteren Stränge eindringe. n—die feinen varikösen Fasern des grauen Nervennetzes, welches an dem Schnitte vollständig gefärbt ist. Die schwach braun angedeuteten queren Fasern, welche von beiden Strängen ausgehen, sind nur durch Ueberosmiumsäure gefärbte collaterale Nerven. own, uwn—die Nervenfasern der beiden Wurzeln, namentlich die collateralen Fasern, welche mit den Fasern des Nervennetzes in Verbindung stehen. Die Fortsätze einiger Nervenzellen gehen auch deutlich in die Fasern beider Wurzeln über. Vergr. 300.
Lavdowsky, M. (1891) Vom Aufbau des Rückenmarks. Histologisches über die Neuroglia und die Nervensubstanz. *Arch. Mikrosk. Anat.* 38, 264–301.

22. Tafel V. Alle Figuren sind nach Präparaten, die nach Alkoholhärtung mit Toluidinblau gefärbt sind, mit Zeiβ' homogener Immersion 1/13, Okular 6 gezeichnet. FIG. 4. Schnitt aus dem Nucleus dentatus des Kleinhirns. *a*, *b* Ganglienzellen; *c* eine diesen ähnliche Gliazelle, als solche besonders durch den 2. kleinen Kern erkennbar; *d* Anhäufung basophiler Körnchen; *e* mit grünlichen lipoiden Abbaustoffen beladene Gliazellen.
von Hoesslin, C., and Alzheimer, A. (1912) Ein Beitrag zur Klinik und pathologischen Anatomie der Westphal-Strümpellschen Pseudosklerose. *Zeitschr. Ges. Neurol. Psych.* 8, 183–209.

23. FIG. 4. Distribución de la microglía en la corteza cerebral del conejo. Véase la forma variada de los corpúsculos microgliales y, sobre todo, las relaciones que tienen con los vasos (satélites vasculares) y con las células nerviosas (satélites neuronales). (Coloración: técnica II).

Del Río-Hortega, P. (1920) Estudios sobre la neuroglia: La microglía y su transformación en células en bastoncito y cuerpos gránulo-adiposos. *Trab. Lab. Invest. Biol. Univ. Madrid* 18, 37–82.

24. FIG. 2. Bulbo olfativo humano. Método áurico de Cajal, previa fijación en nitrato de urea.—A, subestrato superficial de la zona molecular, con numerosas células de forma *cefalopódica*; B, subestrato profundo; C, capa de las células mitrales; D, zona de los granos.

de Castro, F. (1920) Estudios sobre la neuroglia de la corteza cerebral del hombre y de los animales: I. La arquitectonia neuróglica y vascular del bulbo olfativo. *Trab. Lab. Invest. Biol. Univ. Madrid* 18, 1–35.

25. Lámina II. Esquema de la retina y centros ópticos de la mosca azul. *Acg'*: Arborizaciones de una célula gangliónica colosal en la retina profunda; *Apc*: Amacrina de arborización terminal localizada en el plexo difuso cuarto; *App*: Amacrina de arborización terminal localizada en el plexo difuso primero; *Apr*: Amacrina de penacho recurrente periférico; *Aps*: Amacrina de arborización terminal localizada en el plexo difuso segundo; *Apt*: Amacrina de arborización terminal localizada en el plexo difuso tercero; *Arp*: Amacrina de arborización terminal retrógrada profunda; *Asp*: Amacrina de arborización terminal localizada en el plexo difuso primero; *Cai*: Células de asociación interfocal; *Cc*: Célula centrífuga corta; *Cg, Cg', C'g," C'''*: Células gangliónicas con dos ramas terminales, una para el lóbulo óptico y otra para el segmento laminar del mismo; Cg^{IV}: Células gangliónicas con una sola rama terminal destinada al primer plexo difuso del lóbulo óptico; *Cmp, Cmp', Cmp''*: Células monopolares pequeñas; *Cpa, Cpa'*: Centrífugas profundas arciformes; *Crp*: Célula centrífuga para la retina profunda; *Fcl*: Fibra centrífuga larga que termina en la frontera externa de la retina intermediaria; *Fph*: Fibra centrípeta terminada por amplio penacho horizontal en el segundo plexo difuso de la retina profunda; *Lsp*: Lámina serpenteante primera del epióptico; *Lss*: Lámina serpenteante segunda del epióptico; *Lst*: Lámina serpenteante tercera del epióptico; *Pdc*: Plexo difuso cuarto del epióptico; *Pdp*: Plexo difuso primero del epióptico; *Pds*: Plexo difuso segundo del epióptico; *Pdt*: Plexo difuso tercero del epióptico; *Tcd*: Terminación centrípeta difusa en la retina profunda; Tcg^{IV}: Terminación en el primer plexo difuso del lóbulo óptico de la expansión no bifurcada de ciertas células gangliónicas (Cg^{IV}); *Tcm, Tcm'*: Terminaciones de monopolares gigantes; *Tfl, Tfl', Tfl''*: Terminaciones de fibras ópticas largas; *Tgl*: Terminaciones de células gangliónicas en el foco laminar del lóbulo óptico; *Tpr*: Terminación en la retina intermediaria de la expansión periférica de una célula de mango retrógrado de la corteza ganglionar anterior; *Tpr'*: Terminación en la retina intermediaria de la expansión periférica de una célula de mango retrógrado de la corteza ganglionar posterior.

Cajal, S. R., and Sánchez, D. (1915) Contribución al conocimiento de los centros nerviosos de los insectos. *Trab. Lab. Invest. Biol. Univ. Madrid* 13, 1–164.

26. Explanation of the figures. All the illustrations have been drawn from preparations of spinal ganglion cells of the pigeon. Camera lucida, Zeiss apochromatic objective 1·5 mm, and compensating ocular 6 were used for all except Figures 15 and 18 (vide infra). They were reduced by one third in reproduction, giving a magnification of 1067 diameters as they now appear on the plates. This magnification does not however obtain for Figures 15 and 18. Unless stated to the contrary, all the sections were cut 4 μm in thickness. *Plate XV.* FIG. 3. Fixed in Meves' fluid and stained with iron hematoxylin according to his directions. Mitochondria black and Nissl substance gray (page 481). FIG. 4. Fixed and stained by Benda's method. Mitochondria blue, Nissl substance reddish brown and the canals as clear uncolored spaces (page 481). FIG 8. Fixed in Carnoy's 6:3:1 fluid, impregnated with silver after Cajal, toned with gold chloride, counterstained in a saturated aqueous solution of safranin and differentiated in 95% alcohol. Neurofibrils blue–black, canals as clear space, and the ground substance red (page 497). FIG. 9. Same, counterstained in 1% aqueous solution of toluidine blue and differentiated in 95% alcohol. Neurofibrils dark blue and the Nissl substance light blue (page 497). FIG. 10. Fixed in chrome-sublimate at 40° C, stained with iron hematoxylin and counterstained by the application of Held's erythrosine–methylene blue method (i.e., his first method for neurosomes). Mitochondria black, neurosomes of Held type 1 red, and the Nissl substance red with a tinge of purple. Section 3 μm (page 488). FIG. 11. Fixed in chrome sublimate at 40° C, and stained by Bensley's neutral safranin method. Mitochondria and neurosomes of Held type I bluish green, and the Nissl substance red with a tinge of purple (page 485). FIG. 12. Fixed in Carnoy's 6:3:1 fluid and stained by Held's erythrosine–methylene blue method (i.e., his first method for neurosomes). Neurosomes type I red, Nissl substance blue (page 477). FIG. 16. Prepared by Kopsch's method. Shows excentric type of blackened canalicular apparatus. Section 5 μm (page 493). FIG. 17. Same. Shows circumnuclear type of blackened canalicular apparatus. Section 6 μm (page 493). FIG. 18. Stained intravitam with a l:10,000 solution of Janus green in 75% sodium chloride solution. Mitochondria bluish green. Zeiss apochromatic objective 3 mm, compensating ocular 4, and camera lucida. Magnification 380 diameters (page 481).

Cowdry, E. V. (1913) The relations of mitochondria and other cytoplasmic constituents in spinal ganglion cells of the pigeon. *Int. Monatsschr. Anat. Physiol.* 29, 473–504.

27. Tafel IV. 4. Gliabeizegefrierschnitte. Weigertsche Gliafaserfärbung. Homogen. Inmers. Zeiβ 1/13. Fig. 1 mit 140 Tubuslänge, Fig. 2 mit 160 Tubuslänge, Kompensationsokular 4 gezeichnet. *gaz.* Ganglienzelle, *glz.* Gliazelle. *P* zentraler Teil (Kern) der Plaque, P_2 peripherer Teil, Hof der Plaque. FIG. 1: Verhältnis der faserbildenden Gliazellen zu einer Plaque. Oberes Scheitelläppchen rechts. Im Kern der Plaque ein ganz kleiner, offenbar durch das Jod dunkelbraun gefärbter zentraler Teil, um den sich ein dunkler und dann hellerer Ring anschlieβen. Der periphere Teil ist von auβerordentlich zahlreichen, ungemein feinen Gliafäserchen durchzogen, welche von den groβen, am Rande des Hofes gelegenen faserbildenden Gliazellen herstammen.
Alzheimer, A. (1911) Über eigenartige Krankheitsfälle des späteren Alters. *Z. Gesamte Neurol. Psychiatr.* 4, 356–385.

28. Sphaerotichiebildungen gefärbt mit Carbol-Methylenblau-Methylenviolett. Fig. 2. Formolfixierung und Paraffineinbettung.
Fischer, O. (1912) Ein weiterer Beitrag zur Klinik und Pathologie der presbyophrenen Demenz. *Z. Gesamte Neurol. Psychiatr.* 12, 99–135.

29. Taf. XIII–XXII. (Die Fig. 1–14 stammen von dem ersten, 15–30 von dem zweiten Falle.) FIG. 15. Plasmareiche Gliazellenwucherung um eine alte Plaque. Die meisten Fortsätze durchziechen die Plaque. Die mit *a* und *b* bezeichneten Körperchen sind besonders bemerkenswert.
Marinesco, G., and Minea, J. (1912) Untersuchungen über die "senilen Plaques." *Monatsschr. Psychiatr. Neurol.* 31, 79–133.

30. Tavole VIII. Tutte le figure furono disegnate a luce artificiale con apparecchio di Abbe, microscopio Leitz, obb. 1/12 imm. om., oculare comp. 4 (le figg. 4 e 11 furono disegnate con oc. comp. 6). FIGG. 1–4. Metodo Mann-Alzheimer. FIGG. 5–6. Metodo Alzheimer-Mallory. FIG. 7. Metodo Bielschowscky. FIGG. 8–9. Metodo Weigert per la nevroglia. FIGG. 10–11. Metodo Daddi-Herxheimer. La spiegazione dettagliata delle figure si trova nel testo.
Rezza, A. (1913) Alterazioni delle cellule gangliari del bulbo in un caso di demenza precoce con morte improvvisa. *Riv. Patol. Nerv. Ment.* 18, 426–429.

31. Tafel XIV. Fig. 1–4, 7–10 Scharlachrotfärbung nach HERXHEIMER, Fig. 5, 6, 11 bis 15 Methylblau-Eosinfärbung nach ALZHEIMER. Zeiss' homog. Immersion 2 mm, Apert. 1.30, Fig. 1, 2, 4, 7, 8 Okul. 8, die übrigen Okul. 4. FIG. 1, 2. Ganglienzellen aus dem Ammonshorn eines 22 jährigen Pferdes. Die lipoiden Körnchen finden sich fast ausschlieβlich im Spitzenfortsatz in einer zusammenliegenden Reihe angehäuft. FIG. 3. Ganglienzelle aus dem Ammonshorn einer Dementia senilis. Die lipoiden Körnchen liegen im Zelleib und in der ganzen Ausdehnung des sichtbaren Spitzenfortsatzes.
Simchowicz, T. (1911) Histologische Studien über die senile Demenz. In: *Histologische und histopathologische Arbeiten über die Grosshirnrinde*, vol. 4, ed. F. Nissl and A. Alzheimer, 267–444. Jena: Gustav Fischer.

32. Tafel XXI. FIG. 27. Glia limitans externa. *a* = Rindenschicht; *b* = Grenzschicht (HELD); *c* = Radiärfasern; *F.x.* = Form *x*, kleines Gebilde, vermutlich Teilstück eines karyorrhektisch veränderten Gliaelements. *M.* = Mitose im Stadium des Tochtersterns; *Sp.* = Spirem. Nicht ganz ausgetragenes Kaninchen. MANNsches Gemisch.
Spatz, H. (1918) Beiträge zur normalen Histologie des Rückenmarks des neugeborenen Kaninchens. In: *Histologische und his-topathologische Arbeiten über die Grosshirnrind*, vol. 6, ed. F. Nissl and A. Alzheimer, 477–604. Jena: Gustav Fischer.

33. Tafel XV. Fig. 1. Degeneration feiner nervöser Strukturen (Achsenzylinder, eventuell feine Dendriten) in Randpartie eines Vorderhornherdes (Längsschnitt). *cap* Kapillare; *ax* Achsenzylinder, *deg ax* degenerierender Achsenzylinder (eosinfarbig), *deg ax′*, *deg ax″* desgleichen mit einem eosingefärbten Tropfen als Zerfallsprodukt. *varic ax* varikös gequollener Achsenzylinder, degenerierend. *gaz* Ganglienzellen. *gaz′* (etwas links unten von der Mitte) Querschnitt durch den einen Pol einer solchen. *glz* kleinere Gliazellen. *Glz* stark gewucherte Gliazellen. *tr* tropfiges Degenerationsprodukt (leuchtend eosinfarbig) im gittrigen Plasma einer gewucherten Gliazelle. *tr′* ebensolche Tröpfchen. *Den* Dendrit von *gaz′*. Grundgewebe im ganzen aufgelockert, feinmaschig, plasmatisches Glianetzwerk gewuchert, in das perinukleäre Plasma der Gliazellen übergehend. Markscheiden infolge starker Differenzierung fast ganz entfärbt. Tier 9 (16. Tag). Zeiss (hier wie überall), Imm. 1/12. Komp. Ok. 6. MANN. S. auch S. 318 ff.
Lotmar, F. (1918) Beiträge zur Histologie der akuten Myellitis und Encephalitis, sowie verwandter Prozesse. In *Histologische und histopathologische Arbeiten über die Grosshirnrinde*, vol. 6, ed. F. Nissl and A. Alzheimer, 245–432. Jena: Gustav Fischer.

34. Tafel XVIII. Fig. 49. Achsenzylinderquellung, Übersichtsbild aus Querschnitt durch Randpartie eines Herdes in der weiβen Substanz des Rückenmarkes. (Die Verweiselinie *c* müβte bis zu dem in der Mitte der Figur gelegenen, von einer groβen Lichtung umgebenen

unregelmäßigen Achsenzylinderquerschnitt weitergeführt sein.) *gl* Gliazellen. Übrige Erklärungen S. 333 Kleindruck. Tier II (8. Tag). Imm. 1/12. Ok. 2. Fuchsinlichtgrün.
Lotmar, F. (1918) Beiträge zur Histologie der akuten Myellitis und Encephalitis, sowie verwandter Prozesse. In *Histologische und histopathologische Arbeiten über die Grosshirnrinde*, vol. 6, ed. F. Nissl and A. Alzheimer, 245–432. Jena: Gustav Fischer.

35. Tafel II. Fig. 14–20 und 24, 25, 27 sind nach HERXHEIMER-Präparaten gezeichnet und mit dem ABBEschen Zeichenapparat. Vergrößerung Zeiss homog. Immersion 1/12, und Kompensations-Okular 4. Fig. 21, 26, 28 nach ALZHEIMER-VI-Präparaten. Vergrößerung Zeiss homog. Immers. 1/12, Kompensations-Okular 6. FIG. 26. Diffuse Veränderung der Zellen der dritten Schicht. Fuchsinophile Granula zentral verändert und kleiner, bei der rechten Zelle osmophile Granula und Randansammlung der fuchsinophilen Granula, während die Zellmitte sie weniger enthält. FIG. 27. Windungsmark. Fettbedeckter Achsenzylinder, von Gliakern begleitet. FIG. 28. Achsenzylinderschwellung und Achsenzylinderschlängelung. *axq* = geschwollener Kolben.
Creutzfeldt, H. G. (1921) Über eine eigenartige herdförmige Erkrankung des Zentralnervensystems. In *Histologische und his-topathologische Arbeiten über die Grosshirnrind*, ed. F. Nissl and A. Alzheimer, 1–48. Jena: Gustav Fischer.

36. With limited tools, Cajal's original drawings and descriptions allowed him to simplify and understand cerebellar structure and function. Today, various techniques exist for labeling and visualizing individual neurons throughout the nervous system. This color image of the cerebellum was taken from a mouse that was genetically modified to express fluorescent proteins in subsets of cells throughout the nervous system. Neurons are colorfully labeled because they express different combinations of yellow, blue, or red fluorescent proteins (YFP, CFP, or RFP). Shown here coursing through the internal granular layer of the cerebellum are the axons of neurons that reside in other parts of the nervous system and project into the cerebellum. These axonal projections, or "mossy fibers" as Cajal named them, carry crucial information into the cerebellum from regions such as the cerebral cortex, thalamus, spinal cord, and brainstem. The image also shows that each thin mossy fiber has enlarged and complex specializations. Cajal described this elaboration as a "short, delicate stem like a flower," and called them "mossy fiber rosettes." In his work, Cajal included many detailed drawings of mossy fiber rosettes. He correctly predicted that these rosettes are actually enlarged presynaptic terminals onto cerebellar granule cells, and thus represent the point of entry for information into the cerebellum. We owe much of our understanding of this fundamental neural structure to Cajal's original descriptions and pioneering neuroanatomical work. I thank Judy Tollett for her work in generating this triple transgenic mouse.

37. It is intriguing to wonder how Cajal might further his discoveries with the many techniques available today for labeling and visualizing individual cells. *Hippocampus with Cerebral Cortex* is an image taken from a mouse that was genetically modified to express fluorescent proteins in subsets of cells. Neurons are colorfully labeled because they express different combinations of yellow, blue, or red fluorescent proteins (YFP, CFP, or RFP). The center of this image displays the curved hippocampal formation, whereas the upper portion shows neurons in the cerebral cortex. In the hippocampus, cells are labeled to different extents within the dentate gyrus and CA1, CA2, and CA3 regions. Curving around the hippocampus, fibers can be seen coursing through both the corpus callosum (red), which carries information between the cerebral hemispheres, and the alveus (green), which transmits information from the hippocampus into the entorhinal cortex. In the medial cortex, many deep-layer pyramidal neurons are visible with their apical dendrites projecting toward the dorsal surface of the brain. We now know that the cortex and hippocampus are crucial for memory formation and cognition. We owe much of our understanding of cortical and hippocampal circuitry to Cajal's original descriptions and pioneering neuroanatomical work. I thank Judy Tollett for her work in generating this triple transgenic mouse.

38. A large part of our understanding of the organization and functioning of the brain is based on techniques that allow us to label individual brain cells and describe their anatomy. More than a century ago, one of these techniques, the Golgi staining method, allowed Santiago Ramón y Cajal to make an astonishingly accurate description of the brain and its neuronal components. Today, advances in microscopy and genetic techniques open new access to the brain. In particular, one can express fluorescent proteins within neuron or glial cells to label them, achieving, in effect, a multicolor Golgi-like staining of the brain. This image is taken from a Brainbow transgenic mouse that has been genetically engineered to express red, yellow, and cyan fluorescent proteins in a "mosaic" pattern. In this picture of the hippocampus, neurons have typical long dendritic processes, whereas astrocytes (one of the glial cell types of the brain) have a spongy appearance. The picture was acquired using a confocal microscope. Each of the

round cell bodies are about 10 μm in diameter. For maximum contrast, the yellow protein is shown as green, and the cyan protein is displayed as blue.

39. In the adult human brain, a population of multipotent, self-renewing neural stem cells exists within the subventricular zone, which lines the lateral walls of the lateral ventricles. Interestingly, these stem cells have the phenotypic and ultrastructural characteristics of astrocytes. When placed in a culture system supplemented with growth factors such as epidermal growth factor (EGF) and fibroblast growth factor (FGF), these single astrocytic neural stem cells proliferate into floating spheres called *neurospheres*. When allowed to differentiate in vitro, each neurosphere differentiates into the three cell types of the central nervous system. In this figure, these progeny are immunostained in red (neuron), green (astrocyte), and blue (oligodendrocyte).
40. A parsec (symbol: pc) is a unit of length used to measure large distances to objects outside the solar system. A parsec is equal to about 3.26 light-years (31 trillion kilometers in length); 1 mpc is equal to 10^6 pc. A micrometer is equal to 1×10^{-6} of a meter.

REFERENCES

Alonso-Nanclares, L., Gonzalez-Soriano, J., Rodriguez, J. R., and DeFelipe, J. (2008) Gender differences in human cortical synaptic density. *Proc. Natl. Acad. Sci. USA* 105, 14615–14619.

Alzheimer, A. (1911) Über eigenartige Krankheitsfälle des späteren Alters. *Z. Gesamte Neurol. Psychiatr.* 4, 356–385.

Andersen, P., Morris, R., Amaral, D., Bliss, T., and O'Keefe. J., eds. (2007) *The Hippocampus Book.* New York: Oxford University Press.

Angulo, R. E., Springel, V., White, S. D. M., Jenkins, A., Baugh, C. M., and Frenk, C. S. (2012) Scaling relations for galaxy clusters in the Millennium-XXL simulation. *Mon. Not. R. Astron. Soc.* 426, 2046–2062.

Antón-Fernández, A., Rubio-Garrido, P., DeFelipe, J., and Muñoz, A. (2015) Selective presence of a giant saccular organelle in the axon initial segment of a subpopulation of layer V pyramidal neurons. *Brain Struct. Funct.* 220, 869–884.

Arellano, J. I., Espinosa, A., Fairen, A., Yuste, R., and DeFelipe, J. (2007) Non-synaptic dendritic spines in neocortex. *Neuroscience* 145, 464–469.

Ascoli, G. A., Alonso-Nanclares, L., Anderson, S. A., Barrionuevo, G., Benavides-Piccione, R., Burkhalter, A., Buzsaki, G., Cauli, B., DeFelipe, J., Fairén, A., Feldmeyer, D., Fishell, G., Fregnac, Y., Freund, T. F., Karube, F., Gardner, D., Gardner, E. P., Goldberg, J. H., Helmstaedter, M., Hestrin, S., Kisvarday, Z., Lambolez, B., Lewis, D., Marín, O., Markram, H., Muñoz, A., Packer, A., Petersen, C., Rockland, K., Rossier, J., Rudy, B., Somogyi, P., Staiger, J. F., Tamas, G., Thomson, A. M., Toledo-Rodríguez, M., Wang, Y., West, D. C., and Yuste, R. (2008). Petilla terminology: Nomenclature of features of GABAergic interneurons of the cerebral cortex. *Nat. Neurosci.* 9, 557–568.

Barker, L. F. (1899) *The Nervous System and Its Constituent Neurones.* New York: D. Appleton and Company.

Bell, F. J. (1908) National Antarctic expedition 1901–04: Echinoderma. *Nat. History Zool.* (*London*) IV, 1–16.

Bethe, A. (1895) Studien über das Centralnervensystem von Carcinus maenas nebst Angaben über ein neues Verfahren der Methylenblaufixation. *Arch. Mikrosk. Anat.* 44, 579–622.

Bethe, A. (1901) Ueber die Regeneration peripherischen Nerven. *Arch. Psychiatr. Nervenkr.* 34, 1066–1073.

Bethe, A. (1903a) *Allgemeine Anatomie und Physiologie des Nervensystems.* Leipzig: Thieme.

Bethe, A. (1903b) Zur Frage von der autogenen Nervenregeneration. *Neurol. Centralbl.* 22, 60–62.

Bidder, F. H., and Kupffer, C. (1857) *Untersuchungen über die Textur des Rückenmarks und die Entwicklung seiner Formelemente.* Leipzig: Breitkopf & Härtel.

Blanes, T. (1898) Sobre algunos puntos dudosos de la estructura del bulbo olfativo. *Rev. Trim. Micrograf. Madrid* 3, 99–127.

Blazquez-Llorca, L., Garcia-Marin, V., Merino-Serrais, P., Avila, J., and DeFelipe, J. (2011) Abnormal tau phosphorylation in the thorny excrescences of CA3 hippocampal neurons in patients with Alzheimer's. *J. Alzheimers Dis.* 26, 683–698.

Bosch, C., Martínez, A., Masachs, N., Teixeira, C. M., Fernaud, I., Ulloa, F., Pérez-Martínez, E., Lois, C., Comella, J. X., DeFelipe, J., Merchán-Pérez, A., and Soriano, E. (2015). FIB/SEM technology and high-throughput 3D reconstruction of dendritic spines and synapses in GFP-labeled adult-generated neurons. *Front. Neuroanat.* 9, 60. doi: 10.3389/fnana.2015.00060.

Brazier, M. A. B. (1988) *A History of Neurophysiology in the 19th Century.* New York: Raven Press.

Bullock, T. H. (1959). Neuron doctrine and electrophysiology. *Science* 129, 997–1002.

Bullock, T. H., Bennett, M. V., Johnston, D., Josephson, R., Marder, E., and Fields, R. D. (2005) The neuron doctrine, redux. *Science* 310, 791–793.

Cajal, S. R. (1888). Estructura de los centros nerviosos de las aves. *Rev. Trim. Histol. Norm. Patol.* 1, 1–10.

Cajal, S. R. (1889a). Conexión general de los elementos nerviosos. *Medicina Práctica* 88, 341–346.

Cajal, S. R. (1889b). *Manual de histología normal y de técnica micrográfica.* Valencia: Librería de Pascual Aguilar.
Cajal, S. R. (1889c). Nuevas aplicaciones del método de coloración de Golgi. *Gac. Méd. Catalana* 12, 613–616, 643–644.
Cajal, S. R. (1890a) Notas anatómicas: I. Sobre la aparición de las expansiones celulares en la médula embrionaria. *Gac. Sanit. Barcelona* 2, 413–418.
Cajal, S. R. (1890b) Textura de las circunvoluciones cerebrales de los mamíferos inferiores: Nota preventiva. *Gac. Méd. Catalana* 1, 22–31.
Cajal, S. R. (1891a) Significación fisiológica de las expansiones protoplásmicas y nerviosas de las células de la substancia gris. *Rev. Ciencias Méd. Barcelona* 17, 673–679, 715–723.
Cajal, S. R. (1891b) Sur la structure de l´écorce cérébrale de quelques mammifères. *La Cellule* 7, 1–54.
Cajal, S. R. (1892a) El plexo de Auerbach de los batracios: Nota sobre el plexo de Auerbach de la rana. *Trab. Lab. Histol. Fac. Med. Barcelona* February, 23–38.
Cajal, S. R. (1892b) Nuevo concepto de la histología de los centros nerviosos. *Rev. Ciencias Méd. Barcelona* 18, 363–376, 457–476, 505–520, 529–540.
Cajal, S. R. (1893a) Estructura del asta de Ammon y fascia dentate. *Anales Soc. Esp. Hist. Nat.* 22, 53–114.
Cajal, S. R. (1893b) La rétine des vertébrés. *La Cellule* 9, 121–255.
Cajal, S. R. (1893c) *Manual de histología normal y de técnica micrográfica.* 2nd ed. Valencia: Librería de Pascual Aguilar.
Cajal, S. R. (1894a) Estructura íntima de los centros nerviosos. *Rev. Ciencias Méd. Barcelona* 20, 145–160. [Text of the Cronian Lecture in Spanish].
Cajal, S. R. (1894b) The Croonian Lecture: La fine structure des centres nerveux. *Proc. R. Soc. Lond.* 55, 444–468.
Cajal, S. R. (1896) Las espinas colaterales de las células del cerebro teñidas por el azul de metileno. *Rev. Trim. Micrográf. Madrid* 1, 123–136.
Cajal, S. R. (1897a) *Fundamentos racionales y condiciones técnicas de la investigación biológica.* Madrid: L. Aguado.
Cajal, S. R. (1897b) Leyes de la morfología y dinamismo de las células nerviosas. *Rev. Trimest. Micrográf.* 2, 1–28.
Cajal, S. R. (1899) Estudios sobre la corteza cerebral humana: II. Estructura de la corteza motriz del hombre y mamíferos superiores. *Rev. Trim. Micrográf. Madrid* 4, 117–200.
Cajal, S. R. (1899–1904) *Textura del sistema nervioso del hombre y de los vertebrados.* Madrid: Moya,. [This book was revised and extended in the French version: Cajal (1909). English translations: (1995) *Histology of the Nervous System of Man and Vertebrates,* trans. N. Swanson and L. W. Swanson. New York: Oxford University Press, 1995. (2000–2001) *Texture of the Nervous System of Man and the Vertebrates.* New York: Springer Wien (an annotated and edited translation of the original Spanish text with the additions of the French version by P. Pasik and T. Pasik).]
Cajal, S. R. (1900) Estudios sobre la corteza cerebral humana: III. Corteza acústica. *Rev. Trimest. Micrograf.* 5, 129–183
Cajal, S. R. (1901a) *Recuerdos de mi vida, vol.1: Mi infancia y juventud.* Madrid: Fortanet.
Cajal, S. R. (1901b) Textura del lóbulo olfativo accesorio. *Trab. Lab. Invest. Biol. Univ. Madrid* 1, 141–150.
Cajal, S. R. (1901–1902) Estudios sobre la corteza cerebral humana: IV. Estructura de la corteza cerebral olfativa del hombre y mamíferos. *Trab. Lab. Invest. Biol. Univ. Madrid* 1, 1–140.
Cajal, S. R. (1903a) Plan de estructura del tálamo óptico. *Revista de Medicina y Cirugía Prácticas.* May, 1–24.
Cajal, S. R. (1903b) Sobre un sencillo proceder de impregnación de las fibrillas interiores del protoplasma nervioso. *Archivos Latinos de Medicina y Biología* 1, 3–8.
Cajal, S. R. (1904) Neuroglia y neurofibrillas del Lumbricus. *Trab. Lab. Invest. Biol. Univ. Madrid* 3, 277–285.
Cajal, S. R. (1905) Sobre la degeneración y regeneración de los nervios. *Boletín del Instituto de Sueroterapia, Vacunación y Bacteriología de Alfonso XIII* 1, 49–60, 113–119. [This is a summary of the main results later published in Cajal, S. R. (1906) Mecanismo de la regeneración de los nervios. *Trab. Lab. Invest. Biol. Univ. Madrid* 4, 119–210.]
Cajal, S. R. (1907a) Note sur la dégénérescence traumatique des fibres nerveuses du cervelet et du cerveau. *Trav. Lab. Recherches Biol. Univ. Madrid* 5, 105–116.
Cajal, S. R. (1907b) *Structure et connexions des Neurones: Conference de Nobel faite à Stockholm le 12 Décembre 1906.* Stockholm: Imprimeire Royale, P. A. Norstedt & Fils.
Cajal, S. R. (1909) Nota sobre la estructura de la retina de la mosca (*M. vomitoria L.*). *Trab. Lab. Invest. Biol. Univ. Madrid* 7, 217–257.
Cajal, S. R. (1909–1911). *Histologie du système nerveux de l'homme et des vertébrés,* trans. L. Azoulay. Paris: Maloine.
Cajal, S. R. (1910a) Algunas observaciones favorables a la hipótesis neurotrópica. *Trab. Lab. Invest. Biol. Univ. Madrid* 8, 63–135.
Cajal, S. R. (1910b) El núcleo de las células pyramidales del cerebro humano y de algunos mamíferos. *Trab. Lab. Invest. Biol. Univ. Madrid* 8, 27–62.
Cajal, S. R. (1911a) Alteraciones de la substancia gris provocadas por conmoción y aplastamiento. *Trab. Lab. Invest. Biol. Univ. Madrid* 9, 217–253
Cajal, S. R. (1911b) Fibras nerviosas conservadas y fibras nerviosas degeneradas. *Trab. Lab. Invest. Biol. Univ. Madrid* 9, 181–215.

Cajal, S. R. (1911c) Los fenómenos precoces de la degeneración neuronal en el cerebelo. *Trab. Lab. Invest. Biol. Univ. Madrid* 9, 1–38
Cajal, S. R. (1912) *La fotografía de los colores: Fundamentos científicos y reglas prácticas*. Madrid: Moya.
Cajal, S. R. (1913) Contribución al conocimiento de la neuroglia del cerebro humano. *Trab. Lab. Invest. Biol. Univ. Madrid* 11, 255–315.
Cajal, S. R. (1913–1914) *Estudios sobre la degeneración y regeneración del sistema nervioso*. Madrid: Moya. [Reprinted and edited with additional translations by DeFelipe, J., and Jones, E. G. (1991) *Cajal's Degeneration and Regeneration of the Nervous System*. New York: Oxford University Press.]
Cajal, S. R. (1914) *Manual de histología normal y de técnica micrográfica*. 6th ed. Madrid: Imprenta y Librería de Nicolás Moya.
Cajal, S. R. (1917a) Contribución al conocimiento de la retina y centros ópticos de los cefalópodos. *Trab. Lab. Invest. Biol. Univ. Madrid* 15, 1–82.
Cajal, S. R. (1917b) *Recuerdos de mi vida, vol. 2: Historia de mi labor científica*. Madrid: Moya.
Cajal, S. R. (1918) Observaciones sobre la estructura de los ocelos y vías nerviosas ocelares de algunos insectos. *Trab. Lab. Invest. Biol. Univ. Madrid* 16, 109–139.
Cajal, S. R. (1920) Algunas consideraciones sobre la mesoglia de Robertson y Río-Hortega. *Trab. Lab. Invest. Biol. Univ. Madrid* 18, 109–127.
Cajal, S. R. (1921) Textura de la corteza visual del gato. *Trab. Lab. Invest. Biol. Univ. Madrid* 19, 113–146.
Cajal, S. R. (1925) Contribution à la connaissance de la névroglie cérébrale et cérébelleuse dans la paralysie générale progressive. *Trav. Lab. Recherches Biol. Univ. Madrid* 23, 157–216.
Cajal, S. R. (1933) ¿Neuronismo o reticularismo? Las pruebas objetivas de la unidad anatómica de las células nerviosas. Madrid: Góngora. [Reprint of the article published in *Arch. Neurobiol.* 13, 217–291, 579–646, 1933. English translation: Cajal, S. R. (1954) *Neuron Theory or Reticular Theory? Objective Evidence of the Anatomical Unity of Nerve Cells*, trans. M. Ubeda-Purkiss and C. A. Fox. Madrid: Consejo Superior de Investigaciones Científicas.]
Cajal, S. R., and de Castro, F. (1933) *Elementos de técnica micrográfica del sistema nervioso*. Madrid: Tipografía Artística.
Cajal, S. R., and Sala, C. (1891) Terminaciones de los nervios y tubos glandulares del páncreas de los vertebrados. *Trab. Lab. Histol. Fac. Med. Barcelona*, December, 1–15.
Cajal, S. R., and Sánchez, D. (1915) Contribución al conocimiento de los centros nerviosos de los insectos. *Trab. Lab. Invest. Biol. Univ. Madrid* 13, 1–164.
Cajal, S. R., and Tello, J. F. (1933) *Histology*. Baltimore: Williams Wood & Company.
Calleja, C. (1893) *La región olfatoria del cerebro*. Madrid: Moya.
Chang, H. T. (1952) Cortical neurons with particular reference to the apical dendrites. *Cold Spring Harb. Symp. Quant. Biol.* 17, 189–202.
Clarke, E., and Jacyna L. S. (1987) *Nineteenth-Century Origins of Neuroscientific Concepts*. Berkeley: University of California Press.
Cowdry, E. V. (1913) The relations of mitochondria and other cytoplasmic constituents in spinal ganglion cells of the pigeon. *Int. Monatsschr. Anat. Physiol.* 29, 473–504.
Cox, W. H. (1891) Impregnation des centralen Nervensystems mit Quecksilber–salzen. *Arch. Mikr. Anat.* 37, 16–21.
Creutzfeldt, H. G. (1921) Über eine eigenartige herdförmige Erkrankung des Zentralnervensystems. In *Histologische und his-topathologische Arbeiten über die Grosshirnrind*, ed. F. Nissl and A. Alzheimer, 1–48. Jena: Gustav Fischer.
Crous, J. (1878) *Tratado Elemental de Anatomía y Fisiología Normal y Patológica del Sistema Nervioso*. Valencia: Librería de Pascual Aguilar.
de Castro, F. (1920) Estudios sobre la neuroglia de la corteza cerebral del hombre y de los animales: I. La arquitectonia neuróglica y vascular del bulbo olfativo. *Trab. Lab. Invest. Biol. Univ. Madrid* 18, 1–35.
de Castro. F. (1926) Sobre la fina anatomía de los ganglios simpáticos, vertebrales y prevertebrales de los simios. *Bol. Soc. Esp. Biol.* XI, 171–177.
de Castro, F. (1928) Sur la structure et l'innervation du sinus carotidien de l'homme et des mammifères: Nouveaux faits sur l'innervation et la fonction du glomus caroticum. *Trav. Lab. Recherches Biol. Univ. Madrid* 25, 331–380.
DeFelipe, J. (2002a) Cortical interneurons: From Cajal to 2001. *Prog. Brain Res.* 136, 215–238.
DeFelipe, J. (2002b) Sesquicentennial of the birthday of Santiago Ramón y Cajal (1852–2002), the father of modern neuroscience. *Trends Neurosci.* 25, 481–484.
DeFelipe, J. (2006) Brain plasticity and mental processes: Cajal again. *Nat. Rev. Neurosci.* 7, 811–817.
DeFelipe, J. (2010a) *Cajal's Butterflies of the Soul: Science and Art*. New York: Oxford University Press.
DeFelipe, J. (2010b) From the connectome to the synaptome: An epic love history. *Science* 330, 1198–1201.
DeFelipe, J. (2013) Cajal and the discovery of a new artistic world: The neuronal forest. *Prog. Brain Res.* 203, 201–220.
DeFelipe, J. (2014) *El Jardín de la Neurología: Sobre lo bello, el arte y el cerebro*. Madrid: Boletín Oficial del Estado and Consejo Superior de Investigaciones Científicas.
DeFelipe, J. (2015a) The anatomical problem posed by brain complexity and size: A potential solution. *Front. Neuroanat.* 9, 104. doi: 10.3389/fnana.2015.00104.

DeFelipe, J. (2015b) The dendritic spine story: an intriguing process of discovery. *Front. Neuroanat.* 9, 14. doi: 10.3389/fnana.2015.00014.

DeFelipe, J., Garrido, E., and Markram, H. (2014) The death of Cajal and the end of scientific romanticism and individualism. *Trends Neurosci.* 37, 525–527.

DeFelipe, J., and Jones, E. G. (1988) *Cajal on the Cerebral Cortex.* New York: Oxford University Press.

DeFelipe, J., and Jones, E. G. (1991) *Cajal's Degeneration and Regeneration of the Nervous System.* New York: Oxford University Press.

DeFelipe, J., and Jones, E. G. (1992) Santiago Ramón y Cajal and methods in neurohistology. *Trends Neurosci.* 15, 237–246.

DeFelipe, J., Markram, H., and Wagensberg, J. (2007) *Paisajes Neuronales: Homenaje a Santiago Ramón y Cajal.* Madrid: Consejo Superior de Investigaciones Científicas.

Deiters, O. F. K. (1865) *Untersuchungen über Gehirn und Rückenmark des Menschen und der Säugethiere*, ed. M. Schultze. Braunschweig: F. Vieweg und Sohn.

de la Villa, J. (1952) Cajal, observado por un disector. In *Primer Centenario del Nacimiento del Excmo. Señor Don Santiago Ramón y Cajal: Discursos leídos en la Junta solemne conmemorativa de 25 de octubre de 1952*, 19–25. Madrid: Instituto de España.

Del Río-Hortega, P. (1920) Estudios sobre la neuroglia: La microglía y su transformación en células en bastoncito y cuerpos gránulo-adiposos. *Trab. Lab. Invest. Biol. Univ. Madrid* 18, 37–82.

Del Río-Hortega, P. (1925) Algunas observaciones acerca de la neuroglia perivascular. *Bol. Soc. Esp. Hist. Nat.*, April, 184–210.

Del Río-Hortega, P. (1933) Arte y artificio de la ciencia histológica. *Revista de la Residencia de Estudiantes, Madrid* 4, 191–206.

Demoor, J. (1896) La plasticité morphologique des neurones cérébraux. *Arch. Biol. Bruxelles* 14, 723–752.

De Robertis, E. (1959) Submicroscopy morphology of the synapse. *Int. Rev. Cytol.* 8, 61–96.

De Robertis, E., and Bennett, H. S. (1955) Some features of the submicroscopic morphology of synapses in frog and earthworm. *J. Biophys. Biochem. Cytol.* 1, 47–58.

Dogiel, A. S. (1891). Ueber die nervösen Elemente in der Retina des Menschen. *Arch. Mikrosk. Anat.* 38, 317–344.

Dogiel, A. S. (1893) Zur Frage über das Verhalten der Nervenzellen zu einander. *Arch. Anat. Physiol. Anat. Abt.* 429–434.

Dogiel, A.S. (1896) Die Nervenelemente in Kleinhirne der Vögel und Säugethiere. *Arch. mikrosk. Anat.* 47, 707–718.

Dogiel, A. S. (1899) Ueber den Bau der Ganglien in den Geflechten des Darmes und der Gallenblase des Menschen und der Säugethiere. *Arch. Anat. Entwicklungsgesch.* 130–158.

Edinger, L. (1893) Vergleichend-entwickelungsgeschichtliche und anatomische Studien im Bereiche der Hirnanatomie. *Anat. Anz.* 8, 305–321.

Ehrlich, P. (1881) Ueber das Methylenblau und seine klinisch-bakterioskopische Verwerthung. *Z. Klin. Med.* 2, 710–713.

Ehrlich, P. (1886) Ueber die Methyllenblau-reaction der lebenden Nervensubstanz. *Dtsch. Med. Wochenschr.* 12, 49–52.

Fairén, A., Peters, A., and Saldanha, J. (1977) A new procedure for examining Golgi impregnated neurons by light and electron microscopy. *J. Neurocytol.* 6, 311–337.

Feng, G., Mellor, R. H., Bernstein, M., Keller-Peck, C., Nguyen, Q. T., Wallace, M., Nerbonne, J. M., Lichtman, J. W., and Sanes, J. R. (2000) Imaging neuronal subsets in transgenic mice expressing multiple spectral variants of GFP. *Neuron* 28, 41–51.

Fernandez, N., and Breathnach, C. S. (2001) Luis Simarro Lacabra [1851–1921]: From Golgi to Cajal through Simarro, via Ranvier? *J. Hist. Neurosci.* 10, 19–26.

Fischer, O. (1912) Ein weiterer Beitrag zur Klinik und Pathologie der presbyophrenen Demenz. *Z. Gesamte Neurol. Psychiatr.* 12, 99–135.

Forel, A. H. (1887) Einige hirnanatomische Betrachtungen und Ergebnisse. *Arch. Psychiat. Nervenkr.* 18, 162–198.

Forel, A. H. (1890–1891) Ueber das Verhältniss der experimentellen Atrophie und Degenerationsmethode zur Anatomie und Histologie des Centralnervensystems, *Ursprung des ix., x. und xii. Hirnnerven. Festschrift zur Feier des Fünfzigjährigen Doktorjubiläums der Herren Prof. Dr Karl. v. Nägeli u Prof. A. v. Kölliker*, pp. 37–50.

Foster, M., and Sherrington, C. S. (1897) *A Text-Book of Physiology: Part III: The Central Nervous System.* London: Macmillan.

Frotscher, M., and Léránth, C. (1986) The cholinergic innervation of the rat fascia dentata: Identification of target structures on granule cells by combining choline acetyltransferase immunocytochemistry and Golgi impregnation. *J. Comp. Neurol.* 243, 58–70.

Garcia-Lopez, P., Garcia-Marin, V., and Freire, M. (2010) The histological slides and drawings of Cajal. *Front. Neuroanat.* 4, 9. doi: 10.3389/neuro.05.009.2010.

Giepmans, B. N., Adams, S. R., Ellisman, M. H., and Tsien, R. Y. (2006) The fluorescent toolbox for assessing protein location and function. *Science* 312, 217–224.

Globus, A., and Scheibel, A. (1967) The effect of visual deprivation on cortical neurons: A Golgi study. *Exp. Neurol.* 19, 331–345.

Golgi, C. (1873) Sulla struttura della sostanza grigia del cervello (Comunicazione preventiva). *Gazzetta Medica Italiana* 33, 244–246.

Golgi, C. (1875) *Sulla fina struttura del bulbi olfattorii.* Reggio-Emilia: Printer Stefano Calderini.[Reprinted

from Golgi, C. (1875). Sulla fina struttura dei bulbi olfactorii. *Riv. Sper. Freniatr. Med. Leg.* 1, 405–425.]
Golgi, C. (1882–1883) Sulla fina anatomia degli organi centrali del sistema nervoso: Rivista sperimentale di Freniatria, anni 1882–1883 . In *Opera Omnia,* vol. I. *Istologia Normale* (1870–1883) 1903, 295–393. Milano: Ulrico Hoepli.
Golgi, C. (1883) Sulla fina anatomia degli organi centrali del sistema nervoso: Rivista sperimentale di Freniatria, anni 1883. In *Opera Omnia*, vol. II. *Istologia Normale* (1883–1902) 1903, 397–536. Milano: Ulrico Hoepli.
Golgi, C. (1885a) *Sulla fina anatomia degli organi centrali del sistema nervoso*. Reggio Emilia:Tipografia di Stefano Calderini e Figlio.
Golgi, C. (1885b) Sulla fina anatomia degli organi centrali del sistema nervoso. *Riv. Sper. Fremiat. Med. Leg. Alienazioni Ment.* 11, 72–123.
Golgi, C. (1898) Intorno alla struttura delle cellule nervose. *Boll. Soc. Med-Chir. Pavia* 13, 1–14.
Golgi, C. (1901) Sulla fina anatomia degli organi centrali del sistema nervoso. Lettera al Prof. Luigi Luciani [(1901) La lettera fu pubblicata in parte nel Trattato di fisiologia dell'uomo del Professore Luigi Luciani ordinario di Fisiologia nell'Universita di Roma. Milan: Societa editrice libraria.]. In *Opera Omnia*. Vol. II. *Istologia Normale* (1883–1902) 1903, 721–733. Milano: Ulrico Hoepli.
Golgi, C. (1929) *La dottrina del neurone: Teoria e fati*. In *Opera Omnia*. Vol. IV. *Scritti su argomenti varii*, 1259–1291. Milano: Ulrico Hoepli. [Chapter 30, Nobel Prize Lecture].
Gray, E. G. (1959a) Axo-somatic and axo-dendritic synapses of the cerebral cortex: An electron microscopic study. *J. Anat.* 93, 420–433.
Gray, E. G. (1959b) Electron microscopy of synaptic contacts on dendrite spines of the cerebral cortex. *Nature* 183, 1592–1593.
Guerra, C. (2009) *Los códices del vino*. Las Palmas de Gran Canaria: CICCA.
Hatai, S. (1903) The finer structure of the neurones in the nervous system of the white rat. *Univ. Chicago. Dec. Publ.* 10 (ser 1), 170–190.
Heck, N., and Benavides-Piccione, R., eds. (2016) *Dendritic Spines: From Shape to Function*. Lausanne: Frontiers Media.
Held, H. (1895) Beiträge zur Structur der Nervenzellen und ihrer Fortsätze. *Arch. Anat. Phys. Anat. Abt.* 396–416.
Held, H. (1897a) Beiträge zur Structur der Nervenzellen und ihrer Fortsätze: Zweite Abhandlung. *Arch. Anat. Phys. (Anat. Abt.)* 2, 204–294.
Held, H. (1897b) Beiträge zur Structur der Nervenzellen und ihrer Fortsätze" Dritte Abhandlung. *Arch. Anat. Phys.* (Anat. Abt.) 2, 273–312.
Held, H. (1902) Ueber den Bau der grauen und weissen Substanz. *Arch. Anat. Phys. (Anat. Abt.)* 189–224.
Held, H. (1904) Zur weiteren Kenntniss der Nervenendfüsse und zur Struktur der Sehzellen. *Abhandl Math-phys. K.l königl. sächs Ges. Wissensch.* 29, 143–185.
Held, H. (1905) Zur Kenntniss einer neurofibrillären Continuität im Centralnervensystem der Wirbelthiere. *Arch. Anat. Phys. (Anat. Abt.)* 55–78.
Held, H. (1929) Die Lehre von den Neuronen und von Neurencytium und ihr heutiger Stand. In *Fortschritte der naturwissenschftl*, ed. E. Abderhalden and N. F. Forschung, 1–72. Berlin: Urban und Schwarzenberg.
Hendry, S. H. C., Jones, E. G., DeFelipe, J., Schmechel, D., Brandon, C., and Emson, P. C. (1984) Neuropeptide-containing neurons of the cerebral cortex are also GABAergic. *Proc. Natl. Acad. Sci. USA* 81, 6526–6530.
Hensen, V. (1864) Zur Entwickelung des Nervensystems. *Arch. Pathol. Anat. Physiol. Klin. Med.* 30, 176–186.
His, W. (1886) Zur Geschichte des menschlichen Rückenmarks und der Nervenwurzeln. *Abhandl. Math.- Phys. Klass. Königl. Sächs. Gesellsch. Wiss.* 13, 147–209, 477–513.
His, W. (1889) Die Neuroblasten und deren Entstehung im embryonalen Mark. *Abhandl. Math.- Phys. Klass. Königl. Sächs. Gesellsch. Wiss.* 15, 313–372.
Hubbard, E .M. (2007) Neurophysiology of synesthesia. *Curr. Psychiatry Rep.* 9, 193–199.
Hughes, A. (1959) *A History of Cytology*. New York: Abelard-Schuman.
Jones, E. G. (1994). The neuron doctrine. *J. Hist. Neurosci.* 3, 3–20.
Jones, E. G. (2007) Neuroanatomy: Cajal and after Cajal. *Brain Res. Rev.* 55, 248–255.
Jones, E. G., and Powell, T. P. S. (1969) Morphological variations in the dendritic spines of the neocortex. *J. Cell Sci.* 5, 509–529.
Keele, K., and Pedretti, C. (1979) *Leonardo da Vinci: Corpus of the anatomical drawings in the Collection of Her Majesty the Queen at Windsor Castle*. 4 vols. London.
Kölliker, A. von (1852) *Handbuch der Gewebelehre des Menschen*. Leipzig: Engelmann.
Kölliker, A. von (1856) *Éléments d'histologie humaine*. Paris: Victor Masson.
Kölliker, A. von (1893) *Handbuch der Gewebelehre des Menschen*. Vol. II. *Nervensystem des Menschen und der Thiere*. Leipzig: Engelmann.
Kölliker, A. von (1896) *Handbuch der Gewebelehre des Menschen*, 6th ed. Vol. II, *Nervensystem des Menschen und der Thiere*. Leipzig: Engelmann.
Kupffer, G. (1859) *De cornus ammonis textura disquisitiones praecipue in cuniculis institutae. Dissertatio Inauguralis.* Universitate Literarum Caesarea Dorpatensi. Dorpati Livonorum. Typis Viduae (J.C. Schünmanni et C. Mattieseni).
Kuwajima, M., Spacek, J., and Harris, K. M. (2013) Beyond counts and shapes: Studying pathology of dendritic

spines in the context of the surrounding neuropil through serial section electron microscopy. *Neuroscience* 251, 75–89.

Kuypers, H. G., Bentivoglio, M., Catsman-Berrevoets, C. E., and Bharos, A. T. (1980) Double retrograde neuronal labeling through divergent axon collaterals, using two fluorescent tracers with the same excitation wavelength which label different features of the cell. *Exp. Brain Res.* 40, 383–392.

Lavdowsky, M. (1891) Vom Aufbau des Rückenmarks. Histologisches über die Neuroglia und die Nervensubstanz. *Arch. Mikrosk. Anat.* 38, 264–301.

Lichtman, J. W., Livet, J., and Sanes, J. R. (2008) A technicolour approach to the connectome. *Nat. Rev. Neurosci.* 9, 417–422.

Livet, J., Weissman, T. A., Kang, H., Draft, R. W., Lu, J., Bennis, R. A., Sanes, J. R., and Lichtman, J. W. (2007) Transgenic strategies for combinatorial expression of fluorescent proteins in the nervous system. *Nature* 450, 56–62.

Lorente de Nó, R. (1922) La corteza cerebral del ratón. (Primera contribución— La corteza acústica). *Trab. Lab. Invest. Biol. Univ. Madr.* 20, 41–78.

Lorente de Nó. R. (1933) Studies on the structure of the cerebral cortex: I. Area entorhinalis. *J. Psychol. Neurol.* 45, 381–438.

Lorente de Nó. R. (1934). Studies on the structure of the cerebral cortex: II. Continuation of the study of the Ammonic system. *J. Psychol. Neurol.* 46, 113–177.

Lotmar, F. (1918) Beiträge zur Histologie der akuten Myellitis und Encephalitis, sowie verwandter Prozesse. In *Histologische und histopathologische Arbeiten über die Grosshirnrinde*, vol. 6, ed. F. Nissl and A. Alzheimer, 245–432. Jena: Gustav Fischer.

Maestre de San Juan, A. (1879) *Tratado de Histología Normal y Patológica*. Madrid: Moya y Plaza.

Marinesco, G., and Minea, J. (1912) Untersuchungen über die "senilen Plaques." *Monatsschr. Psychiatr. Neurol.* 31, 79–133.

Marín-Padilla, M. (1972) Structural abnormalities of the cerebral cortex in human chromosomal aberrations: A Golgi study. *Brain Res.* 44, 625–629.

Mazzarello, P. (1999) *The Hidden Structure. A Scientific Biography of Camillo Golgi.* Oxford: Oxford University Press.

Merchán, M. A., DeFelipe, J., and de Castro, F. (2016) *Cajal and de Castro's Neurohistological Methods*. New York: Oxford University Press.

Merchán-Pérez, A. (2001) *Santiago Ramón y Cajal: Discurso de doctorado y trabajos de juventud.* Madrid: Universidad Europea-CEES.

Merino-Serrais, P., Benavides-Piccione, R., Blázquez-Llorca, L., Kastanauskaite, A., Rábano, A., Avila, J., and DeFelipe, J. (2013) The influence of phosphotau on dendritic spines of cortical pyramidal neurons in Alzheimer's disease patients. *Brain* 136, 1913–1928.

Meyer, S. (1895) Die Subcutane Methylenblauinjektion ein Mittel zur Darstellung der Elemente des Centralnervensystems von Säugethieren. *Arch. Mikrosk. Anat.* 46, 282–290.

Meyer, S. (1896) Ueber eine Verbindungsweise der Neurone. Nebst Mitteilungen über die Technik und die Erfolge der Methode der subcutanen Methylenblauinjection. *Arch. Mikrosk. Anat.* 47, 734–748.

Meyer, S. (1897) Ueber die Funktion der Protoplasmafortsätze der Nervenzellen. *Bericht. Math.-Phys. Cl. Königl. Sächs. Gesells. Wiss., Leipzig* 49, 475–495.

Meynert, T. (1874). Skizze des menschlichen Grosshirnstammes nach seiner Aussenform und seinem inneren Bau. *Arch. Psychiatr. Nervenkr.* 4, 387–431.

Müller, J. (1841) *Monatsb. k. preuss. Akad. Wiss.*, 1841, p. 185; *Archiv Naturg.*, 1841, vol. 1, p. 144; *Die Gattung Comatula*, p. 257.

Nabokov, V. (1955) *Lolita*. Paris: Olympia Press.

Nabokov, V. (1974) *Look at the Harlequins!* New York: McGraw-Hill.

Nansen, F. (1887) *The structure and combination of the histological elements of the central nervous system.* Bergen: J. Grieg. [Reprinted from Bergens Museums Aarsberetning for 1886.]

Nissl, F. (1903) *Die Neuronenlehre und ihre Anhänger.* Jena: Verlag von Gustav Fischer.

Palade, G. E., and Palay, S. L. (1954) Electron microscope observations of interneuronal and neuromuscular synapses. *Anat. Rec.* 118, 335–336.

Palay, S. L. (1956) Synapses in the central nervous system. *J. Biophys. Biochem. Cytol. Suppl.* 2, 193–202.

Penzes, P., Cahill, M. E., Jones, K. A., VanLeeuwen, J. E., and Woolfrey, K. M. (2011) Dendritic spine pathology in neuropsychiatric disorders. *Nat. Neurosci.* 14, 285–293.

Peters, A., and Kaiserman-Abramof, I. R. (1969) The small pyramidal neuron of the rat cerebral cortex: The synapses upon dendritic spines. *Z. Zellforsch.* 100, 487–506.

Peters, A., and Kaiserman-Abramof, I. R. (1970) The small pyramidal neuron of the rat cerebral cortex: The perikaryon, dendrites and spines. *Am. J. Anat.* 127, 321–355.

Peters, A., Palay, S. L., and Webster, H. deF. (1991). *The Fine Structure of the Nervous System: Neurons and Their Supporting Cells.* New York: Oxford University Press.

Pevsner, J. (2002) Leonardo da Vinci's contributions to neuroscience. *Trends Neurosci.* 25, 217–220.

Purkinje, J. E. (1838) Bericht über die Versammlung deutscher Naturforscher und Ärzte in Prag im September, 1837. pt. 3, sec. 5, A. *Anatomisch-physiologische Verhandlungen* 177–180.

Purpura, D. (1974) Dendritic spine "dysgenesis" and mental retardation. *Science* 186, 1126–1128.
Rácz, B., and Weinberg, R. J. (2013) Microdomains in forebrain spines: An ultrastructural perspective. *Mol. Neurobiol.* 47, 77–89.
Ramón, P. (1896) Estructura del encéfalo del camaleón. *Rev. Trimest. Micrograf.* 1, 46–82.
Ramón, P. (1898) Centros ópticos de las aves. *Rev. Trim. Micrograf. Madrid* 3, 141–197.
Ramón, P. (1899) El lóbulo óptico de los peces (teleosteos). *Rev. Trim. Micrograf. Madrid* 4, 87–107.
Ramón y Cajal-Junquera, M. A. (2007) Cajal, artista. In *Paisajes neuronales: Homenaje a Santiago Ramón y Cajal*, ed. J. DeFelipe, H. Markram, and J. Wagensberg, 29–40. Madrid: Consejo Superior de Investigaciones Científicas.
Ranvier, L. (1878) *Leçons sur l'histologie du système nerveux*. Paris: Savy.
Remak, R. (1838) *Observationes Anatomicae et Microscopicae de Systematis Nervosi Structura*. Berlin: Reimer.
Retzius, G. (1891a) Ueber den Bau der Oberflächeschicht der Grosshirnrinde beim Menschen und bei den Säugethieren. *Biologiska Föreningens Förhandlingar* 3, 90–102.
Retzius, G. (1891b) Zur Kenntniss des centralen Nervensystems der Würmer. *Biol. Untersuch. Neue Folge* 2, 1–28.
Rezza, A. (1913) Alterazioni delle cellule gangliari del bulbo in un caso di demenza precoce con morte improvvisa. *Riv. Patol. Nerv. Ment.* 18, 426–429.
Robertson, J. D. (1953) Ultrastructure of two invertebrate synapses. *Proc. Soc. Exp. Biol. Med.* 82, 219–223.
Rochefort, N. L., and Konnerth, A. (2012) Dendritic spines: From structure to in vivo function. *EMBO Rep.* 13, 699–708.
Russo, S. J., Dietz, D. M., Dumitriu, D., Morrison, J. H., Malenka, R. C., and Nestler, E. J. (2010) The addicted synapse: Mechanisms of synaptic and structural plasticity in nucleus accumbens. *Trends Neurosci.* 33, 267–276.
Sánchez-Ponce, D., DeFelipe, J., Garrido, J. J., and Muñoz, A. (2011) In vitro maturation of the cisternal organelle in the hippocampal neuron's axon initial segment. *Mol. Cell. Neurosci.* 48, 104–116.
Schaffer, K. (1892) Beitrag zur Histologie der Ammonshornformation. *Arch. Mikrosk. Anat.* 39, 611–632.
Segal, M. (2016) Dendritic spines: Morphological building blocks of memory. *Neurobiol. Learn Mem.* 138, 3–9.
Shepherd, G. M. (1991) *Foundations of the Neuron Doctrine*. New York: Oxford University Press.
Shepherd, G. M. (2010) *Creating Modern Neuroscience: The Revolutionary 1950s*. New York: Oxford University Press.
Shepherd, G. M. (2016). *Foundations of the Neuron Doctrine: 25th Anniversary edition.* New York: Oxford University Press.
Sherrington, C. S. (1947) *The Integrative Action of the Nervous System*. Cambridge: University Press.
Simchowicz, T. (1911) Histologische Studien über die senile Demenz. In *Histologische und histopathologische Arbeiten über die Grosshirnrinde*, vol. 4, ed. F. Nissl and A. Alzheimer, 267–444. Jena: Gustav Fischer.
Skirboll, L., Hökfelt, T., Norell, G., Phillipson, O., Kuypers, H. G., Bentivoglio, M., Catsman-Berrevoets, C. E., Visser, T. J., Steinbusch, H., Verhofstad, A., Cuello, A. C., Goldstain, M., and Brownstein, M. (1984) A method for specific transmitter identification of retrogradely labeled neurons: Immunofluorescence combined with fluorescence tracing. *Brain Res.* 320, 99–127.
Smith, J. (1854) *Fruits and Farinacea, the Proper Food of Man: Being an Attempt to Prove, from History, Anatomy, Physiology, and Chemistry, That the Original, Natural, and Best Diet of Man Is Derived from the Vegetable Kingdom*. New York: Fowlers and Wells.
Smith, P. D. (1962) Vladimir Nabokov on his life and work: A BBC television interview with Peter Duval Smith. *The Listener* 22, 856–888.
Soukhanoff, S., Geier, F., and Gourévitsch, M. (1904) Contribution á l'étude de l'aspect externe des prolongements protoplasmatiques des cellules nerveuses colorés par le bleu de méthilène. *Névraxe* 6, 117–122.
Spatz, H. (1918) Beiträge zur normalen Histologie des Rückenmarks des neugeborenen Kaninchens. In *Histologische und his-topathologische Arbeiten über die Grosshirnrind*, vol. 6, ed. F. Nissl and A. Alzheimer, 477–604. Jena: Gustav Fischer.
Spires-Jones, T., and Knafo, S. (2012) Spines, plasticity, and cognition in Alzheimer's model mice. *Neural Plast.* 319836, 1–10.
Stefanowska, M. (1897) Les appendices terminaux des dendrites cérébraux et leur différents états physiologiques. *Ann. Soc. R. Sc. Méd. Nat. Bruxelles* 6, 351–407.
Stefanowska, M. (1901) Les appendices terminaux des dendrites cérébraux et leur différents états physiologiques. *Arch. Sci. Phys. Nat.* 11, 1–25.
Tsien, R. Y. (1998) The green fluorescent protein. *Annu. Rev. Biochem.* 67, 509–544.
Turner, J., and Aber, M. B. (1900) A note on the staining of brain in a mixture of methylene blue and peroxide of hydrogen: A *vital* reaction in *post-mortem* tissue. *Brain* 23, 524–529.
Valverde, F. (1971) Rate and extent of recovery from dark rearing in the visual cortex of the mouse. *Brain Res.* 33, 1–11.
Van der Loos, H. (1967) The history of the neuron. In *The Neuron,* ed. H. Hydén, 1–47. Amsterdam: Elsevier.
van Gehuchten, A. (1913) *Le Névraxe: Livre Jubilaire dédié a M.A. van Gehuchten*, vol. 12–13, pp. 29–45. Louvain: A. Uystpruyst (Librairie Universitaire).

von Gerlach, J. (1872). Über die struktur der grauen Substanz des menschlichen Grosshirns. *Zentralbl. Med. Wiss.* 10, 273–275.

von Gudden, B. (1870) Experimentaluntersuchungen über das peripherische und centrale Nervensystem. *Arch. Psychiat. Nervenkr.* 2, 693–723.

von Hoesslin, C., and Alzheimer, A. (1912) Ein Beitrag zur Klinik und pathologischen Anatomie der Westphal-Strümpellschen Pseudosklerose. *Zeitschr. Ges. Neurol. Psych.* 8, 183–209.

Waldeyer-Hartz, W. von (1891) Über einige neuere Forschungen im Gebiete der Anatomie des Centralnervensystems. *Deutsche Medizinische Wochenschrift* 17, 1213–1218, 1244–1246, 1267–1269, 1287–1289, 1331–1332, 1352–1356.

Waller, A. V. (1850) Experiments on the section of the glosso-pharyngeal and hypoglossal nerves of the frog, and observations of the alterations produced thereby in the structure of their primitive fibres. *Phil. Trans. R. Soc. Lond.* 140, 423–429.

Waller, A. V. (1852) Sur la reproduction des nerfs et sur la structure et les fonctions des ganglions spinaux. *Arch. Anat. Physiol.* (*Liepzig*) 11, 392–401.

Yuste R. (2010) *Dendritic spines*. Cambridge, MA: MIT Press.

PART II

GALLERY OF CAJAL'S DRAWINGS

SECTION A

Spinal Cord

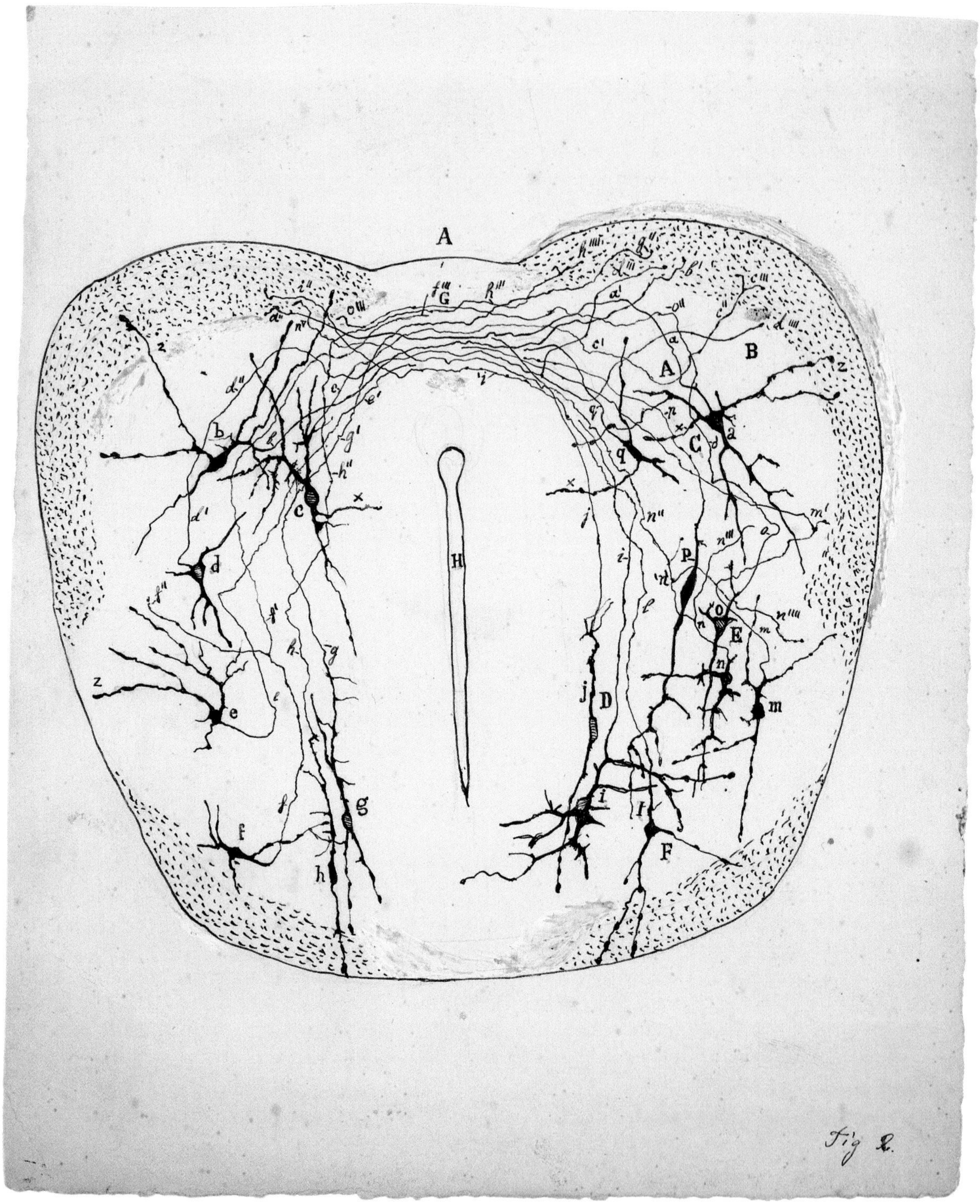

FIGURE 1. Commissural cells of the spinal cord in a chick embryo.

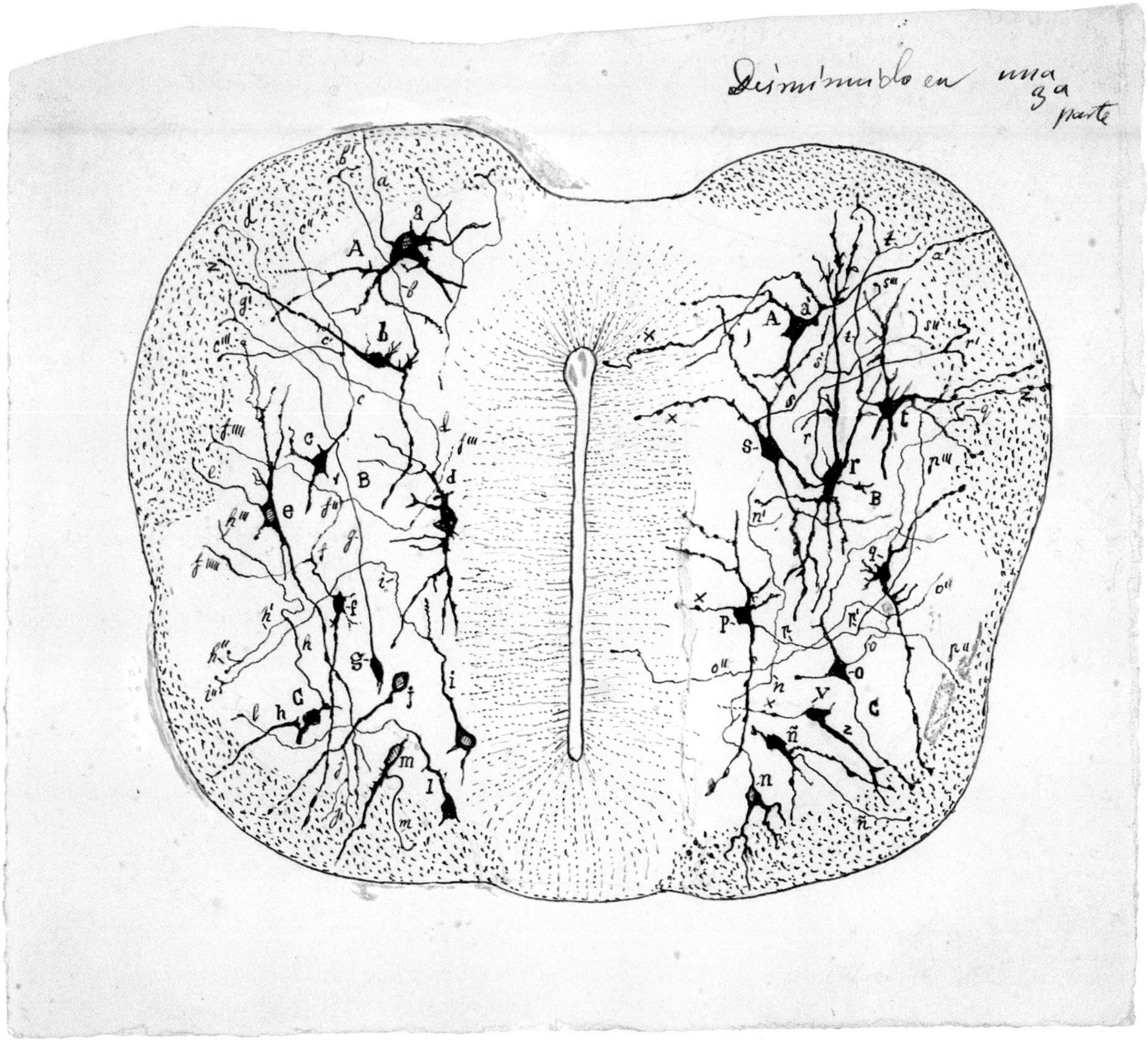

FIGURE 2. Funicular cells of the spinal cord in a chick embryo.

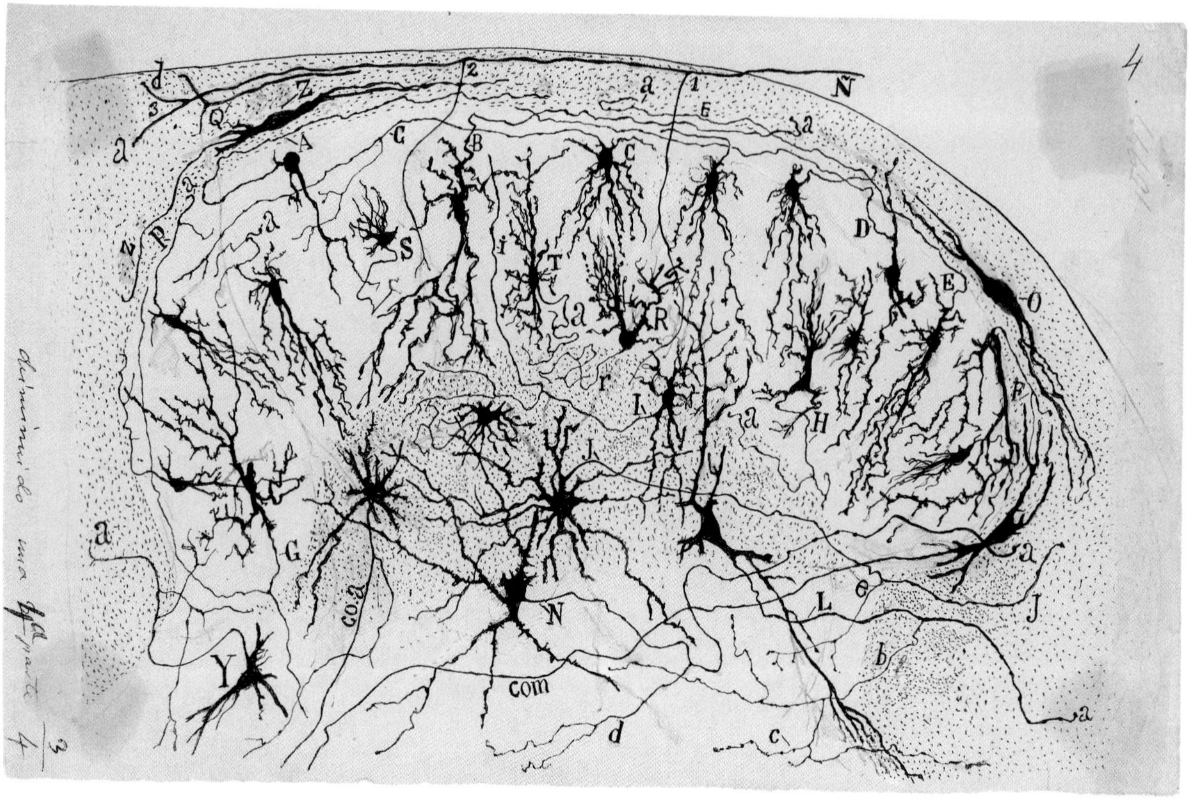

FIGURE 3. Head of the dorsal horn and substancia gelatinosa of the spinal cord in a newborn dog.

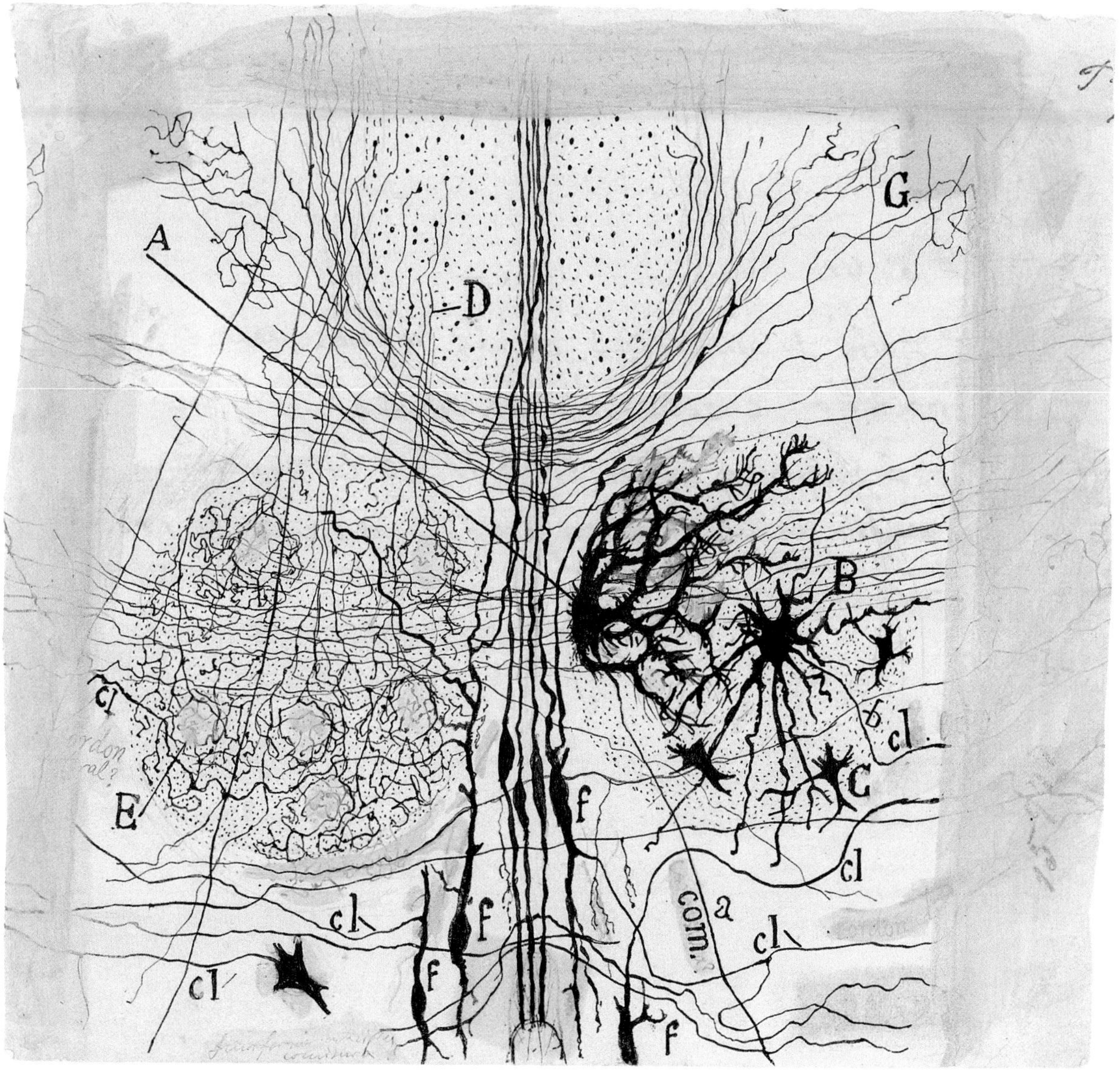

FIGURE 4. Dorsal middle region and column of Clarke of the spinal cord.

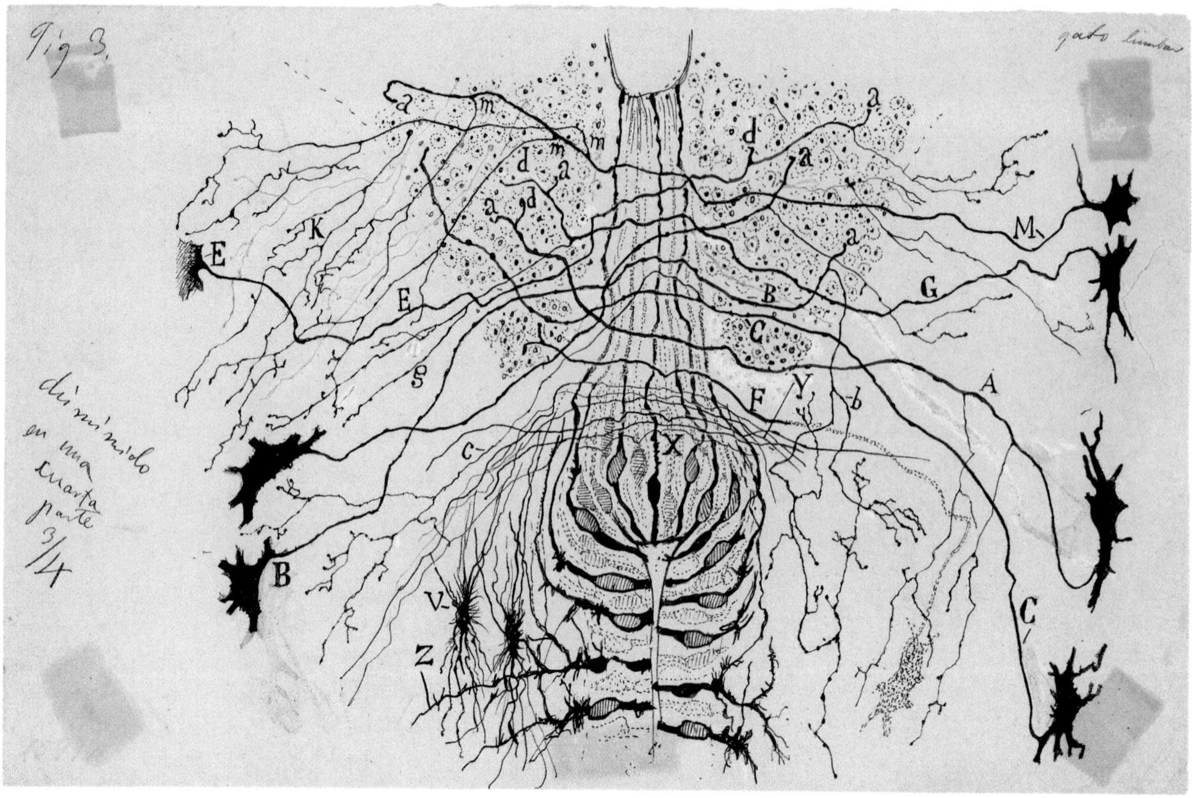

FIGURE 5. Ventral commissure of the spinal cord in a cat a few days old.

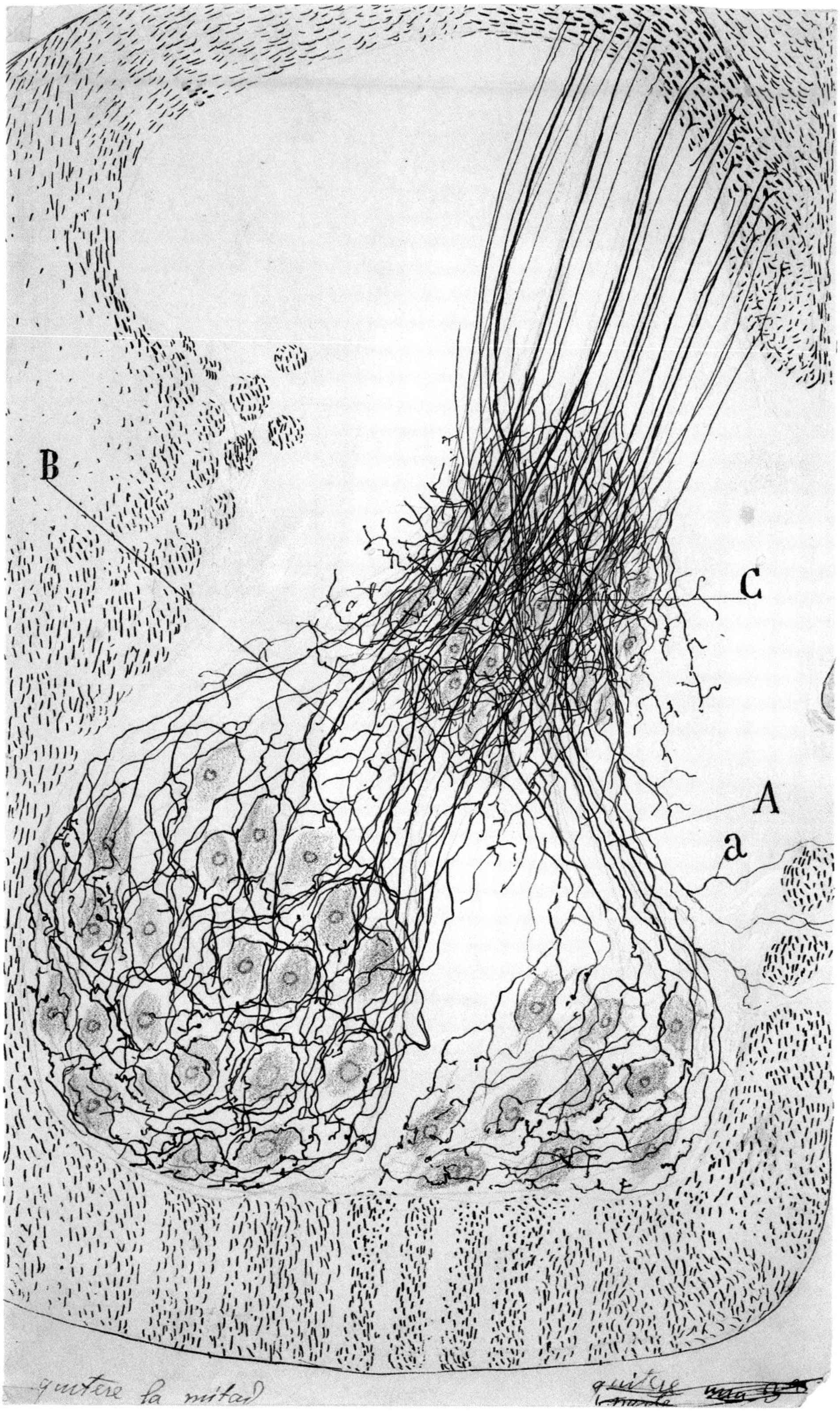

FIGURE 6. Spinal cord in a cat at the level of the cervical enlargement.

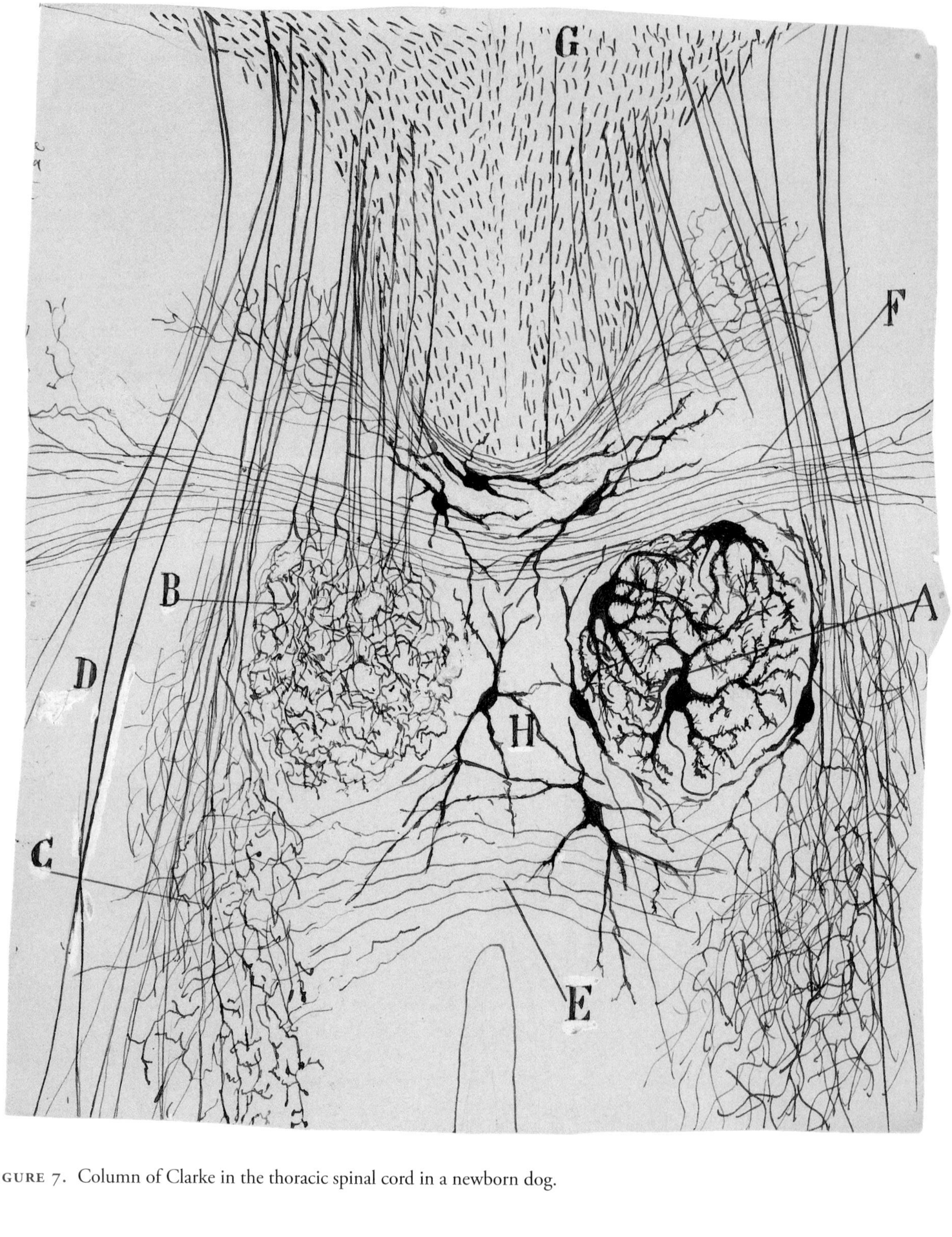

FIGURE 7. Column of Clarke in the thoracic spinal cord in a newborn dog.

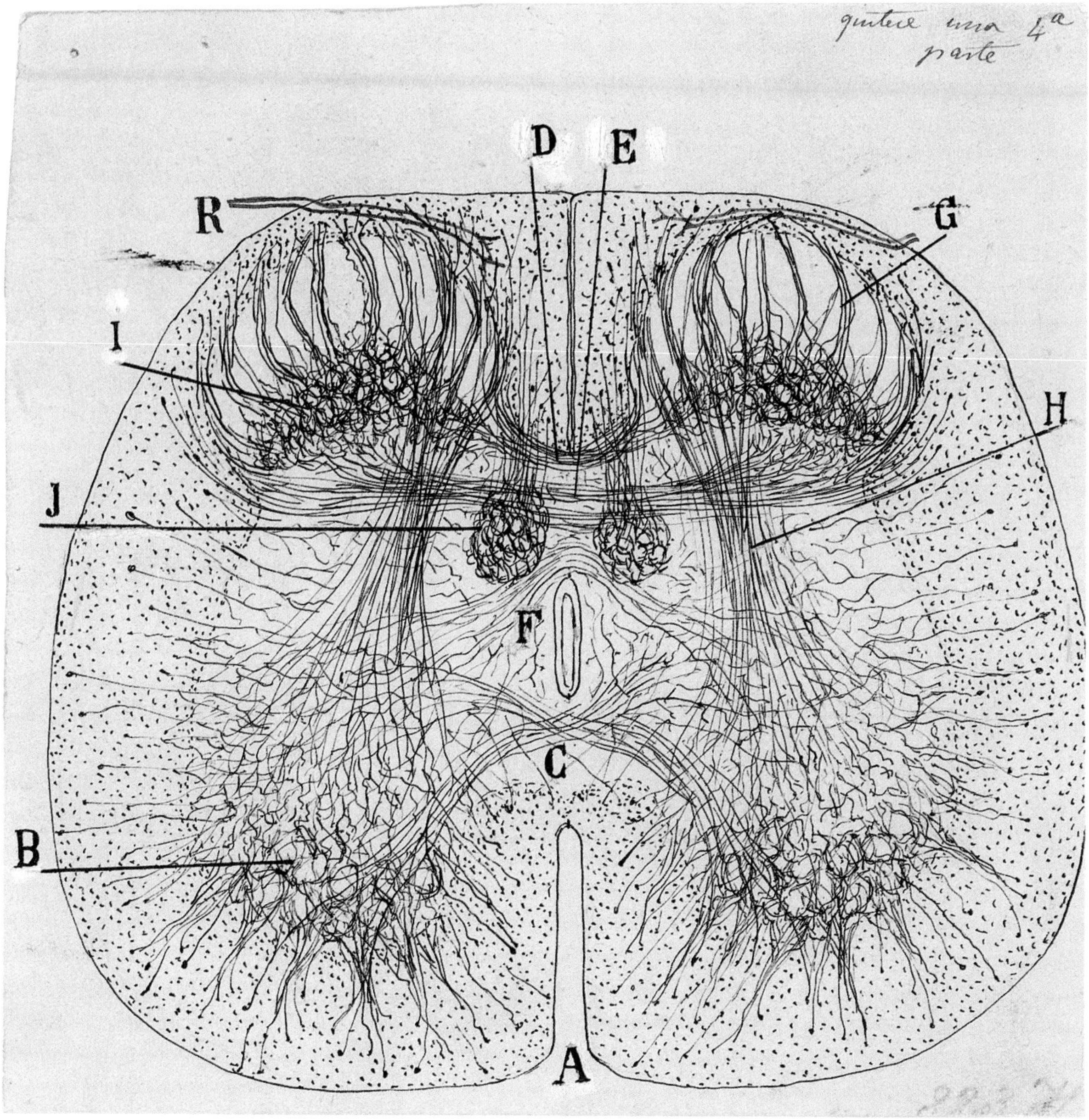

FIGURE 8. Collateral fibers in the thoracic spinal cord of the newborn dog.

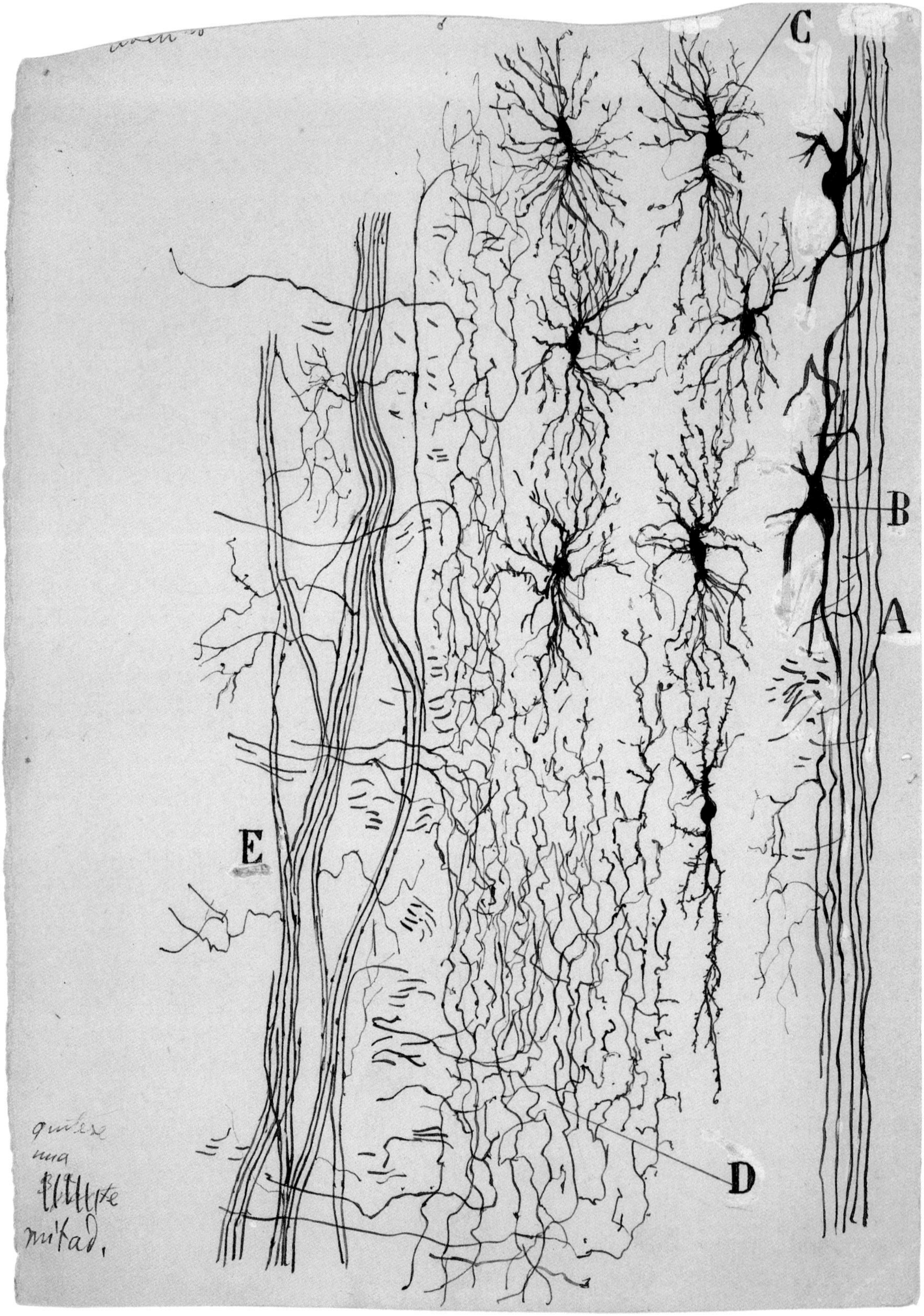

FIGURE 9. Longitudinal section of the substantia gelatinosa and head of the dorsal horn.

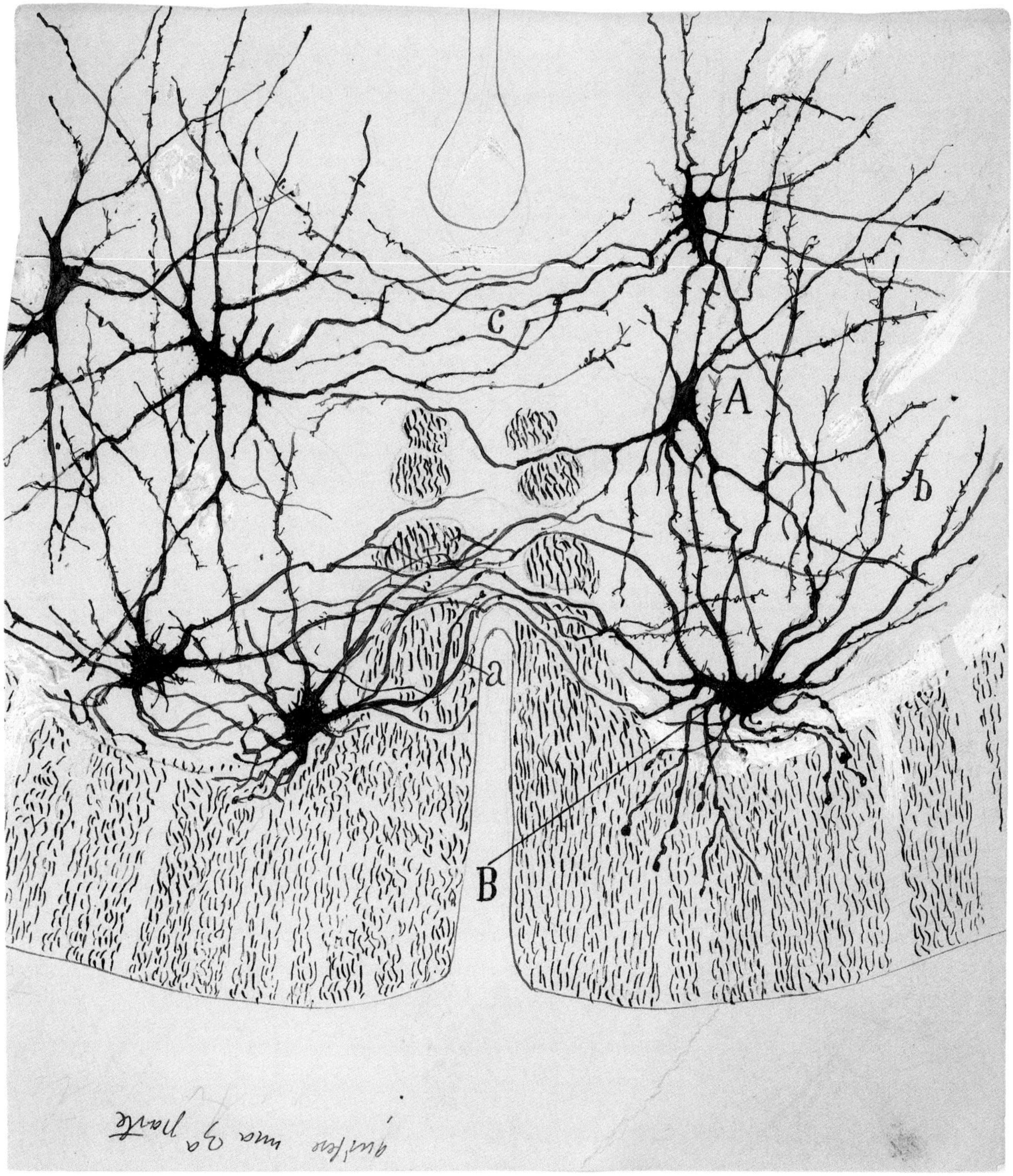

FIGURE 10. Radicular and commissural cells of the thoracic spinal cord in a cat fetus.

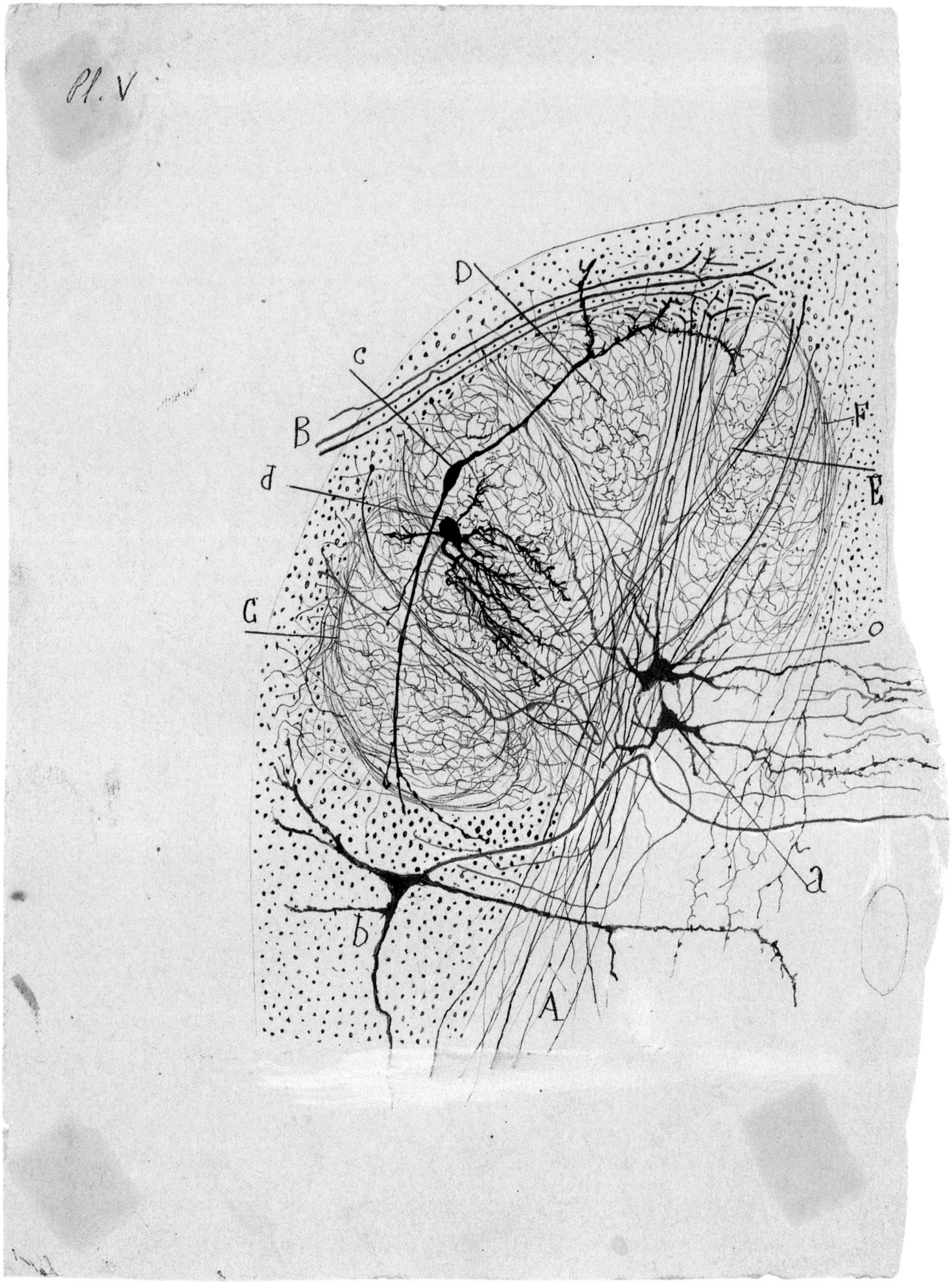

FIGURE 11. Cells of the dorsal horn in a chick embryo on day 15 of incubation.

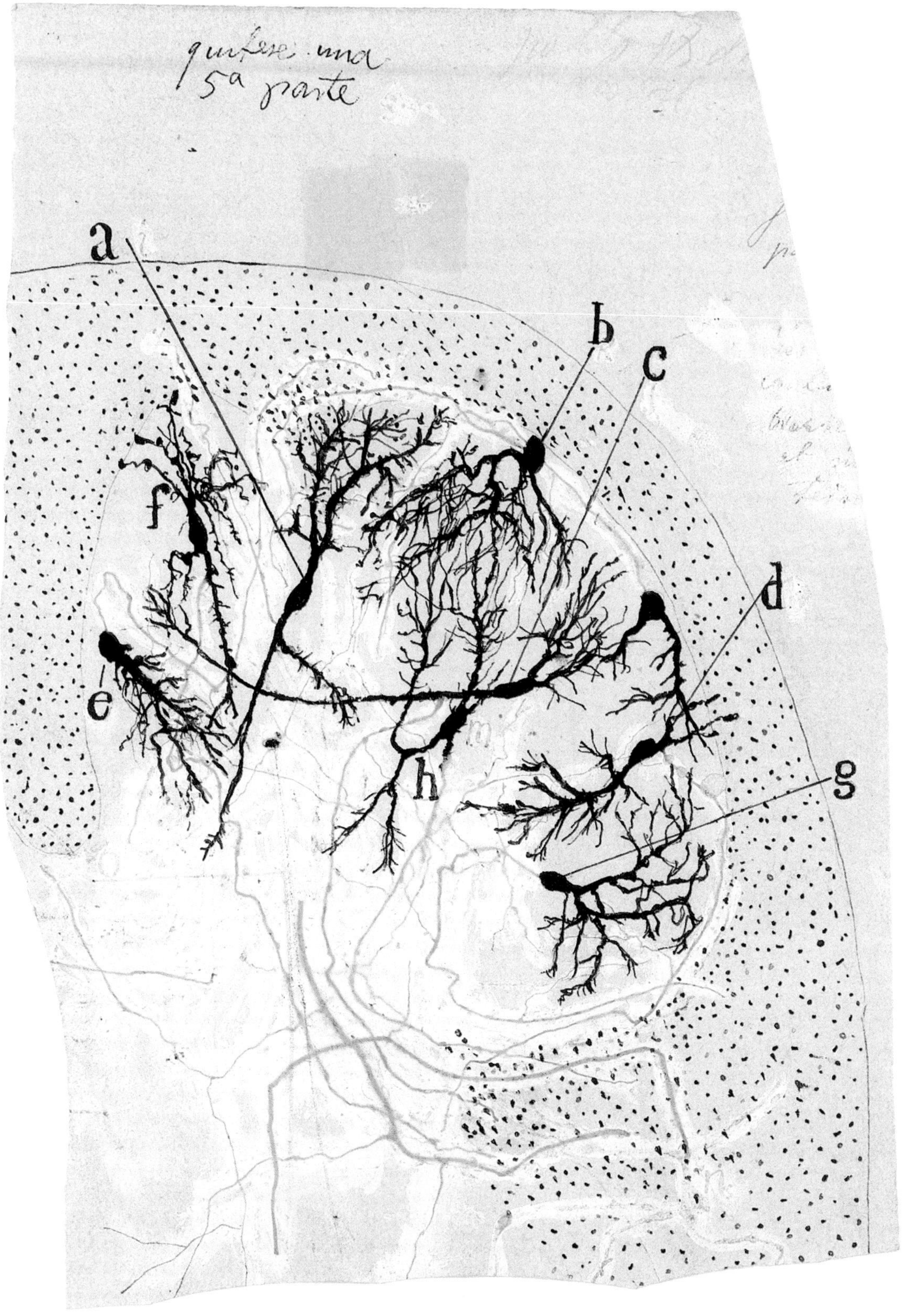

FIGURE 12. Cells of the substantia gelatinosa from a chick embryo on day 19 of incubation.

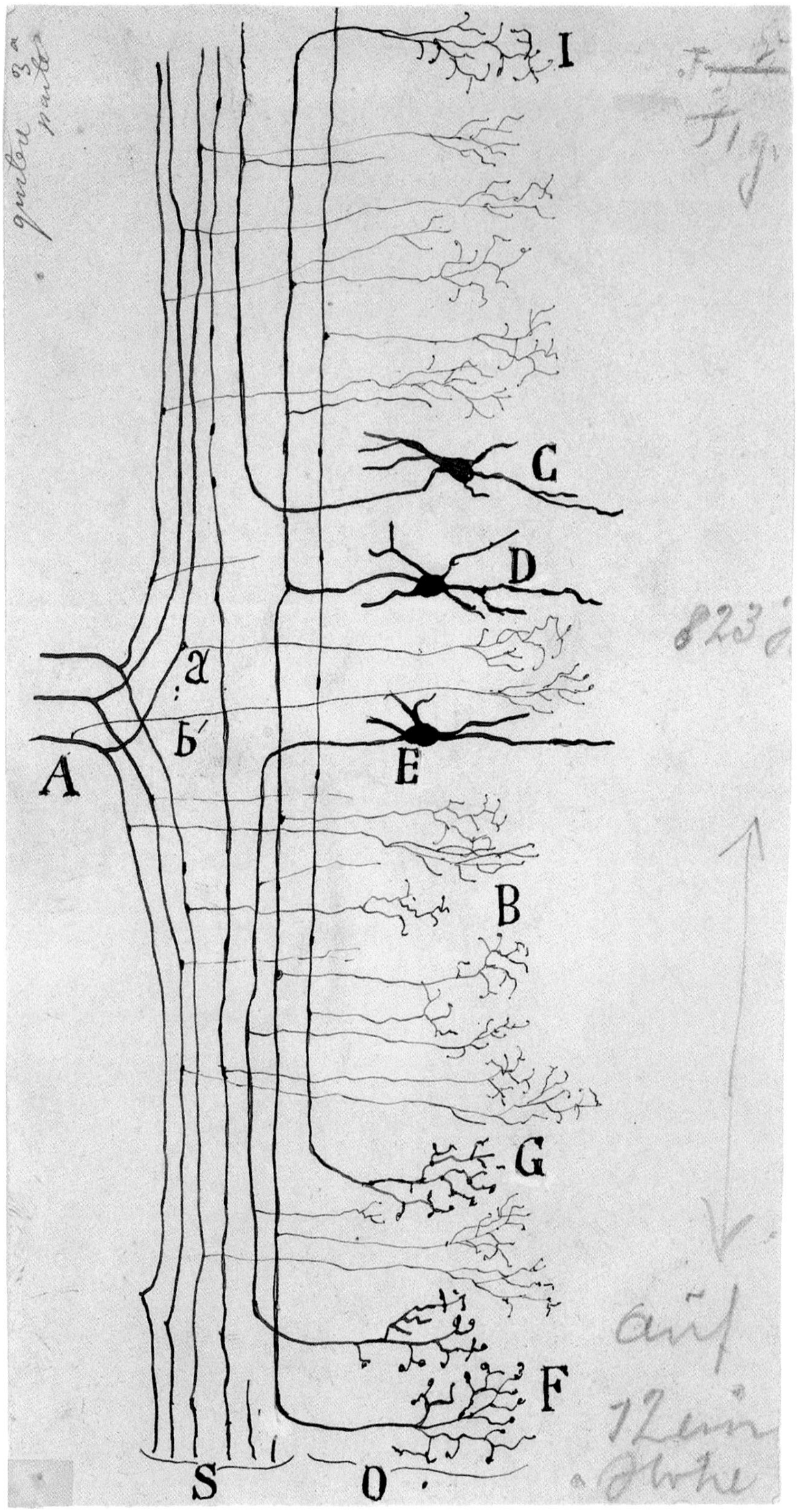

FIGURE 13. Bifurcations of radicular fibers in the dorsal horn in a chick embryo.

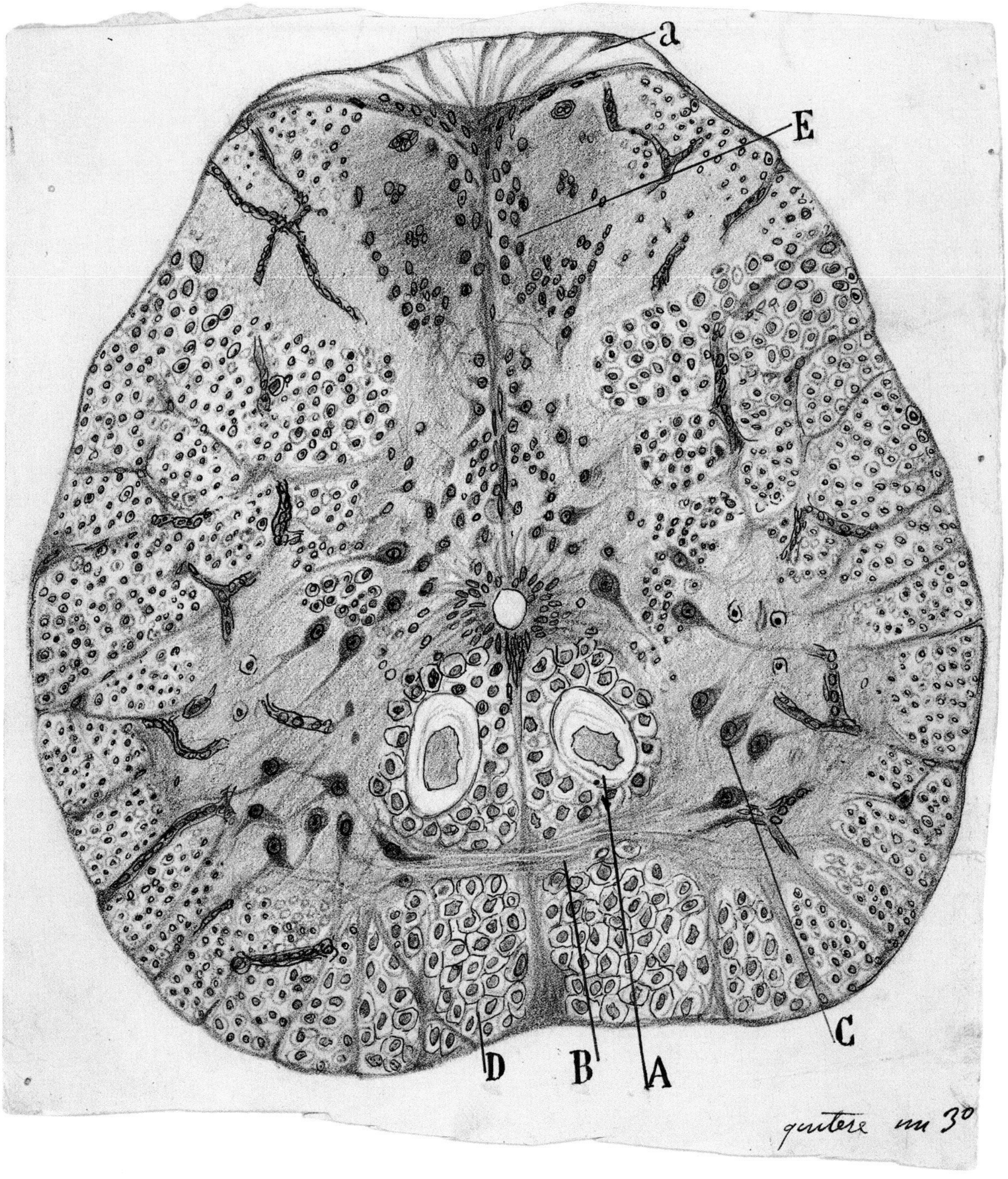

FIGURE 14. Spinal cord in a young teleost.

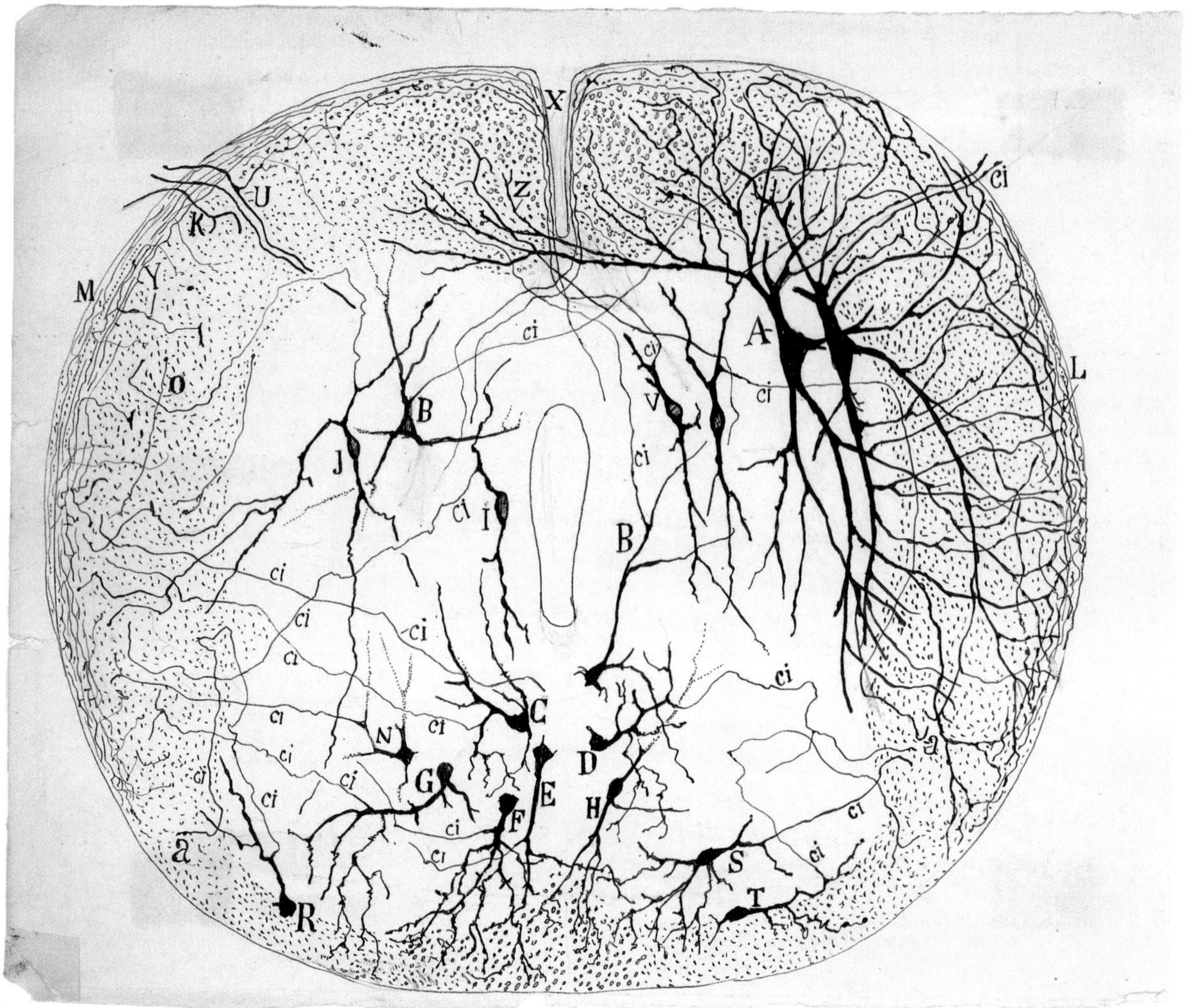

FIGURE 15. Spinal cord of near-term larval stage in a toad.

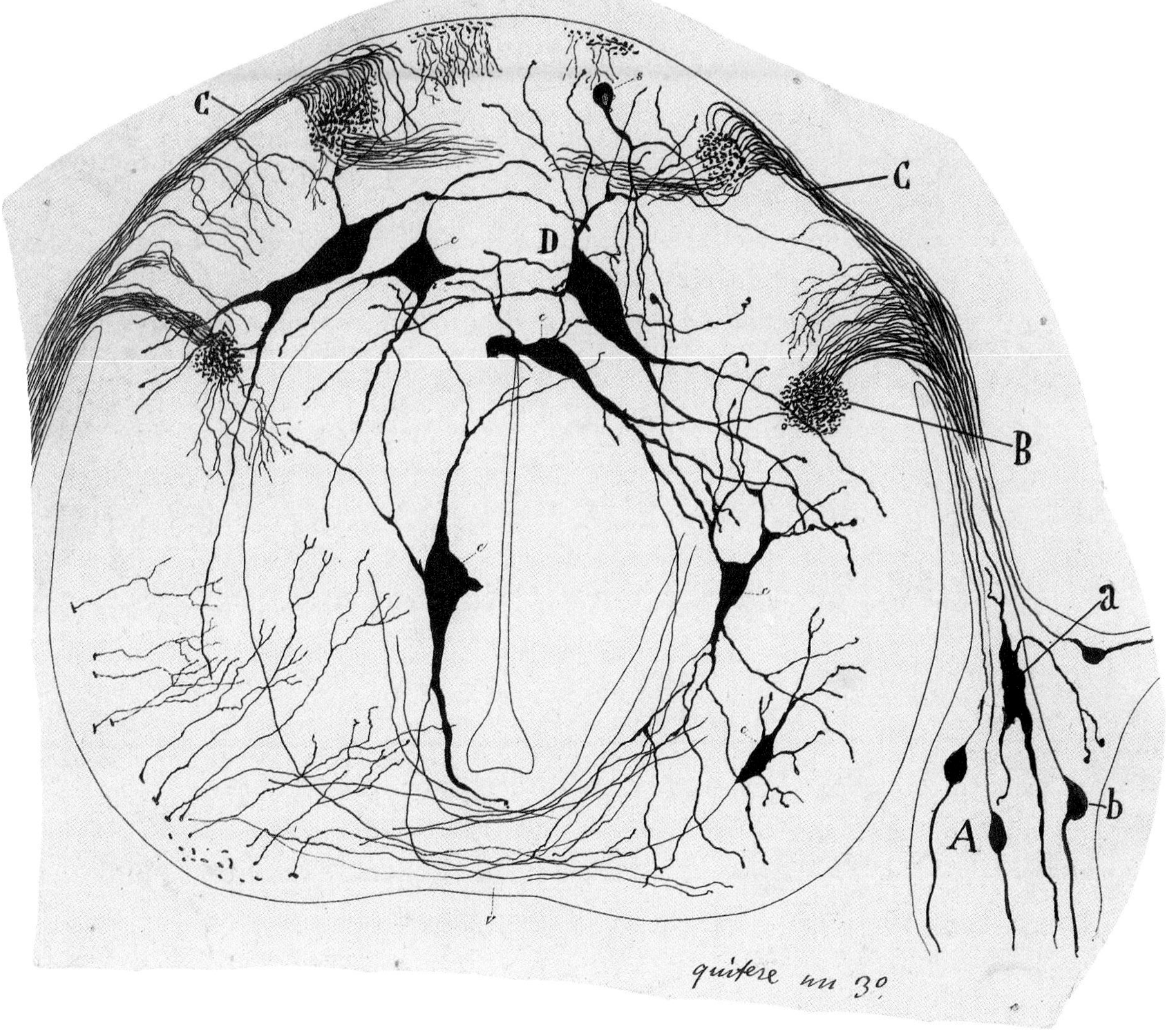

FIGURE 16. Spinal cord in a grass snake embryo.

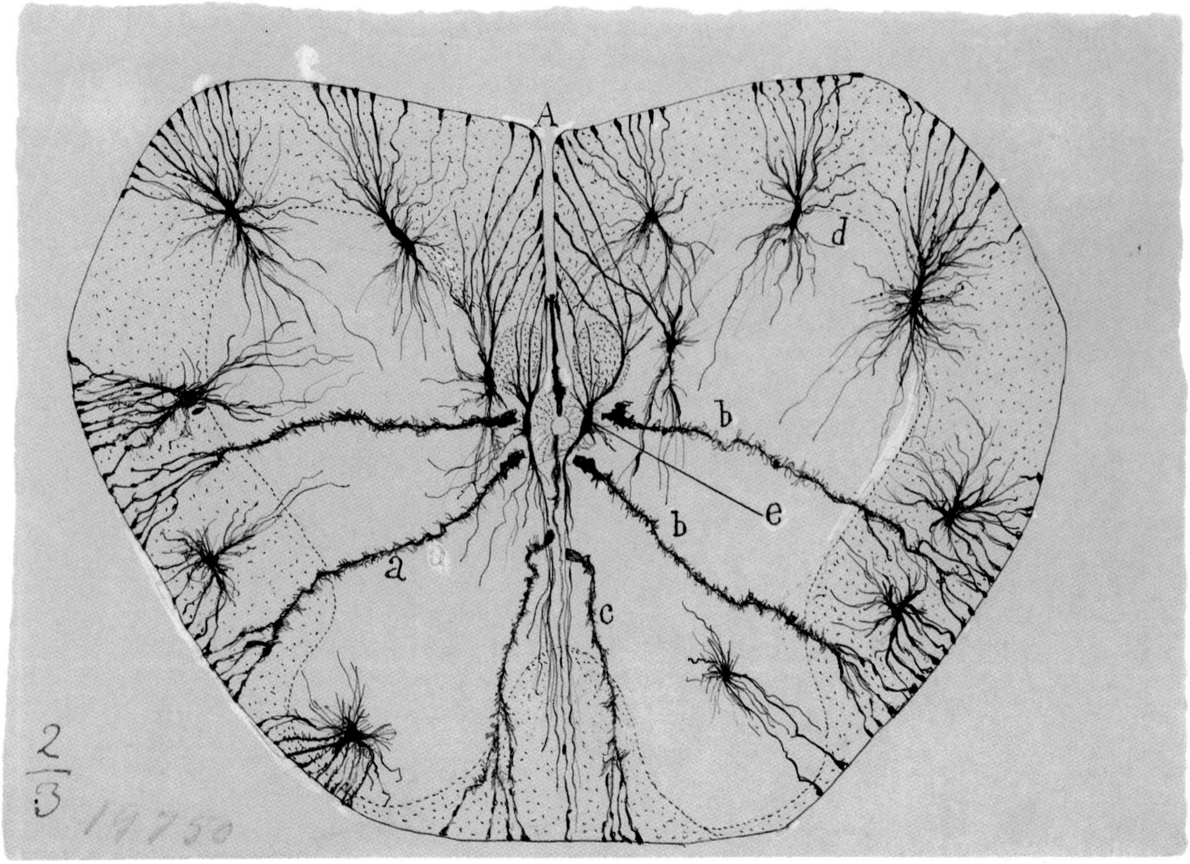

FIGURE 17. Spinal cord in a sand lizard.

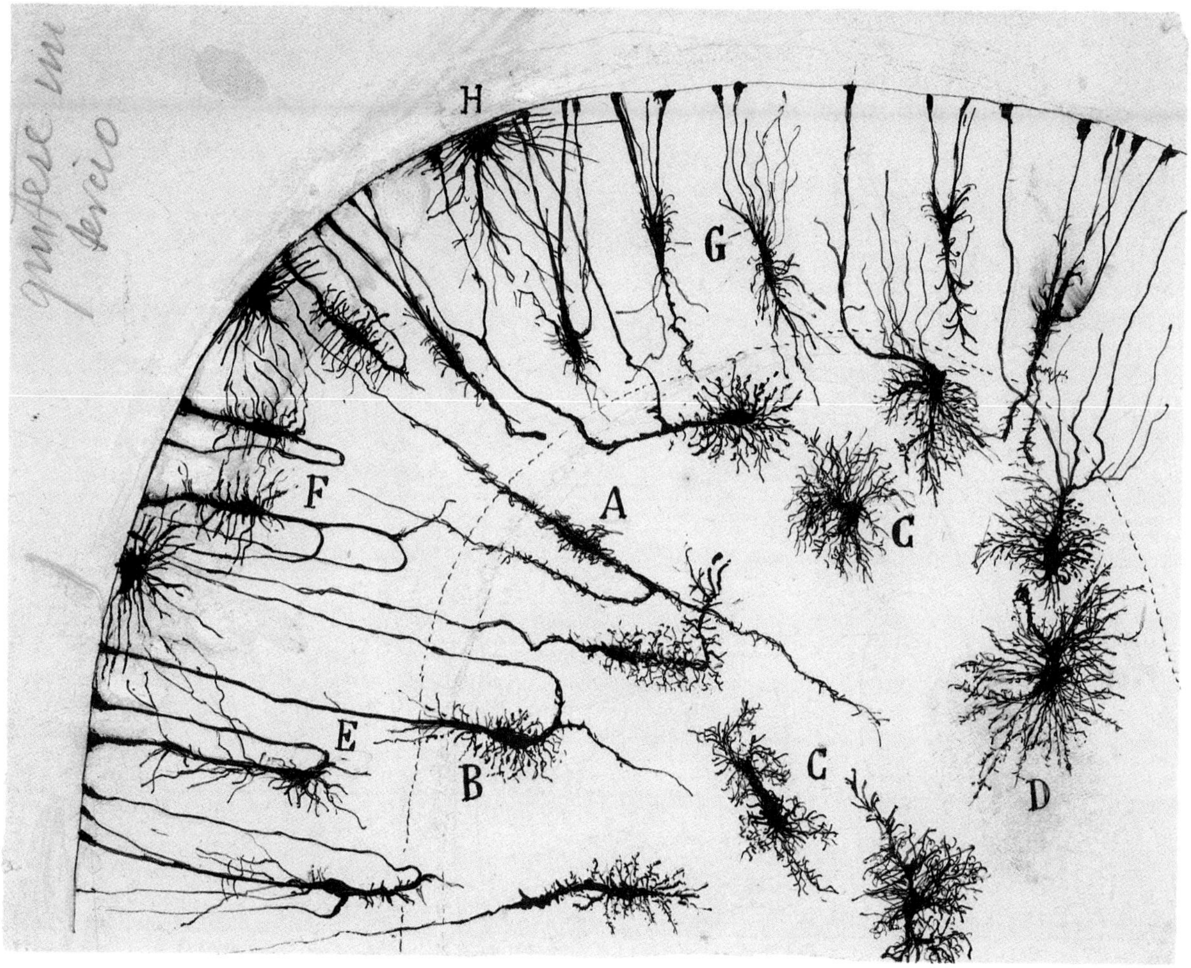

FIGURE 18. Neuroglia in the ventral horn and ventral funiculus in a cat embryo.

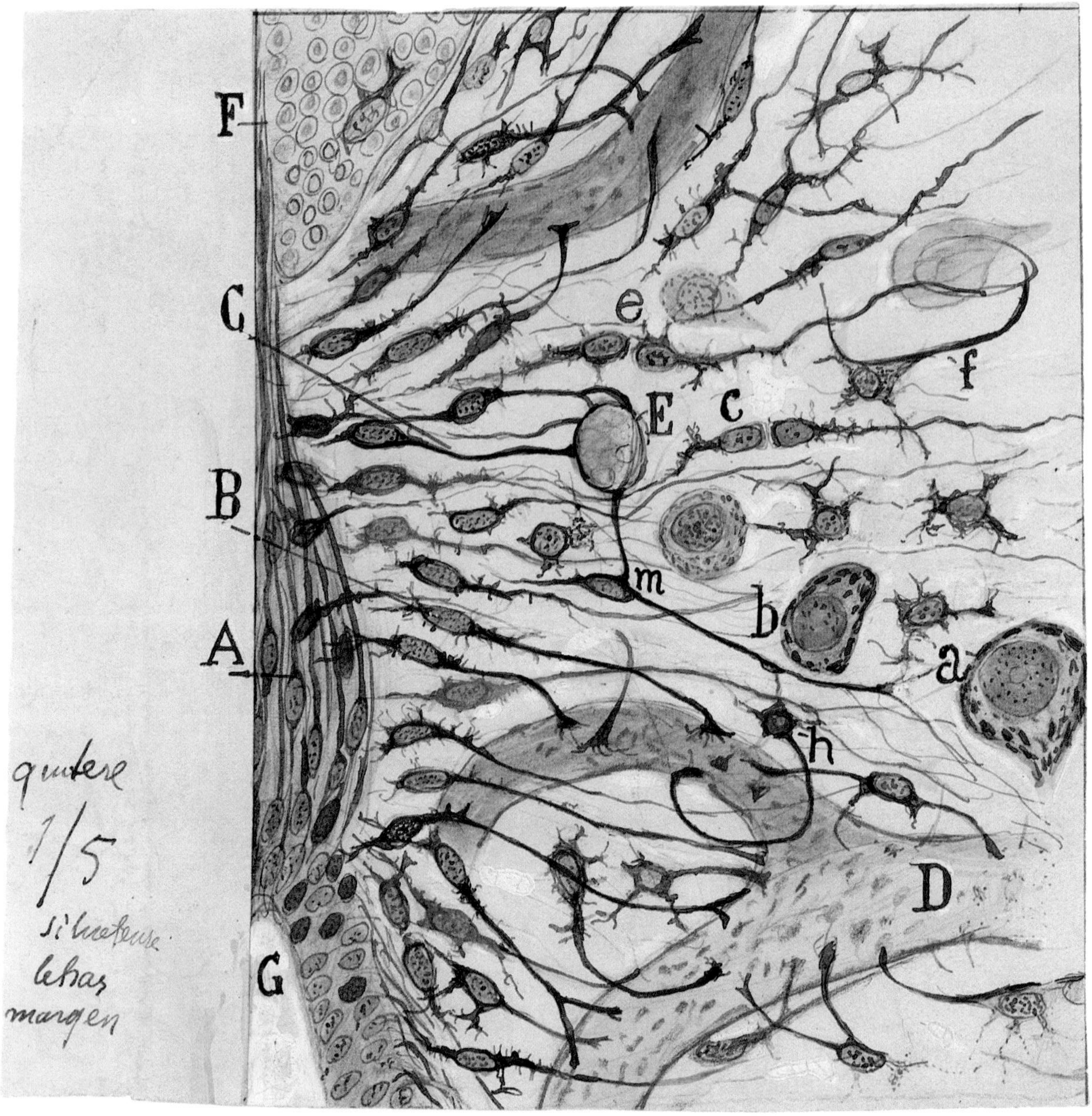

FIGURE 19. Transverse section of the spinal cord in an eight-day-old kitten.

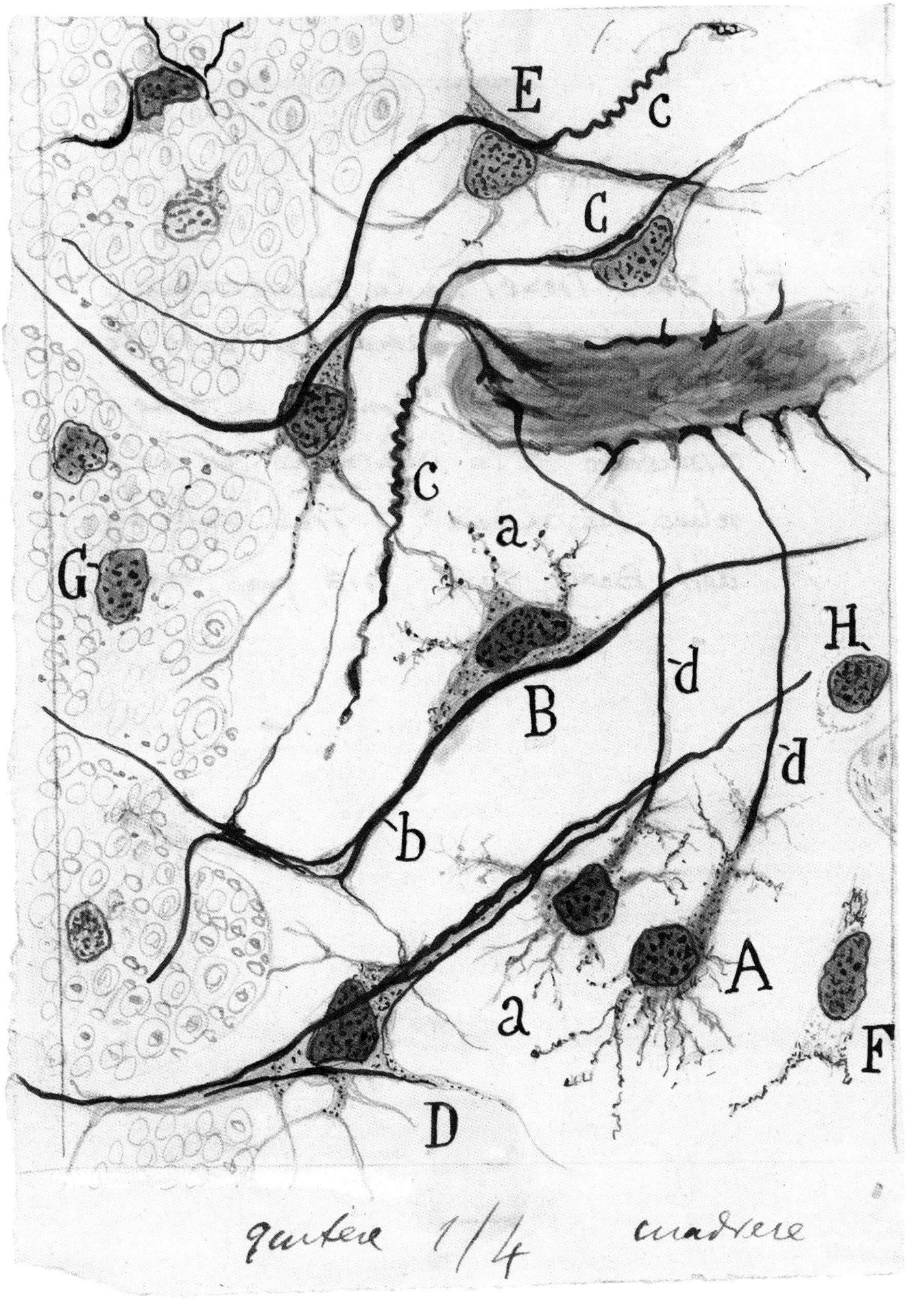

FIGURE 20. Glial cells of the ventral horn in an eight-day-old kitten.

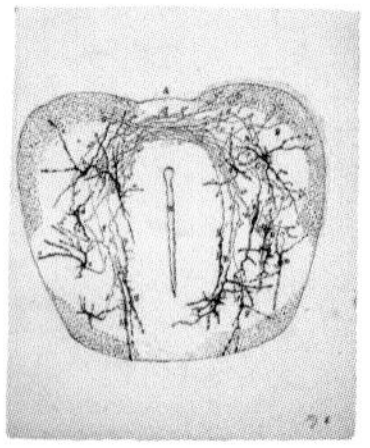

FIGURE 1.

Commissural cells of the spinal cord in a chick embryo.

This figure was published in Cajal, S. R. (1889) Contribución al estudio de la estructura de la médula espinal. *Rev. Trim. Histol. Norm. Patol.* 1, 79–106 (Figure 4).

FIGURE LEGEND: Commissural cells of the spinal cord of the chick embryo on day 7 of incubation. *A*, Ventromedian fissure; *B*, ventral horn; *D, E,* and *F*, cells of the dorsal horn.

Original text: Células comisurales de la médula embrionaria del pollo de 7 días de incubación. *A*, surco anterior de la médula; *B*, asta anterior; *D, E* y *F*, células del asta posterior.

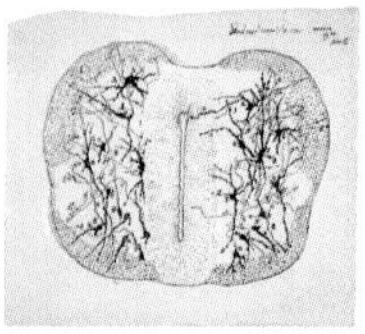

FIGURE 2.

Funicular cells of the spinal cord in a chick embryo.

This figure was published in Cajal, S. R. (1889) Contribución al estudio de la estructura de la médula espinal. *Rev. Trim. Histol. Norm. Patol.* 1, 79–106 (Figure 5).

FIGURE LEGEND: Funicular cells of the spinal cord of the chick embryo on day 7 of incubation. Golgi method. In this figure, cells scattered in various preparations have been collected. *A*, Ventral horn; *B*, central gray region; *C*, dorsal horn. *a*, anterior radicular motor cell; *b*, cell with an axon that is incorporated to the ventral funiculus; *f*, cell with an axon that branches and goes to the lateral funiculus; *m, i, j*, cells with axons that go to the dorsal funiculus. NOTE: Every axon carries in this figure the same letter as the cell from which it arises, but they have been italicized to distinguish them from the normal letters used to indicate the cells.

Original text: Células de los cordones de una médula fetal de pollo de 7 días de incubación. Coloración por el método de Golgi. En esta figura se han reunido células esparcidas en varias preparaciones. *A*, asta anterior; *B*, región gris central; *C*, asta posterior. *a*, célula radicular anterior; *b*, célula cuyo *cilinder* se incorpora al cordón anterior; *f*, célula cuyo *cilinder* se ramifica y marcha al cordón lateral; *m, i, j*, células cuyos cilindros van al cordón posterior. NOTA: todo *cilinder* lleva en esta figura, la misma letra que la célula de que procede, sólo que se ha dibujado cursiva, para distinguirla de las letras de las células.

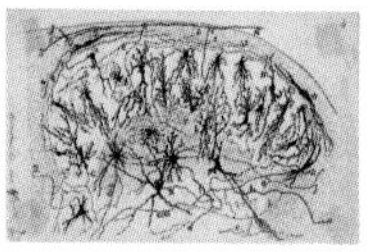

FIGURE 3.

Head of the dorsal horn and substancia gelatinosa of the spinal cord in a newborn dog.

This figure was published in Cajal, S. R. (1890) Nuevas observaciones sobre la estructura de la médula espinal de los mamíferos. *Trab. Lab. Anat. Fac. Med. Barcelona*, April, 1–27 (Figure 3).

FIGURE LEGEND: Transverse section of the dorsal horn head and substancia gelatinosa of Rolando of the spinal cord in a newborn dog. In this figure the cellular elements of various sections have been gathered, and for the sake of clarity in the illustration, many dendritic processes, especially at the head of the dorsal horn, have not been included. *A, B, D, F*, Axons of small dorsal cells of the substancia gelatinosa that were disposed in the transversal direction and took an ascending direction in *a*, (this letter always indicates the longitudinal direction of the fiber that is indicated with this letter); *C*, cell with an axon that is branched during its transversal trajectory; *F*, cell with an axon that showed a dichotomy after a short trajectory; *G*, very irregular cell with an axon that gave rise to a collateral ramification and later took a ventroposterior and marginal direction; *P*, another cell with an axon showing a division; *R, S, T, H*, cells located more ventrally, some of them oriented from top to bottom, with axonal processes that become longitudinal and more or less ventral, ending up by complicated arborizations with an uncertain course. 1, Cell of the head of the dorsal horn with an axon that seemed to go backward, (*i*); *J, L, N*, cells of the head of the dorsal horn with axons that went to the lateral funiculus, after they gave rise in *e, b*, and *d* collaterals to the gray matter. *Y*, Cell with an axon that was bending in the fasciculus cuneatus (fasciculus of Burdach). *O* and *Z*, Robust, marginal fusiform cells; *Q* and *Ñ*, Two radicular fibers ending by bifurcation, after emitting collaterals in 1 and 2; *com.*, axon of marginal cells that seem to go to the dorsal commissure; *coa.*, axon that could be followed up to near the ventral commissure. NOTE: All these cells were copied rigorously from very clear preparations. What is represented here must not be viewed as a schematic, but as an absolute, positive fact.

Original text: Corte transversal del vértice del asta posterior y sustancia de Rolando de la médula del perro recíen nacido. En esta figura se han reunido elementos de diversos cortes, y para que no se perjudicara la claridad se ha prescindido de la representación de muchas ramas protoplasmáticas, sobre todo en el vértice del asta posterior. *A, B, D, F*, Cilindros-ejes de pequeñas células posteriores de la sustancia de Rolando los cuales se disponían en dirección transversal y tomaban dirección ascendente en *a*, (esta letra indica siempre dirección longitudinal en la fibra que la lleve); C, Célula cuyo cilindro-eje se arborizaba durante su trayecto transversal; *F*, Célula cuyo cilindro-eje sufría á poco una dicotomia; *G*, Célula muy irregular cuyo cílindro-eje daba una ramificación colateral para luego tornarse antero-posterior y marginal; *P*, Otra célula cuyo *cilinder* ofrecía una dívisión; *R, S, T, H*, Células situadas más anteriormente, algunas dirigidas de arriba abajo, cuyas espansiones nerviosas venían á hacerse longitudinales y más ó menos anteriores, terminándose por arborizaciones complicadas de curso algo incierto. 1, Célula del vértice del asta posterior cuyo *cilinder* parecía ir hacia atrás, (i); *J, L, N*, Células del vértice del asta posterior cuyos cilindros iban al cordón lateral, después de emitir en *e, b* y *d*, colaterales para la sustancia gris. *Y*, Célula cuyo cilindro-eje se acodaba en el cordón de Burdach. *O* y *Z*, Células fusiformes recias marginales; *Q* y *Ñ*, Dos fibras radiculares terminadas por bifurcación, después de dar en 1 y 2, colaterales; *com.*, cilindro-eje de una célula marginal que parecía ir á la comisura posterior; *coa.*, cilindro-eje que pudo seguirse hasta cerca de la comisura anterior. NOTA: Todas estas células están rigurosamente copiadas de preparaciones clarísimas; lo que aquí se representa es preciso no tomarlo por esquemas, sino por hechos absolutamente positivos.

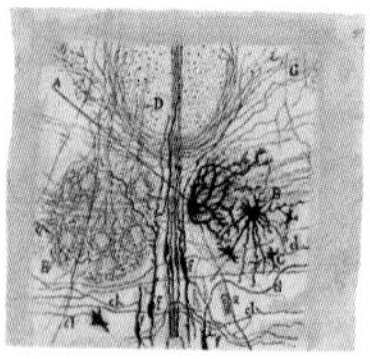

FIGURE 4.

Dorsal middle region and column of Clarke of the spinal cord.

This figure was published in Cajal, S. R. (1890) Nuevas observaciones sobre la estructura de la médula espinal de los mamíferos. *Trab. Lab. Anat. Fac. Med. Barcelona*, April, 1–27 (Figure 4).

FIGURE LEGEND: Transverse section of the dorsal middle region and column of Clarke. On the right, the cellular types of the column of Clarke are represented in *A, B,* and *C*. On the left, the column of Clarke shows connecting fibers that end in this column in the spaces destined to lodge some cells. *D*, Connecting fibers of the fasciculus cuneatus (fasciculus of Burdach); *E*, termination of one of these fibers by means of a free arborization around one cell of this fasciculus; *G*, terminal arborization of the arcuate fibers of the dorsal commissure. *F*, Epithelial cells situated adjacent to the epithelium of the midline line and with axons *cl* that go to the lateral funiculus. These two letters, *cl*, always indicate that it is possible to follow the axon up to this funiculus. The letters *com.* indicate a commissural axon.

Original text: Corte transversal de la región media posterior y columna de Clarke. A la derecha se han representado en *A, B* y *C*, los tipos celulares de la columna de Clarke. A la izquierda, la columna Clarke, presenta las fibras de conexión que en ella se terminan con los huecos ó reservas destinados á algunas células. *D*, fibras de conexión del cordón de Burdach; *E*, Terminacion de una de estas fibras, por arborización libre en torno de una célula de dicha columna: *G*, Arborizaciones terminales de las fibras arciformes de la comisura posterior: *F*, Células fusiformes situadas junto al epitelio de la línea media y cuyos cilindros-ejes *cl*, marchan al cordón lateral. Estas dos letras *cl*, indican siempre, que el cilindro-eje se logró seguir hasta dicho cordón. Las letras *com.*, señalan un cilindro comisural.

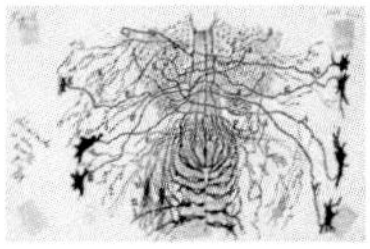

FIGURE 5.

Ventral commissure of the spinal cord in a cat a few days old.

This figure was published in Cajal, S. R. (1890) Nuevas observaciones sobre la estructura de la médula espinal de los mamíferos. *Trab. Lab. Anat. Fac. Med. Barcelona*, April, 1–27 (Figure 5).

FIGURE LEGEND: Section of the ventral commissure region of the spinal cord in a cat a few days old. In this drawing, the commissural axons that have been better impregnated from numerous histological sections of the spinal cord are presented. *A*, Axon that is bifurcated at its termination in ascending (*a*) and descending (*d*) after giving rise to some collaterals near its origin. *B*, Cell with an axon that is bending at its termination (*a*) after giving rise to a large collateral in the other side (*b*), and is represented in detail. *C*, Another axon that, in the midline, supplies a magnificent collateral (*c*) to the gray matter of the other side; *G*, another similar axon. *E*, Another axon that was divided into two branches, one ascending and the other with a longer horizontal trajectory (*a*) with one collateral. *M*, Another axon with three collaterals in the opposite side (*m*); *K*, small branches of ventral connections; *V*, ventrodorsal neuroglia cells; *X*, ventrodorsal bundles of epithelial cells; *Y*, group of fine commissural fibers; *Z*, external poles of the lateral cells of the ependyma. NOTE: For clarity, the dendritic processes of the cells have been removed.

Original text: Corte de la región de la comisura anterior de la médula del gato de pocos días. En esta preparación se han reunido los cilindros-ejes comisurales más correctamente impregnados de numerosos cortes medulares. *A*, Cilindro-eje bifurcado a su terminación en rama ascendente (*a*) y descendente (*d*) después de dar algunas colaterales cerca de su origen; B, Célula cuyo cilindro-eje se acoda al terminar (a), después de dar una hermosa colateral en el otro lado (b), que se ba representado detalladamente; C, Otro cilindro, que suministra en la línea media una magnífica colateral (c), para la sustancia gris del otro lado; G, Otro *cilinder* análogo; E, Otro que se dividía en dos ramas, una descendente y otra de trayecto horizontal más largo (*a*), con una colateral; *M*, Otro *cilinder* con tres colaterales en el opuesto lado (*m*); *K*, ramitas de conexión anteriores; *V*, Células neuróglicas antero-posteriores; *X*, manojo antero-posterior de células epileliales; *Y*, Grupo de finas fibras comisurales; *Z*, Extremos externos de las células laterales del epéndimo. NOTA: Para mayor claridad se han suprimido las expansiones protoplasmáticas de las células.

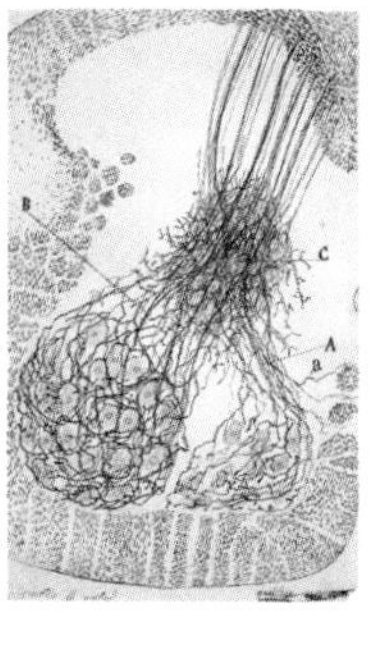

FIGURE 6.

Spinal cord in a cat at the level of the cervical enlargement.

This figure was published in Cajal, S. R. (1899–1904) *Textura del sistema nervioso del hombre y de los vertebrados*. Madrid: Moya (Figure 84).

FIGURE LEGEND: Transverse section of the cat spinal cord at the level of the cervical enlargement (near-term fetus). Golgi method. *A*, Bundle destined to the medial motor nucleus; *B*, thicker and broader bundle for the lateral motor nucleus; *C*, plexus of the intermediate nucleus; *a*, some collaterals directed toward the dendritic commissure.

Original text: Corte transversal de la médula de gato al nivel del engrosamiento cervical (feto casi de término). Método de Golgi. *A*, manojo destinado al foco motor interno; *B*, manojo más grueso y ancho consagrado al foco externo; *C*, plexo del foco gris intermediario; *a*, algunas colaterales para la comisura protoplásmica.

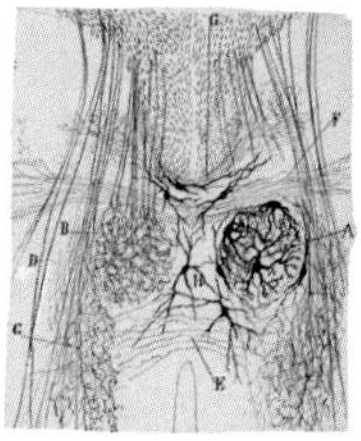

FIGURE 7.

Column of Clarke in the thoracic spinal cord in a newborn dog.

This figure was published in Cajal, S. R. (1899–1904) *Textura del sistema nervioso del hombre y de los vertebrados*. Madrid: Moya (Figure 86).

FIGURE LEGEND: Horizontal section of the region of Clarke's column in a newborn dog (thoracic spinal cord). Golgi method. *A*, Cells of Clarke's column; *B*, arborizations of collaterals destined to Clarke's column; *C*, collaterals in the intermediate nucleus; *D*, long or reflexomotor collaterals; *E*, ventral commissural bundle; *F*, intermediate commissural bundle; *G*, dorsal commissural bundle; *H*, cells of the dorsal commissure.

Original text: Corte horizontal de la región de la columna de Clarke del perro recien nacido (médula dorsal). Método de Golgi. *A*, células de la columna de Clarke; *B*, arborizaciones de sus colaterales; *C*, colaterales del foco gris intermediario; *D*, colaterales largas ó reflejo-motrices; *E*, manojo comisural anterior; *F*, manojo comisural medio; *G*, manojo comisural posterior; *H*, células de la comisura posterior.

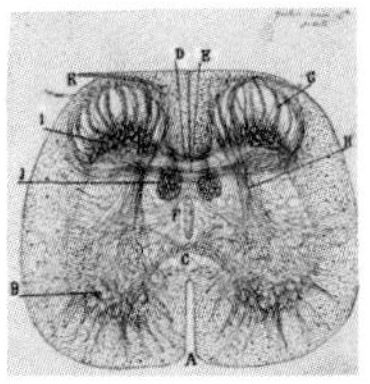

FIGURE 8.

Collateral fibers in the thoracic spinal cord in a newborn dog.

This figure was published in Cajal, S. R. (1899–1904) *Textura del sistema nervioso del hombre y de los vertebrados*. Madrid: Moya (Figure 88).

FIGURE LEGEND: Composite of collateral fibers in the thoracic spinal cord in a newborn dog. Golgi method. *A*, Ventral median fissure of the spinal cord; *B*, collaterals of the ventral funiculus; *C*, collaterals of the ventral commissure; *D*, dorsal bundle of the dorsal commissure; *E*, middle bundle of the dorsal commissure; *F*, ventral bundle of the dorsal commissure; *G*, arcuate collaterals of the dorsal funiculus that cross the substancia gelatinosa in arcs; *H*, sensorimotor; *I*, collaterals ramified in the dorsal horn; *J*, collaterals destined to Clarke's column; *R*, dorsal root.

Original text: Conjunto de las fibras colaterales de la médula espinal dorsal del perro recién nacido. Método de Golgi. *A*, surco anterior de la médula; *B*, colaterales del cordón anterior; *C*, colaterales de la comisura anterior; *D*, manojo posterior de la comisura posterior; *E*, manojo medio de ésta; *F*, manojo anterior de la misma; *G*, colaterales [arciformes] del cordón posterior que cruzan en arcos la substancia de Rolando; *H*, manojo sensitivo-motor; *I*, colaterales ramificadas en el asta posterior; *J*, colaterales para la columna de Clarke; *R*, raíz posterior.

Note from the author (J. D.): In brackets is the text added in the French version of the *Textura*: Cajal, S. R. (1909–1911) *Histologie du système nerveux de l'homme et des vertébrés*, trans. L. Azoulay. Paris: Maloine. This drawing is very similar to Figure 6 in Cajal, S. R. (1890) Nuevas observaciones sobre la estructura de la médula espinal de los mamíferos. *Trab. Lab. Anat. Fac. Med. Barcelona*, April, 1–27.

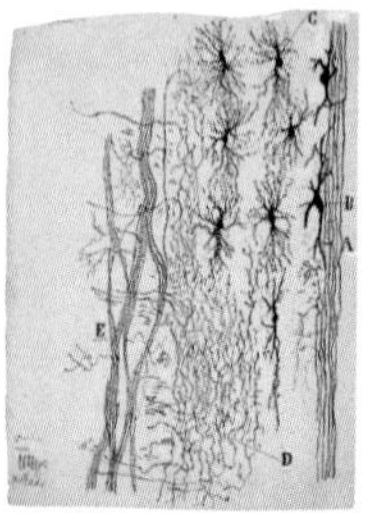

FIGURE 9.

Longitudinal section of the substantia gelatinosa and head of the dorsal horn.

This figure was published in Cajal, S. R. (1899–1904) *Textura del sistema nervioso del hombre y de los vertebrados*. Madrid: Moya (Figure 97 and Figure 119).

FIGURE LEGEND: Longitudinal section that is slightly obliquely lateral to the substantia gelatinosa and head of the dorsal horn. Newborn dog. Golgi method. *A*, Fibers of the dorsal funiculus; *B*, border cells of the substantia gelatinosa; *C*, cells of the substantia gelatinosa; *D*, longitudinal plexus of collaterals in the head of the dorsal horn; *E*, longitudinal fibers that are probably sensory collaterals in the head of the dorsal horn.

Original text: Corte antero-posterior vertical y algo oblicuo hacia afuera de la substancia de Rolando y vértice del asta posterior. Perro recién nacido. Método de Golgi. *A*, fibras del cordón posterior; *B*, células limitantes de la substancia de Rolando; *C*, células de esta substancia; *D*, plexo longitudinal de colaterales del vértice del asta posterior; *E*, fibras longitudinales, probablemente colaterales sensitivas del vértice del asta posterior.

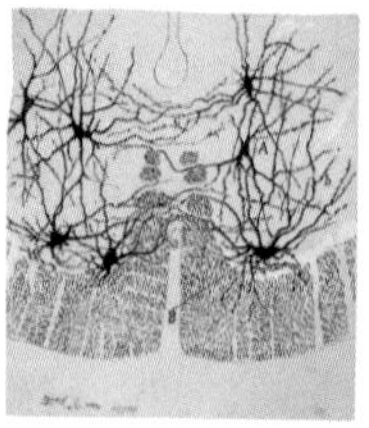

FIGURE 10.

Radicular and commissural cells of the thoracic spinal cord in a cat fetus.

This figure was published in Cajal, S. R. (1899–1904) *Textura del sistema nervioso del hombre y de los vertebrados*. Madrid: Moya (Figure 98).

FIGURE LEGEND: Radicular and commissural cells of the thoracic spinal cord in a cat fetus. Golgi method. *A*, Commissural cell; *B*, motor cell of the medial nucleus; *a*, commissural dendritic processes; *b*, dorsal dendritic processes; *c*, commissure formed by dendrites of commissural cells. Fibers in red are axons.

Original text: Células radiculares y comisurales de la médula dorsal del feto de gato. Método de Golgi. *A*, célula comisural; *B*, célula motriz del foco interno; *a*, expansiones dendritas comisurales; *b*, expansiones posteriores; *c*, comisura de dendritas emanadas de células funiculares. Las fibras en rojo son cilindros-ejes.

Note from the author (J. D.): The fibers in red (see Supplementary Figure S1) were added in the publication of *Textura*: Cajal, S. R. (1909–1911) *Histologie du système nerveux de l'homme et des vertébrés*, trans. L. Azoulay. Paris: Maloine.

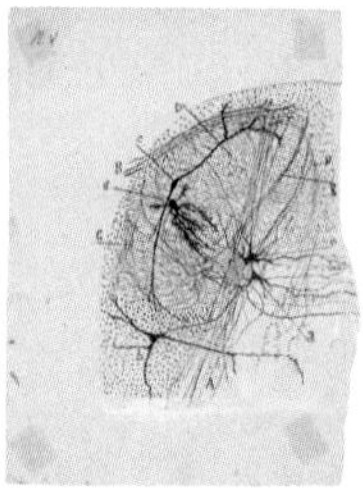

FIGURE 11.

Cells of the dorsal horn in a chick embryo on day 15 of incubation.

This figure was published in Cajal, S. R. (1895) L'anatomie fine de la moelle epinière. In *Atlas der Pathologischen Histologie des Nervensystems. IV. Lieferung*, ed. V. Babes, Berlin: Verlag von August Hirschwald (part of Figure 5). This figure was modified and reproduced as Figure 116 (see Supplementary Figure S2) in Cajal, S. R. (1899–1904) *Textura del sistema nervioso del hombre y de los vertebrados*. Madrid: Moya.

FIGURE LEGEND: Some cells of the dorsal horn of the chick embryo on day 15 of incubation. Golgi method. *A*, Dorsal root; *B*, fusiform cell of the substantia gelatinosa; *C*, another cell of this substance; *D*, cell of the dorsal horn with an axon directed to the dorsal commissure; *E*, cell of the interstitial nucleus with an axon directed to the dorsal commissure; *F*, dorsal dendritic commissure.

Original text: Algunas células del asta posterior del embrión de pollo de quince días. Método de Golgi. *A*, raíz posterior; *B*, célula transversal de la substancia de Rolando; C, célula de esta substancia; *D*, célula del centro del asta posterior cuyo axon iba á la comisura posterior; *E*, célula intersticial también comisural posterior; *F*, comisura protoplásmica posterior.

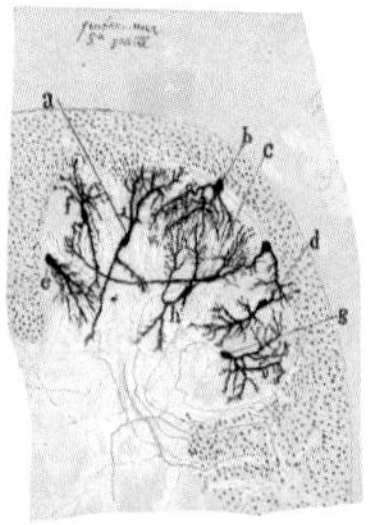

FIGURE 12.

Cells of the substantia gelatinosa from a chick embryo on day 19 of incubation.

This figure was published in Cajal, S. R. (1895) L'anatomie fine de la moelle epinière. In *Atlas der Pathologischen Histologie des Nervensystems. IV. Lieferung*, ed. V. Babes. Berlin: Verlag von August Hirschwald (part of Figure 5). This figure was modified and reproduced as Figure 121 (see Supplementary Figure S3) in Cajal, S. R. (1899–1904) *Textura del sistema nervioso del hombre y de los vertebrados*. Madrid: Moya.

FIGURE LEGEND: Almost fully developed cells of the substantia gelatinosa from a chick embryo on day 19 of incubation. Golgi method. *A, D, E*, Cells with axons that are going to the bundle of the dorsal horn; *C*, *F*, border cells with axons that are going first in a tangential direction; *B*, transverse cell; *G, I*, cells with axons going to the dorsal funiculus.

Original text: Células de la substancia de Rolando casi adultas tomadas de la médula del embrión de pollo del décimonoveno día de incubación. Método de Golgi. *A, D, E*, células cuyo axon iba al manojo del asta posterior; *C, F*, células limitantes cuyos axones marchaban primero en dirección tangencial; *B*, célula transversal; *G, I*, células cuyo axon iba al cordón posterior.

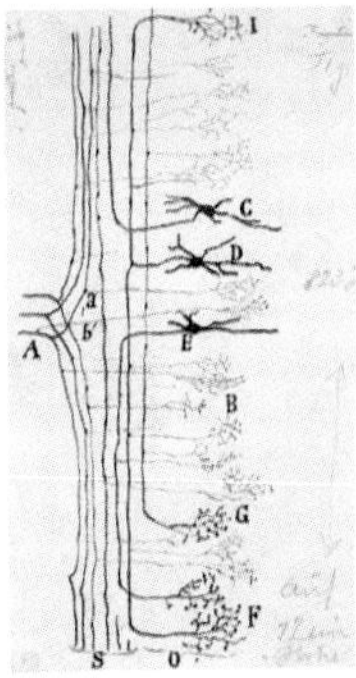

FIGURE 13.

Bifurcations of radicular fibers in the dorsal horn in a chick embryo

This figure was published in Cajal, S. R. (1892) Nuevo concepto de la histología de los centros nerviosos. *Rev. Ciencias Méd. Barcelona* 18, 363–376, 457–476, 505–520, 529–540 (Figure 4). It has also been reproduced as Figure 200 in Cajal, S. R. (1899–1904) *Textura del sistema nervioso del hombre y de los vertebrados*. Madrid: Moya.

FIGURE LEGEND: Bifurcations of some radicular fibers in the dorsal horn in a chick embryo. Golgi method. *a*, Collateral of ascending and descending branches; *b*, collateral of the radicular fiber trunk. **A*, Dorsal root; S, white matter; *O*, gray matter; *C*, cell of the dorsal funiculus with a bending axon; *D*, another cell with axon bifurcated in ascending and descending branches; *E*, another cell with a bending descending axon; *G, F*, axon terminal arborizations; B, terminal arborizations of collaterals of the gray matter.*

Original text: Bifurcación, en el cordón posterior del embrión de pollo, de algunas radiculares. *a*, colateral de las ramas ascendente ó descendente; *b*, colateral del tallo. **A*, raíz posterior; *S*, substancia blanca; *O*, substancia gris; *C*, célula del cordón posterior con cilindro acodado; *D*, otra con cilindro-eje bifurcado en rama ascendente y descendente; *E*, otra célula de cilindro acodado descendente; *G* y *F*, arborizaciones finales de cilindros-eje; *B*, arborizaciones finales de colaterales de la substancia blanca.*

Note from the author (J. D.): The text between asterisks appears in the original publication only.

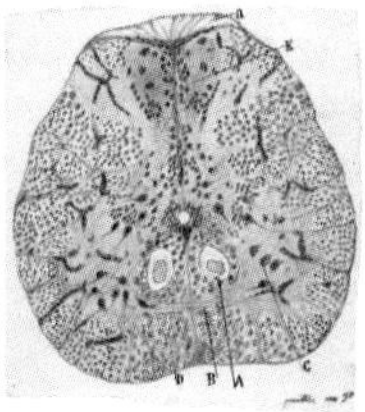

FIGURE 14.

Spinal cord in a young teleost.

This figure was published in Cajal, S. R. (1899–1904) *Textura del sistema nervioso del hombre y de los vertebrados*. Madrid: Moya (Figure 169).

FIGURE LEGEND: Transverse section of the spinal cord in a young teleost (*Cyprinus carpio*). Hematoxylin staining. *A*, Colossal or Mauthner fiber; *B*, accessory commissure; *D*, robust fibers of the ventral funiculus (ventral portion); *C*, pyriform motor cells; *E*, small neurons in the medial part of the substantia gelatinosa; *a*, salient endings of ependymal cells.

Original text: Corte transversal de la médula espinal de un teleosteo joven (*Cyprinus carpio*). Coloración con hematoxilina. *A*, Tubo colosal ó de Mauthner; *B*, comisura accesoria; *D*, tubos robustos del cordón ventral (porción anterior); *C*, células motrices piriformes; *E*, pequeñas neuronas de la parte interna de la substancia de Rolando; *a*, cabos salientes de las células epiteliales.

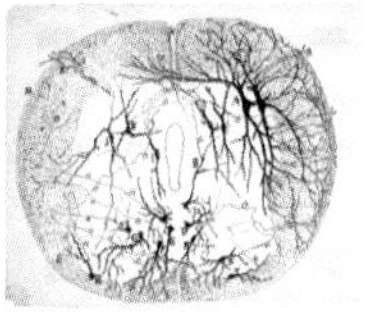

FIGURE 15.

Spinal cord of near-term larval stage in a toad.

This figure was published in Sala y Pons, C. (1892) Estructura de la médula espinal de los batracios. *Trab. Lab. Histol. Fac. Med. Barcelona*, 1–22 (Figure 5). It has also been reproduced as Figure 173 in Cajal, S. R. (1899–1904) *Textura del sistema nervioso del hombre y de los vertebrados*. Madrid: Moya.

FIGURE LEGEND: Transverse section of the spinal cord in a near-term larval stage of the toad (*Bufo vulgaris*) after C. Sala. Golgi method. *A*, Motor cells; *B*, commissural neurons; *I, J*, lateral funicular neurons; *D, G, S, T, R*, cells of the dorsal horn with axons directed to the dorsal horn bundle; *L*, perimedular *dendritic* plexus; *K, U*, collaterals of radicular motor fibers; *X*, axons for the perimedular plexus; *ci*, axons; **N, G, S*, cells in the head of the dorsal horn with axons were seen to enter in the lateral funiculus; *V*, commissural cell with an axon that is sliding through the ventral cleft to reach the perimedular plexus; *M*, axonal perimedular plexus; *O*, interstitial colateral to the white matter; *Y*, peripheral collateral.*

Original text: Corte transversal de la médula de una larva casi de término (*Bufo vulgaris*) según Cl. Sala. Método de Golgi. *A*, células motrices; *B*, neuronas comisurales; *I, J*, neuronas del cordón lateral; *D, G, S, T, R*, corpúsculos del asta posterior, cuyo axon va al manojo del asta dorsal; *L*, plexo *protoplasmático* perimedular; *K, U*, colaterales motrices; *X*, axones para el plexo perimedular; *ci*, cilindros-ejes; **N, G, S*, células del vértice del asta posterior cuyas espansiones nerviosas se vieron ingresar en el cordón lateral; V, célula comisural cuyo cilindro-eje se deslizaba por la hendidura anterior llegando al plexo perimedular; *M*, plexo nervioso perimedular; *O*, colateral intersticial ó para la sustancia blanca; *Y*, colateral periférica.*

Note from the author (J. D.): The text between asterisks appears in the original publication only.

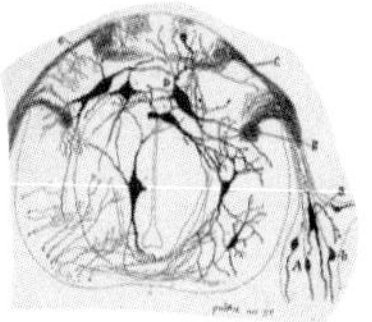

FIGURE 16.

Spinal cord in a grass snake embryo.

This figure was published in Cajal, S. R. (1899–1904) *Textura del sistema nervioso del hombre y de los vertebrados*. Moya, Madrid (Figure 180).

FIGURE LEGEND: Spinal cord in a [grass snake] (*Tropidonotus natrix*) embryo, after Retzius. Método de Golgi. *A*, Spinal ganglion; *B*, ventral bundles of the sensory root; *C*, dorsal bundle; *D*, dorsal cells; *a*, robust multipolar cell of the spinal ganglion; *b*, common bipolar type; *c*, commissural cells.

Original text: Médula del embrión de [la culebra de collar] (*Tropidonotus natrix*) según Retzius. Método de Golgi. *A*, ganglios raquídeos; *B*, manojo anterior de la raíz sensitiva; *C*, manojo posterior; *D*, células dorsales; *a*, robusta célula multipolar de los ganglios raquídeos; *b*, tipo bipolar común; *c*, células comisurales.

Note from the author (J. D.): In brackets is the text added in the French version of the *Textura: Cajal, S. R. (1909–1911) Histologie du système nerveux de l'homme et des vertébrés*. Paris, Maloine.

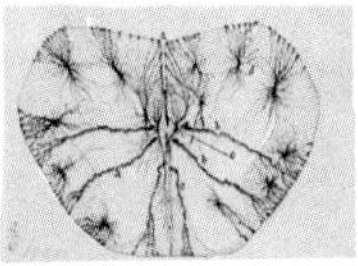

FIGURE 17.

Spinal cord in a sand lizard.

This figure was published in Cajal, S. R. (1891) Pequeñas contribuciones al conocimiento del sistema nervioso. *Trab. Lab. Histol. Fac. Med. Barcelona. Imprenta de la Casa Provincial de Caridad*, August, 1–56 (Figure 12). It has also been reproduced as Figure 181 in Cajal, S. R. (1899–1904) *Textura del sistema nervioso del hombre y de los vertebrados*. Madrid: Moya.

FIGURE LEGEND: Transverse section of the spinal cord in a twenty-day old sand lizard (*Lacerta agilis*). Only ependymal and neuroglia cell are represented in the figure. [Golgi method.] *a, b, c,* Ependymal cells with the inner ends that do not reach the central canal; *d,* neuroglia cells that send processes to the surface of the spinal cord; *e,* ventrodorsal neuroglia cells. *A,* ventromedial fissure of the spinal cord.

Original text: Corte transversal de la médula espinal de la lagartija (*Lacerta agilis*) de veinte días. En él sólo se han representado las células epiteliales y neuróglicas. [Método de Golgi]. *a, b, c,* células epiteliales que no llegan por dentro al epéndimo; *d,* células neuróglicas que envían fibras á la superficie medular; *e,* células neuróglicas anteroposteriores. *A,* surco anterior de la médula.

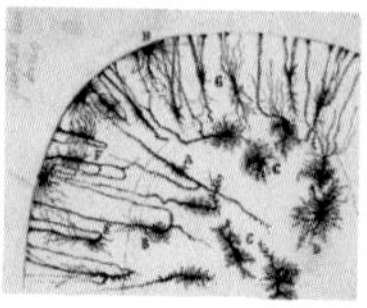

FIGURE 18.

Neuroglia in the ventral horn and ventral funiculus in a cat embryo.

This figure was published in Cajal, S. R. (1899–1904) *Textura del sistema nervioso del hombre y de los vertebrados*. Moya, Madrid (Figure 200).

FIGURE LEGEND: Neuroglia in the ventral horn and ventral funiculus in a cat embryo. Golgi method. *A* and *B,* Arcuate cells near the white matter; *C,* young neuroglia of the gray matter; *E, F,* young neuroglia of the ventral funiculus; *H,* marginal cells.

Original text: Neuroglia del asta y cordón anterior del embrión de gato. Método de Golgi. *A* y *B,* células arciformes vecinas de la substancia blanca; *C,* neuroglia joven de la substancia gris; *E, F,* neuroglia joven del cordón anterior; *H,* células marginales.

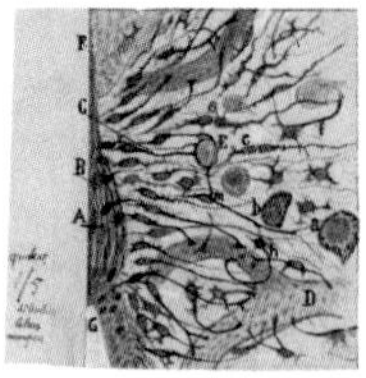

FIGURE 19.

Transverse section of the spinal cord in an eight-day-old kitten.

This figure was published in Cajal, S. R. (1913) Contribución al conocimiento de la neuroglia del cerebro humano. *Trab. Lab. Invest. Biol. Univ. Madrid* 11, 255–315 (Figure 25).

FIGURE LEGEND: Transverse section of the spinal cord in an eight-day-old cat. *A,* Epithelium of the dorsal raphe; *B, C,* displaced epithelial cells with a peripheral process ending in a capillary; *D,* capillary that attracts processes of young astrocytes; *E,* another capillary on which converge several end-feet and collaterals; *e,* twin astrocytes.

Original text: Corte transversal de la médula espinal del gato de ocho días. *A,* epitelio del rafe posterior; *B, C,* corpúsculos epiteliales dislocados cuya expansión periférica se fija en un capilar; *D,* capilar que atrae apéndices de astrocitos jóvenes; *E,* otro capilar al cual convergen varios pedículos terminales y colatarales; *e,* astrocitos gemelos.

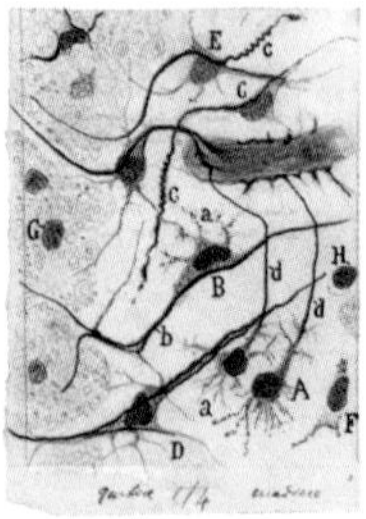

FIGURE 20.

Glial cells of the ventral horn in an eight-day-old kitten.

This figure was published in Cajal, S. R. (1913) Contribución al conocimiento de la neuroglia del cerebro humano. *Trab. Lab. Invest. Biol. Univ. Madrid* 11, 255–315 (Figure 27).

FIGURE LEGEND: Portion of the gray matter of the ventral horn in an eight-day-old kitten. *A,* Cells with almost all processes that are granular, except one (*d*), where the fiber appears; *B, C,* astrocytes provided with robust cortical fiber; *D,* another with various differentiated fibers; *F,* cells from which rudimentary processes emanate; *G, H,* adendritic cells; *a,* granular processes; *b,* fibrous processes; *c,* helical fibers.

Original text: Trozo de la substancia gris del asta anterior del gato de ocho días. *A,* células en que casi todas las expansiones son granulosas, menos una (*d*), donde aparece la fibra; *B, C,* astrocitos provistos de robusta fibra cortical; *D,* otro con varias fibras diferenciadas; *F,* células de que emanan expansiones rudimentarias; *G, H,* elementos adendríticos; *a,* expansiones granulosas; *b,* expansiones fibrosas; *c,* fibras helicoidales.

SECTION B

Medulla Oblongata

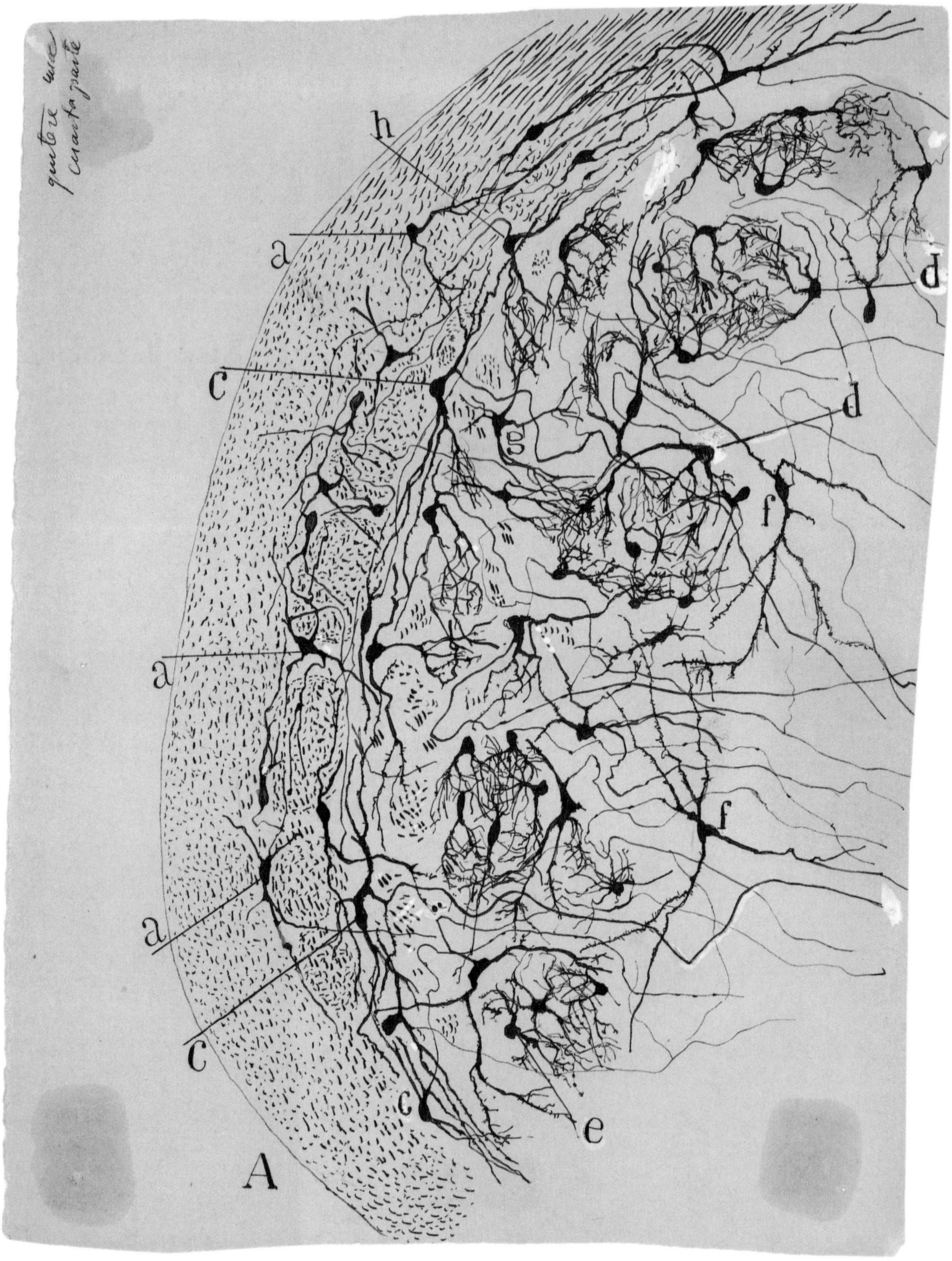

FIGURE 21. Spinal tract of the trigeminal nerve in a newborn rabbit.

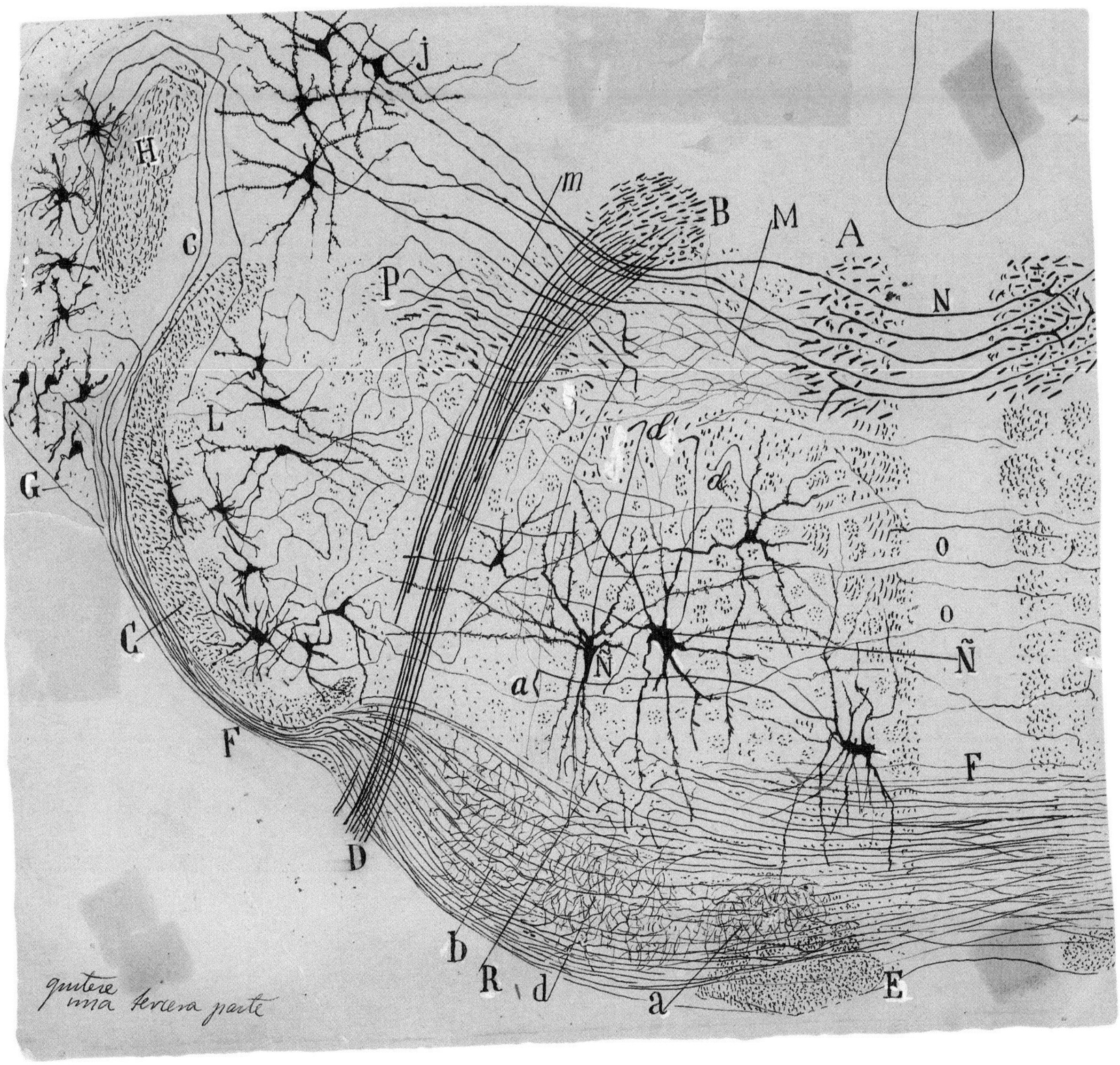

FIGURE 22. Medulla in a newborn mouse at the level of the emergence of the facial nerve and plane of the trapezoid body.

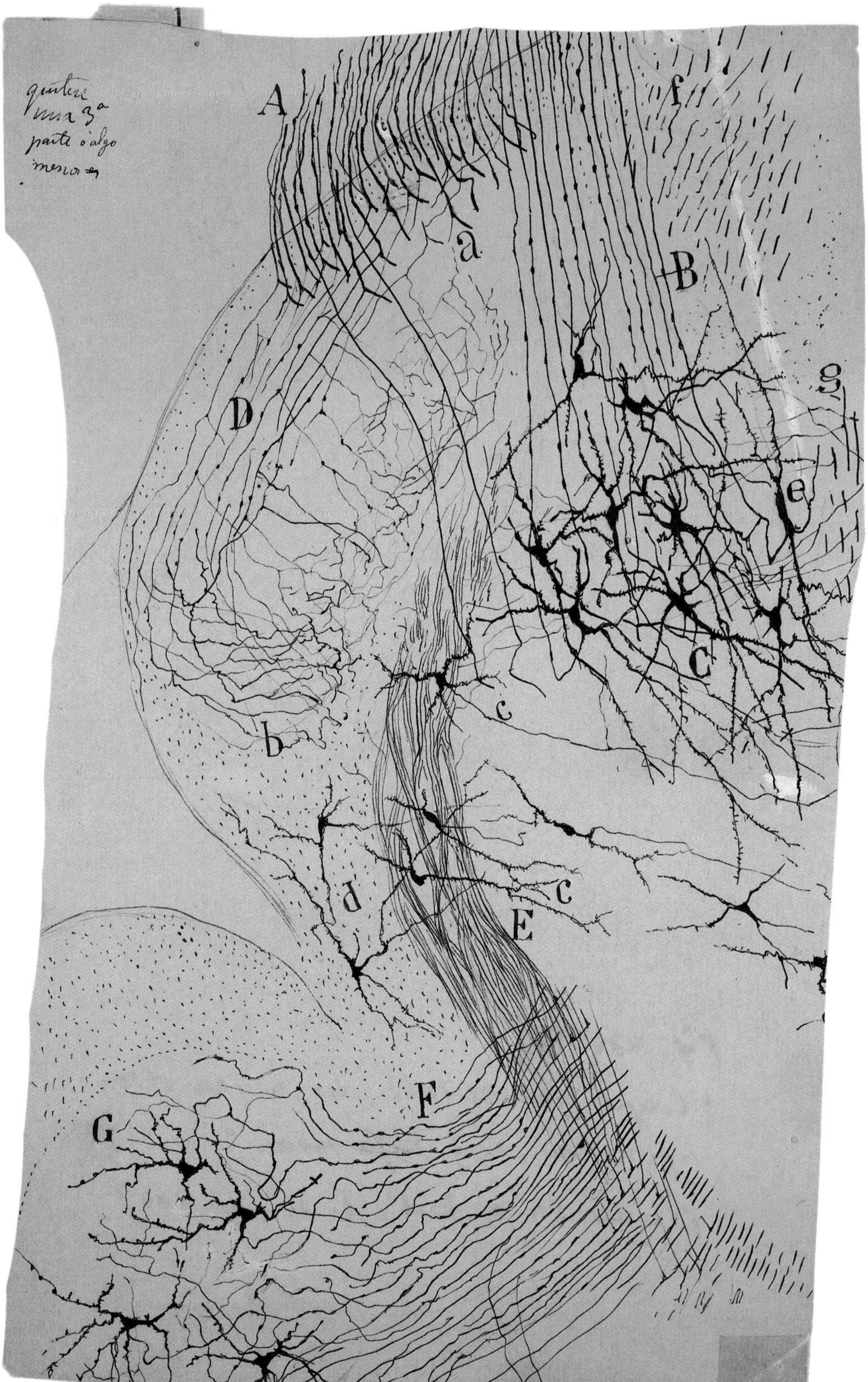

FIGURE 23. Nuclei of the trigeminal nerve in a mouse fetus.

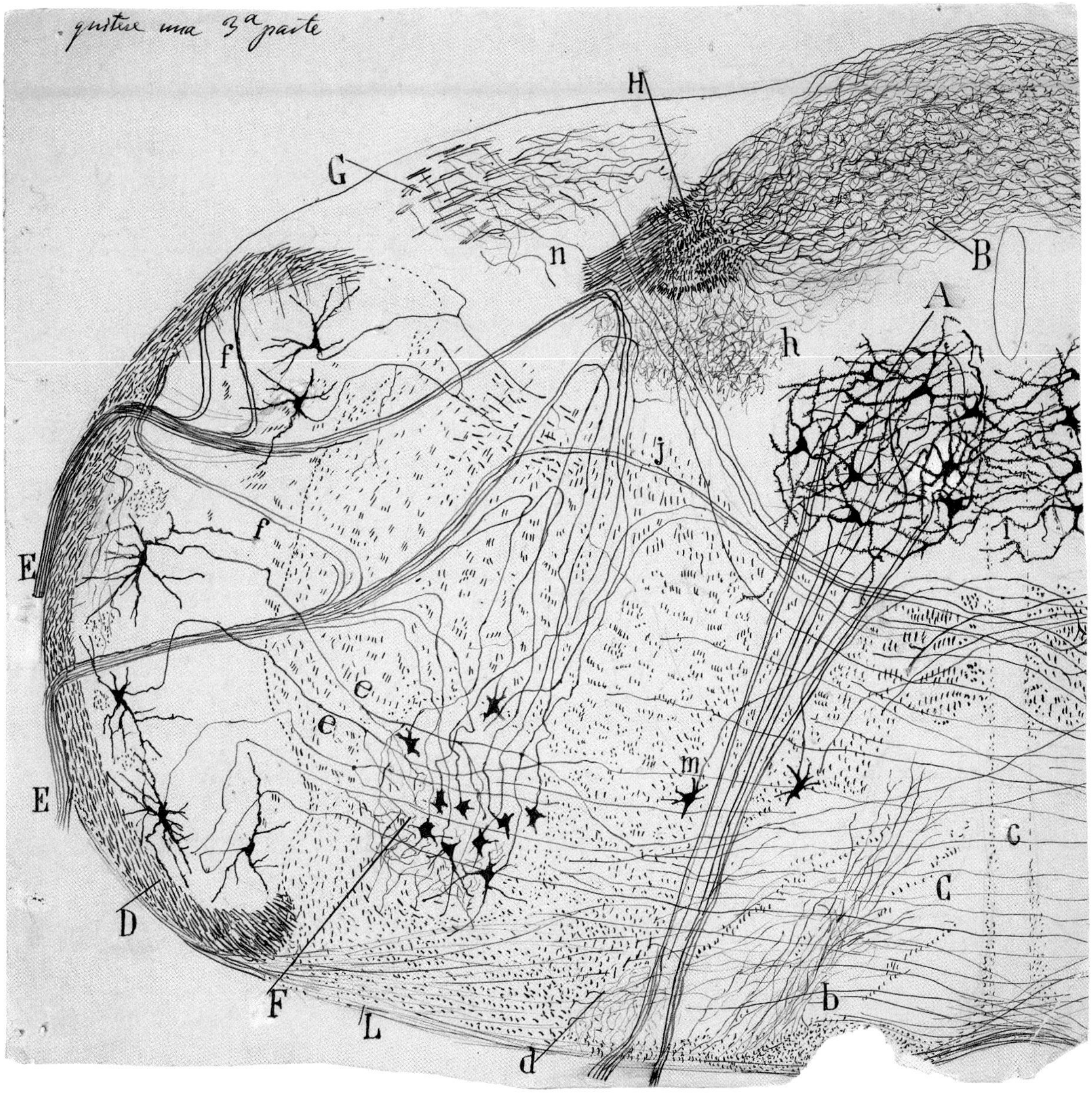

FIGURE 24. Transverse section of the medulla in a four-day-old mouse.

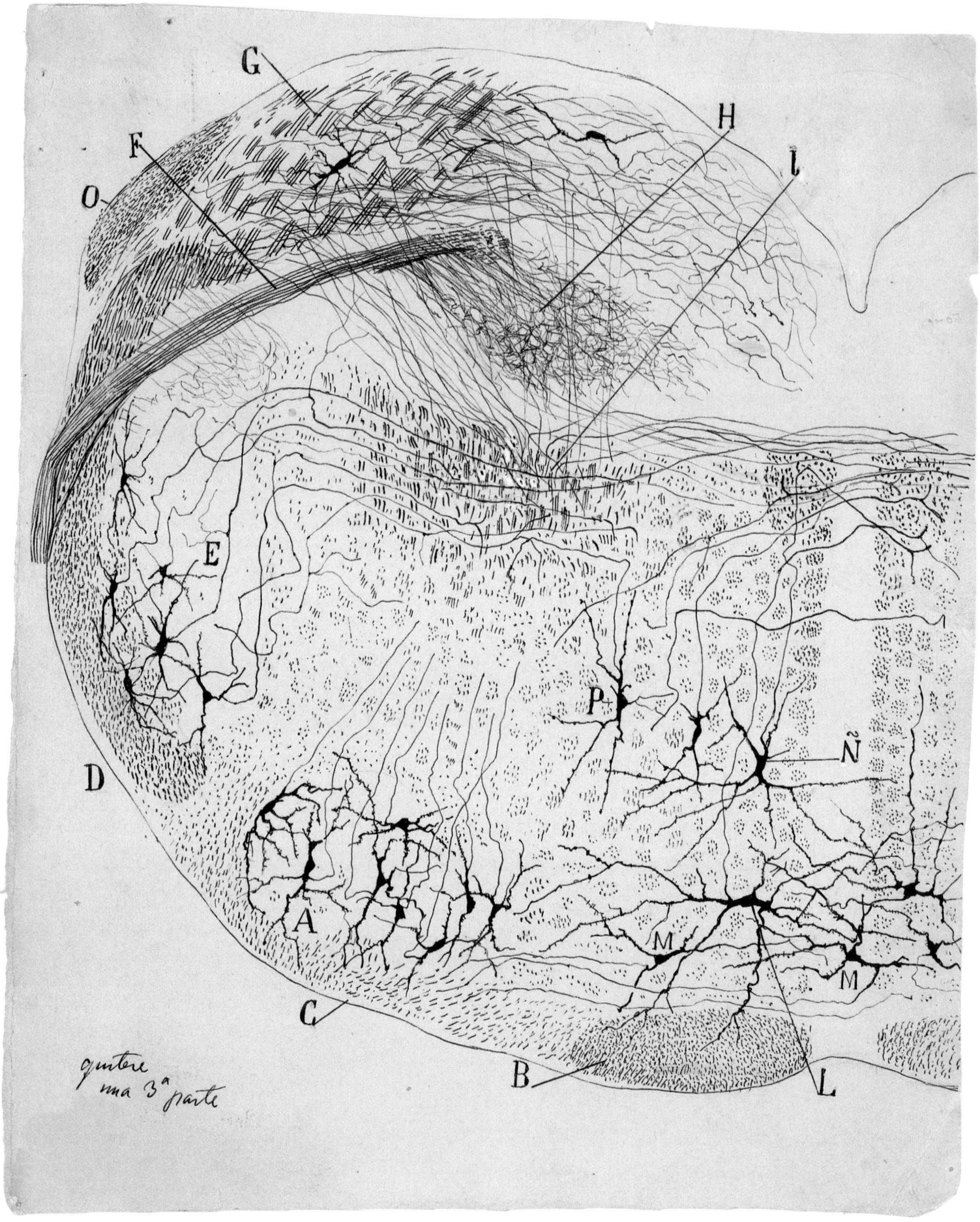

FIGURE 25. Medulla in a newborn mouse.

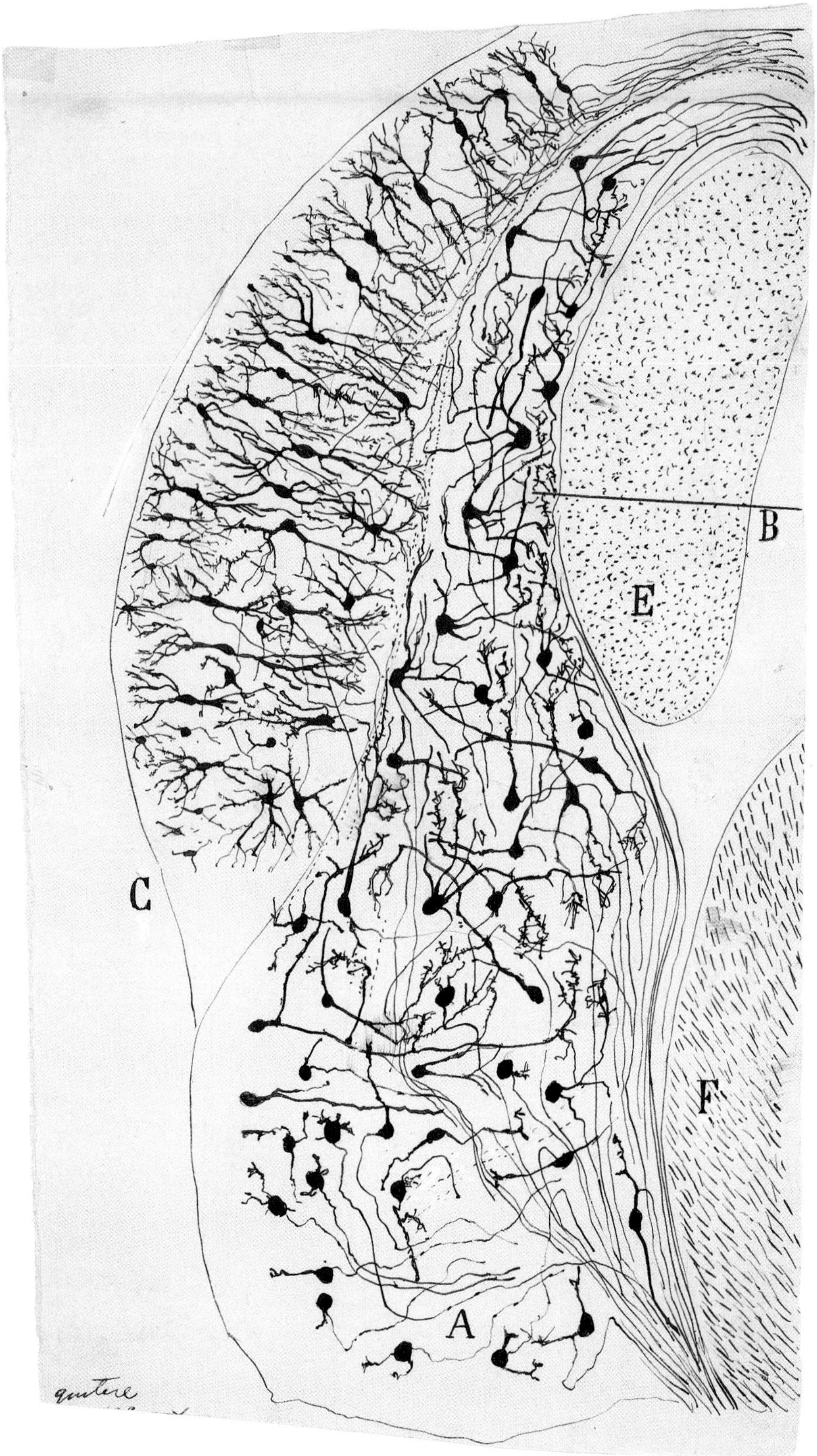

FIGURE 26. Neurons of the ventral and dorsal cochlear nuclei in a rabbit.

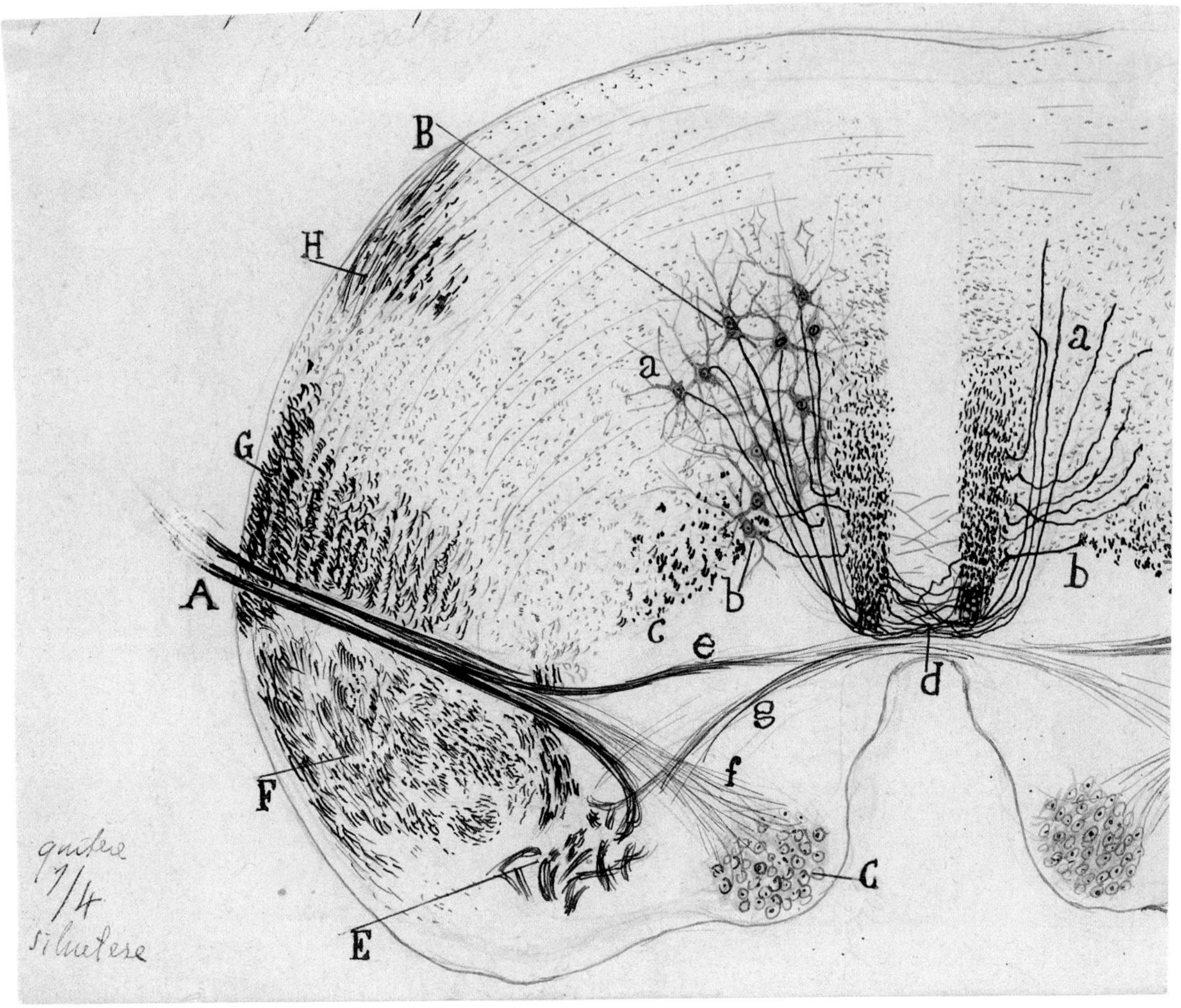

FIGURE 27. Medulla at the level of the glossopharyngeal nucleus in a chick embryo.

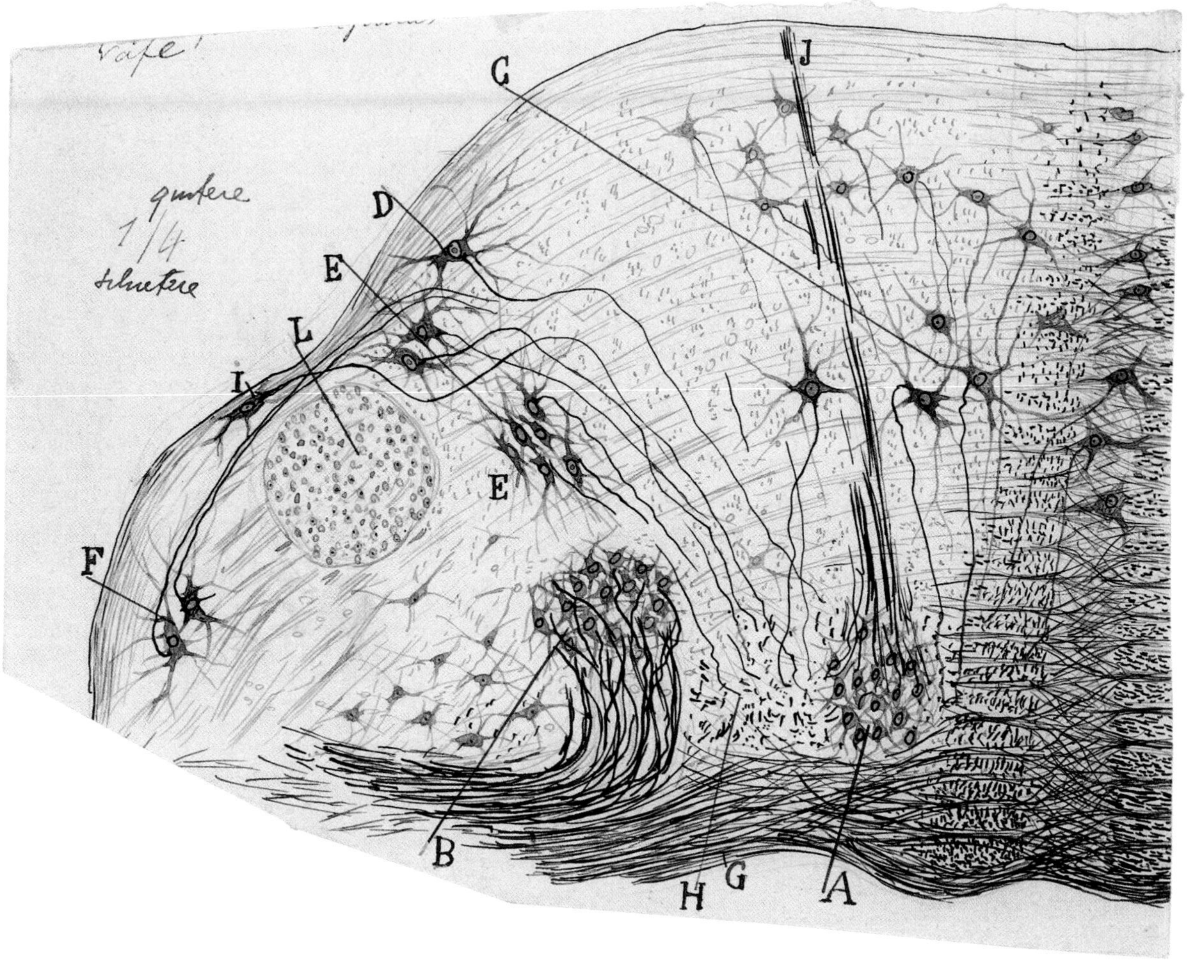

FIGURE 28. Medulla in a newborn bird.

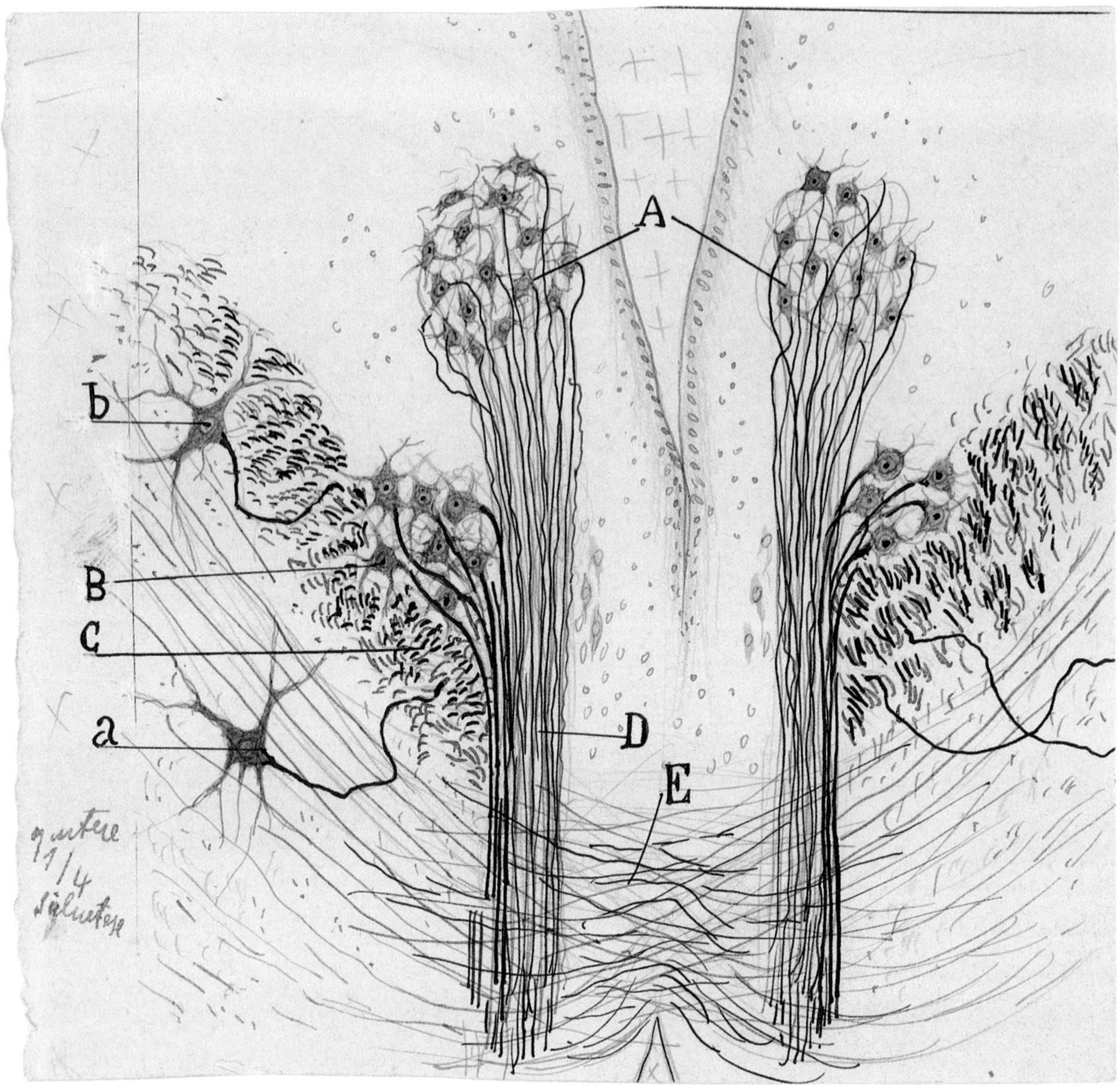

FIGURE 29. Midbrain in a chick embryo.

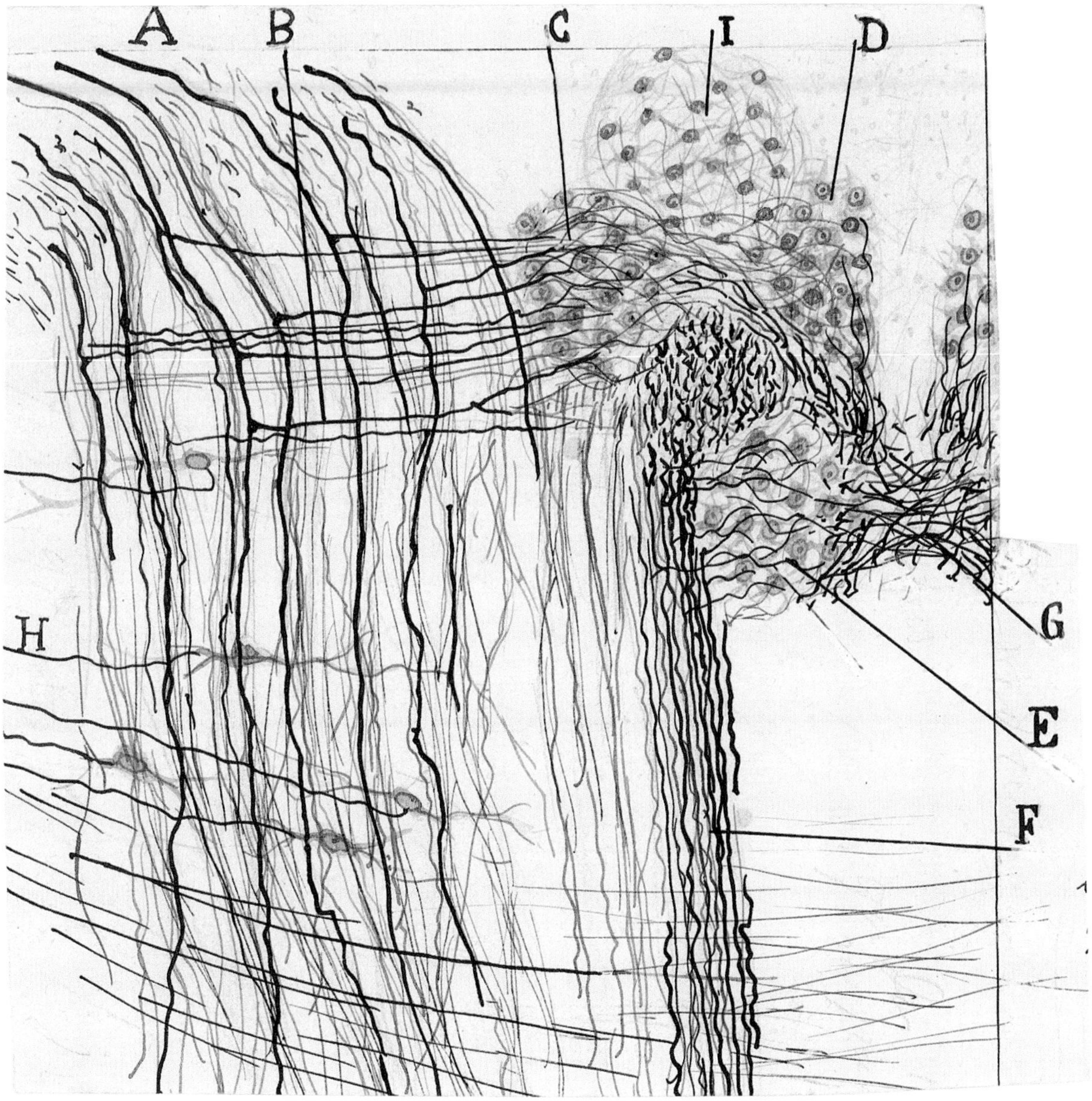

FIGURE 30. Oculomotor nucleus in a chick embryo.

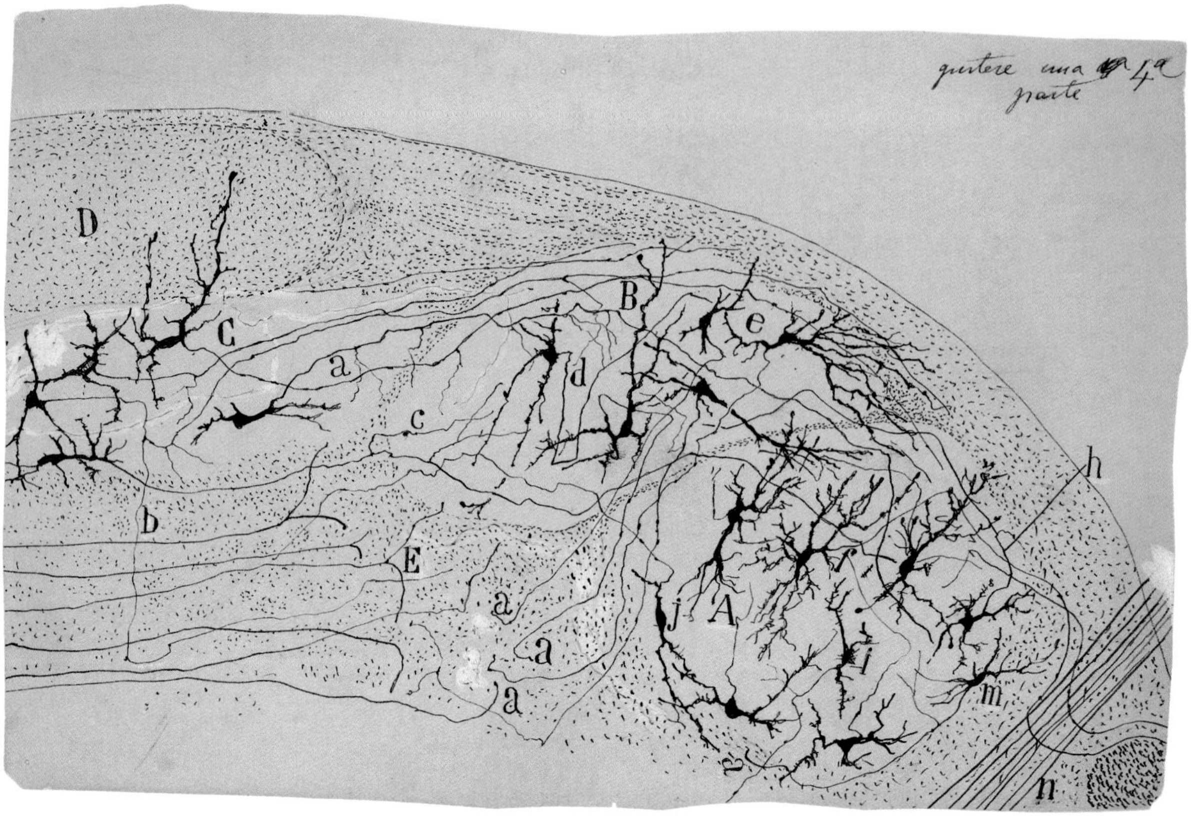

FIGURE 31. Transverse section of the trapezoid body in a newborn mouse.

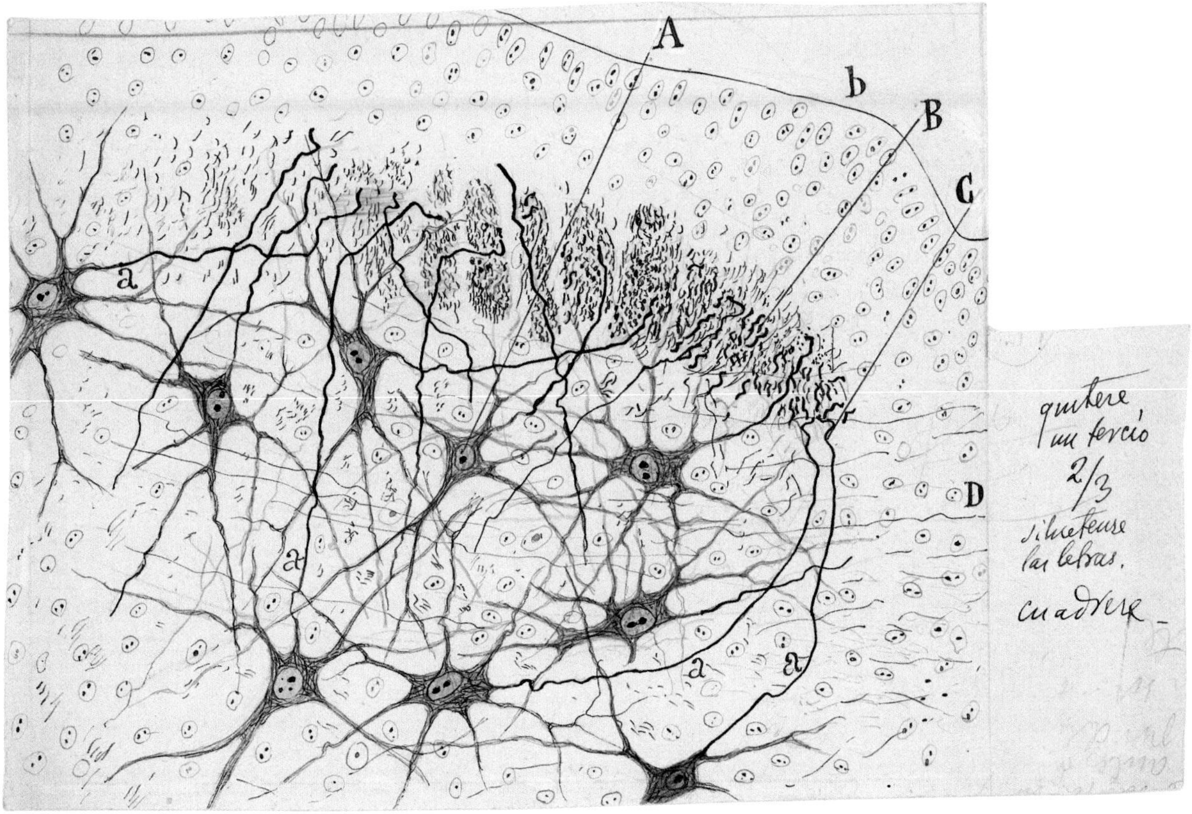

FIGURE 32. Transverse section of the tegmentum in a human embryo.

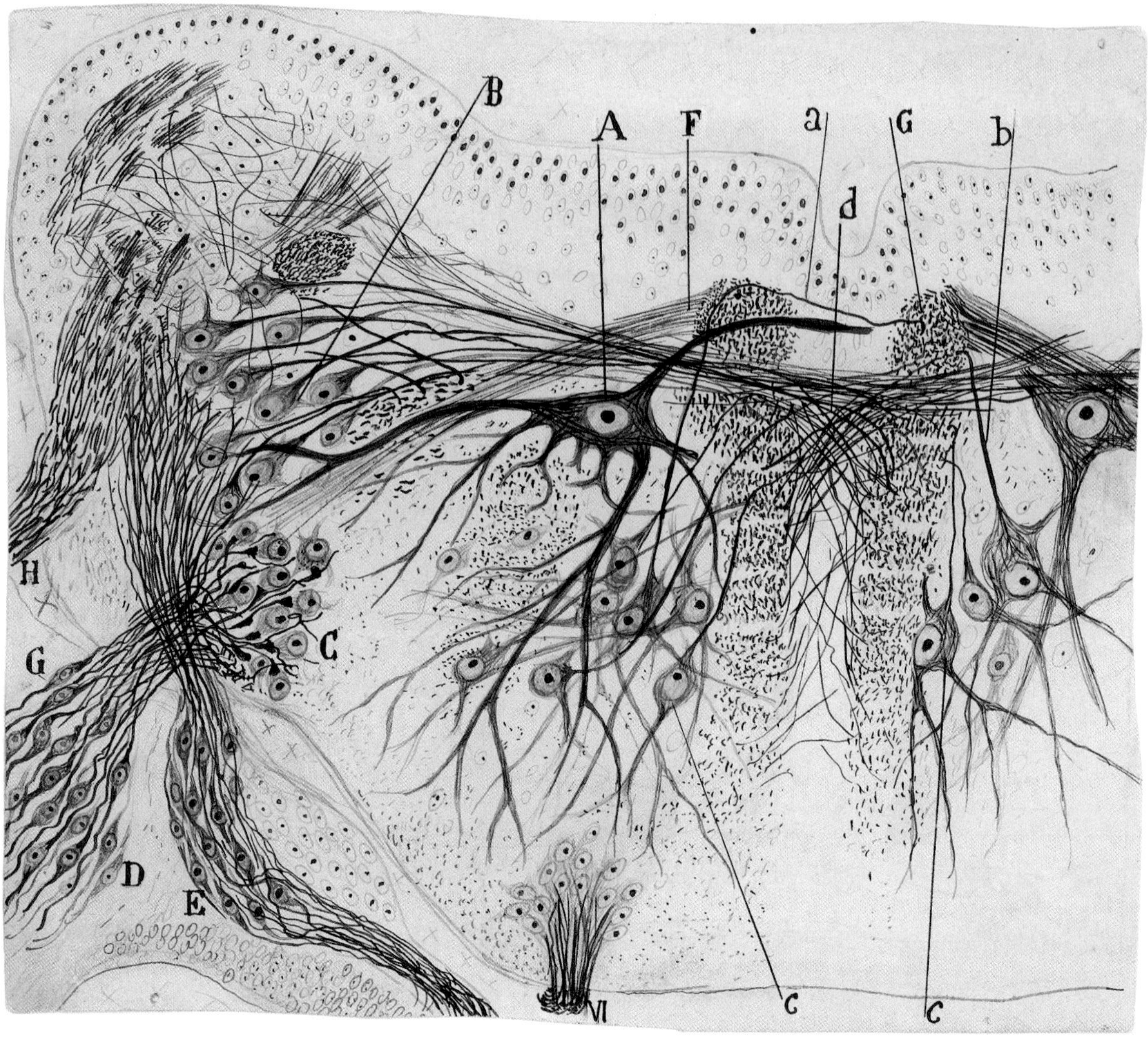

FIGURE 33. Section of the medulla at the level of the auditory region in a trout.

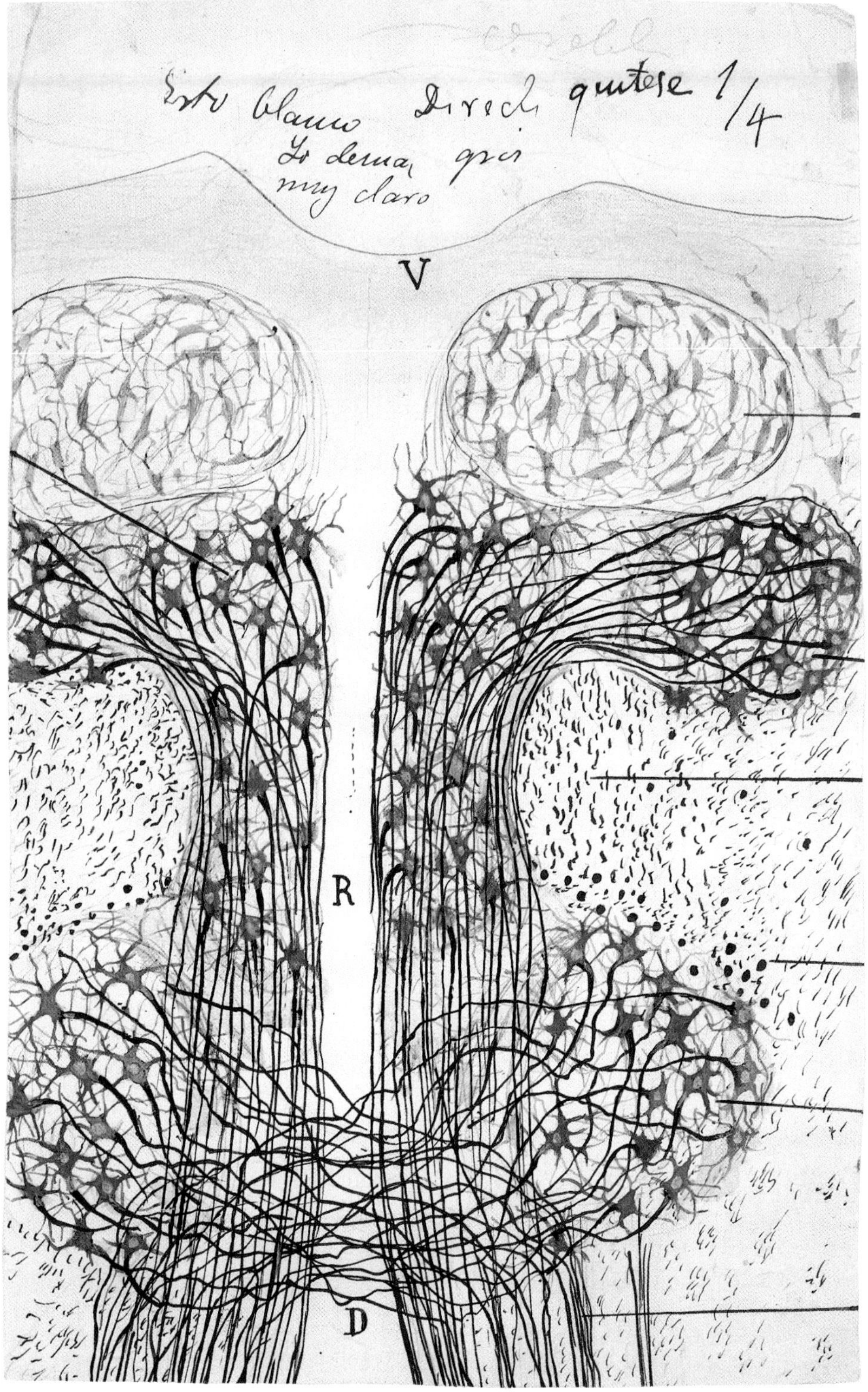

FIGURE 34. Section through cell groups forming the oculomotor nucleus in a kite.

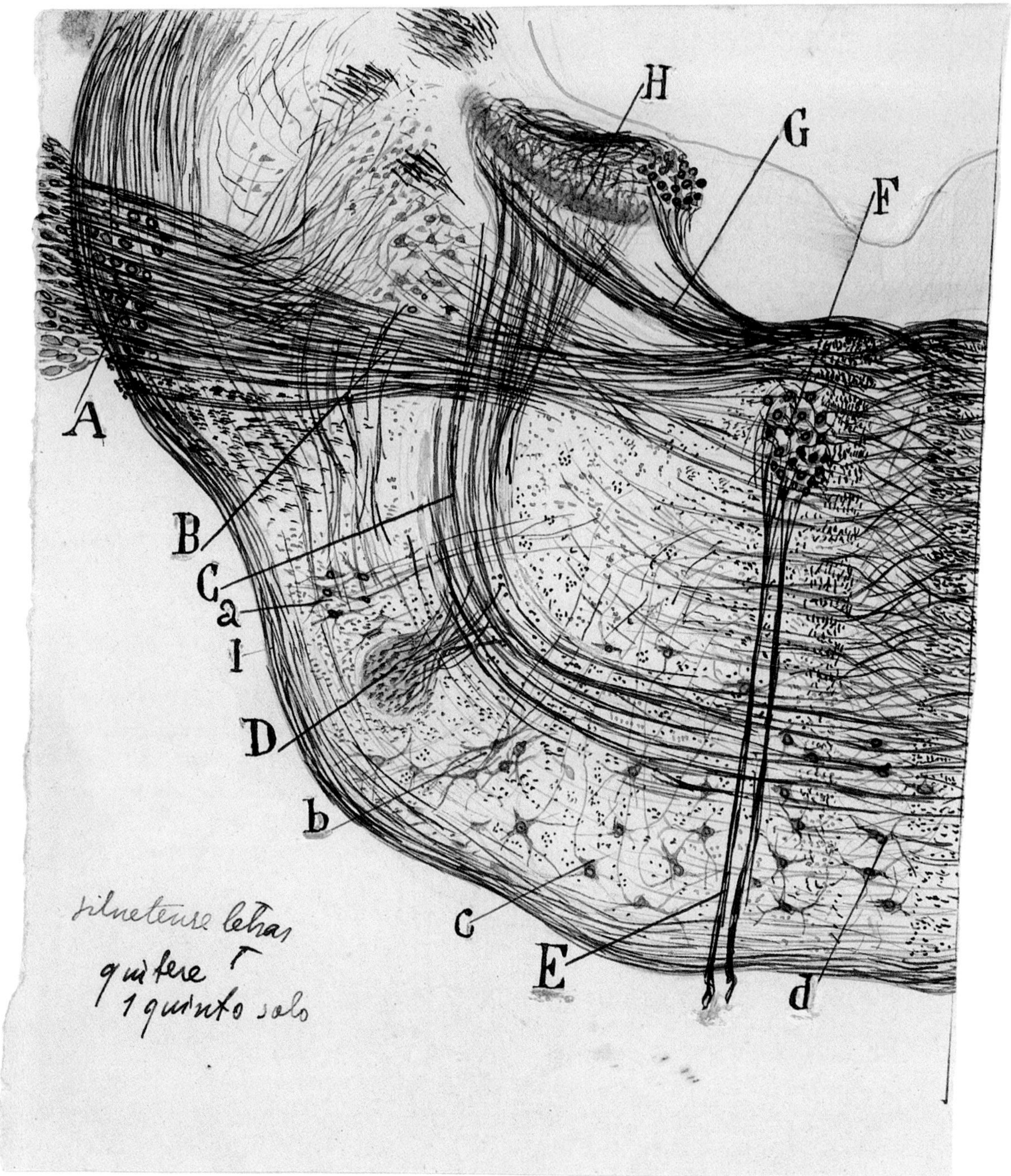

FIGURE 35. Section of the medulla in a sparrow a few days old.

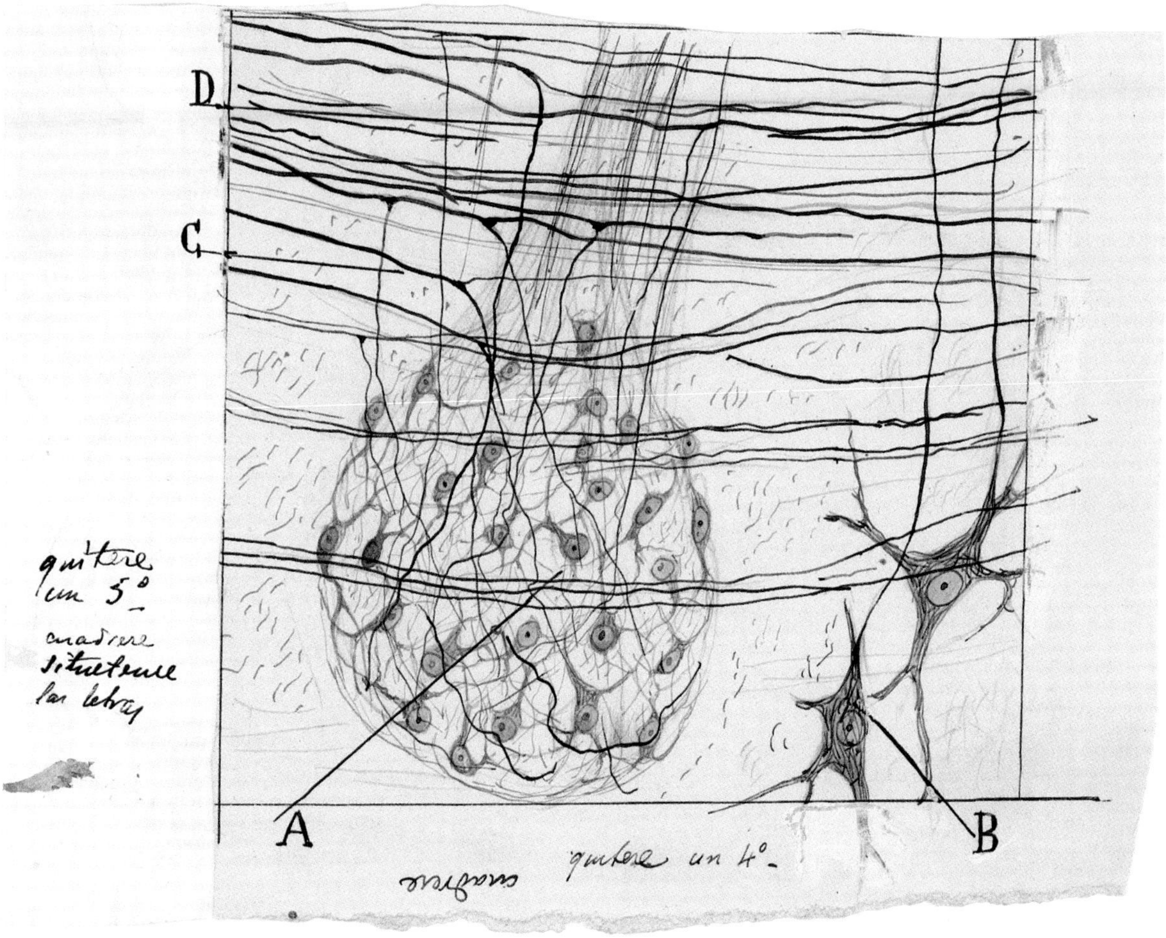

FIGURE 36. Section at the level of the superior olive and trapezoid body in a bird.

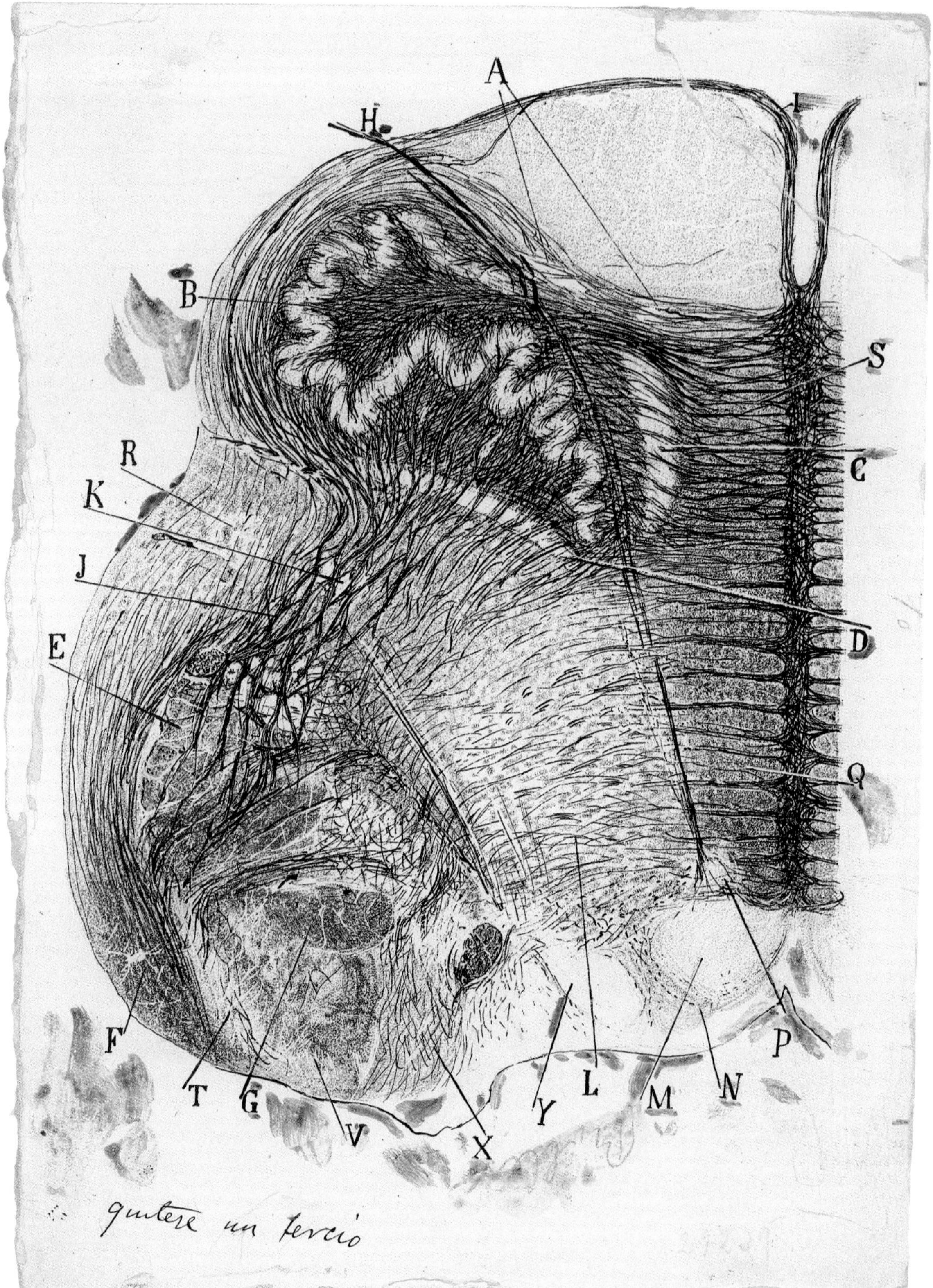

FIGURE 37. Medulla in a hemiplegic individual.

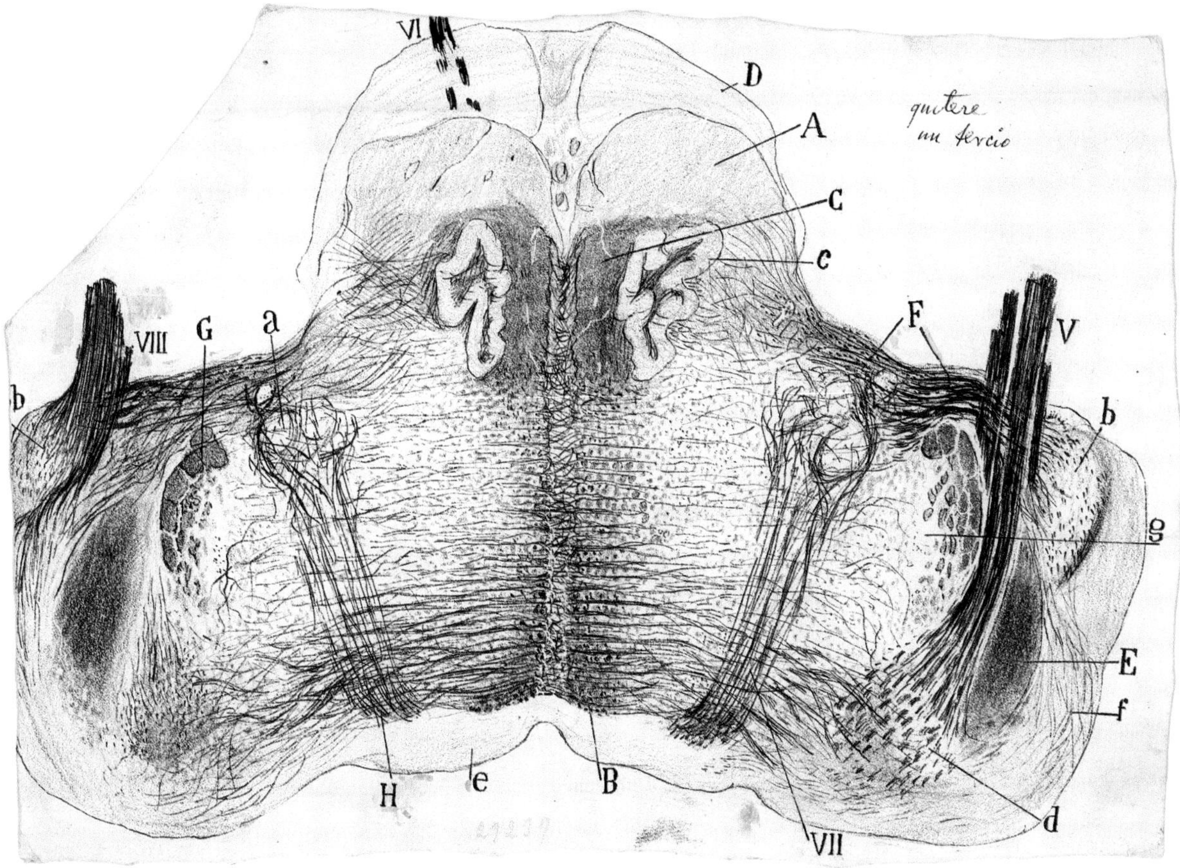

FIGURE 38. Medulla in a fifteen-day-old child at the level of the caudal border of the pons.

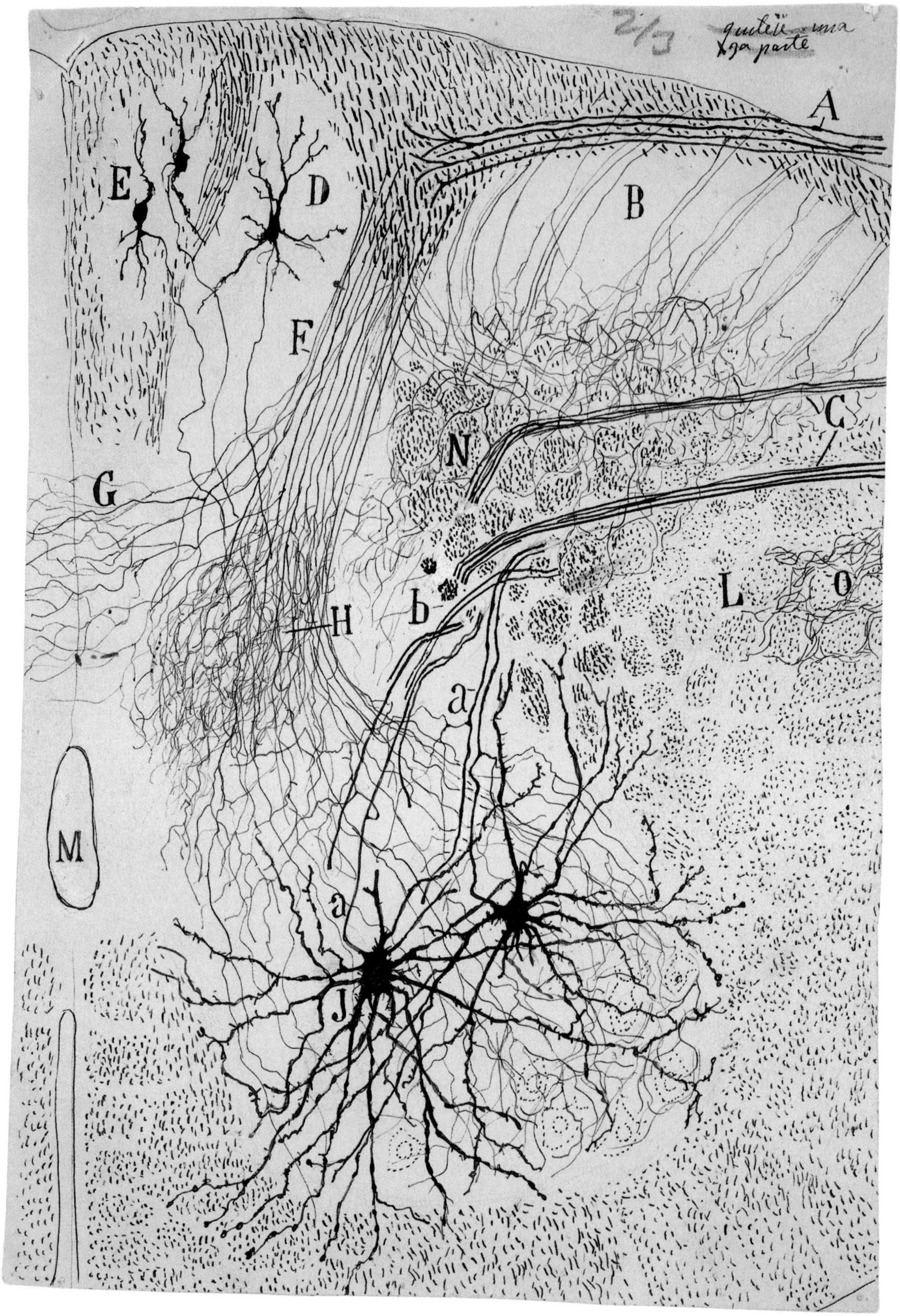

FIGURE 39. Section of the medulla caudal to the pyramid decussation in a cat fetus.

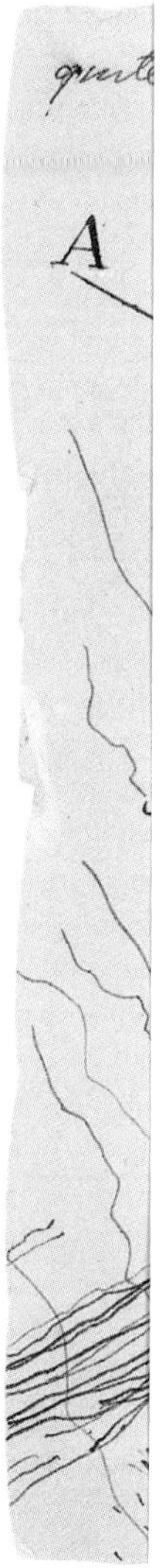

FIGURE 42.

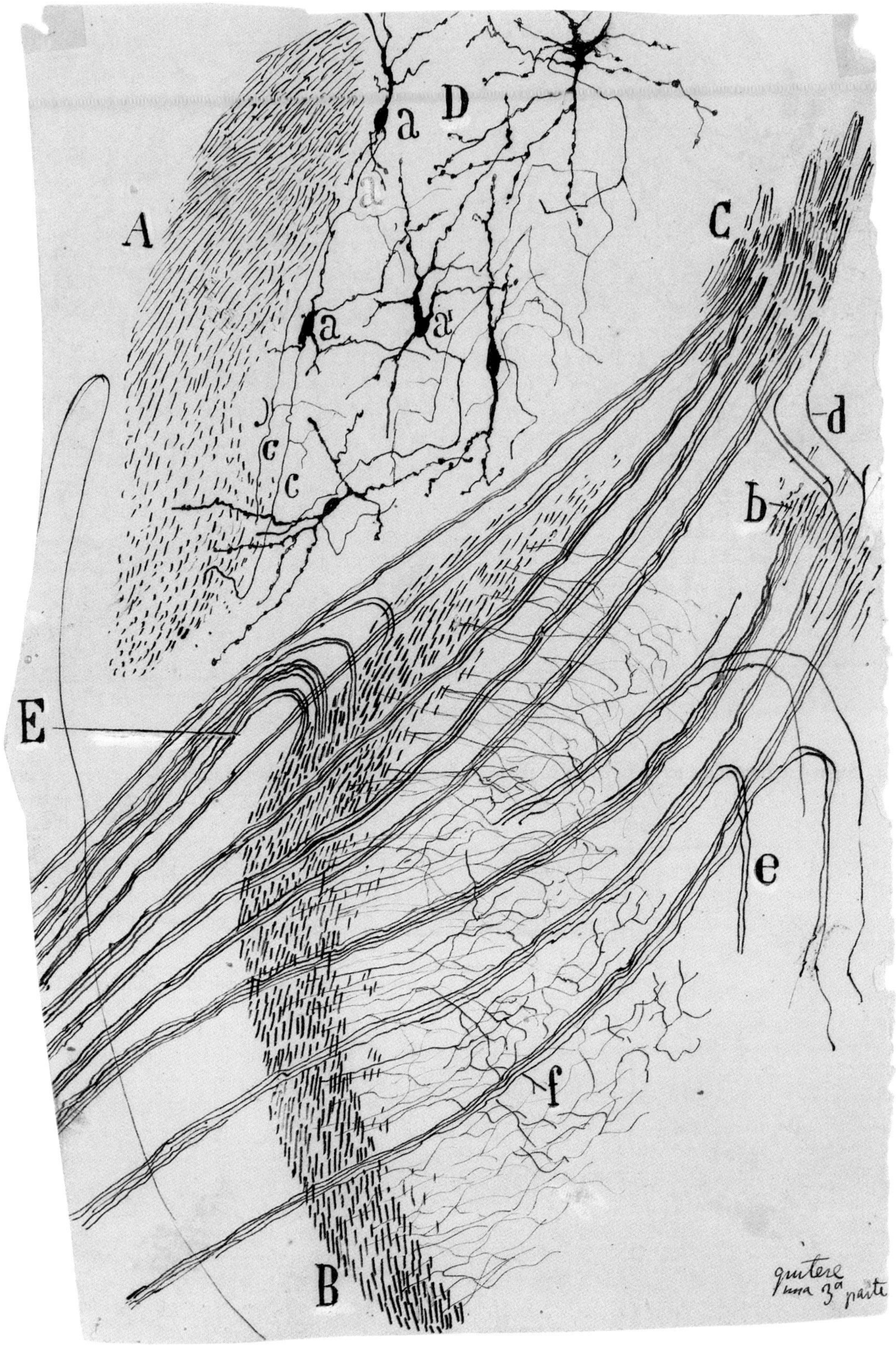

FIGURE 40. Medulla in a cat fetus.

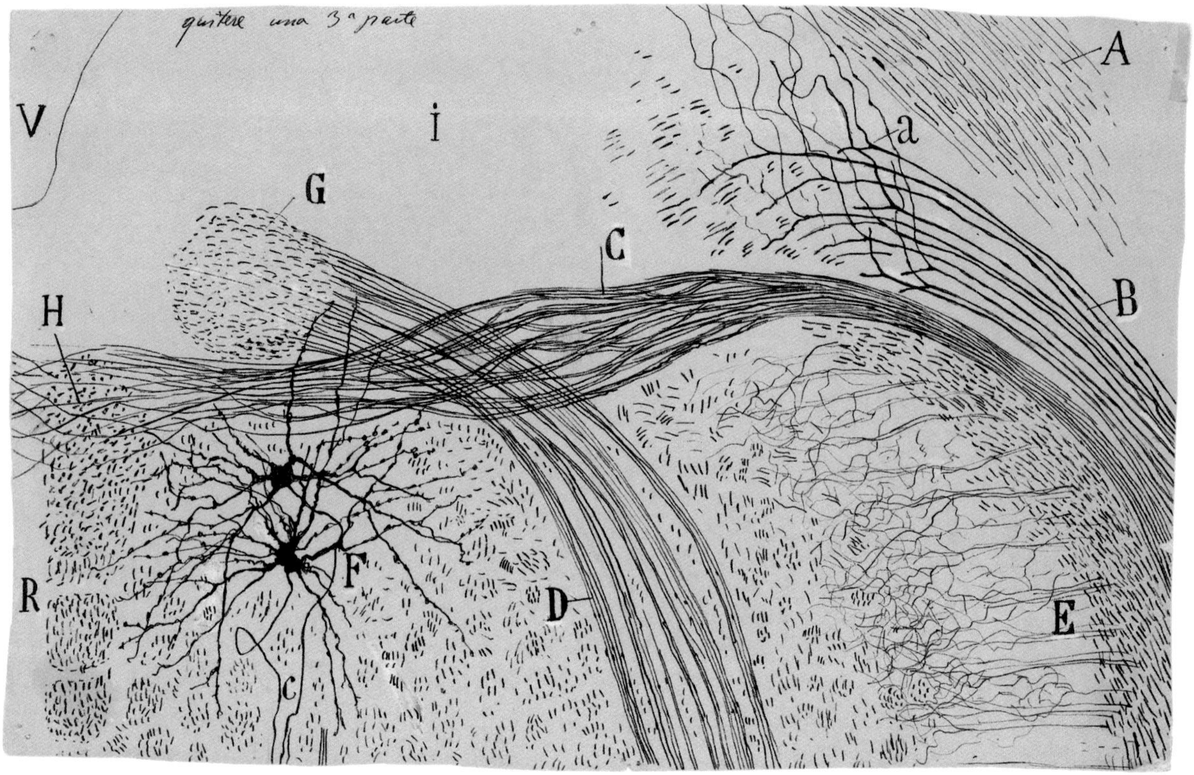

FIGURE 43. Transverse section of the medulla in a cat fetus.

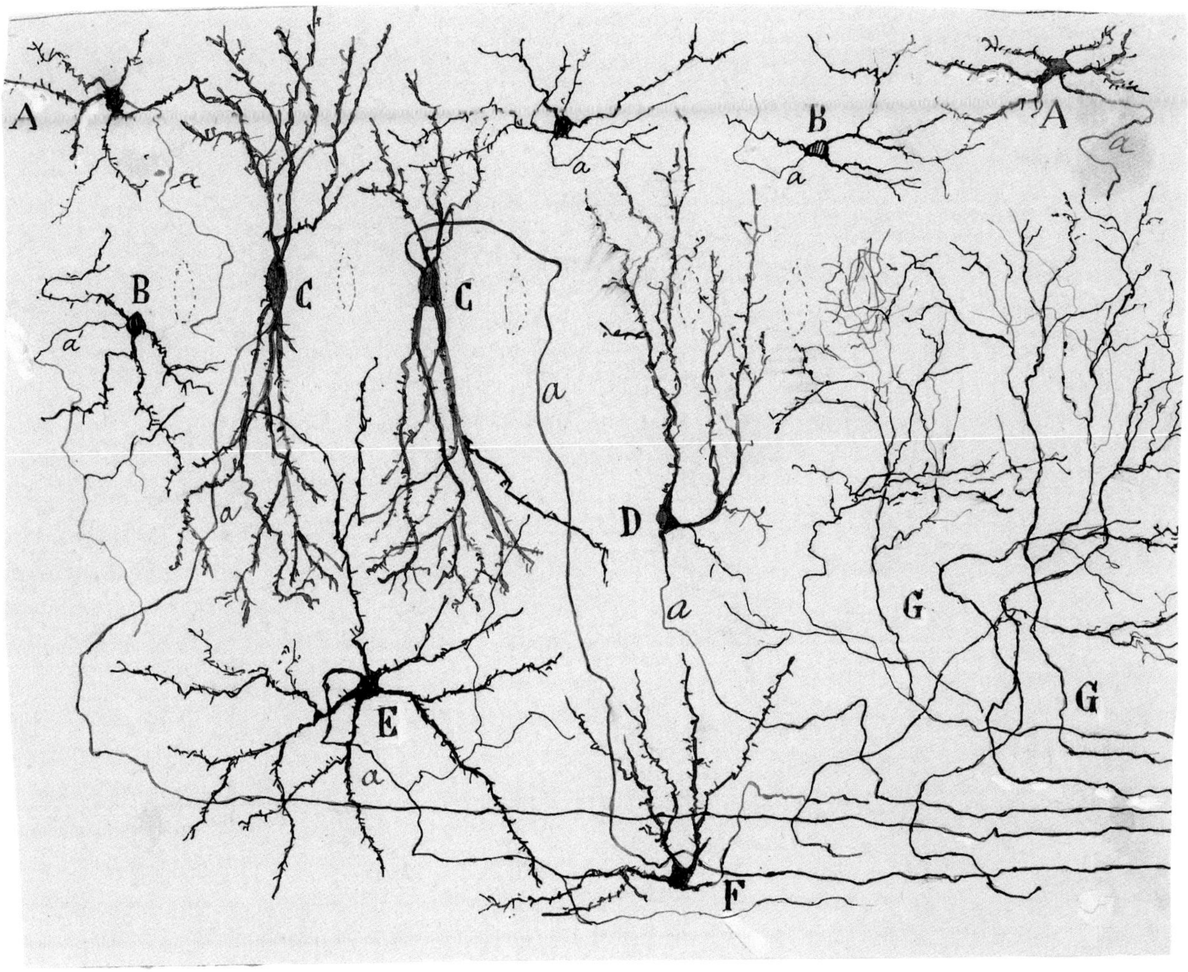

FIGURE 44. Principal cellular types in the dorsal cochlear nucleus in a kitten.

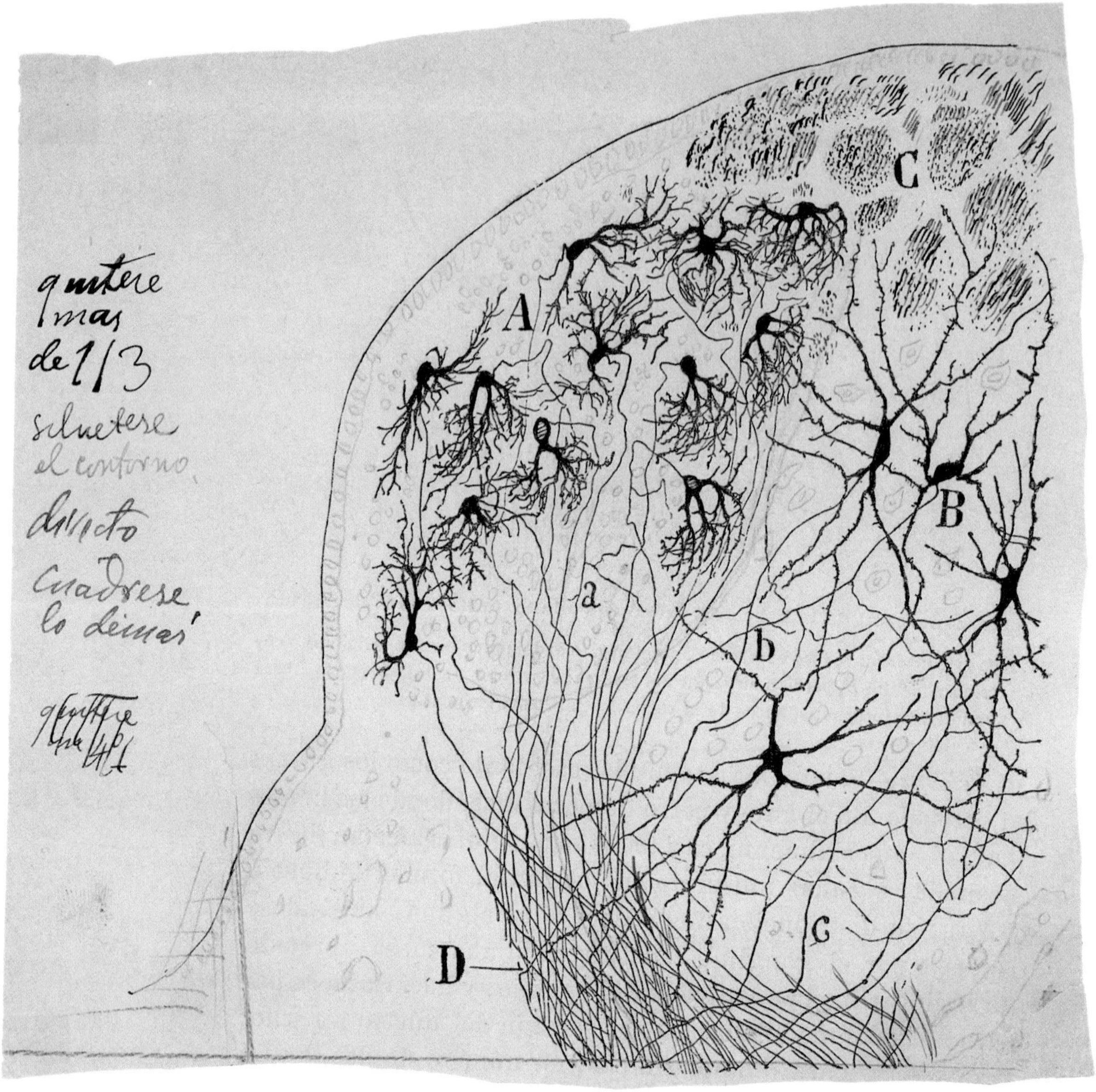

FIGURE 45. Nucleus of the habenula in a newborn dog.

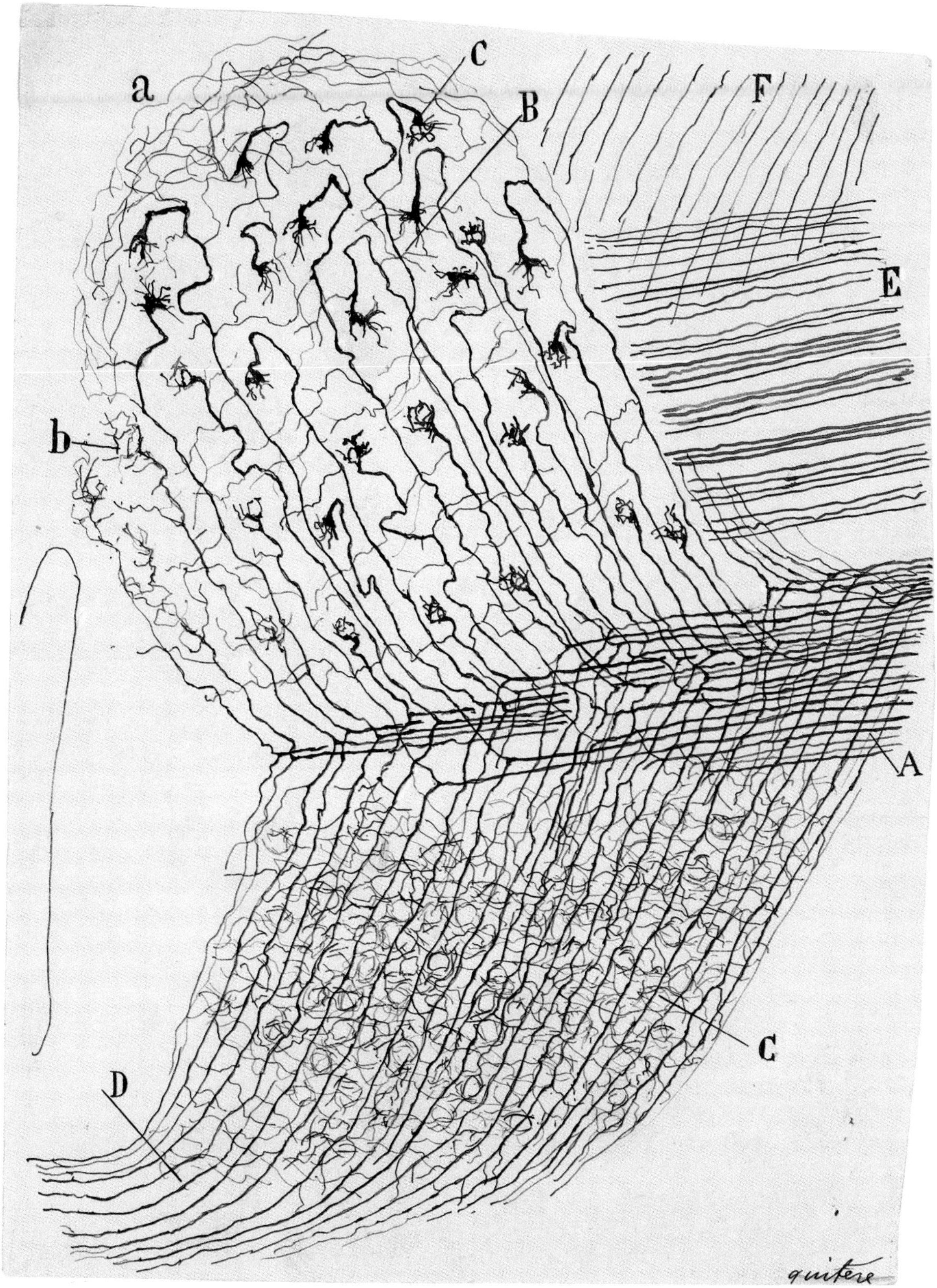

FIGURE 46. Ventral cochlear nucleus in a newborn dog.

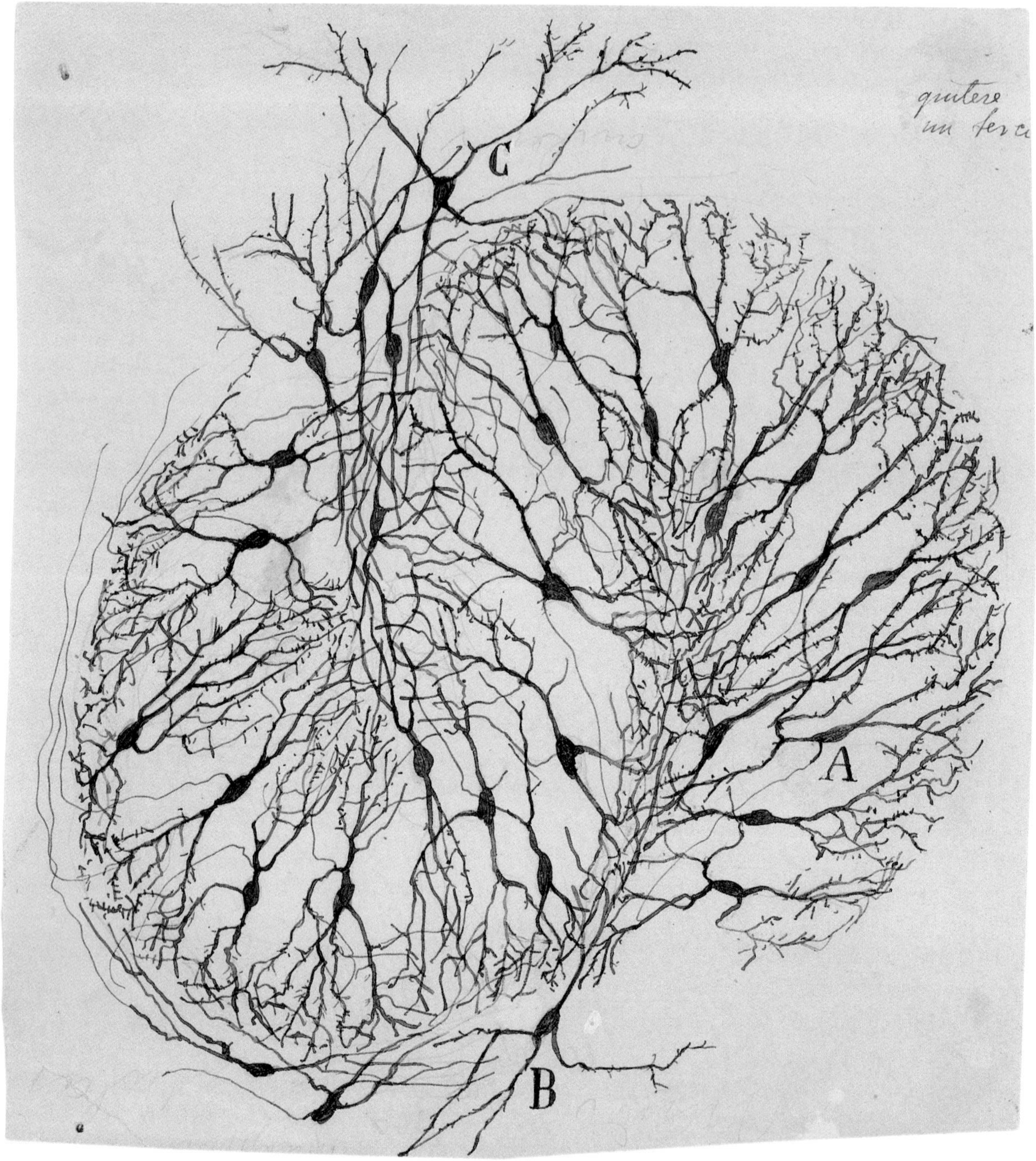

FIGURE 47. Assembly of superior olive cells in a kitten.

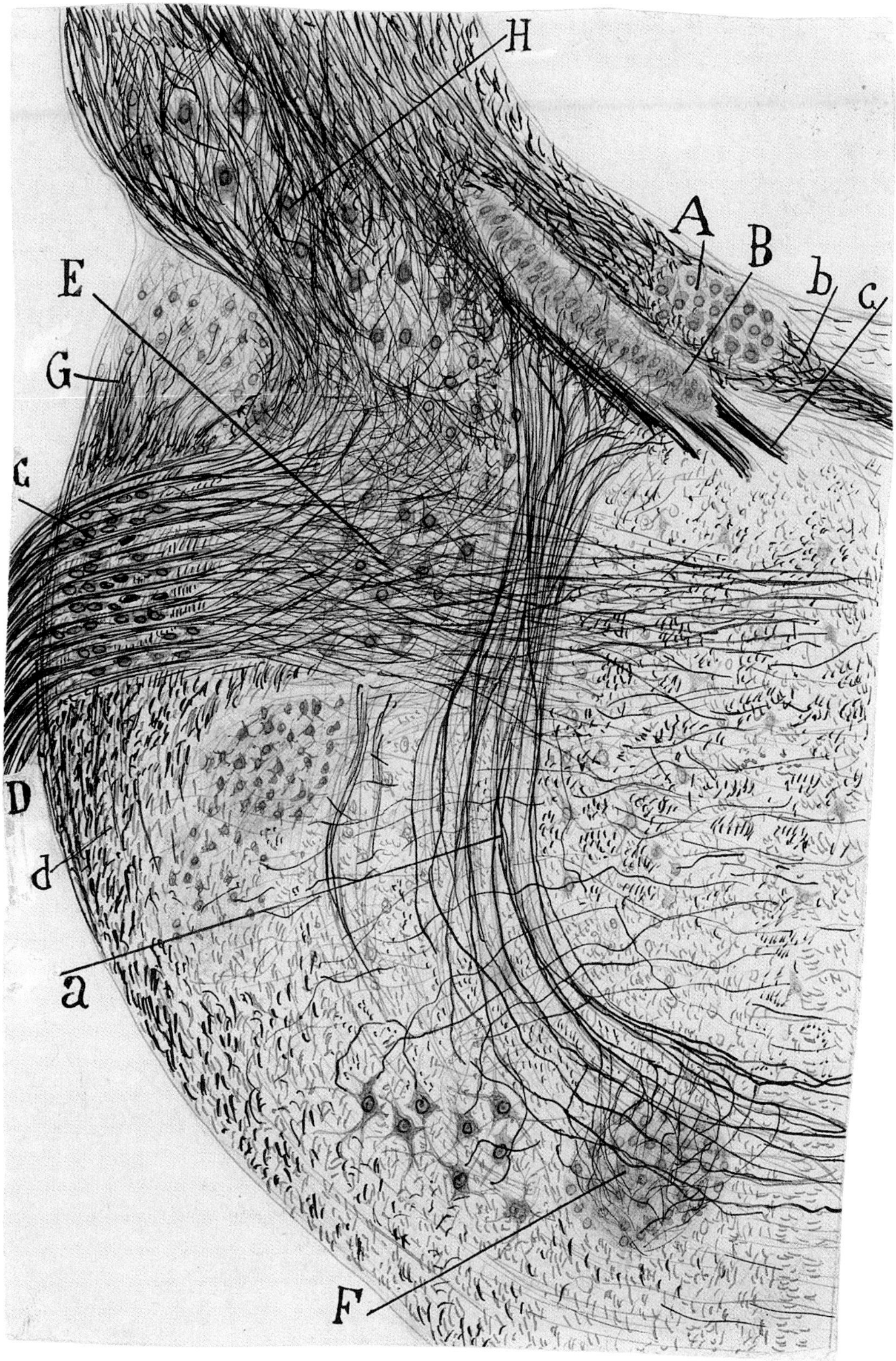

FIGURE 48. Medulla in a kite a few days old.

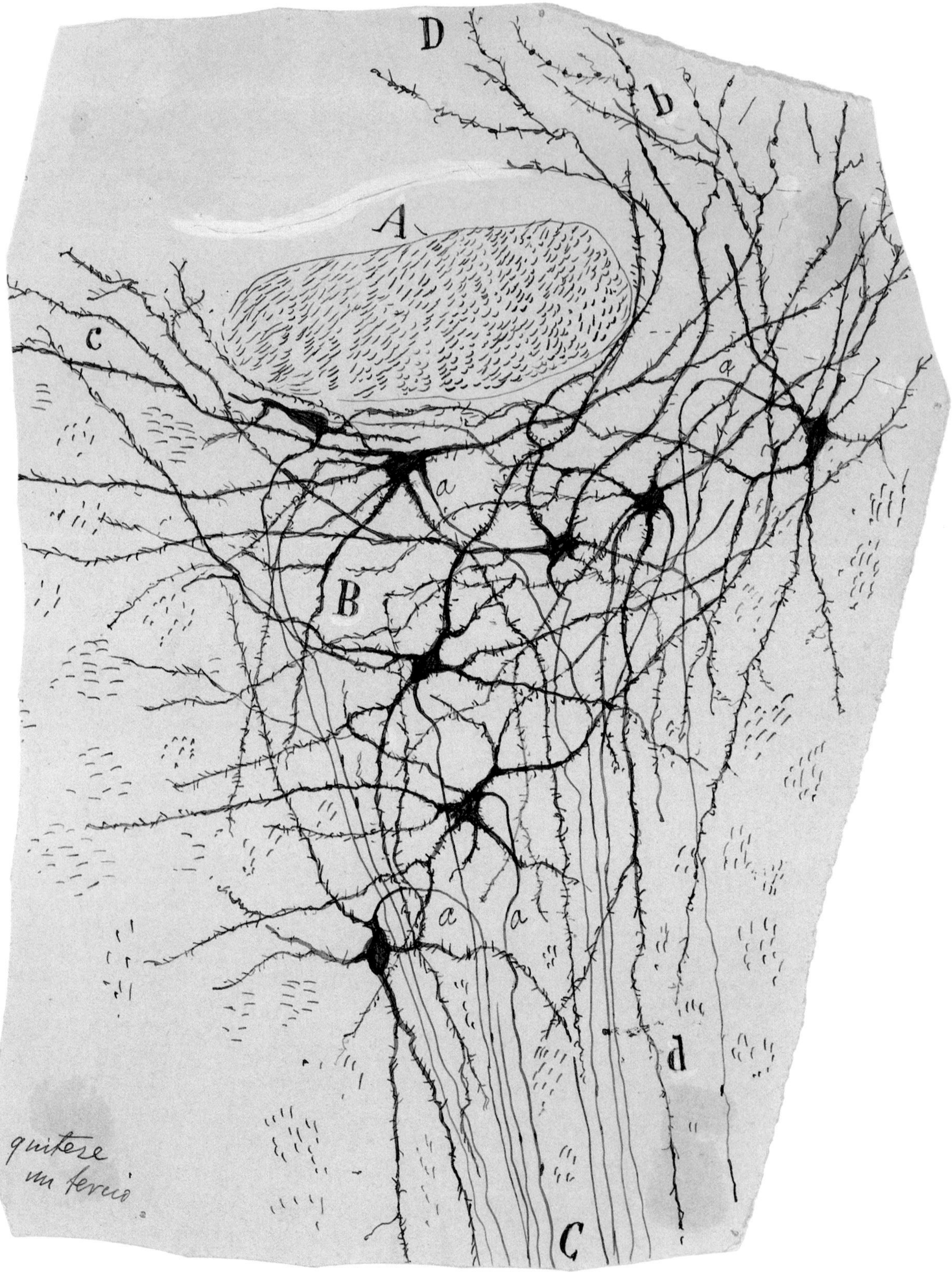

FIGURE 49. Abducens nucleus in a kitten.

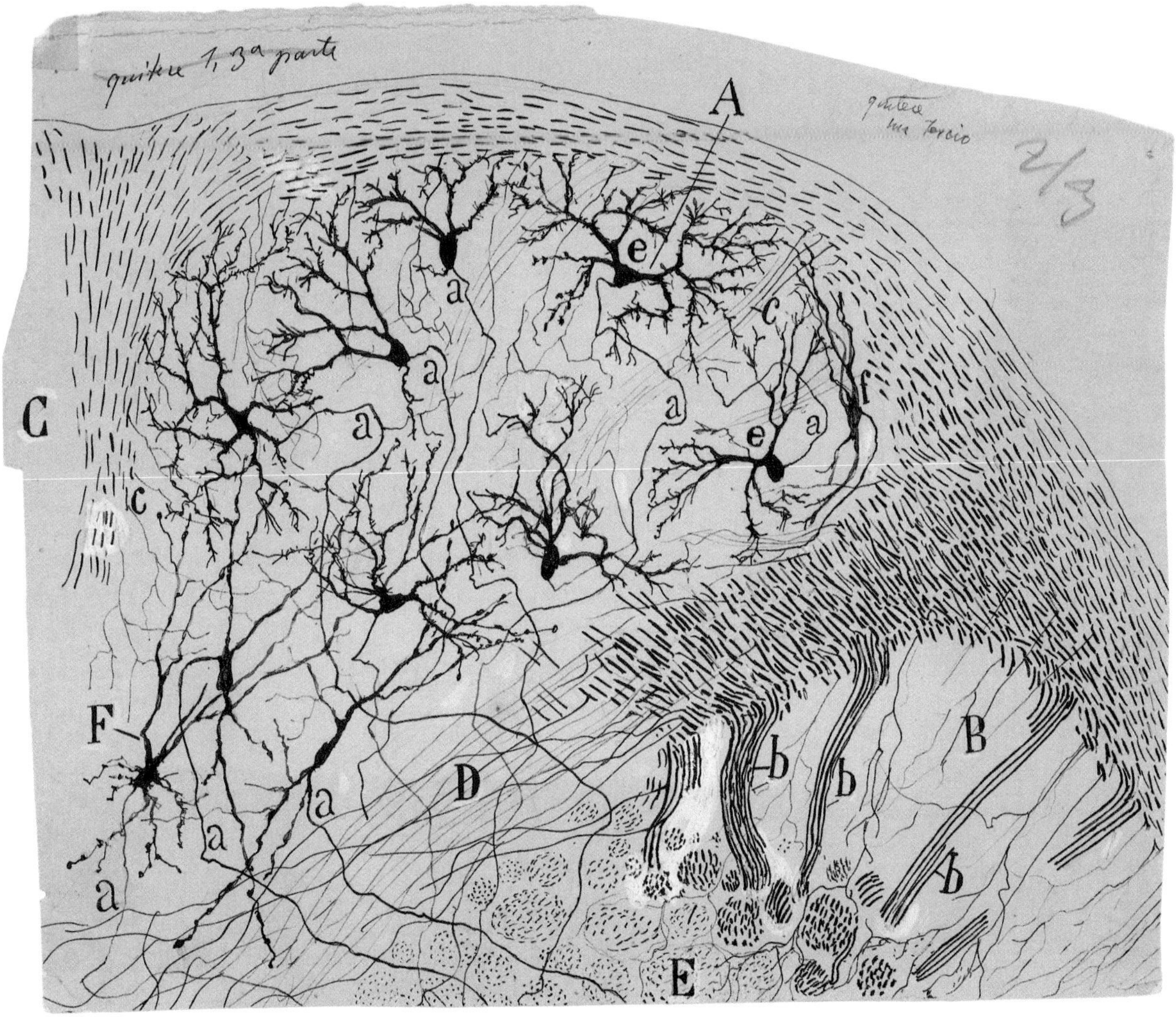

FIGURE 50. Section of the medulla at the level of the nucleus cuneatus in a kitten.

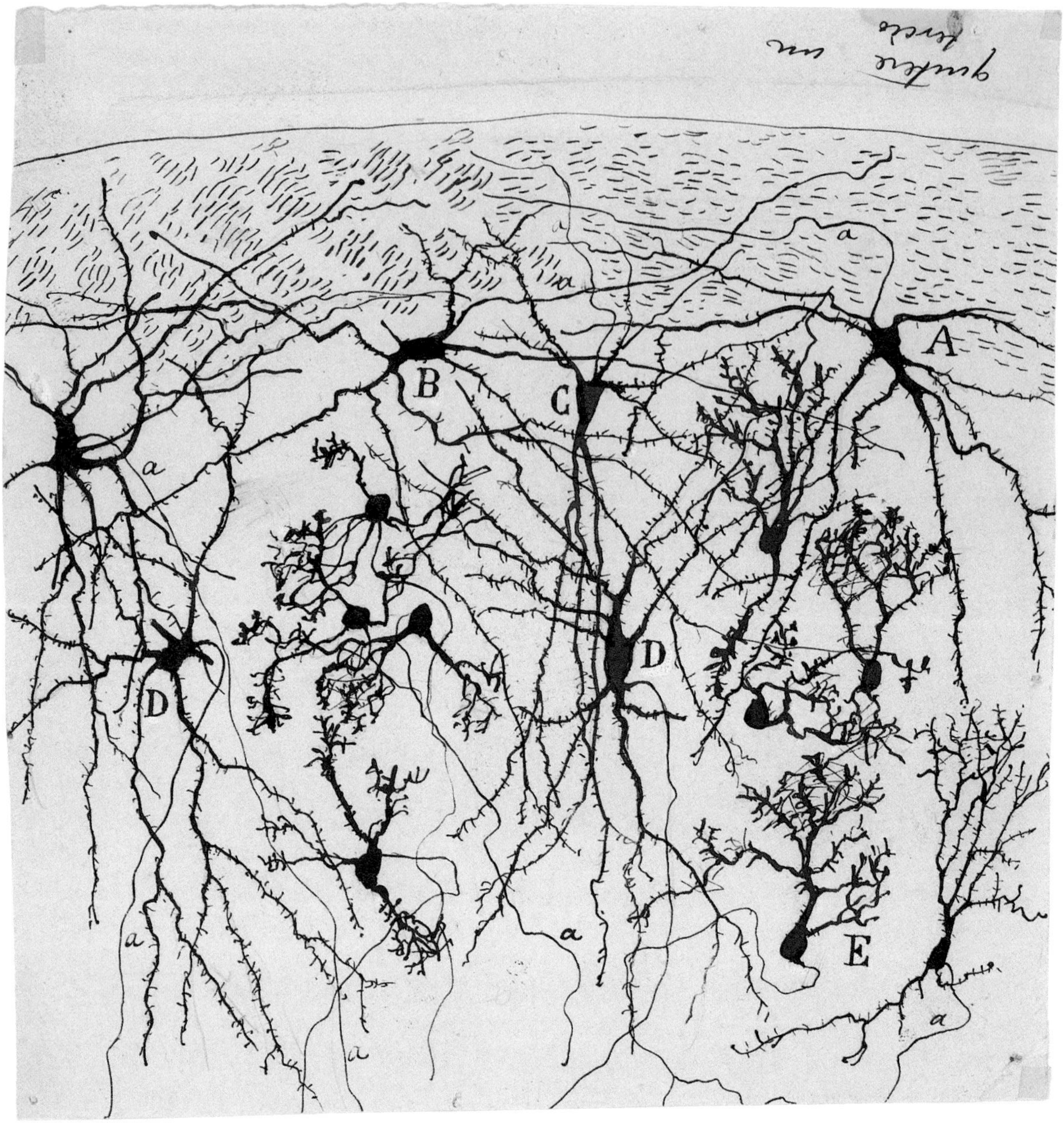

FIGURE 51. Section of the rostral region of the nucleus cuneatus in a kitten.

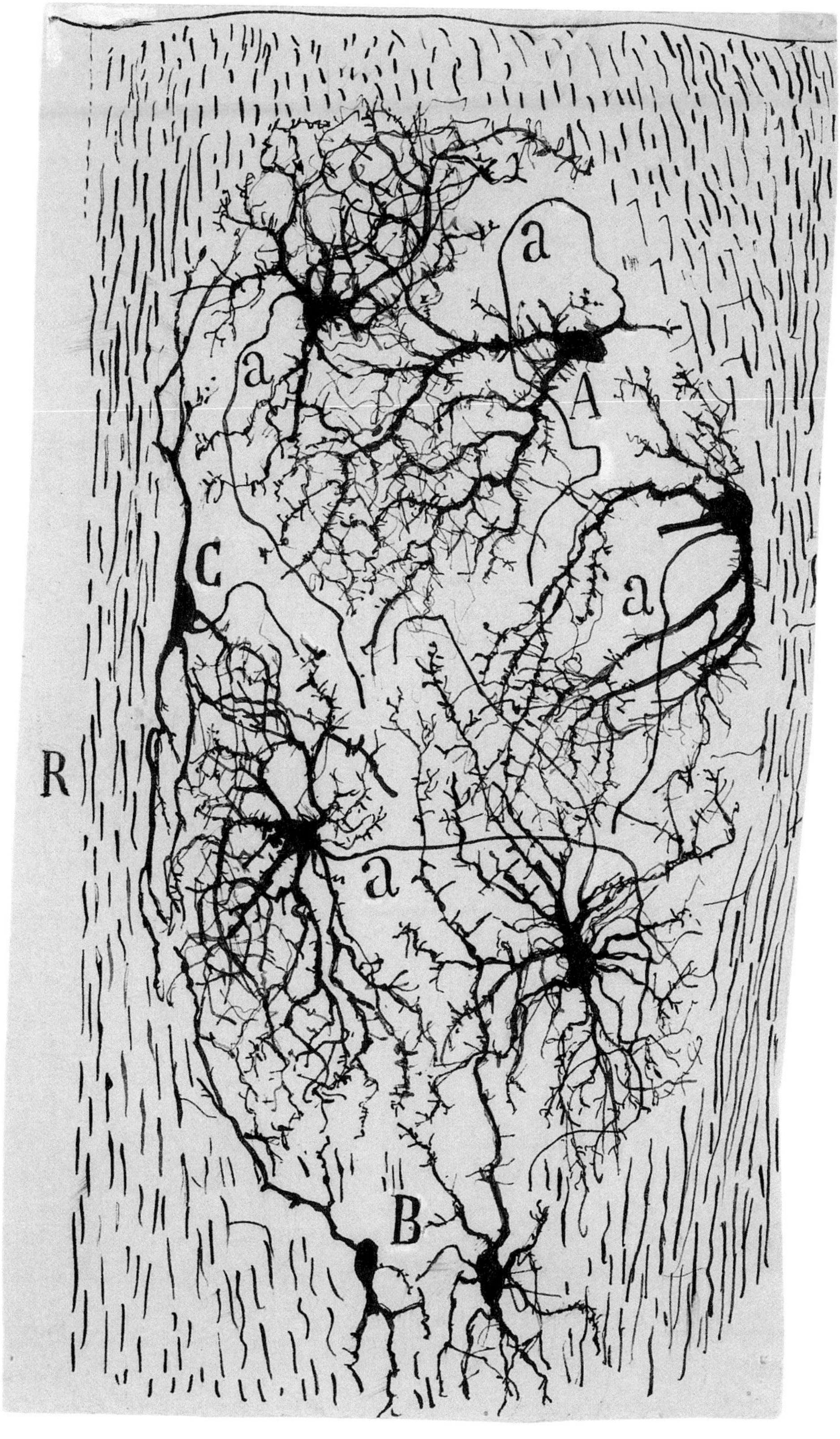

FIGURE 52. Transverse section of the nucleus gracilis in a kitten.

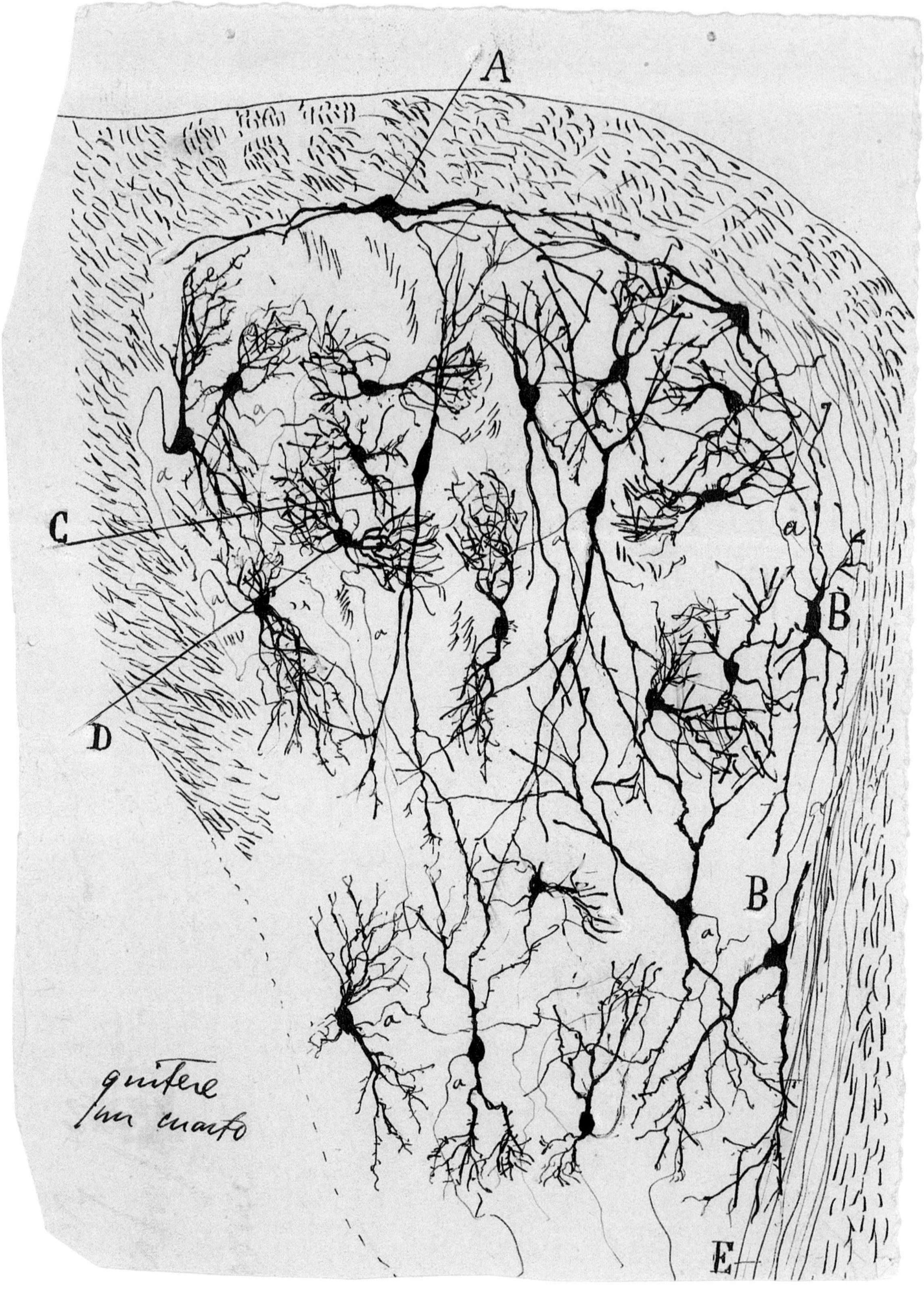

FIGURE 53. Section of the nucleus gracilis in a human fetus.

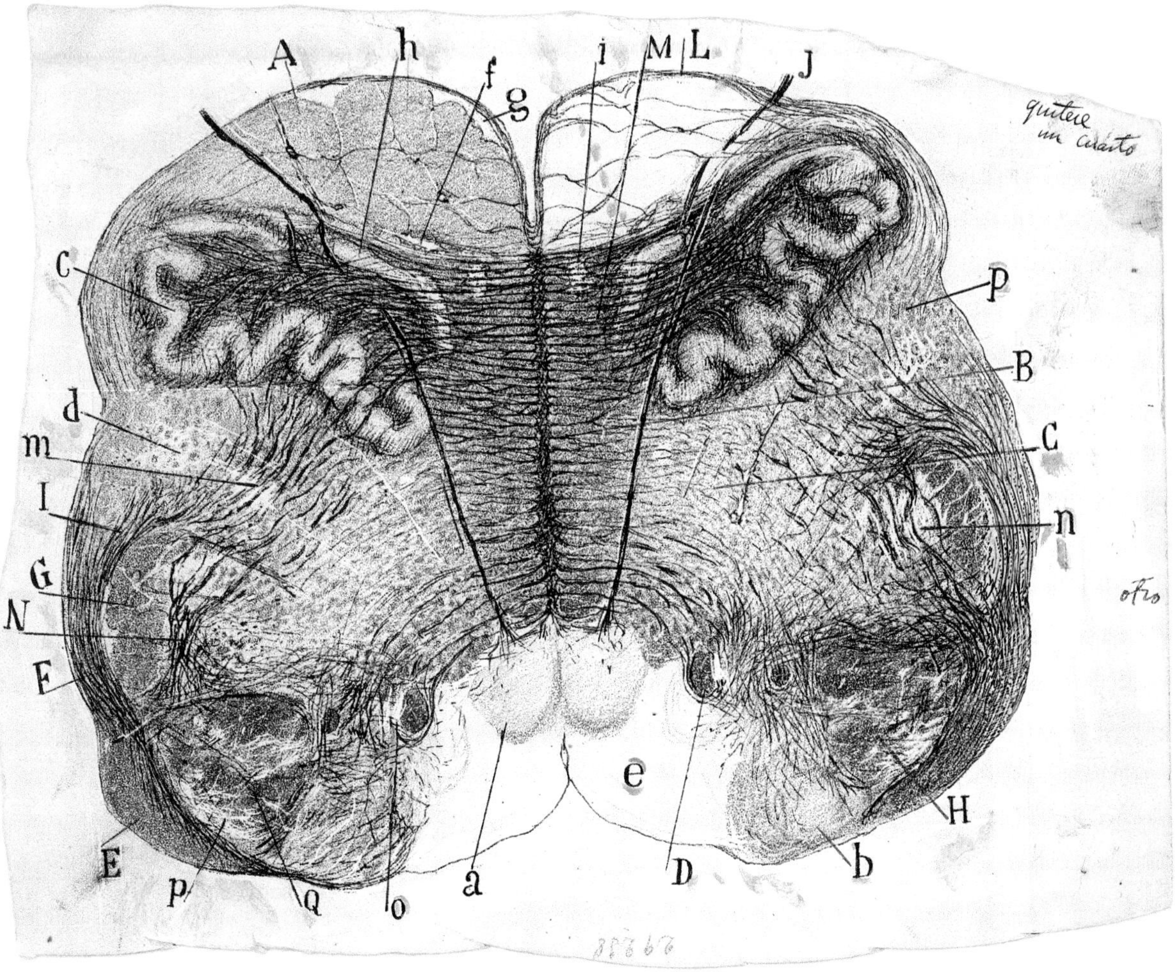

FIGURE 54. Medulla of a hemiplegic individual at the level of the caudal third of the olive.

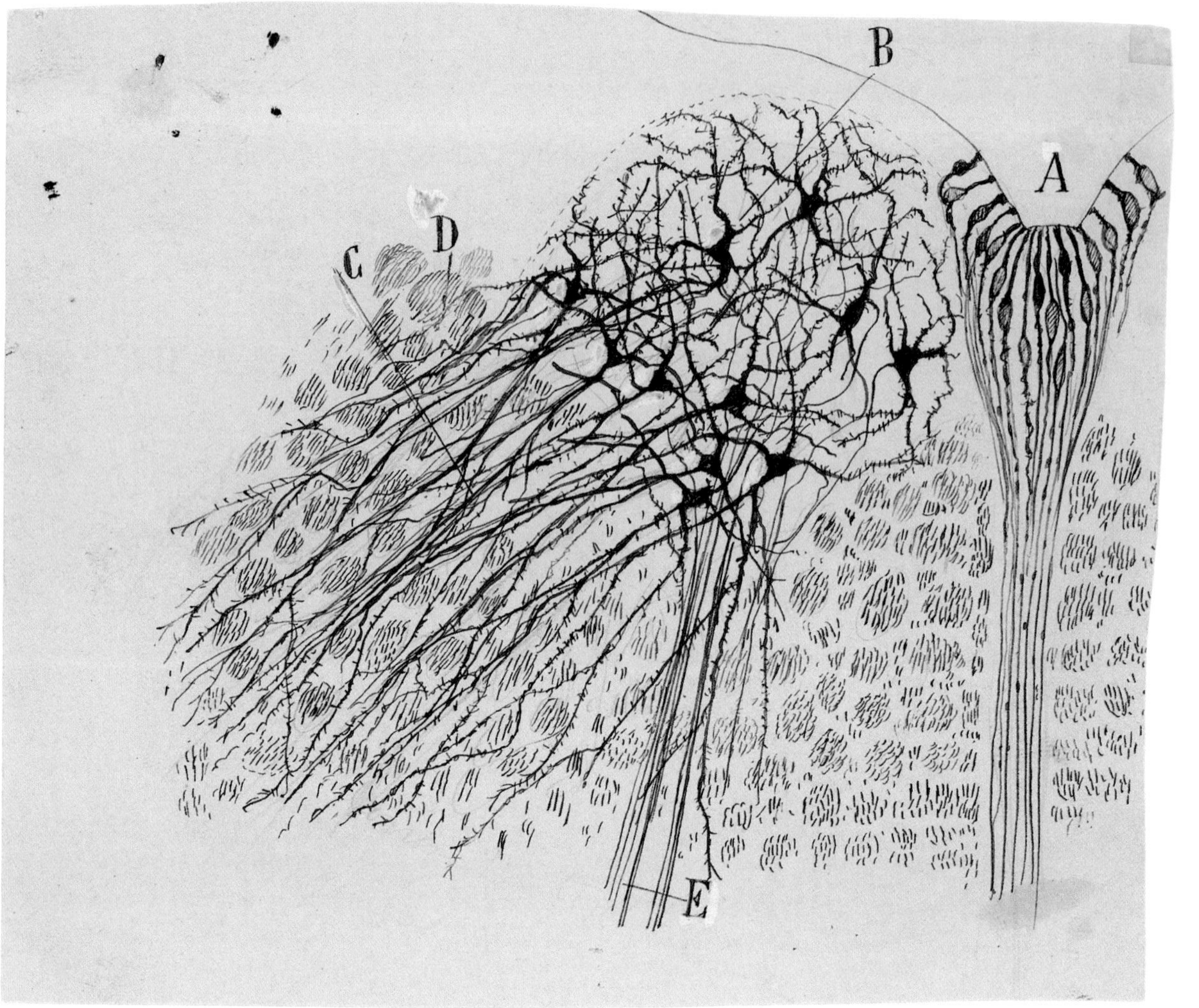

FIGURE 55. Hypoglossal nucleus at the level of the rostral third in a kitten.

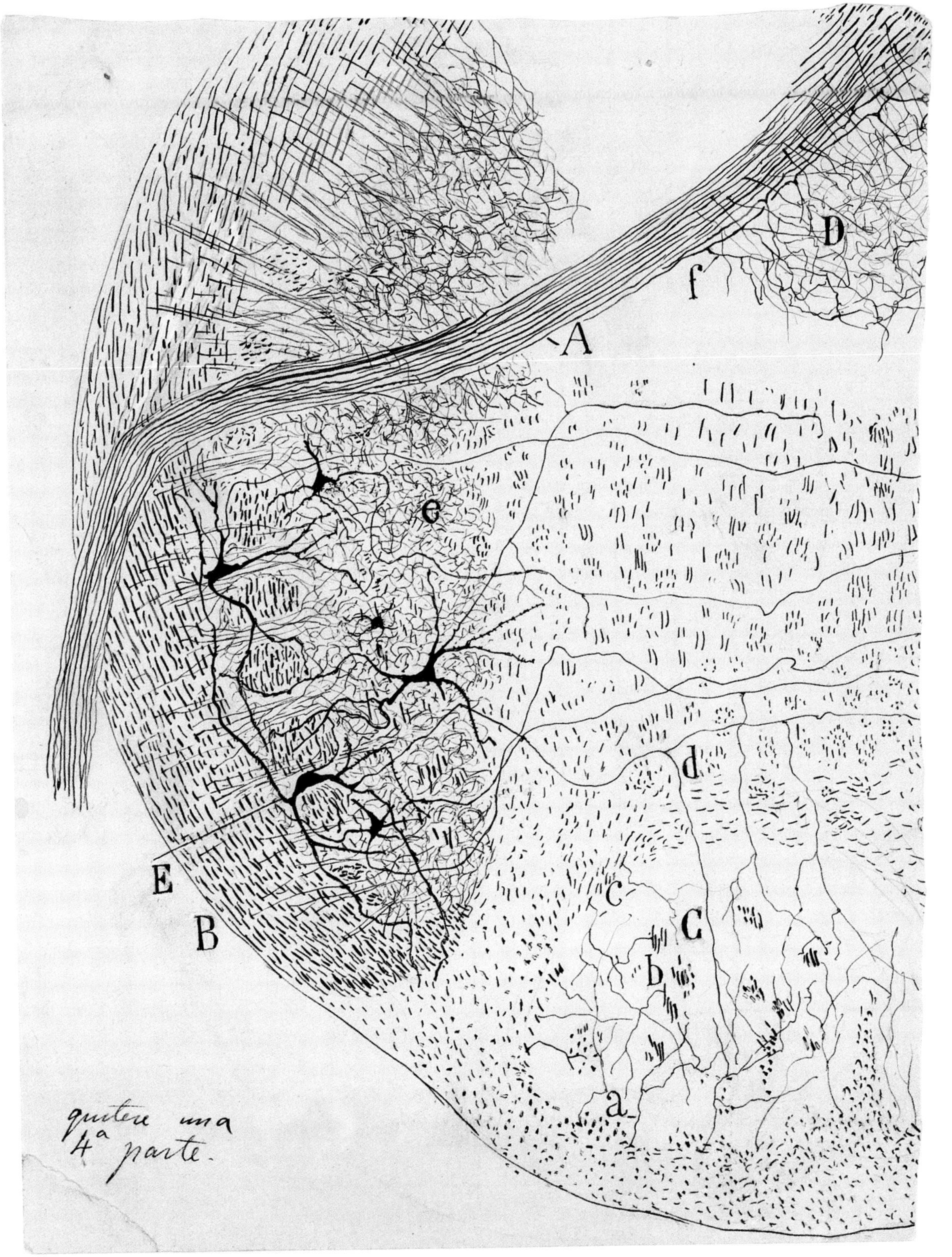

FIGURE 56. Section of the medulla at the level of the facial nucleus in a mouse.

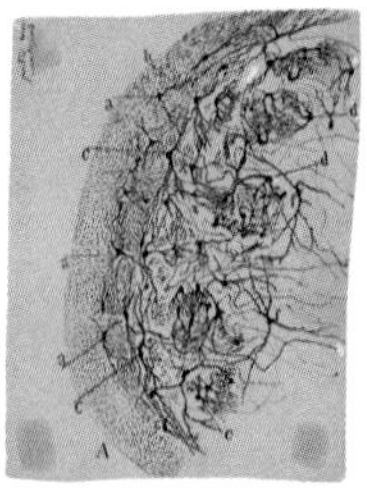

FIGURE 21.

Spinal tract of the trigeminal nerve in a newborn rabbit.

This figure was published in Cajal, S. R. (1895) Apuntes para el estudio del bulbo raquídeo, cerebelo y origen de los nervios encefálicos. *An. Soc. Españ. Hist. Nat.* 24, 1–118 (Figure 2). It has also been reproduced as Figure 303 in Cajal, S. R. (1899–1904) *Textura del sistema nervioso del hombre y de los vertebrados*. Madrid: Moya.

FIGURE LEGEND: Transverse section through the spinal tract of the trigeminal nerve in a newborn rabbit. Golgi method. *A*, Ventral part of the tract; *a*, interstitial cells; *c*, marginal cells; *d*, cellular islands of the substantia gelatinosa at the level of the spinal nucleus; *e*, small cells of these islands; *f*, large, stellate cells that do not form islands; *g*, cells between islands; *h*, a marginal cell with an axon that seems to go toward the white matter or ventral region of the root.

Original text: Corte transversal de la raíz sensitiva descendente del trigémino del conejo recién nacido. Método de Golgi. *A*, parte anterior de la raíz; *a*, células intersticiales; *c*, células marginales; *d*, islotes celulares de la substancia gelatinosa; *e*, células pequeñas de estos islotes; *f*, células grandes, estrelladas, no dispuestas en islotes; *g*, células intercoloniales; *h*, una célula marginal, cuyo cilindro-eje parecía ir hacia la substancia blanca ó región anterior de la raíz.

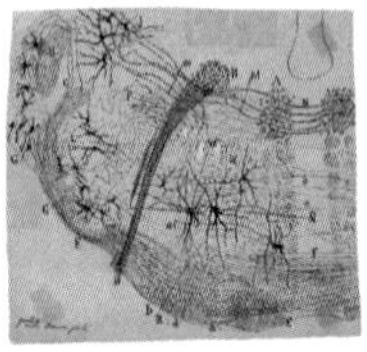

FIGURE 22.

Medulla in a newborn mouse at the level of the emergence of the facial nerve and plane of the trapezoid body.

This figure was published in Cajal, S. R. (1895) Apuntes para el estudio del bulbo raquídeo, cerebelo y origen de los nervios encefálicos. *An. Soc. Españ. Hist. Nat.* 24, 1–118 (Figure 3). It has also been reproduced as Figure 304 in Cajal, S. R. (1899–1904) *Textura del sistema nervioso del hombre y de los vertebrados*. Madrid: Moya.

FIGURE LEGEND: Transverse section of the medulla in a newborn mouse at the level of the emergence of the facial nerve and plane of the trapezoid body. Golgi method. *A*, Medial longitudinal fasciculus at the level where it is incorporating the crossed vestibular pathway; *B*, genu of the facial nerve; *C*, descending root of the trigeminal nerve; *D*, emergence of the facial nerve; *E*, pyramid; *F*, ventral trapezoid fibers; *G*, ventral cochlear nucleus; *H*, dorsal cochlear nucleus; *J*, lateral vestibular nucleus (Deiter's nucleus); *L*, nucleus of the spinal tract of the trigeminal nerve showing its giant cells and the course of their axons, many of which form a longitudinal pathway in *P* whereas others cross the raphe; *M*, nucleus of the sixth cranial nerve with collaterals received from the medial longitudinal fasciculus; *O*, trapezoid fibers originating in the dorsal cochlear nucleus; *N*, axons from the lateral vestibular nucleus (Deiter's nucleus) forming the central crossed vestibular pathway; *P*, uncrossed central trigeminal pathway.

Original text: Corte transversal del bulbo de ratón recién nacido, á la altura de la emergencia del facial y en el plano del cuerpo trapezoide. Método de Golgi. *A*, fascículo longitudinal posterior donde ingresa la vía vestibular cruzada; *B*, [rodilla del] facial; *C*, [raíz descendente del] trigémino; *D*, emergencia del facial; *E*, pirámide; *F*, fibras trapezóideas anteriores; *G*, ganglio ventral del vestibular; *H*, tubérculo acústico; *J*, ganglio de Deiters; *L*, substancia gelatinosa del trigémino [en donde se muestra sus células gigantes y la marcha de sus cilindros-ejes, muchos de ellos forman una vía longitudinal en *P* pero otros cruzan el rafe]; *M*, foco del sexto par, con las colaterales recibidas del haz longitudinal posterior; *O*, fibras trapezóideas nacidas del tubérculo acústico; *N*, axones llegados del ganglio de Deiters y formadores de la vía vestibular lateral central; *P*, vía lateral central del trigémino.

Note from the author (J. D.): In brackets is the text added in the French version of the *Textura*: Cajal, S. R. (1909–1911) *Histologie du système nerveux de l'homme et des vertébrés*, trans. L. Azoulay. Paris: Maloine. In G, "vestibular" in the original Spanish text should be "cochlear." *D, H, G, M, N, O*, and *P* are not described in the legend of the figure in *Histologie*.

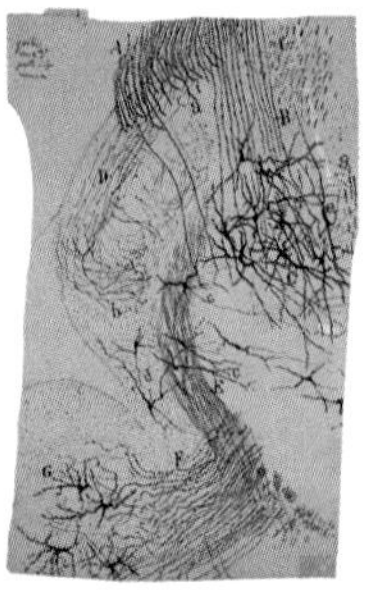

FIGURE 23.

Nuclei of the trigeminal nerve in a mouse fetus.

This figure was published in Cajal, S. R. (1895) Apuntes para el estudio del bulbo raquídeo, cerebelo y origen de los nervios encefálicos. *An. Soc. Españ. Hist. Nat.* 24, 1–118 (Figure 5). It has also been reproduced as Figure 307 in Cajal, S. R. (1899–1904) *Textura del sistema nervioso del hombre y de los vertebrados*. Madrid: Moya.

FIGURE LEGEND: Transverse section through the nuclei of the fifth cranial nerve in a mouse fetus. Golgi method. *A*, Sensory root of the trigeminal nerve; *B*, masticatory nerve (or motor root); *C*, masticatory nucleus; *D*, ascending branch of the sensory root; *F*, superior cerebellar peduncle; *E*, bundle of collaterals of this peduncle; **G*, dentate nucleus; *a*, bifurcation of sensory fibers of the trigeminal nerve; *b*, endings of small ascending sensory fibers; *c*, cells located within the descending cerebellar bundle; *e*, cell of the masticatory nucleus; *g*, fibers of the lateral central pathways of the trigeminal and glossopharyngeal nerves that provide collaterals to the masticatory nucleus.*

Original text: Corte transversal de los focos de origen del quinto par del feto de ratón. Método de Golgi. *A*, raíz sensitiva del trigémino; *B*, nervio masticador; *C*, foco masticador; *D*, rama ascendente de la raíz sensitiva; *F*, pedúnculo cerebeloso superior; *E*, haz de colaterales del pedúnculo; **G*, oliva cerebelosa; *a*, bifurcación de las fibras sensitivas del trigémino; *b*, terminación de las ramillas sensitivas ascendentes; *c*, células colocadas en el espesor de dicho fascículo cerebeloso descendente; *e*, célula del núcleo masticador; *g*, fibras de la vía sensitiva central lateral del trigémino y glosofaríngeo que suministran colaterales al núcleo masticador.*

Note from the author (J. D.): The text between asterisks appears in the original publication only.

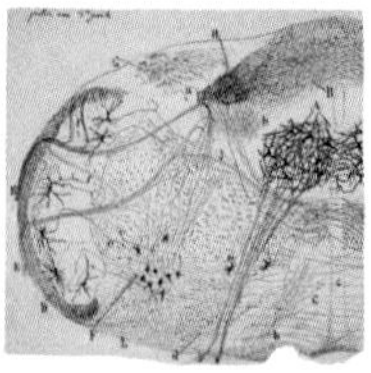

FIGURE 24.

Transverse section of the medulla in a four-day-old mouse.

This figure was published in Cajal, S. R. (1895) Apuntes para el estudio del bulbo raquídeo, cerebelo y origen de los nervios encefálicos. *An. Soc. Españ. Hist. Nat.* 24, 1–118 (Figure 13). It has also been reproduced as Figure 242 in Cajal, S. R. (1899–1904) *Textura del sistema nervioso del hombre y de los vertebrados*. Madrid: Moya.

FIGURE LEGEND: Transverse section of the medulla in a four-day-old mouse. Golgi method. *A*, Hypoglossal nucleus; *B*, commissural nucleus; *C*, inferior olive; *D*, descending root of the trigeminal nerve; *E*, motor roots of the vagus and glossopharyngeal nerves; *F*, nucleus ambiguus; *G*, terminal portion of the inferior vestibular nucleus; *H*, transverse section of the solitary tract; *L*, fibers that go to the olive; *a*, pyramid; *b*, collaterals of the white matter located lateral to the pyramid and from the pyramid itself; *d*, collaterals from remnants of the lateral funiculus; *e*, sensory collaterals for the nucleus ambiguus; *f*, recurrent fibers of the motor root entering the trigeminal spinal tract; *j*, crossed motor radicular fibers of the vagus and glossopharyngeal nerves; *h*, collaterals of sensory roots of the vagus and glossopharyngeal nerves for the solitary tract nucleus.

Original text: Corte transversal del bulbo de ratón de cuatro días. Método de Golgi. *A*, núcleo del hipogloso; *B*, ganglio comisural; *C*, oliva bulbar; *D*, raíz descendente sensitiva del trigémino; *E*, raíces motrices del vago y gloso-faríngeo; *F*, núcleo ambiguo; *G*, porción terminal del ganglio vestibular descendente; *H*, corte transversal del fascículo solitario; *L*, fibras que van á la oliva; *a*, pirámides; *b*, colaterales de la substancia blanca situada por fuera de las pirámides y de las pirámides mismas; *d*, colaterales del resto del cordón lateral; *e*, colaterales sensitivas para el núcleo ambiguo; *f*, fibras recurrentes de la raíz motora que iban á la raíz del trigémino; *j*, radiculares motrices cruzadas del vago y gloso-faríngeo; *h*, colaterales de la raíz sensitiva de estos nervios para el núcleo que acompaña al fascículo solitario.

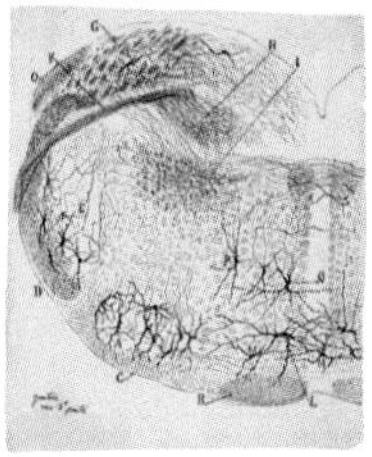

FIGURE 25.

Medulla in a newborn mouse.

This figure was published in Cajal, S. R. (1895) Apuntes para el estudio del bulbo raquídeo, cerebelo y origen de los nervios encefálicos. *An. Soc. Españ. Hist. Nat.* 24, 1–118 (Figure 16). It has also been reproduced as Figure 292 in Cajal, S. R. (1899–1904) *Textura del sistema nervioso del hombre y de los vertebrados*. Madrid: Moya.

FIGURE LEGEND: Section of the medulla in a newborn mouse at the level of the facial nucleus. Golgi method. *A*, Facial nucleus; *E*, pyramidal pathway; *C*, remnants of the lateral funiculus; *D*, *spinal tract of* the trigeminal nerve; *E*, spinal nucleus of the trigeminal nerve; *F*, vagus nerve; *G*, inferior vestibular nucleus; *H*, medial gray column of the solitary tract; *J*, central vestibular pathway; *O*, restiform body. **I*, lateral central pathway of the vestibular, trigeminal, vagal, and glossopharyngeal nerves; *L*, *Ñ*, giant cells with axons going to the medial longitudinal fasciculus; *M*, cells with axons going to remnants of the lateral funiculus; *P*, cell with axon going to the gray reticular formation.*

Original text: Corte de bulbo de ratón recién nacido á la altura del núcleo del facial. Método de Golgi. *A*, núcleo del facial; *E*, vía piramidal; *C*, resto del cordón lateral; *D*, *sección de la raíz descendente del* trigémino; *E*, substancia gelatinosa de éste; *F*, vago; *G*, foco descendente del vestibular; *H*, columna gris interna del cordón solitario; *J*, vía central del vestibular; *O*, cuerpo restiforme. **I*, vía lateral central del vestibular, del trigémino y del vago y glosofaríngeo; *L*, *Ñ*, células gigantes cuyos cilindros-ejes van al fascículo longitudinal posterior; *M*, células cuyo cilindro-eje iba al resto del cordón lateral; *P*, célula cuya expansión funcional iba á la substancia reticular gris.*

Note from the author (J. D.): The text between asterisks appears in the original publication only.

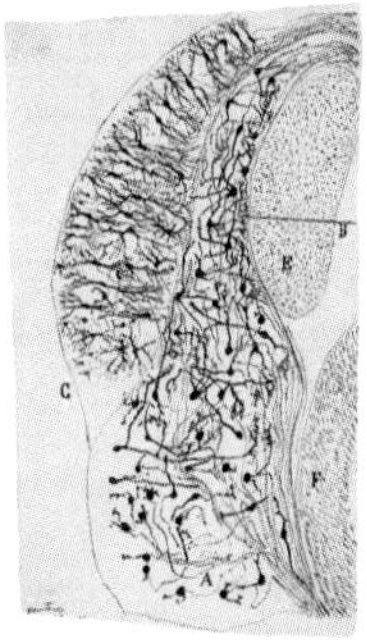

FIGURE 26.

Neurons of the ventral and dorsal cochlear nuclei in a rabbit.

This figure was published in Cajal, S. R. (1895) Apuntes para el estudio del bulbo raquídeo, cerebelo y origen de los nervios encefálicos. *An. Soc. Españ. Hist. Nat.* 24, 1–118 (Figure 22). It has also been reproduced as Figure 265 in Cajal, S. R. (1899–1904) *Textura del sistema nervioso del hombre y de los vertebrados*. Madrid: Moya.

FIGURE LEGEND: Lateral part of a transverse pontomedullary section showing the assembly of neurons of the ventral and dorsal cochlear nuclei in an eight-day-old rabbit. Golgi method. *A*, Ventral cochlear nucleus; *B*, tail of the ventral cochlear nucleus; *C*, acoustic tubercle or dorsal cochlear nucleus; *E*, restiform body; *F*, trigeminal nerve.

Original text: [Parte lateral de un corte transversal bulbo-protuberancial mostrando] el conjunto de las células nerviosas de los ganglios ventral y lateral del coclear, en el conejo de ocho días. Método de Golgi. *A*, ganglio ventral; *B*, cola del ganglio ventral; *C*, tubérculo acústico [ó ganglio lateral]; *E*, cuerpo restiforme; *F*, trigémino.

Note from the author (J. D.): In brackets is the text added in the French version of the *Textura*: Cajal, S. R. (1909–1911) *Histologie du système nerveux de l'homme et des vertébrés*, trans. L. Azoulay. Paris: Maloine.

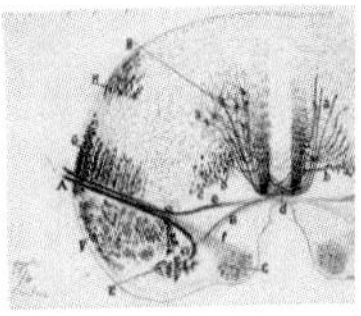

FIGURE 27.

Medulla at the level of the glossopharyngeal nucleus in a chick embryo.

This figure was published in Cajal, S. R. (1909) Contribución al estudio de los ganglios de la substancia reticular del bulbo, con algunos detalles concernientes a los focos motores y vías reflejas. *Trab. Lab. Invest. Biol. Univ. Madrid* 7, 259–284 (Figure 3).

FIGURE LEGEND: Transverse section of the medulla at the level of the glossopharyngeal nucleus. Chick embryo on day 10 of incubation. *A*, Radicular fibers of the glossopharyngeal nerve; *B*, inferior magnocellular nucleus; *C*, motor nucleus of the glossopharyngeal nerve; *E*, dorsal solitary tract; *F*, descending portion of the vestibular nerve; *G*, descending root of the trigeminal nerve; *a*, neurons with crossed axons; *b*, neurons with uncrossed axons that are incorporated to the fibrillar medial wall; *e*, crossed radicular fibers of the glossopharyngeal nerve; *d*, chiasm of the axons of the medial magnocellular nucleus.

Original text: Corte frontal del bulbo a la altura del gloso-faríngeo. Embrión del pollo del 10º. día. *A*, radiculares del gloso-faríngeo; *B*, foco magno-celular inferior; *C*, foco motor del gloso-faríngeo; *E*, fascículo solitario dorsal; *F*, porción descendente del vestibular; *G*, raíz descendente sensitiva del trigémino; *a*, neuronas de axon cruzado; *b*, neuronas de axon directo incorporado al muro fibrilar interno; *e*, radiculares cruzadas del gloso-faríngeo; *d*, quiasma de los axones del foco magno-celular inferior.

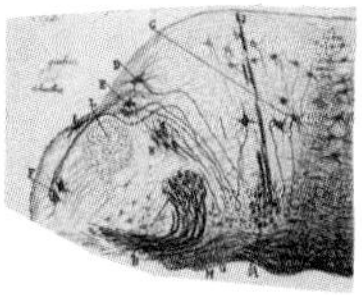

FIGURE 28.

Medulla in a newborn bird.

This figure was published in Cajal, S. R. (1909) Contribución al estudio de los ganglios de la substancia reticular del bulbo, con algunos detalles concernientes a los focos motores y vías reflejas. *Trab. Lab. Invest. Biol. Univ. Madrid* 7, 259–284 (Figure 4).

FIGURE LEGEND: Section of the medulla in a newborn bird at the level of the facial nucleus (*B*) and abducens nucleus (*A*); *C*, caudal neurons of the superior magnocellular nucleus; *D, E, F*, islands of the scattered nucleus; *H*, pathway of the superior magnocellular nucleus; *G*, crossed auditory pathway; *J*, radicular fibers of the abducens nucleus.

Original text: Corte del bulbo de un pájaro recién nacido. Altura del foco del facial (*B*) y núcleo del motor ocular externo (*A*); *C*, neuronas caudales del núcleo magnocélular superior; *D, E, F*, pléyades del núcleo diseminado; *H*, vía del núcleo magnocelular superior; *G*, vía acústica cruzada; *J*, radiculares del motor ocular externo.

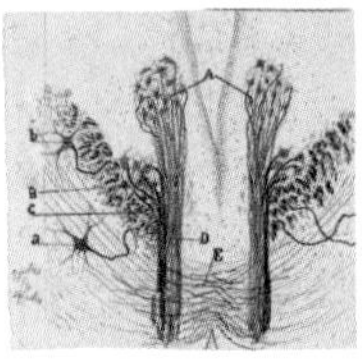

FIGURE 29.

Midbrain in a chick embryo.

This figure was published in Cajal, S. R. (1909) Contribución al estudio de los ganglios de la substancia reticular del bulbo, con algunos detalles concernientes a los focos motores y vías reflejas. *Trab. Lab. Invest. Biol. Univ. Madrid* 7, 259–284 (Figure 9).

FIGURE LEGEND: Transverse section of the mesencephalon in a chick embryo on day 9 of incubation. The section passed through the rostral tip of the principal nucleus of the third cranial nerve. *A*, Edinger-Westphal nucleus; *B*, rostral tip of dorsolateral island; *D*, fibers of the Edinger-Westphal nucleus entering into the roots of the oculomotor nucleus; *C*, medial longitudinal fasciculus; *a, b*, cells of the interstitial nucleus.

Original text: Corte frontal del mesocéfalo del embrión de pollo del 9.º día. La sección pasaba por el cabo anterior del núcleo principal de tercer par. *A*, núcleo de Edinger-Westphal; *B*, cabo anterior de la pléyade supero-externa; *D*, fibras del núcleo de Edinger-Westphal incorporadas á las raíces del motor ocular común; *C*, fascículo longitudinal posterior; *a, b*, células del foco intersticial.

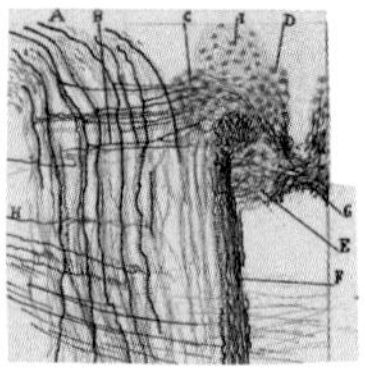

FIGURE 30.

Oculomotor nucleus in a chick embryo.

This figure was published in Cajal, S. R. (1909) Contribución al estudio de los ganglios de la substancia reticular del bulbo, con algunos detalles concernientes a los focos motores y vías reflejas. *Trab. Lab. Invest. Biol. Univ. Madrid* 7, 259–284 (Figure 10).

FIGURE LEGEND: Almost horizontal section of the region of the oculomotor nucleus. Chick embryo on day 9 of incubation. *A*, Thick fibers that descend from the nucleus of colossal cells of the posterior commissure; *B*, collaterals of these fibers coursing to the oculomotor nucleus; *C*, laterorostral island of this nucleus; *D*, rostromedial island; *E*, medial island; *F*, medial longitudinal fasciculus; *I*, nucleus of Edinger-Westphal; *H*, axons of the cells of the tegmental reticular substance.

Original text: Corte casi horizontal de la región del motor ocular común. Embrión de pollo del 9.º día. *A*, fibras gruesas que bajan del ganglio de células colosales de la comisura posterior; *B*, colaterales de estas fibras para el foco del motor ocular común; *C*, pléyade externa y superior de este núcleo; *D*, pléyade supero-interna; *E*, pléyade interior; *F*, fascículo longitudinal posterior; *I*, foco de Edinger-Westphal; *H*, axones de células de la substancia reticular de la calota.

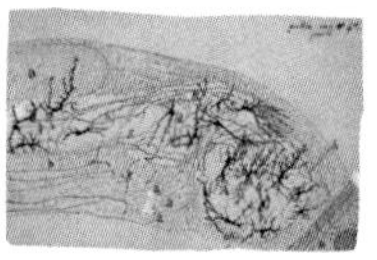

FIGURE 31.

Transverse section of the trapezoid body in a newborn mouse.

This figure was published in Cajal, S. R. (1895) Apuntes para el estudio del bulbo raquídeo, cerebelo y origen de los nervios encefálicos. *An. Soc. Españ. Hist. Nat.* 24, 1–118 (Figure 23).

FIGURE LEGEND: Transverse section of the trapezoid body in a newborn mouse. *A*, Superior olive; *B*, preolivary nucleus; *C*, nucleus of the trapezoid body; *D*, cross-cut pyramid; *E*, central auditory pathway or origin of the lateral lemniscus, where the trapezoidal fibers become vertical; *a*, cell of nucleus of the trapezoid body with an axon that gives collaterals for this nucleus and for the preolivary nucleus; *b*, another similar bifurcating fiber; *c*, collateral of another similar fiber coursing to the preolivary nucleus; *d*, cell of the preolivary nucleus with axons that seem to go laterally; *e*, cells with an axon that went to the white matter to form a central ascending pathway (*a, a, a*); *f, m, j*, cells of the olive; *n*, facial nerve.

Original text: Corte transversal de la región del cuerpo trapezoide en el ratón recién nacido. *A*, oliva superior; *B*, núcleo preolivar; *C*, núcleo del cuerpo trapezoide; *D*, pirámide cortada de través; *E*, vía central acústica ú origen del lemnisco externo, donde las fibras trapezoideas se hacen verticales; *a*, célula del núcleo del cuerpo trapezoide, cuyo cilindro-eje daba colaterales para dicho núcleo y para el preolivar; *b*, otra fibra análoga que se bifurcaba; *c*, colateral de otra fibra semejante para el foco preolivar; *d*, célula del foco preolivar, cuya expansión parecía ir hacia afuera; *e*, células cuya expansión iba á la substancia blanca á formar una vía central ascendente (*a, a, a*); *f, m, j*, células de la oliva; *n*, facial.

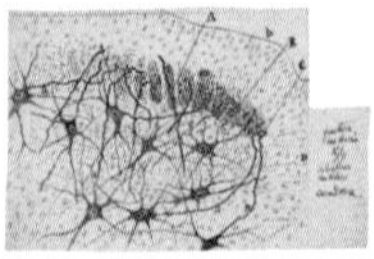

FIGURE 32.

Transverse section of the tegmentum in a human embryo.

This figure was published in Cajal, S. R. (1908) El ganglio intersticial del fascículo longitudinal posterior en el hombre y diversos vertebrados. *Trav. Lab. Recherches Biol. Univ. Madrid* 6, 145–160 (Figure 1). It has also been reproduced as Figure 170 in Cajal, S. R. (1909–1911) *Histologie du système nerveux de l'homme et des vertébrés*, trans. L. Azoulay. Paris: Maloine.

FIGURE LEGEND: Portion of a transverse section of the tegmentum. Human embryo at 7 weeks' gestation. Reduced silver nitrate method. *A*, Voluminous cells of the interstitial nucleus; *B*, medial longitudinal fasciculus; *C*, thick axons of cells of the interstitial nucleus; *D*, raphe; *a*, axons.

Original text: Trozo de un corte frontal de la calota; embrión humano de 7 semanas. Método del nitrato de plata reducido. *A*, células voluminosas del núcleo intersticial; *B*, fascículo longitudinal posterior; *C*, axones gruesos de las células del núcleo intersticial; *D*, rafe; *a*, axones.

Note from the author (J. D.): This figure is not included in Cajal, S. R. (1899–1904) *Textura del sistema nervioso del hombre y de los vertebrados*. Madrid: Moya.

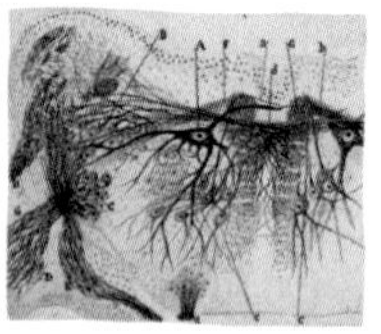

FIGURE 33.

Section of the medulla at the level of the auditory region in a trout.

This figure was published in Cajal, S. R. (1908) El ganglio intersticial del fascículo longitudinal posterior en el hombre y diversos vertebrados. *Trav. Lab. Recherches Biol. Univ. Madrid* 6, 145–160 (Figure 5).

FIGURE LEGEND: Transverse section of the medulla at the level of the auditory region in a fifteen-day-old trout. *A*, Cell of Mauthner; *B*, nucleus of Deiters; *D, E*, lobules of the vestibular nucleus; *a, b*, axons of the cells of the reticular substance that are incorporated in the medial longitudinal fasciculus; *F*, direct pathway of the vestibular nucleus associated with this fascicle.

Original text: Corte transversal del bulbo raquídeo de la trucha de quince días al nivel de la región acústica. *A*, célula de Mauthner; *B*, ganglio de Deiters; *D, E*, lóbulos del ganglio del vestíbular; *a, b*, axones de células de la substancia reticular, incorporados al fascículo longitudinal posterior; *F*, vía directa del vestibular asociada á este fascículo.

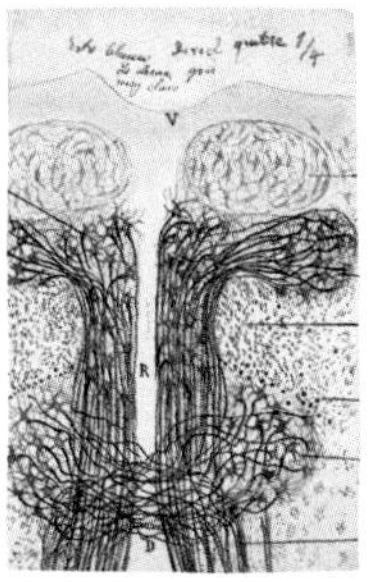

FIGURE 34.

Section through cell groups forming the oculomotor nucleus in a kite.

This figure was published in Cajal, S. R. (1904). Asociación del método de nitrato de plata con el embrionario para el estudio de los focos motores y sensitivos. *Trab. Lab. Invest. Biol. Univ. Madrid* 3, 65–96 (Figure 2). It has also been reproduced as Figure 159 in Cajal, S. R. (1909–1911) *Histologie du système nerveux de l'homme et des vertébrés*, trans. L. Azoulay. Paris: Maloine.

FIGURE LEGEND: Transverse section through cell groups forming the oculomotor nucleus. Kite (a few days of age) (*Milvus regalis*, Briss). Reduced silver nitrate method. *A*, Dorsolateral cell group; *B*, dorsomedial cell group; *C*, ventral cell group; *D*, crossing of radicular fibers; *E*, dorsal nucleus of small cells (Edinger-Westphal nucleus?); *F*, medial longitudinal fasciculus; *G*, its very thick fibers arising in the interstitial nucleus; *H*, radicular fibers of the oculomotor nerve; *V*, ventricle.

Original text: Corte transversal de los focos componentes del núcleo motor ocular común; milano de algunos días (*Milvus regalis*, Briss). Método del nitrato de plata reducido. *A*, grupo celular súpero-externo; *B*, grupo súpero-interno; *C*, grupo inferior; *D*, cruzamiento de sus radiculares; *E*, núcleo superior de células pequeñas (núcleo de Edinger-Westphal?); *F*, fascículo longitudinal posterior; *G*, sus tubos muy gruesos, salidos del núcleo intersticial; *H*, radiculares del motor ocular común; *V*, ventrículo.

Note from the author (J. D.): This figure is not included in Cajal, S. R. (1899–1904) *Textura del sistema nervioso del hombre y de los vertebrados*. Madrid: Moya. The letters that should appear at the end of indicating lines in the figure are missing. In Supplementary Figure S4, the missing letters A, B, C, E, F, G, and H are included.

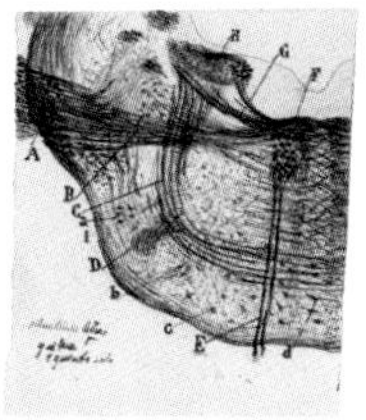

FIGURE 35.

Section of the medulla in a sparrow a few days old.

This figure was published in Cajal, S. R. (1908) Les ganglions terminaux du nerf acoustique des oiseaux. *Trav. Lab. Recherches Biol. Univ. Madrid* 6, 195–226 (Figure 1).

FIGURE LEGEND: Transverse section of the medulla in a sparrow a few days old. *A*, Vestibular nerve and tangential nucleus; *B*, fascicle from this nucleus; *C*, trapezoid body; *D*, superior olive; *E*, abducens nerve; *F*, nucleus of this nerve; *G*, dorsal crossed auditory pathway; *H*, parvocellular nucleus; *a, b*, magnocellular nuclei with cells that had axons coursing dorsally.

Original text: Coupe frontale du bulbe rachidien d'un moineau âgé de quelques jours. *A*, nerf vestibulaire et noyau tangentiel; *B*, faisceau provenant de ce noyan; *C*, corps trapézoïde; *D*, olive supérieure; *E*, nerf oculaire externe; *F*, noyau de ce nerf; *G*, voie acoustique dorsale croisée; *H*, noyau lamellaire ou à petites cellules; *a, b*, noyaux à cellules géantes dont les axones marchent en arrière.

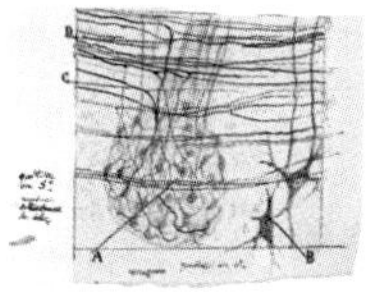

FIGURE 36.

Section at the level of the superior olive and trapezoid body in a bird.

This figure was published in Cajal, S. R. (1908) Les ganglions terminaux du nerf acoustique des oiseaux. *Trav. Lab. Recherches Biol. Univ. Madrid* 6, 195–226 (Figure 2).

FIGURE LEGEND: Portion of a transverse section of an eight-day-old bird. *A*, Superior olive; *D*, trapezoid body; *C*, branched collaterals in the superior olive; *B*, giant cells of the reticular substance close to the olive.

Original text: Morceau d'une coupe frontale d'un oiseau âgé de 8 jours. *A*, olive supérieure; *D*, corps trapézoïde; *C*, collatérales ramifiées dans l'olive supérieure; *B*, cellules géantes de la substance reticulaire voisine de l'olive.

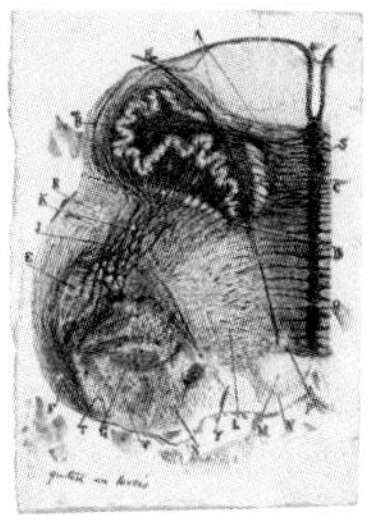

FIGURE 37.

Medulla in a hemiplegic individual.

This figure was published in Cajal, S. R. (1899–1904) *Textura del sistema nervioso del hombre y de los vertebrados*. Madrid: Moya. (Figure 215).

FIGURE LEGEND: Section of the medulla in a hemiplegic individual at the level of the middle third of the olive (Weigert-Pal method). *A*, Postpyramidal nuclei *B*, olive; *C*, medial accessory olive; *D*, lateral accessory olive; *E*, spinal tract of the trigeminal nerve; *F*, restiform body; *G*, thick bundle of the tract of Burdach (fasciculus cuneatus); *H*, hypoglossal nerve; *I*, ventral arcuate fibers; *J*, intermediate or olivary arcuate fibers; *K*, nucleus ambiguus; *L*, gray reticular substance; *Q*, white reticular substance; *M*, hypoglossal nucleus; *N*, intercalated nucleus; *P*, nucleus of Roller; *R*, lateral reticular nucleus; *S*, region of the medial lemniscus; *T*, nucleus accessory cuneatus; V, nucleus cuneatus; *X*, remnants of nucleus gracilis; *Y*, dorsal motor nucleus of the vagus nerve.

Original text: Corte del bulbo [de un hemipléɡico,] por el tercio medio de la oliva. (Método de Weigert-Pal). *A*, núcleos post-piramidales; *B*, oliva; *C*, oliva accesoria interna; *D*, oliva accesoria externa; *E*, porción descendente del trigémino; *F*, cuerpo restiforme; *G*, grueso manojo del cordón de Burdach; *H*, hipogloso; *I*, fibras arciformes anteriores; *J*, fibras [arciformes medias u] olivares; *K*, núcleo ambiguo; *L*, substancia reticular gris; *Q*, substancia reticular blanca; *M*, núcleo del hipogloso; *N*, núcleo intercalado; *P*, núcleo de Roller; *R*, núcleo del cordón lateral; *S*, región del lemnisco interno; *T*, núcleo accesorio del cordón de Burdach; [V, núcleo de Burdach]; *X*, resto del núcleo del cordón de Goll; *Y*, núcleo dorsal del vago.

Note from the author (J. D.): In brackets is the text added in the French version of the *Textura*: Cajal, S. R. (1909–1911) *Histologie du système nerveux de l'homme et des vertébrés*, trans. L. Azoulay. Paris: Maloine.

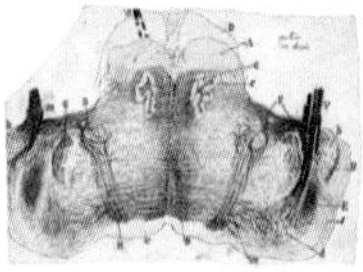

FIGURE 38.
Medulla in a fifteen-day-old child at the level of the caudal border of the pons.

This figure was published in Cajal, S. R. (1899–1904) *Textura del sistema nervioso del hombre y de los vertebrados*. Madrid: Moya. (Figure 217).

FIGURE LEGEND: Section of the medulla in a fifteen-day-old child at the level of the caudal border of the pons (Weigert-Pal method). *A*, Pyramid; *B*, medial longitudinal fasciculus; *C*, sensory pathway; *D*, pons; *E*, inferior cerebellar; *F*, fibers of the trapezoid body; *G*, descending root of the trigeminal; *H*, fibers of the facial nerve; *a*, facial nucleus; *b*, ventral cochlear nucleus; *c*, olive; *d*, inferior vestibular nucleus; *e*, central gray matter; *f*, auditory tubercle (dorsal cochlear nucleus); *g*, spinal nucleus of the fifth cranial nerve; *VI*, abducens nerve; *VII*, facial nerve; *V*, vestibular nerve; *VIII*, cochlear nerve.

Original text: Corte del bulbo del niño de quince días al nivel del borde posterior de la protuberancia. (Weigert-Pal). *A*, pirámides; *B*, cordón longitudinal posterior; *C*, vía sensitiva; *D*, protuberancia; *E*, pedúnculo cerebeloso inferior; *F*, fibras del cuerpo trapezoide; *G*, porción descendente del trigémino; *H*, fibras del facial; *a*, núcleo del facial; *b*, núcleo ventral del nervio coclear; *c*, oliva; *d*, núcleo descendente del nervio vestibular; *e*, substancia gris central; *f*, tubérculo acústico; *g*, substancia gelatinosa del quinto par; *VI*, motor ocular externo; *VII*, facial; *V*, nervio vestibular; *VIII*, nervio coclear.

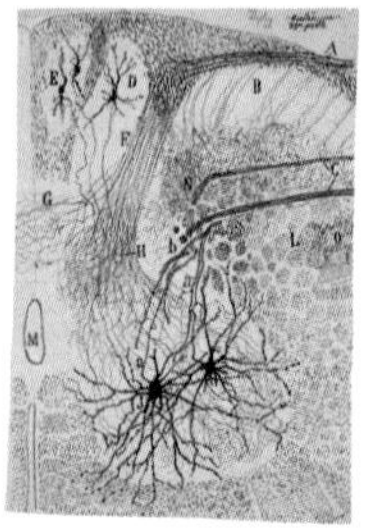

FIGURE 39.
Section of the medulla caudal to the pyramid decussation in a cat fetus.

This figure was published in Cajal, S. R. (1897) Nueva contribución al estudio del bulbo raquídeo. *Rev. Trim. Micrograf. Madrid* 2, 67–99 (Figure 1). It has also been reproduced as Figure 226 in Cajal, S. R. (1899–1904) *Textura del sistema nervioso del hombre y de los vertebrados*. Madrid: Moya.

FIGURE LEGEND: Section of the medulla caudal to the pyramid decussation. Cat fetus of *seven centimeters*. Golgi method. *A*, Dorsal roots; *B*, substantia gelatinosa of Rolando; *C*, radicular fibers of the spinal accessory nerve; *D*, nucleus cuneatus; *E*, nucleus gracilis; *F*, sensory-motor bundle; *J*, cells of the spinal accessory nucleus; *G, dorsal commissure; *H*, plexus of the intermediate nucleus; *L*, lateral corticospinal tract; *a*, axons; *b*, cross-cut radicular fibers of the spinal accessory nerve*.

Original text: Corte del bulbo por debajo del cruce de las pirámides. Feto de gato *de 7 centímetros*. Método de Golgi. *A*, raíces posteriores; *B*, substancia gelatinosa de Rolando; *C*, radiculares del espinal; *D*, ganglio del cordón de Burdach; *E*, ganglio de Goll; *F*, manojo reflejo-motor; *J*, células del espinal; *G, comisura posterior; *H*, plexo del foco gris intermediario; *L*, haces de la vía piramidal; *a*, axones; *b*, radiculares del espinal cortadas de través.*

Note from the author (J. D.): The text between asterisks appears in the original publication only.

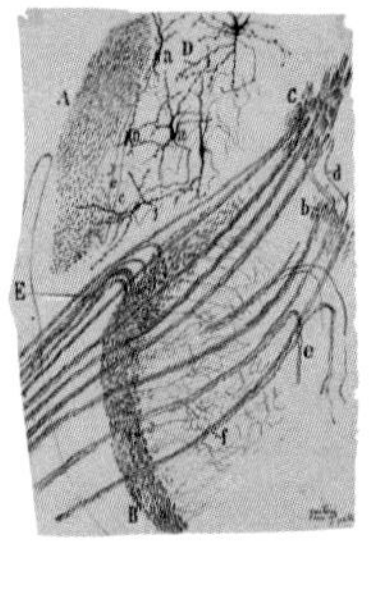

FIGURE 40.
Medulla in a cat fetus.

This figure was published in Cajal, S. R. (1897) Nueva contribución al estudio del bulbo raquídeo. *Rev. Trim. Micrograf. Madrid* 2, 67–99 (Figure 9). It has also been reproduced as Figure 234 in Cajal, S. R. (1899–1904) *Textura del sistema nervioso del hombre y de los vertebrados*. Madrid: Moya.

FIGURE LEGEND: Medulla in a cat fetus. Golgi method. *A*, Restiform body; *B*, trigeminal spinal tract; *C*, solitary tract; *D*, vestibular nucleus; *E*, trigeminal portion of the vagus and glossopharyngeal nerves; *e*, motor fibers of the ninth and tenth cranial nerves originating in the nucleus ambiguus; *b*, accessory fascicles of the solitary tract; **a*, cells with axons going to the restiform body; *d*, fibers that pass from one to another fascicle of the solitary tract.*

Original text: Bulbo de feto de gato. Método de Golgi. *A*, cuerpo restiforme; *B*, porción descendente del trigémino; *C*, haz solitario; *D*, foco del vestibular; *E*, porción trigeminal del vago gloso faríngeo; *e*, fibras motrices del noveno y décimo par destinadas al núcleo ambiguo; *b*, haces accesorios del cordón solitario; **a*, células cuyos axones iban al cuerpo restiforme; *d*, fibras que pasan de uno á otro fascículo solitario.*

Note from the author (J. D.): The text between asterisks appears in the original publication only.

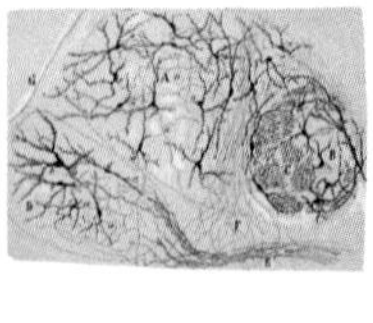

FIGURE 41.
Sagittal section of the medulla, lateral to the hypoglossal nucleus, in a newborn kitten.

This figure was published in Cajal, S. R. (1899–1904) *Textura del sistema nervioso del hombre y de los vertebrados*. Madrid: Moya. (Figure 238).

FIGURE LEGEND: Sagittal section of the medulla, lateral to the hypoglossal nucleus, and showing various nuclei at the floor of the fourth ventricle. Region of the ventricular floor in a newborn kitten. Golgi method. *A*, Medial or descending nucleus of the solitary tract; *B*, lateral or interstitial nucleus of the solitary tract; *C*, solitary tract; *D*, dorsal motor nucleus of the vagus nerve; *E*, radicular fibers of the vagus nerve; *F*, axons of the central pathway of the vagus and glossopharyngeal nerves; *G*, fourth ventricle; *a*, axon; *b*, motor cell of the vagus nerve; *d, c*, small cells of the dorsal motor nucleus of the tenth cranial nerve.

Original text: [Corte sagital del bulbo pasando por fuera del núcleo del hipogloso y mostrando diversos focos subyacentes al cuarto ventrículo]. Región del suelo ventricular del gato recién nacido. Método de Golgi. *A*, foco gris interno [o ganglio descendente] del haz solitario; *B*, núcleo externo ó intersticial; *C*, haz solitario; *D*, foco dorsal del vago; *E*, radiculares de éste; *F*, axones de la vía central del vago y gloso-faríngeo; *G*, [cuarto] ventrículo; *a*, axon; *b*, célula motriz del vago; *d, c*, células pequeñas del citado núcleo dorsal del décimo par.

Note from the author (J. D.): In brackets is the text added in the French version of the *Textura:* Cajal, S. R. (1909–1911) *Histologie du système nerveux de l'homme et des vertébrés*, trans. L. Azoulay. Paris: Maloine.

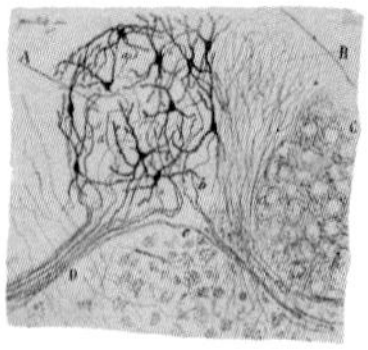

FIGURE 42.
Hypoglossal nucleus and dorsal motor nucleus of the vagus nerve in a kitten.

This figure was published in Cajal, S. R. (1899–1904) *Textura del sistema nervioso del hombre y de los vertebrados*. Madrid: Moya. (Figure 240).

FIGURE LEGEND: Hypoglossal nucleus and dorsal motor nucleus of the vagus nerve in a kitten (a few days of age). Golgi method. *A*, Motor nucleus of the vagus nerve; *B*, intercalated nucleus; *C*, hypoglossal nucleus; *D*, motor root of the vagus nerve; *a*, axons; *b*, fibers that seem to course toward the raphe.

Original text: Ganglios del hipogloso y motor dorsal del vago del gato de pocos días. Método de Golgi. *A*, foco motor del vago; *B*, núcleo intercalado; *C*, núcleo del hipogloso; *D*, raíz motriz del vago; *a*, axones; *b*, fibras que parecen ir al rafe.

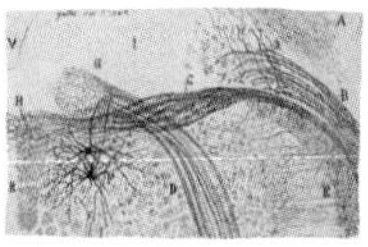

FIGURE 43.

Transverse section of the medulla in a cat fetus.

This figure was published in Cajal, S. R. (1899–1904) *Textura del sistema nervioso del hombre y de los vertebrados*. Madrid: Moya. (Figure 249).

FIGURE LEGEND: Transverse section of the medulla in a cat fetus. Golgi method. *A*, Restiform body; *B*, principal, uncrossed part of the vestibular nerve; *C*, crossed bundle; *D*, facial nerve; *F*, abducens nucleus.

Original text: Corte transversal del bulbo del feto de gato. Método de Golgi. *A*, cuerpo restiforme; *B*, porción principal no decusada del vestibular; *C*, manojo cruzado; *D*, facial; *F*, foco del motor ocular externo.

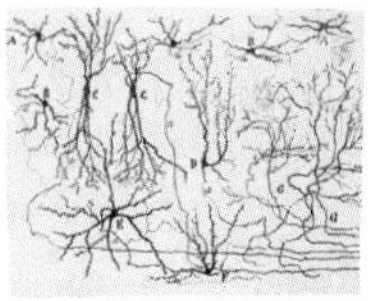

FIGURE 44.

Principal cellular types in the dorsal cochlear nucleus in a kitten.

This figure was published in Cajal, S. R. (1899–1904) *Textura del sistema nervioso del hombre y de los vertebrados*. Madrid: Moya. (Figure 268).

FIGURE LEGEND: Principal cellular types found in the dorsal cochlear nucleus of in an eight-day-old kitten. Golgi method. *A, B*, Cells of the plexiform layer; *C*, fusiform cells of the granular zone; *B*, granule cells; *D, E, F*, cells of the zone of ganglion cells; *G*, free terminal arborizations of the cochlear nerve.

Original text: Principales tipos celulares hallados en el tubérculo acústico del gato de ocho días. Método de Golgi. *A, B*, células de la capa plexiforme; *C*, células fusiformes de la zona de los granos; *B*, [granos]; *D, E, F*, corpúsculos de la zona de los elementos gangliónicos; *G*, arborizaciones [terminales] libres del [nervio] coclear.

Note from the author (J. D.): In brackets is the text added in the French version of the *Textura*: Cajal, S. R. (1909–1911) *Histologie du système nerveux de l'homme et des vertébrés*, trans. L. Azoulay. Paris: Maloine.

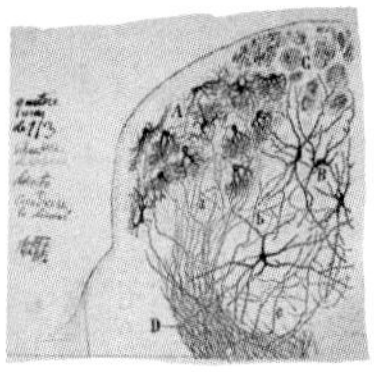

FIGURE 45.

Nucleus of the habenula in a newborn dog.

This figure was published in Cajal, S. R. (1894) Estructura del ganglio de la habénula de los mamíferos. *Anales Soc. Esp. Hist. Nat.* 23, 185–194 (Figure 2).

FIGURE LEGEND: Nucleus of the habenula in a newborn dog. *A*, Cells of the medial nucleus; *B*, cells of the lateral nucleus; *C*, transverse section of the fibers of the *stria medullaris; D*, fasciculus retroflexus; *a*, axons of the cells of the medial nucleus; *b*, axons of the cells of the lateral nucleus.

Original text: Ganglio de la habenula del perro recién nacido. *A*, células del foco interno; *B*, células del foco externo; *C*, corte transversal de las fibras de la *stria medullaris; D*, fascículo retro-reflejo; *a*, cilíndros-ejes de las células del foco interno; *b*, cilindros-ejes de las del externo.

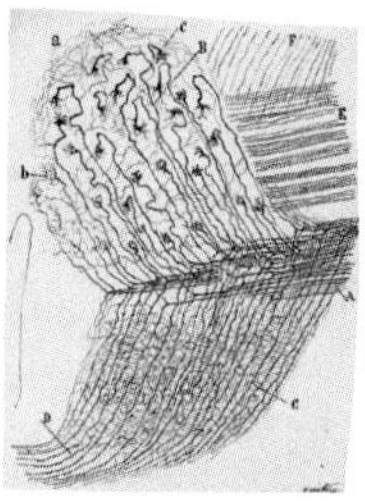

FIGURE 46.

Ventral cochlear nucleus in a newborn dog.

This figure was published in Cajal, S. R. (1900). Disposición terminal de las fibras del nervio coclear. *Rev. Trim. Micrograf. Madrid* 5, 111–127 (Figure 1). It has also been reproduced as Figure 260 in Cajal, S. R. (1899–1904) *Textura del sistema nervioso del hombre y de los vertebrados*. Madrid: Moya.

FIGURE LEGEND: Rostrocaudal longitudinal section of the ventral cochlear nucleus in a newborn dog. Golgi method. *A*, Cochlear nerve; *B*, rostral portion of the ventral nucleus where the ascending branch of the cochlear nerve terminates; *C*, caudal portion of the same nucleus where endings of the descending branch of the cochlear nerve are found; *D*, bundle of fibers destined to the tail of the ventral nucleus and dorsal cochlear nucleus; *a*, rostral marginal plexus; *b*, terminal arborizations of the ascending branch of the cochlear nerve; *c*, pericellular nets formed by collateral fibers of the descending branch.

Original text: Corte longitudinal y antero-posterior del ganglio ventral del acústico del perro recién nacido. Método de Golgi. *A*, [nervio] coclear; *B*, porción superior del ganglio ventral donde acaba la rama ascendente [del nervio coclear]; *C*, porción del mismo [parte inferior] donde se arboriza la descendente [del nervio coclear]; *D*, manojo destinado á la cola del ganglio [ventral] y tubérculo acústico; *a*, plexo limitante superior; *b*, arborizaciones terminales de la rama ascendente [del nervio coclear]; *c*, nidos pericelulares formados por colaterales de la descendente.

Note from the author (J. D.): In brackets is the text added in the French version of the *Textura*: Cajal, S. R. (1909–1911) *Histologie du système nerveux de l'homme et des vertébrés*, trans. L. Azoulay. Paris: Maloine.

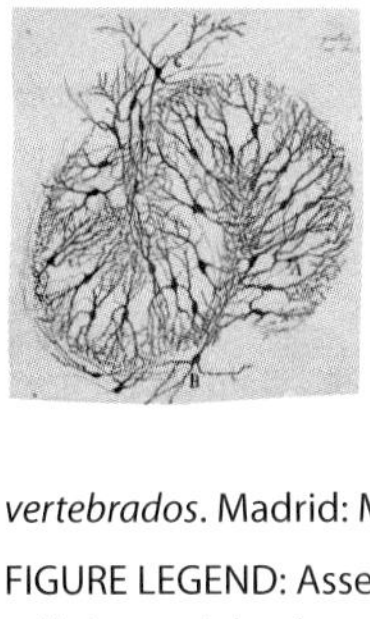

FIGURE 47.

Assembly of superior olive cells in a kitten.

This figure was published in Cajal, S. R. (1899–1904) *Textura del sistema nervioso del hombre y de los vertebrados*. Madrid: Moya. (Figure 271).

FIGURE LEGEND: Assembly of superior olive cells in an eight-day-old kitten. Golgi method. *A*, Intranuclear fusiform cells; *B*, marginal cells of the ventral border; *C*, marginal cells of the dorsal hilus.

Original text: Conjunto de las células de la oliva superior del gato de ocho días. Método de Golgi. *A*, células fusiformes intrafocales; *B*, células limitantes del contorno anterior; *C*, células limitantes del híleo posterior.

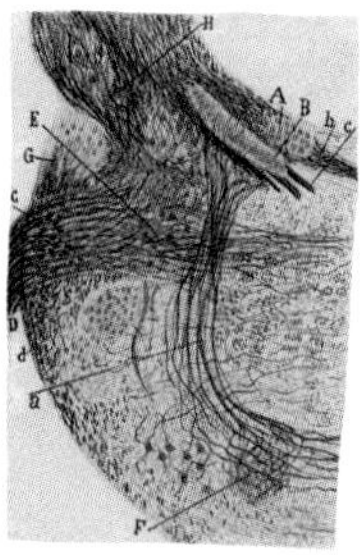

FIGURE 48.

Medulla in a kite a few days old.

This figure was published in Cajal, S. R. (1908) Sur un noyau spécial du nerf vestibulaire des poissons et des oiseaux. *Trav. Lab. Recherches Biol. Univ. Madrid* 6, 1–20 (Figure 1). It has also been reproduced as Figure 365 in Cajal, S. R. (1909–1911) *Histologie du système nerveux de l'homme et des vertébrés*, trans. L. Azoulay. Paris: Maloine.

FIGURE LEGEND: Portion of a transverse section of the acoustic region of the medulla in a kite several days old (*Milvus regalis*, Briss.). Reduced silver nitrate method. *A*, Magnocellular acoustic nucleus; *B*, parvocellular nucleus; *C*, vestibular root of the vestibulocochlear nerve; *D*, tangential or interstitial nucleus; *E*, lateral vestibular nucleus (nucleus of Deiters); *F*, superior olive; *a*, trapezoid body.

Original text: Morceau d'une coupe transversale de la región acoustique bulbaire d'un oiseau âgé de quelques jours (milan). [*Milvus regalis*, Briss. Méthode du nitrate d'argent réduit]. *A*, noyau acoustique à grosses cellules; *B*, noyau lamellaire [noyau acoustique à petites cellules]; *C*, [racine] vestibulaire [du nerf acoustique]; *D*, ganglion tangentiel [ou interstitiel]; *E*, noyau de Deiters[; *F*, olive supérieure; *a*, corps trapézoide.]

Note from the author (J. D.): This figure is not included in Cajal, S. R. (1899–1904) *Textura del sistema nervioso del hombre y de los vertebrados*. Madrid: Moya. The text between brackets was added in Cajal, S. R. (1909–1911) *Histologie du système nerveux de l'homme et des vertébrés*, trans. L. Azoulay. Paris: Maloine.

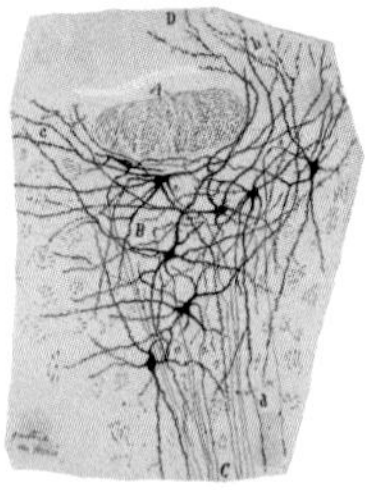

FIGURE 49.

Abducens nucleus in a kitten.

This figure was published in Cajal, S. R. (1899–1904) *Textura del sistema nervioso del hombre y de los vertebrados*. Madrid: Moya. (Figure 298).

FIGURE LEGEND: Abducens nucleus in a kitten a few days of age. Golgi method. *A*, Section of the ascending portion of the facial root; *B*, nucleus of the sixth cranial nerve (or lateral oculomotor nucleus); *C*, radicular fibers; *D*, medial nucleus of the vestibular nerve; *a*, axon; *b*, dorsal dendrites; *c*, medial dendrites.

Original text: Núcleo del motor ocular externo del gato de pocos días. Método de Golgi. *A*, corte de la porción ascendente del facial; *B*, foco del sexto par [ó núcleo oculomotor externo]; *C*, fibras radiculares; *D*, núcleo dorsal del [nervio] vestibular; *a*, axon; *b*, dendritas posteriores; *c*, dendritas internas.

Note from the author (J. D.): In brackets is the text added in the French version of the *Textura*: Cajal, S. R. (1909–1911) *Histologie du système nerveux de l'homme et des vertébrés*, trans. L. Azoulay. Paris: Maloine.

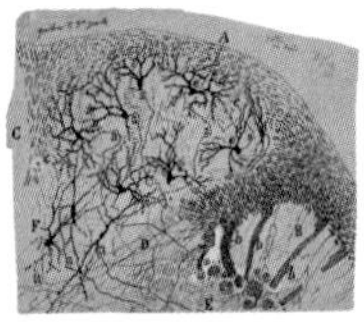

FIGURE 50.

Section of the medulla at the level of the nucleus cuneatus in a kitten.

This figure was published in Cajal, S. R. (1897) Nueva contribución al estudio del bulbo raquídeo. *Rev. Trim. Micrograf. Madrid* 2, 67–99 (Figure 8). It has also been reproduced as Figure 320 in Cajal, S. R. (1899–1904) *Textura del sistema nervioso del hombre y de los vertebrados*. Madrid: Moya.

FIGURE LEGEND: Transverse section of the medulla at the level of the caudal third of the nucleus cuneatus in a kitten a few days old. Golgi method. *A*, Nucleus cuneatus; *B*, substantia gelatinosa of the dorsal horn; *D*, sensorimotor bundle of fibers; *C*, nucleus gracilis; *E*, fasciculus proprius of the lateral funiculus; *F*, pedicle of the nucleus cuneatus; *a*, axons; *b*, bundle of ascending sensory radicular fibers, which pass into the region of the head of the dorsal horn.

Original text: Sección transversal, al nivel del tercio inferior del núcleo del cordón de Burdach del gato de pocos días. Método de Golgi. *A*, núcleo de Burdach; *B*, substancia [gelatinosa] de Rolando del asta posterior; *D*, haz sensitivo de colaterales; *C*, núcleo [del cordón] de Goll; *E*, porción limitante del cordón lateral; *F*, mango del foco de Burdach; *a*, axones; *b*, haces de radiculares sensitivas ascendentes que pasan á la región del vértice del asta posterior.

Note from the author (J. D.): In brackets is the text added in the French version of the *Textura*: Cajal, S. R. (1909–1911) *Histologie du système nerveux de l'homme et des vertébrés*, trans. L. Azoulay. Paris: Maloine.

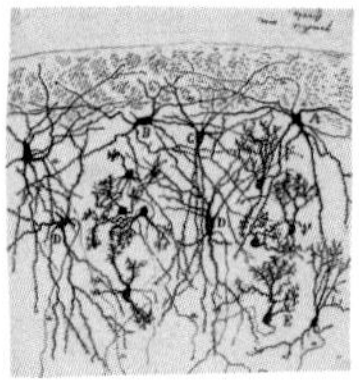

FIGURE 51.

Section of the rostral region of the nucleus cuneatus in a kitten.

This figure was published in Cajal, S. R. (1899–1904) *Textura del sistema nervioso del hombre y de los vertebrados*. Madrid: Moya. (Figure 322).

FIGURE LEGEND: Portion of a transverse section of the rostral region of the nucleus cuneatus in an eight-day-old kitten. Golgi method. *A, B, C*, Marginal cells with an axon coursing dorsally; *D*, cells of the partitions; *E*, cells of islands.

Original text: Trozo de un corte transversal de la porción superior del núcleo de Burdach del gato de ocho días. Método de Golgi. *A, B, C*, células marginales cuyo axon iba hacia atrás; *D*, células de los tabiques; *E*, células de los islotes.

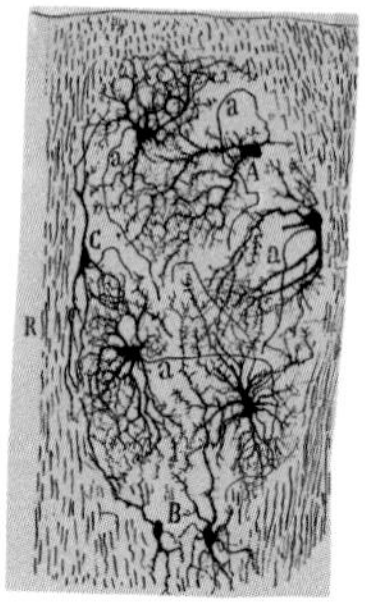

FIGURE 52.

Transverse section of the nucleus gracilis in a kitten.

This figure was published in Cajal, S. R. (1897) Nueva contribución al estudio del bulbo raquídeo. *Rev. Trim. Micrograf. Madrid* 2, 67–99 (Figure 7). It has also been reproduced as Figure 323 in Cajal, S. R. (1899–1904) *Textura del sistema nervioso del hombre y de los vertebrados*. Madrid: Moya.

FIGURE LEGEND: Transverse section of the nucleus gracilis in a *four-day-old* kitten. Caudal region of the nucleus. Golgi method. *B*, **C**, Marginal cells; *R*, raphe; *a*, axon.

Original text: Corte transversal del núcleo de Goll del gato recién nacido *(de cuatro días).* Porción inferior del núcleo. Método de Golgi. *B*, **C**, células limitantes; *R*, rafe; *a*, axon.

Note from the author (J. D.): The text between asterisks appears in the original publication only.

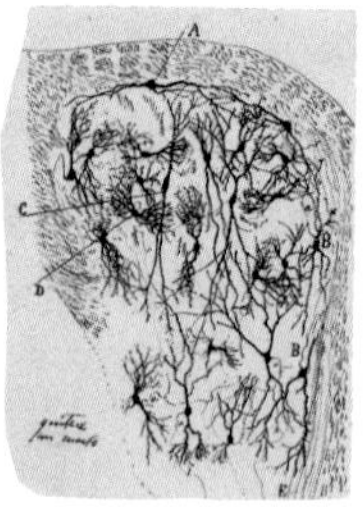

FIGURE 53.

Section of the nucleus gracilis in a human fetus.

This figure was published in Cajal, S. R. (1899–1904) *Textura del sistema nervioso del hombre y de los vertebrados*. Madrid: Moya. (Figure 324).

FIGURE LEGEND: Transverse section of the nucleus gracilis in a seven-month human fetus. Golgi method. *A*, Marginal cells; *B*, cells with an axon coursing dorsomedially to join the superficial white matter; *C*, fusiform cells of partitions; *D*, bramble cells within the islands.

Original text: Corte transversal del núcleo de Goll del feto humano de siete meses. Método de Golgi. *A*, células marginales; *B*, células cuyo axon iba hacia adentro y atrás incorporándose á la corteza blanca; *C*, células fusiformes de los tabiques; *D*, células de zarzal de las pléyades.

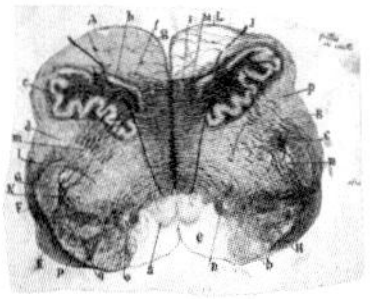

FIGURE 54.
Medulla of a hemiplegic individual at the level of the caudal third of the olive.

This figure was published in Cajal, S. R. (1899–1904) *Textura del sistema nervioso del hombre y de los vertebrados*. Madrid: Moya. (Figure 214).

FIGURE LEGEND: Section of the medulla of a hemiplegic individual at the level of the caudal third of the olive (Weigert-Pal method). *A*, Pyramid; *B*, white reticular substance; *C*, gray reticular substance; *D*, solitary tract; *E*, restiform body; *F*, olivary or intermediate arcuate fibers; *G*, spinal tract of the trigeminal nerve; *H*, remnants of the fasciculus cuneatus ; *J*, hypoglossal nerve; *L*, ventral arcuate fibers; *M*, transverse bundles of interolivary fibers; *N*, intermediate arcuate or retrotrigeminal olivary fibers; *P*, remnant of the lateral funiculus; *a*, hypoglossal nucleus; *b*, nucleus gracilis; *c*, olive; *d*, lateral reticular nucleus; *e*, vagospinal nucleus or dorsal motor nucleus of the vagus nerve; *f*, retropyramidal nucleus; *h*, medial accessory olive; *i*, displaced foci of the arcuate nucleus; *g*, principal part of the arcuate nucleus or prepyramidal nucleus; *m*, nucleus ambiguus or innominata *n*, nucleus of the fifth cranial nerve; *o*, interstitial or lateral column of the solitary tract nucleus; *p*, nucleus accessory cuneatus.

Original text: Corte del bulbo [de un hemipléjico] al nivel del tercio inferior de la oliva. (Weigert-Pal). *A*, pirámide; *B*, substancia reticular blanca; *C*, substancia reticular gris; *D*, cordón solitario; *E*, cuerpo restiforme; *F*, fibras olivares [ó arciformes medias]; *G*, raíz descendente del trigémino; *H*, restos del cordón de Burdach; *J*, hipogloso; *L*, fibras arciformes anteriores; *M*, haces transversales de fibras interolivares; *N*, fibras olivares [ó arciformes medias] post-trigeminales; *P*, resto del cordón lateral; *a*, núcleo del hipogloso; *b*, núcleo de Goll; *c*, oliva; *d*, núcleo del cordón lateral; *e*, foco vago-espinal [ó núcleo dorsal del vago]; *f*, núcleo postpiramidal; *h*, oliva accesoria interna; *i*, focos [grises] erráticos del núcleo arciforme; *g*, núcleo arciforme principal [ó pre-piramidal]; *m*, núcleo ambiguo [ó innominado]; *n*, foco del quinto par; [*o*, núcleo intersticial ó columna gris externa del fascículo solitario; *p*, núcleo accesorio del ganglio de Burdach].

Note from the author (J. D.): In brackets is the text added in the French version of the *Textura*: Cajal, S. R. (1909–1911) *Histologie du système nerveux de l'homme et des vertébrés*, trans. L. Azoulay. Paris: Maloine.

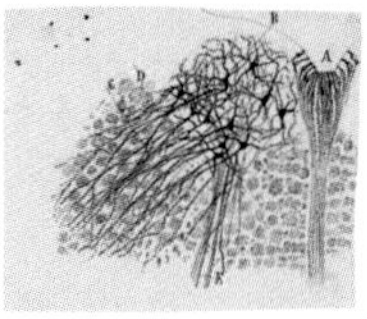

FIGURE 55.
Hypoglossal nucleus at the level of the rostral third in a kitten.

This figure was published in Cajal, S. R. (1899–1904) *Textura del sistema nervioso del hombre y de los vertebrados*. Madrid: Moya. (Figure 223).

FIGURE LEGEND: Section through the rostral third of the hypoglossal nucleus in an eight-day-old kitten. Golgi method. *A*, Raphe with epithelial barrel; *B*, cells of the hypoglossal nucleus; *C*, lateral dendrite; *D*, central pathways of the trigeminal, glossopharyngeal and vagus nerves; *E*, radicular fibers of the twelfth cranial nerve.

Original text: Núcleo del hipogloso (tercio superior) del gato de ocho días. Método de Golgi. *A*, Rafe [medio] con el tonel epitelial; *B*, células del hipogloso; *C*, dendritas externas; *D*, vía central del trigémino, gloso-faríngeo y vago; *E*, radicular del duodécimo par.

Note from the author (J. D.): In brackets is the text added in the French version of the *Textura*: Cajal, S. R. (1909–1911) *Histologie du système nerveux de l'homme et des vertébrés*, trans. L. Azoulay. Paris: Maloine.

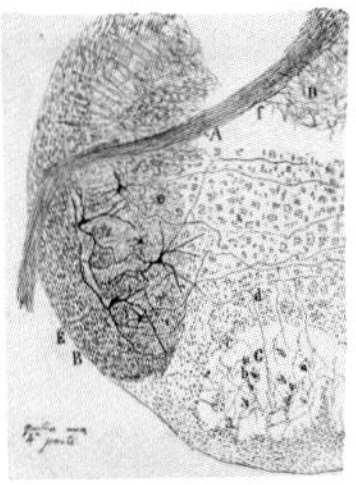

FIGURE 56.
Section of the medulla at the level of the facial nucleus in a mouse.

This figure was published in Cajal, S. R. (1899–1904) *Textura del sistema nervioso del hombre y de los vertebrados*. Madrid: Moya. (Figure 233).

FIGURE LEGEND: Transverse section of the medulla at the level of the facial nucleus. A mouse a few days old. Golgi method. *A*, Sensory root of the glossopharyngeal nerve; *B*, transverse section of the descending sensory root of the trigeminal nerve; *C*, facial nucleus; *D*, rostral region of the nucleus of the solitary tract where fibers of the vagus and glossopharyngeal nerves terminate; *E*, giant cell of the nucleus of the spinal tract of the trigeminal nerve; *a*, collaterals arising from remnants of the lateral funiculus and coursing to the facial nucleus; *b*, interstitial bundles of the lateral funiculus with their collaterals; *d*, collateral arising from second-order sensory fibers destined to the facial nucleus; *f*, collaterals of the radicular fibers of the vagus and glossopharyngeal nerves; *c*, plexus of the substantia gelatinosa.

Original text: Corte frontal del bulbo á la altura del núcleo del facial. Ratón de pocos días. Método de Golgi. *A*, raíz sensitiva del gloso-faríngeo; *B*, corte transversal de la raíz sensitiva descendente del trigémino; *C*, núcleo del facial; *D*, núcleo terminal superior del vago y glosofaríngeo; *E*, célula gigante de la substancia gelatinosa del trigémino; *a*, colaterales para el facial del resto del cordón lateral; *b*, haces intersticiales de este mismo cordón con colaterales; *d*, colaterales para el facial, procedentes de fibras sensitivas de segundo orden; *f*, colaterales de las fibras radiculares del vago y gloso-faríngeo; *c*, plexo de la substancia gelatinosa.

SECTION C

Cerebellum and Deep Cerebellar Nuclei

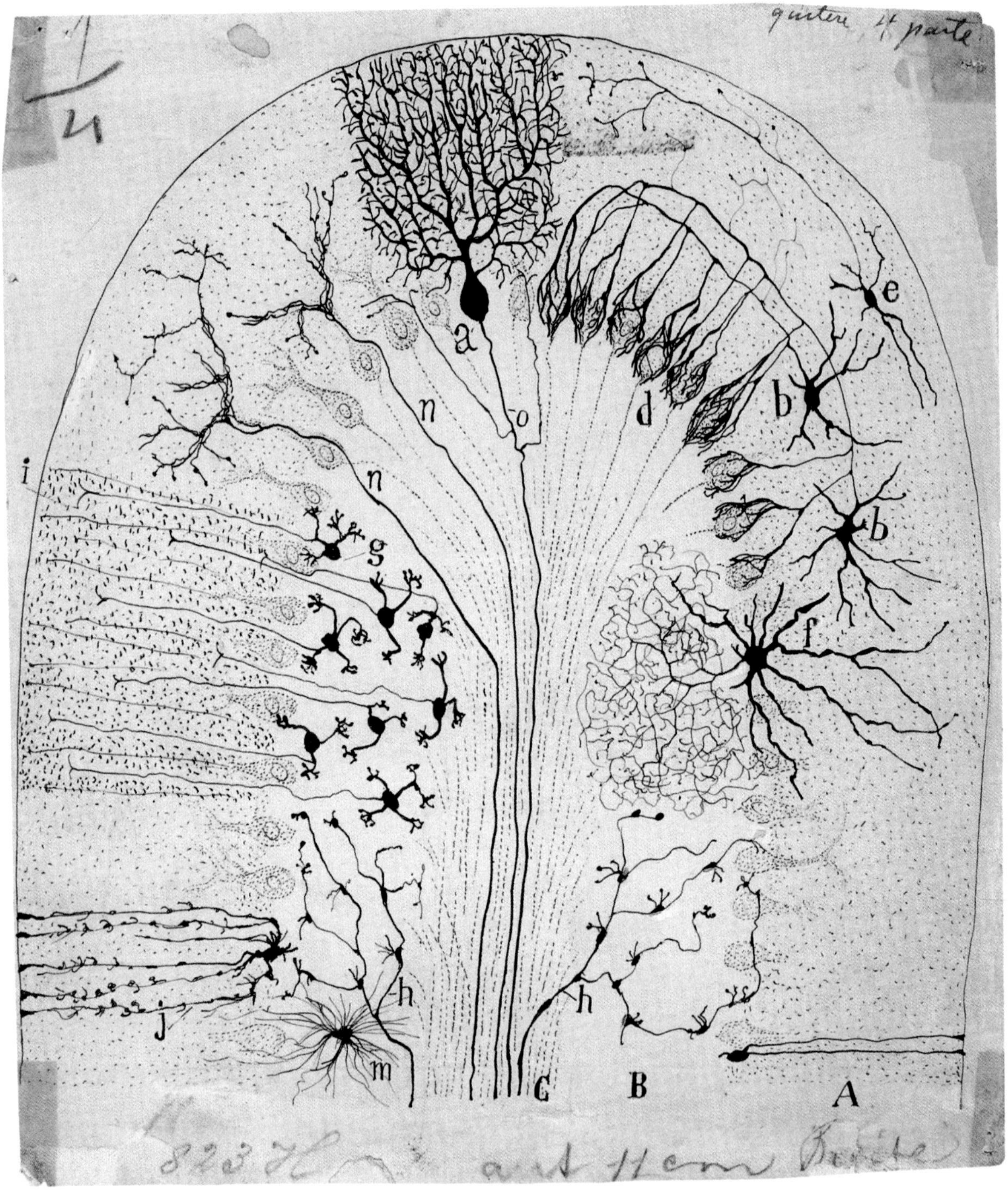

FIGURE 57. Semischematic transverse section of a cerebellar folium in mammals.

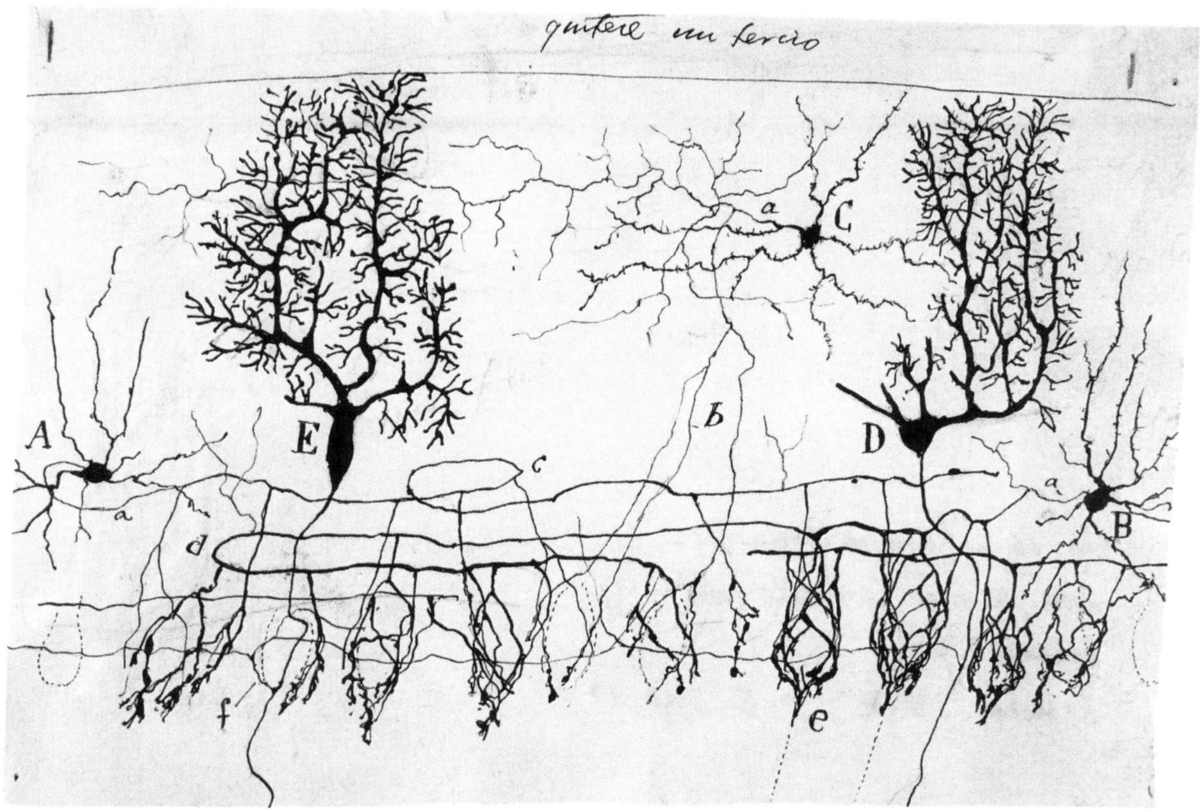

FIGURE 58. Transverse section of a cerebellar folium in a one-month-old guinea pig.

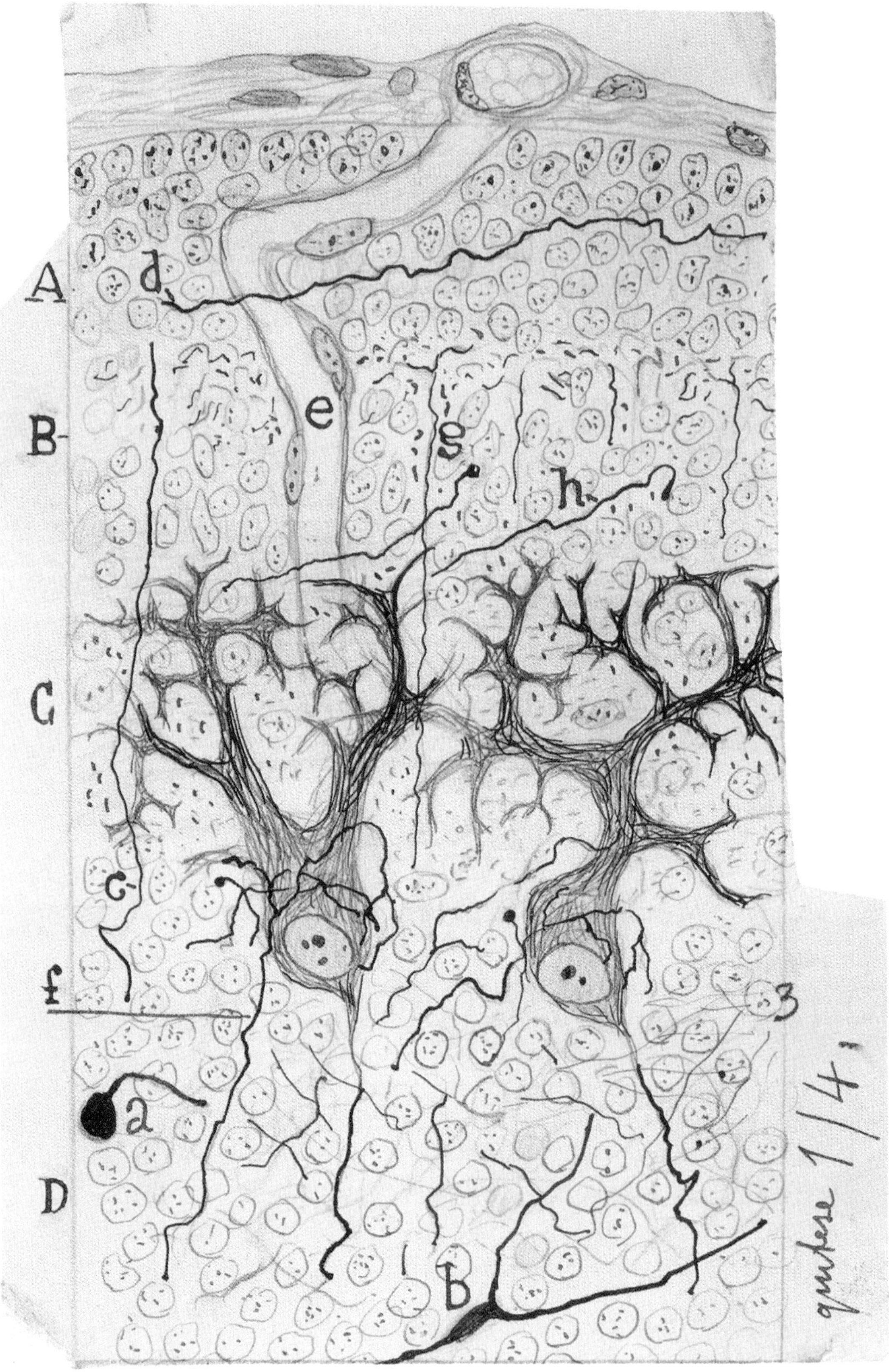

FIGURE 59. Section of the cerebellum in an eight-day-old dog.

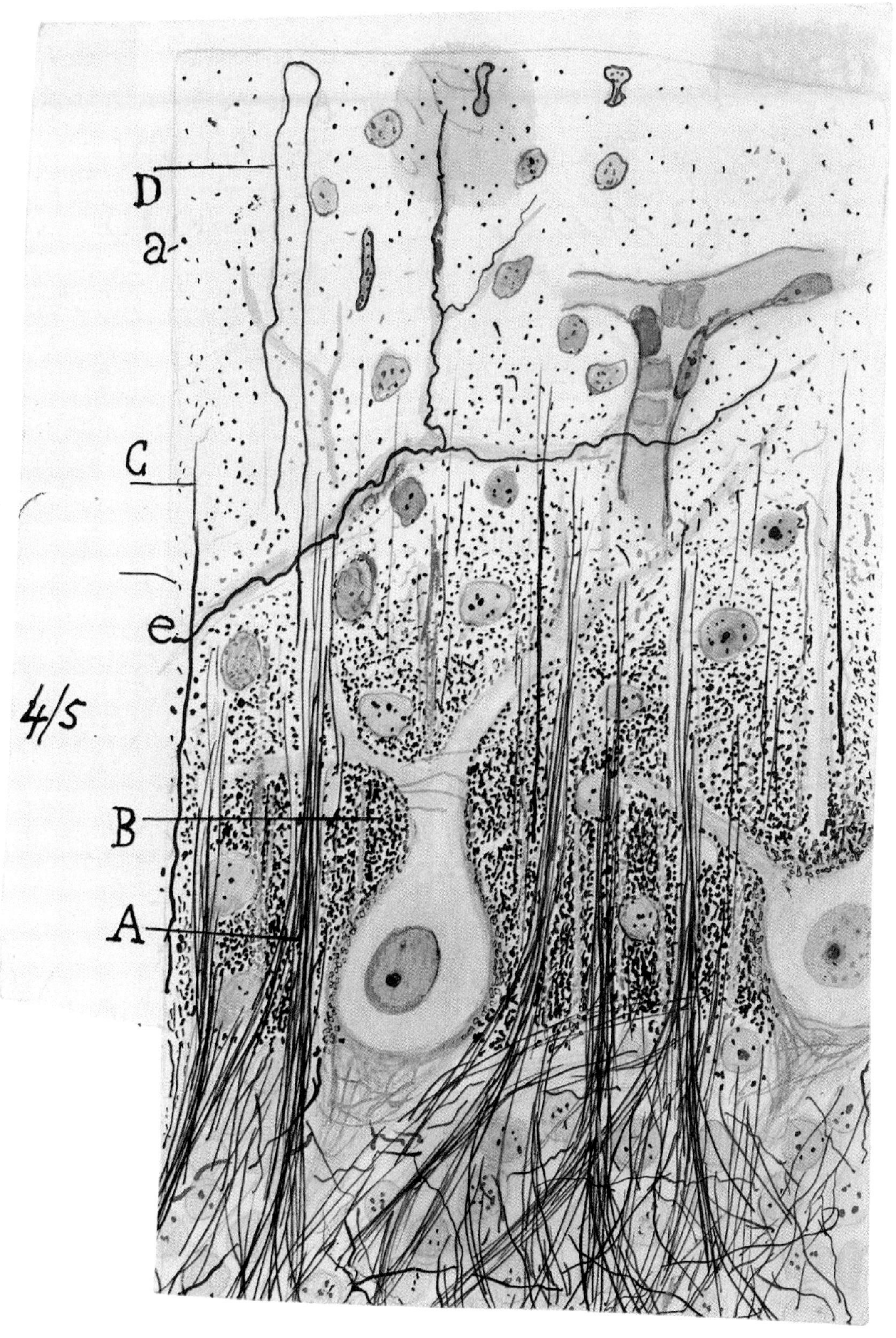

FIGURE 60. Parallel fibers of a near-adult cat.

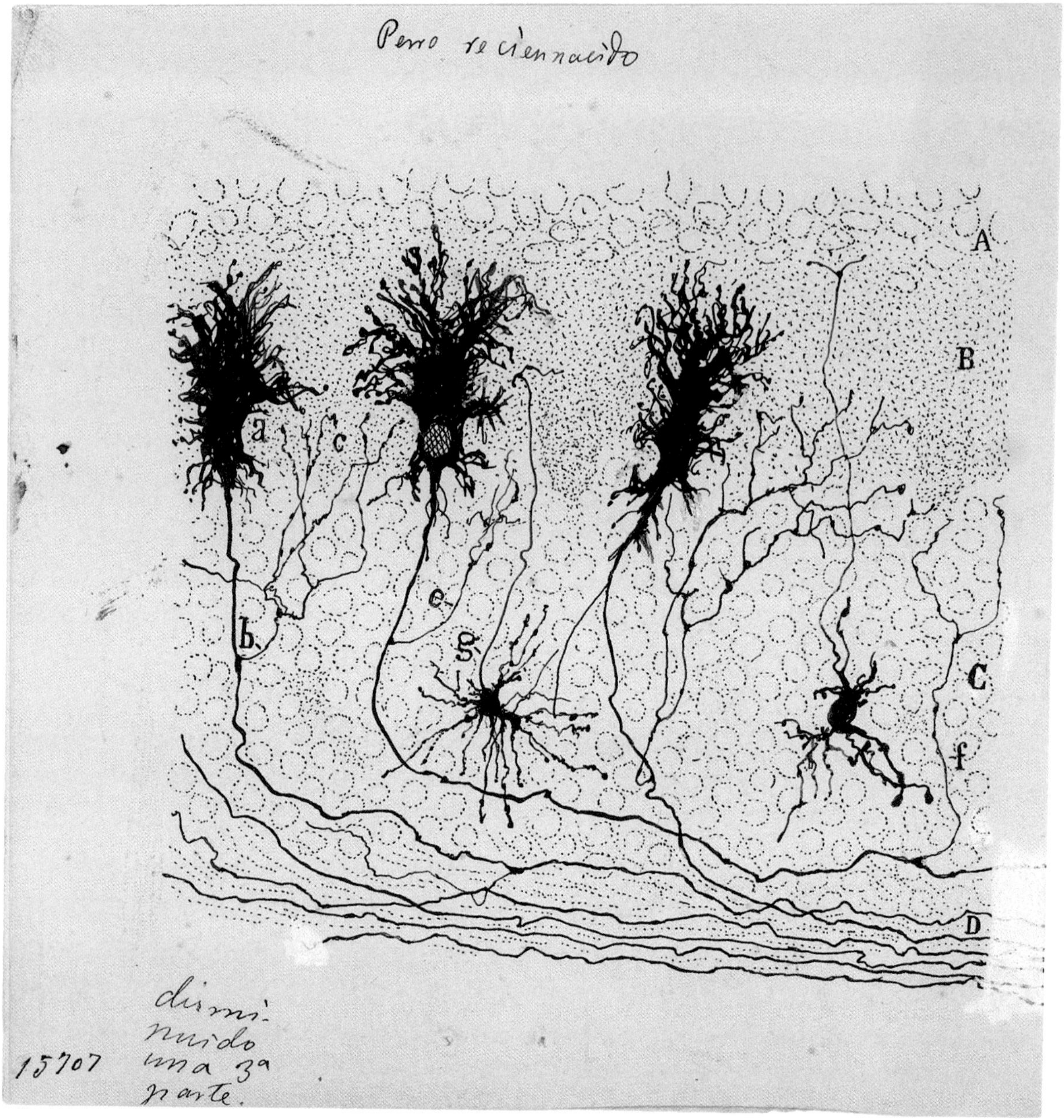

FIGURE 61. Purkinje cells in a newborn dog.

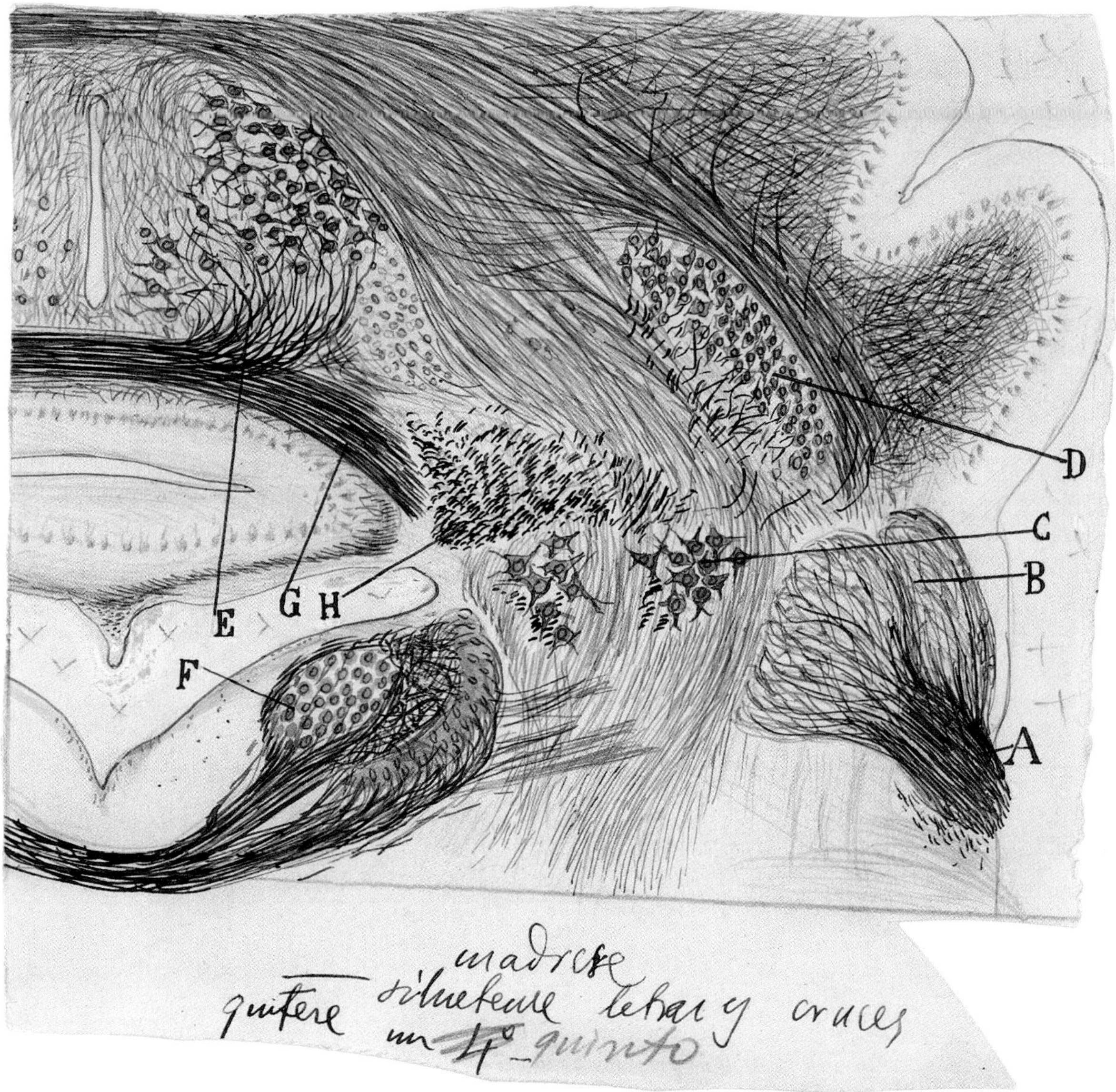

FIGURE 62. Section of the cerebellum and medulla in a newborn bird.

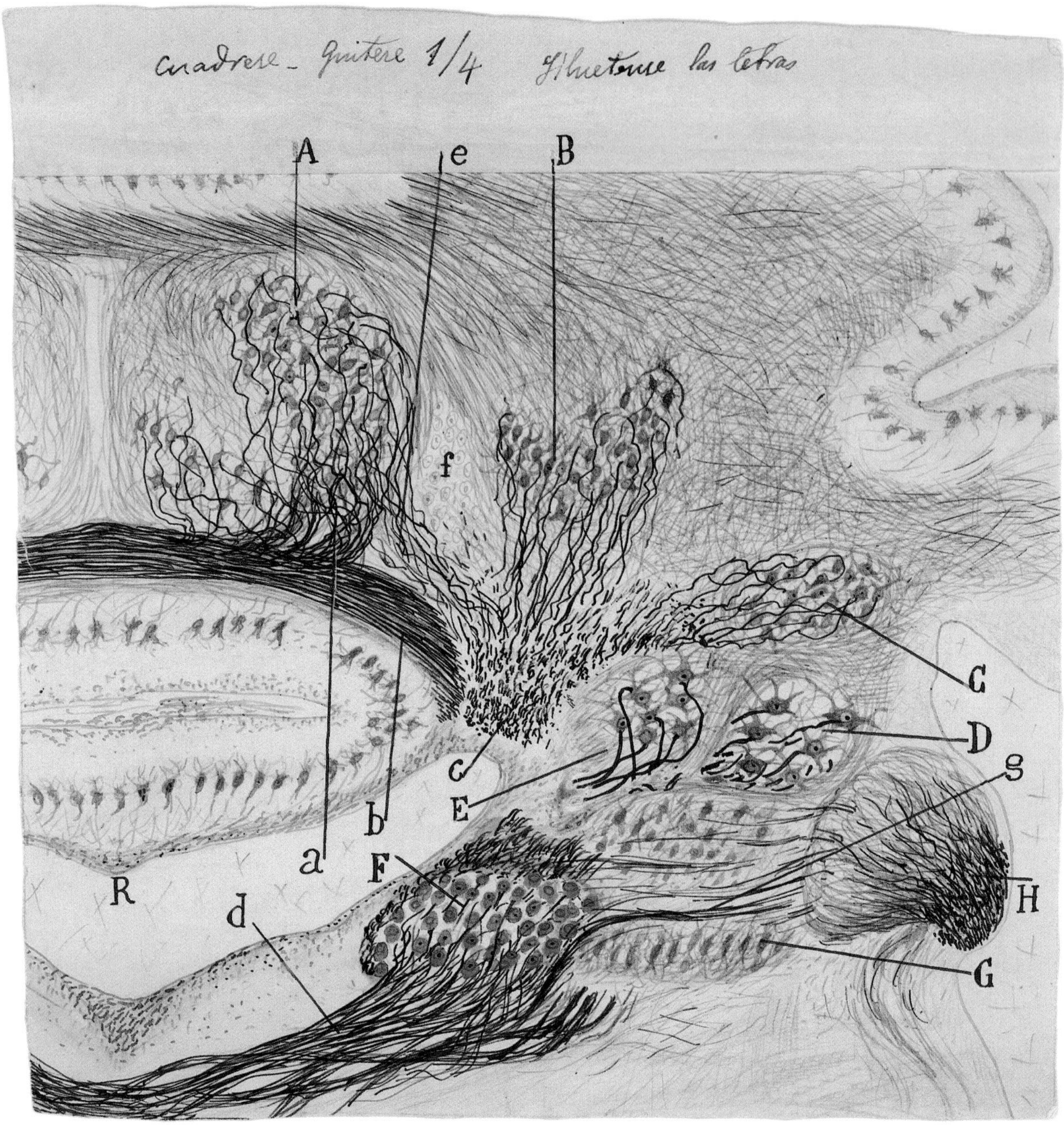

FIGURE 63. Frontal section of the cerebellum and vestibulocochlear nuclei in a newborn sparrow.

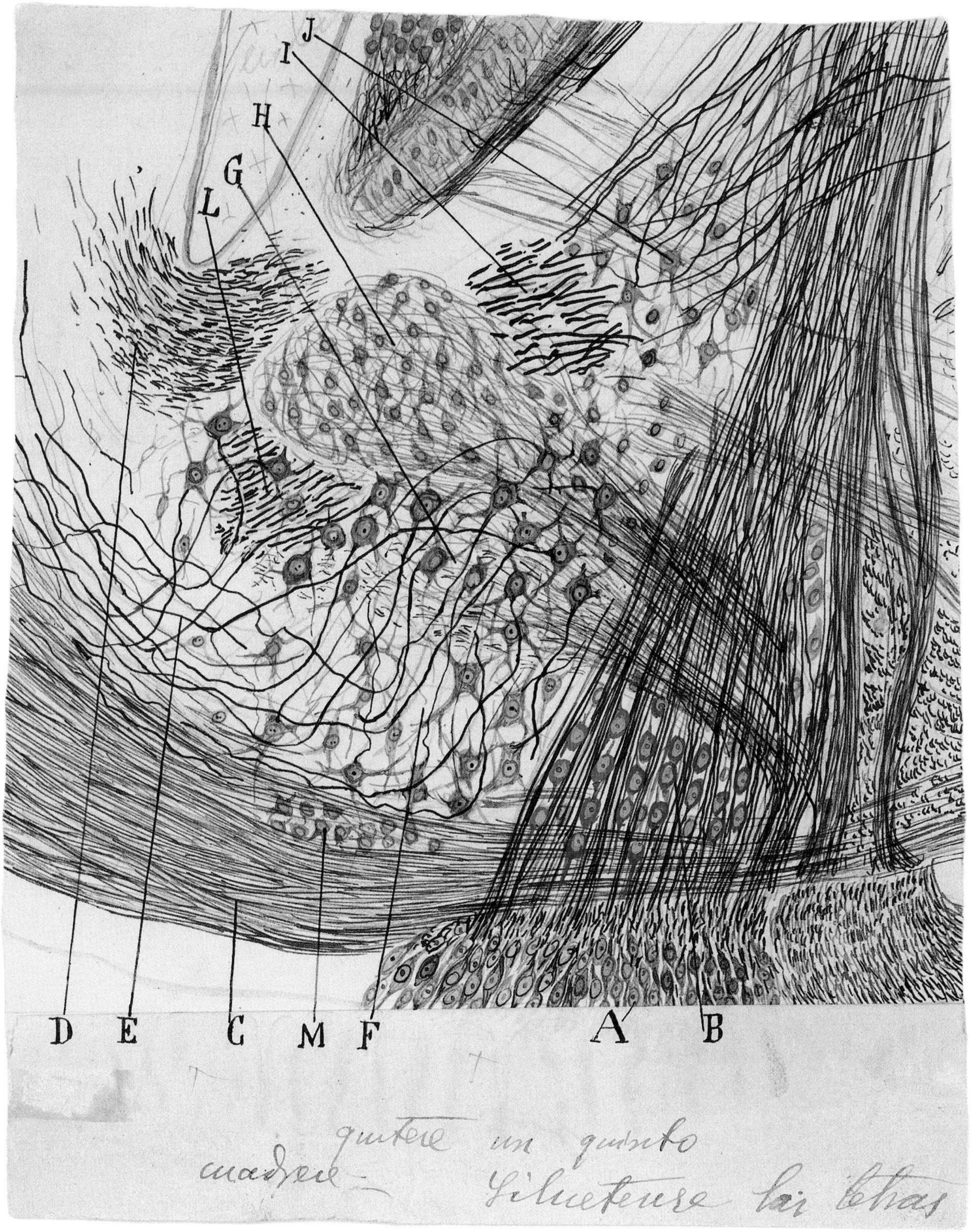

FIGURE 64. Terminal region of the vestibular nerve in an eight-day-old sparrow.

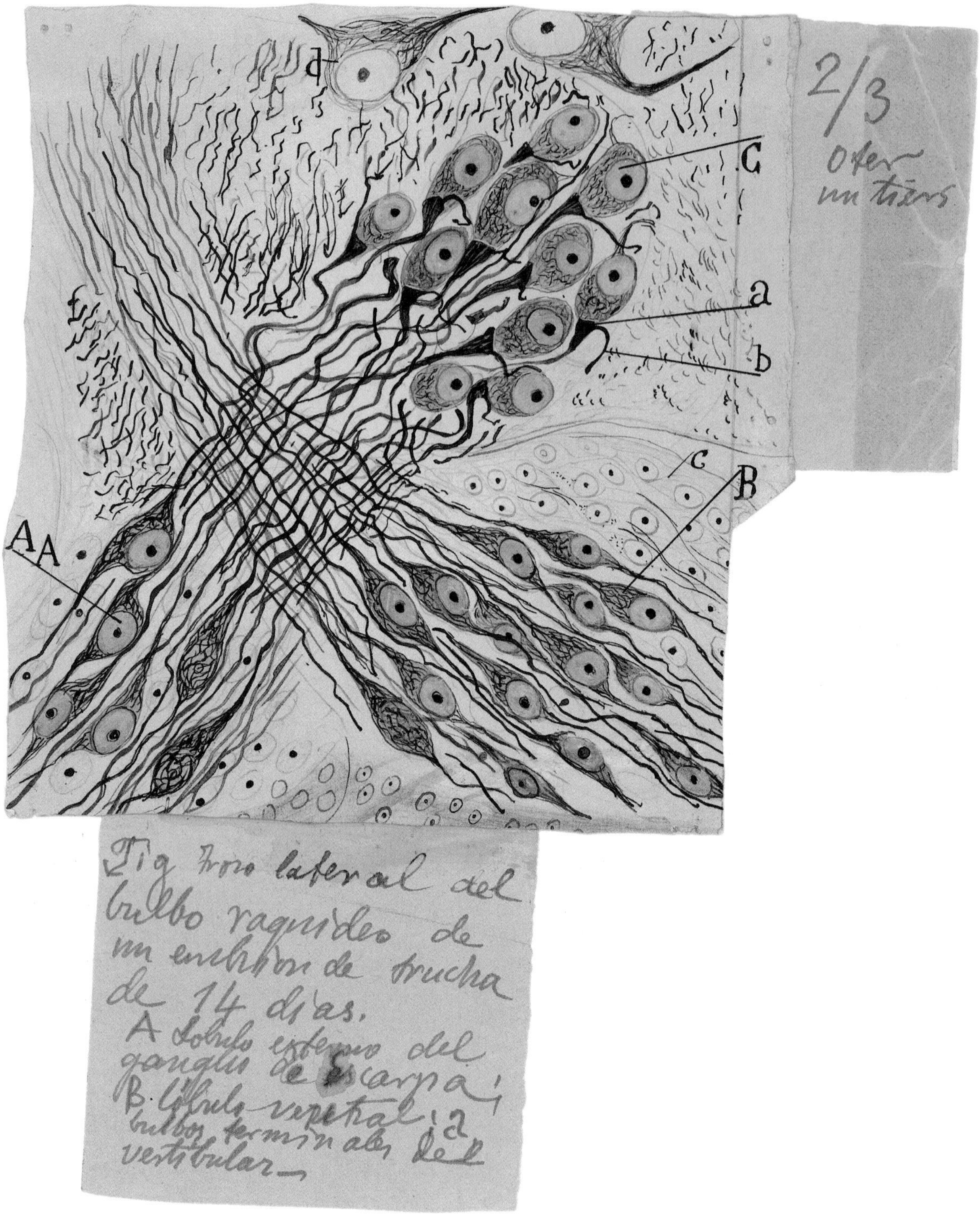

FIGURE 65. Medulla in a trout embryo.

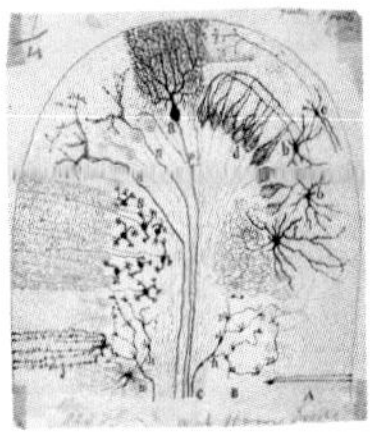

FIGURE 57.

Semischematic transverse section of a cerebellar folium in mammals.

This figure was originally published in Cajal, S. R. (1892) Nuevo concepto de la histología de los centros nerviosos. *Rev. Ciencias Méd. Barcelona* 18, 363–376, 457–476, 505–520, 529–540 (Figure 5). It has also been reproduced as Figure 369 in Cajal, S. R. (1899–1904) *Textura del sistema nervioso del hombre y de los vertebrados*. Madrid: Moya.

FIGURE LEGEND: Semischematic representation of a transverse section of a cerebellar folium in mammals, according to information provided by the Golgi method. *A*, Molecular layer; *B*, granule cell layer; *C*, layer of white matter; *a*, Purkinje cell as seen in a frontal view; *b*, small stellate cells of the molecular layer; *d*, descending terminal axonal arborizations from stellate cells that form baskets around Purkinje cell bodies; *e*, outer stellate cells; *g*, granule cells with ascending axons that bifurcate at *i*; *h*, mossy fibers; *j*, epithelial cell or tufted neuroglia cell; *n*, climbing fibers; *m*, neuroglia cell of the granule layer; *f*, large stellate cells of the granule layer.

Original text: Corte transversal semi-esquemático de una circunvolución cerebelosa de mamífero, [según las enseñanzas suministradas por el método de Golgi]. *A*, zona molecular; *B*, zona de los granos; *C*, zona de substancia blanca; *a*, célula de Purkinje vista de plano; *b*, células estrelladas pequeñas de la zona molecular; *d*, arborizaciones [axónicas] finales descendentes que [provienen de las células estrelladas y forman las cestas que] rodean las células de Purkinje; *e*, células estrelladas superficiales; *g*, granos con sus cilindros ejes ascendentes bifurcados en *i*; *h*, fibras musgosas; *j*, [célula epitelial o] célula neuróglica en penacho; *n*, fibras trepadoras; *m*, célula neuróglica de la zona de los granos; *f*, células estrelladas grandes de la zona de los granos.

Note from the author (J. D.): In brackets is the text added in the French version of the *Textura*: Cajal, S. R. (1909–1911) *Histologie du système nerveux de l'homme et des vertébrés*, trans. L. Azoulay. Paris: Maloine.

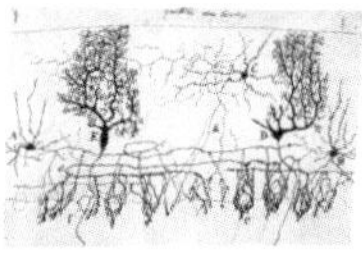

FIGURE 58.

Transverse section of a cerebellar folium in a one-month-old guinea pig.

This figure was published in Cajal, S. R. (1899–1904) *Textura del sistema nervioso del hombre y de los vertebrados*. Madrid: Moya. (Figure 372).

FIGURE LEGEND: Transverse section of a cerebellar folium in a one-month-old guinea pig. Golgi method. *A*, Basket cell with an axon tracing an initial loop; *B*, another basket cell with an axon following a final recurrent course; *C*, cell with a tangential axon that sends a single, thin descending collateral for the baskets; *E, D*, displaced Purkinje cells; *e*, brush-tips of baskets.

Original text: Corte transversal de una lámina cerebelosa del cobaya de un mes. Método de Golgi. *A*, célula de cesta cuyo axon daba una revuelta; *B*, otra cuyo axon tenía una curva final; *C*, célula de axon horizontal que enviaba á las cestas una sola colateral descendente delgada; *E, D*, células de Purkinje dislocadas; *e*, punta de las cestas.

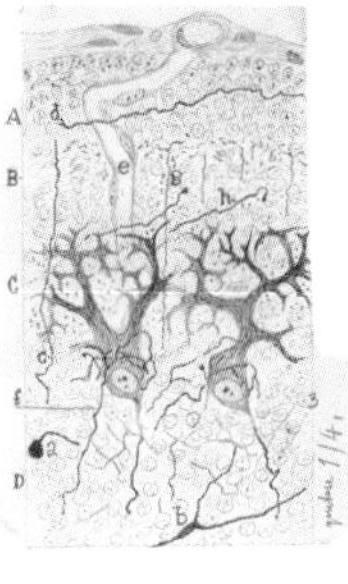

FIGURE 59.

Section of the cerebellum in an eight-day-old dog.

This figure was published in Cajal, S. R. (1926) Sur les fibres mousseuses et quelques points douteux de la texture de l´écorce cérébelleuse. *Trav. Lab. Recherches Biol. Univ. Madrid* 24, 215–251. (Figure 16).

FIGURE LEGEND: Section of the cerebellum in an eight-day-old dog: *A*, Layer of germinal or granule cells; *B*, layer of fusiform cells (granule cells in the process of development); *C*, molecular layer; *D*, deep or migrated granules; *a*, fiber ending in a ball; *b*, varicosity of the trajectory of a probably mossy fiber; *c*, meandering or Cajal-Smirnow fiber; *d*, another with a tangential trajectory; *e*, capillary; *g*, granule cell axon; *h*, another meandering fiber terminating with a button.

Original text: Coupe du cervelet de chien âgé de huit jours: *A*, couche des cellules ou grains germinaux; *B*, couche des corpuscules fusiformes (grains en voie d'évolution); *C*, couche moléculaire; *D*, grains profonds ou émigrés; *a*, fibre se terminant en boule; *b*, renflement de trajet d'une fibre probablement mousseuse; *c*, fibre égarée ou de Cajal-Smirnow; *d*, une autre à trajet tangentiel; *e*, capillaire; *g*, axone de grain; *h*, une autre fibre égarée se terminant au moyen d'un bouton.

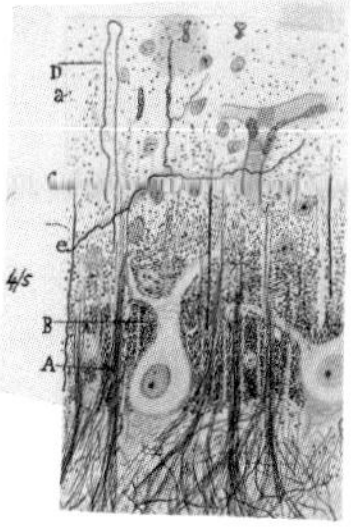

FIGURE 60.

Parallel fibers in a near-adult cat.

This figure was published in Cajal, S. R. (1926) Sobre las fibras musgosas y algunos puntos dudosos de la textura de la corteza cerebelosa. *Arch. Neurobiol.* 6, 77–101 (Figure 6).

FIGURE LEGEND: Parallel fibrils in a near-adult cat (four months) stained using the formalin–uranyl nitrate method (formula III of the technical indications). *A*, Ascending fascicles formed by axons of granule cells; *B*, transverse section of the lower parallel fibers, which are strongly impregnated with silver; *a*, superior parallel fibers, which are much more scarce; *c*, solitary radial fibers; *D*, loop of an aberrant parallel fiber; *e*, climbing fiber.

Original text: Fibrillas paralelas del gato casi adulto (cuatro meses) teñidas por el proceder del nitratoformol (fórmula III de las indicaciones técnicas); *A*, Fascículos ascendentes constituídos por axones de granos; *B*, Corte transversal de las fibrillas paralelas inferiores, las cuales atraen con energía la plata; *a*, Paralelas superiores mucho más escasas; *c*, Fibras radiales solitarias; *D*, Asa de fibra paralela aberrante; *e*, Fibra trepadora.

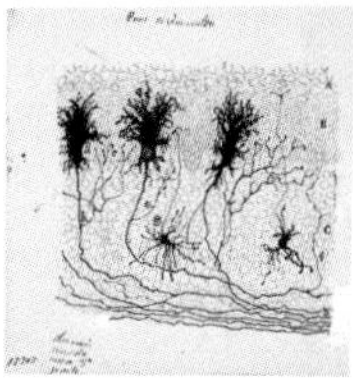

FIGURE 61.

Purkinje cells in a newborn dog.

This figure was originally published in Cajal, S. R. (1890) Sobre ciertos elementos bipolares del cerebelo joven y algunos detalles más acerca del crecimiento y evolución de las fibras cerebelosas. *Gac. Sanit. Barcelona* 2, 1–20 (Figure 3). It has also been reproduced as Figure 416 in Cajal, S. R. (1899–1904) *Textura del sistema nervioso del hombre y de los vertebrados*. Madrid: Moya.

FIGURE LEGEND: *Transverse section of a cerebellar folium* in a newborn dog. Golgi method. Very embryonic Purkinje cells (a); *b and e*, collaterals of the axon of *these cells*; *g*, embryonic granule cell *with its ascending axon*; *A*, superficial granule cells; *B*, molecular layer; *C*, *layer of * deep granule cells; *D*, white matter; **f*, collateral originating from a great distance, almost in the white matter*.

Original text: *Corte transversal de una circunvolución del cerebelo* del perro recién nacido. Método de Golgi. Células de Purkinje muy embrionarias (a); *b* *y e,* colaterales del axon *de estas células*; *g*, grano embrionario *con su fibra ascendente*; *A*, granos superficiales; *B*, capa plexiforme; *C*, *capa de* granos profundos; *D*, substancia blanca; **f*, colateral originada á gran distancia casi en la sustancia blanca.*

Note from the author (J. D.): The text between asterisks appears in the original publication only.

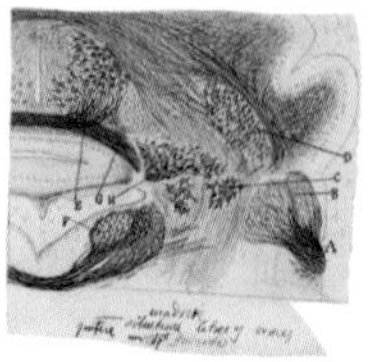

FIGURE 62.

Section of the cerebellum and medulla in a newborn bird.

This figure was published in Cajal, S. R. (1908) Los ganglios centrales del cerebelo de las aves. *Trav. Lab. Recherches Biol. Univ. Madrid* 6, 177–194 (Figure 3).

FIGURE LEGEND: Section of the cerebellum and medulla in a newborn bird. *A*, Cochlear nerve; *B*, angular nucleus; *C*, twin nuclei of large cells; *D*, superior lateral nucleus of the cerebellum; *E*, fastigial nucleus; G, crossed tectobulbar pathway; *H*, superior cerebellar peduncle.

Original text: Corte del cerebelo y bulbo de un pájaro recién nacido. *A*, Nervio coclear; *B*, Foco angular; *C*, Focos gemelos de gruesas células; *D*, Núcleo lateral superior del cerebelo; *E*, Ganglio tectal; G, Vía tecto-bulbar cruzada; *H*, pedúnculo cerebeloso superior.

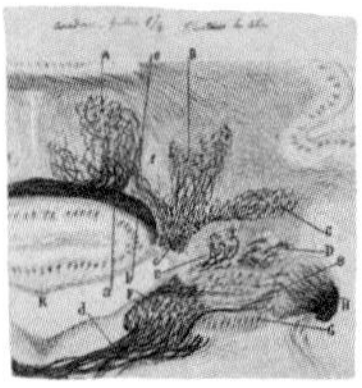

FIGURE 63.

Frontal section of the cerebellum and vestibulocochlear nuclei in a newborn sparrow.

This figure was originally published in Cajal, S. R. (1908) Los ganglios centrales del cerebelo de las aves. *Trav. Lab. Recherches Biol. Univ. Madrid* 6, 177–194 (Figure 1). It has also been reproduced as Figure 86 in Cajal, S. R. (1909–1911) *Histologie du système nerveux de l'homme et des vertébrés*, trans. L. Azoulay. Paris, Maloine.

FIGURE LEGEND: Frontal section of the cerebellum and vestibulocochlear nuclei. Newborn sparrow *(eight days old)* (*Passer domesticus*). Reduced silver nitrate method. *A*, Fastigial nucleus; *B*, intermediate nucleus; *C*, *inferior* lateral nucleus; *D, E*, *twin* nuclei of giant cells (superior vestibular nucleus?); *F*, nucleus of large cells, terminal station of the cochlear nerve descending branch; *G*, nucleus of small cells; *H*, cochlear nerve and angular nucleus; *a*, origin of the cerebello-bulbar fascicle; *b*, fibers of this fascicle after their decussation; *c*, superior cerebellar peduncle containing axons originating in the lateral and intermediate nuclei; **d*, crossed auditory pathway; *e*, ipsilateral tectobulbar fibers; *f*, intercalated nucleus; *R*, lingula of the cerebellum*.

Original text: Corte frontal del cerebelo y de los núcleos acústicos: gorrión recién nacido *ocho días* (*Passer domesticus*). Método del nitrato de plata reducido. *A*, núcleo del techo; *B*, núcleo intermedio; *C*, núcleo lateral *inferior*; *D, E*, núcleos *gemelos* de células gigantes (núcleo de Betcherew?); *F*, núcleo de grandes células, estación terminal de la rama descendente del coclear; *G*, núcleo de células pequeñas; *H*, nervio coclear y núcleo angular; *a*, origen del fascículo cerebelo-bulbar; *b*, fibras de este fascículo después de su entrecruzamiento; *c*, pedúnculo cerebeloso superior al que se incorporan los axones nacidos en los núcleos lateral e intermedio; **d*, Vía acústica cruzada; *e*, Fibras tecto-bulbares homolaterales; *f*, núcleo intercalado; *R*, lingula cerebelosa.*

Note from the author (J. D.): This figure is not included in the *Textura del sistema nervioso del hombre y de los vertebrados*. The text between asterisks appears in the original publication only.

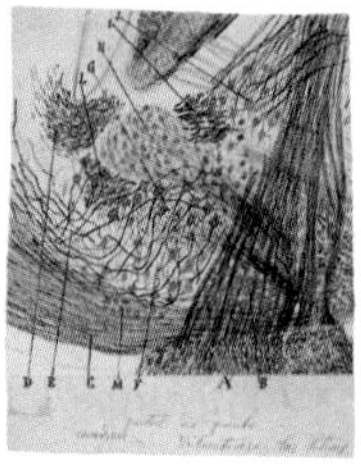

FIGURE 64.

Terminal region of the vestibular nerve in an eight-day-old sparrow.

This figure was published in Cajal, S. R. (1908) Los ganglios centrales del cerebelo de las aves. *Trav. Lab. Recherches Biol. Univ. Madrid* 6, 177–194 (Figure 6).

FIGURE LEGEND: Section at the level of the terminal region of the vestibular nerve of an eight-day-old bird (sparrow). *A*, Ganglion of Scarpa (vestibular nerve ganglion); *B*, tangential nucleus; *C*, restiform body; *D*, superior cerebellar peduncle; *F*, quadrangular nucleus; *G*, vestibulo-cerebellar nucleus; *H*, pyriform nucleus; *I*, pathway of the twin nuclei of giant cells; *L*, pathway of the upper cerebellar lateral focus; *J*, accessory nucleus of the nucleus of Deiters.

Original text: Corte de la región de terminación del nervio vestibular en los pájaros de ocho días (gorrión). *A*, Ganglio de Scarpa; *B*, Foco tangencial; *C*, Cuerpo restiforme; *D*, Pedúnculo cerebeloso superior; *F*, Foco cuadrilongo; *G*, Foco vestíbulo-cerebeloso; *H*, Núcleo piriforme; *I*, Vía de los núcleos gemelos de células gigantes; *L*, Vía del foco lateral superior cerebeloso; *J*, Foco accesorio del núcleo de Deiters.

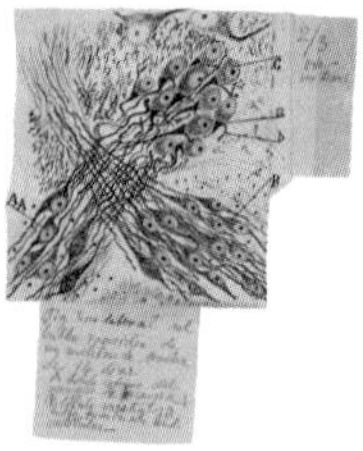

FIGURE 65.

Medulla in a trout embryo.

This figure was published in Cajal, S. R. (1908) Sur un noyau spécial du nerf vestibulaire des poissons et des oiseaux. *Trav. Lab. Recherches Biol. Univ. Madrid* 6, 1–20 (Figure 4).

FIGURE LEGEND: Lateral portion of a section of the medulla in a trout (fourteen-day-old embryo). *A*, External lobule of the ganglion of Scarpa (vestibular nerve ganglion), giving rise to the colossal fibers of the tangential nucleus; *B*, ventral lobule; *C*, tangential ganglion; *a*, excrescence of connection; *b*, descending branch of the vestibular nerve; *c*, not-yet-mature cells of the ganglion of Scarpa.

Original text: Morceau latéral d'une coupe du bulbe de la truite (embryon âgé de 14 jóurs). *A*, Lobule externe du ganglion de Scarpa donnant origine aux fibres colossales du noyau tangentiel; *B*, lobule ventral; *C*, ganglion tangentiel; *a*, excroissance de connexion; *b*, branche descendante du nerf vestibulaire; *c*, cellules non encore mûres du ganglion de Scarpa.

SECTION D

Midbrain and Thalamus

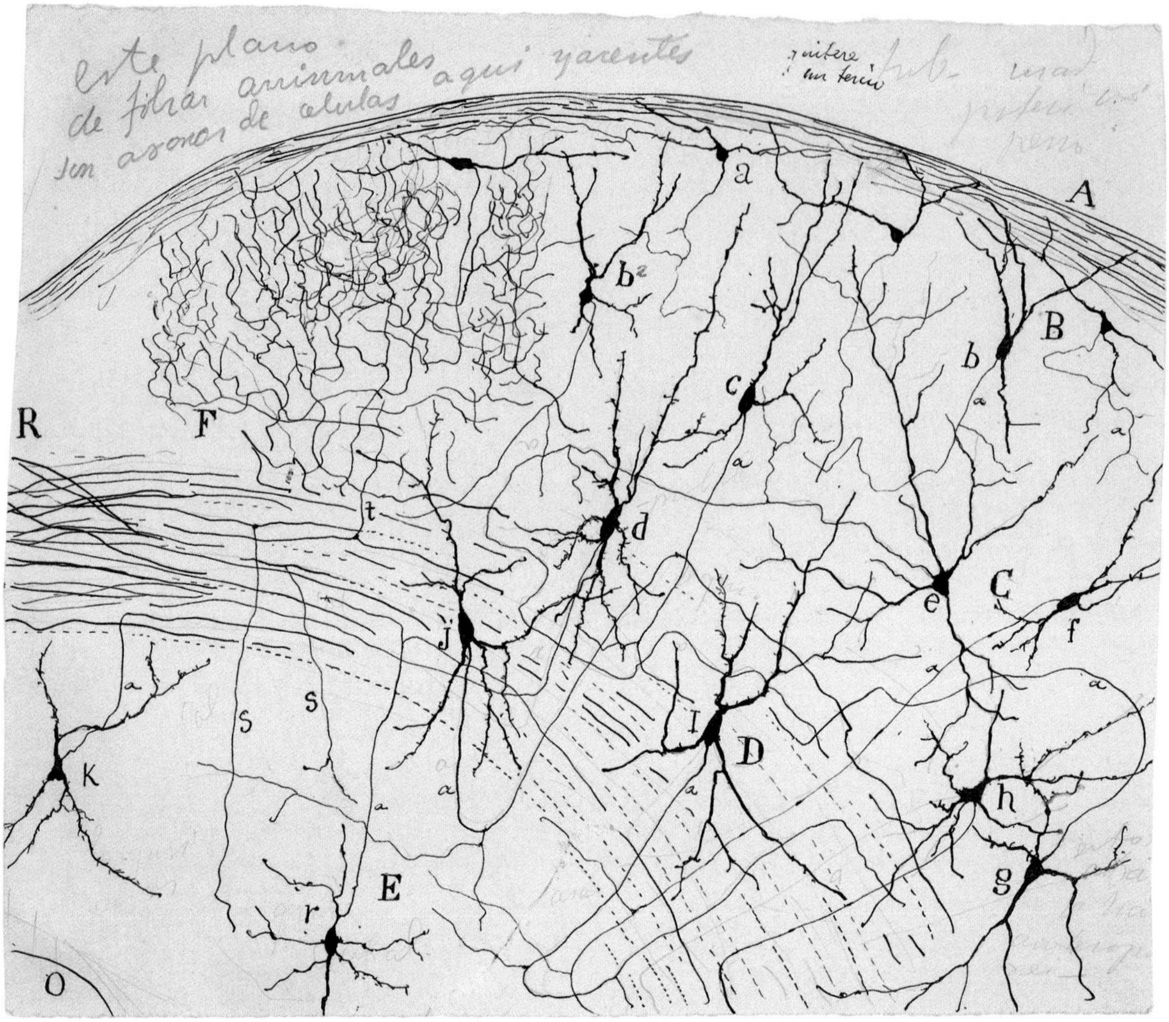

FIGURE 66. Section of the dorsomedial region of the inferior colliculus in a newborn dog.

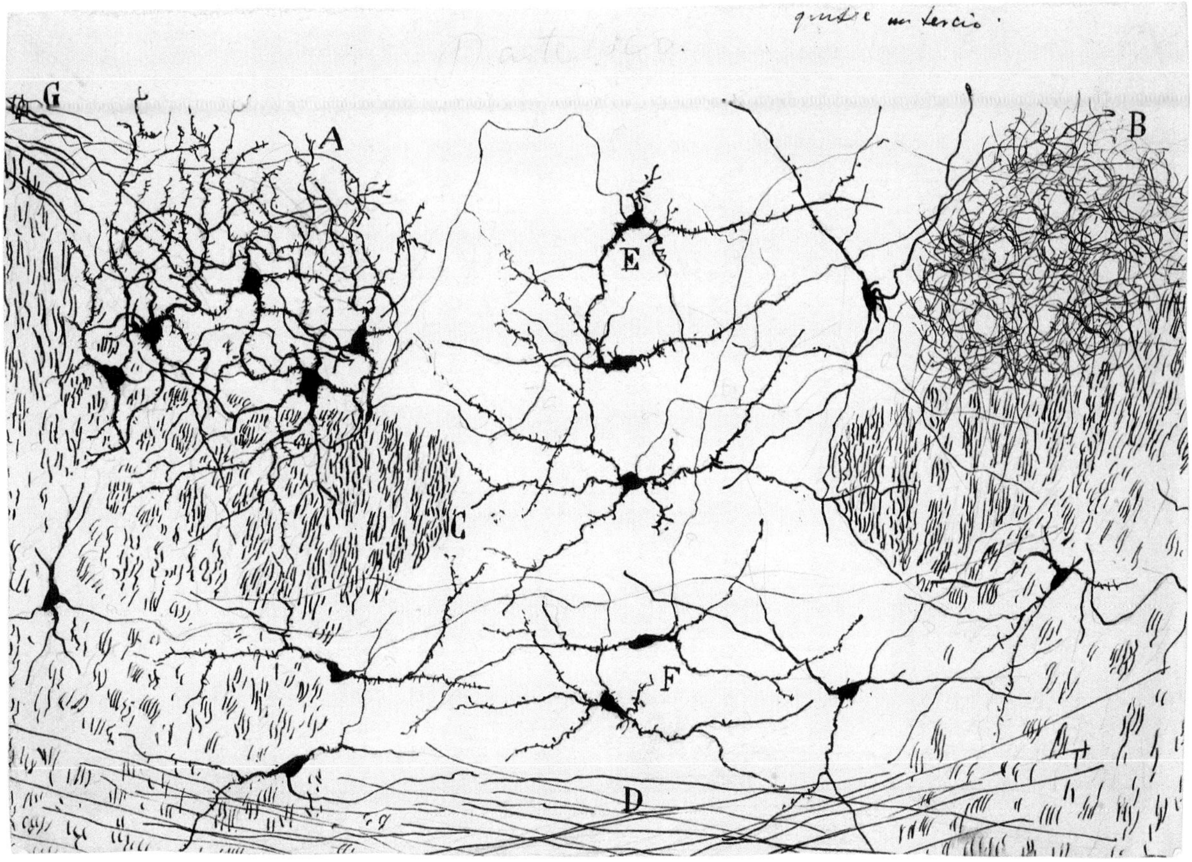

FIGURE 69. Superior colliculus in a kitten.

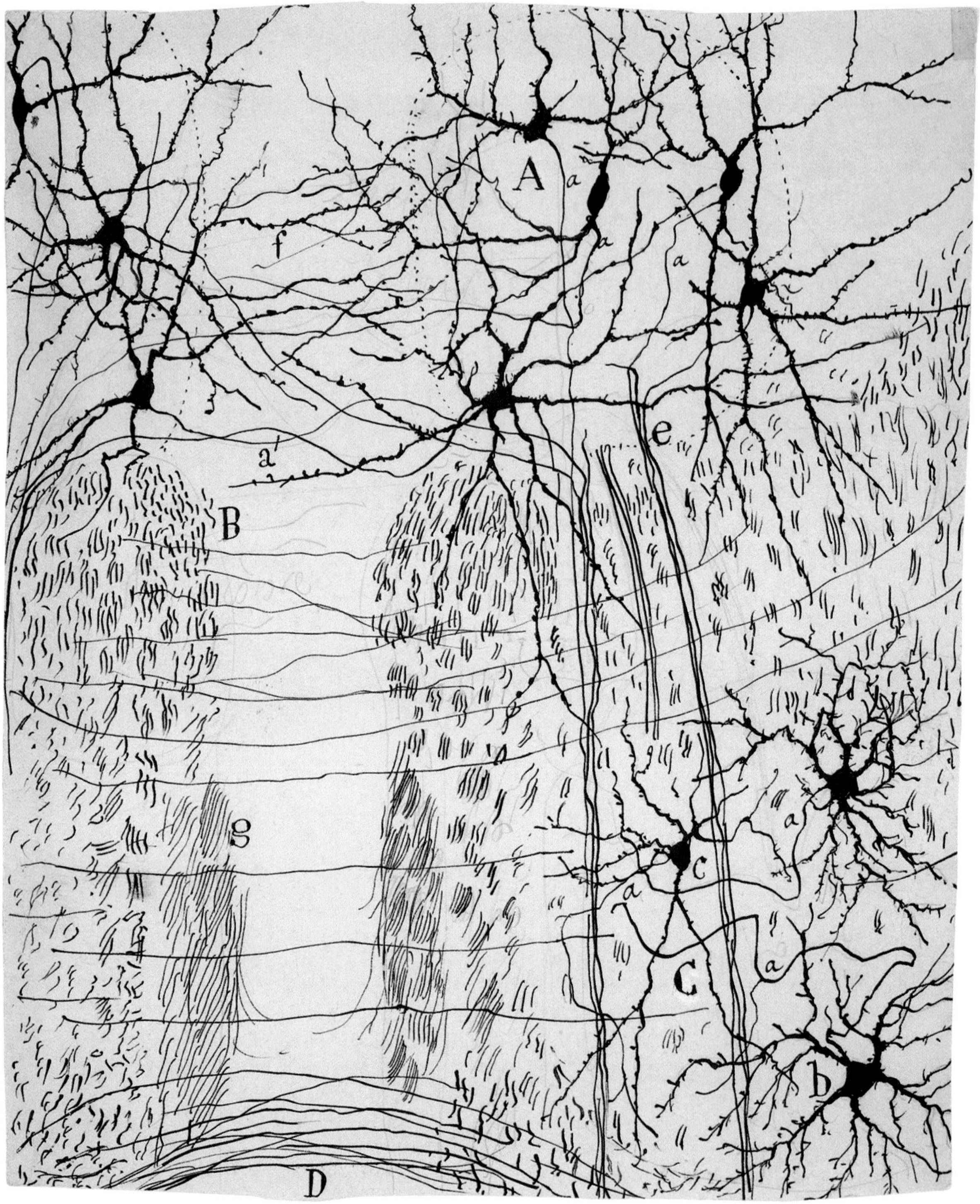

FIGURE 70. Section of the oculomotor nucleus in a mouse a few days old.

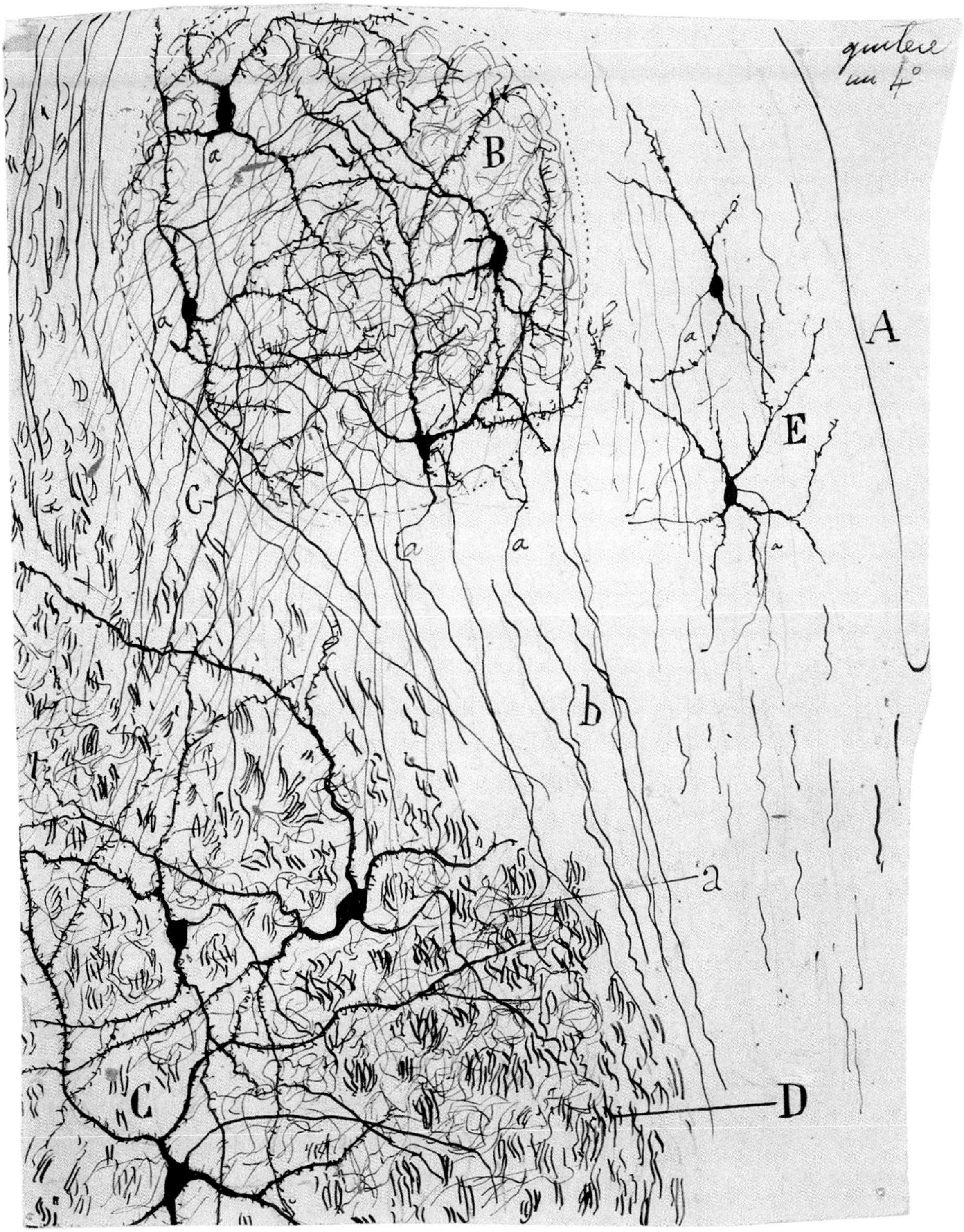

FIGURE 71. Section of the central gray matter and nucleus of Darkschewitsch in a kitten.

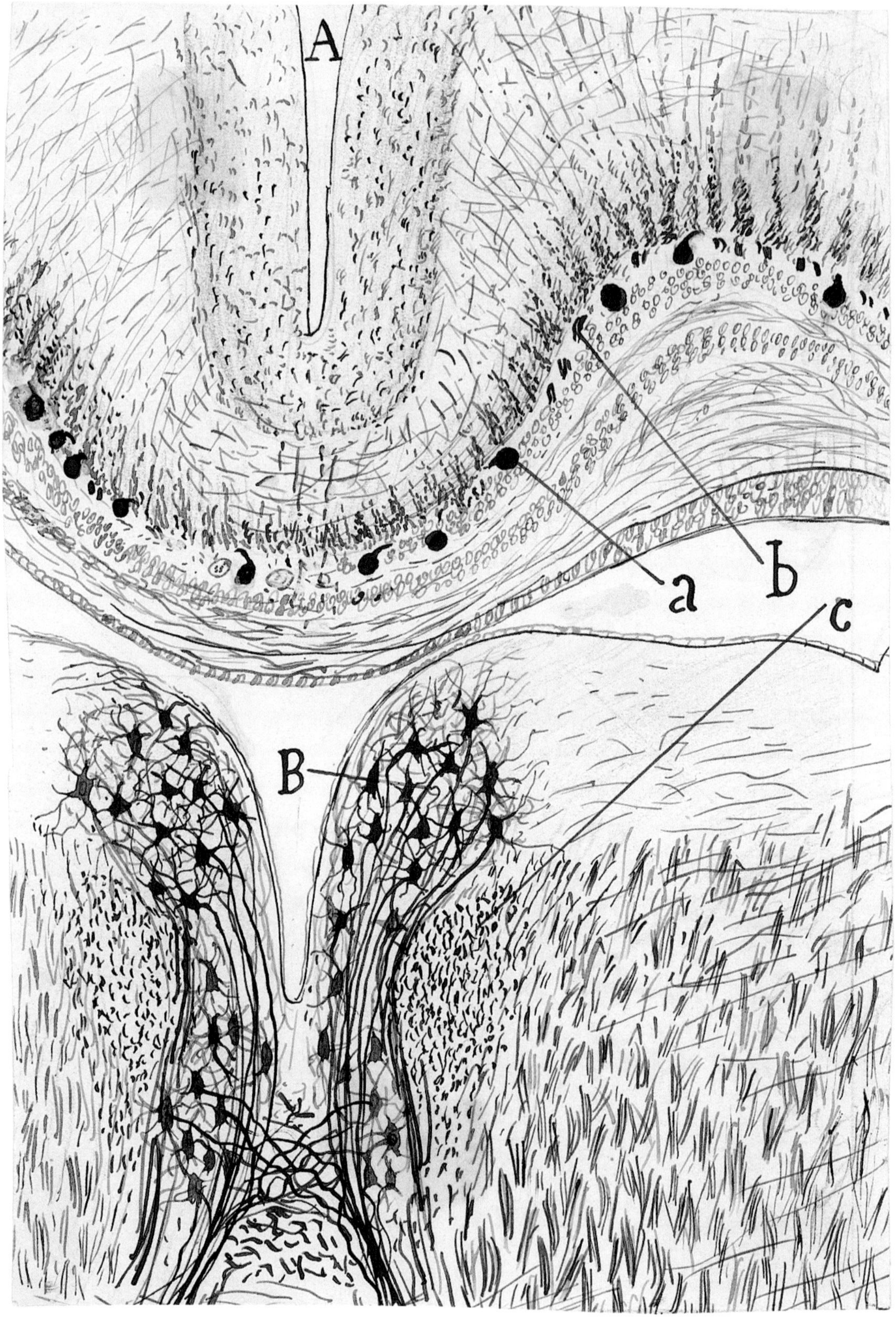

FIGURE 72. Section of the midbrain in a sand lizard.

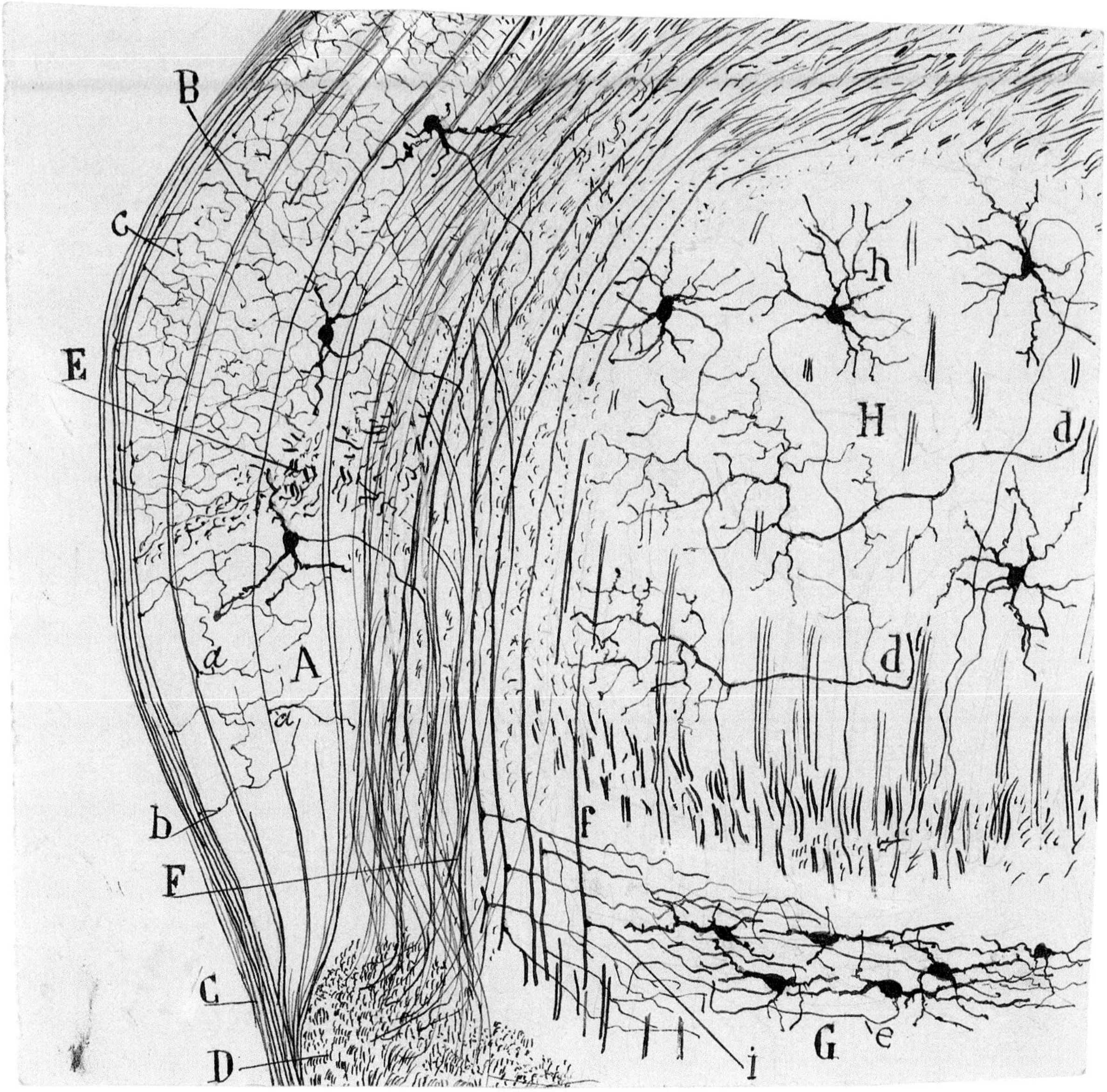

FIGURE 73. Coronal section of the thalamus in a kitten a few days old.

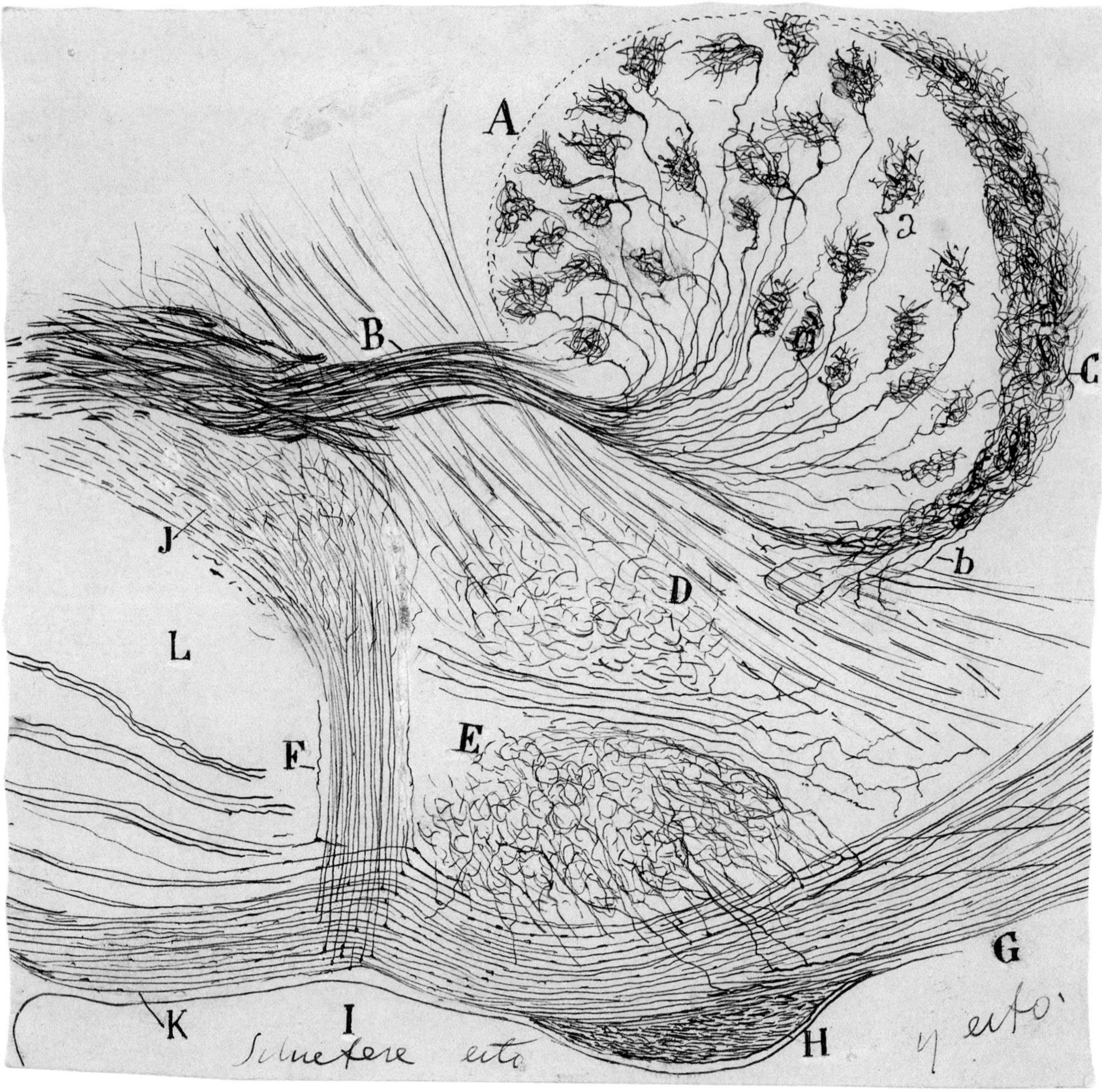

FIGURE 74. Penduncular and ventral thalamic regions in a twenty-day-old mouse.

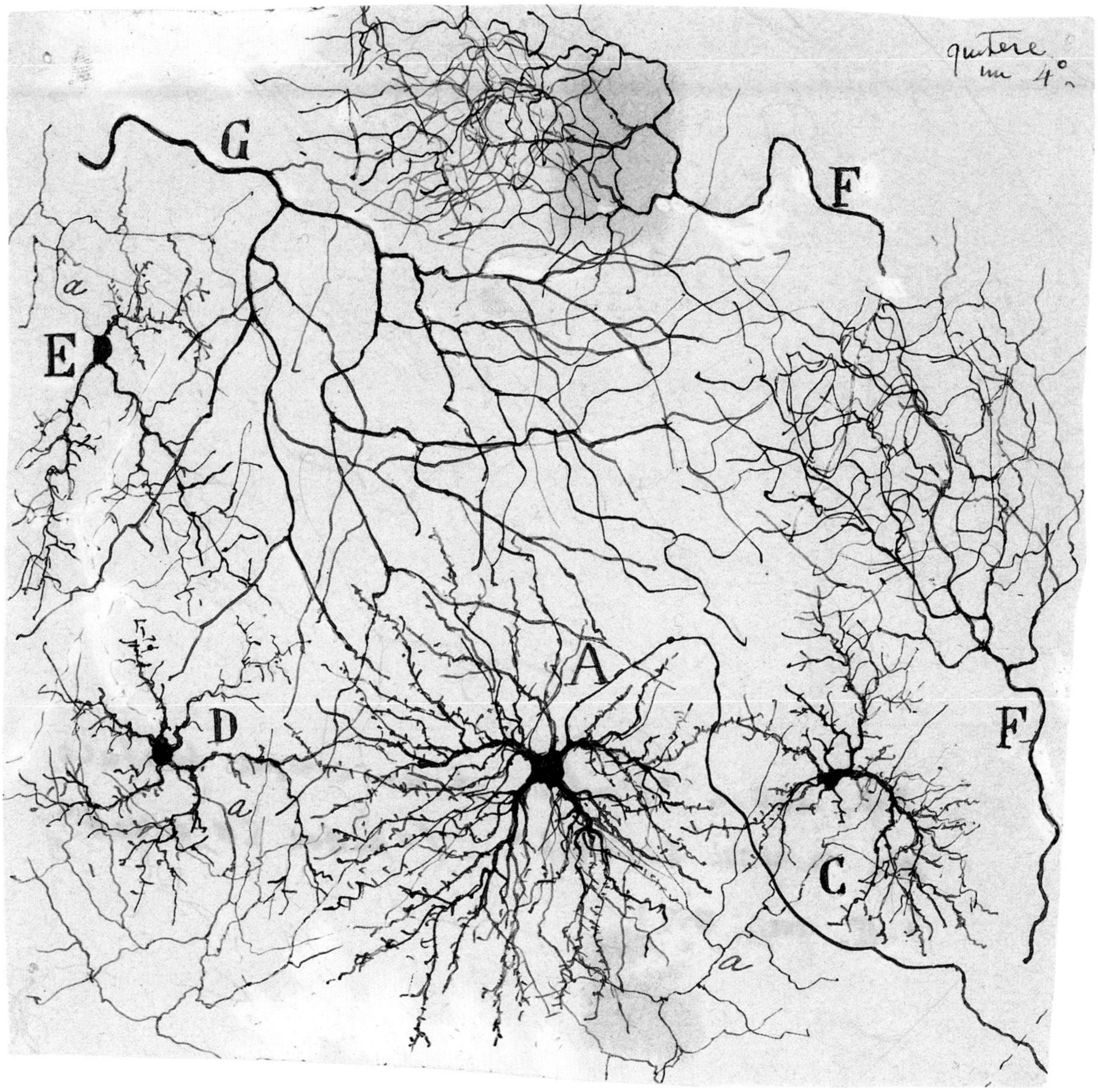

FIGURE 75. Coronal section of the sensory nucleus in a kitten a few days old.

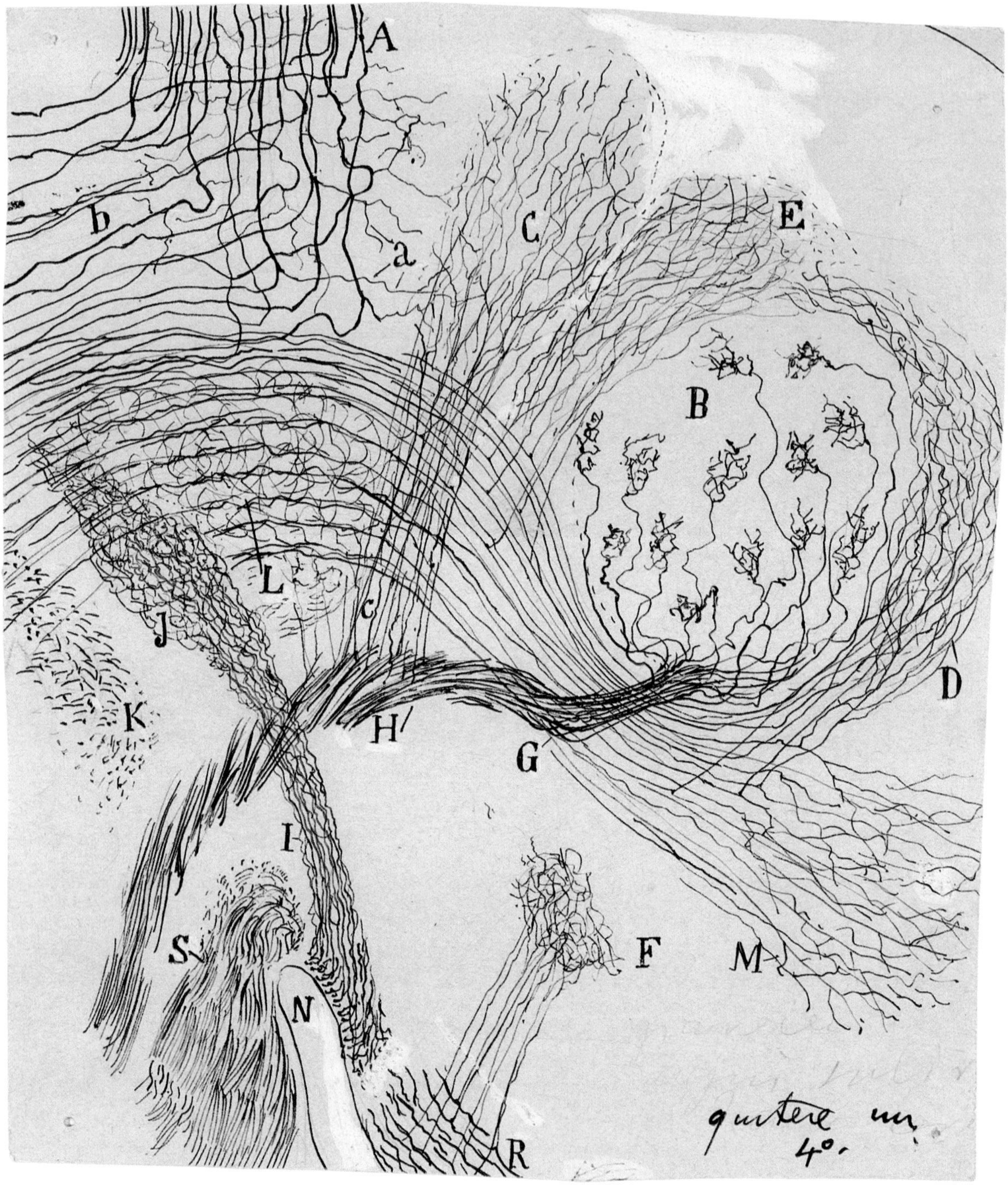

FIGURE 76. Section of the thalamus and part of the mesencephalon in an eight-day-old mouse.

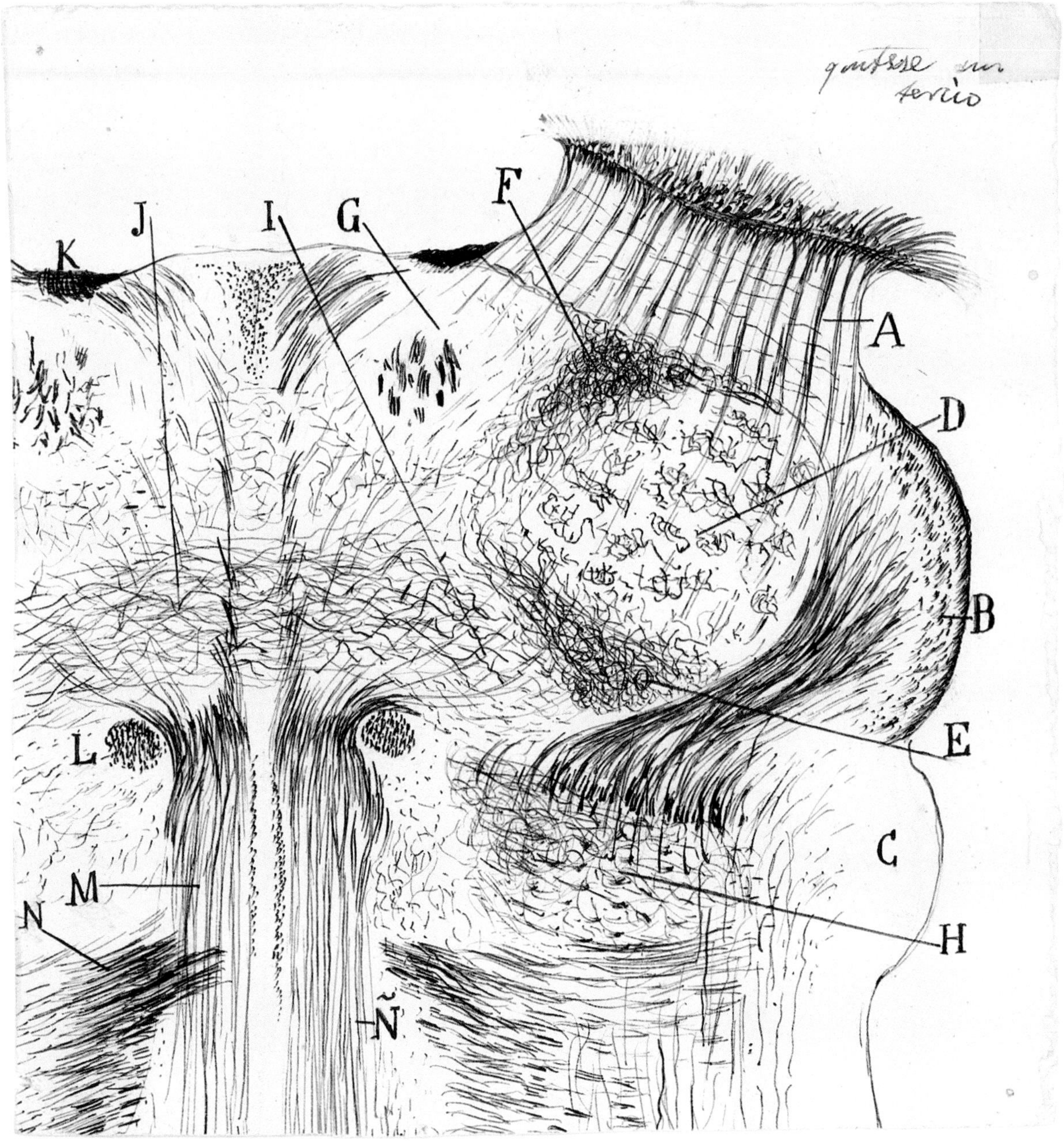

FIGURE 77. Horizontal section of the thalamus in a twenty-day-old mouse.

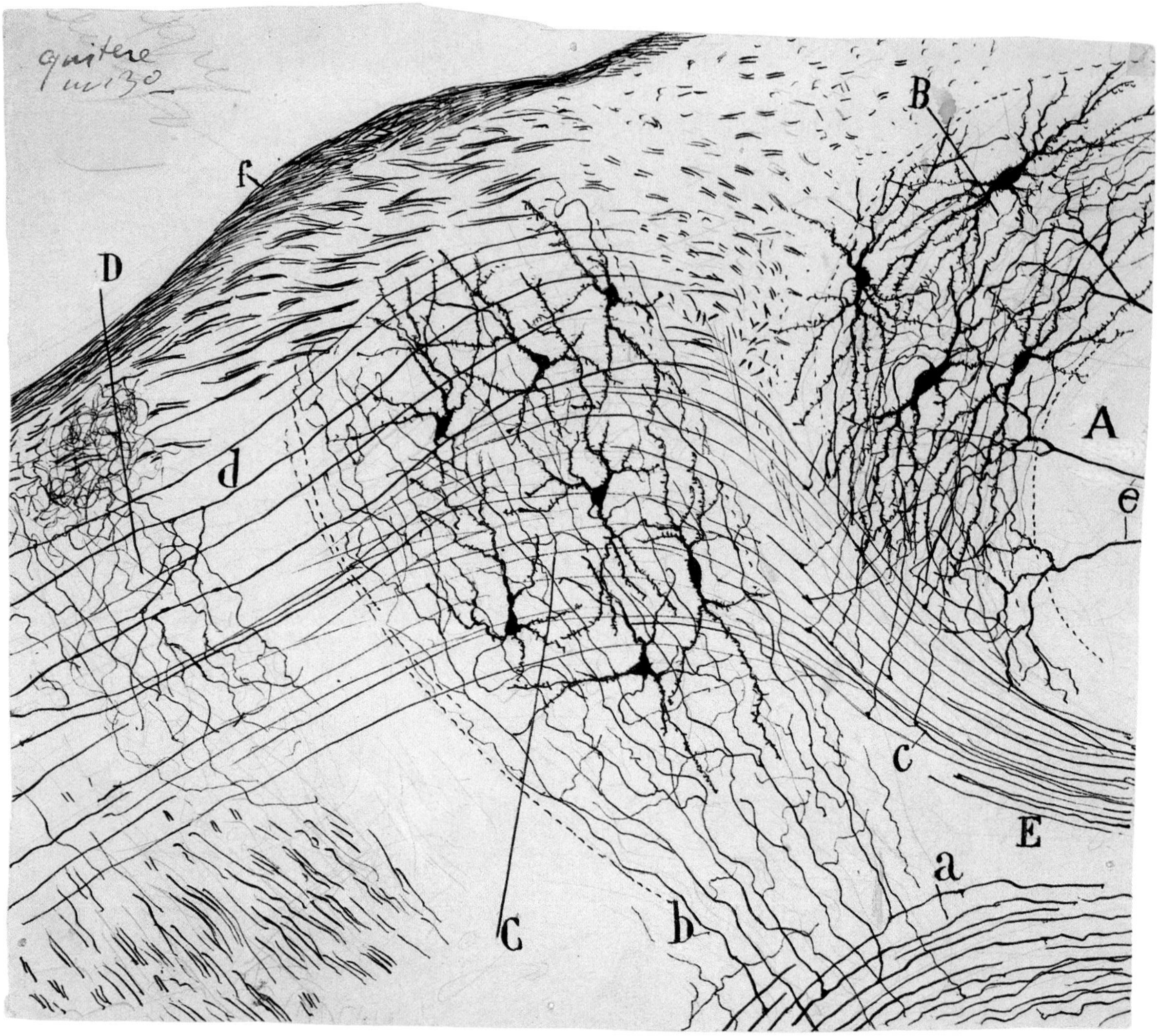

FIGURE 78. Sagittal section of the thalamus in a nineteen-day-old mouse.

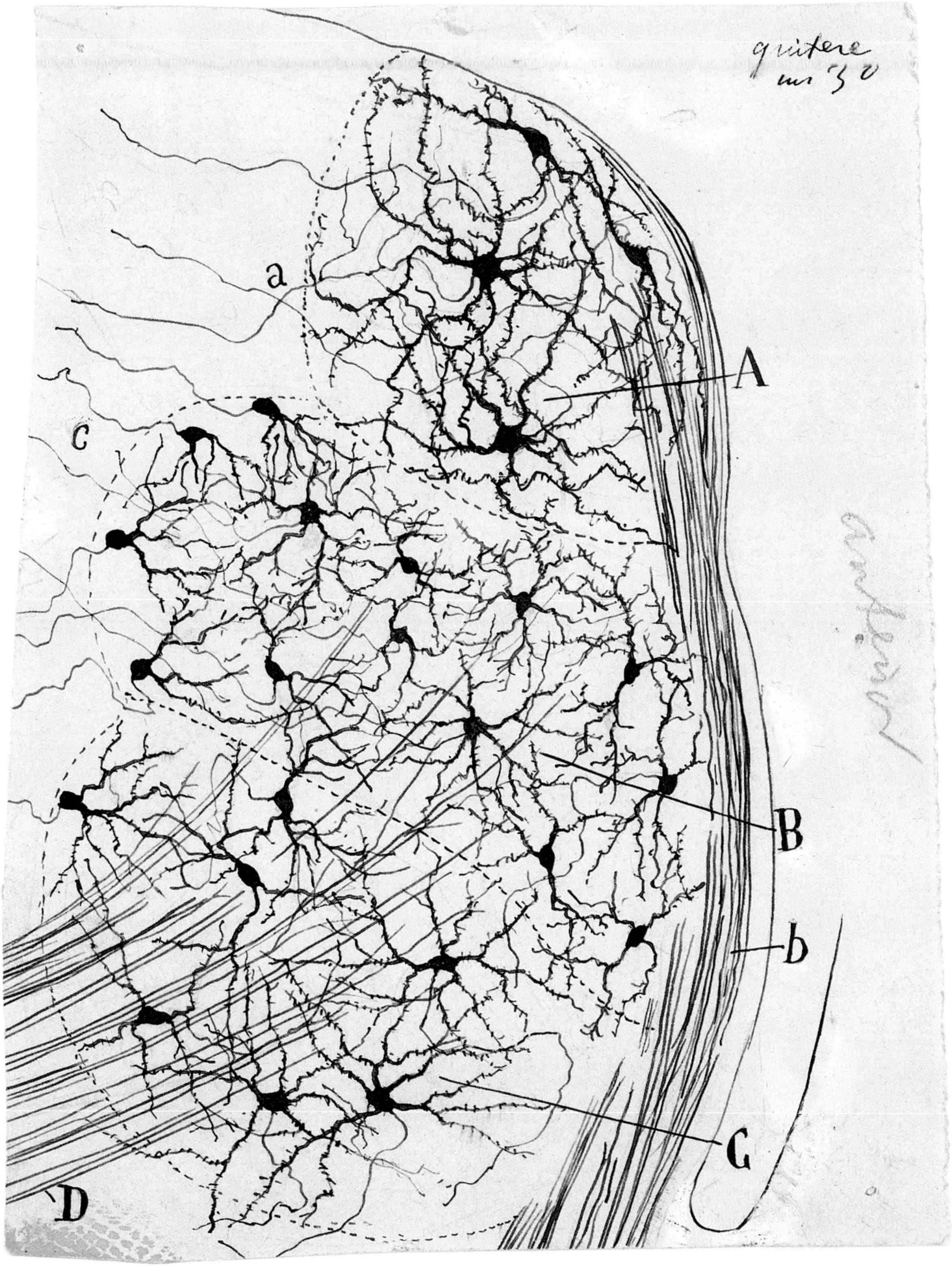

FIGURE 79. Rostral pole of the thalamus parallel to the stria medullaris in a mouse.

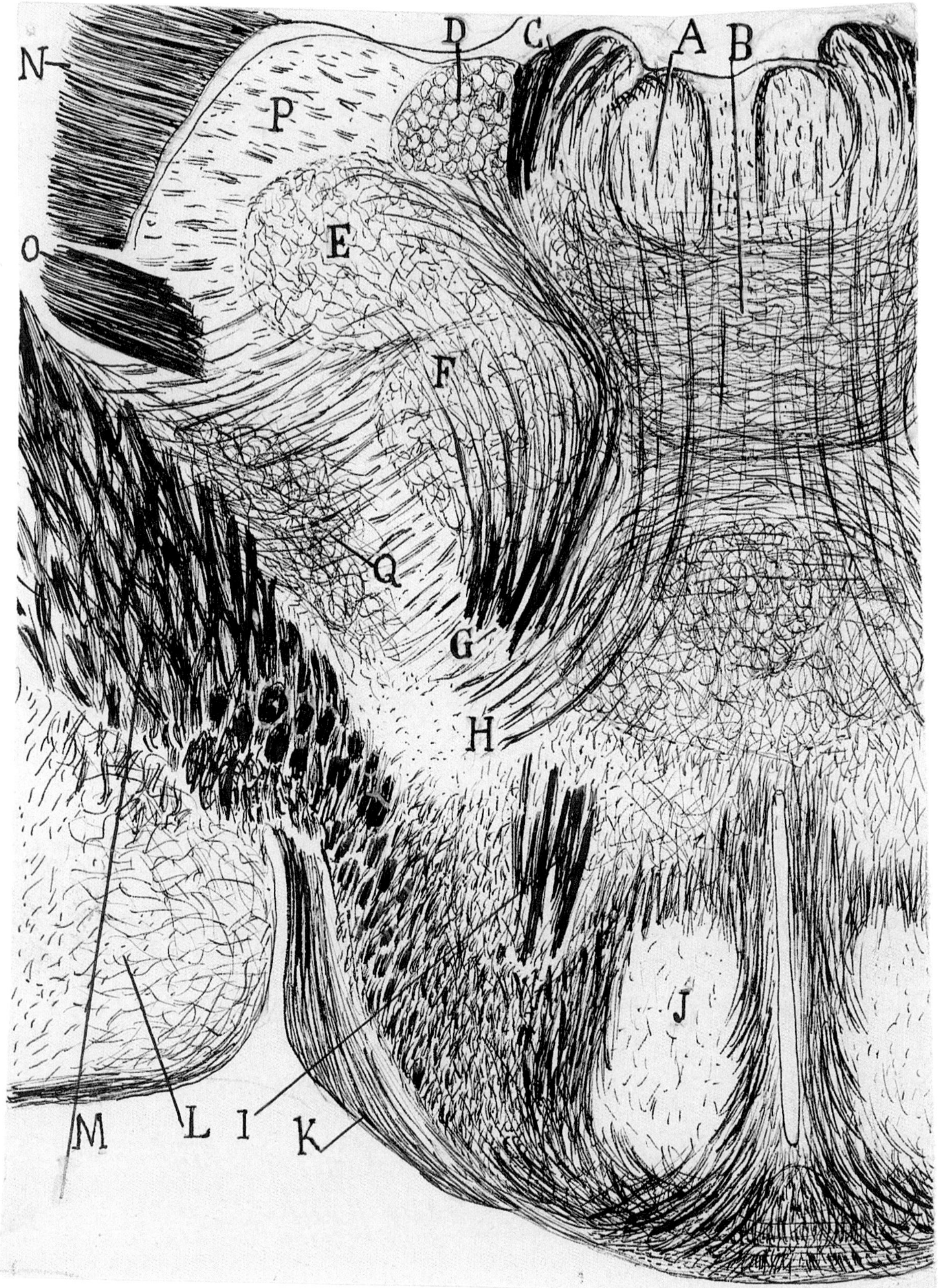

FIGURE 80. Coronal section of the thalamus in a mouse.

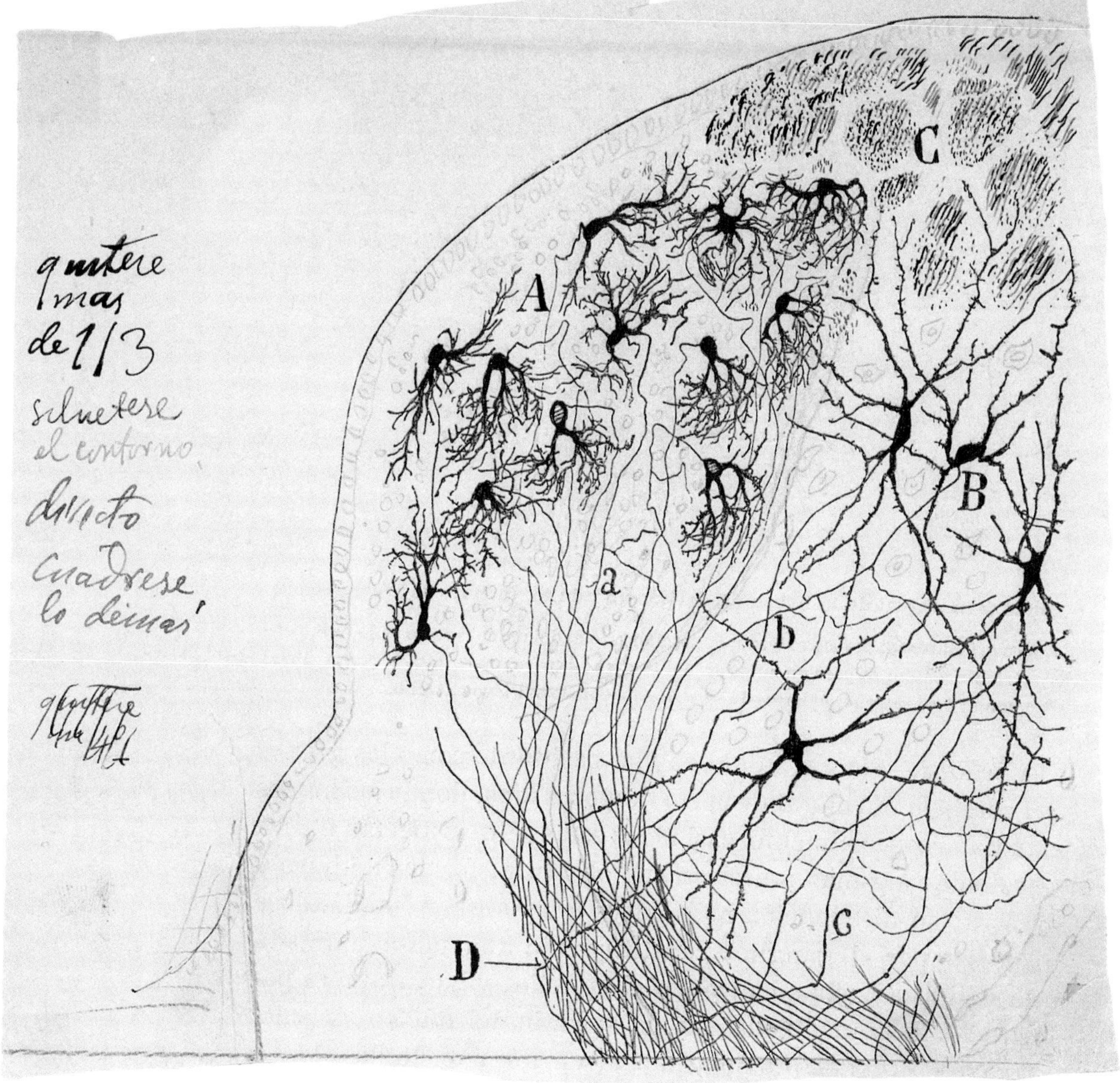

FIGURE 81. Coronal section of the two habenular nuclei in a dog.

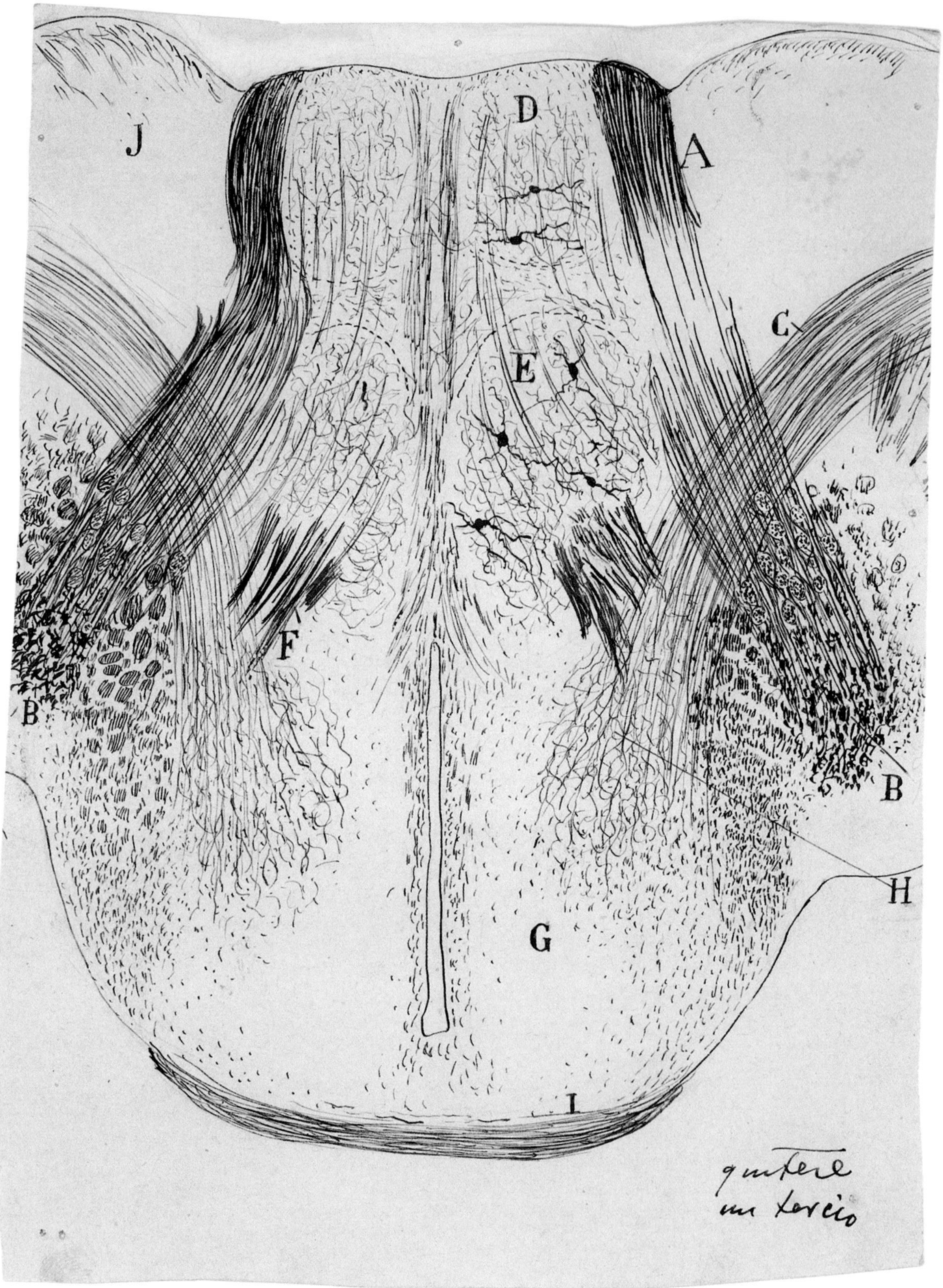

FIGURE 82. Rostral pole of the thalamus in a ten-day-old mouse, I.

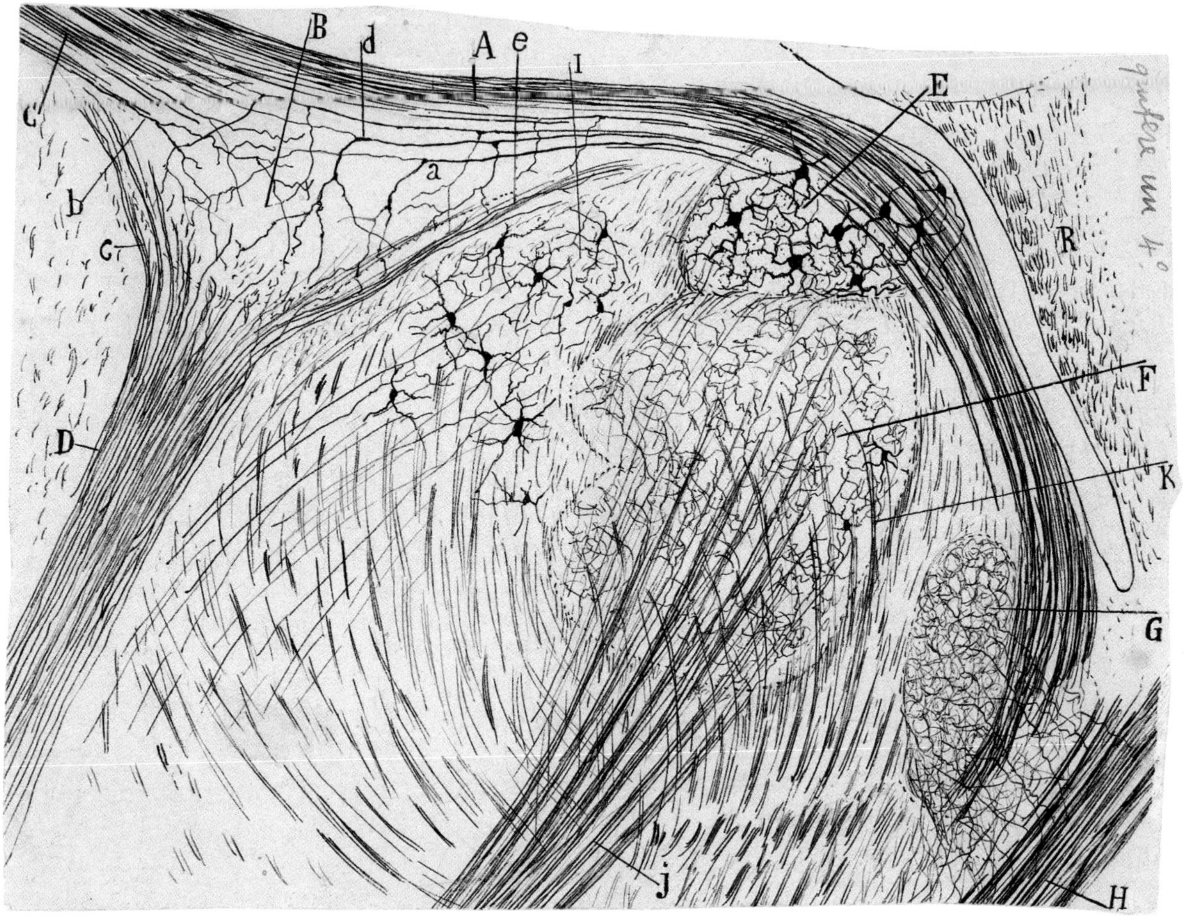

FIGURE 83. Section of the thalamus in a mouse.

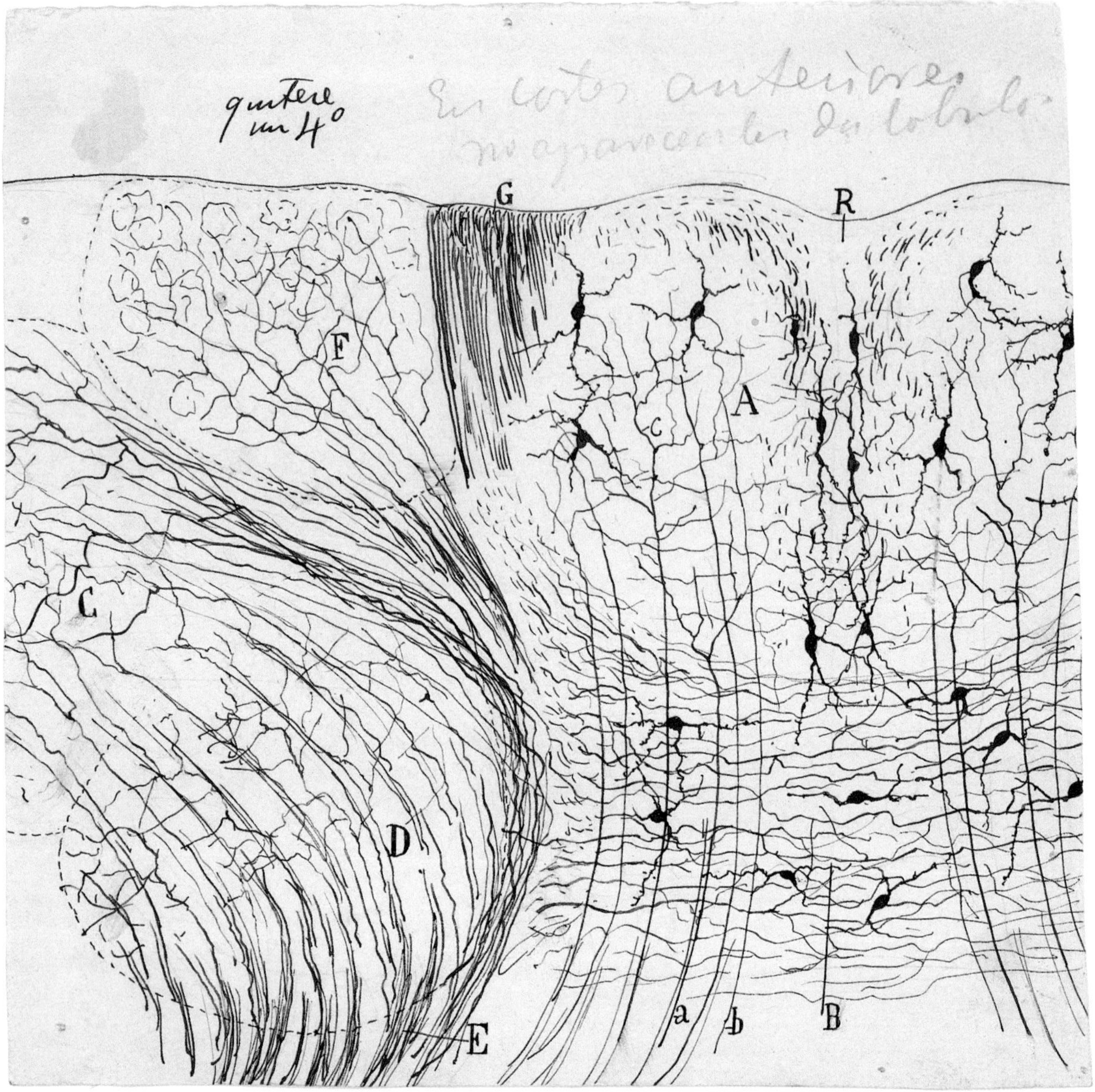

FIGURE 84. Rostral pole of the thalamus in a ten-day-old mouse, II.

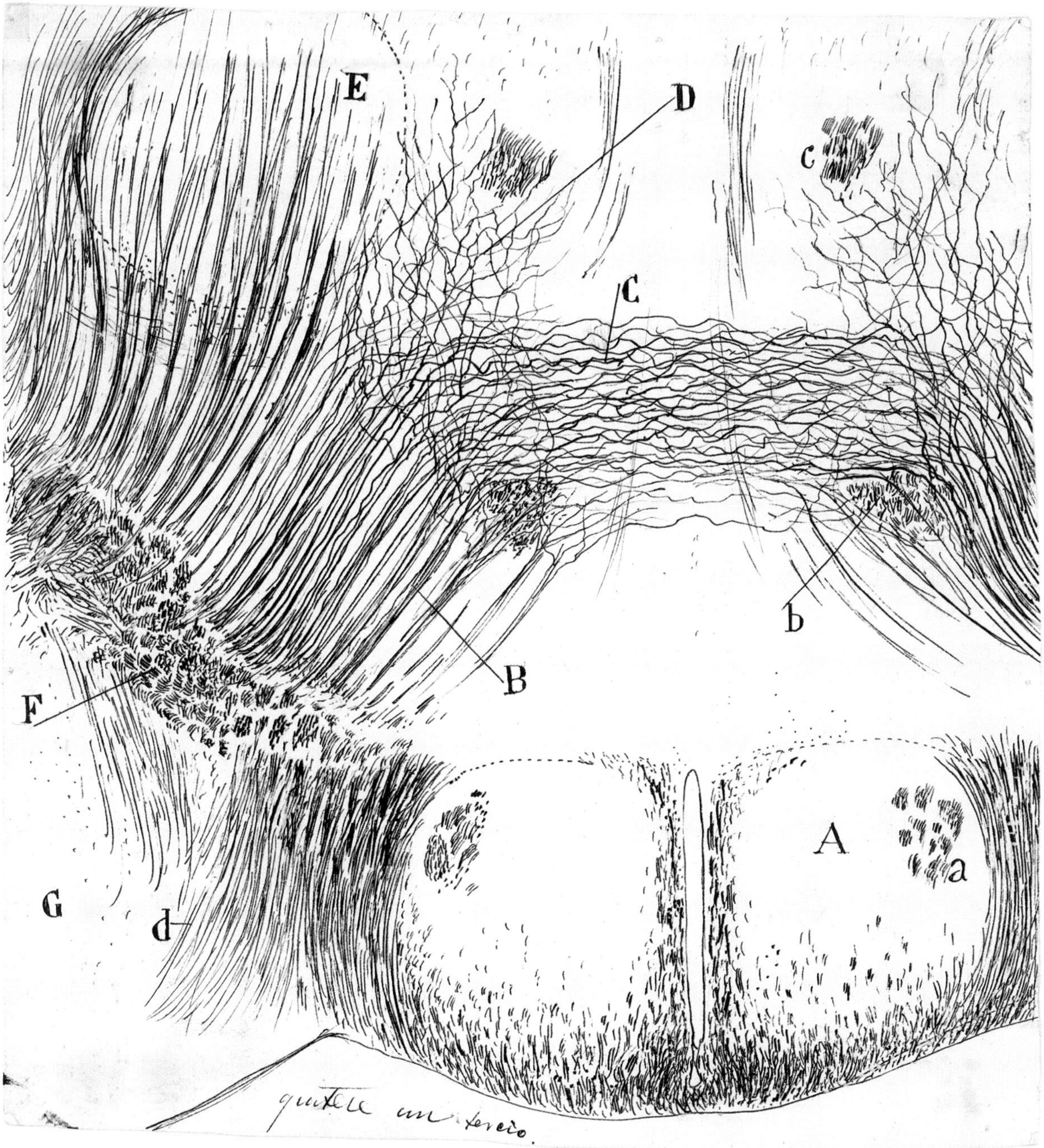

FIGURE 85. Section of the optic thalamus in a mouse.

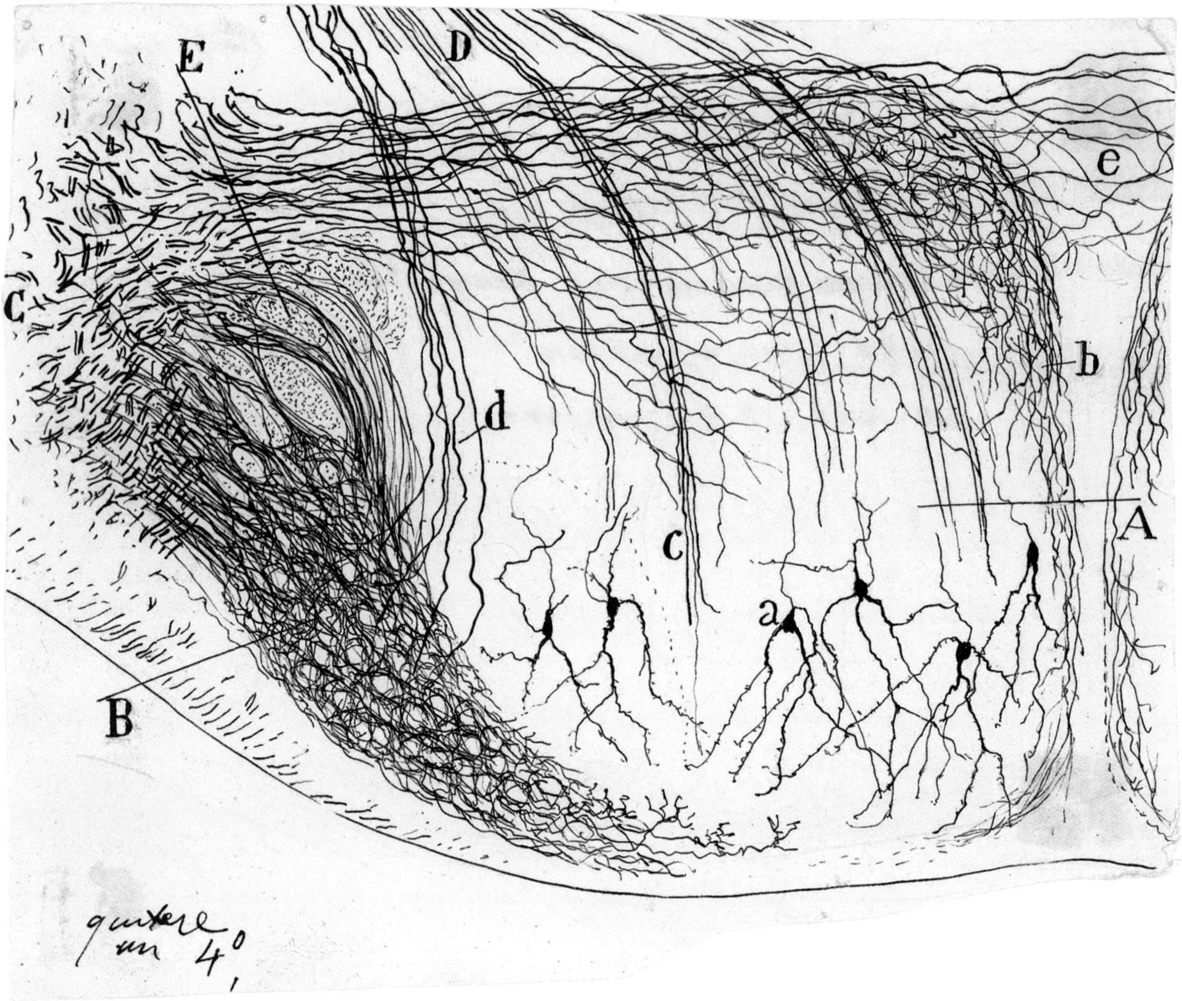

FIGURE 86. Coronal section of the two mammillary nuclei in a kitten.

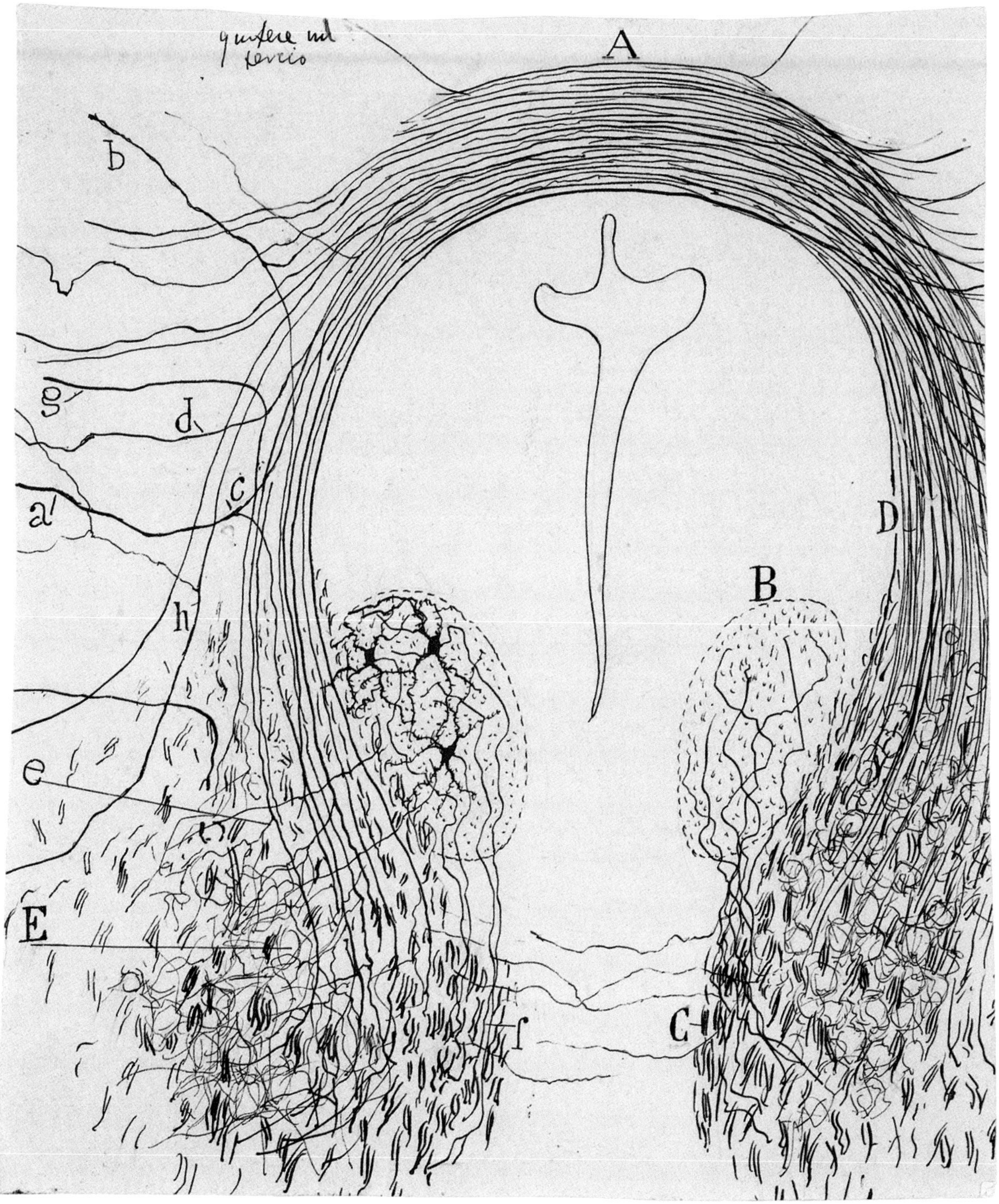

FIGURE 87. Coronal section of the posterior commissure in an eight-day-old kitten.

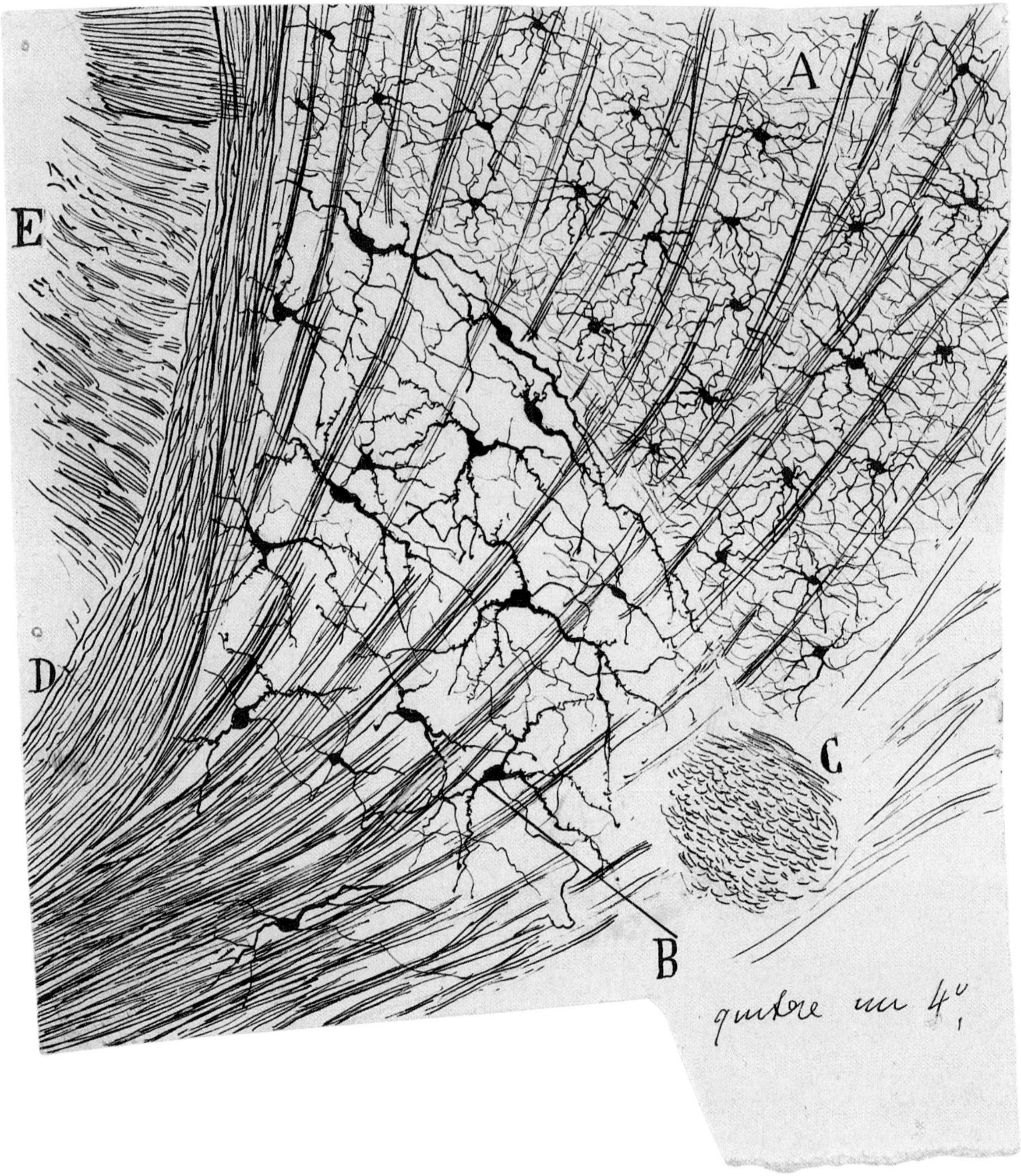

FIGURE 88. Sagittal section of the brain in a twenty-day-old mouse.

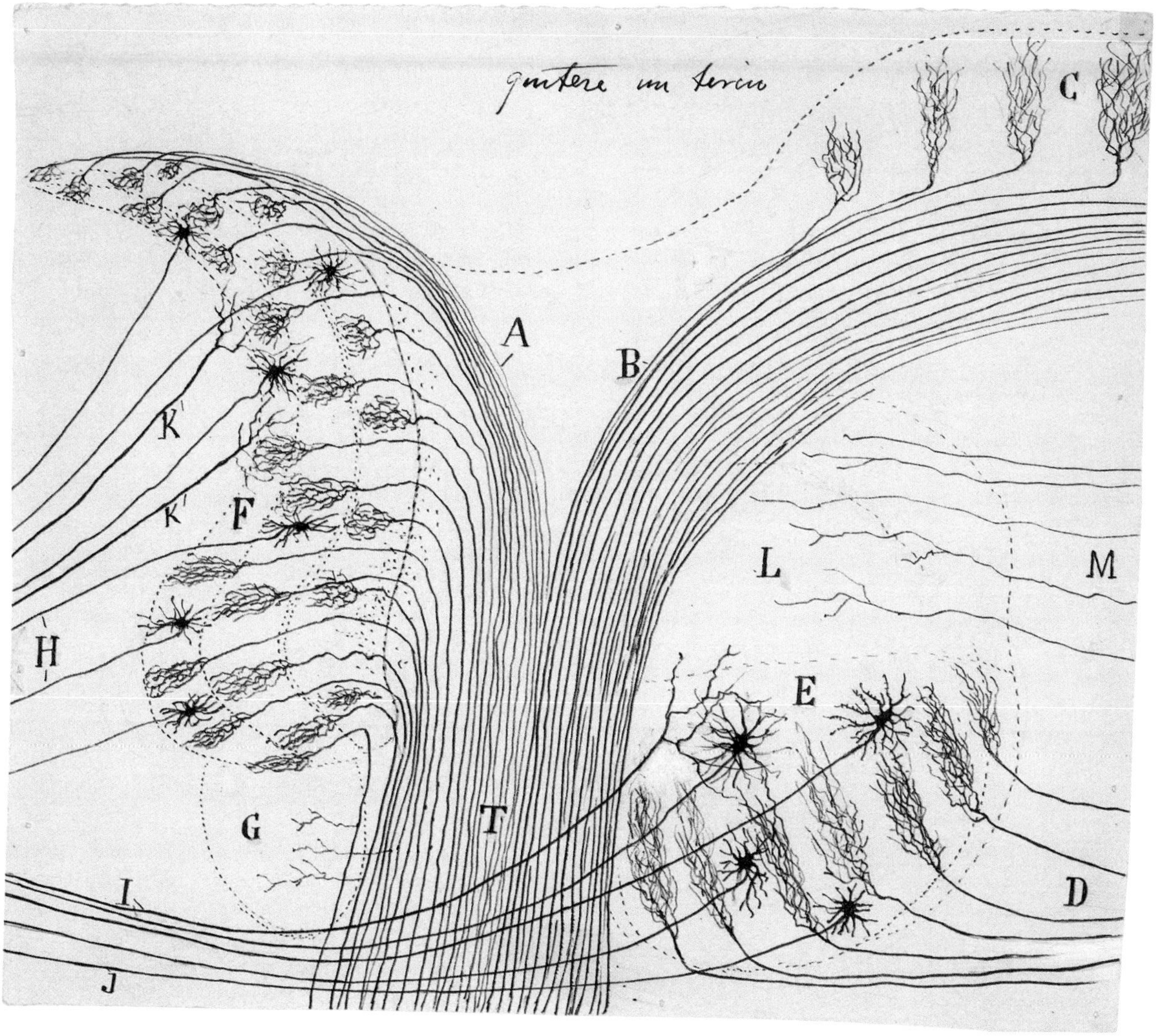

FIGURE 89. Diagram of the termination of the optic nerve in a cat.

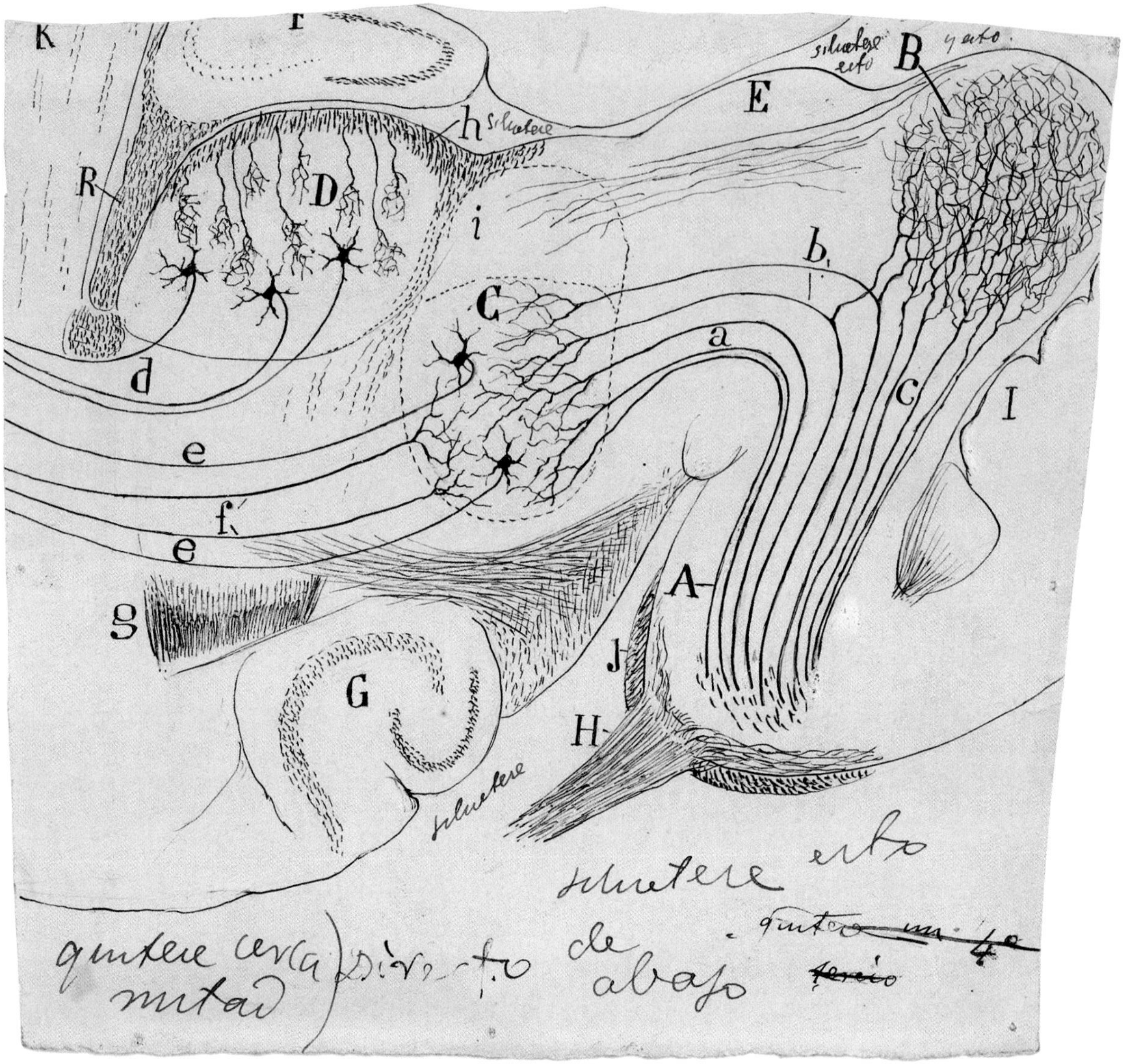

FIGURE 90. Diagram of the auditory pathways in a rabbit and a mouse.

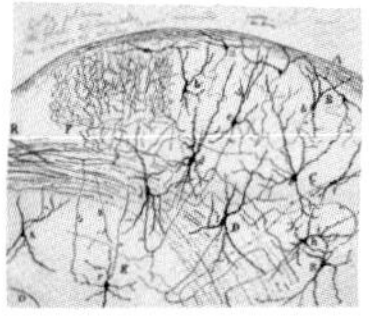

FIGURE 66.

Section of the dorsomedial region of the inferior colliculus in a newborn dog.

This figure was published in Cajal, S. R. (1902) Estructura del tubérculo cuadrigémino posterior, cuerpo geniculado interno y vías acústicas centrales. *Trab. Lab. Invest. Biol. Univ. Madrid* 1, 207–227 (Figure 6). It has also been reproduced as Figure 454 in Cajal, S. R. (1899–1904) *Textura del sistema nervioso del hombre y de los vertebrados*. Madrid: Moya.

FIGURE LEGEND: Transverse section of the dorsomedial region of the inferior colliculus in a newborn dog. Golgi method. *A*, Peripheral fibrillar layer; *B*, cells of the second layer; *C*, stellate and fusiform neurons of the third layer; *D*, fibro-cellular layer with its neurons *I* and *J*; *E*, central gray matter; *R*, axonal commissure; *F*, axonal plexuses of the second layer.

Original text: Corte frontal de la porción superior é interna del tubérculo cuadrigémino posterior del perro recién nacido. Método de Golgi. *A*, capa fibrilar periférica; *B*, células de la capa segunda; *C*, corpúsculos estrellados y fusiformes de la zona tercera; *D*, capa fibrocelular con sus neuronas *I*, *J*; *E*, substancia gris central; *R*, comisura nerviosa; *F*, plexo nervioso de la zona segunda.

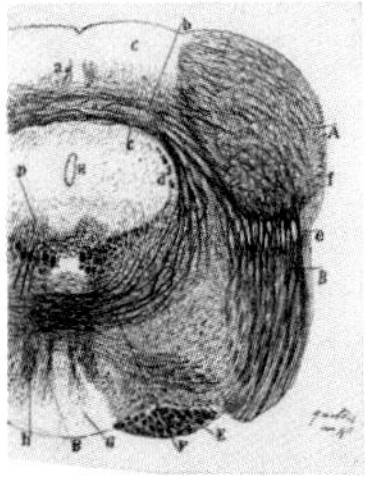

FIGURE 67.

Section of the inferior colliculus in an adult mouse.

This figure was published in Cajal, S. R. (1899–1904) *Textura del sistema nervioso del hombre y de los vertebrados*. Madrid: Moya. (Figure 455 and Figure 469).

FIGURE LEGEND: Transverse, slightly oblique section of the inferior colliculus and tegmental region in an [adult] mouse. Weigert-Pal method. *A*, Nucleus of the inferior colliculus; *B*, lateral lemniscus; *C*, caudal region of the superior colliculus [, which is still visible at this level thanks to the obliqueness of the section]; *D*, nucleus of the oculomotor [nerve]; *E*, cerebral peduncle; *F*, descending optic–auditory reflex pathway decussating ventral to the medial longitudinal fasciculus; *G*, interpeduncular nucleus; *a*, optic fibers; *b* and *c*, two planes of axons of the transverse fiber layer of the superior colliculus.

Original text: Corte frontal algo oblicuo del tubérculo cuadrigémino anterior del ratón [adulto]. Método de Weigert-Pal. *A*, núcleo del tubérculo cuadrigémino posterior; *B*, lemnisco externo; *C*, parte posterior de la corteza del *nates* [visible aun en el corte merced á su oblicuidad]; *D*, foco del [nervio] motor ocular común; *E*, pedúnculo cerebral; *F*, vía óptico-acústico refleja descendente que se cruza debajo del fascículo longitudinal; *G*, ganglio interpeduncular; *a*, fibras ópticas; *b* y *c*, los dos planos de tubos nerviosos de la capa de fibras transversales del *nates*.

Note from the author (J. D.): In brackets is the text added in the French version of the *Textura*: Cajal, S. R. (1909–1911) *Histologie du système nerveux de l'homme et des vertébrés*, trans. L. Azoulay. Paris: Maloine.

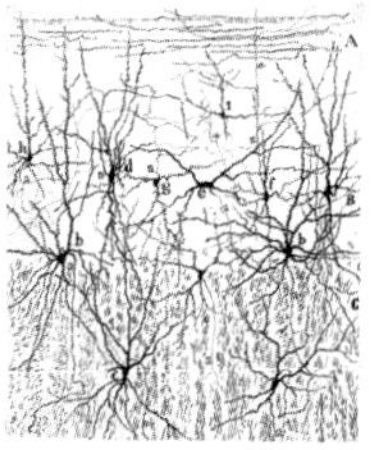

FIGURE 68.

Section of the superior colliculus in a kitten.

This figure was published in Cajal, S. R. (1903) Las fibras nerviosas de origen cerebral del tubérculo cuadrigémino anterior y tálamo óptico. *Trab. Lab. Invest. Biol. Univ. Madrid* 2, 5–21 (Figure 4). It has also been reproduced as Figure 126 in Cajal, S. R. (1909–1911) *Histologie du système nerveux de l'homme et des vertébrés*, trans. L. Azoulay. Paris: Maloine.

FIGURE LEGEND: Portion of a sagittal section of the superior colliculus in an eight-day-old kitten. *A*, Most caudal portion of the optic fibers; *B*, layer of fibers of cerebral origin; *C*, layer of the transverse fibers; *a*, *b*, *c*, large neurons with a long descending axon; *e*, smaller neuron with a long axon; *d*, *h*, *g*, *i*, neurons with a short axon; *f*, fusiform cell with an ascending axon.

Original text: Trozo de un corte sagital del tubérculo cuadrigémino anterior del gato de ocho días. *A*, porción más inferior de las fibras ópticas; *B*, capa de las fibras de origen cerebral; *C*, zona de las fibras transversales; *a*, *b*, *c*, corpúsculos gangliónicos voluminosos de axon largo y descendente; *e*, neurona de axon largo más pequeña; *d*, *h*, *g*, *i*, neuronas de axon corto; *f*, neurona fusiforme de axon ascendente.

Note from the author (J. D.): This figure is not included in Cajal, S. R. (1899–1904) *Textura del sistema nervioso del hombre y de los vertebrados*. Madrid: Moya.

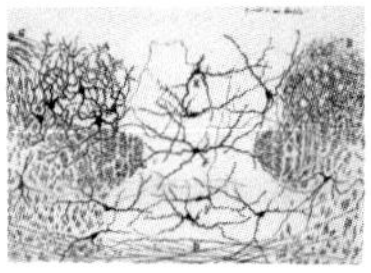

FIGURE 69.

Superior colliculus in a kitten.

This figure was published in Cajal, S. R. (1899–1904) *Textura del sistema nervioso del hombre y de los vertebrados*. Madrid: Moya. (Figure 489).

FIGURE LEGEND: Transverse section through the caudal region of the superior colliculus in a kitten a few days old. Golgi method. *A*, Cells of the trochlear nerve nucleus; *B*, plexus of collaterals within this nucleus; [*C*, medial longitudinal fasciculus]; *D*, crossing fibers of the superior cerebellar peduncle; *E*, cells of the subaqueductal nucleus of the raphe; *F*, ventral cells of the raphe; *G*, radicular fibers of the trochlear nerve.

Original text: Corte frontal de los tubérculos cuadrigéminos (porción posterior) proximales del gato de pocos días. Método de Golgi. *A*, células del foco del [nervio] patético; *B*, Plexo de colaterales de este núcleo; [*C*, fascículo longitudinal posterior]; *D*, fibras cruzadas del pedúnculo cerebeloso superior; *E*, células del foco subacueductal del rafe; *F*, células inferiores del rafe; *G*, radiculares del patético.

Note from the author (J. D.): In brackets is the text added in the French version of the *Textura*: Cajal, S. R. (1909–1911) *Histologie du système nerveux de l'homme et des vertébrés*, trans. L. Azoulay. Paris: Maloine.

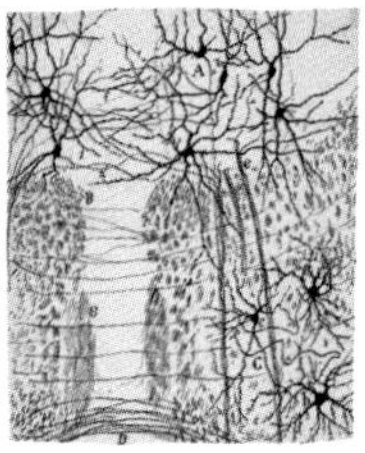

FIGURE 70.

Section of the oculomotor nucleus in a mouse a few days old.

This figure was published in Cajal, S. R. (1899–1904) *Textura del sistema nervioso del hombre y de los vertebrados*. Madrid: Moya. (Figure 492).

FIGURE LEGEND: Transverse section through the caudal region of the oculomotor nucleus in a mouse a few days old. Golgi method. *A*, Motor cells of the nucleus of the third cranial nerve; *B*, medial longitudinal fasciculus; *C*, red nucleus; *D*, ventral tegmental decussation; *a*, crossed radicular fibers; *f*, dendritic commissure.

Original text: Corte frontal del foco del motor ocular común (porción distal) del ratón de pocos días. Método de Golgi. *A*, células motrices [del núcleo del tercer par]; *B*, fascículo longitudinal posterior; *C*, núcleo rojo; *D*, decusación ventral de la calota; *a*, radiculares cruzadas; *f*, comisura protoplásmica.

Note from the author (J. D.): In brackets is the text added in the French version of the *Textura*: Cajal, S. R. (1909–1911) *Histologie du système nerveux de l'homme et des vertébrés*, trans. L. Azoulay. Paris: Maloine.

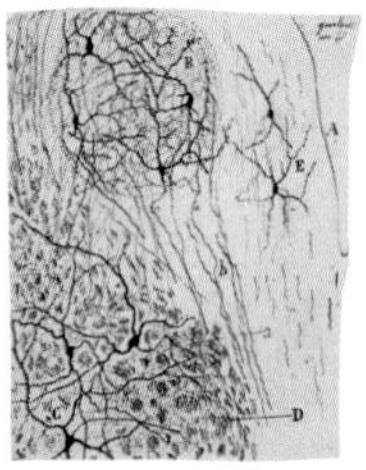

FIGURE 71

Section of the central gray matter and nucleus of Darkschewitsch in a kitten.

This figure was published in Cajal, S. R. (1899–1904) *Textura del sistema nervioso del hombre y de los vertebrados*. Madrid: Moya. (Figure 504).

FIGURE LEGEND: Section of the central gray matter and nucleus of Darkschewitsch in a kitten a few days old. Golgi method. *A*, Aqueduct of Sylvius (cerebral aqueduct); *B*, nucleus of Darkschewitsch; *C*, interstitial nucleus located at the rostral tip of the medial longitudinal fasciculus; *D*, bundles of this fascicle; *a*, pericellular nets of the interstitial nucleus; *b*, axons of the nucleus of Darkschewitsch; *c*, collaterals terminated in this nucleus.

Original text: Corte de la substancia gris central y foco de Darkschewitsch del gato de pocos días. Método de Golgi. *A*, acueducto de Silvio; *B*, foco de Darkschewitsch; *C*, foco intersticial del cabo anterior del fascículo longitudinal posterior; *D*, haces de este fascículo; *a*, nidos pericelulares del foco intersticial; *b*, axones del foco de Darkschewitsch; *c*, colaterales terminadas en éste.

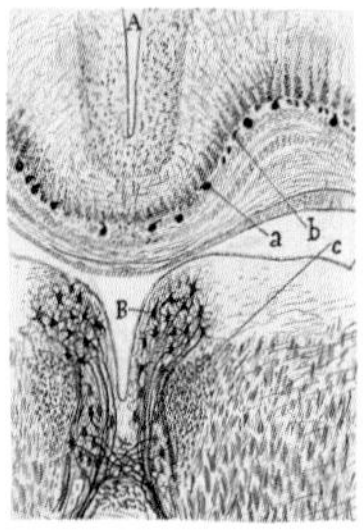

FIGURE 72.

Section of the midbrain in a sand lizard.

This figure was published in Ramón, P. (1904) Origen del nervio masticador en las aves, reptiles y batracios. *Trab. Lab. Invest. Biol. Univ. Madrid* 3, 153–162 (Figure 4). It has also been reproduced as Figure 158 in Cajal, S. R. (1909–1911) *Histologie du système nerveux de l'homme et des vertébrés*, trans. L. Azoulay. Paris: Maloine.

FIGURE LEGEND: Transverse section of the midbrain of the sand lizard (*Lacerta stirpium*). Reduced silver nitrate method. *A*, Interlobular fissure; *B*, oculomotor nucleus; *a*, cell of the nucleus of the mesencephalic root of the masticatory (trigeminal) nerve; *b*, bundle of fibers arising from them.

Original text: Corte frontal del cerebro medio del lagarto de las cepas (*Lacerta stirpium*). Método del nitrato de plata reducido. *A*, cisura interlobular; *B*, núcleo del motor ocular común; *a*, células del núcleo del nervio masticador; *b*, fascículo de fibras que emanan de ellas.

Note from the author (J. D.): This figure is not included in Cajal, S. R. (1899–1904) *Textura del sistema nervioso del hombre y de los vertebrados*. Madrid: Moya.

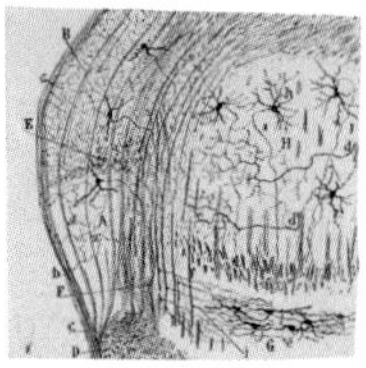

FIGURE 73.

Coronal section of the thalamus in a kitten a few days old.

This figure was published in Cajal, S. R. (1899–1904) *Textura del sistema nervioso del hombre y de los vertebrados*. Madrid: Moya. (Figures 576).

FIGURE LEGEND: Coronal section of part of the thalamus in a kitten a few days old. Golgi method. *A*, Ventral segment of the lateral geniculate body; *B*, dorsal segment of the same body; C, optic tract; *D*, cerebral peduncle; *E*, intermediate white lamina; *F*, central optic pathway; *H*, sensory nucleus.

Original text: Trozo del tálamo del ratón de pocos días. Corte frontal. Método de Golgi. *A*, núcleo inferior del cuerpo geniculado externo; *B*, núcleo superior de éste; C, cinta óptica; *D*, pedúnculo cerebral; *E*, lámina blanca intermediaria; *F*, vía óptica central; *H*, núcleo sensitivo.

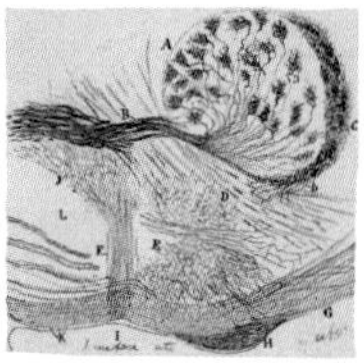

FIGURE 74.

Peduncular and ventral thalamic regions in a twenty-day-old mouse.

This figure was originally published in Cajal, S. R. (1900) Contribución al estudio de la vía sensitiva central y estructura del tálamo óptico. *Rev. Trim. Micrograf. Madrid* 5, 185–198 (Figure 4). It has also been reproduced as Figures 352 and 581 in Cajal, S. R. (1899–1904) *Textura del sistema nervioso del hombre y de los vertebrados*. Madrid: Moya.

FIGURE LEGEND: Sagittal section of the peduncular and ventral thalamic regions in a twenty-day-old mouse. The section is rather lateral and includes the axis of the cerebral peduncle. Golgi method. *A*, Somatosensory nucleus of the thalamus; *B*, somatosensory pathway (medial lemniscus); *C*, semilunar nucleus; *D*, ventral nucleus (*Gitterkern*) of Nissl; *E*, nucleus of Luys (subthalamic nucleus); *F*, fascicle of collaterals of the cerebral peduncle; *G*, peduncle; *H*, optic tract; *I*, Ammon's horn; *J*, field of Forel, the main termination site of the fascicle of peduncular collaterals.

Original text: Corte sagital de la región talámica inferior y penduncular del ratón de veinte días. La sección es bastante lateral y comprende el eje del pedúnculo cerebral. Método de Golgi. *A*, foco lateral del tálamo; *B*, fascículo sensitivo; *C*, foco semilunar; *D*, *Gitterkern* ventral de Nissl; *E*, Ganglio de Luys; *F*, fascículo de colaterales del pedúnculo; *G*, pedúnculo; *H*, tractus óptico; *I*, asta de Ammon; *J*, campo de Forel donde principalmente se termina el haz de colaterales.

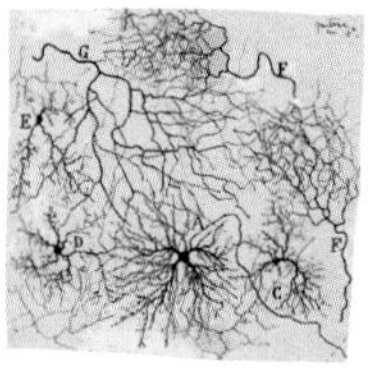

FIGURE 75.

Coronal section of the [thalamic] sensory nucleus in a kitten a few days old.

This figure was published in Cajal, S. R. (1899–1904) *Textura del sistema nervioso del hombre y de los vertebrados*. Madrid: Moya. (Figure 585).

FIGURE LEGEND: Part of a coronal section of the [thalamic] sensory nucleus in a kitten a few days old. Golgi method. *A*, Cell with a long axon; *C*, *D*, *E*, cells with a short axon; *F*, sensory fibers; *G*, centrifugal or cerebral cortical fibers.

Original text: Trozo de un corte frontal del foco sensitivo [del tálamo] del gato de pocos días. Método de Golgi. *A*, célula de axon largo; *C*, *D*, *E*, corpúsculos de axon corto; *F*, fibras sensitivas; *G*, fibras centrífugas ó cerebrales.

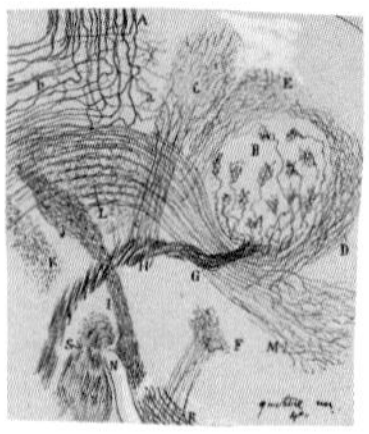

FIGURE 76.

Section of the thalamus and part of the mesencephalon in an eight-day-old mouse.

This figure was published in Cajal, S. R. (1899–1904) *Textura del sistema nervioso del hombre y de los vertebrados*. Madrid: Moya. (Figures 510 and 586).

FIGURE LEGEND: Lateral sagittal section of the thalamus and part of the mesencephalon in an eight-day-old mouse. Golgi method. *A*, Posterior commissure; *B*, thalamic sensory nucleus; *C*, posterior thalamic nucleus; *D* and *E*, [semilunar] or accessory nuclei of the sensory nucleus; *F*, special subthalamic nucleus; *G*, medial lemniscus; *H*, portion of this bundle giving off collaterals; *I*, *tractus peduncularis transversus; J*, nucleus of termination of this tract; *L*, red nucleus; *S*, pyramidal pathway; [*c*, medial lemniscus collaterals for the posterior thalamic nucleus].

Original text: Corte sagital lateral del tálamo y parte del mesencéfalo del ratón de ocho días. Método de Golgi. *A*, comisura posterior; *B*, foco sensitivo del tálamo; *C*, foco talámico posterior; *D* y *E*, núcleos [semilunares] accesorios del foco sensitivo; *F*, núcleo especial subtalámico; *G*, lemnisco interno; *H*, porción de éste de donde brotan colaterales; *I*, *tractus peduncularis transversus; J*, foco de terminación de éste; *L*, núcleo rojo; *S*, vía piramidal; [*c*, colaterales sensitivas para el núcleo prebigeminal].

Note from the author (J. D.): In brackets is the text added in the French version of the *Textura*: Cajal, S. R. (1909–1911) *Histologie du système nerveux de l'homme et des vertébrés*, trans. L. Azoulay. Paris: Maloine.

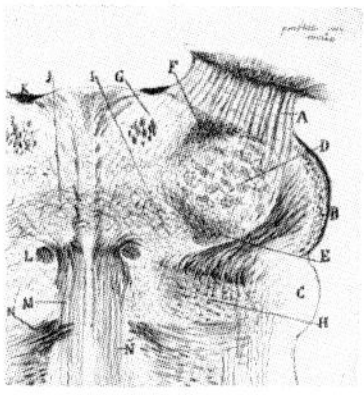

FIGURE 77.

Horizontal section of the thalamus in a twenty-day-old mouse.

This figure was published in Cajal, S. R. (1899–1904) *Textura del sistema nervioso del hombre y de los vertebrados*. Madrid: Moya. (Figure 587).

FIGURE LEGEND: Horizontal section of the thalamus in a twenty-day-old mouse. Golgi method. *A*, Reticular nucleus; *B*, lateral geniculate body; *C*, medial geniculate body; *D*, sensory nucleus; *E, F*, posterior and anterior semilunar nuclei; *H*, posterior nucleus; *G*, anterior nucleus and mammillothalamic track of Vicq d'Azyr; *K*, stria medullaris; *I*, medial dorsal nucleus; *L*, fascicle retroflexus of Meynert; *N*, posterior commissure.

Original text: Corte horizontal del tálamo del ratón de veinte días. Método de Golgi. *A*, foco rayado; *B*, cuerpo geniculado externo; *C*, cuerpo geniculado interno; *D*, núcleo sensitivo; *E, F*, focos semilunares anterior y posterior; *H*, foco posterior; *G*, núcleo dorsal con el haz de Vicq d'Azyr; *K*, estría talámica; *I*, foco mediano; *L*, fascículo [retroflexo] de Meynert; *N*, comisura posterior.

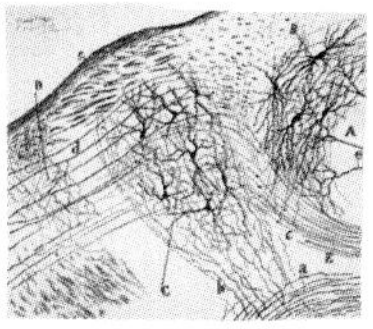

FIGURE 78.

Sagittal section of the thalamus in a nineteen-day-old mouse.

This figure was published in Cajal, S. R. (1899–1904) *Textura del sistema nervioso del hombre y de los vertebrados*. Madrid: Moya. (Figure 589).

FIGURE LEGEND: Sagittal section of the thalamus in a nineteen-day-old mouse. Part of the thalamus adjacent to the superior colliculus. Golgi method. *A*, Caudal pole of the sensory nucleus; *B*, caudal semilunar nucleus; *C*, posterior or prebigeminal nucleus; *D*, nucleus of the bigeminal optic pathway; *E*, central (or internal) medullary lamina of the thalamus; *a*, medial lemniscus; *b*, collaterals to the posterior nucleus; *c*, collaterals from the internal medullary lamina destined to the caudal semilunar nucleus; *d*, centrifugal optic pathway; *e*, centrifugal (corticofugal) fibers for the caudal semilunar nucleus; *f*, optic fibers destined to the superior colliculus.

Original section: Corte sagital del tálamo del ratón de diecinueve días. Porción posterior vecina del tubérculo cuadrigémino anterior. Método de Golgi. *A*, cabo posterior del foco sensitivo; *B*, núcleo semilunar posterior; *C*, foco posterior ó prebigeminal; *D*, foco de la vía óptica bigeminal; *E*, lámina blanca central del tálamo; *a*, lemnisco interno; *b*, colaterales para el núcleo posterior; *c*, colaterales de la lámina blanca para el núcleo semilunar posterior; *d*, vía óptica centrífuga; *e*, fibras centrífugas del foco semilunar posterior; *f*, fibras ópticas destinadas al tubérculo cuadrigémino.

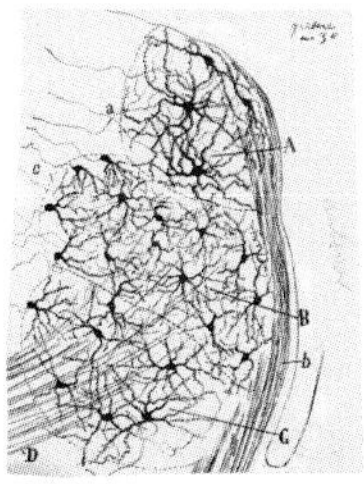

FIGURE 79.

Rostral pole of the thalamus parallel to the *stria medullaris* in a mouse.

This figure was published in Cajal, S. R. (1899–1904) *Textura del sistema nervioso del hombre y de los vertebrados*. Madrid: Moya. (Figure 593).

FIGURE LEGEND: Sagittal section of the rostral pole of the thalamus parallel to the stria medullaris in a fifteen-day-old mouse. Golgi method. *A*, Anterior dorsal nucleus; *B*, anterior ventral nucleus; *C*, anterior medial nucleus; *D*, mammillothalamic tract of Vicq d'Azyr; *a*, axons from the anterior dorsal nucleus; *b*, stria medullaris.

Original text: Corte sagital paralelo á la *stria thalami* del cabo anterior del tálamo del ratón de quince días. Método de Golgi. *A*, foco angular; *B*, lóbulo superior del núcleo dorsal; *C*, lóbulo inferior; *D*, cordón de Vicq d'Azyr; *a*, axones del foco angular; *b*, *stria thalami*.

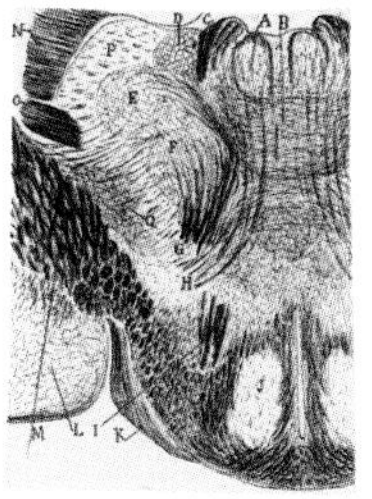

FIGURE 80.

Coronal section of the thalamus in a mouse.

This figure was published in Cajal, S. R. (1899–1904) *Textura del sistema nervioso del hombre y de los vertebrados*. Madrid: Moya. (Figure 594).

FIGURE LEGEND: Coronal section of the thalamus in a mouse. Golgi method. [*A*, Superior (or paraventricular) commissural nucleus]; *B*, interanterior medial nucleus; *C*, stria medullaris; *D*, anterior dorsal nucleus or nucleus of large cells; *E* and *F*, anterior ventral and anterior medial nuclei; *G*, mammillothalamic tract of Vicq d'Azyr; [H, descending fascicles of the paraventricular nucleus; *I*, fornix; *K*, optic chiasm; *L*, cortex of the temporal lobe; *M*, internal capsule; *N*, fimbria of Ammon's horn; *O*, projection tract of the olfactory cortex (stria terminalis)].

Original text: Corte frontal del tálamo del ratón. Método de Golgi. [*A*, núcleo comisural superior]; *B*, foco comisural interdorsal; *C*, estría talámica ó *taenia thalami; D*, foco angular ó de gruesas células; *E* y *F*, lóbulos superior é inferior del núcleo dorsal; *G*, cordón de Vicq d'Azyr; [*H*, fascículos descendentes del núcleo superior del rafe; *I*, trígono cerebral; *K*, kiasma óptico; *L*, corteza del lóbulo temporal; *M*, cápsula interna; *N*, fimbria ó cuerpo bordeando el asta de Ammon; *O*, vía de proyección de la corteza olfativa del cerebro].

Note from the author (J. D.): In brackets is the text added in the French version of the *Textura*: Cajal, S. R. (1909–1911) *Histologie du système nerveux de l'homme et des vertébrés*, trans. L. Azoulay. Paris: Maloine.

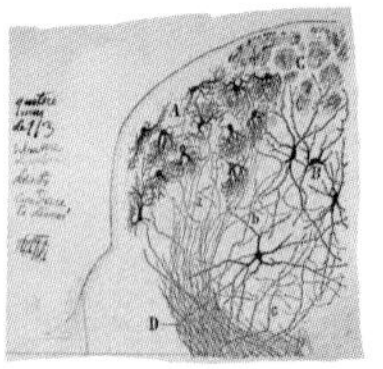

FIGURE 81.

Coronal section of the two habenular nuclei in a dog.

This figure was published in Cajal, S. R. (1899–1904) *Textura del sistema nervioso del hombre y de los vertebrados*. Madrid: Moya. (Figure 597).

FIGURE LEGEND: Coronal section of the two habenular nuclei in a dog. Golgi method. *A*, Medial nucleus; *B*, lateral nucleus; *C, stria medullaris; D*, fasciculus retroflexus of Meynert.

Original text: Corte frontal de los dos focos habenulares del perro. Método de Golgi. *A*, interno; *B*, externo; *C*, estría talámica; *D*, fascículo de Meynert.

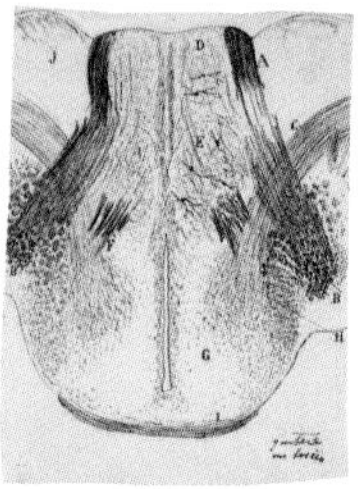

FIGURE 82.

Rostral pole of the thalamus in a ten-day-old mouse.

This figure was published in Cajal, S. R. (1903) Estudios talámicos. *Trab. Lab. Invest. Biol. Univ. Madrid* 2, 31–69 (Figure 15). It has also been reproduced as Figure 599 in Cajal, S. R. (1899–1904) *Textura del sistema nervioso del hombre y de los vertebrados*. Madrid: Moya.

FIGURE LEGEND: Coronal section of the rostral pole of the thalamus in a ten-day-old mouse. Golgi method. *A*, Stria medullaris; *B*, frontal olfactory pathway; *C*, stria terminalis; *F*, column of the fornix; *H*, bed nucleus of the stria terminalis; *J*, Ammon's horn; *I*, chiasm.

Original text: Corte frontal del cabo anterior del tálamo del ratón de diez días. Método de Golgi. *A, stria thalami; B*, vía olfativa frontal; *C, thenia* semicircular; *F*, columnas anteriores del fornix; *H*, foco de la estría semicircular; *J*, asta de Ammon; *I*, kiasma.

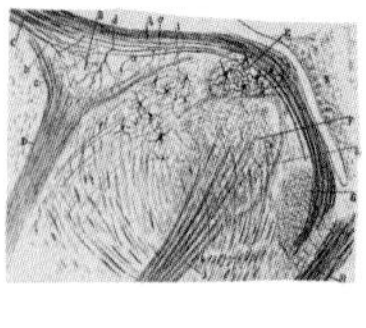

FIGURE 83.

Section of the thalamus in a mouse.

This figure was published in Cajal, S. R. (1899–1904) *Textura del sistema nervioso del hombre y de los vertebrados*. Madrid: Moya. (Figure 602).

FIGURE LEGEND: Sagittal section of the thalamus in a mouse a few days old. Golgi method. *A*, Stria medullaris; *B*, lateral habenular nucleus; *C*, fibers destined to the habenular commissure; *D*, fasciculus retroflexus (fasciculus of Meynert); *J*, mammillothalamic tract (bundle of Vicq d'Azyr); *F, K*, anteroventral and anteromedial nuclei; *G*, nucleus of the stria medullaris; [*H*, columns of the fornix; *I*, rostral pole of the sensory nucleus of the thalamus; *d*, collaterals of the stria medullaris for the habenular nuclei.]

Original text: Corte sagital del tálamo del ratón de pocos días. Método de Golgi. *A, stria thalami; B*, foco habenular externo; *C*, fibras destinadas á la comisura interhabenular; *D*, fascículo de Meynert; *J*, cordón de Vicq d'Azyr; *F, K*, focos del núcleo talámico-dorsal; *G*, núcleo de la *stria thalami*; [*H*, columnas anteriores del fornix; *I*, comienzo del núcleo sensitivo del tálamo; *d*, colaterales de la *stria thalami* para el ganglio de la habénula].

Note from the author (J. D.): In brackets is the text added in the French version of the *Textura*: Cajal, S. R. (1909–1911) *Histologie du système nerveux de l'homme et des vertébrés*, trans. L. Azoulay. Paris: Maloine.

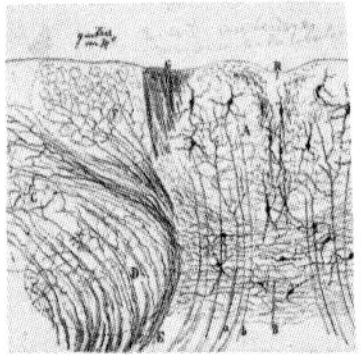

FIGURE 84.

Rostral pole of the thalamus in a ten-day-old mouse.

This figure was published in Cajal, S. R. (1899–1904) *Textura del sistema nervioso del hombre y de los vertebrados*. Madrid: Moya. (Figure 605).

FIGURE LEGEND: Coronal section of the rostral pole of the thalamus in a 10-day-old mouse. *A*, Paraventricular nucleus; *B*, interanterior medial nucleus; *C, D*, anterior ventral and anterior medial nuclei; *E*, mammillothalamic tract of Vicq d'Azyr; *G*, stria medullaris; *F*, anterior dorsal nucleus; *R*, raphe.

Original text: Corte transversal del cabo anterior del tálamo (ratón de diez días). Método de Golgi. *A*, foco comisural superior; *B*, núcleo comisural interdorsal; *C, D*, subfocos del núcleo dorsal; *E*, fibras del cordón de Vicq d'Azyr; *G*, estría talámica; *F*, foco angular; *R*, rafe.

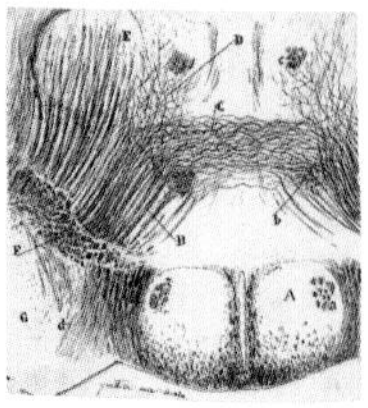

FIGURE 85.

Section of the optic thalamus in a mouse.

This figure was published in Cajal, S. R. (1903) Las fibras nerviosas de origen cerebral del tubérculo cuadrigémino anterior y tálamo óptico. *Trab. Lab. Invest. Biol. Univ. Madrid* 2, 5–21 (Figure 9). It has also been reproduced as Figure 609 in Cajal, S. R. (1899–1904) *Textura del sistema nervioso del hombre y de los vertebrados*. Madrid: Moya.

FIGURE LEGEND: Coronal and rostroventrally oblique section of the optic thalamus in a mouse a few days old. The section is oblique from bottom to top and from front to back. *A*, Principal or ventromedial nucleus of the tuber cinereum; *B*, fibers of cortical origin coursing to the intermedioventral commissure and the ventral medial nucleus; *C*, commissural fibers; *D*, ascending branches; *E*, sensory nucleus; *F*, internal capsule; *a*, column of the fornix; *b*, tract of Vicq d'Azyr (mammillothalamic tract); *c*, fasciculus retroflexus of Meynert.

Original text: Corte frontal del tálamo óptico del ratón de pocos días. El corte es oblicuo de abajo á arriba y de delante á atrás. *A*, foco principal ó anterior del *tuber cinereum; B*, fibras cerebrales para la comisura y foco mediano; *C*, ramas comisurales; *D*, ramas ascendentes; *E*, foco sensitivo; *F*, cápsula interna; *a*, pilar del fornix; *b*, haz de Vicq d'Azyr; *c*, cordón de Meynert.

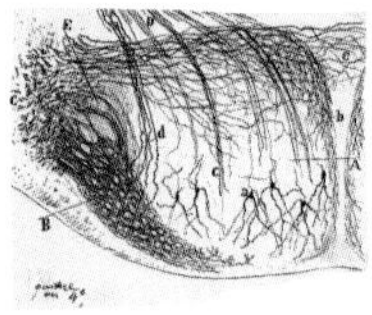

FIGURE 86.

Coronal section of the two mammillary nuclei in a kitten.

This figure was published in Cajal, S. R. (1903) Estudios talámicos. *Trab. Lab. Invest. Biol. Univ. Madrid* 2, 31–69 (Figure 7). It has also been reproduced as Figure 630 in Cajal, S. R. (1899–1904) *Textura del sistema nervioso del hombre y de los vertebrados*. Madrid: Moya.

FIGURE LEGEND: Coronal section of the two mammillary nuclei in a kitten a few days old. *A*, Medial mammillary nucleus; *B*, lateral mammillary nucleus with plexus of arborizations formed by the mammillary peduncle; *C*, trunks of mammillary peduncle fibers cut tangentially; *D*, fascicle of the efferent mammillary pathway; *E*, section of fascicles of the column of the fornix; *a*, cells of the medial mammillary nucleus; *b*, terminal arborizations of medial peduncular branches; *c*, fascicles of efferent axons; *d*, axons arising in the lateral mammillary nucleus; *e*, commissure formed by the decussation of medial peduncular branches.

Original text: Corte frontal de los dos ganglios mamilares del gato de pocos días. *A*, núcleo mamilar interno; *B*, núcleo mamilar externo con su plexo de arborizaciones formadas por el pedúnculo mamilar; *C*, tallos de este pedúnculo cortados de través; *D*, manojos de la vía mamilar eferente; *E*, corte de los haces de la columna anterior del fornix; *a*, células del foco mamilar interno; *b*, ramificaciones terminales de las ramas pedunculares internas; *c*, haces de axones eferentes; *d*, axones nacidos en el foco mamilar externo; *e*, comisura formada por el cruce de ramas pedunculares internas.

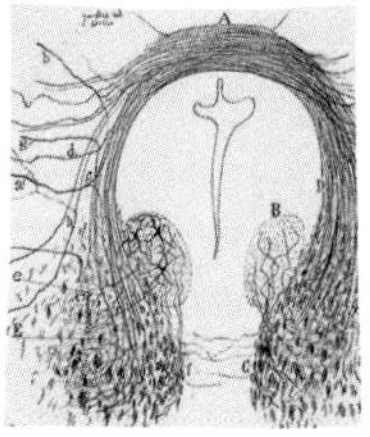

FIGURE 87.

Coronal section of the posterior commissure in an eight-day-old kitten.

This figure was published in Cajal, S. R. (1899–1904) *Textura del sistema nervioso del hombre y de los vertebrados*. Madrid: Moya. (Figure 645).

FIGURE LEGEND: Coronal section of the posterior commissure in an eight-day-old kitten. Golgi method. *A*, Posterior commissure; *B*, nucleus of Darkschewitsch; *C*, remnant of the medial longitudinal fasciculus; *E*, interstitial nucleus; *a, b, c*, fibers entering the commissure; *e*, collaterals arising from these fibers coursing to the interstitial nucleus.

Original text: Corte frontal de la comisura posterior del gato de ocho días. Método de Golgi. *A*, comisura posterior; *B*, foco de Darkschewitsch; *C*, resto del fascículo longitudinal posterior; *E*, foco intersticial; *a, b, c*, fibras que ingresan en la comisura; *e*, colaterales de éstas para el foco intersticial.

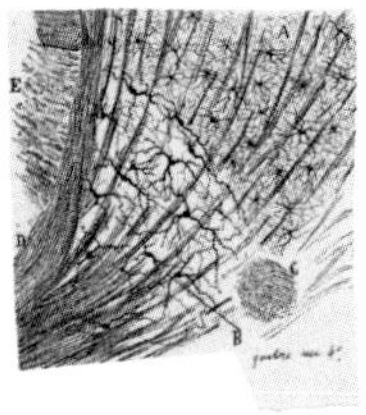

FIGURE 88.

Sagittal section of the brain in a twenty-day-old mouse.

This figure was published in Cajal, S. R. (1899–1904) *Textura del sistema nervioso del hombre y de los vertebrados*. Madrid: Moya. (Figure 653).

FIGURE LEGEND: Portion of a sagittal section of the brain in a twenty-day-old mouse. Golgi method. *A*, Caudate nucleus; *B*, central nucleus or nucleus of giant cells; *D*, internal capsule; *C*, anterior commissure; *E*, stria terminalis.

Original text: Trozo de un corte sagital del cerebro del ratón de veinte días. Método de Golgi. *A*, núcleo caudal; *B*, foco central ó de células gigantes; *D*, cápsula interna; *C*, comisura anterior; *E*, *thænia semicircularis*.

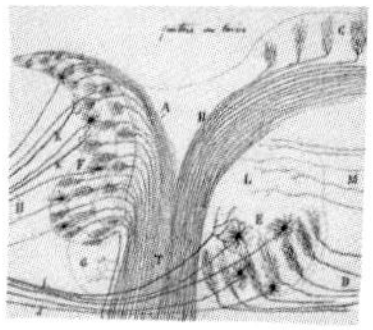

FIGURE 89.

Diagram of the termination of the optic nerve in a cat.

This figure was published in Cajal, S. R. (1903) Plan de estructura del tálamo óptico. *Rev. Med. Cirug. Práct*, May, 1–24 (Figure 1).

FIGURE LEGEND: Diagram of the termination of the optic nerve in a cat. *T*, Optic tract; *A*, bundle for the lateral geniculate body; *B*, optic fibers destined to the superior colliculus; *C*, superior colliculus; *D*, auditory pathway or lateral lemniscus; *E*, inferior segment of the medial geniculate body; *L*, superior segment of the medial geniculate body; *G*, inferior segment of the lateral geniculate body; *F*, principal or dorsal nucleus of the lateral geniculate body; *I*, thalamocortical auditory pathway; *H*, thalamocortical optic pathway. (The figure represents a very lateral sagittal section.)

Original text: Esquema de la terminación del nervio óptico en el gato. *T*, cinta óptica; *A*, haz para el cuerpo geniculado externo; *B*, cordón óptico para el tubérculo cuadrigémino anterior; *C*, tubérculo cuadrigémino; *D*, vía acústica ó lemnisco externo; *E*, foco inferior del cuerpo geniculado interno; *L*, foco superior de éste; *G*, foco inferior del ganglio geniculado externo; *F*, foco principal ó dorsal de éste; *I*, vía acústica tálamo-cortical; *H*, vía óptica tálamo-cortical. (El conjunto representa un corte sagital muy lateral.)

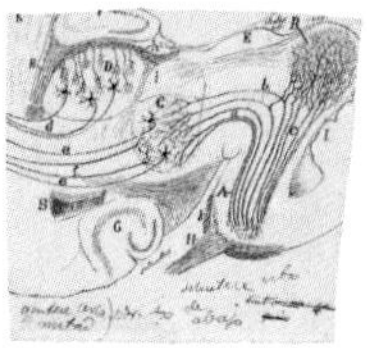

FIGURE 90.

Diagram of the auditory pathways in a rabbit and a mouse.

This figure was published in Cajal, S. R. (1903) Plan de estructura del tálamo óptico. *Rev. Med. Cirug. Práct*, May, 1–24 (Figure 2).

FIGURE LEGEND: Diagram of the auditory pathways in a rabbit and a mouse. *A*, Auditory pathway or lateral lemniscus; *B*, nucleus of the inferior colliculus; *C*, inferior segment of the medial geniculate body; *D*, lateral geniculate body; *E*, superior colliculus; *F, G*, Ammon's horn; *H*, trigeminal nerve; *e*, superior auditory or thalamocortical pathway; *d*, superior visual or thalamocortical pathway; *f*, cortical auditory fibers.

Original text: Conjunto esquemático de las vias acústicas del conejo y ratón. *A*, lemnisco externo ó vía acústica central; *B*, núcleo del tubérculo cuadrigémino posterior; *C*, lóbulo inferior del cuerpo geniculado interno; *D*, cuerpo geniculado externo; *E*, tubérculo cuadrigémino anterior; *F, G*, asta de Ammon; *H*, nervio trigémino; *e*, via acústica superior ó tálamo-cortical; *d*, vía visual superior ó tálamo-cortical; *f*, fibras acústicas cerebrales.

SECTION E

Optic Lobe of Lower Vertebrates

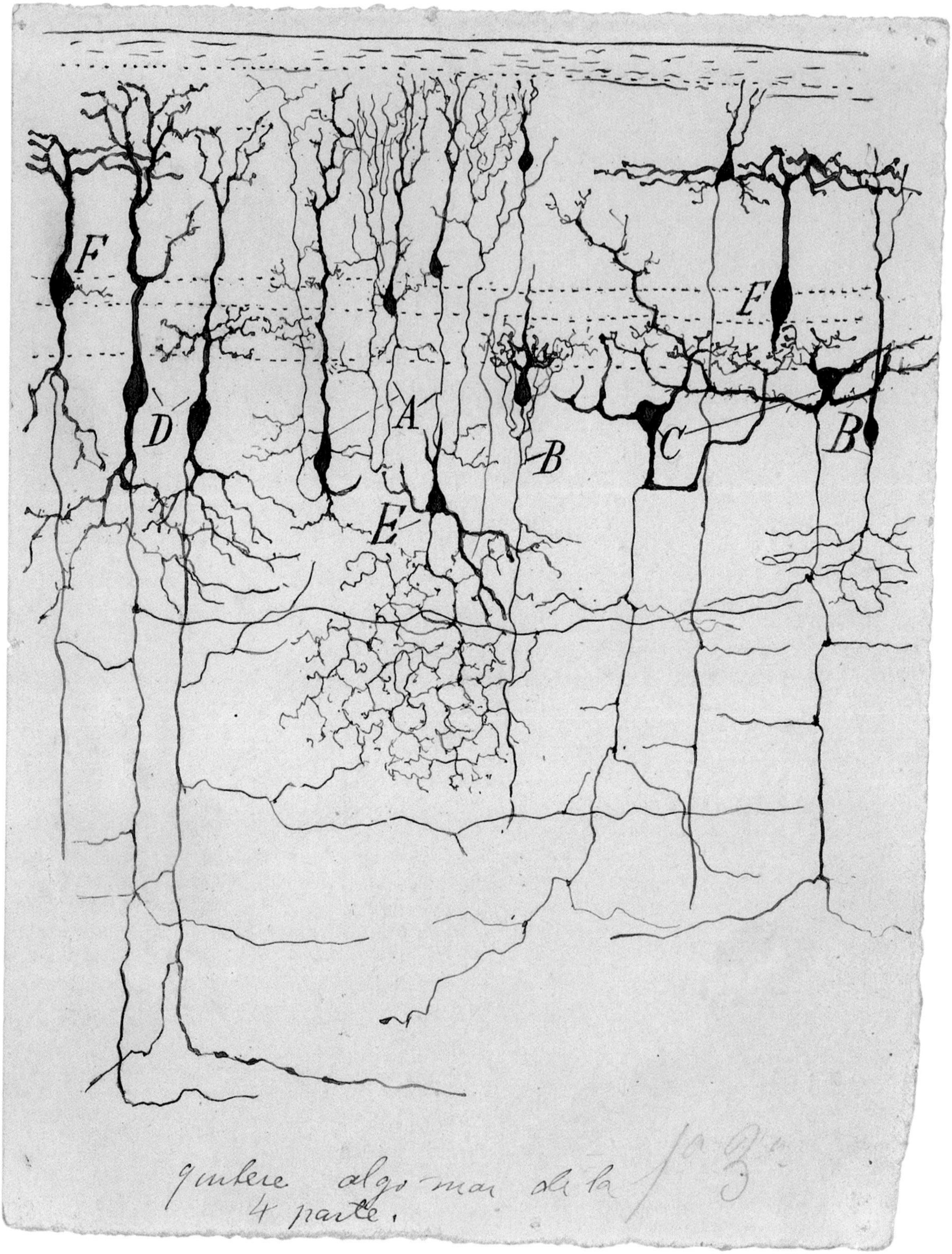

FIGURE 91. Sagittal section of the optic lobe in a young sparrow.

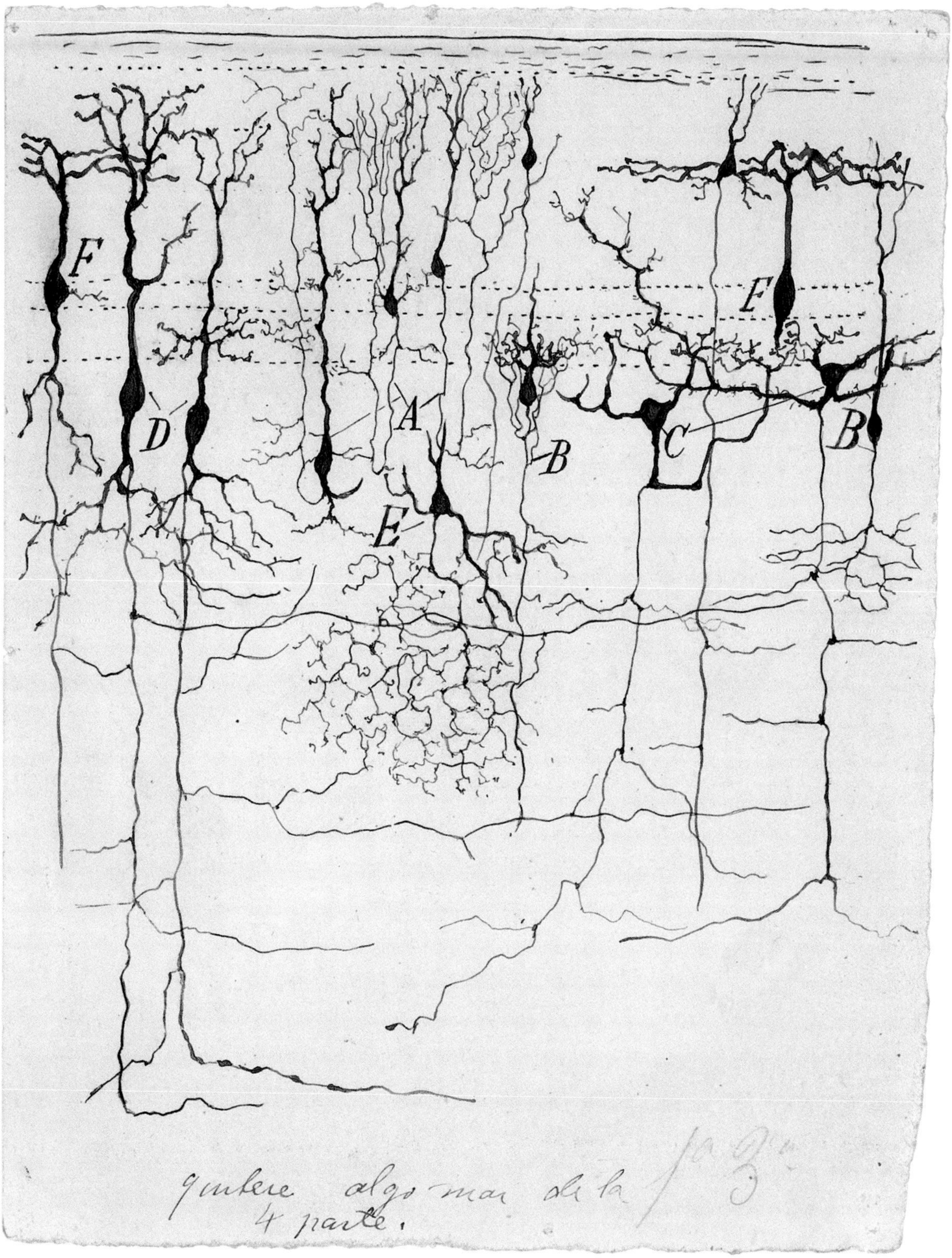

FIGURE 92. Transverse section of the optic tectum in a sparrow.

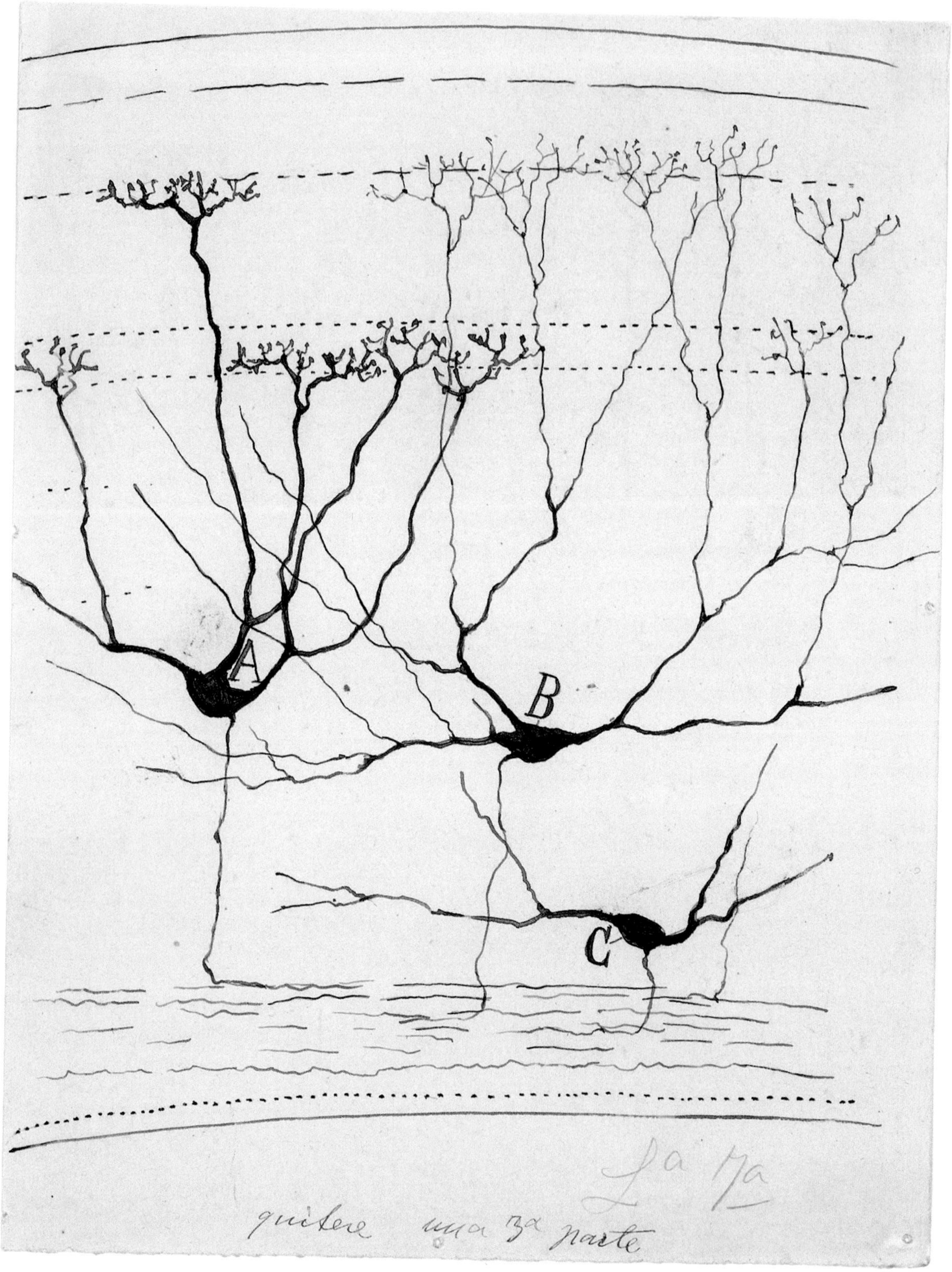

FIGURE 93. Optic tectum in a sparrow.

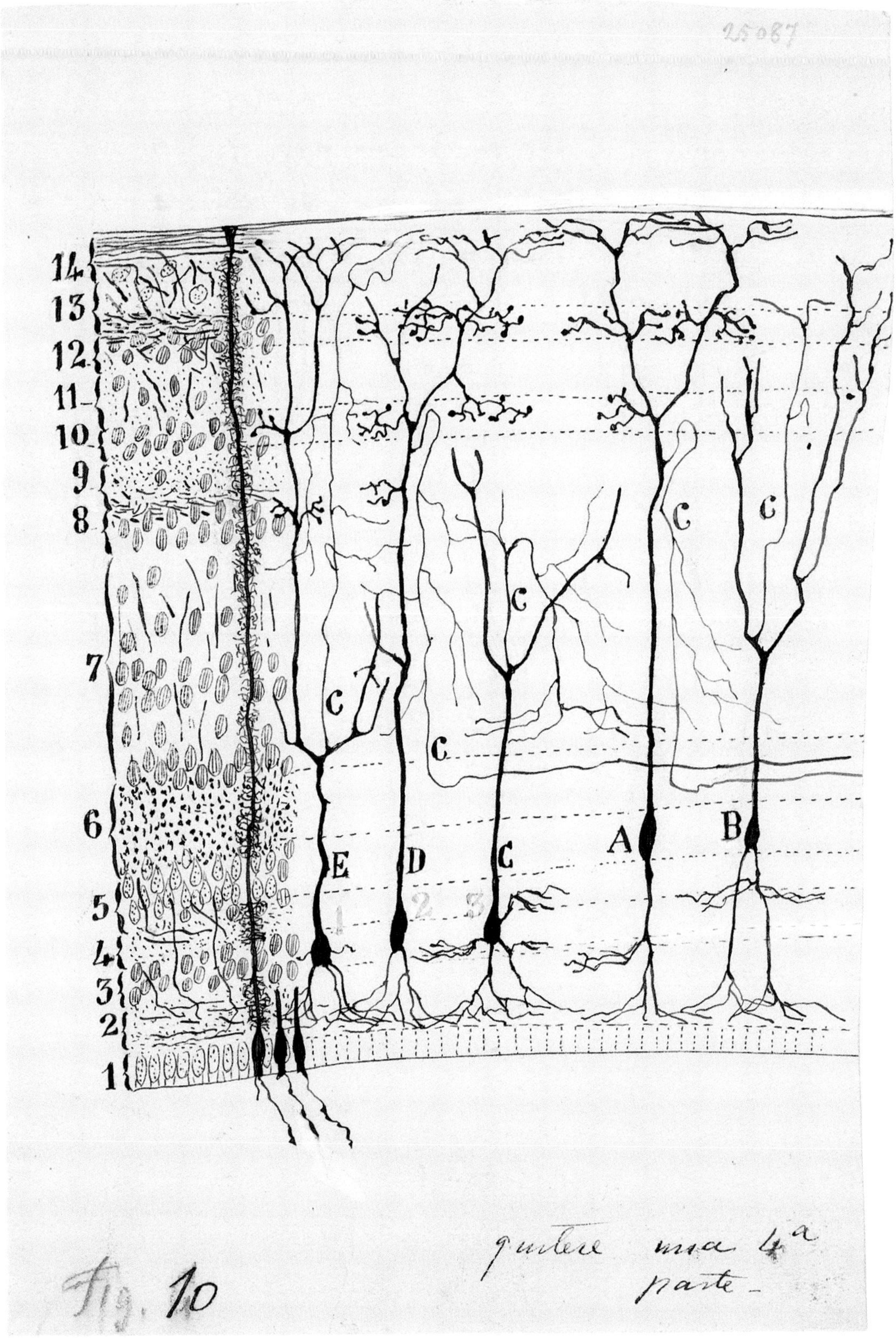

FIGURE 94. Optic lobe in a chameleon.

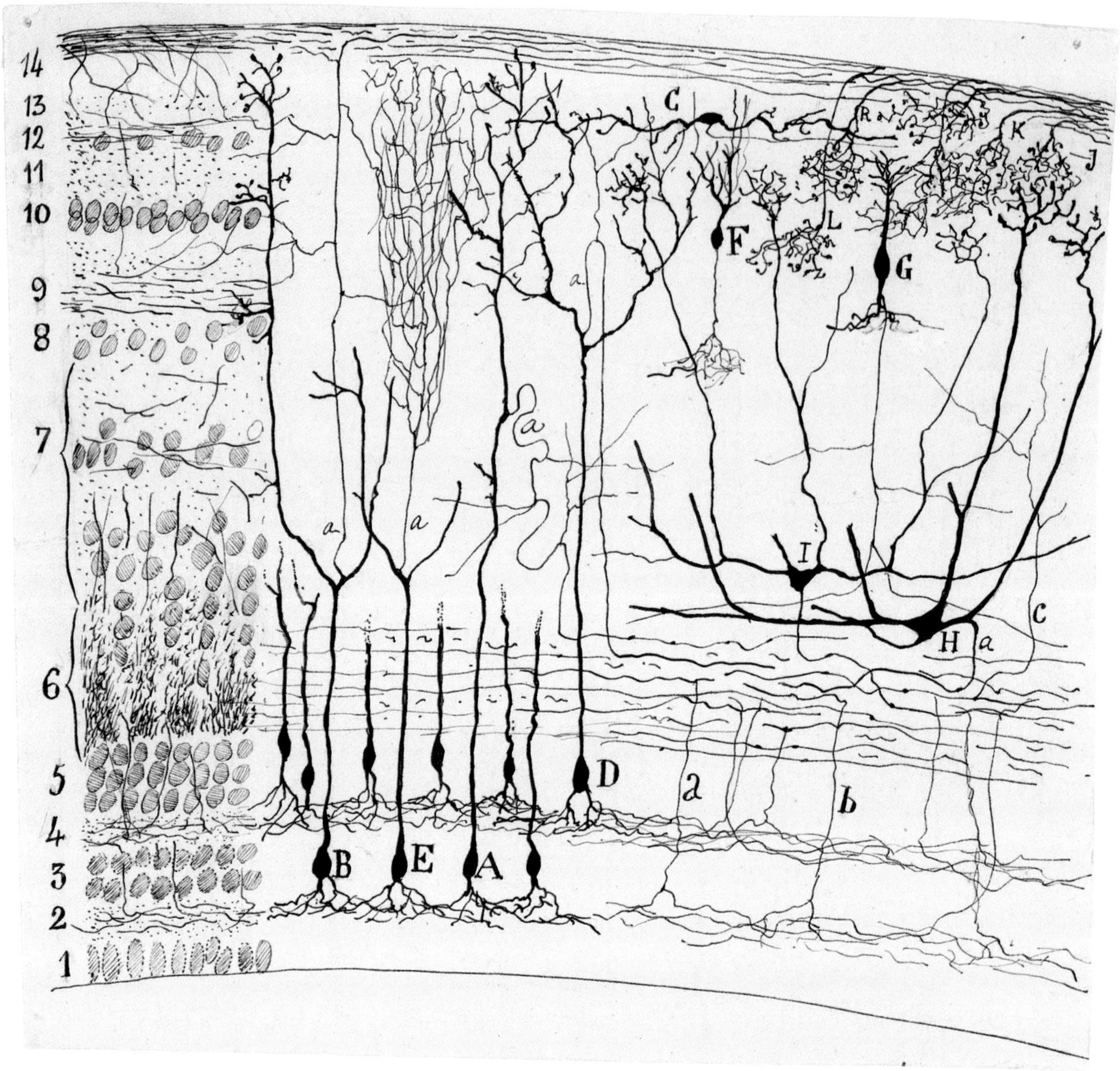

FIGURE 95. Transverse section of the optic lobe in a reptile.

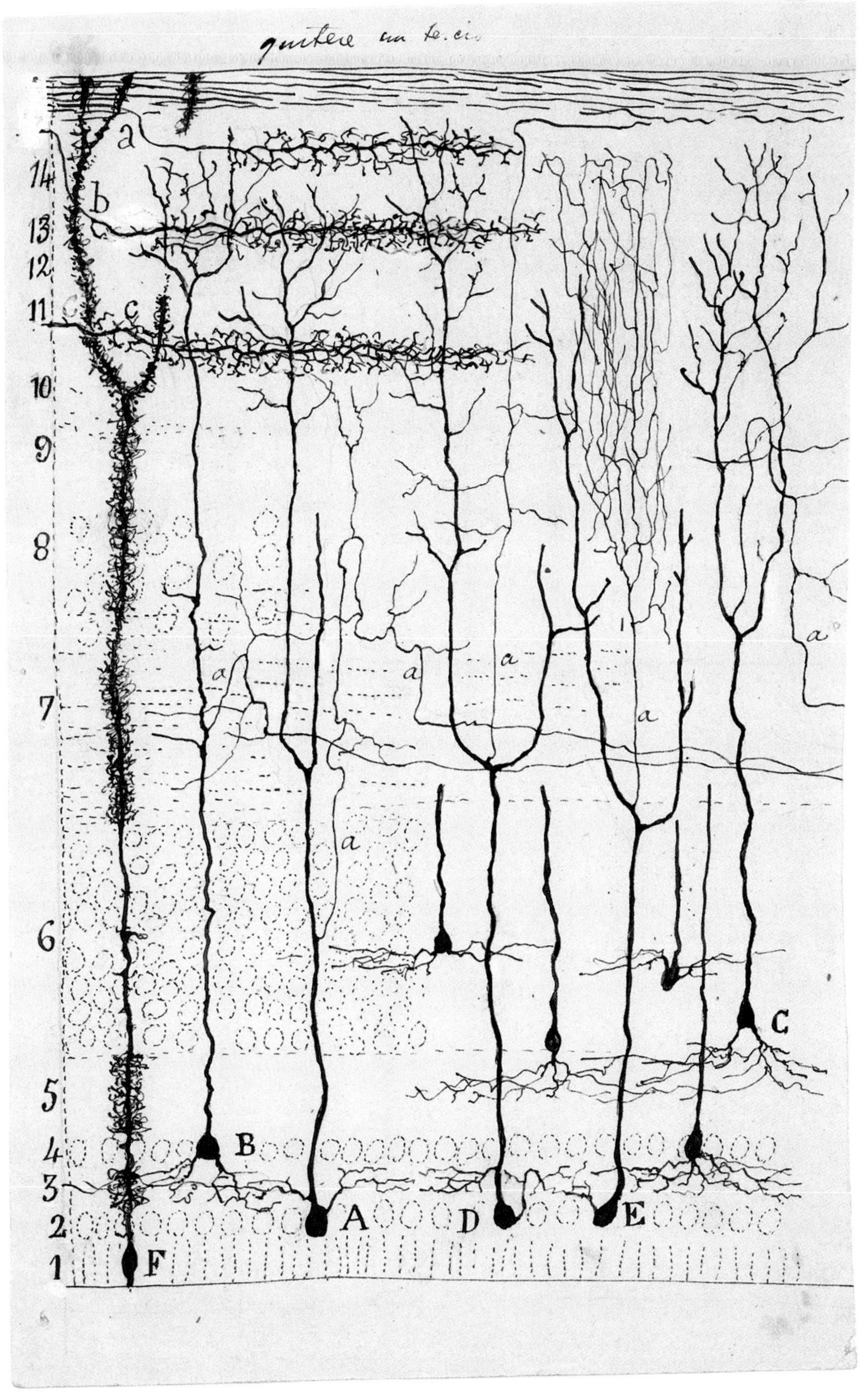

FIGURE 96. Optic tectum in a frog.

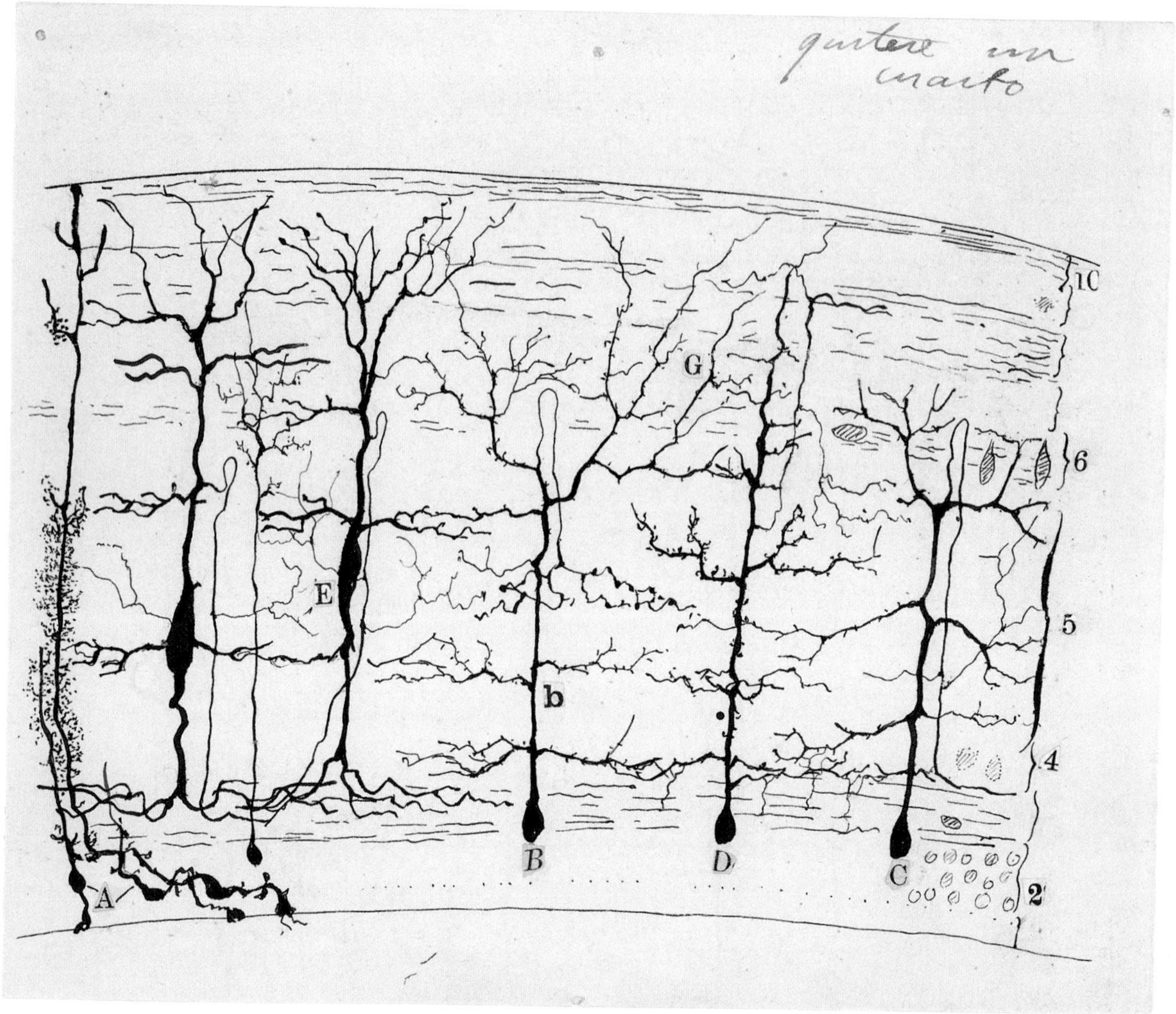

FIGURE 97. Optic tectum in a fish.

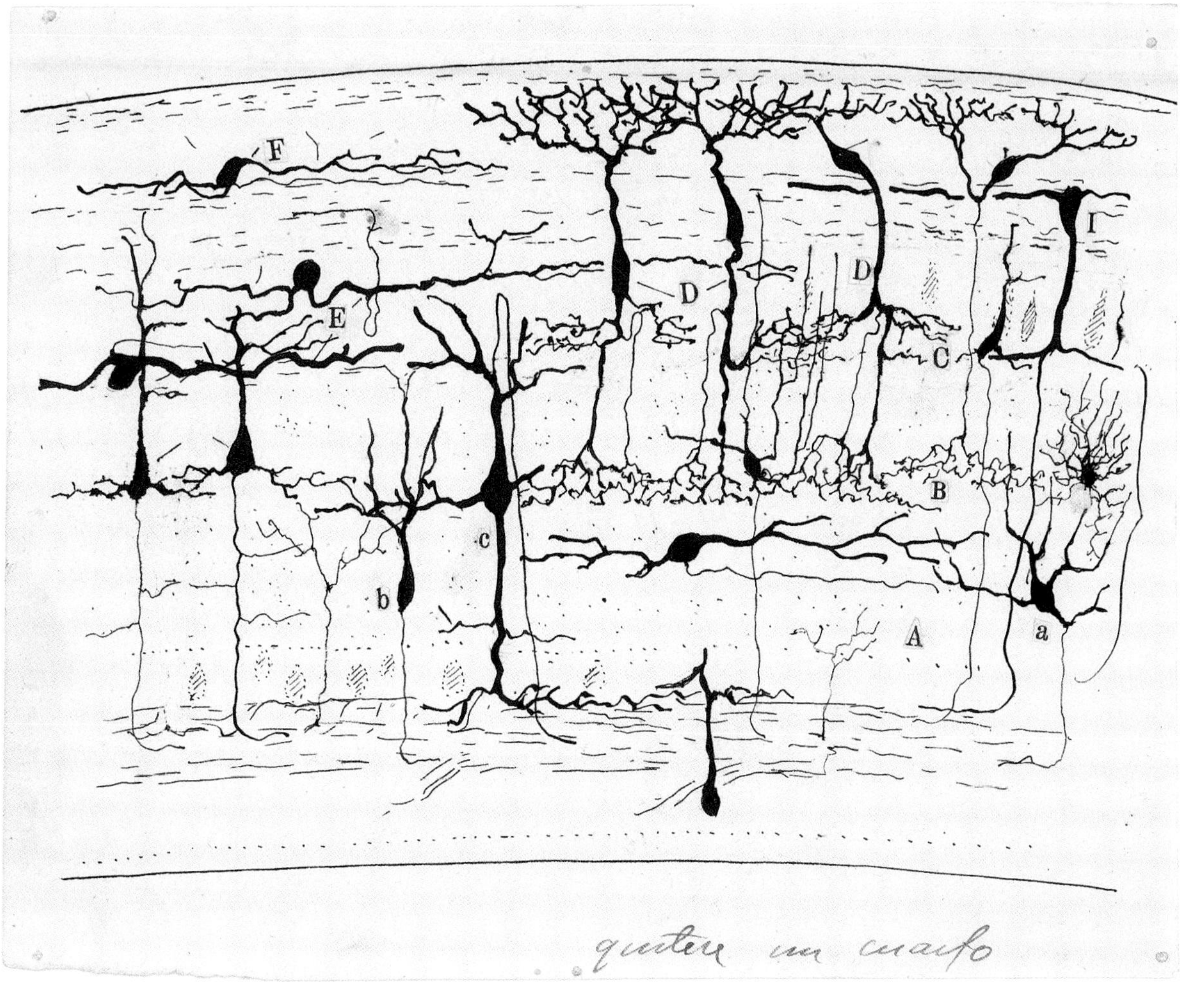

FIGURE 98. Optic lobe in a barb.

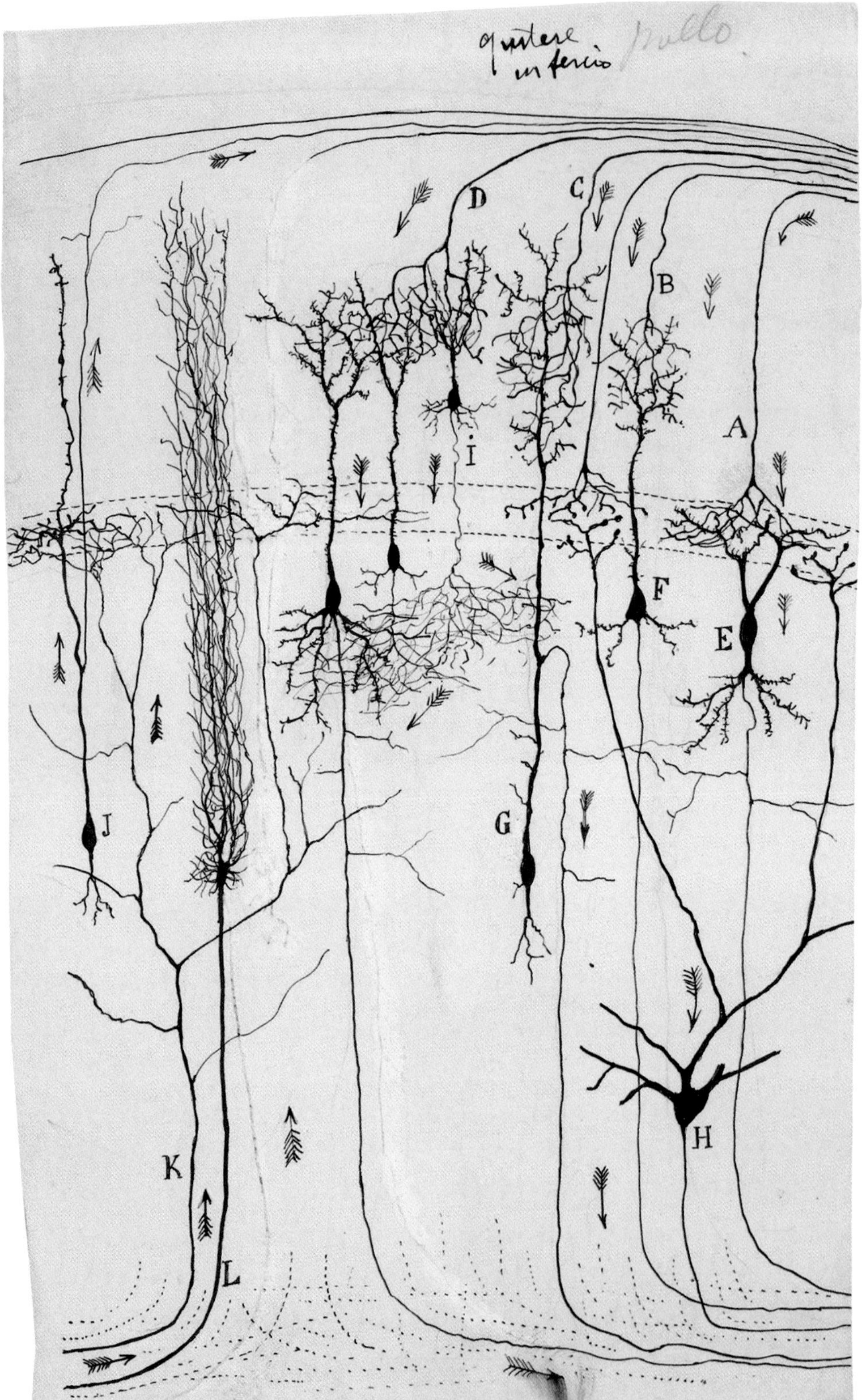

FIGURE 99. Main intercellular connections in the optic lobe of birds.

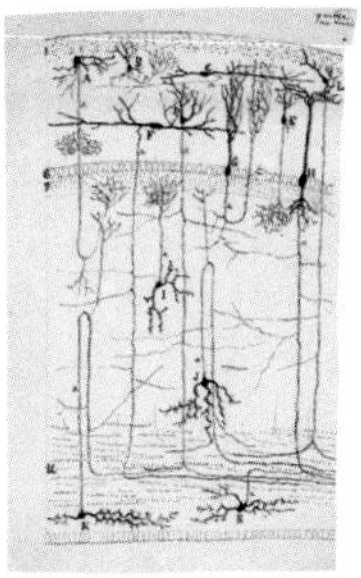

FIGURE 91.

Sagittal section of the optic lobe in a young sparrow.

This figure was published in Cajal, S. R. (1899–1904) *Textura del sistema nervioso del hombre y de los vertebrados*. Madrid: Moya. (Figure 475).

FIGURE LEGEND: Sagittal section of the optic lobe in a sparrow a few days old. After P. Ramón [and according to information provided by the Golgi method]. Numbers indicate the order and numbering of the layers

Original text: Corte antero-posterior del lóbulo óptico del pájaro de pocos días. (Células tomadas de preparados de P. Ramón [y según las enseñanzas del método de Golgi]). Los números marcan los de las capas.

Note from the author (J. D.): In brackets is the text added in the French version of the *Textura*: Cajal, S. R. (1909–1911) *Histologie du système nerveux de l'homme et des vertébrés*, trans. L. Azoulay. Paris: Maloine.

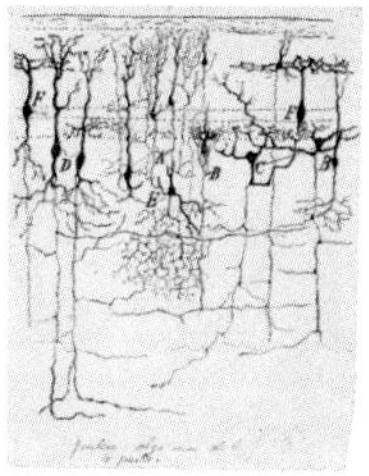

FIGURE 92.

Transverse section of the optic tectum in a sparrow.

This figure was published in Ramón, P. (1898) Centros ópticos de las aves. *Rev. Trim. Micrograf. Madrid* 3, 141–197 (Figure 7). It has also been reproduced as Figure 476 in Cajal, S. R. (1899–1904) *Textura del sistema nervioso del hombre y de los vertebrados*. Madrid: Moya.

FIGURE LEGEND: [Transverse section of the optic tectum. Sparrow, a few days after hatching. Golgi method. *A*, Cells with short, recurrent axons of the fifth, sixth, and eighth layers]; *B*, *E*, short axon cells of the eighth layer; *C*, triangular cells of the eighth layer with spiny ascending processes; *D*, cell with conical soma and a central axon; *F*, cell of the sixth layer with horizontal dendritic tuft.

Original text: [Corte frontal del techo óptico del gorrión de algunos días. Método de Golgi]. *A*, células de cilindro-eje corto y recurrente de las quinta, sexta y octava capas; *B*, célula de cilindro-eje corto de la octava capa; *C*, células triangulares con expansiones espinosas ascendentes de la octava capa; *D*, células de cuerpo cónico con cilindroeje central; *F*, célula de penacho protoplasmático horizontal de la sexta capa; *E*, célula de cilindro-eje corto de la octava capa.

Note from the author (J. D.): In brackets is the text added in the French version of the *Textura*: Cajal, S. R. (1909–1911) *Histologie du système nerveux de l'homme et des vertébrés*, trans. L. Azoulay. Paris: Maloine.

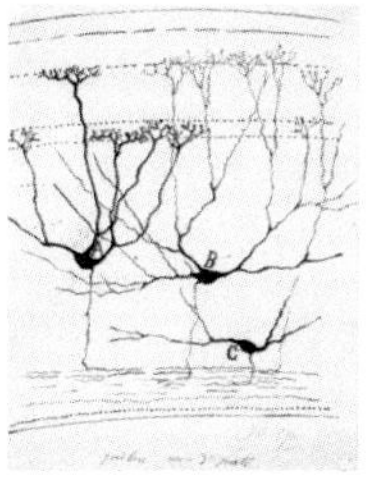

FIGURE 93.

Optic tectum in a sparrow.

This figure was published in Ramón, P. (1898) Centros ópticos de las aves. *Rev. Trim. Micrograf. Madrid* 3, 141–197 (Figure 11). It has also been reproduced as Figure 479 in Cajal, S. R. (1899–1904) *Textura del sistema nervioso del hombre y de los vertebrados*. Madrid: Moya.

FIGURE LEGEND: Transverse section of the optic tectum in a sparrow a few days old. Golgi method. *A*, Ganglion cell with thick dendrites; *B*, ganglion cell with thin dendritic processes; *C*, another ganglion cell of the thirteenth layer. (After P. Ramón).

Original text: [Corte frontal del techo óptico del gorrión de algunos días. Método de Golgi]. *A*, célula ganglionar de ramas [protoplásmicas] gruesas; *B*, célula ganglionar de ramitas [dendríticas] finas; *C*, célula de idéntica clase de la capa décima-tercera. [(Según P. Ramón)].

Note from the author (J. D.): In brackets is the text added in the French version of the *Textura*: Cajal, S. R. (1909–1911) *Histologie du système nerveux de l'homme et des vertébrés*, trans. L. Azoulay. Paris: Maloine.

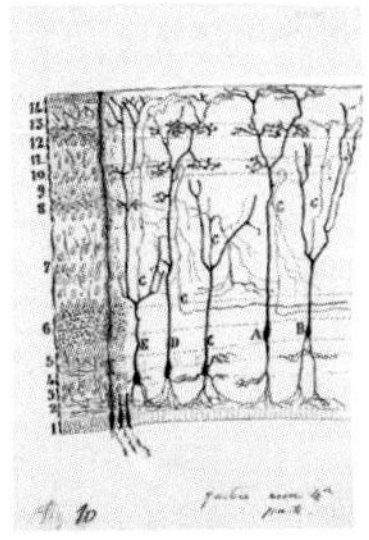

FIGURE 94.

Optic lobe in a chameleon.

This figure was published in Ramón, P. (1896) Estructura del encéfalo del camaleón. *Rev. Trimest. Micrograf.* 1, 46–82 (Figure 9). It has also been reproduced as Figure 24 in Cajal, S. R. (1899–1904) *Textura del sistema nervioso del hombre y de los vertebrados*. Madrid: Moya.

FIGURE LEGEND: Optic lobe in a chameleon. Golgi method. The left side of the drawing shows the fourteen layers that can be outlined in carmine or Weigert-Pal preparations. *A*, *C*, *D*, Varieties of shepherd's crook cells; *B* and *E*, cells with an ascending axon; *c*, axon. (After P. Ramón).

Original text: Lóbulo óptico del camaleón. Método de Golgi. *La porción derecha de la figura presenta las 14 capas que pueden distinguirse en las preparaciones al carmín y en las teñidas por el procedimiento de Weigert-Pal.* *A*, *C*, *D*, variedades de células de cayado; *B* y *E*, células de cilindro-eje ascendente; *c*, cilindro-eje; [los números indican el orden de las capas, de la profundidad a la superficie]. (según P. Ramón).

Note from the author (J. D.): The text between asterisks appears in the original publication only.

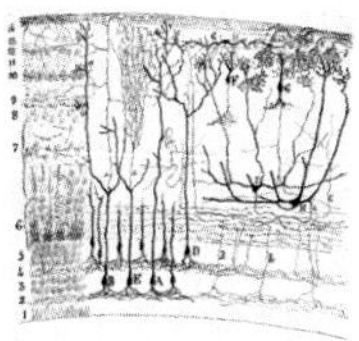

FIGURE 95.

Transverse section of the optic lobe in a reptile.

This figure was published in Cajal, S. R. (1899–1904) *Textura del sistema nervioso del hombre y de los vertebrados*. Madrid: Moya. (Figure 481).

FIGURE LEGEND: [Transverse section of the] optic lobe in a reptile [(*Lacerta muralis*). (After P. Ramón). Golgi method]. The left side of the drawing shows the fourteen layers that can be outlined in carmine or Weigert-Pal preparations. [The numbering of the layers is the reverse as that adopted for birds.] *A*, shepherd's crook cell; *B*, *E*, cells with ascending axons; *H*, ganglion cells.

Original text: [Corte frontal] del segmento del lóbulo óptico de un reptil [(*Lacerta muralis*). (Según P. Ramón). Método de Golgi]. La porción izquierda de la figura presenta las 14 capas que pueden distinguirse en las preparaciones al carmín y en las teñidas por el procedimiento de Weigert- Pal. [La numeración de las capas se ha hecho aquí en sentido inverso al adoptado para los pájaros]. *A*, célula con cilindro-eje en cayado; *B* y *E*, células de cilindro-eje ascendente; *H*, células gangliónicas.

Note from the author (J. D.): In brackets is the text added in the French version of the *Textura*: Cajal, S. R. (1909–1911) *Histologie du système nerveux de l'homme et des vertébrés*, trans. L. Azoulay. Paris: Maloine.

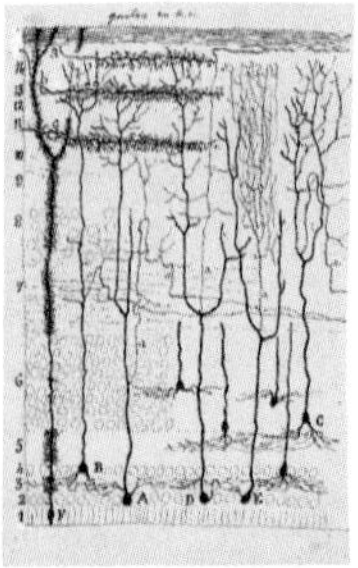

FIGURE 96.

Optic tectum in a frog.

This figure was published in Cajal, S. R. (1899–1904) *Textura del sistema nervioso del hombre y de los vertebrados*. Madrid: Moya. (Figure 484).

FIGURE LEGEND: Transverse section of the optic tectum in a frog. (After P. Ramón.) Golgi method. Figures indicate the numbering of layers starting at the ventricle. *A, B, C*, types of shepherd's crook cells; *D*, cells with centrifugal or peripheral axons coursing to the retina; *E*, short axon cells; *a, b, c*, arborizations of optic fibers coming from the retina.

Original text: Corte del techo óptico de la rana (tomada de preparaciones de P. Ramón). Método de Golgi. Los números señalan el de las capas, á comenzar por la profunda ó epitelial. *a, b, c*, arborizaciones de fibras ópticas ó llegadas de la retina; *A, B, C*, tipos de células de cayado; *D*, células de axon periférico; *E*, otra de axon corto.

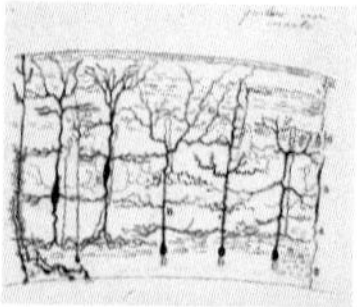

FIGURE 97.

Optic tectum in a fish.

This figure was published in Ramón, P. (1899) El lóbulo óptico de los peces (teleosteos). *Rev. Trim. Micrograf. Madrid* 4, 87–107 (Figure 1). It has also been reproduced as Figure 485 in Cajal, S. R. (1899–1904) *Textura del sistema nervioso del hombre y de los vertebrados*. Madrid: Moya.

FIGURE LEGEND: [Transverse section of] the optic tectum [in a fish (*Barbus fluviatilis*)]. Golgi method. 1, epithelial layer; 2, central gray matter; 3, deep white matter; 4, intermediate gray substance; 5, large plexiform layer; 6, layer of fusiform cells and deep optic fibers; 7, deep plexiform layer of the retinal formation; 8, intermediate optic fiber layer; 9, superficial plexiform layer of the retinal formation; 10, superficial optic fiber layer. *A*, Ependymal cells; *B*, cell with looped axon; *C*, shepherd's crook cell; *D*, cell with centrifugal axon going to the retina; *E*, large shepherd's crook cells of the fifth layer; *F*, cell without axon. [(After P. Ramón.)]

Original text: [Corte frontal del] techo óptico [en los peces (*Barbus fluviatilis*)]. Método de Golgi. 1.ª, capa epitelial; 2.ª, capa de la substancia gris central; 3.ª, capa de la substancia blanca profunda; 4.ª, substancia gris media; 5.ª, capa plexiforme grande; 6.ª, capa de los corpúsculos fusiformes y de las fibras ópticas profundas; 7.ª, capa plexiforme profunda de la región retiniana; 8.ª, capa media de las fibras ópticas; 9.ª, capa plexiforme superficial de la región retiniana; 10.ª, capa cortical de las fibras ópticas. *A*, células epiteliales; *B*, célula de cilindro-eje arqueado; *C*, célula de cilindroeje en cayado; *D*, célula de cilindro-eje retiniano; *E*, corpúsculos grandes en cayado de la capa quinta; *F*, célula sin cilindro-eje. [(Según P. Ramón).]

Note from the author (J. D.): In brackets is the text added in the French version of the *Textura*: Cajal, S. R. (1909–1911) *Histologie du système nerveux de l'homme et des vertébrés*, trans. L. Azoulay. Paris: Maloine.

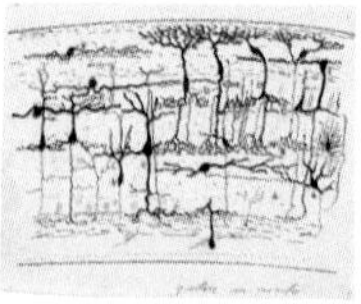

FIGURE 98.

Optic lobe in a barb.

This figure was published in Ramón, P. (1899) El lóbulo óptico de los peces (teleosteos). *Rev. Trim. Micrograf. Madrid* 4, 87–107 (Figure 3). It has also been reproduced as Figure 487 in Cajal, S. R. (1899–1904) *Textura del sistema nervioso del hombre y de los vertebrados*. Madrid: Moya.

FIGURE LEGEND: [Transverse section of the optic lobe in a barb (*Barbus fluviatilis*)]. Golgi method. *A*, Inner region of the fifth layer; *B*, intermediate region of the same with its central plexus; *C*, outer region, formed mainly by dendritic branchlets of fusiform cells; *a*, ganglion cell of the fifth layer; *b*, pyramidal cells with central axons; *c*, shepherd's crook cell with dendrites contributing to the central plexus; *d*, tangential cell of the fifth layer; e, small stellate cell. [(After P. Ramón.)]

Original text: [Corte frontal del techo óptico del barbo (*Barbus fluviatilis*)]. Método de Golgi. *A*, región inferior de la capa quinta; *B*, región media de la misma y plexo central de la misma; *C*, región superior de la misma capa formada principalmente por ramitos protoplásmicos de los corpúsculos fusiformes; *a*, célula ganglionar de esta capa; *b*, corpúsculos piramidales de cilindro-eje central; *c*, célula de cayado con ramas protoplasmáticas para el plexo central; *d*, célula tangencial de la capa quinta; e, célula estelar de pequeño tamaño. [(Según P. Ramón).]

Note from the author (J. D.): In brackets is the text added in the French version of the *Textura*: Cajal, S. R. (1909–1911) *Histologie du système nerveux de l'homme et des vertébrés*, trans. L. Azoulay. Paris: Maloine.

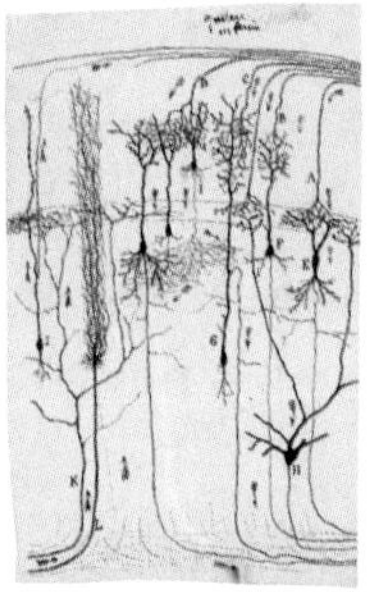

FIGURE 99.

Main intercellular connections in the optic lobe of birds.

This figure was published in Cajal, S. R. (1899–1904) *Textura del sistema nervioso del hombre y de los vertebrados*. Madrid: Moya (Figure 488).

FIGURE LEGEND: Diagram showing the main intercellular connections in the optic lobe of birds. Arrows indicate the direction of current flow. *A, B, C, D*, Afferent optic fibers; *E, F*, long axon cell; *G*, shepherd's crook cell; *J*, cell with centrifugal axon; *K, L*, fibers coming from other centers; *H*, ganglion cell.

Original text: Esquema de las principales articulaciones neuronales del lóbulo óptico de las aves. Las flechas marcan el sentido de las corrientes. *A, B, C, D*, fibras ópticas aferentes; *E, F*, células de axon largo; *G*, célula de cayado; *J*, célula de axon centrífugo; *K, L*, fibras centrífugas; *H*, corpúsculo ganglionar.

SECTION F

Retina of Vertebrates

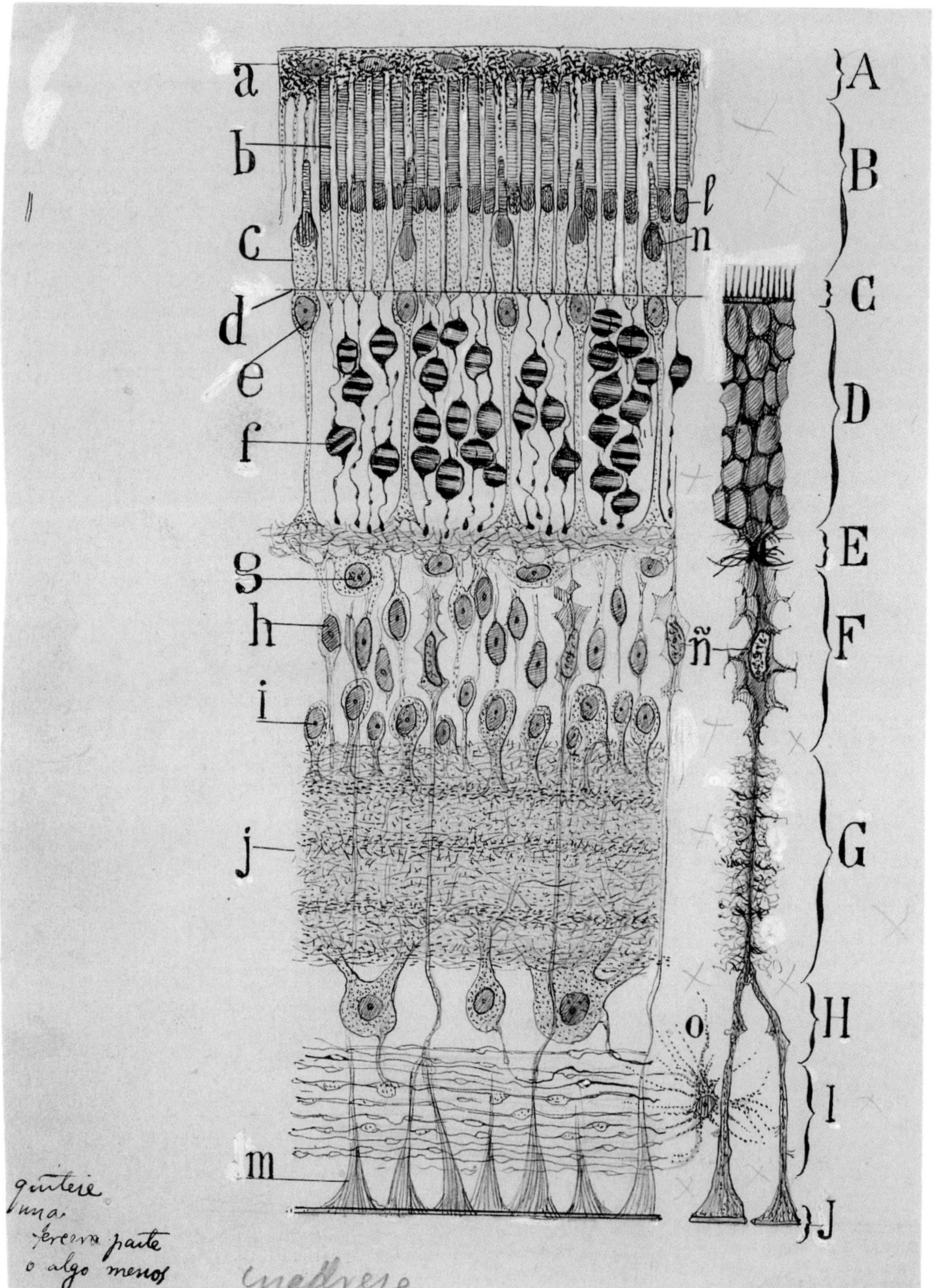

FIGURE 100. Perpendicular section in a dog retina.

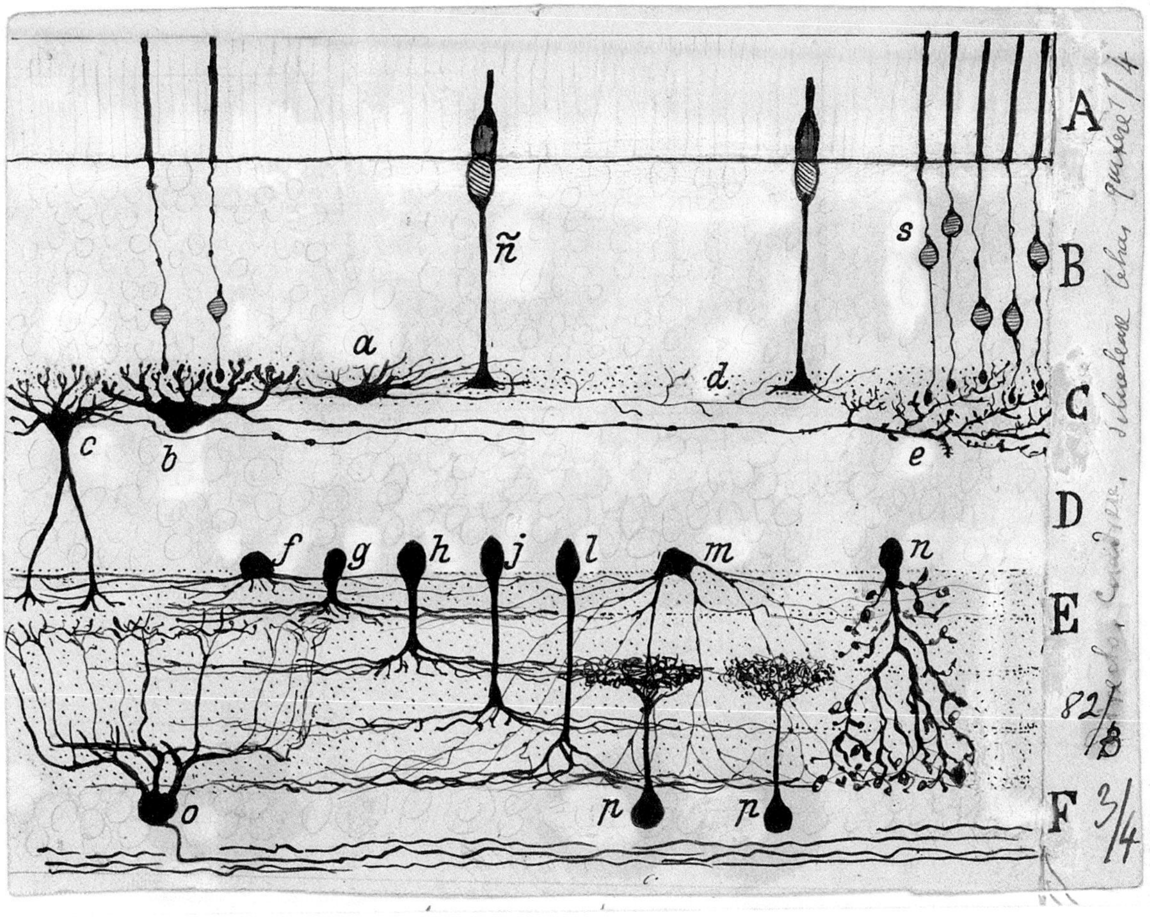

FIGURE 101. Perpendicular section in a mammalian retina.

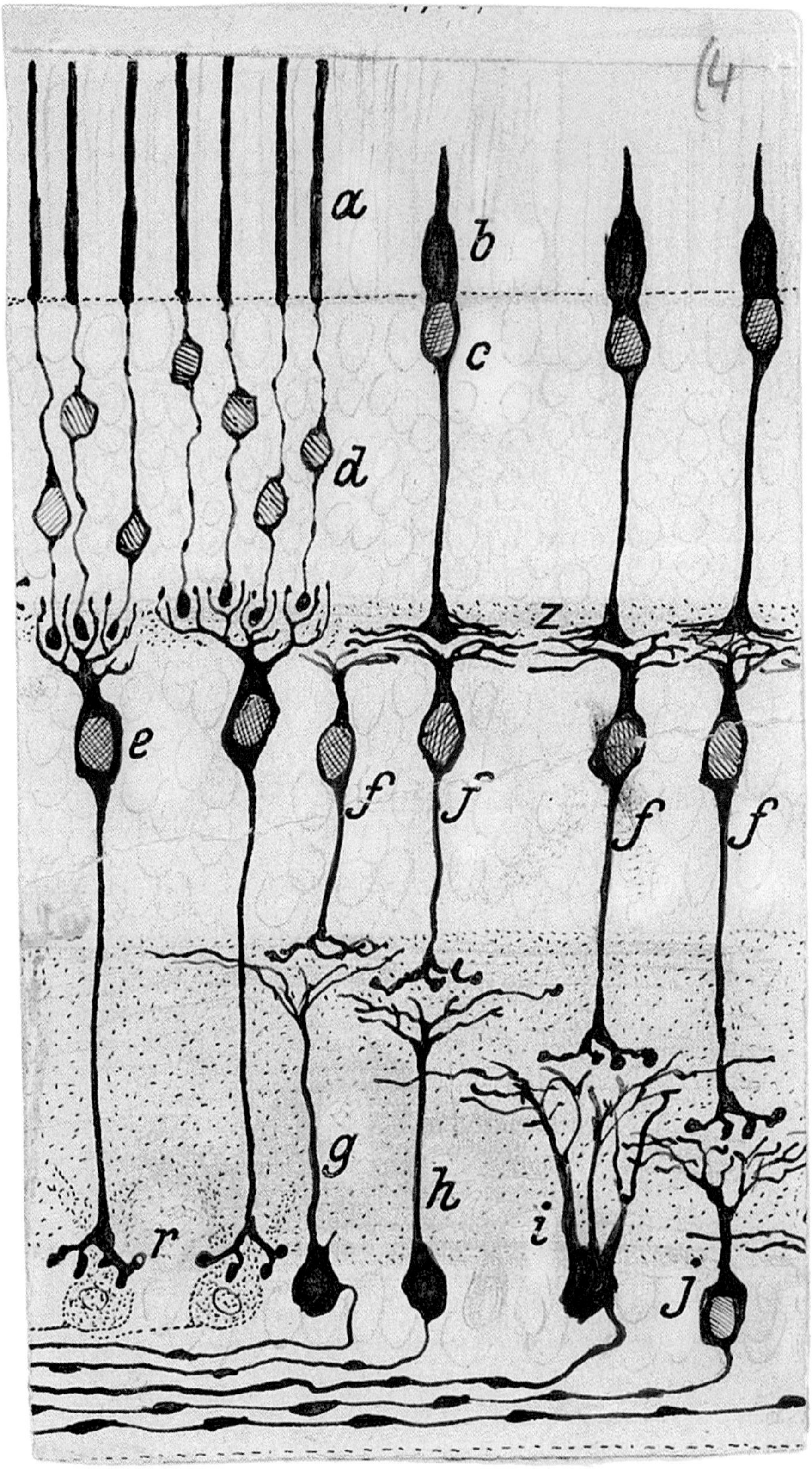

FIGURE 102. Retina in a mammal.

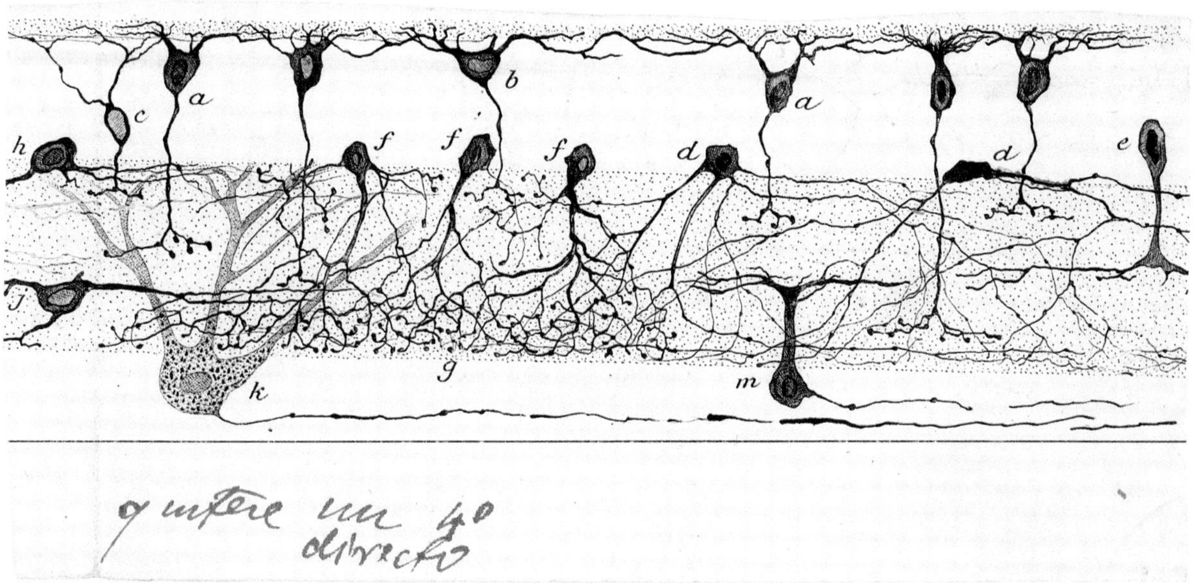

FIGURE 103. Cone bipolars and amacrine cells in a dog retina.

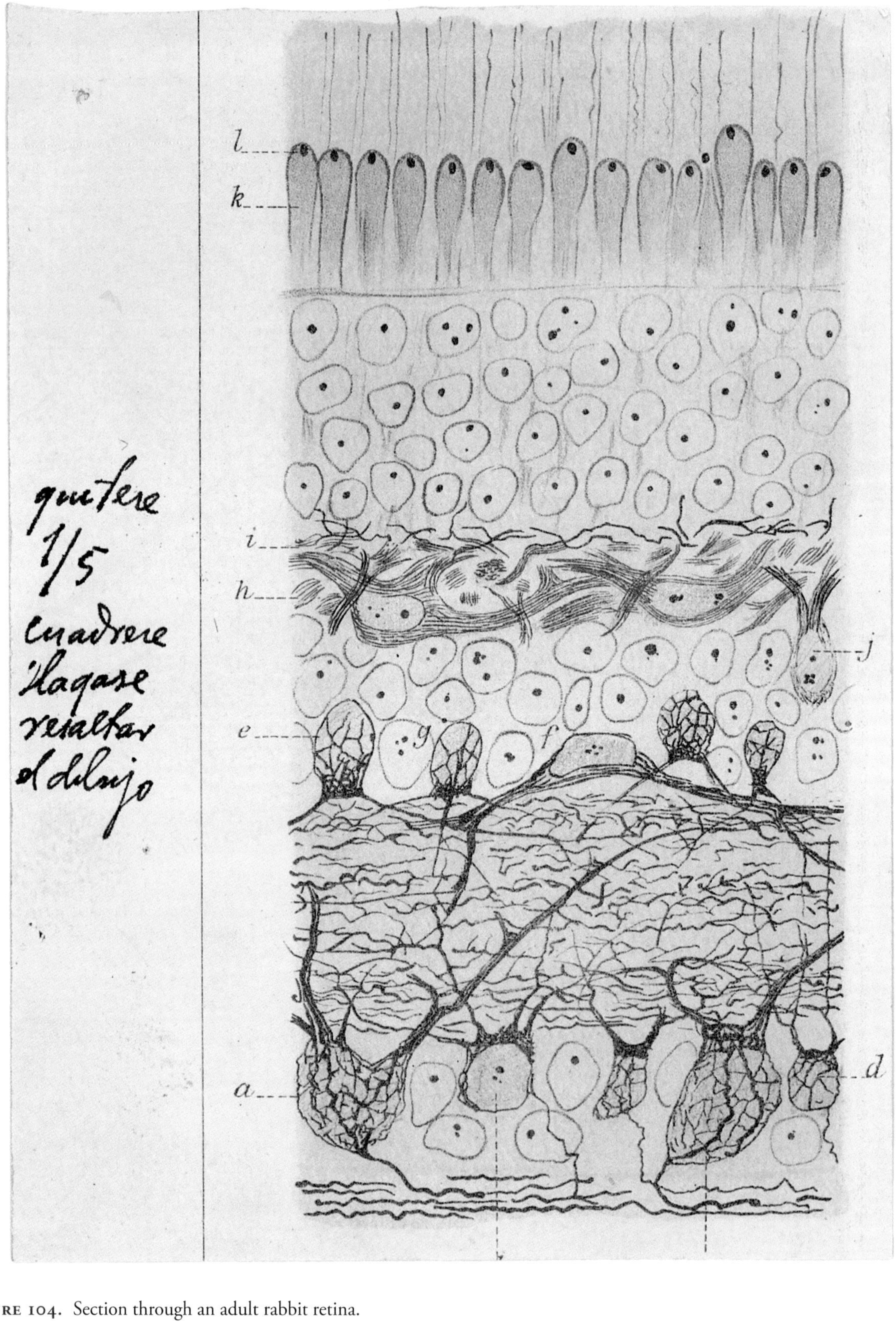

FIGURE 104. Section through an adult rabbit retina.

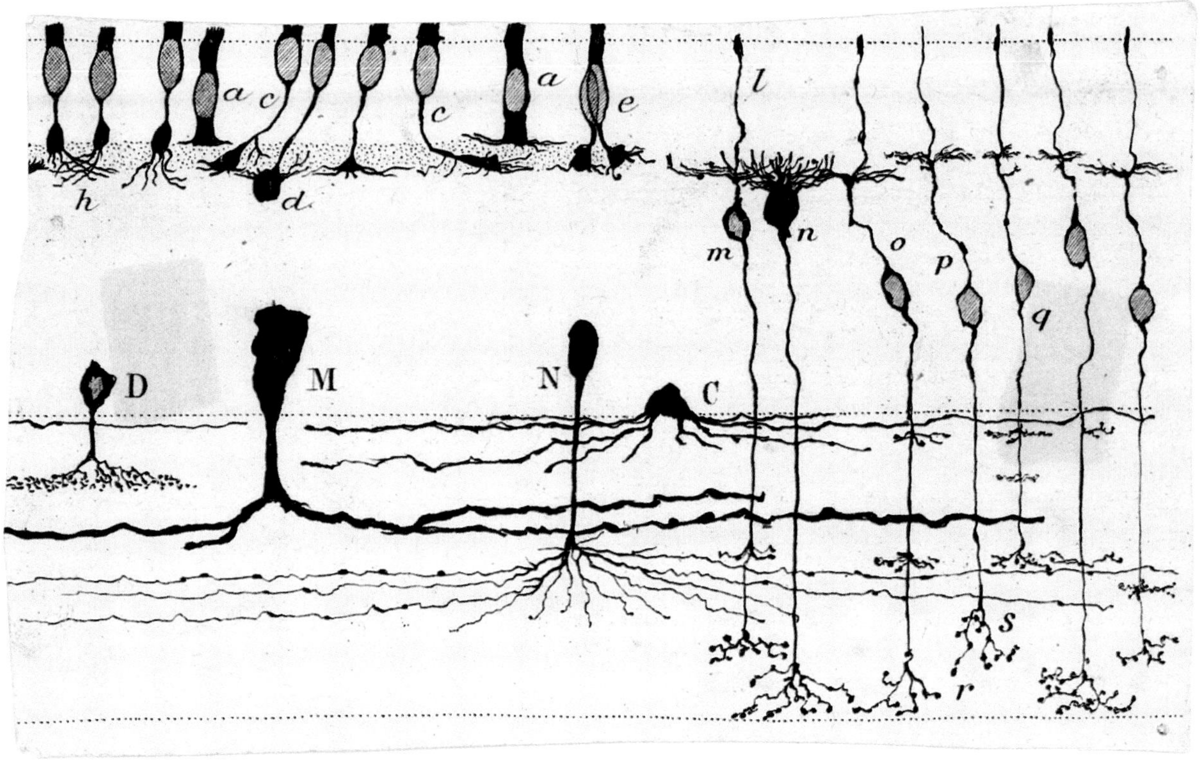

FIGURE 105. Retina in a chicken.

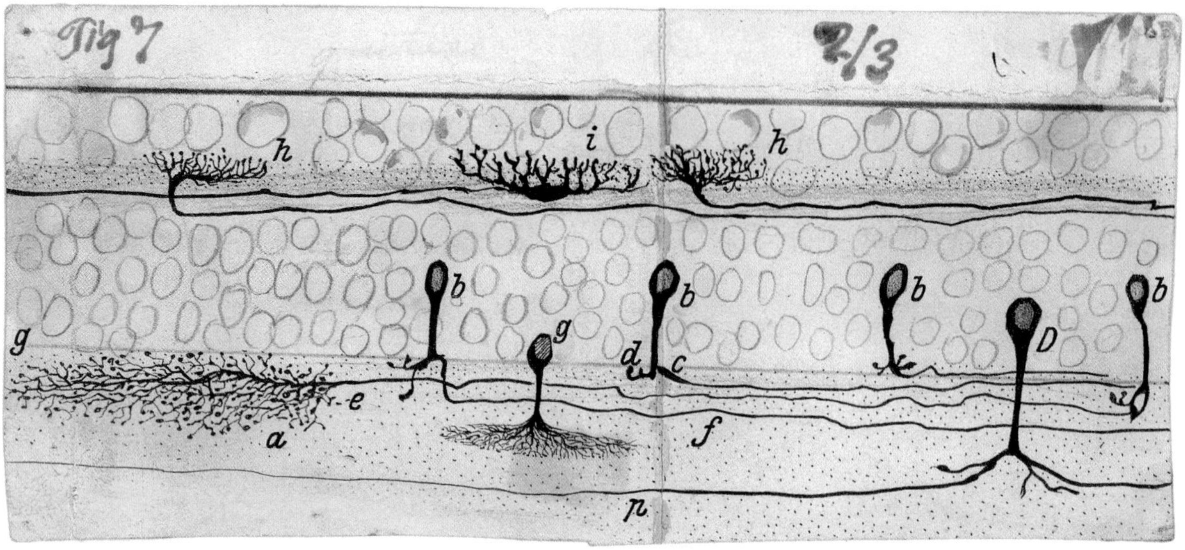

FIGURE 106. Retina in a bird (greenfinch).

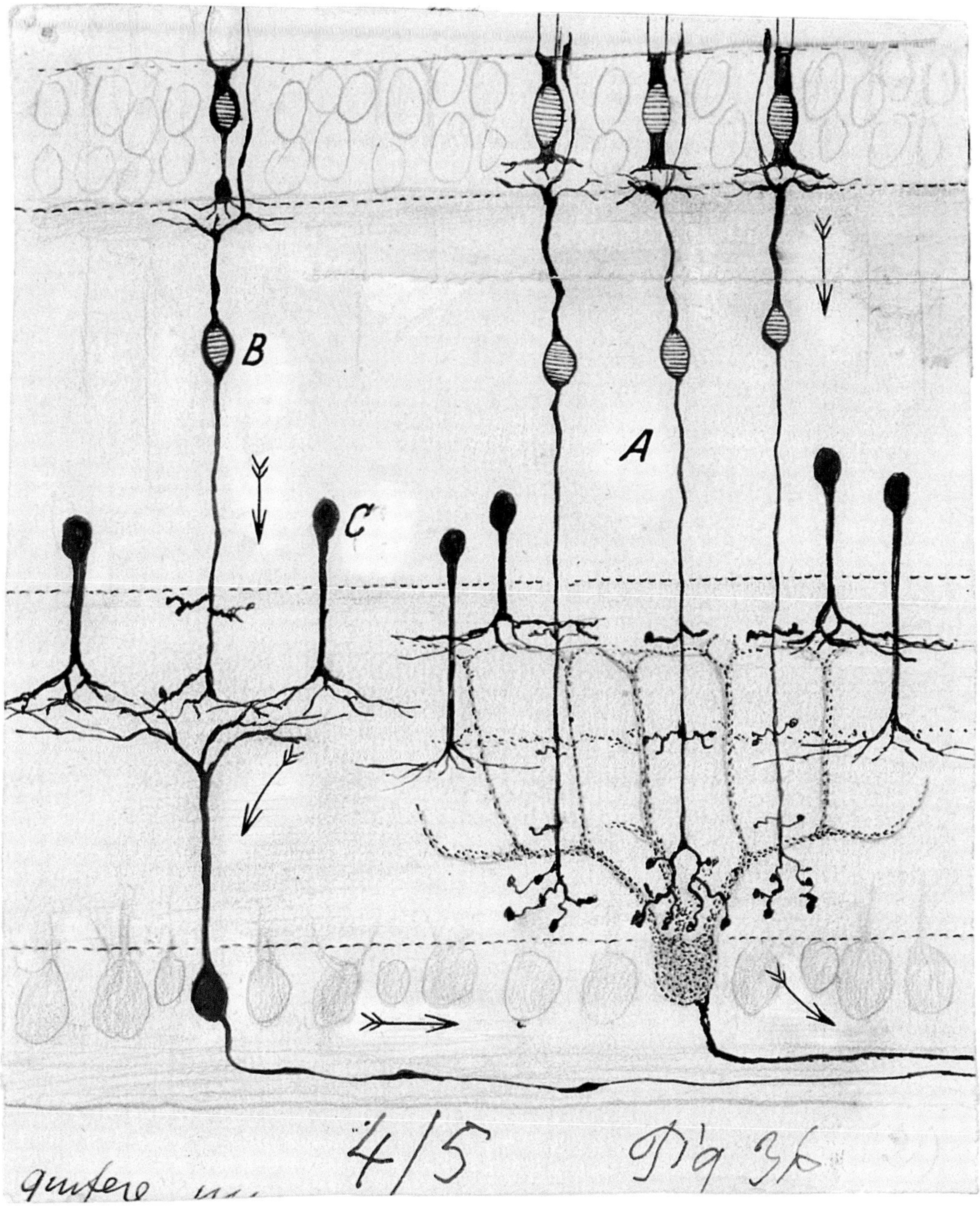

FIGURE 107. Two possible channels for visual stimuli in the retina of birds.

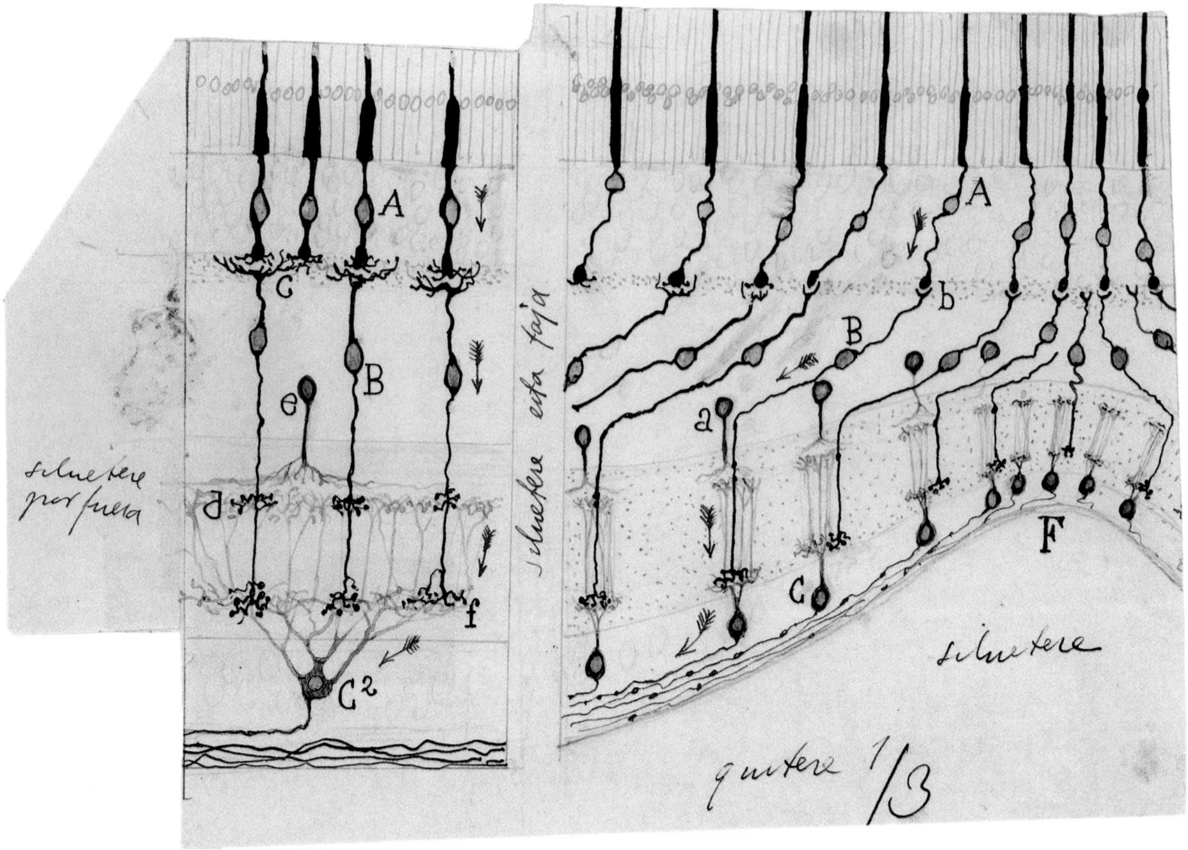

FIGURE 108. Fovea centralis of the retina in a bird.

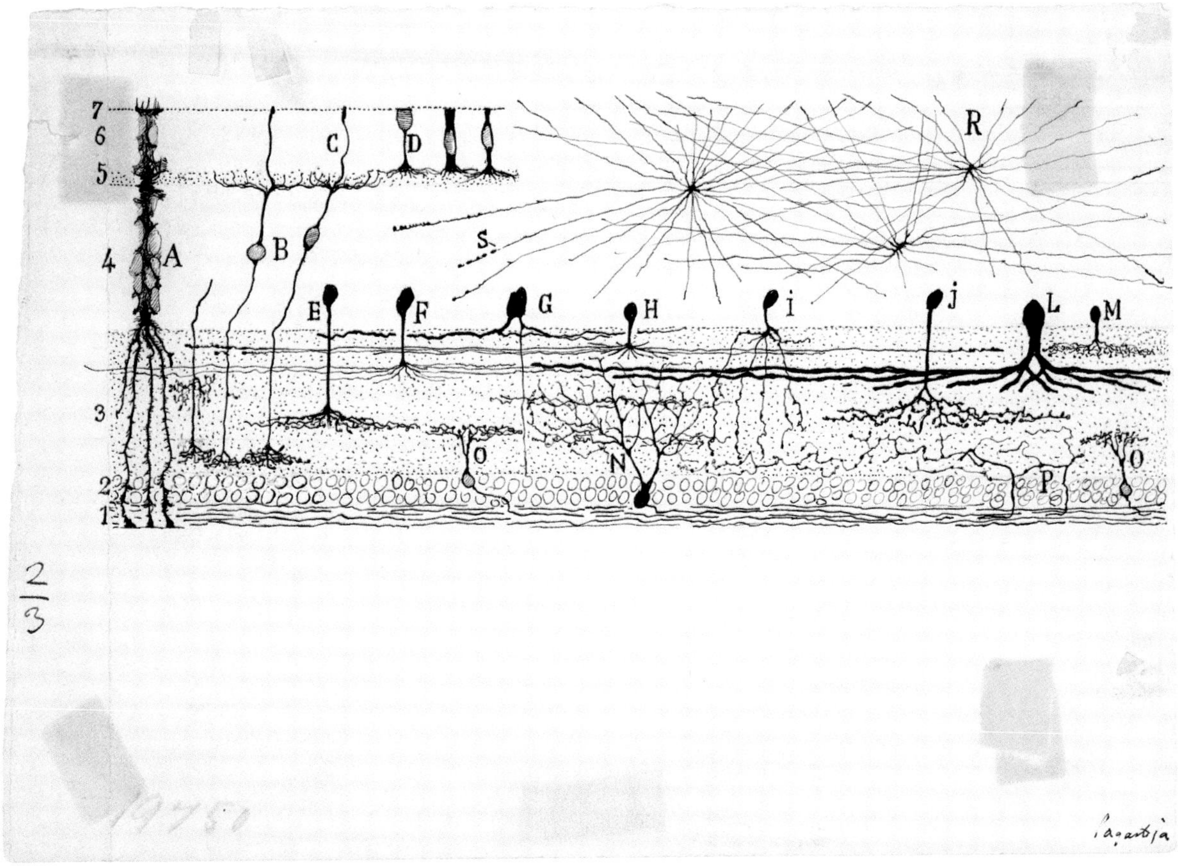

FIGURE 109. Retina in a lizard.

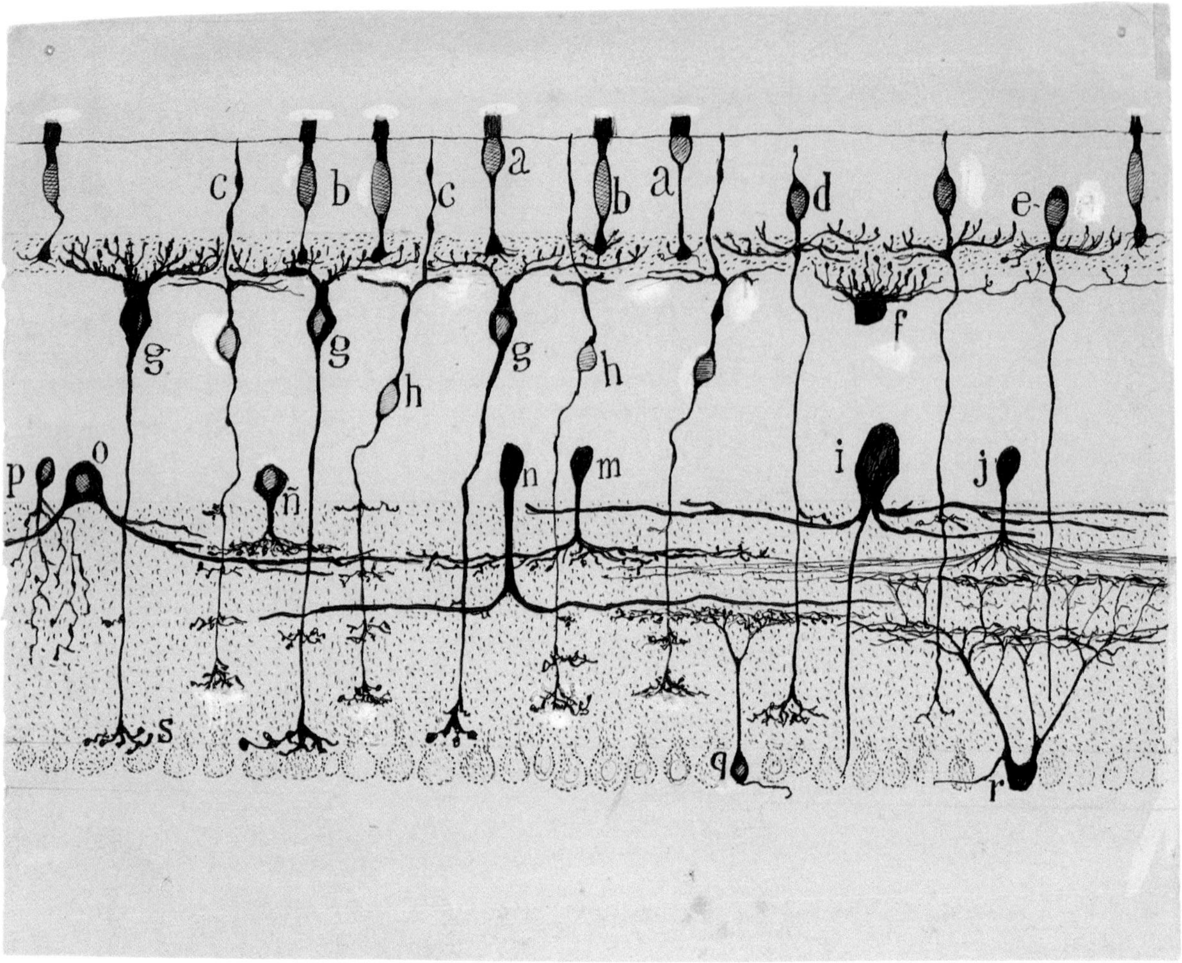

FIGURE 110. Transverse section in a lizard retina.

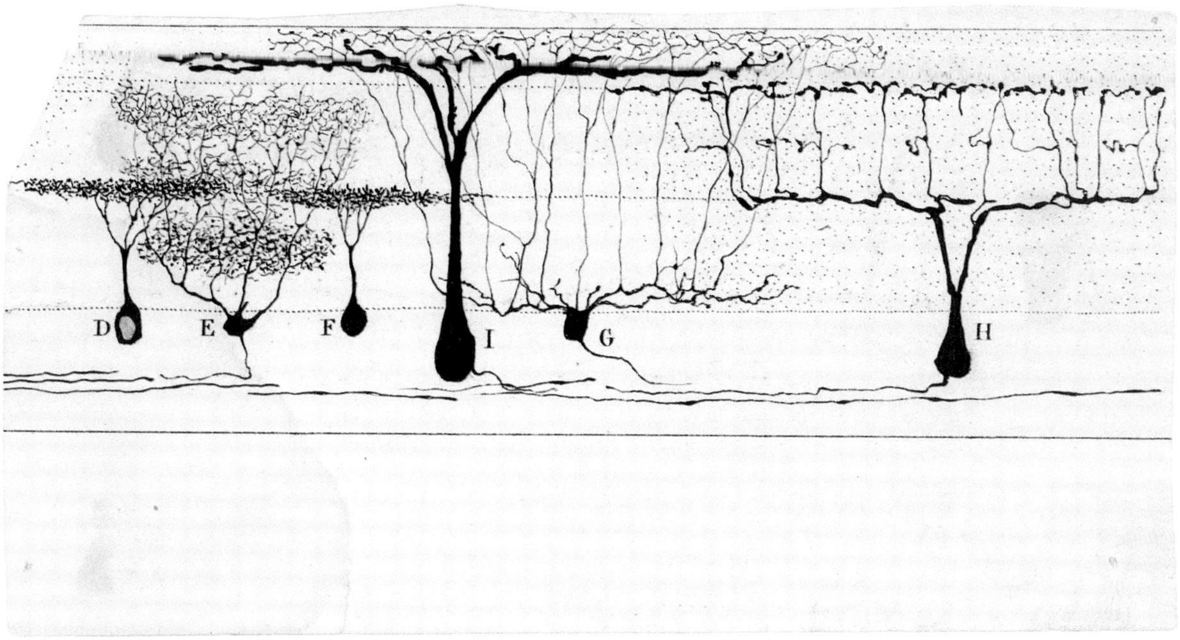

FIGURE III. Ganglion cells in an eyed-lizard retina.

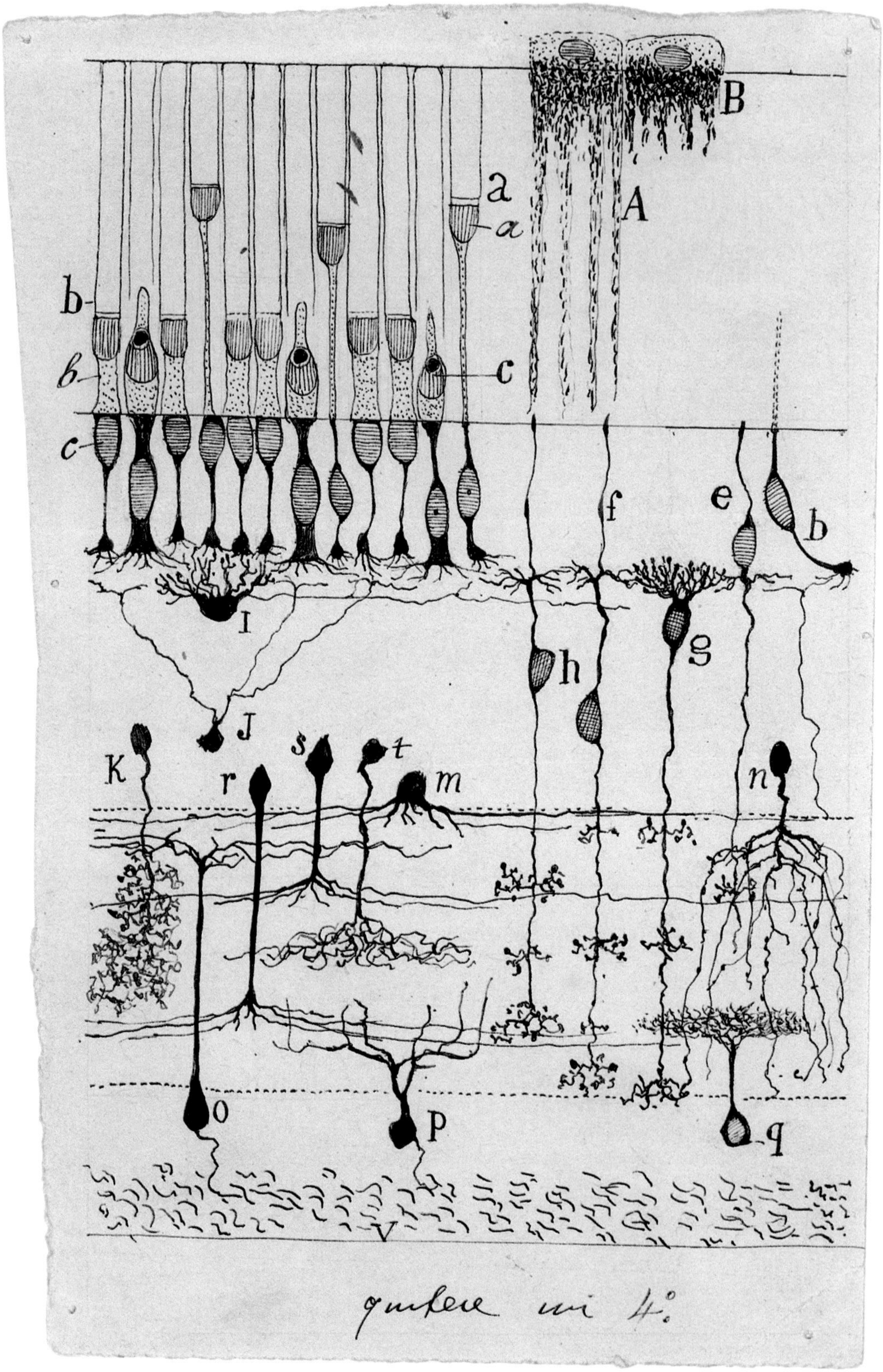

FIGURE 112. Retina in a frog.

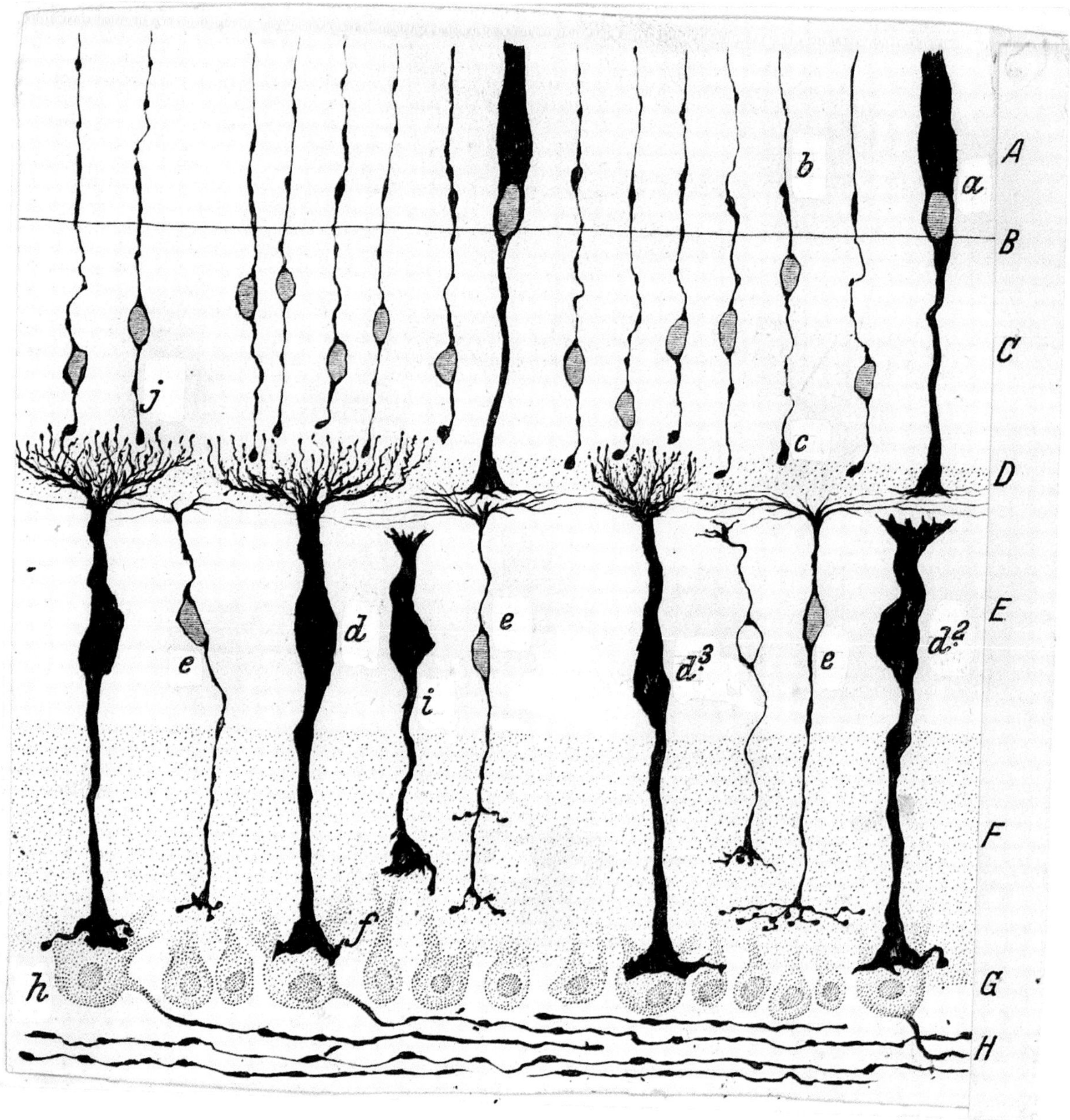

FIGURE 113. Vertical section of the retina in a common barb.

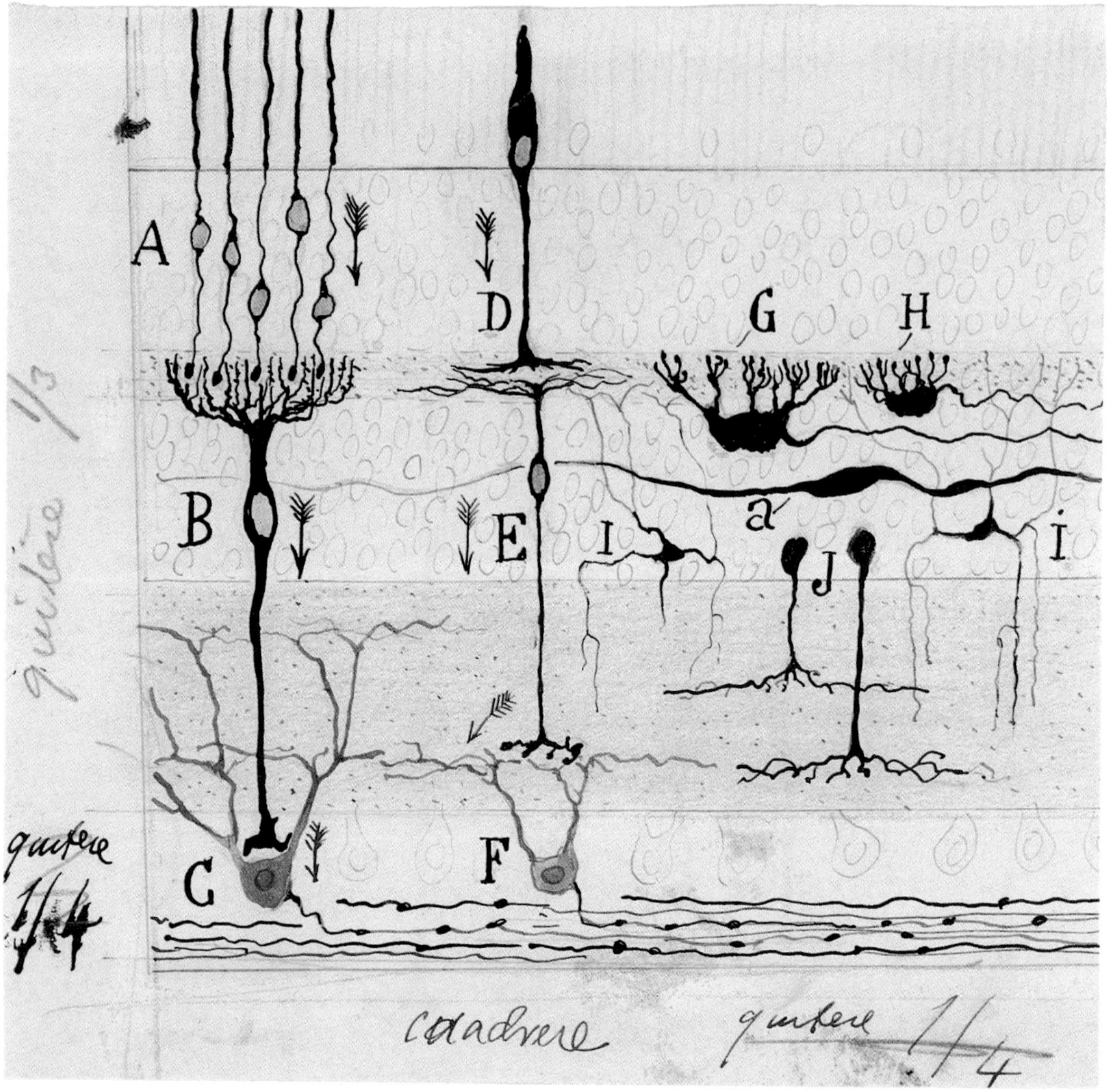

FIGURE 114. Retina in a perch.

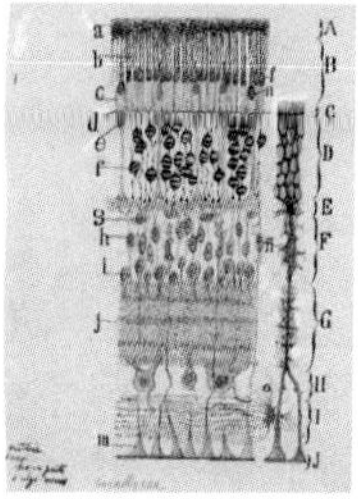

FIGURE 100.

Perpendicular section in a dog retina.

This figure was published in Cajal, S. R. (1899–1904) *Textura del sistema nervioso del hombre y de los vertebrados*. Madrid: Moya. (Figure 520).

FIGURE LEGEND: Perpendicular section of the retina in a dog, [according to information provided by the Golgi method]. *A*, Layer of pigment cells; *B*, layer of the rods and cones; *C*, outer limiting membrane; *D*, layer of the somata of receptor cells (outer nuclear layer); *E*, outer plexiform layer; *F*, layer of the bipolar cells (inner nuclear layer); *G*, inner plexiform layer; *H*, layer of cells with a long axon [or ganglion cells]; *I*, optic fiber layer; *J*, inner limiting membrane. *a*, Pigment cells; *b*, outer segment of a rod; *c*, cone; *d*, outer limiting membrane; *e*, nucleus of a cone cell body; F, nucleus of a rod cell body; *g*, horizontal cell; *h*, bipolar cell; *i*, spongioblasts or amacrine cells; *j*, granular zones or tiers of the inner plexiform layer; *m*, terminal cone-shape enlargement of a Müller fiber; [*n*, ellipsoid or intercalated body of a cone]; *o*, neuroglia cell; *ñ*, nucleus of a Müller fiber. An isolated Müller fiber or epithelial cell is shown at the right of the figure.

Original text: Corte perpendicular de la retina del perro, [según las enseñanzas suministradas por el método de Golgi]. *A*, capa pigmentaria; *B*, de los bastones y conos; *C*, basal externa; *D*, de los cuerpos de las células visuales; *E*, plexiforme externa; *F*, de las células bipolares; *G*, plexiforme interna; *H*, de las células de axon largo [ó ganglionares]; *I*, de las fibras del nervio óptico; *J*, capa basal interna. *a*, células pigmentarias; *b*, segmento externo de un bastón; *c*, cono; *d*, basal externa; *e*, núcleo del cuerpo del cono; *f*, núcleo del cuerpo del bastón; *g*, célula horizontal; *h*, célula bipolar; *i*, espongiablasto ó célula amacrina; *j*, zonas granulosas ó pisos de la plexiforme interna; *m*, cono terminal de una fibra de Müller; [*n*, cuerpo elipsoideo ó intercalar de los conos]; *o*, célula de neuroglia; *ñ*, núcleo de las fibras de Müller. A la derecha de la figura se ve una fibra de Müller ó célula epitelial.

Note from the author (J. D.): In brackets is the text added in the French version of the *Textura*: Cajal, S. R. (1909–1911) *Histologie du système nerveux de l'homme et des vertébrés*, trans. L. Azoulay. Paris: Maloine.

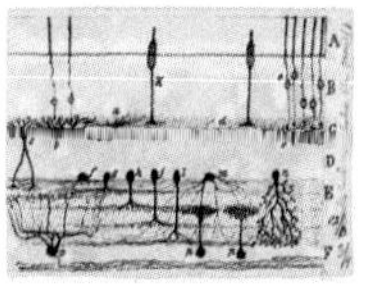

FIGURE 101.

Perpendicular section in a mammalian retina.

This figure was originally published in Cajal, S. R. (1892) Nuevo concepto de la histología de los centros nerviosos. *Rev. Cienc. Méd. Barcelona* 18, 361–376 (Figure 19). It has also been reproduced as Figure 526 in Cajal, S. R. (1899–1904) *Textura del sistema nervioso del hombre y de los vertebrados*. Madrid: Moya.

FIGURE LEGEND: Perpendicular section in a mammalian retina [derived from Golgi preparations] (semischematic figure). *A*, Somata of rods; *B*, somata of cones; *a*, small horizontal cell; *b*, large horizontal cell; *c*, horizontal cell with descending dendrites; *e*, terminal arborization of a horizontal cell axon; *f, g, h, j, l, m, n*, various types of [amacrine cells or] spongioblasts; *o*, bistratified ganglion cell; *1, outer plexiform zone; 2, internal plexiform zone*.

Original text: Corte perpendicular de una retina de mamífero, [según el método de Golgi] (figura semiesquemática). *A*, cuerpo de los bastones; *B*, cuerpo de los conos; *a*, célula horizontal pequeña; *b*, célula horizontal grande; *c*, célula horizontal con expansión protoplásmica descendente; *e*, arborización terminal de un cilindro-eje de célula horizontal; *f, g, h, j, l, m, n*, variedades de [amacrinas ó] espongioblastos; *o*, célula ganglionar bi-estratificada. *1, capa plexiforme externa; 2, capa plexiform interna*.

Note from the author (J. D.): In brackets is the text added in the French version of the *Textura*: Cajal, S. R. (1909–1911) *Histologie du système nerveux de l'homme et des vertébrés*, trans. L. Azoulay. Paris: Maloine. The text between asterisks appears in the original publication only.

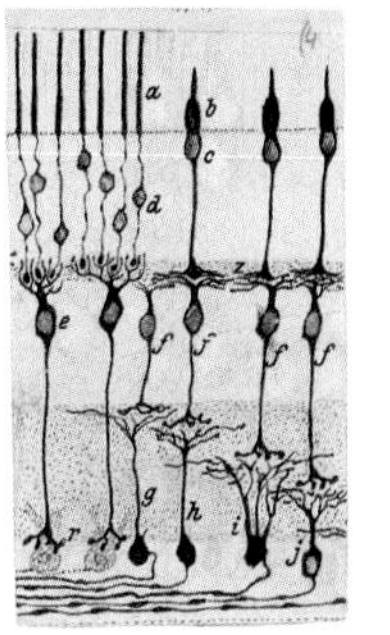

FIGURE 102.

Retina in a mammal.

This drawing was published in Cajal, S. R. (1892) Nuevo concepto de la histología de los centros nerviosos. *Rev. Cienc. Méd. Barcelona* 18, 363–376, 457–476, 505–520, 529–540 (part of Figure 18).

FIGURE LEGEND: Transverse section of the retina in a mammal. *a*, Rod; *b*, cone; *e*, rod bipolar cells; *f*, cone bipolar cells; *r*, lower arborization of bipolar rod cells; *g, h, i, j, k*, ganglion cells with axons that branch in different tiers of the inner plexiform layer; *z*, contact between the cones and the bipolar cone cells.

Original text: Corte transversal de la retina de un mamífero: *a*, bastoncito; *b*, cono; *e*, bipolar para bastones; *f*, bipolares para conos; *r*, arborización inferior de las bipolares de bastón; *g, h, i, j, k*, células ganglionares arborizadas en los distintos pisos de la zona plexiforme interna; *z*, contacto entre los conos y sus bipolares.

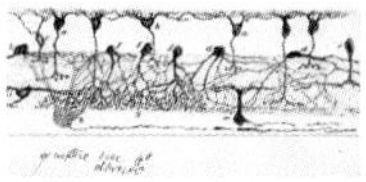

FIGURE 103.

Cone bipolars and amacrine cells in a dog retina.

Part of this figure was published in Cajal, S. R. (1893) La rétine des vertébrés. *Cellule* 9, 121–255 (Figure 8). It has also been reproduced as Figure 530 in Cajal, S. R. (1899–1904) *Textura del sistema nervioso del hombre y de los vertebrados*. Madrid: Moya.

FIGURE LEGEND: Various types of cone bipolars and amacrine cells of the retina in a dog (method of Ehrlich).

Original text: Diversos tipos de bipolares para cono y amacrinas de la retina del perro. (Método de Ehrlich).

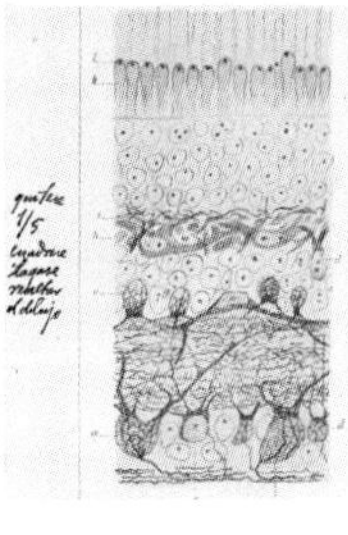

FIGURE 104.

Section through an adult rabbit retina.

This figure was published in Cajal, S. R. (1904) El retículo neurofibrillar en la retina. *Trab. Lab. Invest. Biol. Univ. Madrid* 3, 185–212 (Figure 1). It has also been reproduced as Figure 198 in Cajal, S. R. (1909–1911) *Histologie du système nerveux de l'homme et des vertébrés*, trans. L. Azoulay. Paris: Maloine.

FIGURE LEGEND: Section through an adult rabbit retina. Reduced silver nitrate method. *a*, Large ganglion cell; *b*, small ganglion cell; *c*, neurofibril coursing to the axon; *e*, amacrine cell showing the superficial neurofibrillar net; *h*, large horizontal cells; *i*, dendritic plexus formed by the dendrites of the horizontal cells in the outer plexiform layer; *k*, inner segments of rods; *l*, corpuscle impregnated at the tip of this segment of the rod.

Original text: Corte de la retina del conejo adulto. Método del nitrato de plata reducido. *a*, célula ganglionar grande; *b*, célula ganglionar pequeña; *c*, neurofibrilla yendo al axon; *e*, espongioblasto mostrando su red neurofibrilar superficial; *h*, células horizontales grandes; *i*, plexo dendrítico formado por las expansiones de las células horizontales en la plexiforme externa; *k*, artículo interno de los bastones; *l*, corpúsculo impregnado en la extremidad de este artículo del bastón.

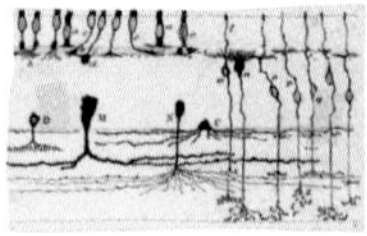

FIGURE 105.

Retina in a chicken.

This drawing was published in Cajal, S. R. (1899–1904) *Textura del sistema nervioso del hombre y de los vertebrados*. Madrid: Moya. (Figure 537).

FIGURE LEGEND: Retina in a chicken. Golgi method. *a*, Rod; *c*, oblique cone; *d*, cone with a displaced foot; *e*, twin cone; *m*, bipolar cell with a club; *n*, large bipolar cell without a club; *l*, Landolt's club; *s*, terminal tuft of bipolar cells; *M, N, D, C*, types of amacrine cells.

Original text: Retina del pollo. Método de Golgi. *a*, bastón; *c*, cono oblícuo; *d*, cono de pié dislocado; *e*, cono gemelo; *m*, bipolar de maza; *n*, bipolar gruesa sin maza; *l*, maza de Landolt; *s*, penacho terminal de las bipolares; *M, N, D, C*, tipos de amacrinas.

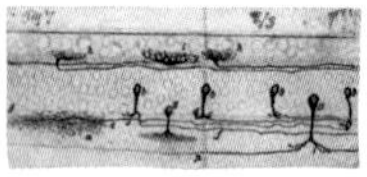

FIGURE 106.

Retina in a bird (greenfinch).

This drawing was published in Cajal, S. R. (1899–1904) *Textura del sistema nervioso del hombre y de los vertebrados*. Madrid: Moya. (Figure 539).

FIGURE LEGEND: Retina in a bird (greenfinch) [(*Ligurinus chloris*, L.)]. Golgi method. *b*, Amacrine cells with a short axon or association amacrine cells; *d*, dendrites of these cells; *c, f*, their horizontal axons; *e*, their terminal axonal arborization; *i*, flattened horizontal cell; *h*, its axonal arborization; *g, n*, amacrine cells.

Original text: Retina de un pájaro (verderón) [*Ligurinus chloris*, L.)]. Método de Golgi. *b*, amacrinas de axon corto ó de asociación; *d*, dendritas; *c, f*, axon horizontal; *e*, arborización final; *i*, célula horizontal aplanada; *h*, arborización nerviosa de éstas; *g, n*, amacrinas.

Note from the author (J. D.): In brackets is the text added in the French version of the *Textura*: Cajal, S. R. (1909–1911) *Histologie du système nerveux de l'homme et des vertébrés*, trans. L. Azoulay. Paris: Maloine.

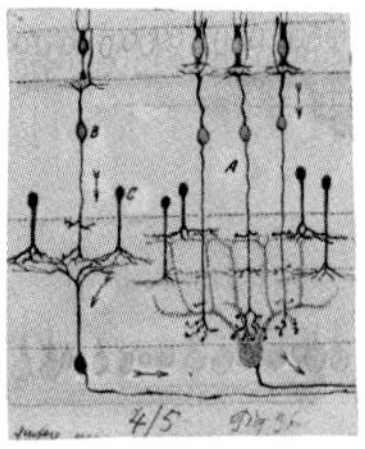

FIGURE 107.

Two possible channels for visual stimuli in the retina of birds,

This figure was published in Cajal, S. R. (1899–1904) *Textura del sistema nervioso del hombre y de los vertebrados*. Madrid: Moya. (Figure 562).

FIGURE LEGEND: The two possible channels for visual stimuli in the retina of birds, individual and collective. *A*, Diffuse channel for reflexes; *B*, individualized channel for the visual mental image. [The arrows indicate the direction of current flow.]

Original text: Los dos cauces posibles, individual y colectivo, de la retina de las aves. *A*, cauce difuso para los reflejos; *B*, Cauce individualizado para la imagen mental. [Las flechas indican el sentido de las corrientes.]

Note from the author (J. D.): In brackets is the text added in the French version of the *Textura*: Cajal, S. R. (1909–1911) *Histologie du système nerveux de l'homme et des vertébrés*, trans. L. Azoulay. Paris: Maloine.

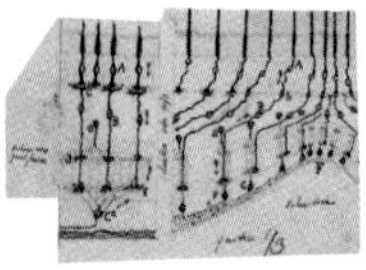

FIGURE 108.

Fovea centralis of the retina in a bird.

This drawing was published in Cajal, S. R., and Tello, J. F. (1928) *Elementos de histología normal y de técnica micrográfica*. 9th ed. Madrid: Tipografía Artística. (Figure 385).

FIGURE LEGEND: Fovea centralis of the retina in a bird. Note the structural differences that exist between the fovea itself (*F*) and the retinal regions somewhat distant from it (figure on the left). *A*, Cones; *B*, bipolar cells; *C*, ganglion cells; *a, e*, amacrine cells.

Original text: Fovea centralis de la retina de un pájaro. Nótese el contraste estructural existente entre la fovea misma (*F*) y las regiones retinianas algo alejadas de ella (figura de la izquierda). *A*, conos; *B*, bipolares; *C*, ganglionares; *a, e*, amacrinas.

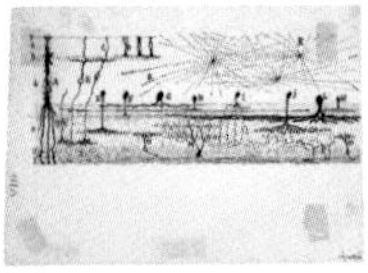

FIGURE 109.

Retina in a lizard.

This figure was published in Cajal, S. R. (1891) Pequeñas contribuciones al conocimiento del sistema nervioso. *Trab. Lab. Histol. Fac. Med. Barcelona. Imprenta de la Casa Provincial de Caridad*, August, 1–56 (Figure 9).

FIGURE LEGEND: Section of the retina in a lizard (*Lacerta agilis*). *A*, Epithelial cell; *B*, bipolar cells; *C*, Landolt's club; *D*, cone; *E*, spongioblast with long shaft (type 1); *F, H*, thin spongioblasts with a shaft that is expanded in a star shape of delicate and horizontal fibrils (type 3); *I*, thin spongioblast with an irregular tuft (type 2); *J*, spongioblast with long shaft (type 4); *L*, giant spongioblast; *M*, dwarf spongioblast with a very small arborization (type 5); *O*, small ganglion cell with a fine and varicose arborization; *N*, large ganglion cell with multistratified arborization; *R*, arborizations of spongioblasts *F* and *H*, as seen in horizontal sections of the retina; *S*, thick and granular tip of their fibers.

Original text: Cortes de la retina de la lagartija (*Lacerta agilis*). *A*, célula epitelial; *B*, bipolares; *C*, maza de Landolt; *D*, cono; *E*, espongioblasto de tallo largo (tipo 1º); *F, H*, espongioblastos finos cuyo tallo se dilata en una estrella de fibrillas delicadísimas y horizontales (tipo 3º); *I*, espongioblasto fino, de penacho irregular (tipo 2º); *J*, espongioblasto de tallo largo (tipo 4º); *L*, espongioblosto gigante; *M*, espongioblasto enano, de arborización minúscula (tipo 5º); *O*, célula ganglionar menuda de arborización fina y varicosa; *N*, célula ganglionar grande de arborización multiestratificada; *R*, arborizaciones de los espongioblastos *F* y *H*, vistas en cortes horizontales de la retina; *S*, extremidad recia y granulosa de sus fibras.

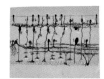

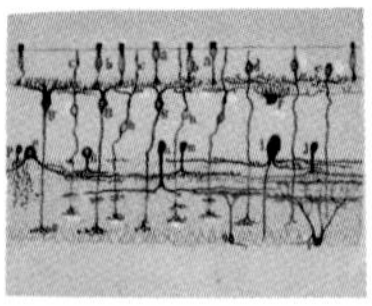

FIGURE 110.

Transverse section in a lizard retina.

This figure was published in Cajal, S. R. (1892) La retina de los teleósteos y algunas observaciones sobre la de los vertebrados superiores. *An. Soc. Españ. Hist. Nat.* 21, 1–29, 281–305 (Figure 5).

FIGURE LEGEND: Transverse section of the retina in a lizard (*Lacerta viridis*). *a, b*, Straight cones: *c*, Landolt's club; *d, e*, displaced bipolar cells; *g*, outer bipolar or giant cells; *h*, thin or typical bipolar cells; *i*, spongioblast; *j*, spongioblast with a starry and fine arborization; *m*, spongioblast with a sinuous ramification; *n*, spongioblast with thick branches; *o*, mitral spongioblast; *q*, unistratified nerve cell; *r*, multistratified ganglion cell; *p*, diffuse spongioblast.

Original text: Corte transversal de la retina del lagarto (*Lacerta viridis*). *a*, *b*, conos rectos: *c*, maza de Landolt; *d*, *e*, bipolares dislocados; *g*, bipolares externas o gigantes; **h**, bipolares ordinarias ó delgadas; *i*, espongioblasto nervioso; *j*, espongioblasto de arborización estrellada y fina; *m*, espongioblasto de ramificación flexuosa; *n*, espongioblasto de ramas gruesas; o, espongioblasto mitral; *q*, célula nerviosa unistratificada; *r*, célula ganglionar poliestratificada; *p*, espongioblasto difuso.

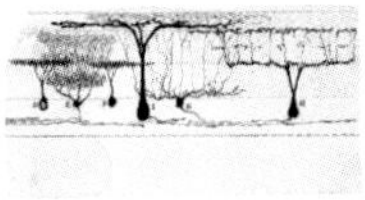

FIGURE 111.

Ganglion cells in an eyed-lizard retina.

Part of this figure was published in Cajal, S. R. (1893) La rétine des vertébrés. *Cellule* 9, 121–255 (Figure 6). It has also been reproduced as Figure 546 in Cajal, S. R. (1899–1904) *Textura del sistema nervioso del hombre y de los vertebrados*. Madrid: Moya.

FIGURE LEGEND: Ganglion cells of unistratified, bistratified, [and multistratified] types of the retina in an eyed-lizard [(*Lacerta ocellata*)]. Golgi method. *D*, *F*, Displaced amacrine cells.

Original text: Tipos de células gangliónicas mono estratificadas, bi-estratificadas [y pluriestratificadas] de la retina del lagarto [ocelado (*Lacerta ocellata*). Método de Golgi.]. *D*, *F*, amacrinas dislocadas.

Note from the author (J. D.): In brackets is the text added in the French version of the *Textura*: Cajal, S. R. (1909–1911) *Histologie du système nerveux de l'homme et des vertébrés*, trans. L. Azoulay. Paris: Maloine.

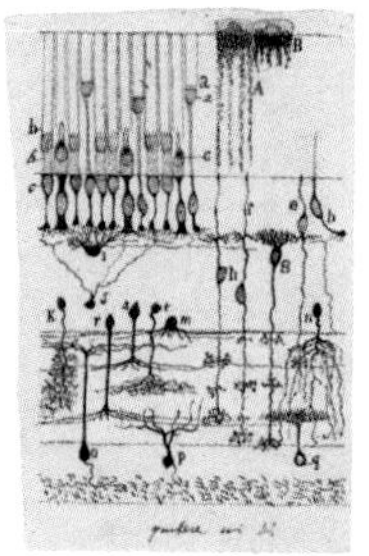

FIGURE 112.

Retina in a frog.

This figure was published in Cajal, S. R. (1899–1904) *Textura del sistema nervioso del hombre y de los vertebrados*. Madrid: Moya. (Figure 548).

FIGURE LEGEND: Retina in a frog [(*Rana esculenta*)]. Semischematic figure according to information provided by the Golgi method. *A*, Pigment epithelial cell with expanded processes; *B*, pigment cell with retracted processes; a, green rods; *b* (left), red rod; [b, inner segment of rods]; c, cones; *a*, ellipsoid body; *c*, rods bodies; [*b* (right), oblique rod]; *e*, displaced bipolar; *f*, Landolt's club; [*g*, large bipolar cell without a club; *h*, thin bipolar cell with a club; *i*, horizontal cell; *J*, stellate cell (?)]; [*k*,] *m*, *n*, [various types of] amacrine cells; *o*, *p*, ganglion cells; *q*, displaced amacrine cells [; *r*, *s*, *t*, various types of common amacrine cells.]

Original text: Retina de la rana. [*Rana esculenta*]. Figura semi-esquemática según el método de Golgi. *A*, célula epitelial con el pigmento relajado; *B*, retraído; a, bastones verdes; b, bastones rojos; [*b*, segmento interno de los bastones]; c, conos; *a*, elipsoide; *c*, cuerpo del bastón; [*b*, bastón oblícuo]; *e*, bipolar dislocada; *f*, maza de Landolt; [*g*, bipolar gruesa sin maza; *h*, bipolar delgada con maza; *i*, célula horizontal; *J*, célula estrellada (?)]; [*k*,] *m*, *n*, [diversos tipos de] amacrinas; *o*, *p*, células gangliónicas; *q*, amacrina dislocada[; *r*, *s*, *t*, células amacrinas normales de diversos tipos.]

Note from the author (J. D.): In brackets is the text added in the French version of the *Textura*: Cajal, S. R. (1909–1911) *Histologie du système nerveux de l'homme et des vertébrés*, trans. L. Azoulay. Paris: Maloine.

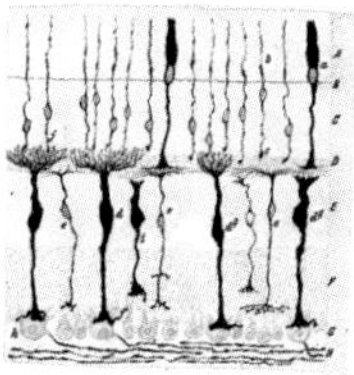

FIGURE 113.

Vertical section of the retina in a common barb.

This figure was published in Cajal, S. R. (1892) La retina de los teleósteos y algunas observaciones sobre la de los vertebrados superiores. *An. Soc. Españ. Hist. Nat.* 21, 1–29, 281–305 (Figure 1). It has also been reproduced as Figure 552 in Cajal, S. R. (1899–1904) *Textura del sistema nervioso del hombre y de los vertebrados*. Madrid: Moya.

FIGURE LEGEND: [Vertical] section of the retina in a common barb [(*Barbus fluviatilis*, Agass)]. Golgi method. *A*, Layer of cones and rods; *B*, outer limiting layer; *D*, outer plexiform layer; [*C*, layer of receptor cell bodies; *E*, bipolar cell layer; *F*, inner plexiform layer; *G*, ganglion cell layer]; *a*, cone; *b*, rod; *c*, rod terminal spherule; *d*, *i*, rod bipolar cells; *e*, cone bipolar cell; *h*, ganglion cells; *j*, synapse between a bipolar cell and a rod cell.

Original text: Corte [vertical] de la retina del barbo común [(*Barbus fluviatilis*, Agass). Método de Golgi]. *A*, capa de conos y bastones; *B*, limitante externa; *D*, plexiforme externa; [*C*, capa de los cuerpos celulares de los receptores; *E*, capa de las bipolares; *F*, plexiforme interna; *G*, capa de las células ganglionares]; *a*, cono; *b*, bastón; *c*, esfera terminal del bastón; *d*, bipolares para bastón; *e*, bipolares para cono; *h*, células gangliónicas; *i*, bipolar para bastón; *j*, articulación de una bipolar con un bastón.

Note from the author (J. D.): In brackets is the text added in the French version of the *Textura*: Cajal, S. R. (1909–1911) *Histologie du système nerveux de l'homme et des vertébrés*, trans. L. Azoulay. Paris: Maloine.

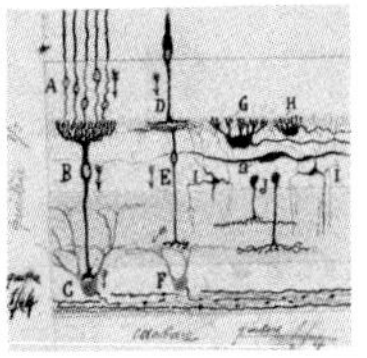

FIGURE 114.

Retina in a perch.

This figure was published in Cajal, S. R. (1933) ¿Neuronismo o reticularismo? Las pruebas objetivas de la unidad anatómica de las células nerviosas. *Arch. Neurobiol.* 13, 217–291, 579–646 (Figure 43).

FIGURE LEGEND: Section of the retina in a perch. Semischematic figure designed to show the main results of my research. *A*, *B*, *C*, Specific channels of the impression collected by the rods; *D*, *E*, *F*, channels of the excitation collected by the cones; *G*, *H*, morphology of the horizontal cells; *a*, *i*, special elements of the retina of the fish.

Original text: Corte de la retina de la perca. Figura semiesquemática destinada a mostrar los principales resultados de mis investigaciones. *A*, *B*, *C*, cauces específicos de la impresión recogida por los bastoncitos; *D*, *E*, *F*, cauces de la excitación recolectada por los conos; *G*, *H*, morfología de las células horizontales; *a*, *i*, elementos especiales de la retina de los peces.

SECTION G

Cerebral Cortex and Olfactory Apparatus

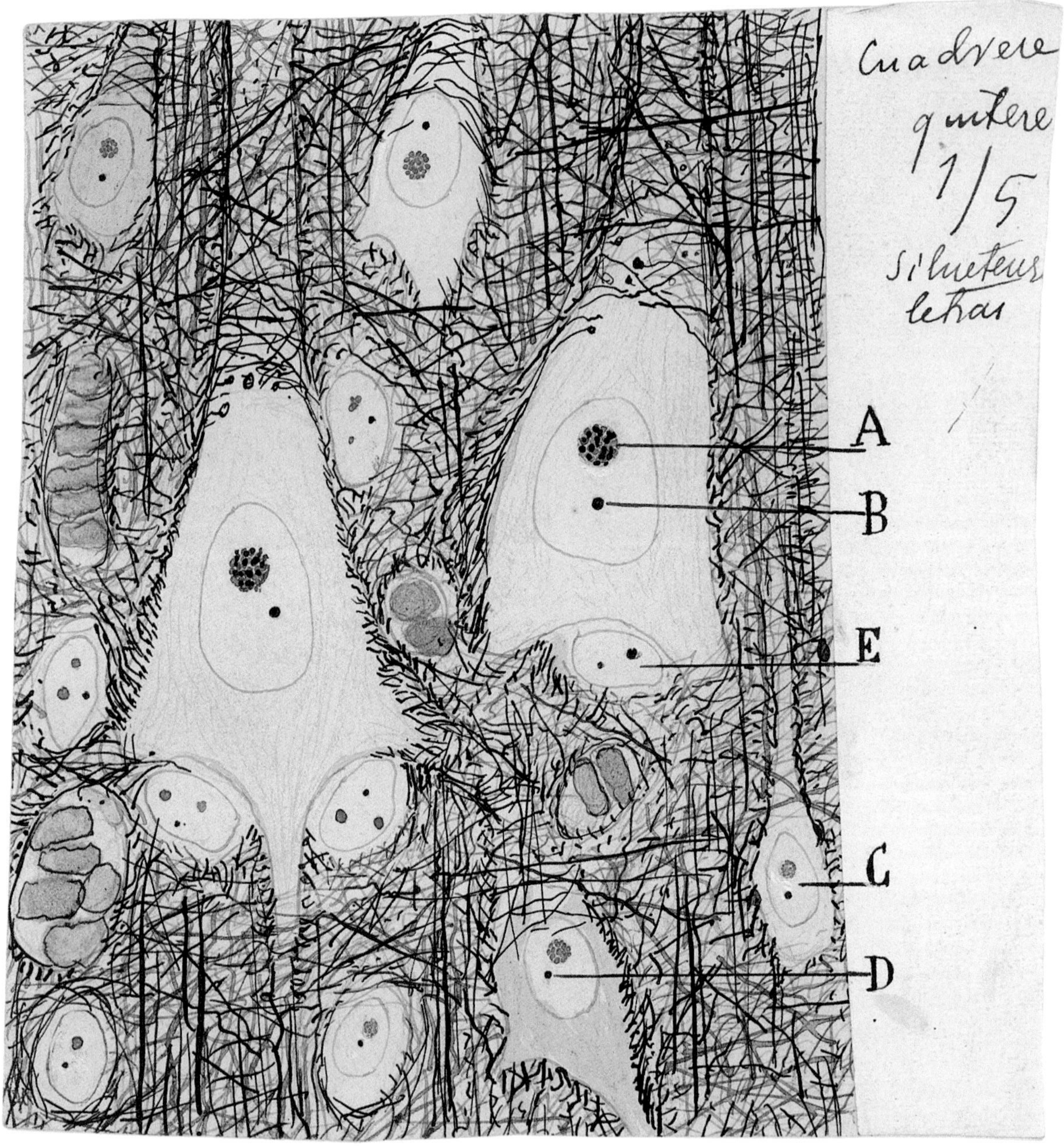

FIGURE 115. The nucleus in human pyramidal cells.

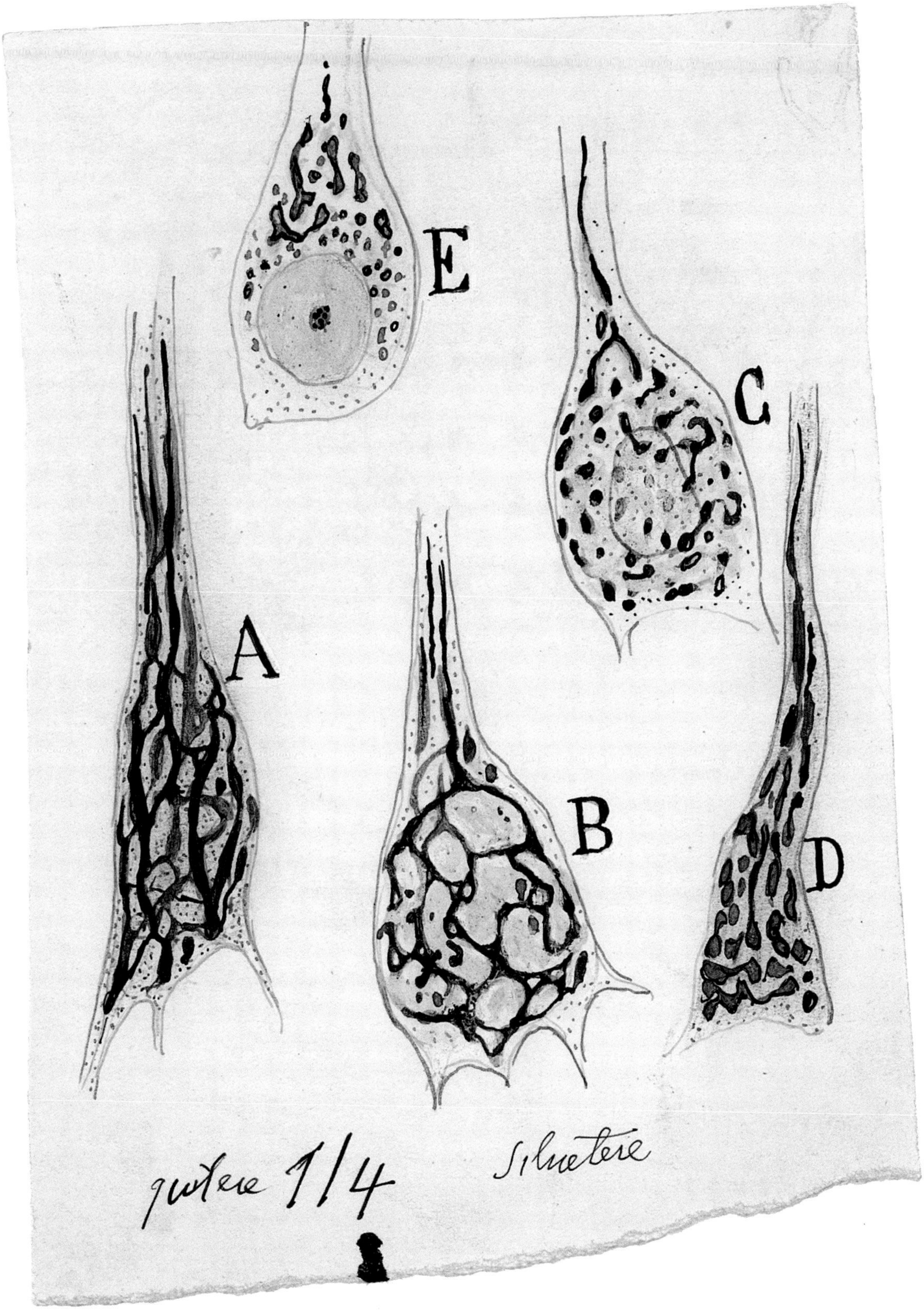

FIGURE 116. Different types of large pyramidal cells of the cerebral cortex in a dog.

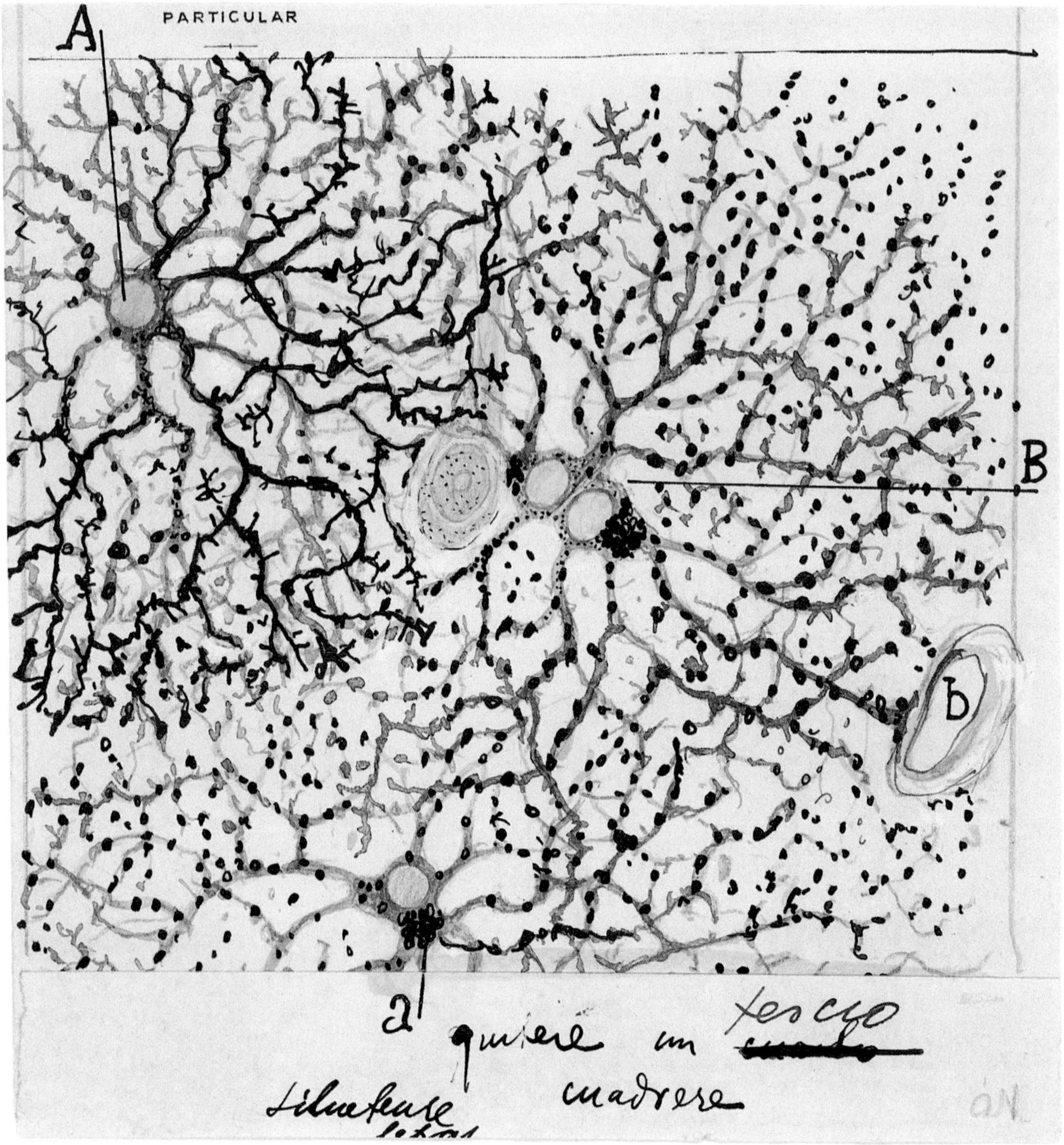

FIGURE 117. Neuroglial plexus of the gray matter in a human brain.

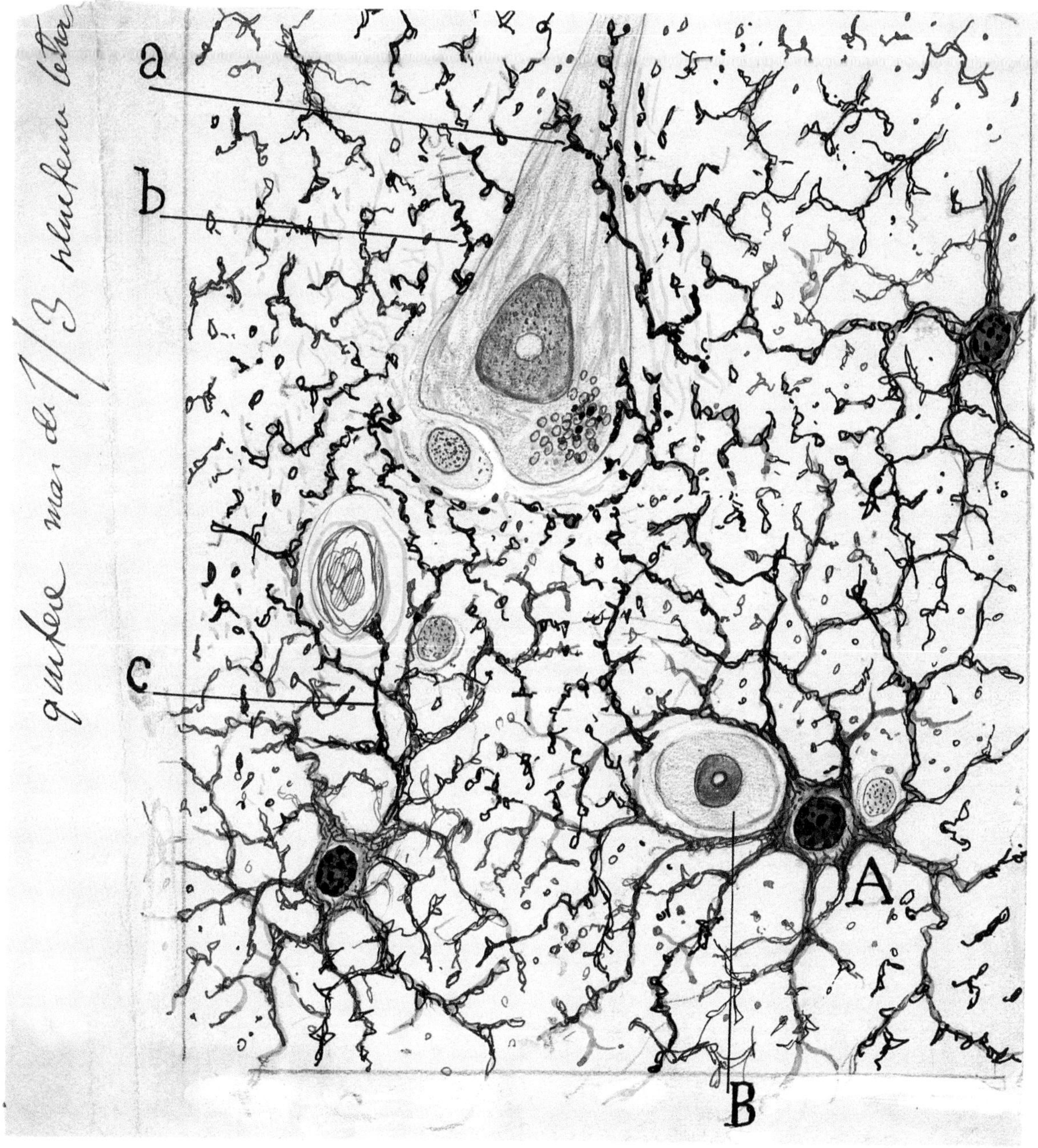

FIGURE 118. Human cerebral cortex.

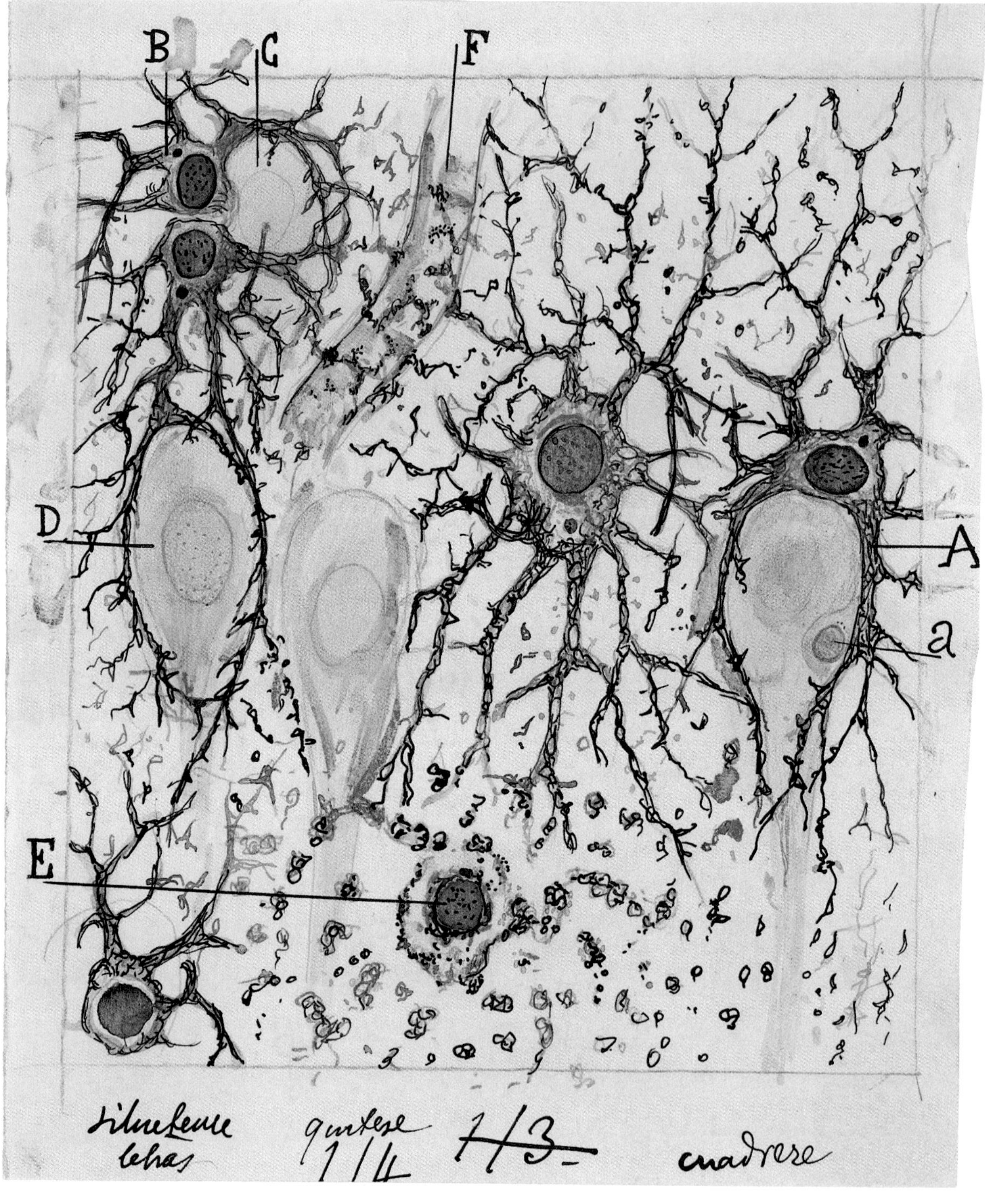

FIGURE 119. Neuroglia of the stratum pyramidale and stratum radiatum of Ammon's horn.

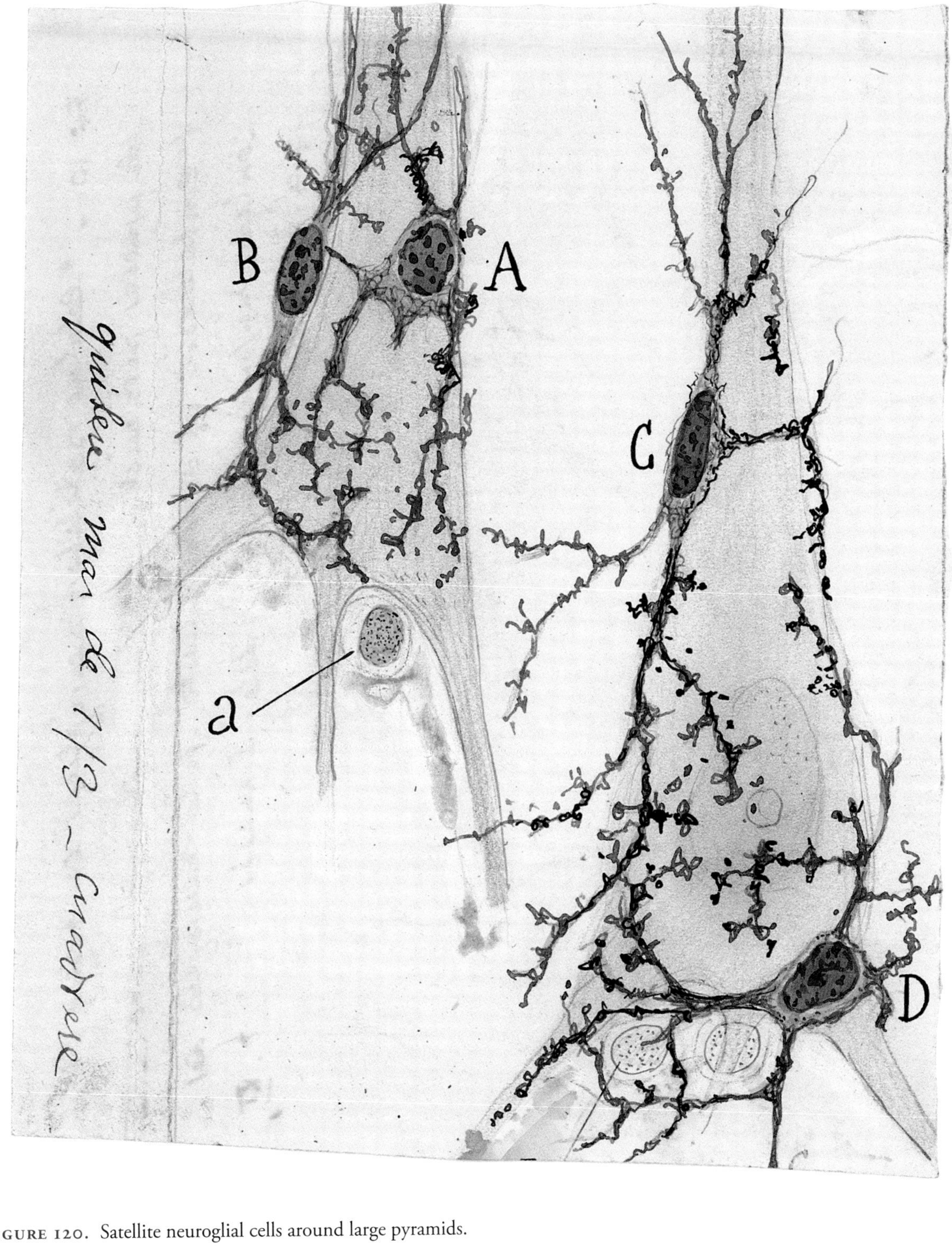

FIGURE 120. Satellite neuroglial cells around large pyramids.

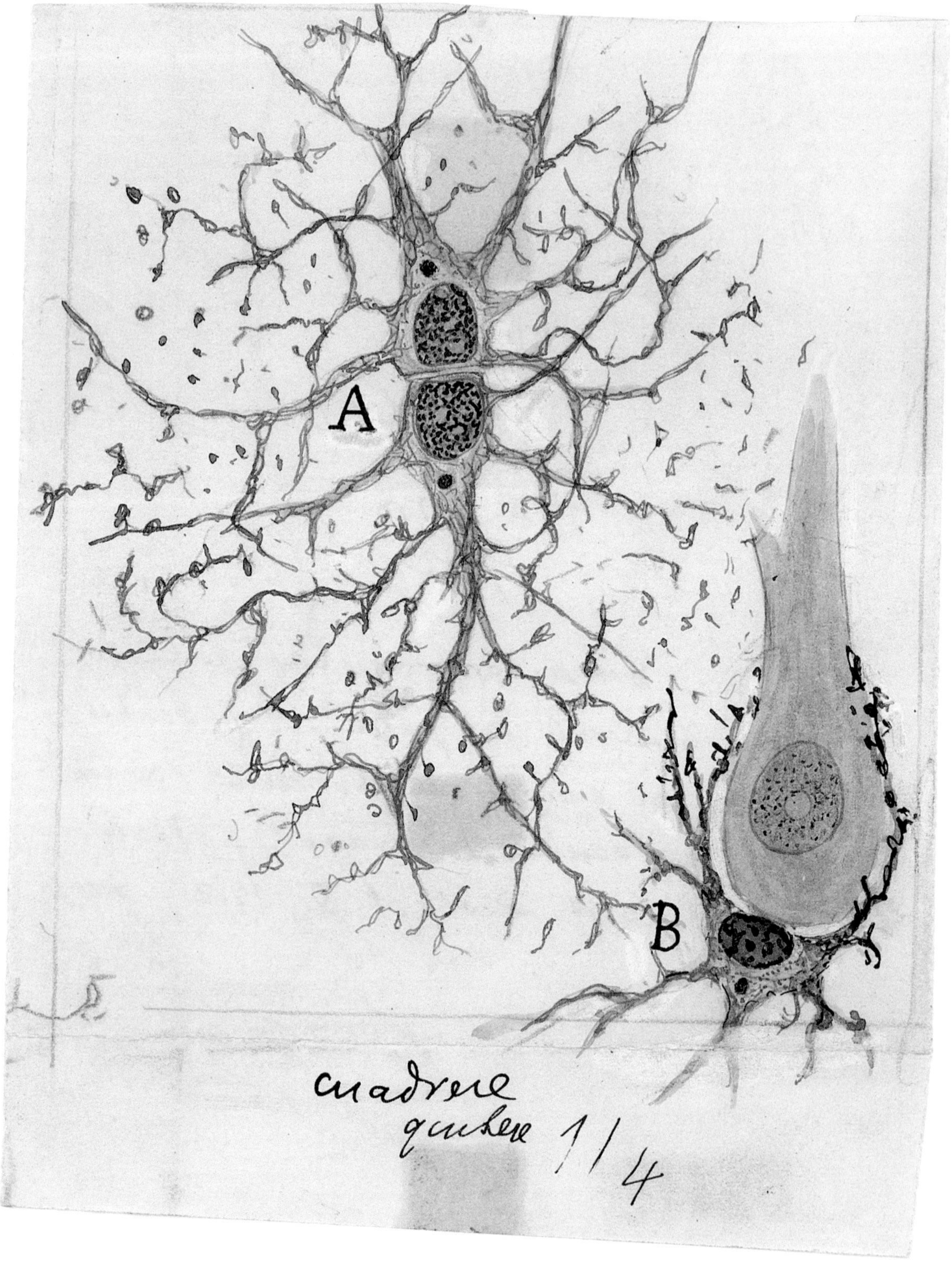

FIGURE 121. Twin astrocytes in the cerebral cortex of an adult dog.

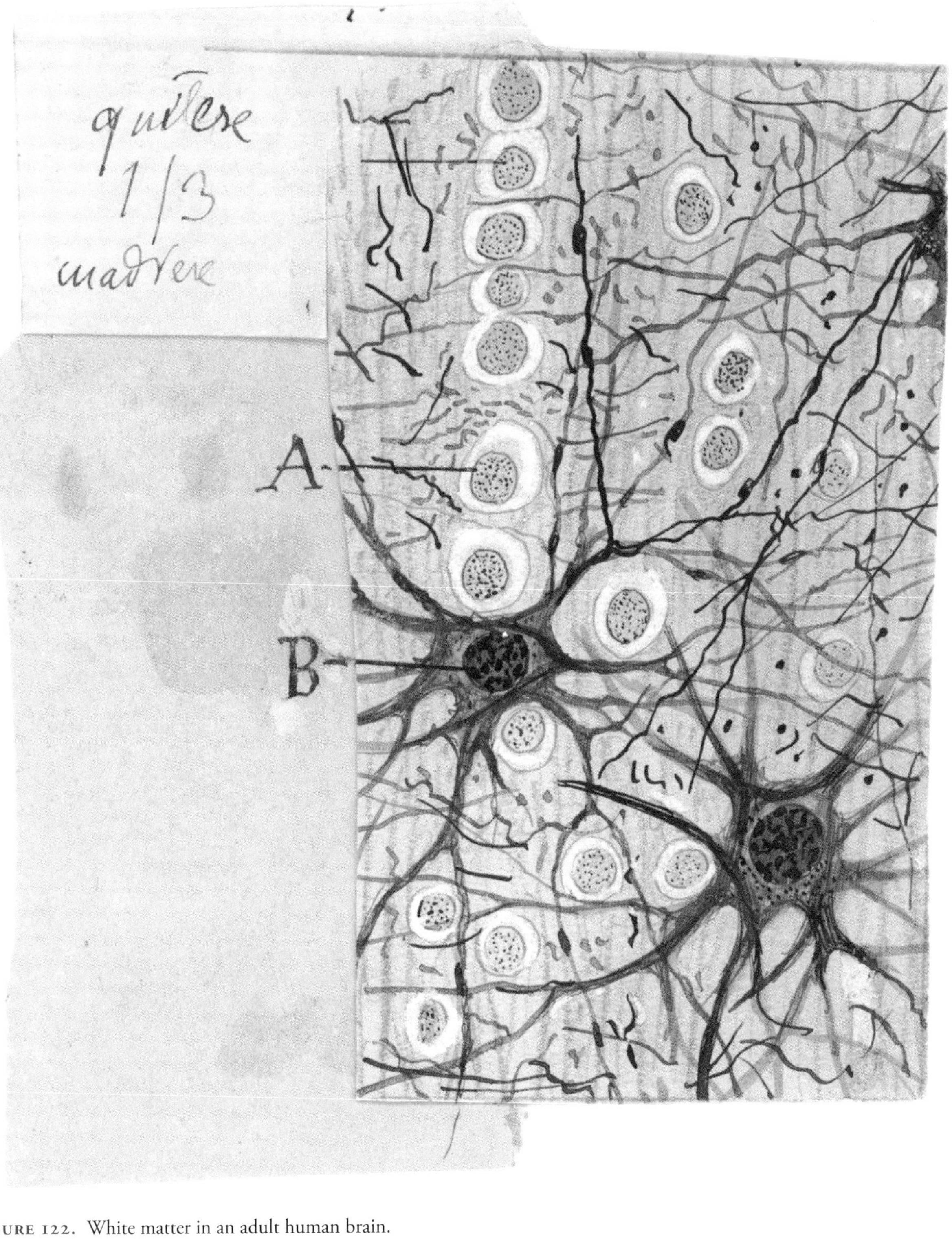

FIGURE 122. White matter in an adult human brain.

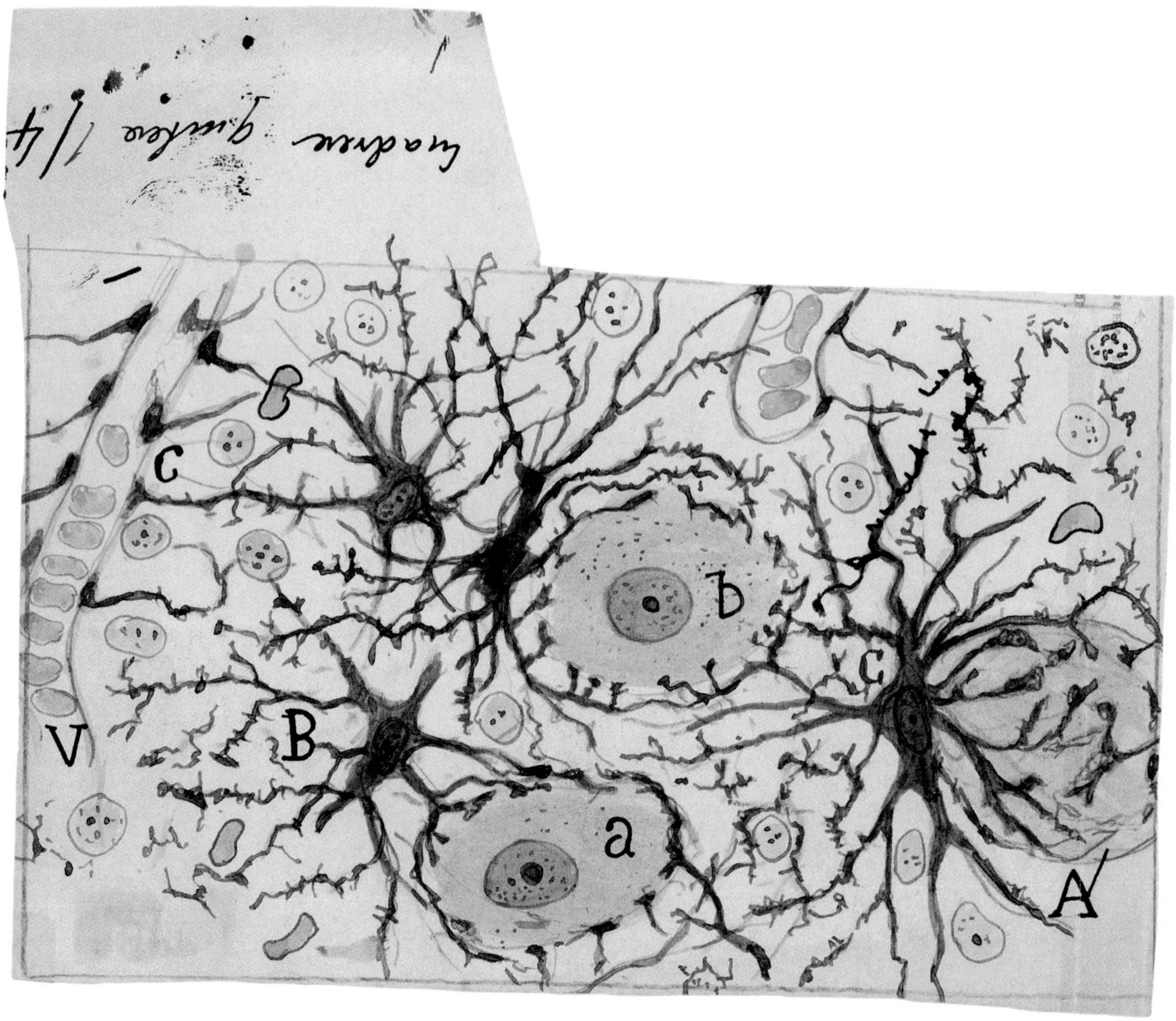

FIGURE 123. Pericellular neuroglial cells of the gray matter of the spinal cord in a cat.

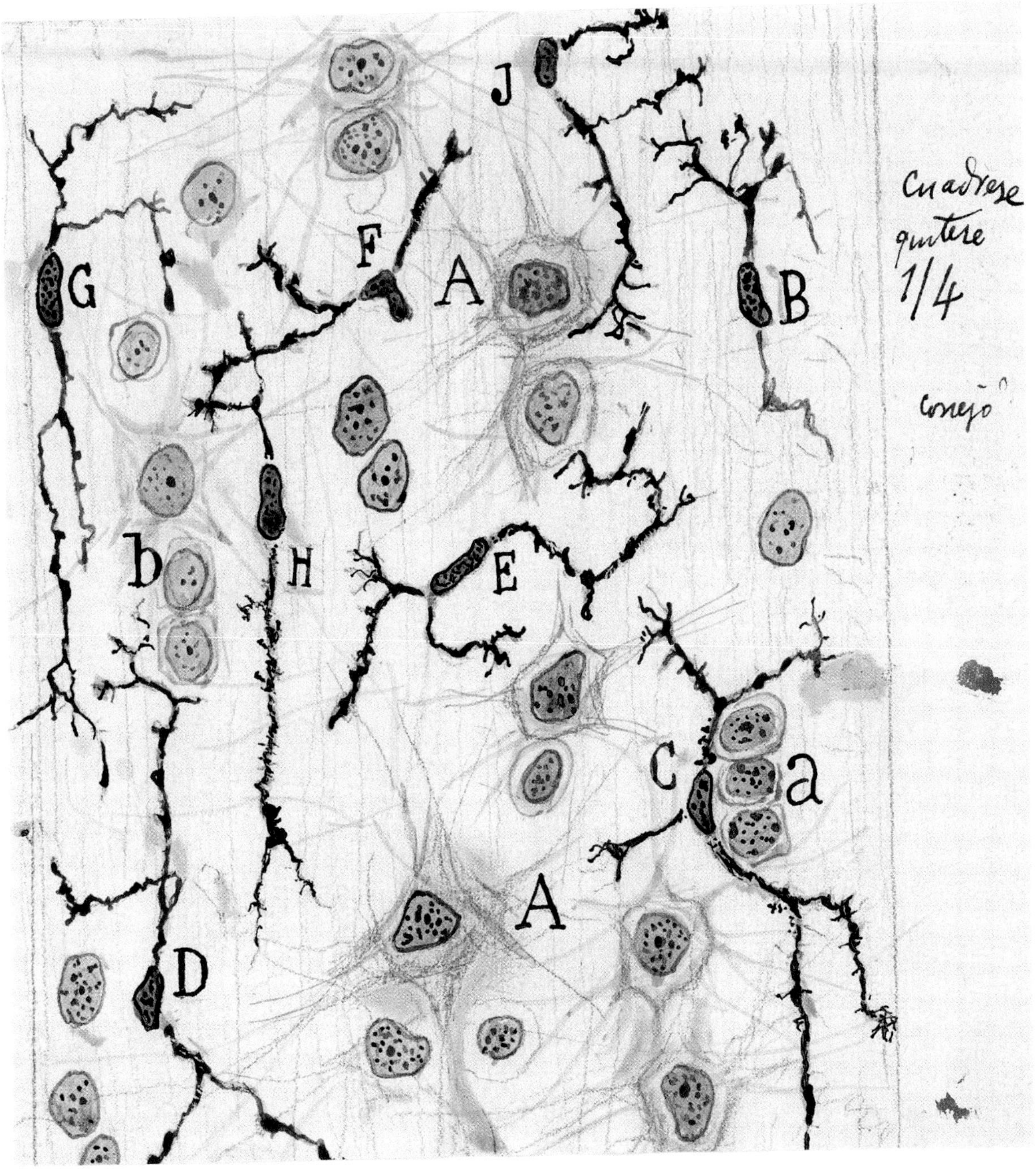

FIGURE 124. Microglia of the white matter of the cerebellum in an adult cat.

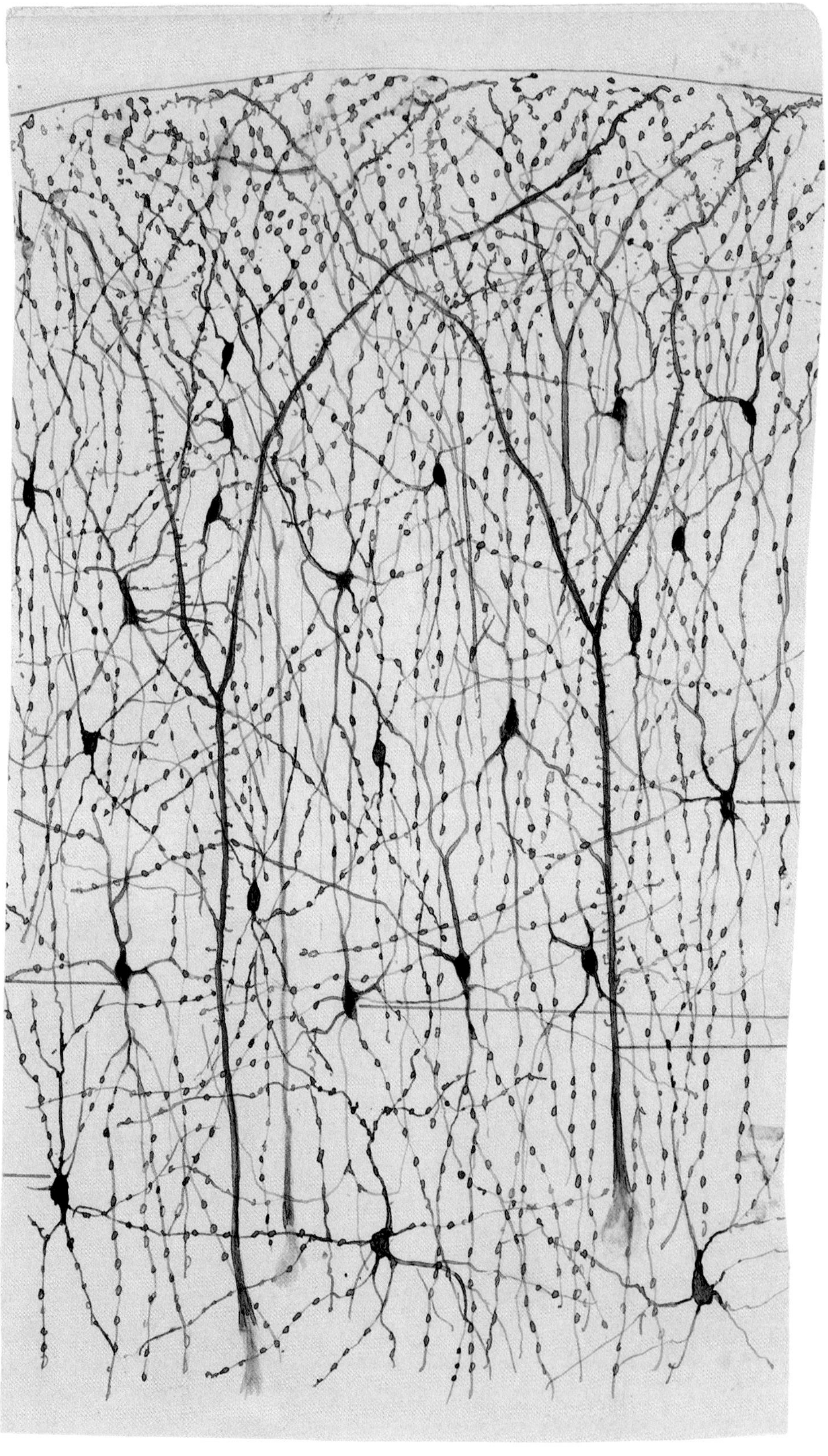

FIGURE 125. Section of a cortical gyrus in an adult cat.

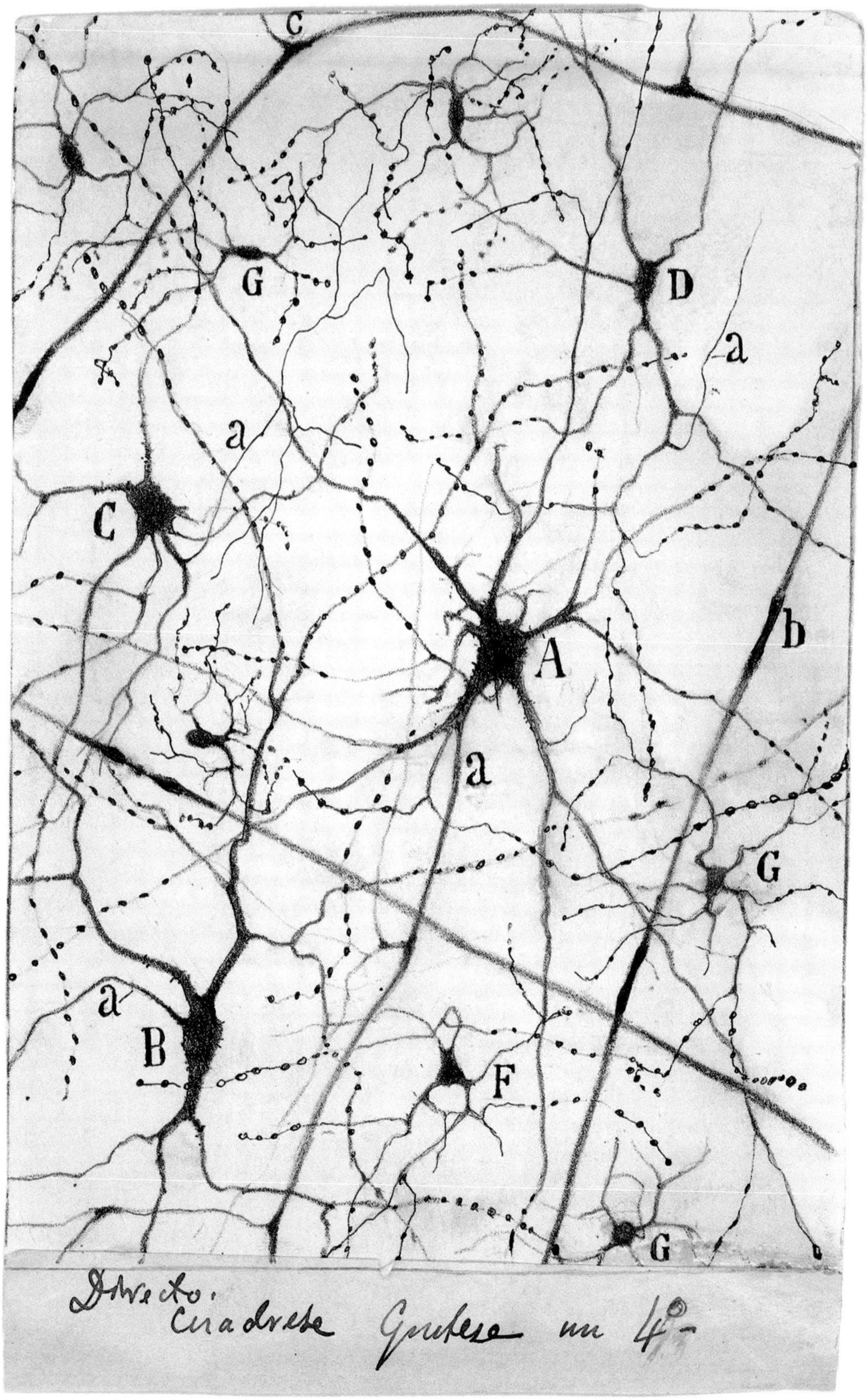

FIGURE 126. Tangential section of the plexiform layer in an adult cat.

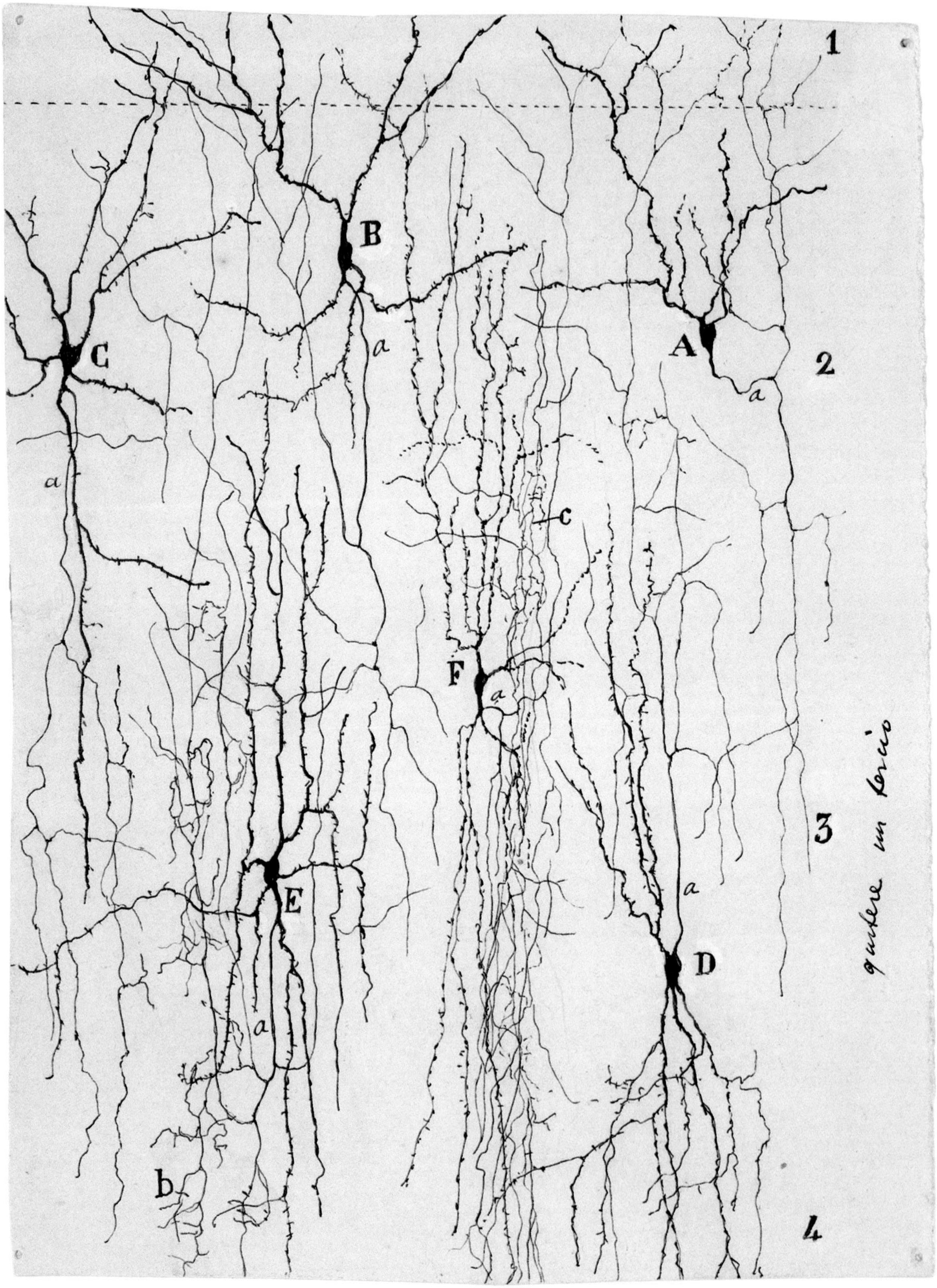

FIGURE 127. Cells with a short axon in the second and third layers of the temporal cortex.

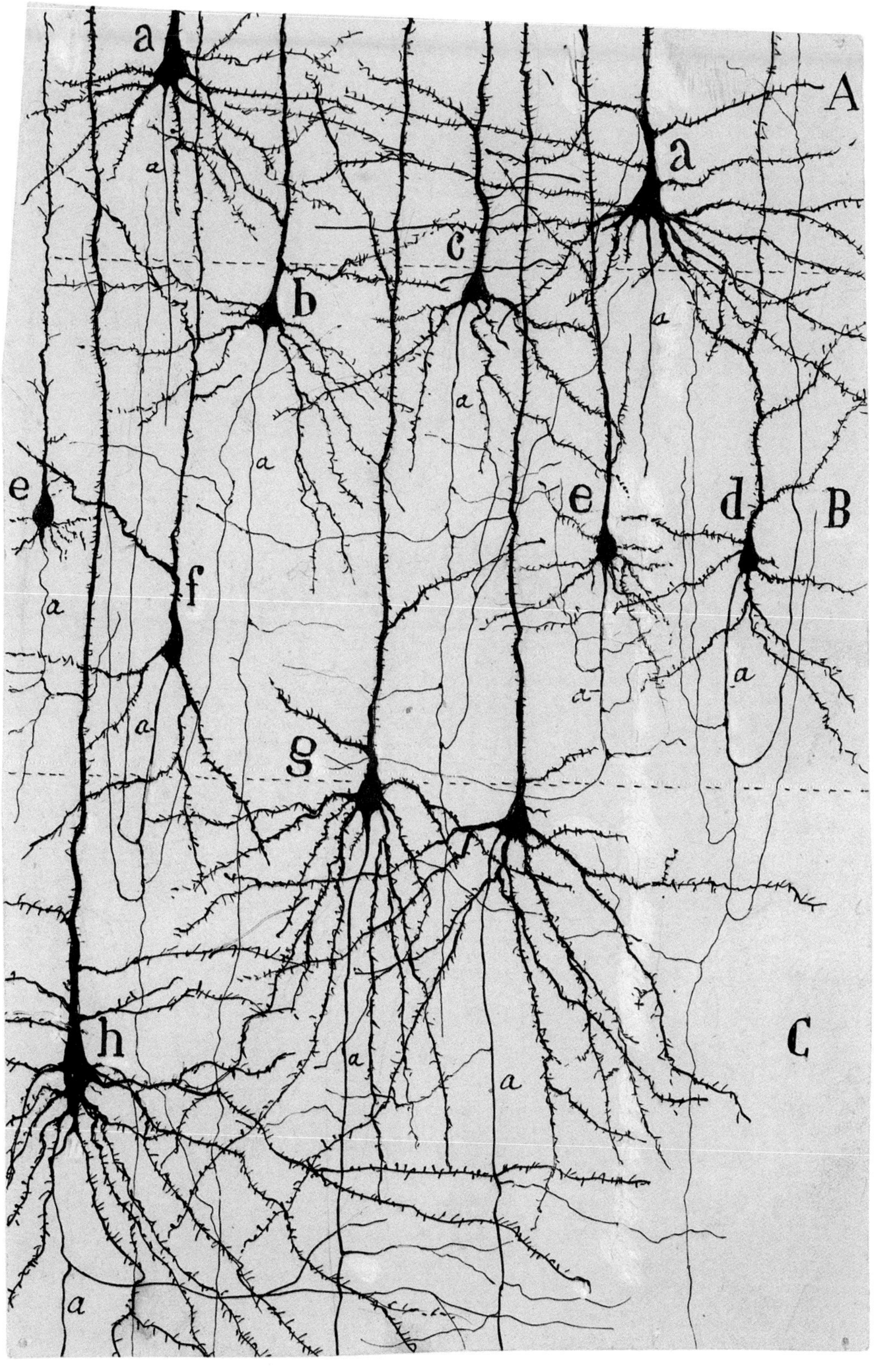

FIGURE 128. Cells of the fourth, fifth, and sixth layers of the superior temporal gyrus in a twenty-five-day-old infant.

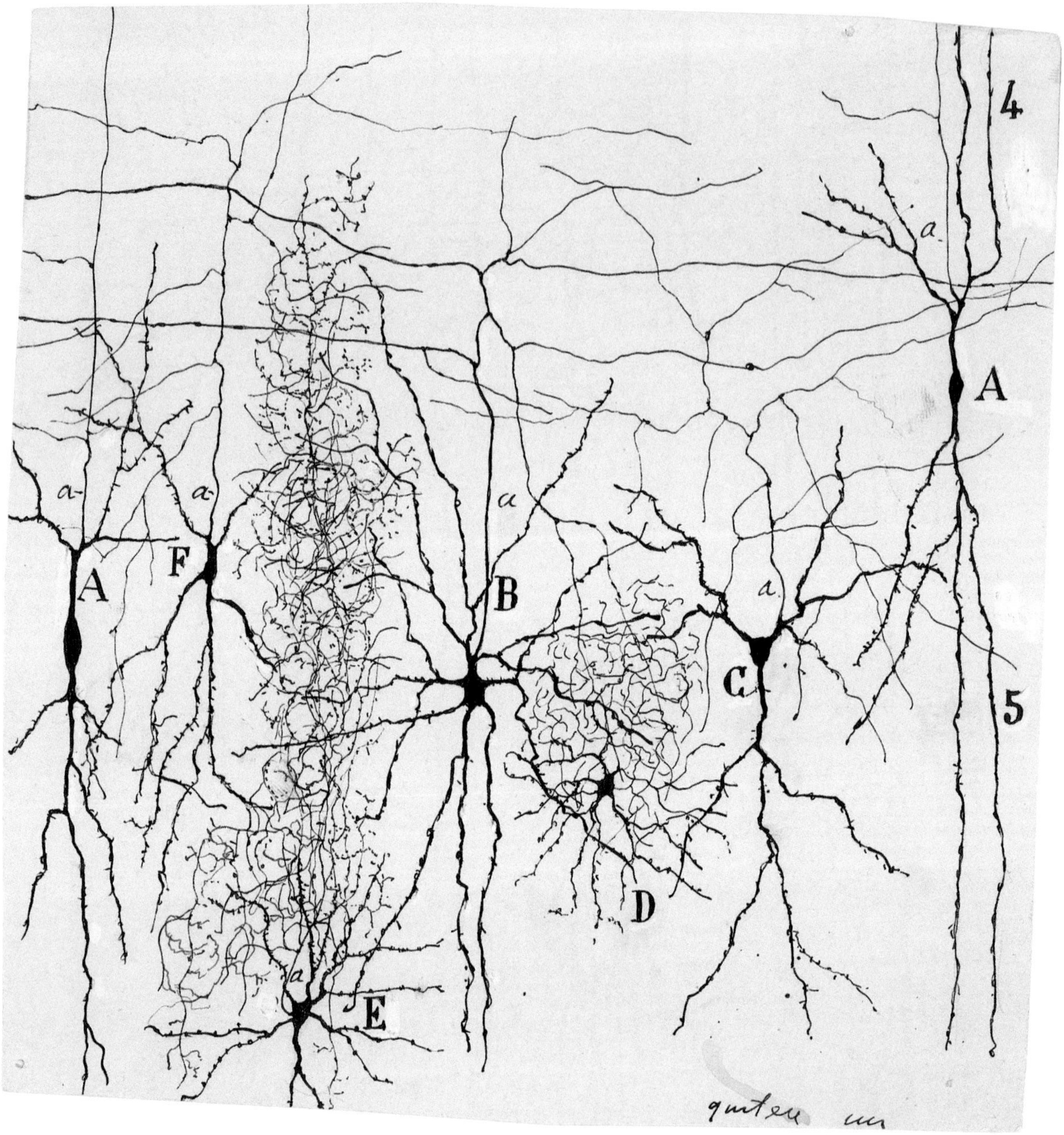

FIGURE 129. Several types of cells with a short axon of the fifth layer in the human temporal cortex.

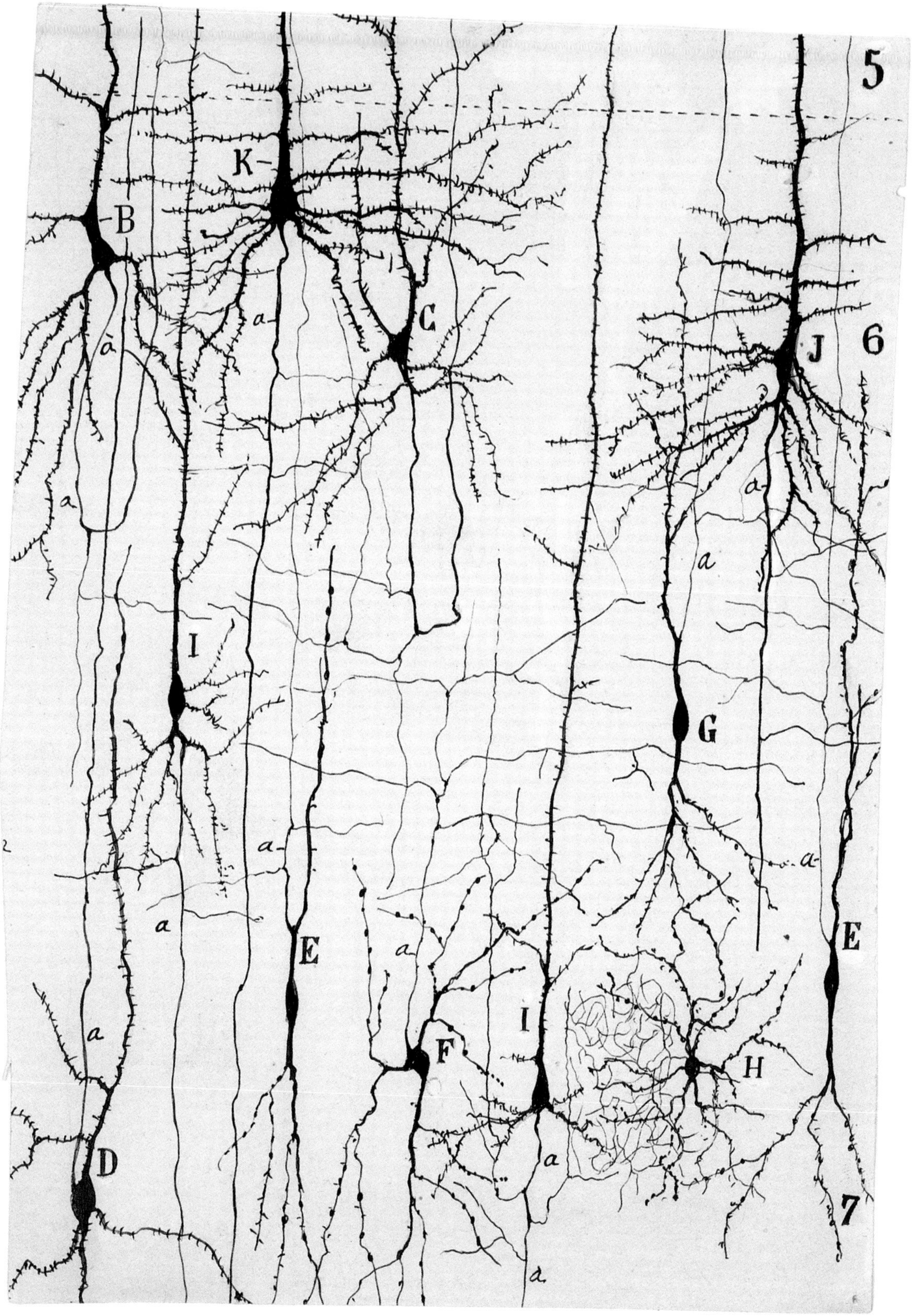

FIGURE 130. Several cellular types of the sixth layer and beginning of the seventh in the human temporal cortex.

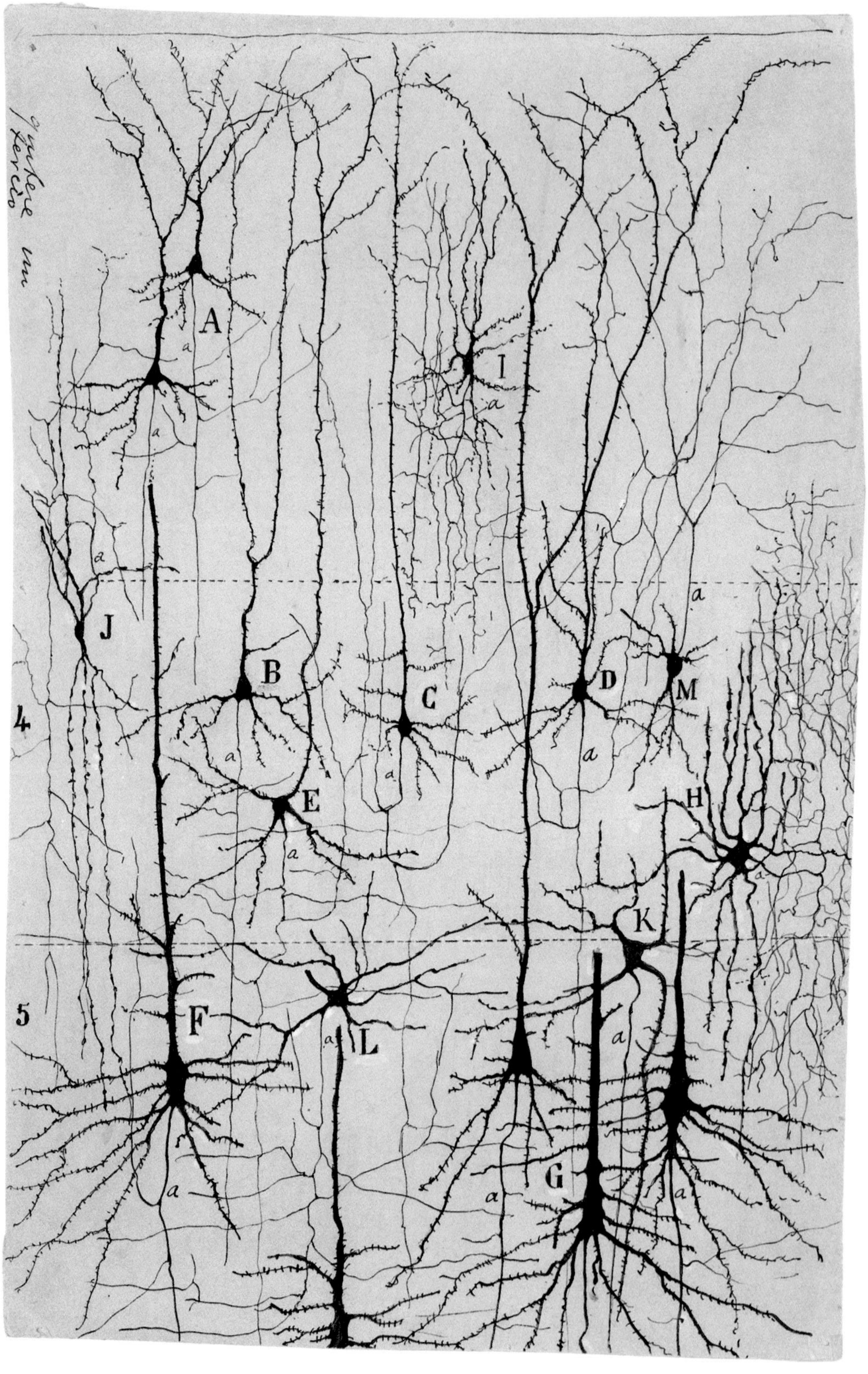

FIGURE 131. Several cellular types of the temporal cortex in a cat.

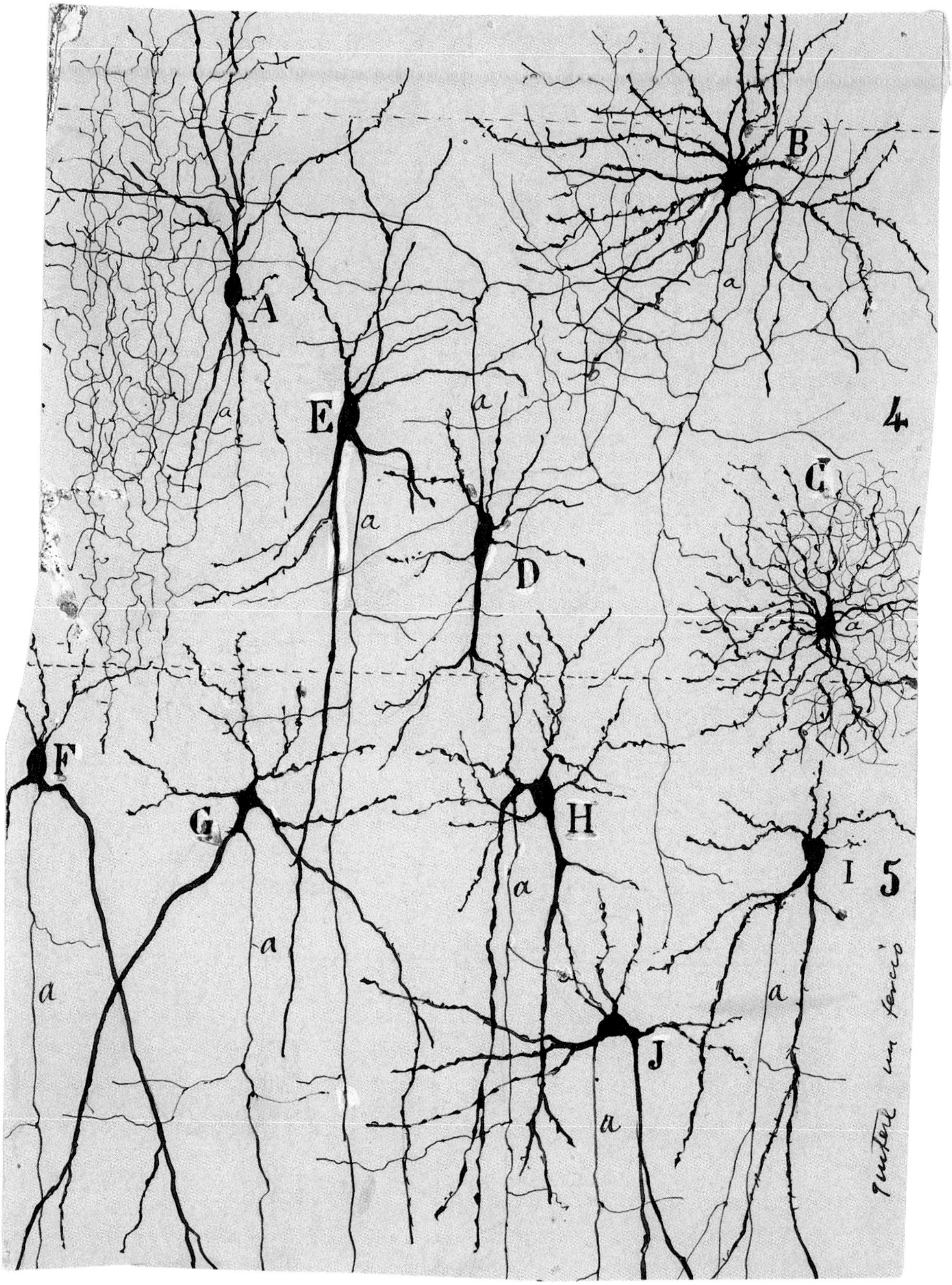

FIGURE 132. Cells of the fourth and fifth layers of the temporal cortex in a cat.

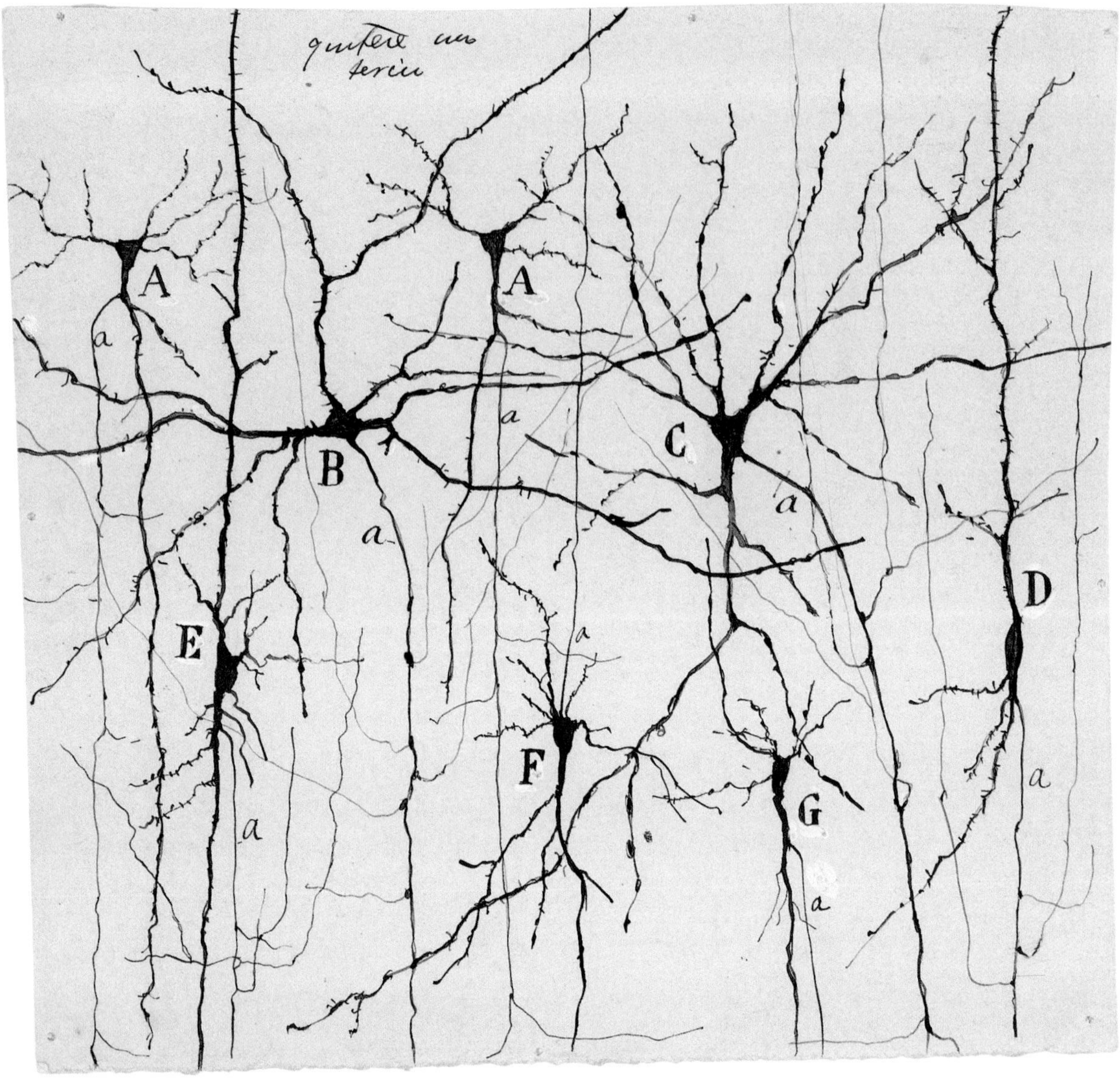

FIGURE 133. Some cellular types of the seventh layer of the temporal cortex in a cat.

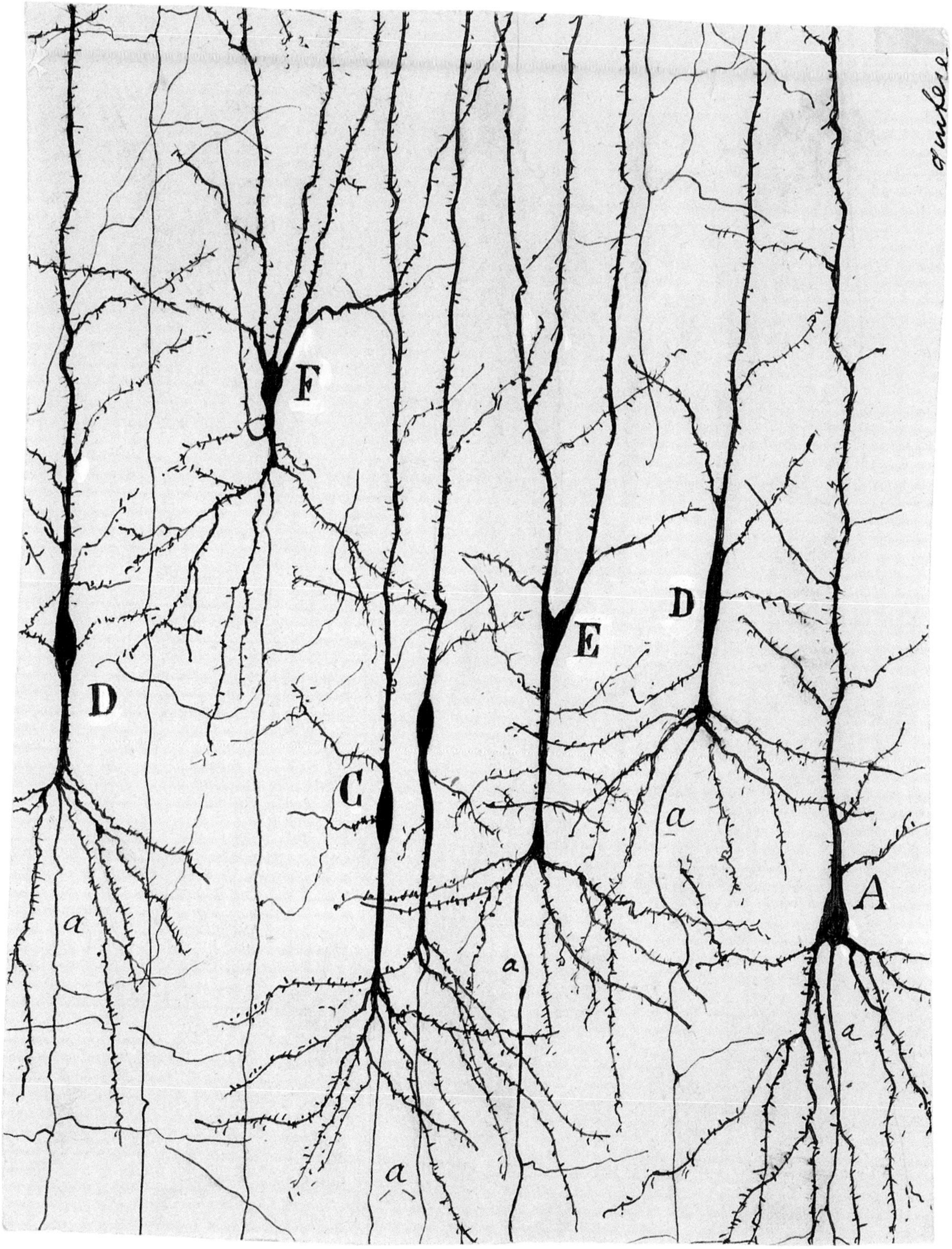

FIGURE 134. Vertical section of the cortex of the insula in a child.

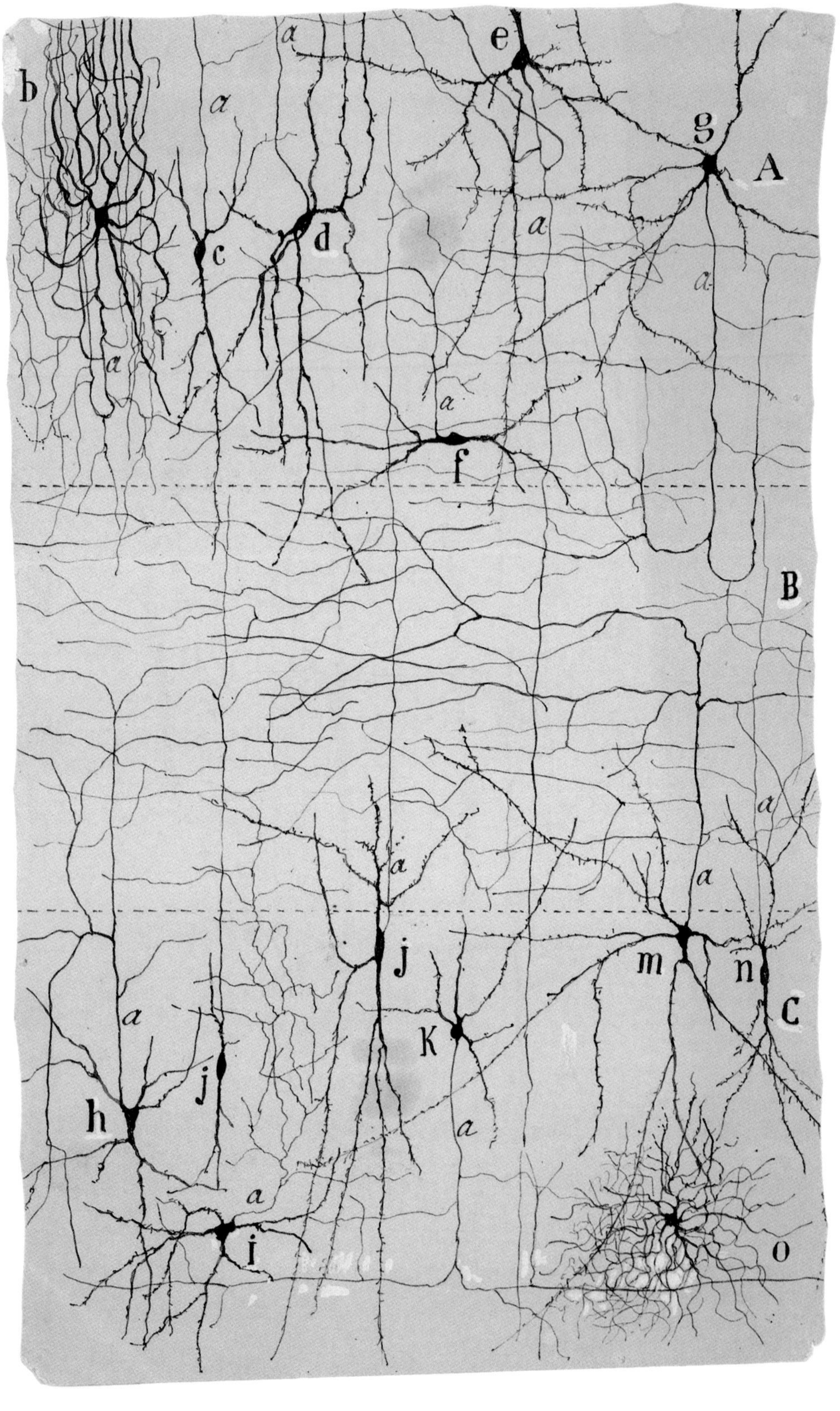

FIGURE 135. Layers that contain small stellate cells of the precentral gyrus in a child.

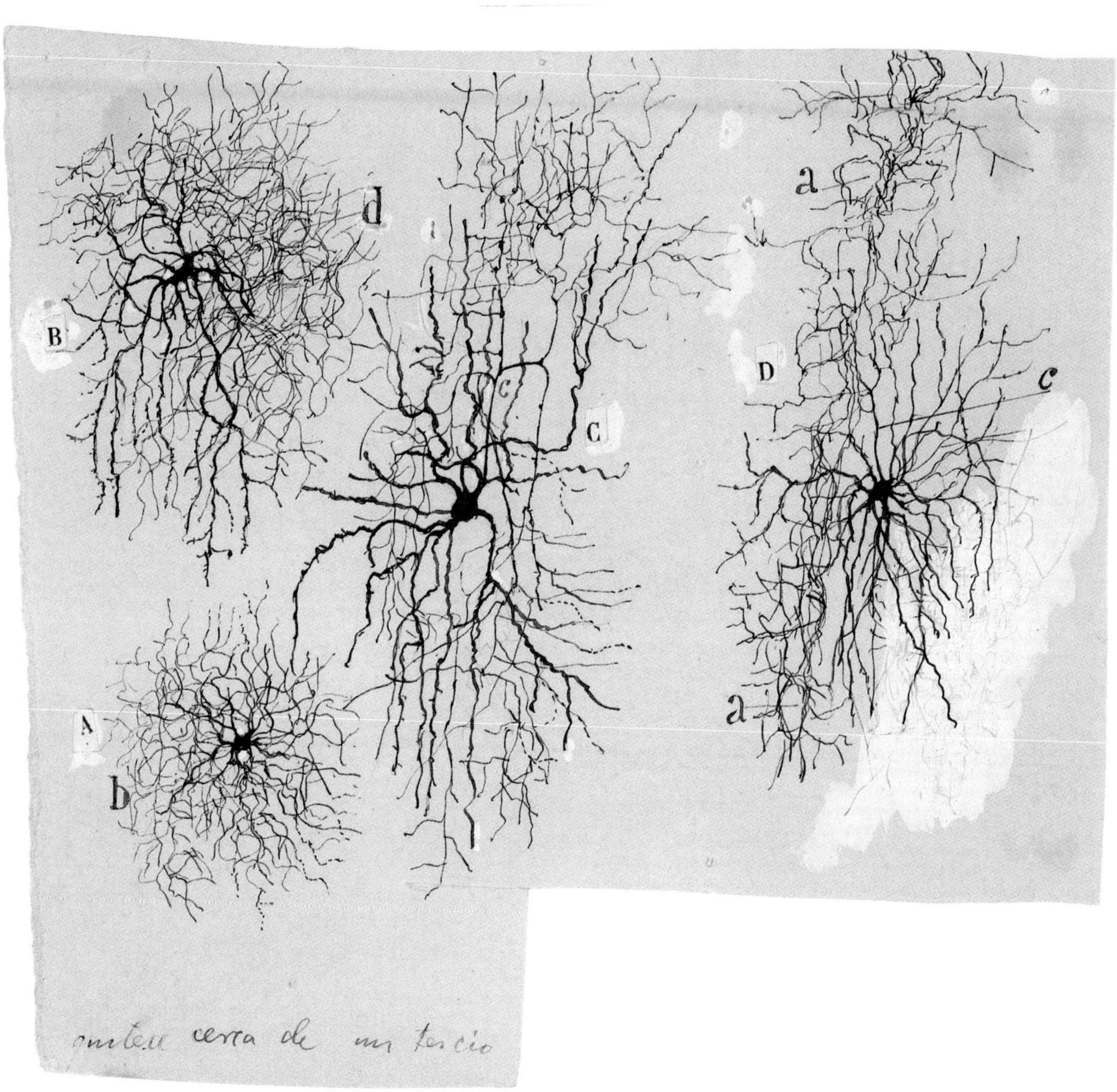

FIGURE 136. Cells with a short axon from the region of the medium and large pyramids in a cat.

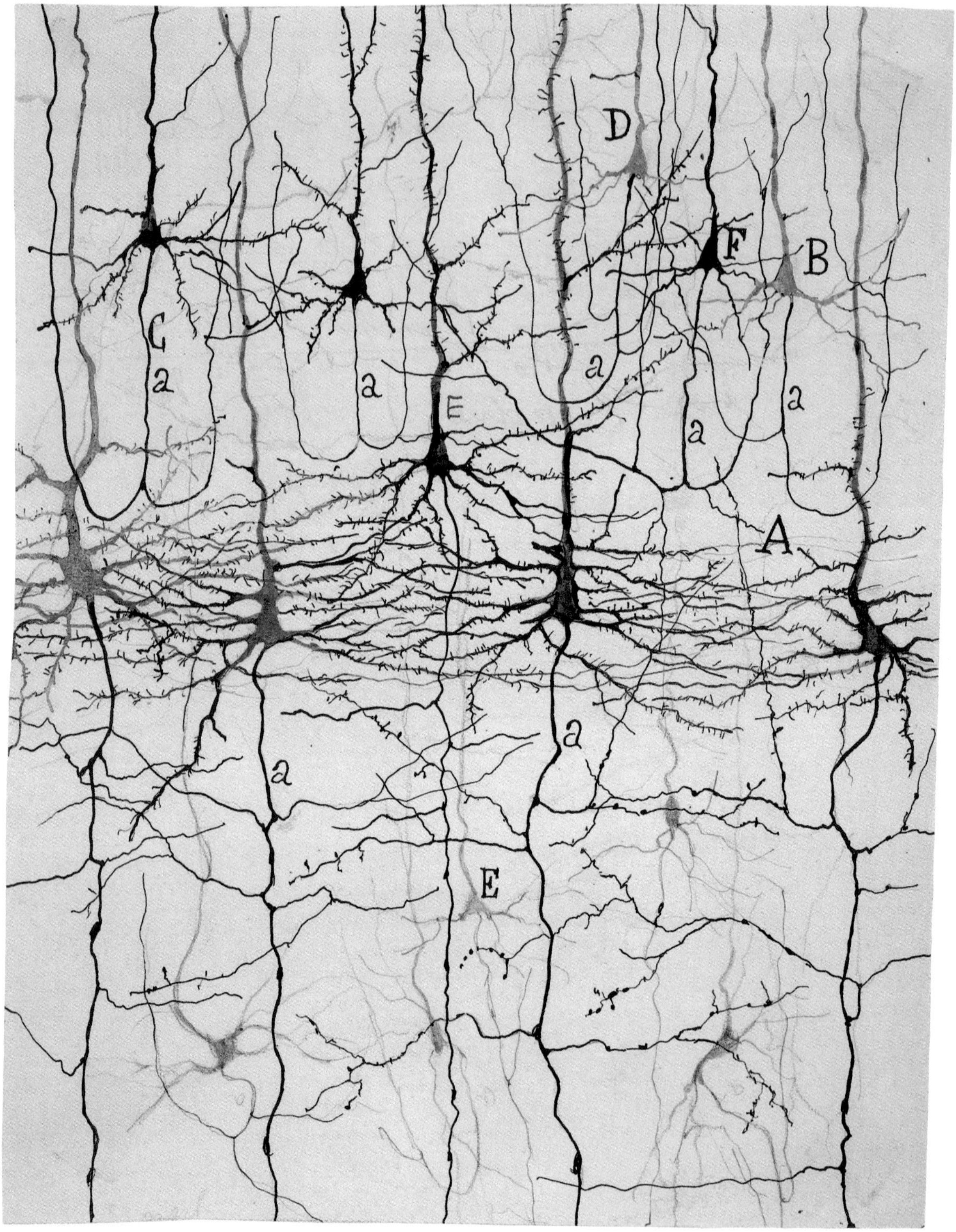

FIGURE 137. Layers 5, 6, and 7 of the visual cortex in a cat.

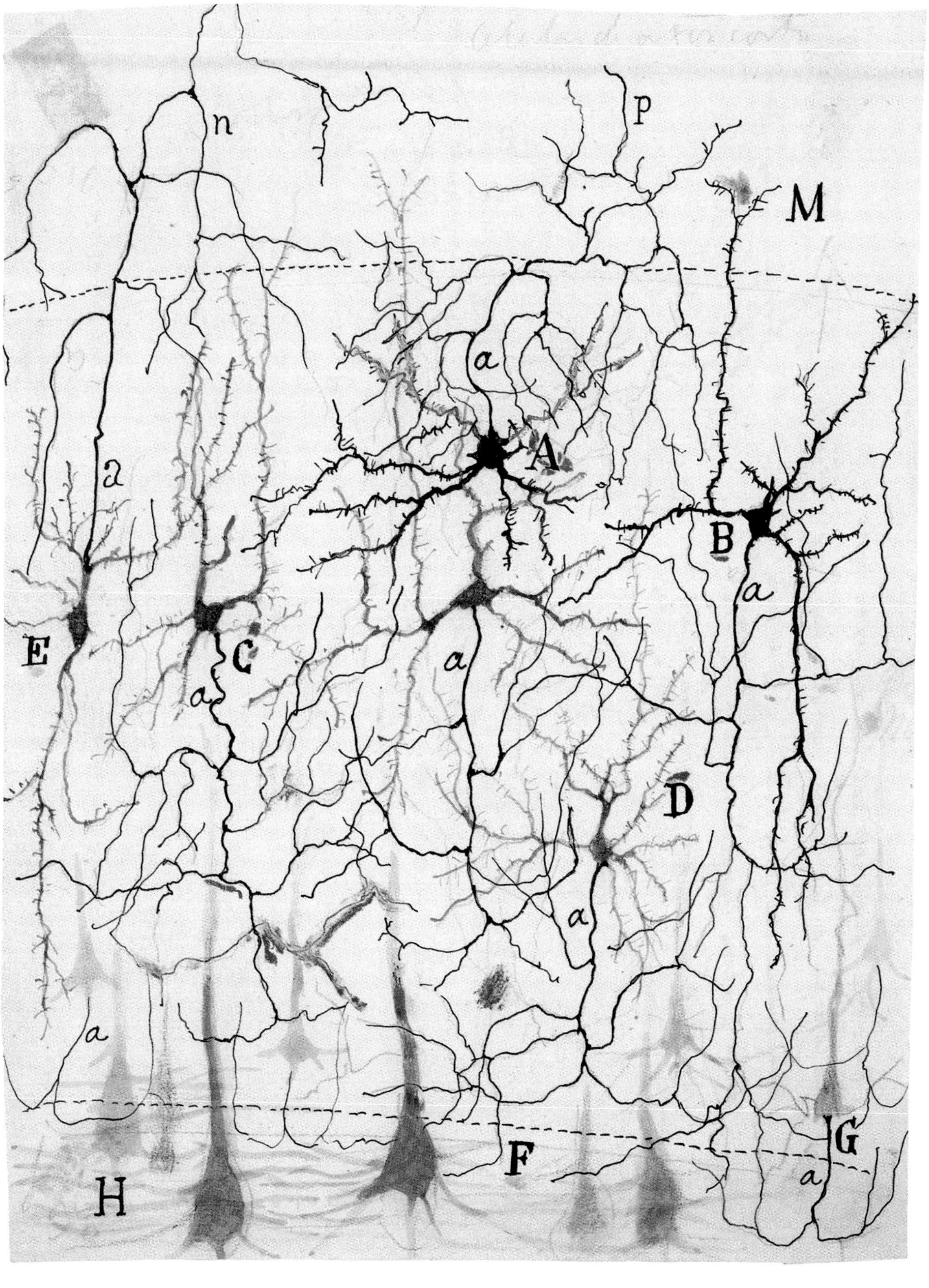

FIGURE 138. Cells with a short axon of the layer of the stellate cells in the cat visual cortex.

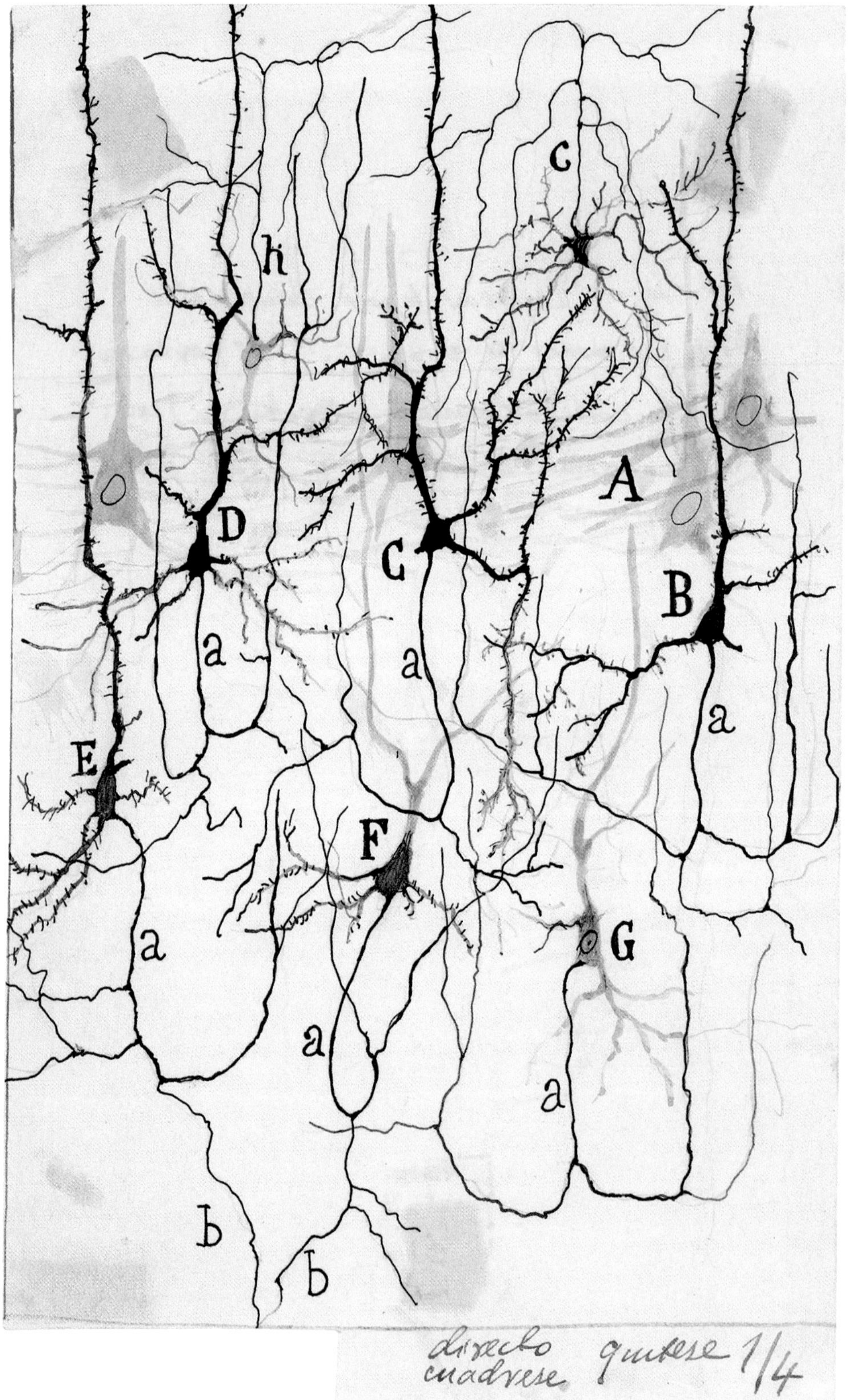

FIGURE 139. Diverse neuronal types of layers 4, 5, and 6 of the visual cortex in a cat.

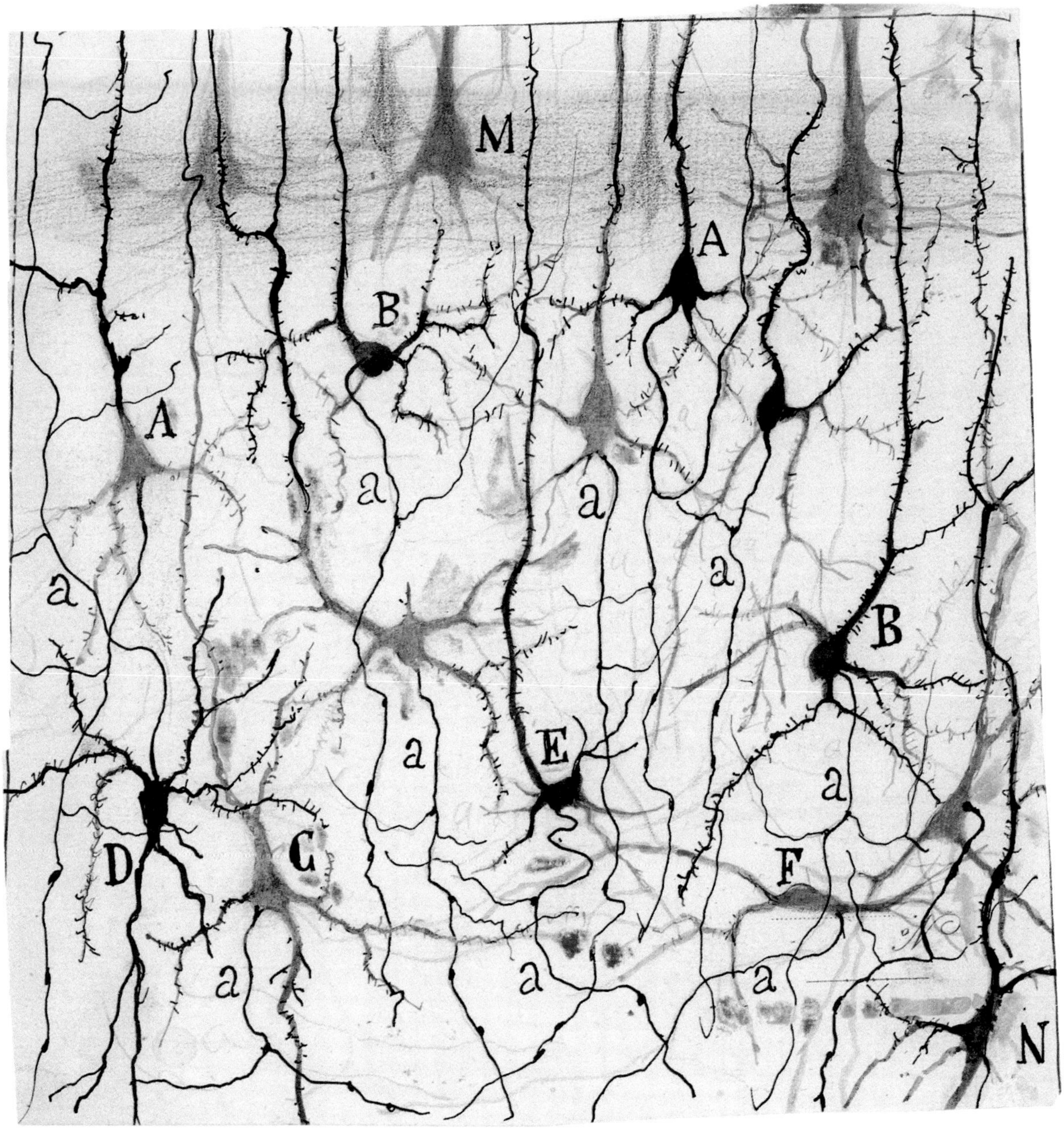

FIGURE 140. Neurons of the layer of the polymorphic cells in the cat visual cortex.

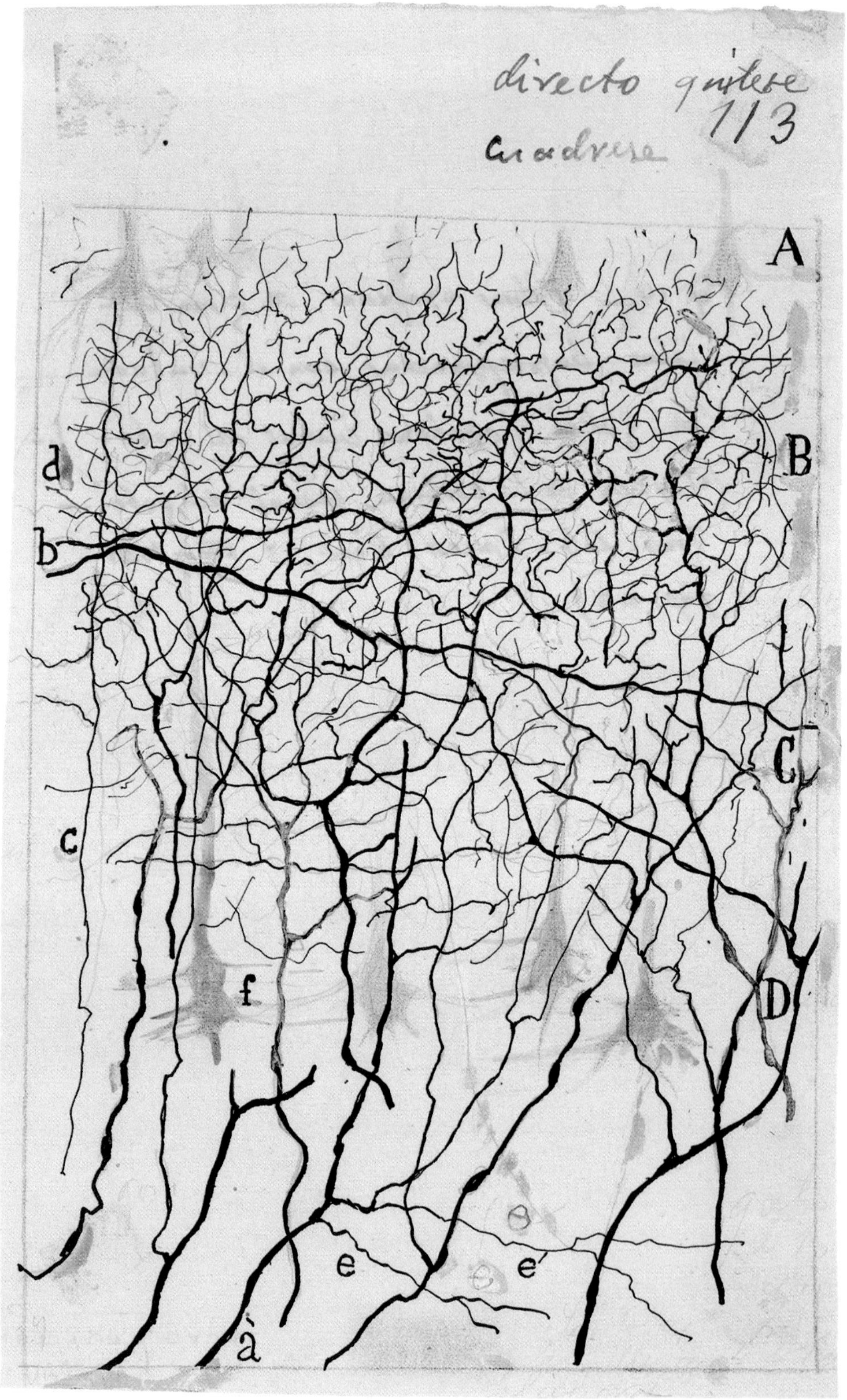

FIGURE 141. Exogenous fibers of large caliber of the visual cortex in a cat.

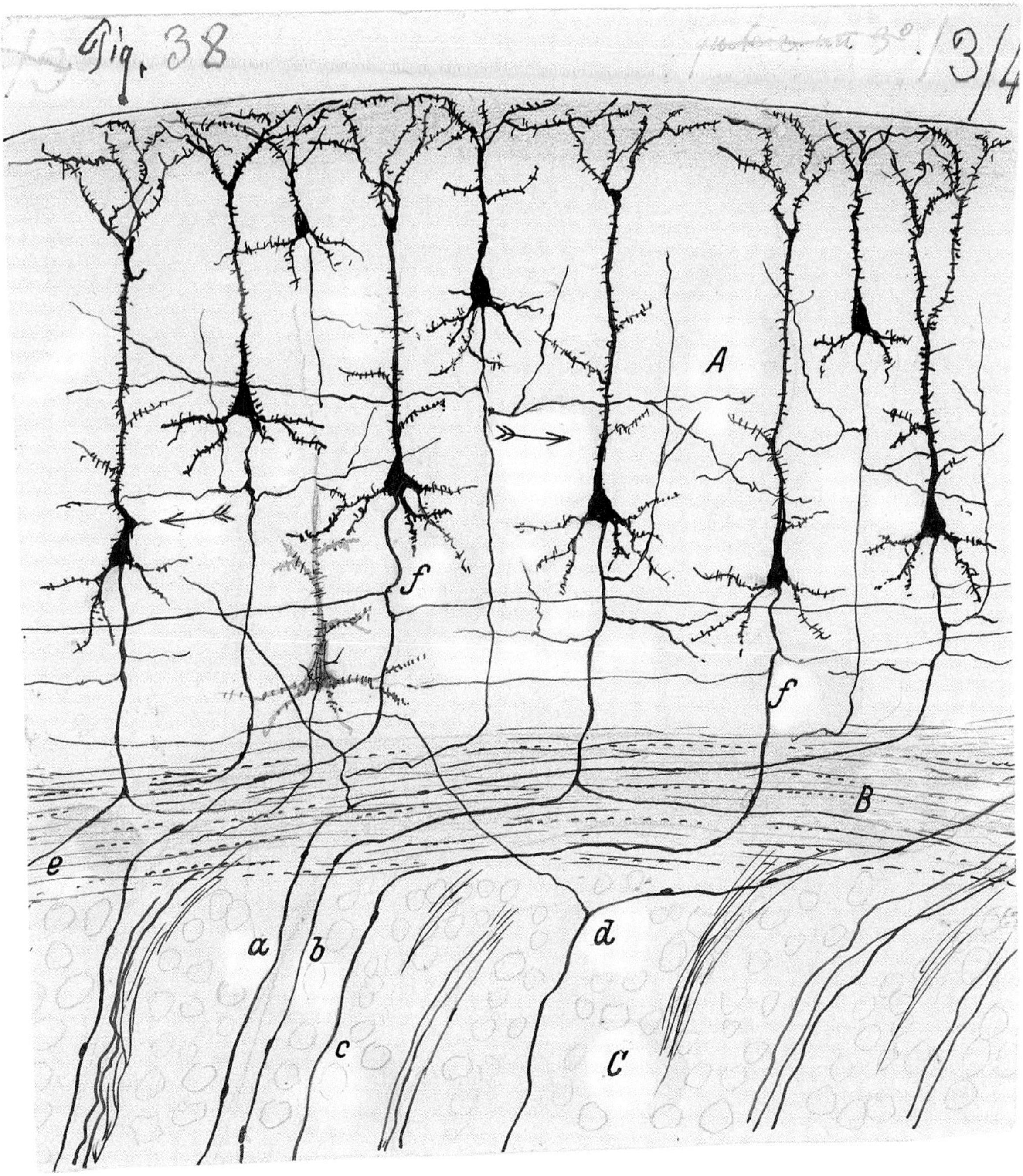

FIGURE 142. Schematic representation of the enormous length of the cerebral axonal collaterals in the mouse.

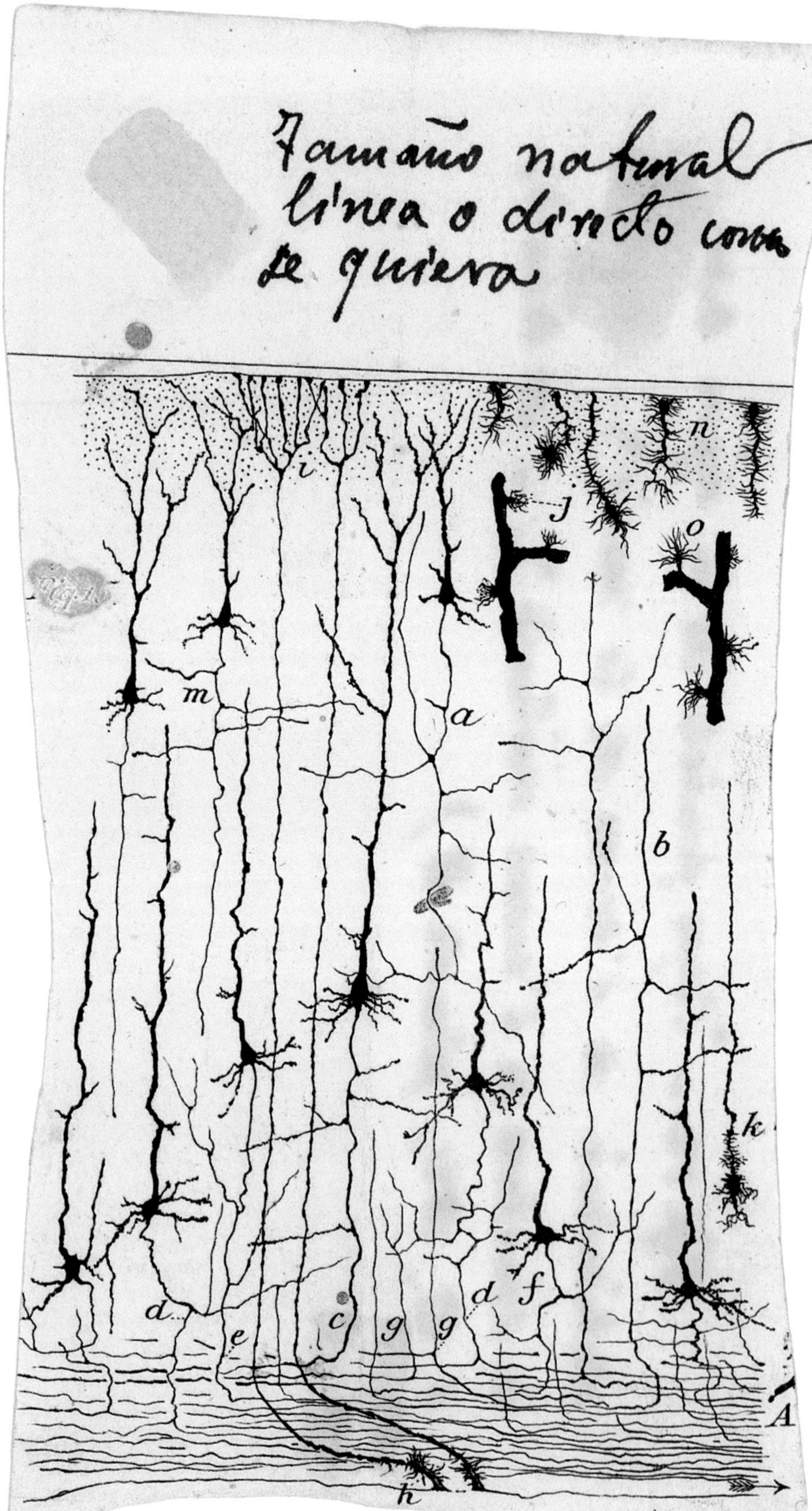

FIGURE 143. Frontal section of the supraventricular region in the mouse cortex.

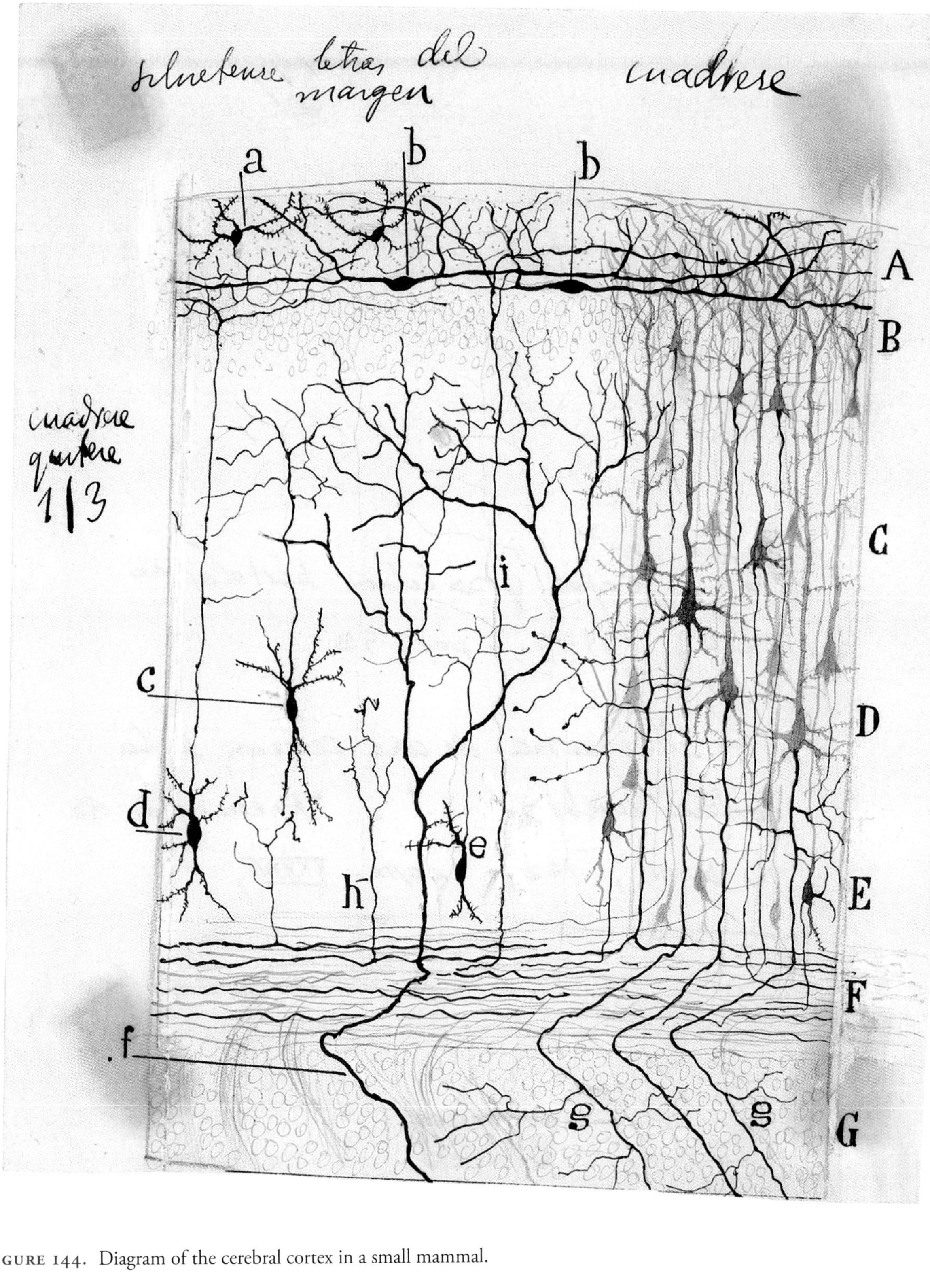

FIGURE 144. Diagram of the cerebral cortex in a small mammal.

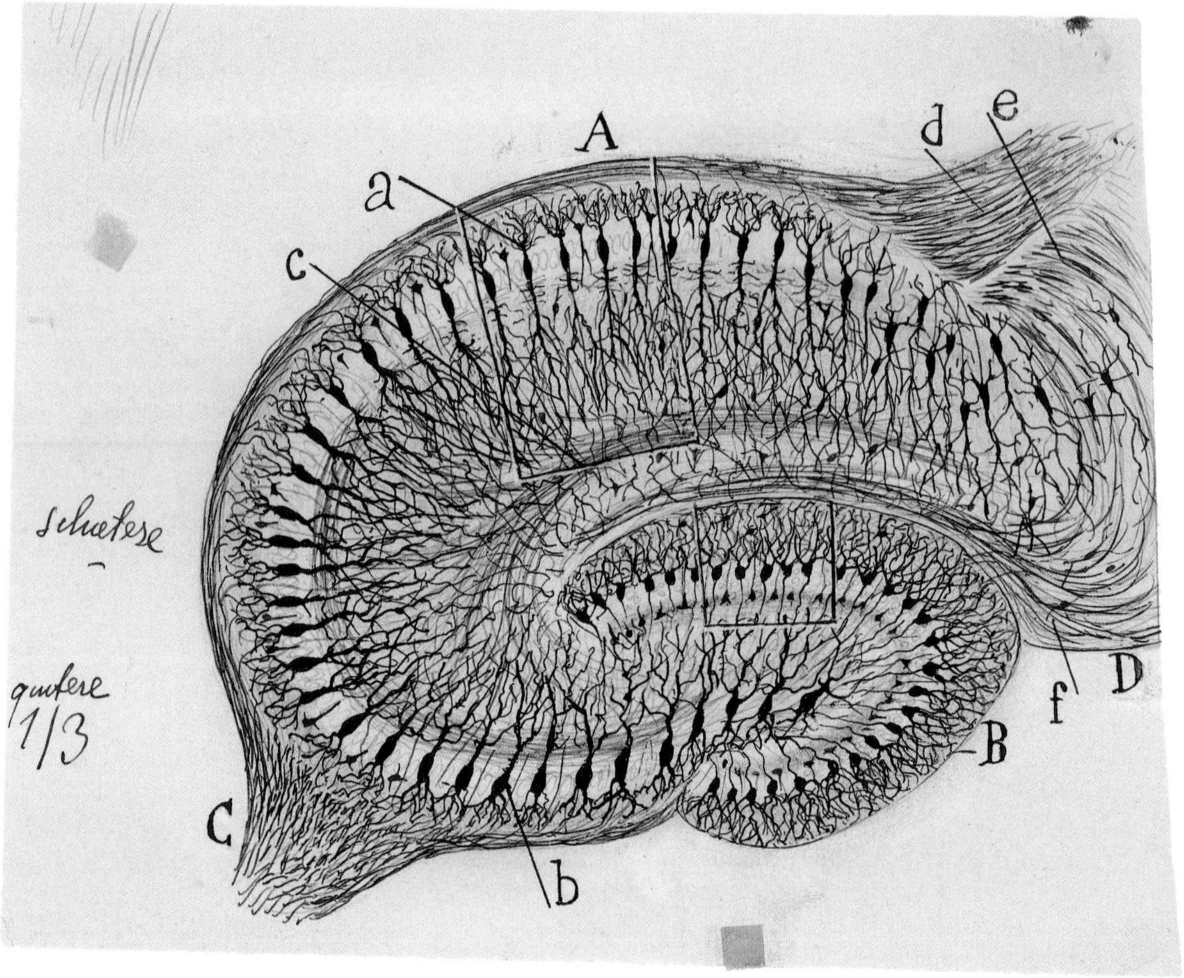

FIGURE 145. Diagram of the architecture of Ammon's horn and fascia dentata.

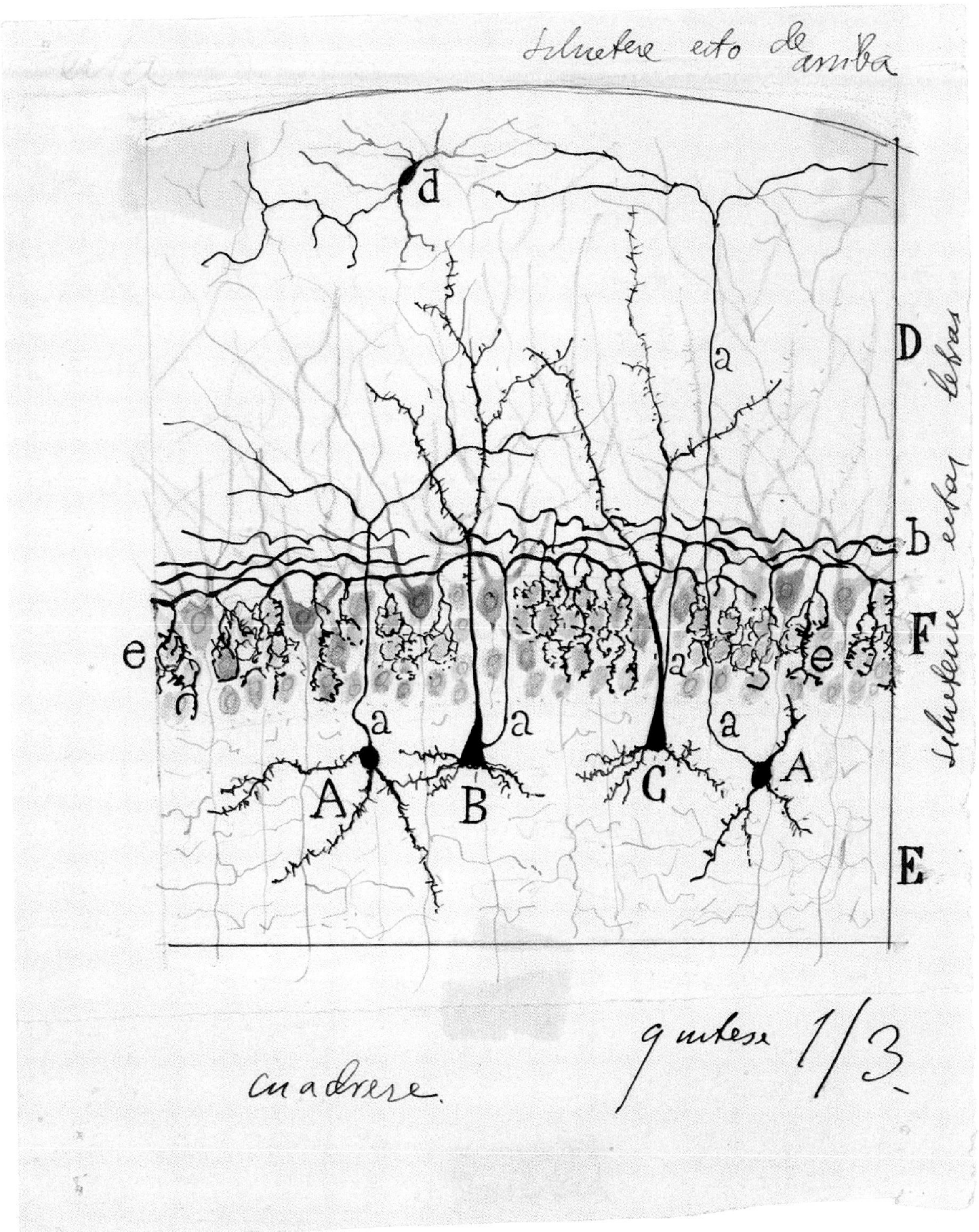

FIGURE 146. Diagram of the fascia dentata.

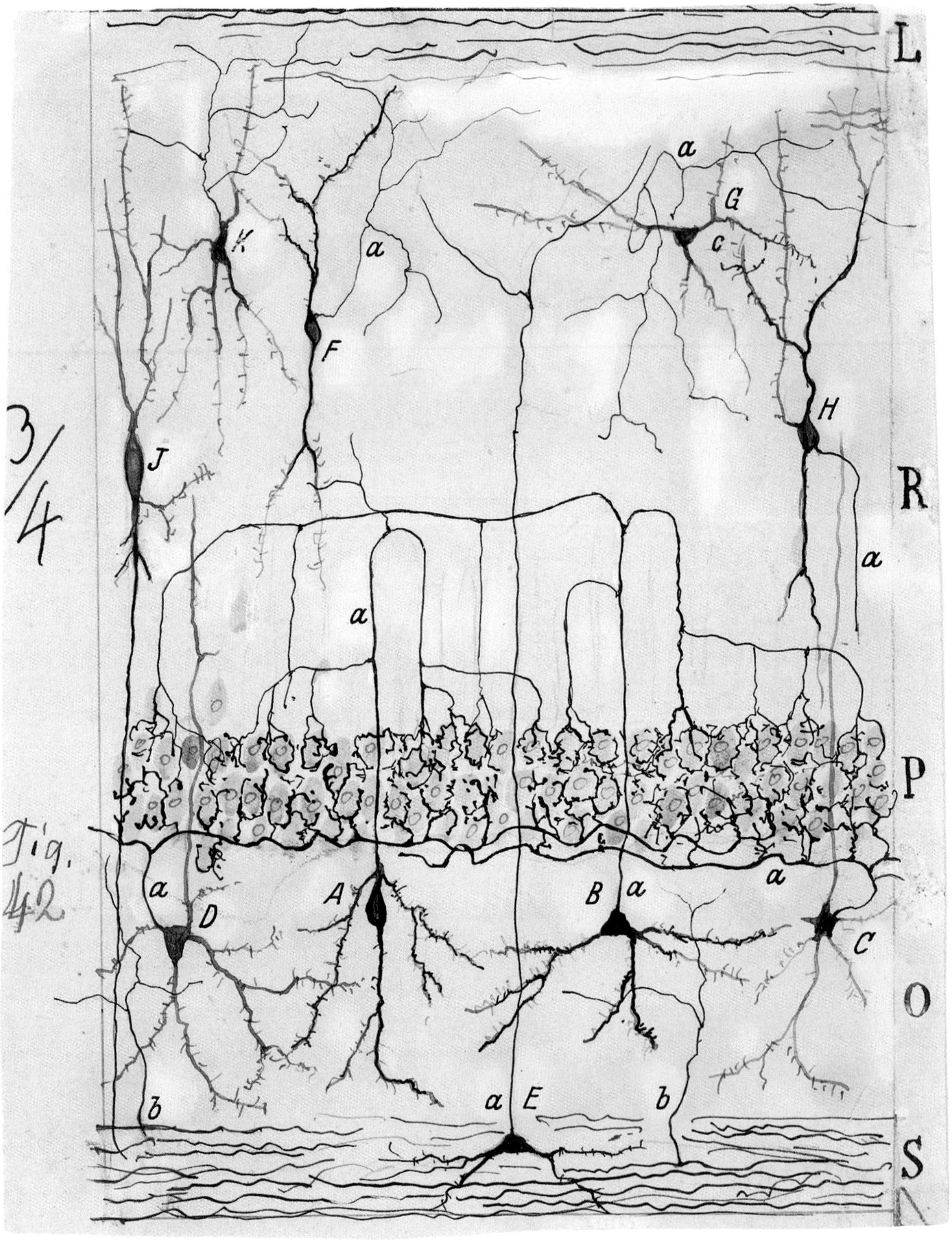

FIGURE 147. Diagram of Ammon's horn.

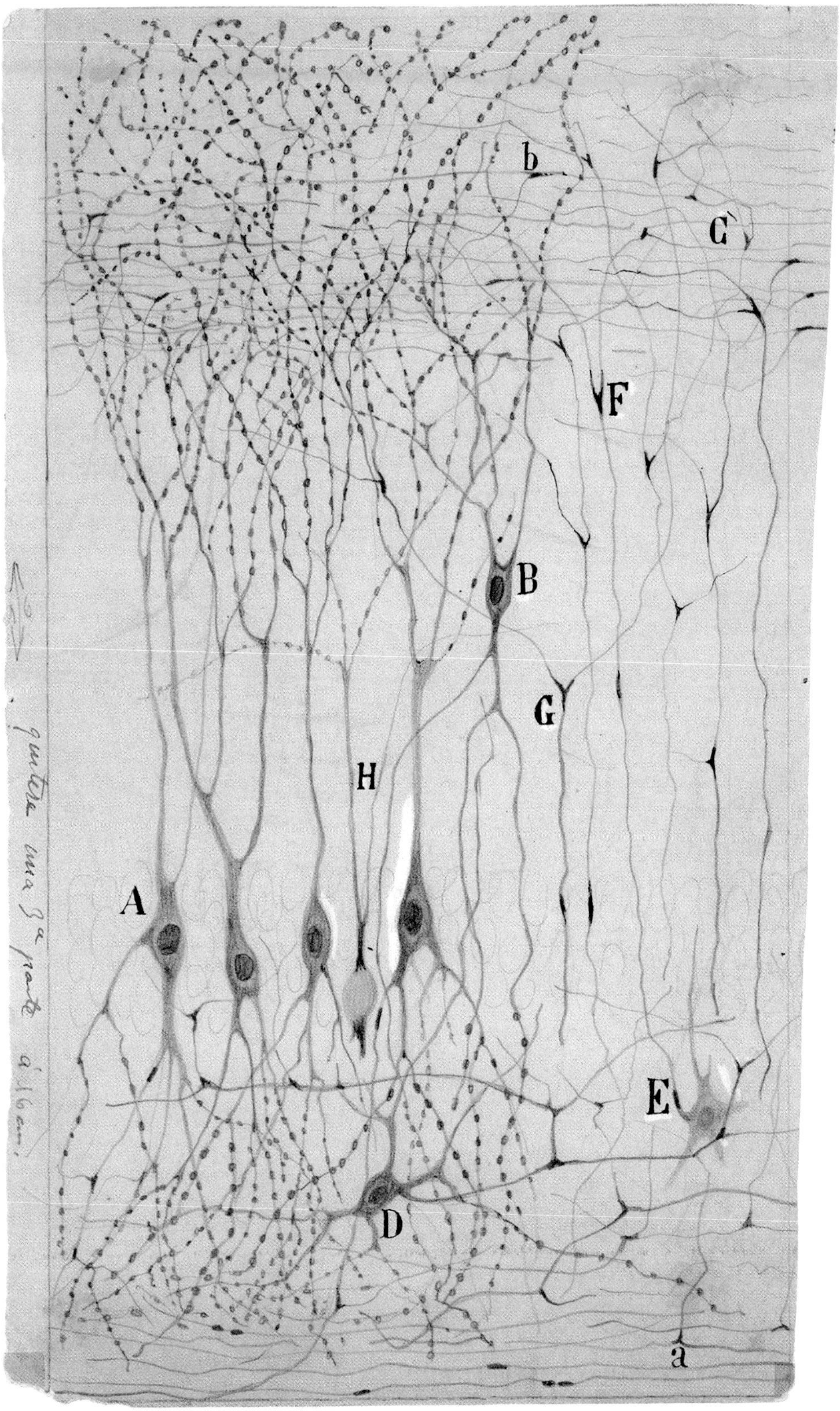

FIGURE 148. Ammon's horn in a one-month-old rabbit.

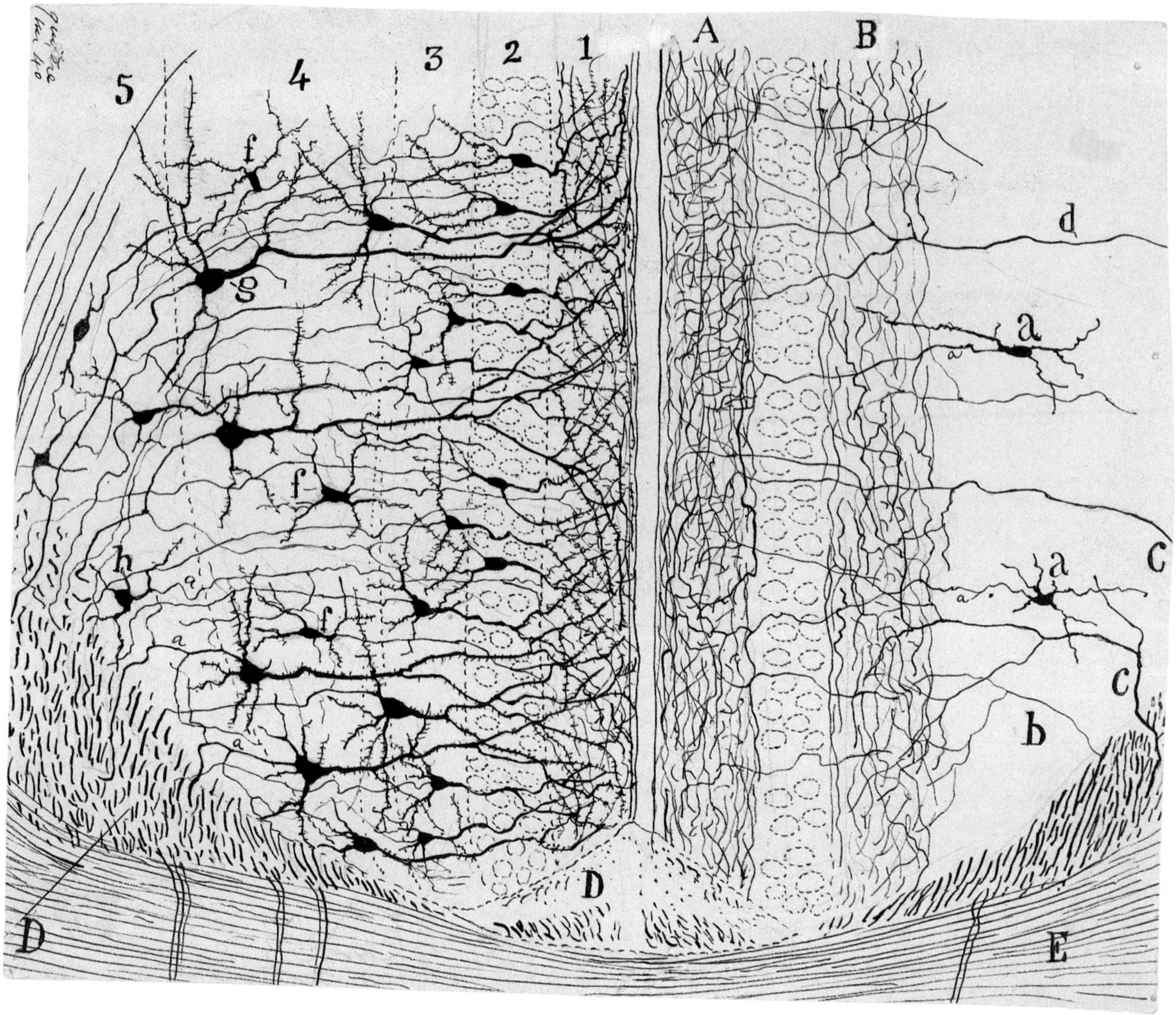

FIGURE 149. Interhemispheric cortex in the mouse.

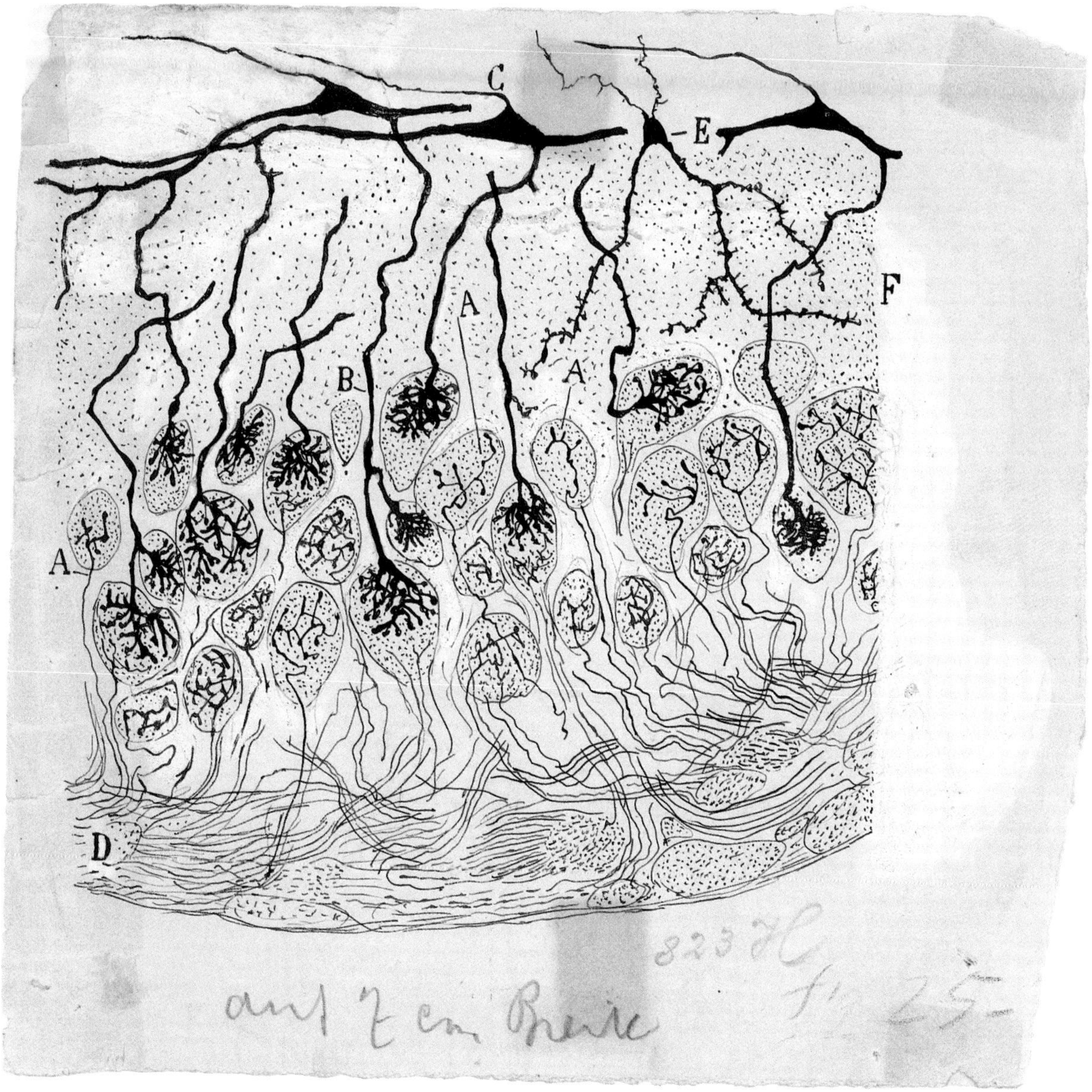

FIGURE 150. Olfactory bulb in a duck.

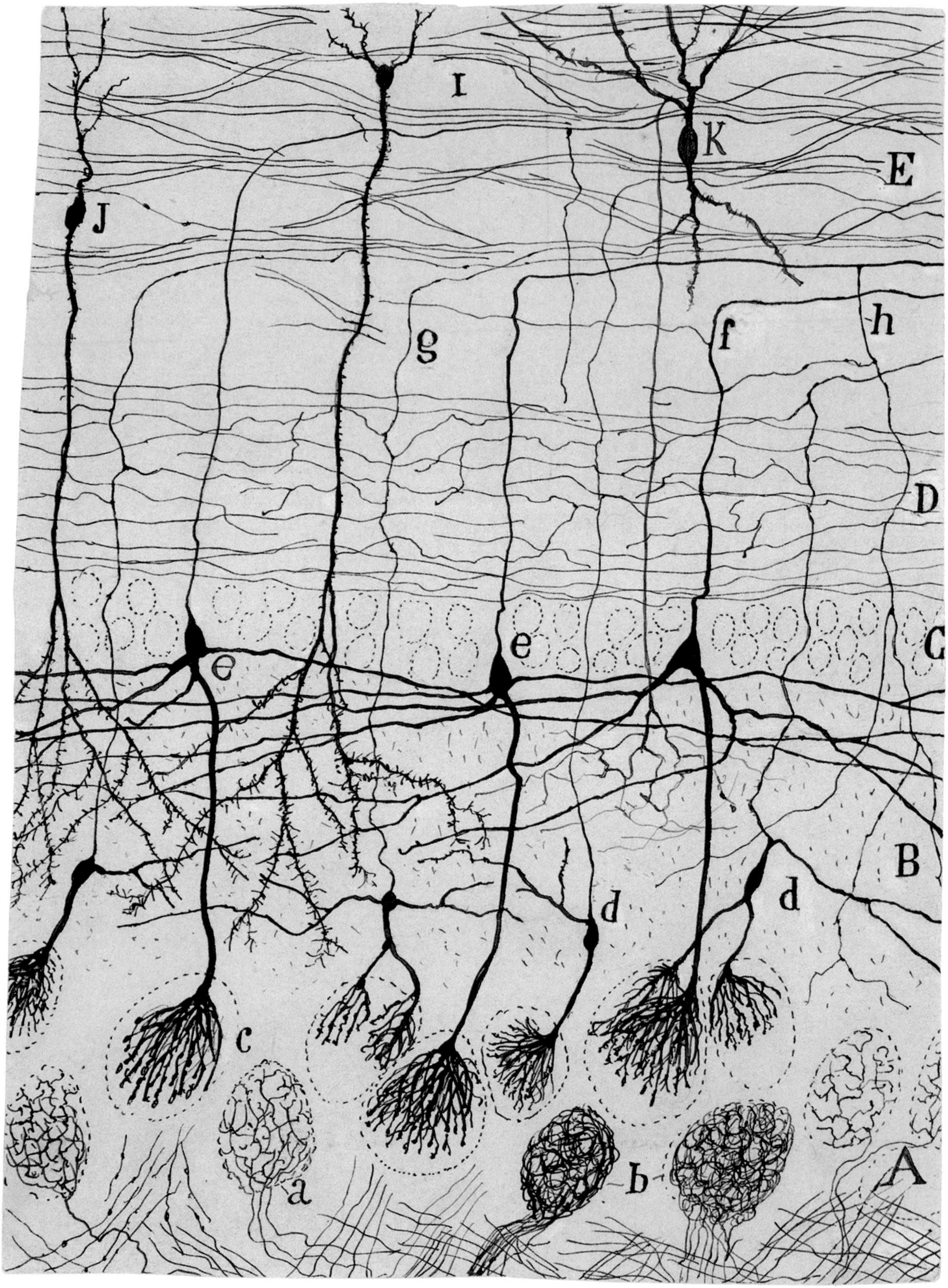

FIGURE 151. Olfactory bulb in a kitten.

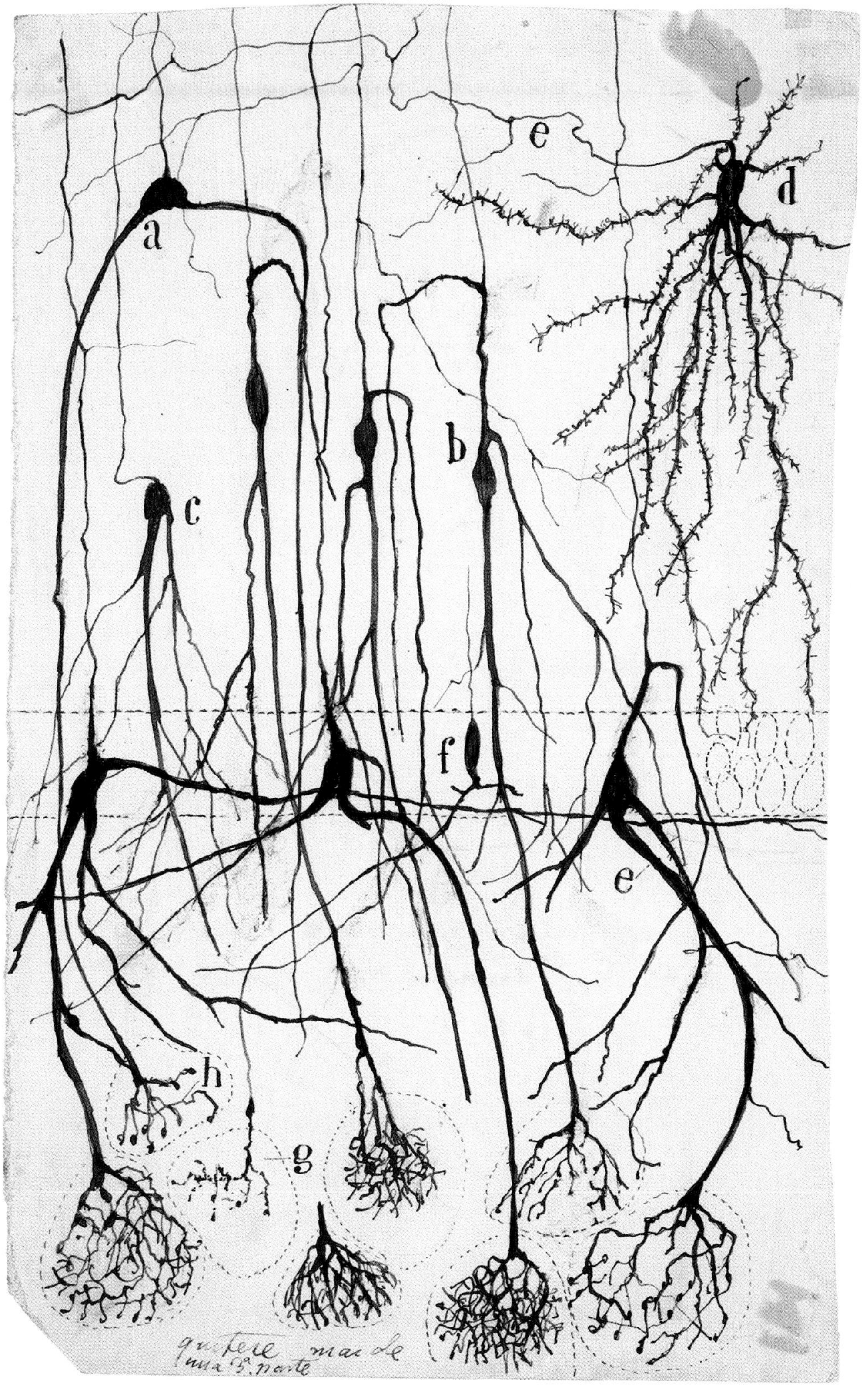

FIGURE 152. Olfactory bulb in a cat.

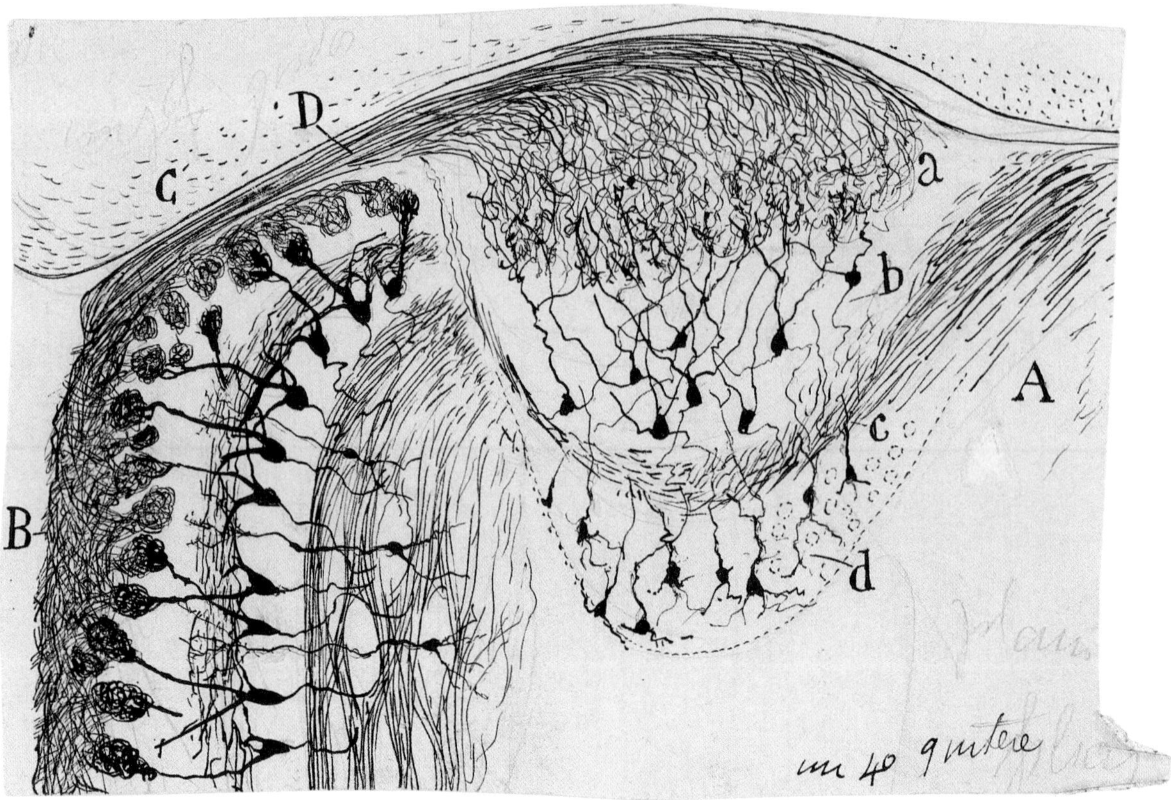

FIGURE 153. Horizontal section of the olfactory bulb in a mouse.

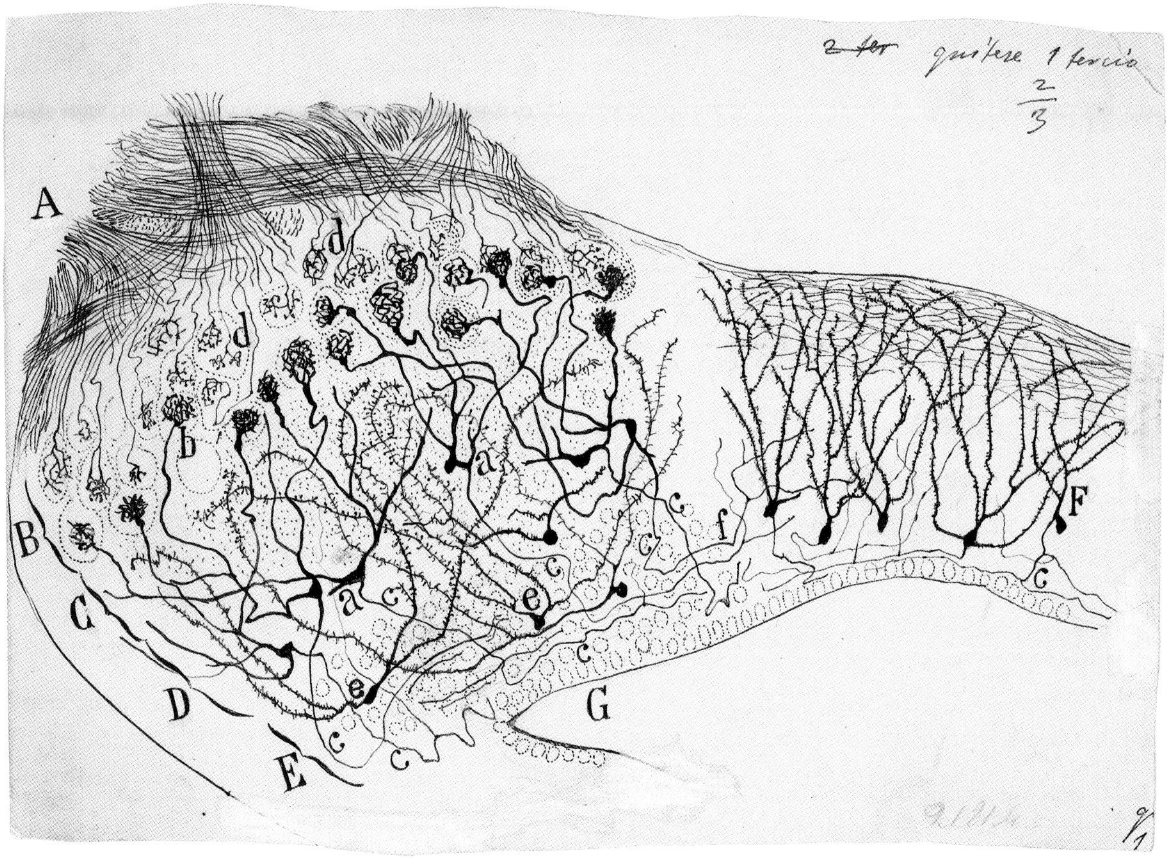

FIGURE 154. Cerebral vesicle in an Iberian ribbed newt.

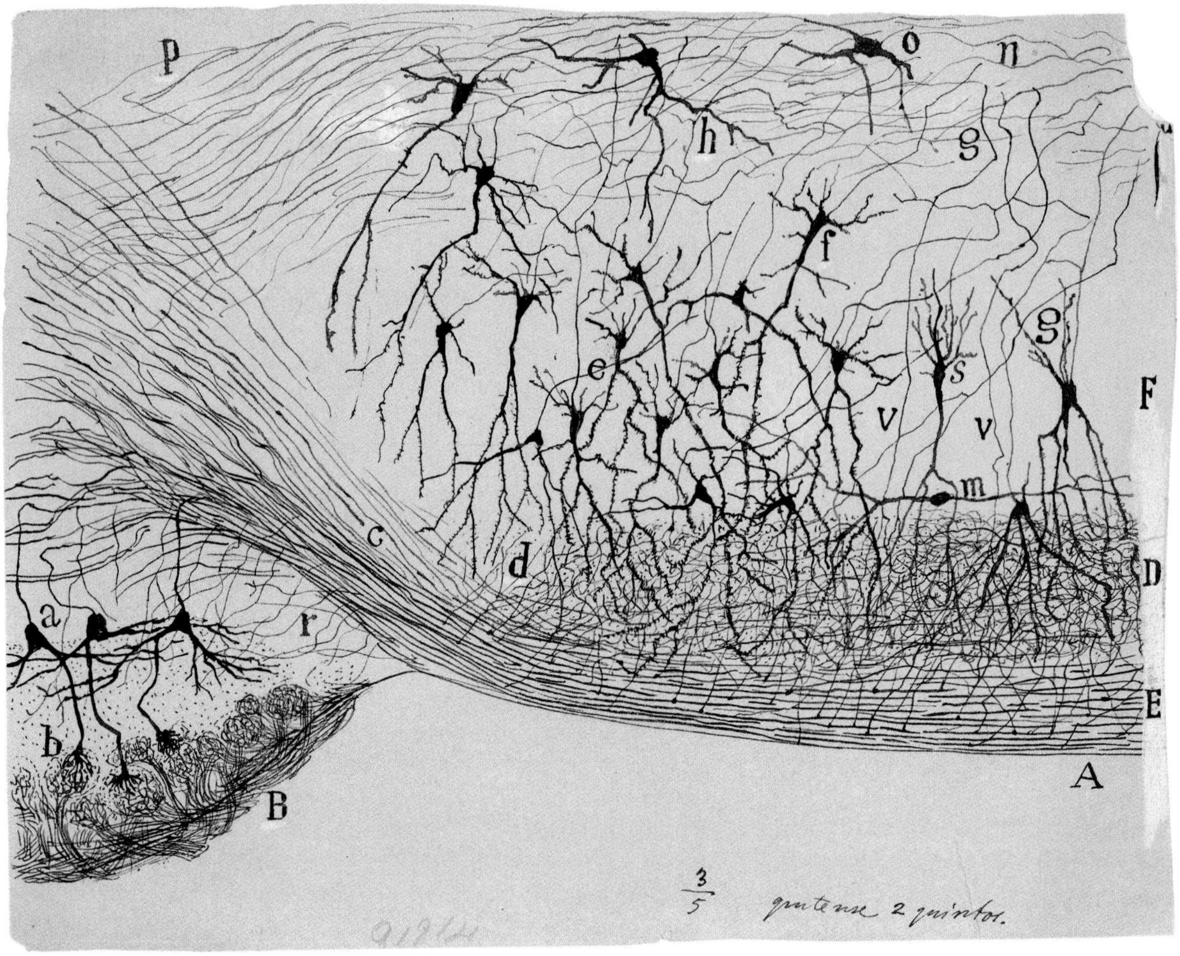

FIGURE 155. Olfactory bulb and tract in a fifteen-day-old mouse.

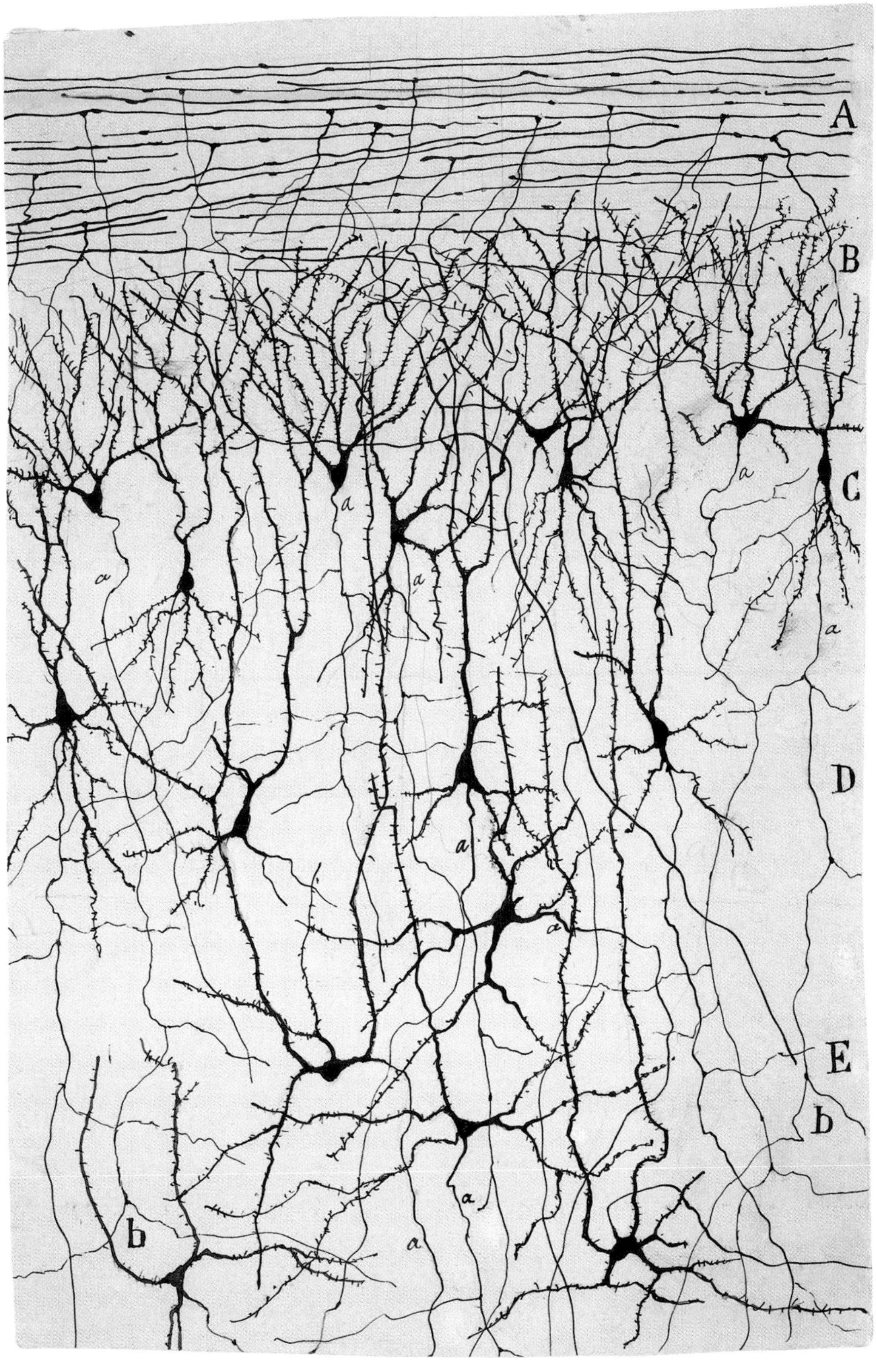

FIGURE 156. Cortex of the frontal lobe covered by the lateral olfactory root.

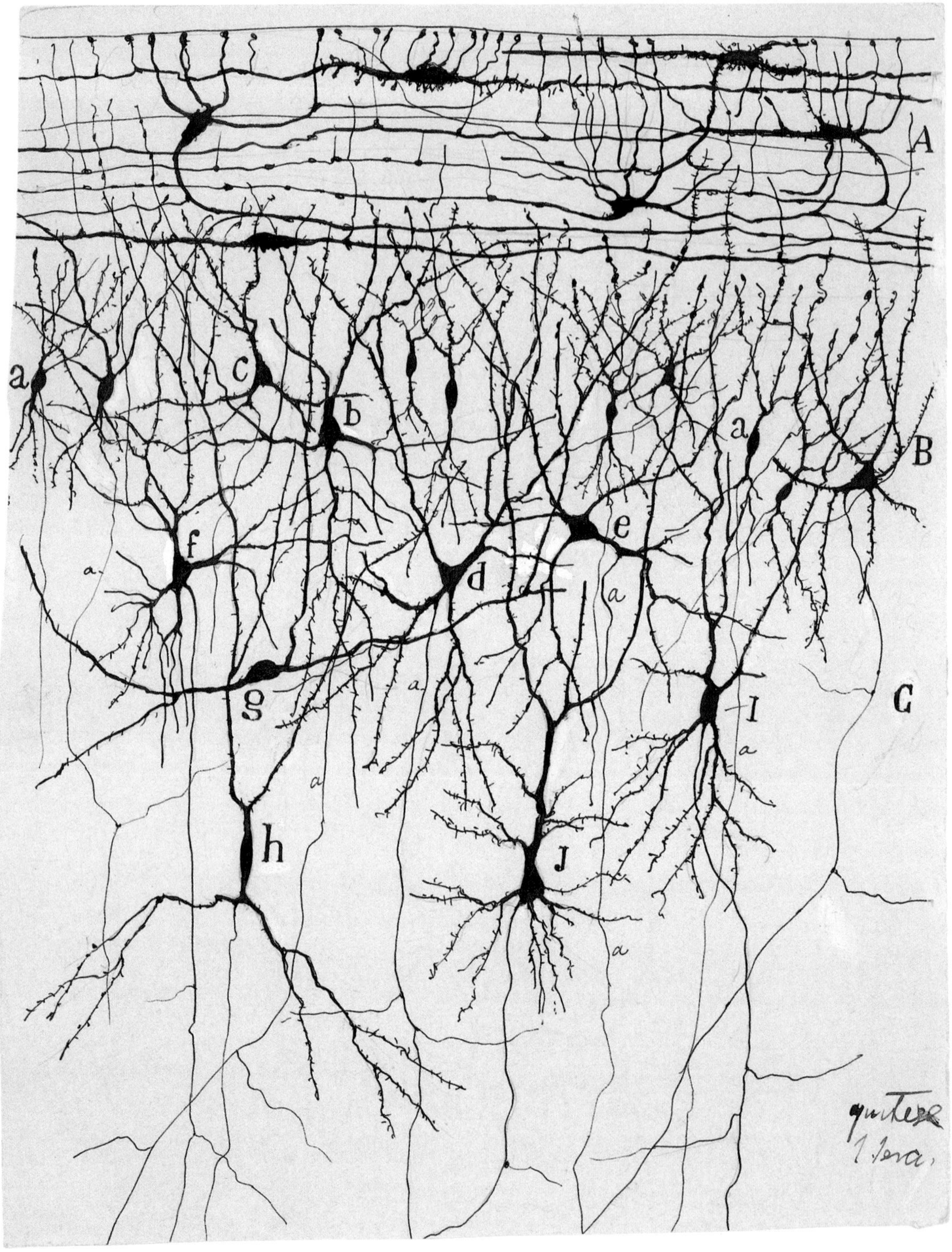

FIGURE 157. Section of the first and second layers of the human entorhinal cortex.

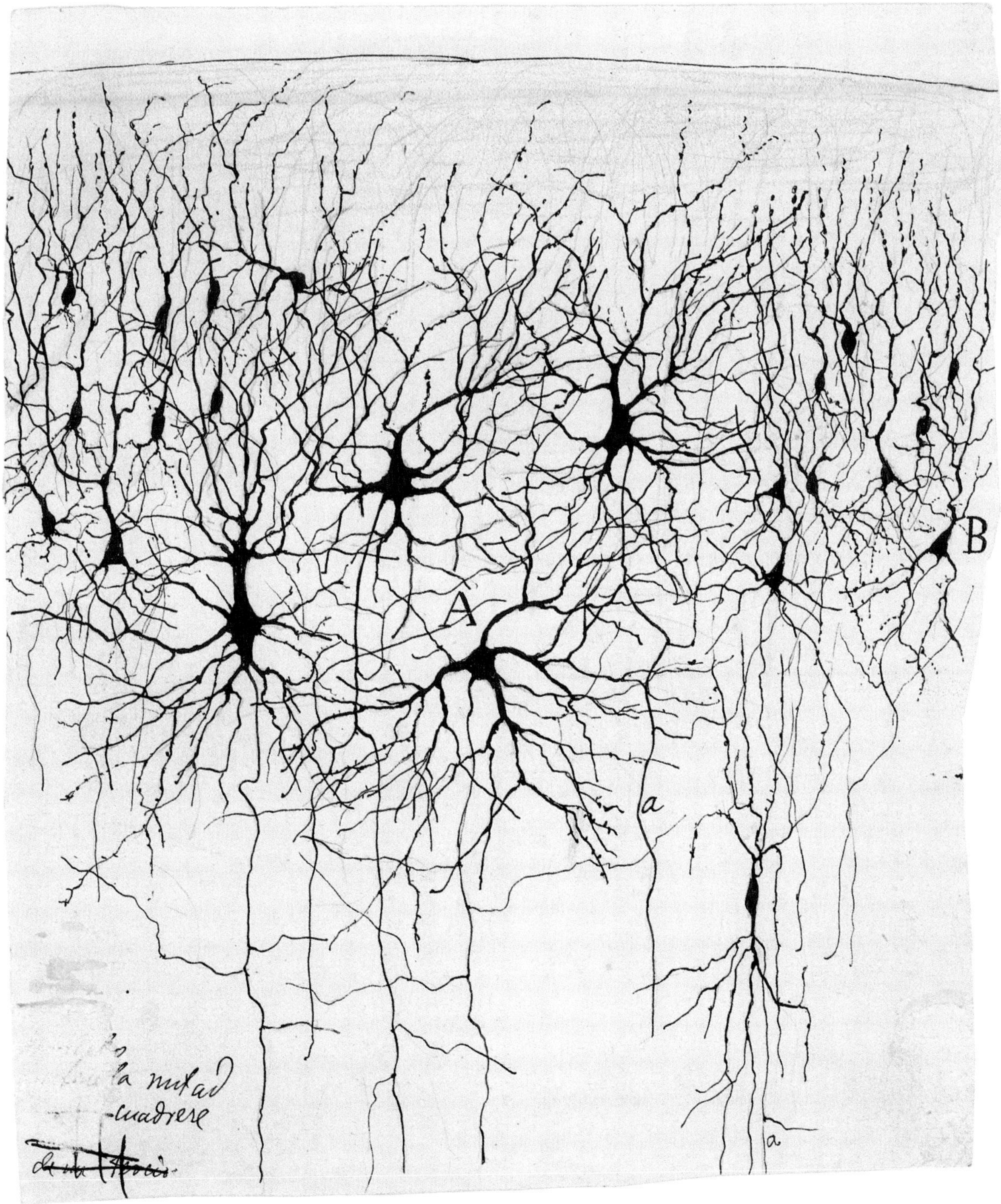

FIGURE 158. Cells of the layer of the giant polymorphic cells of the human entorhinal cortex.

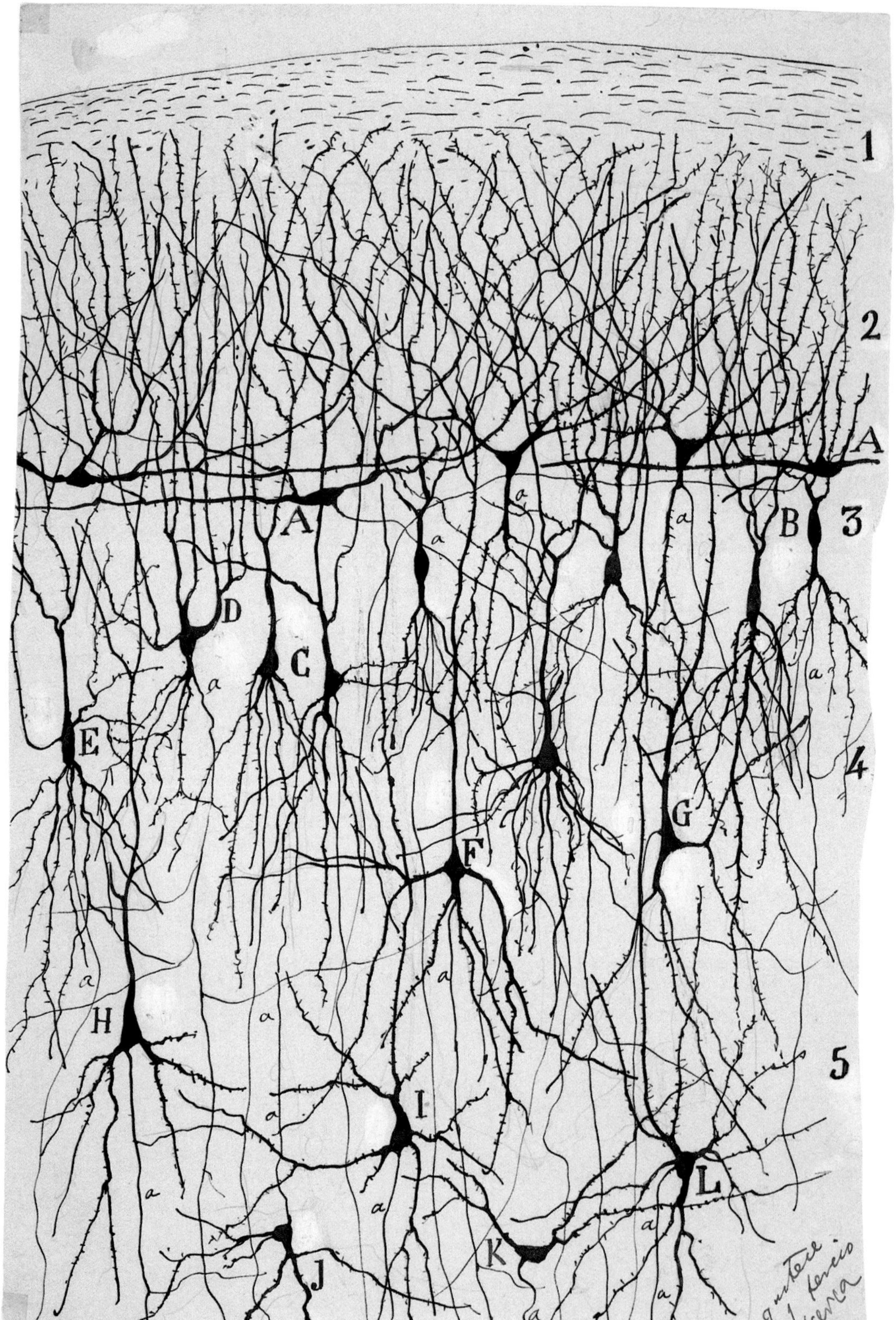

FIGURE 159. Transverse section of the temporal lobe in a cat.

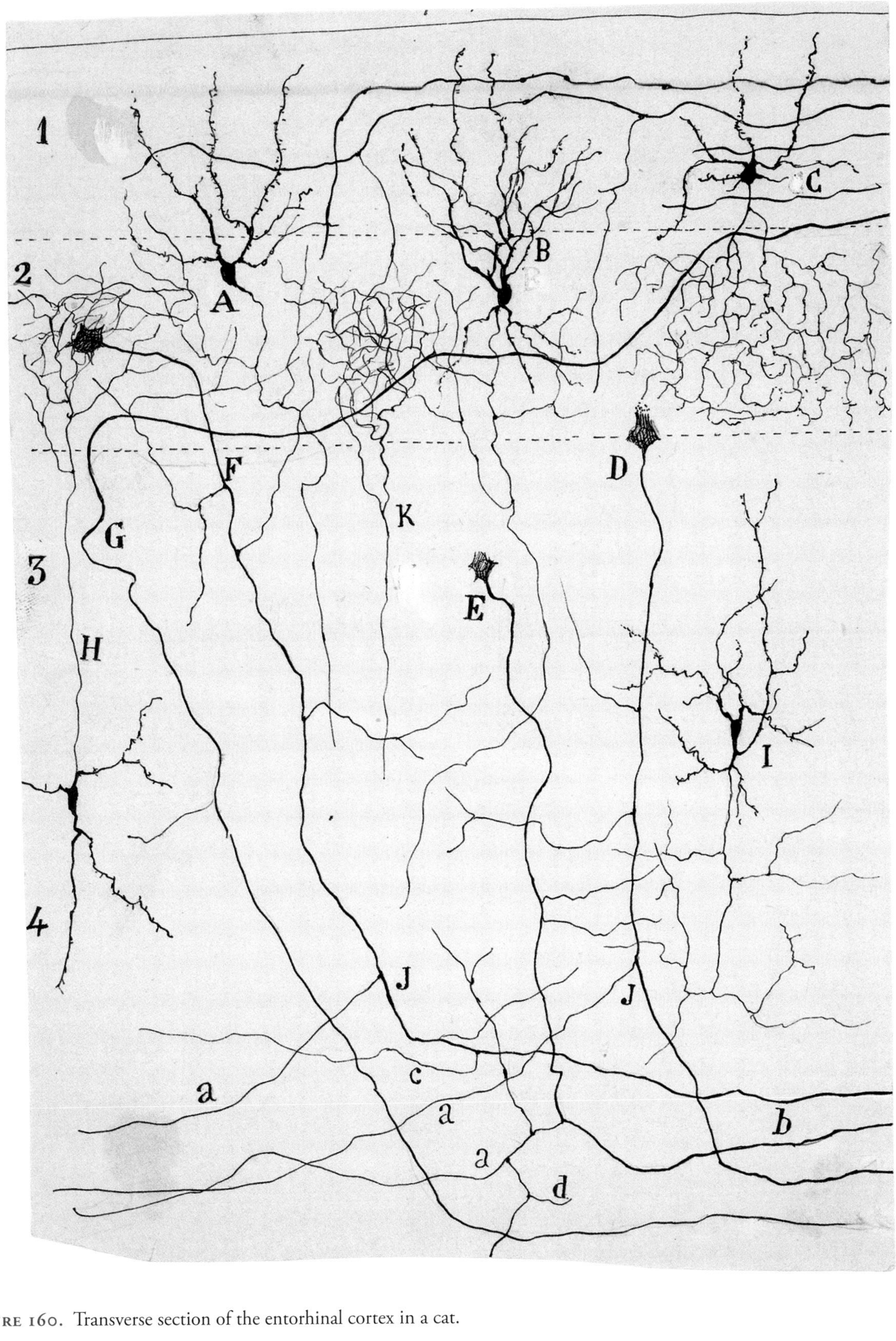

FIGURE 160. Transverse section of the entorhinal cortex in a cat.

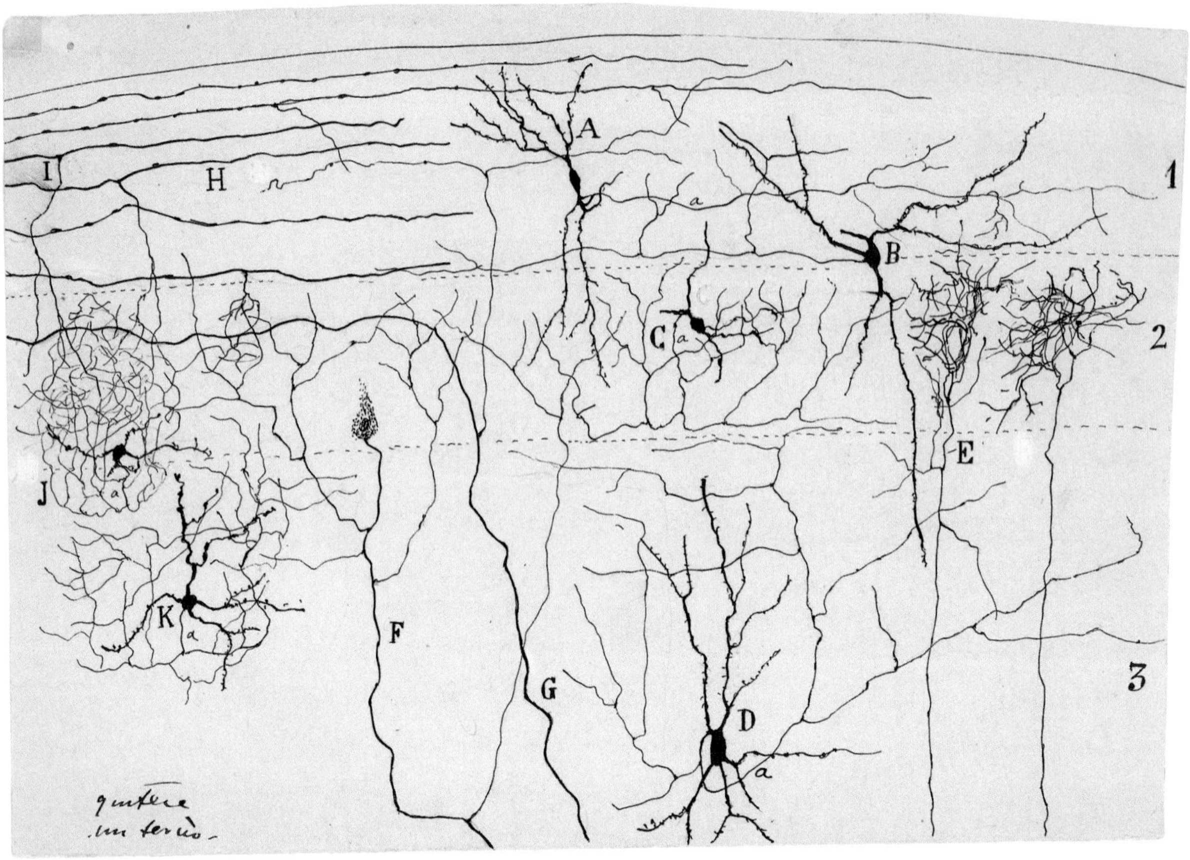

FIGURE 161. Cells with a short axon in the cat entorhinal cortex.

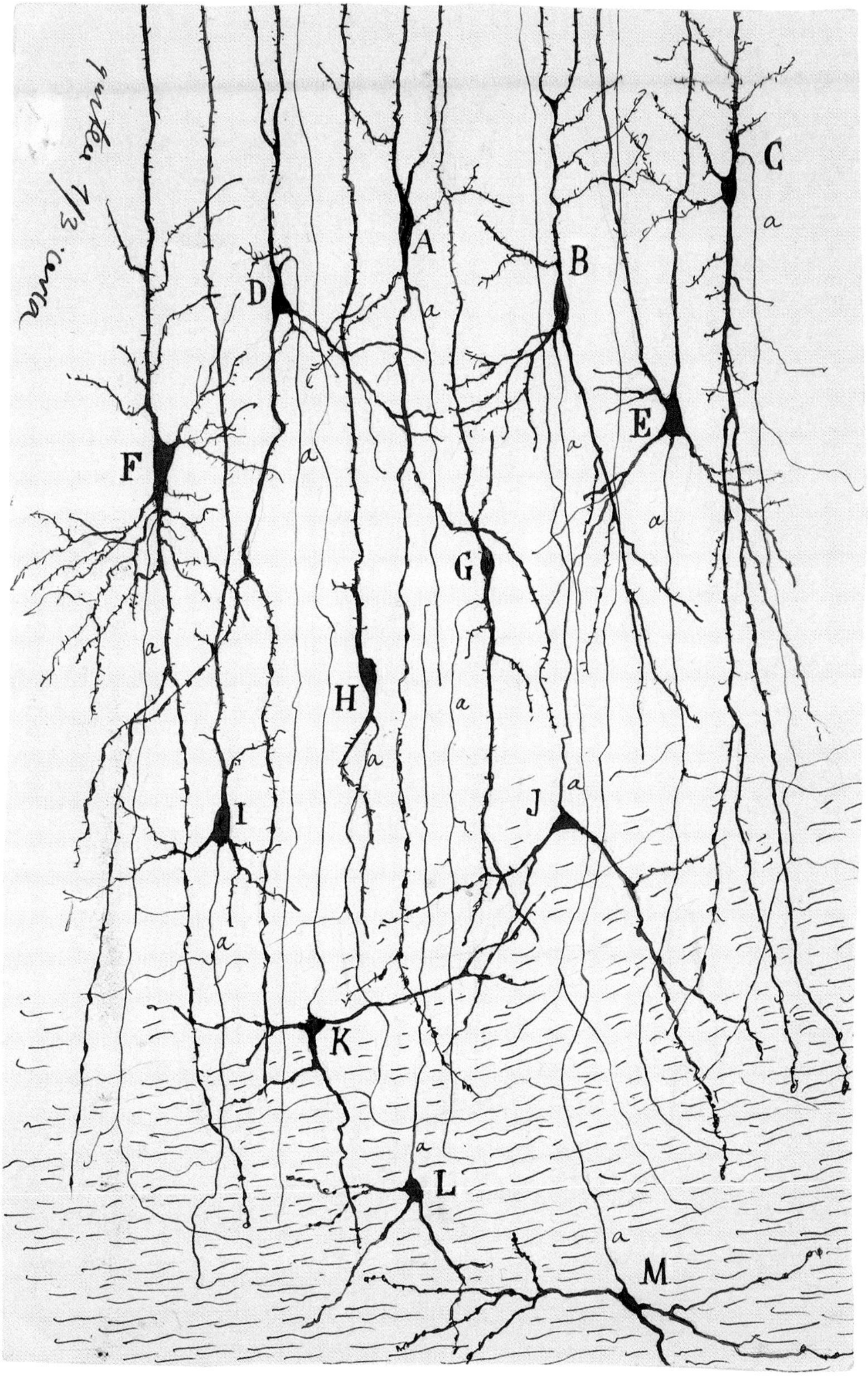

FIGURE 162. Section of the deep layers in the human entorhinal cortex.

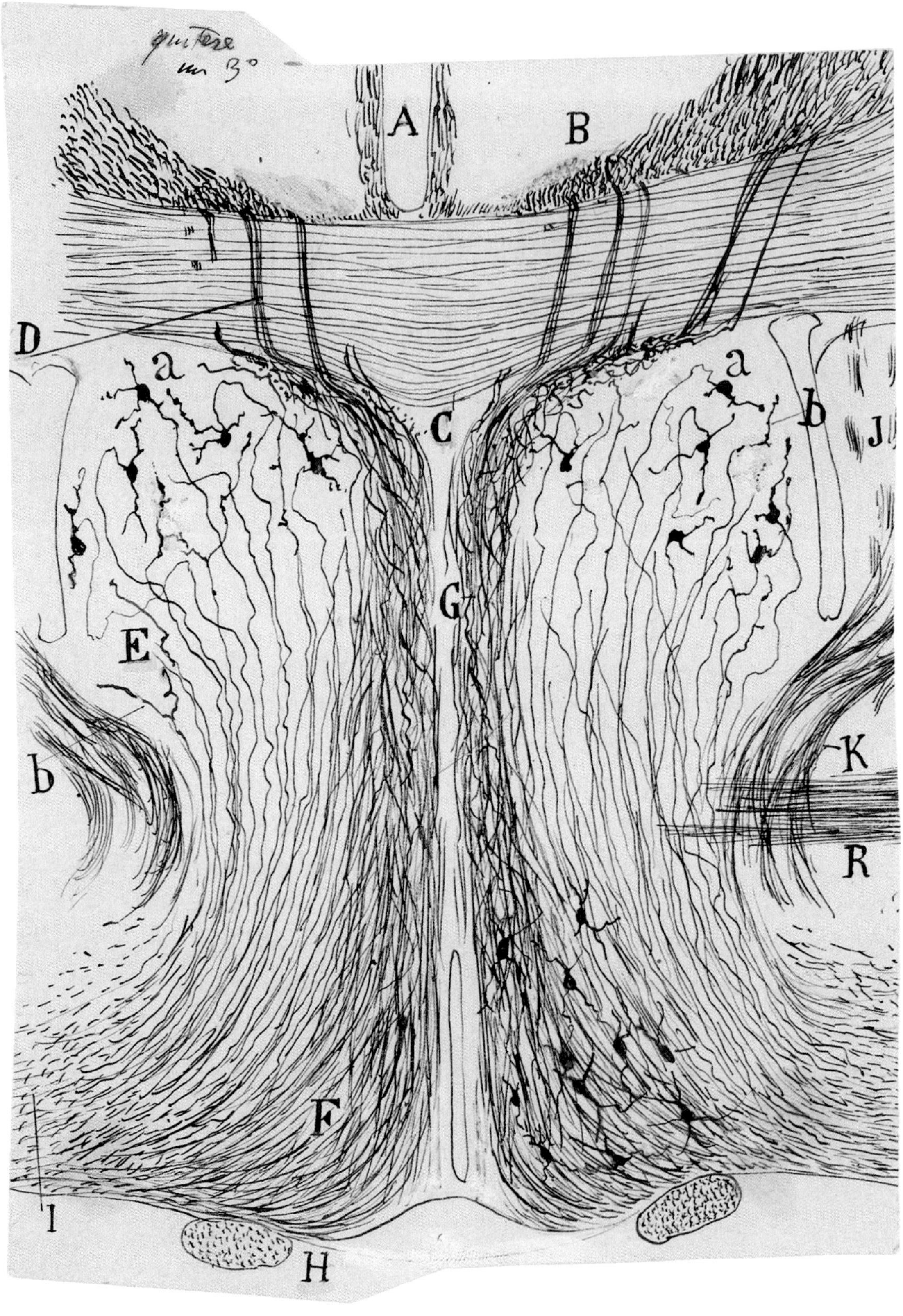

FIGURE 163. Section of the septum in a newborn mouse.

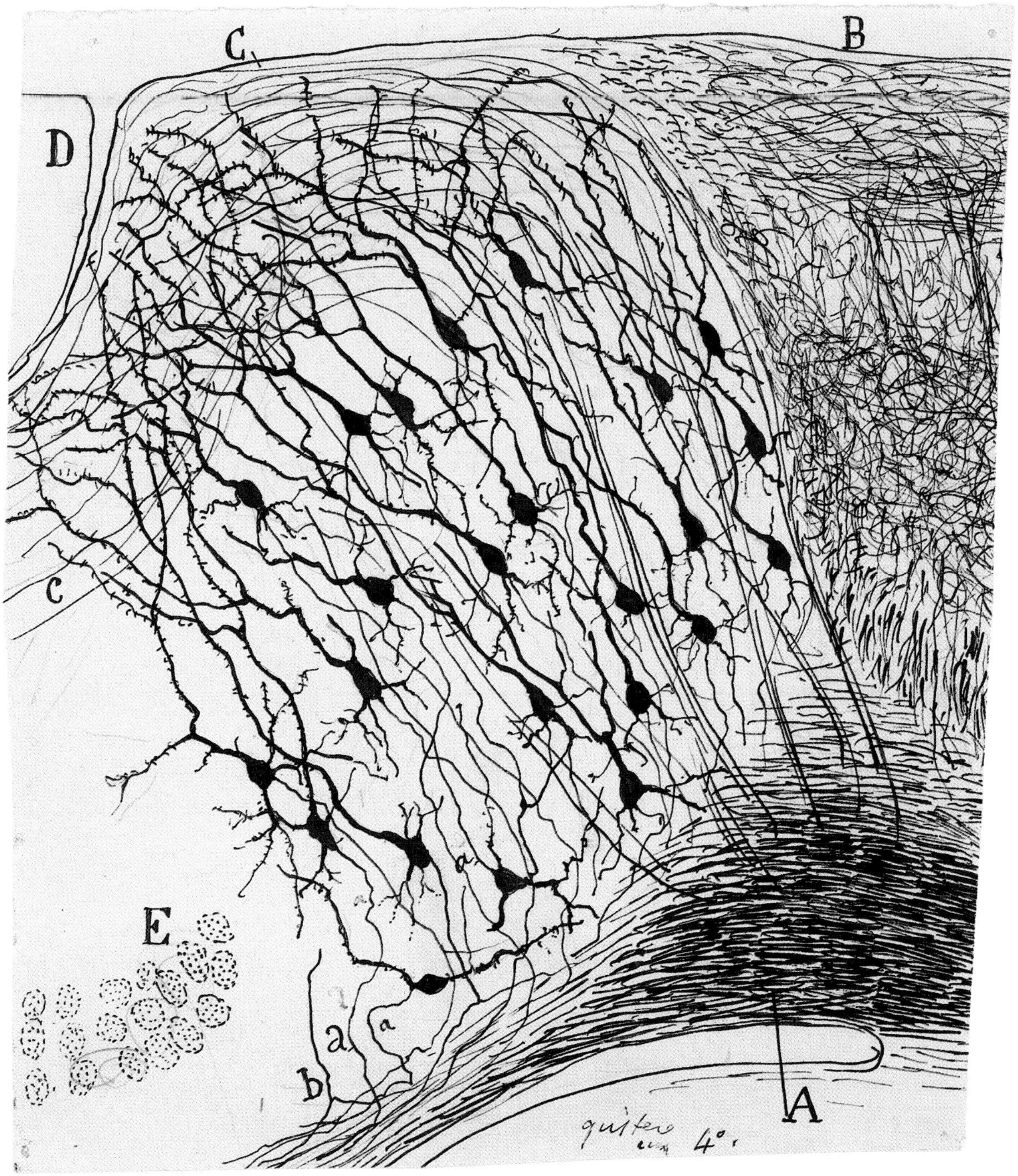

FIGURE 164. Sagittal section of the subiculum in a mouse.

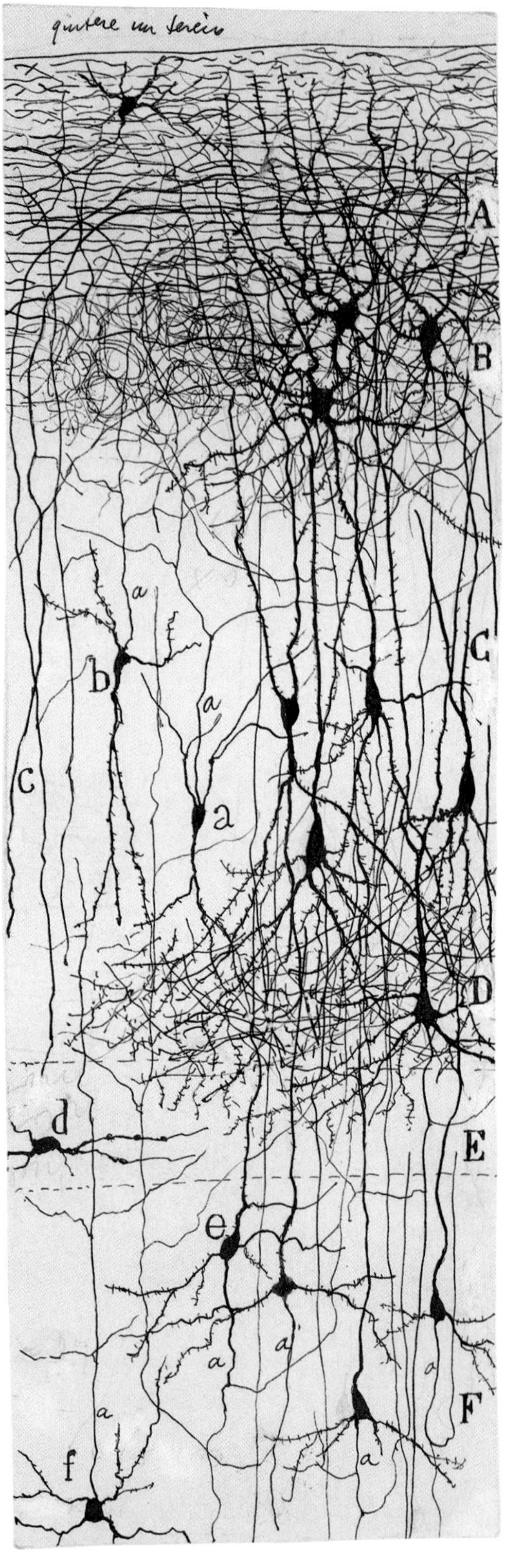

FIGURE 165. Coronal section of the medial entorhinal cortex in a rabbit.

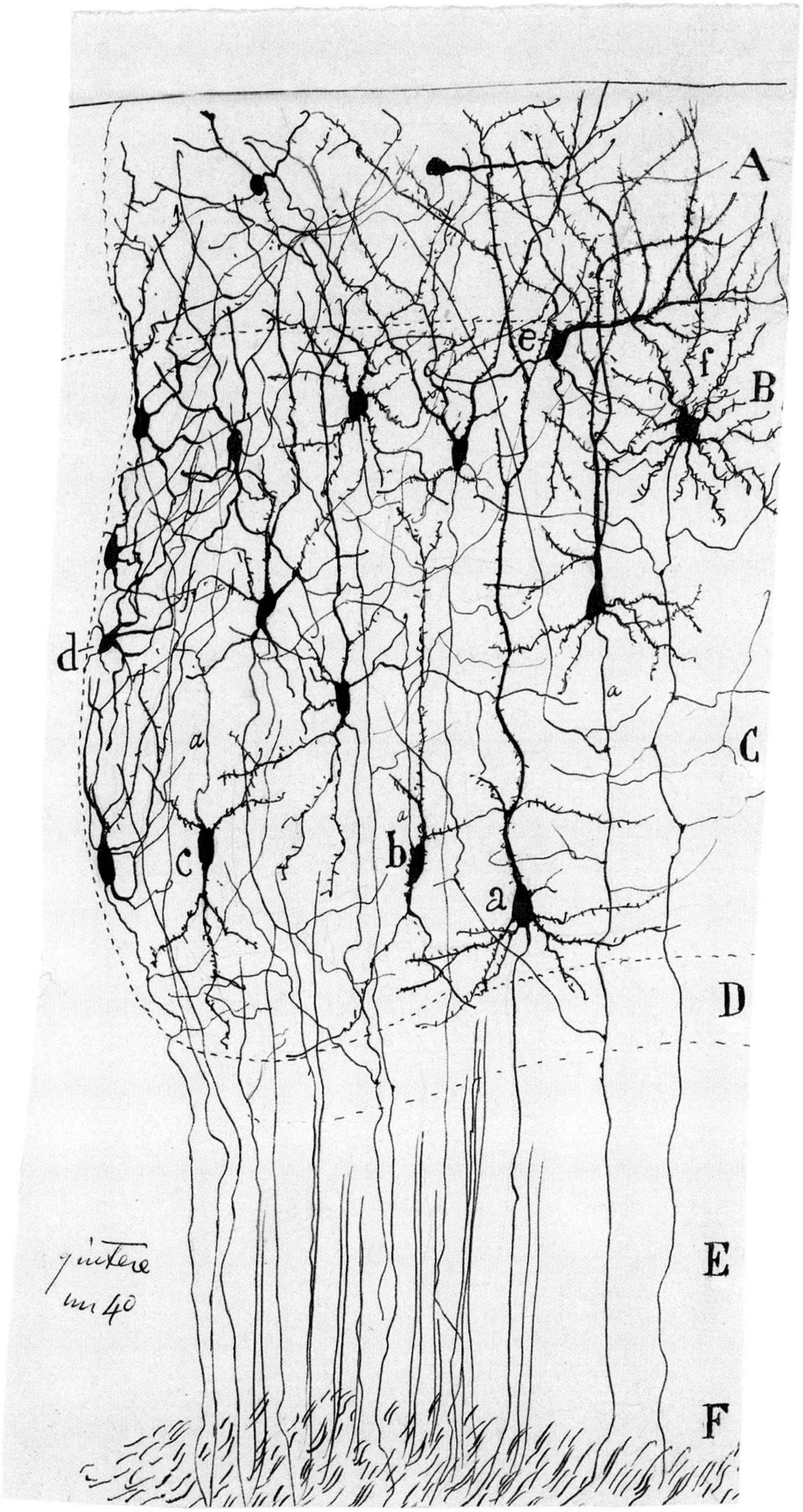

FIGURE 166. Sagittal lateral section of the dorsal limit of the medial entorhinal cortex in a mouse.

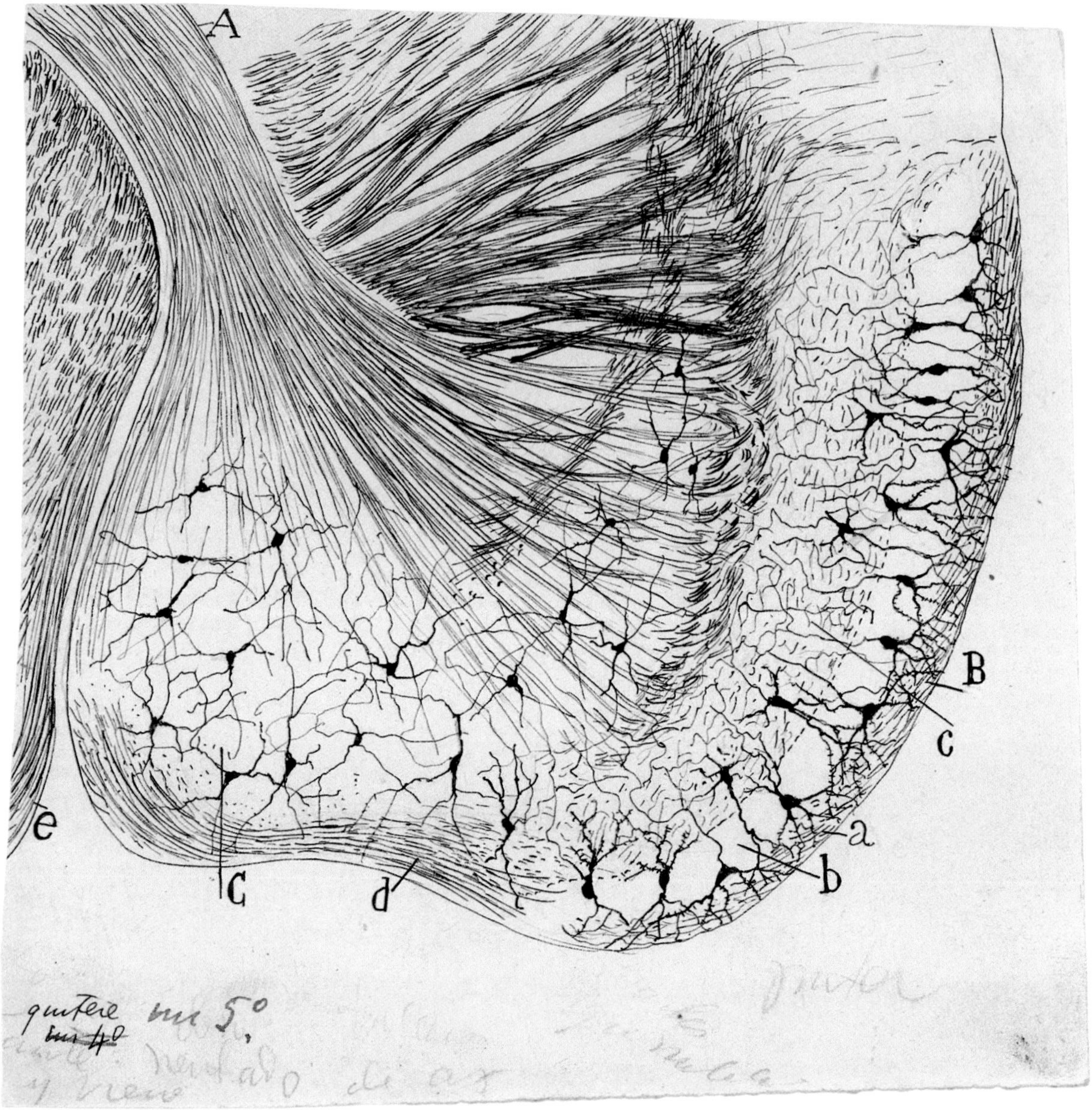

FIGURE 167. Frontal section of the temporal cortex in a mouse.

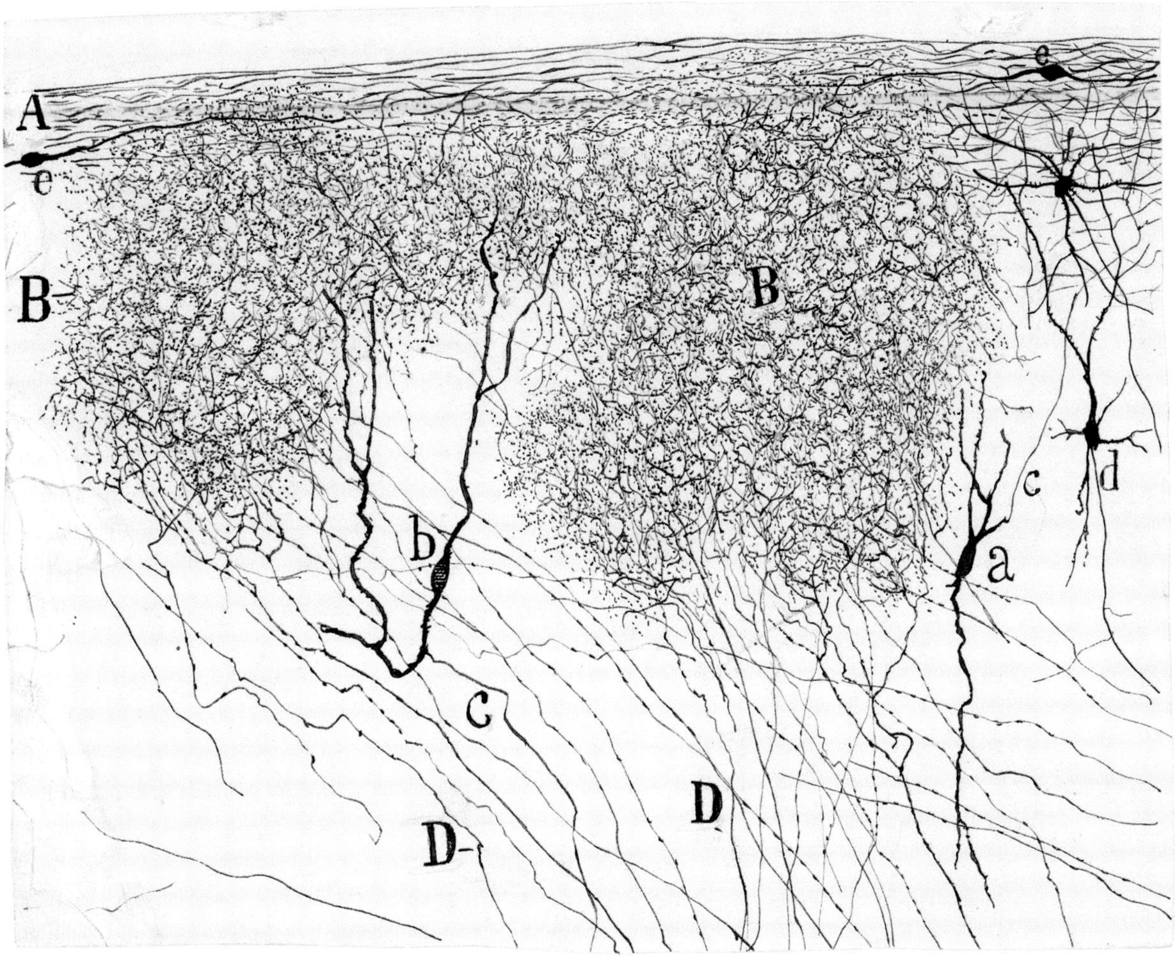

FIGURE 168. Islands of pyramidal cells of the olfactory tubercle in a rabbit.

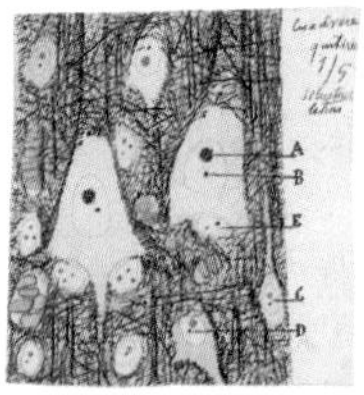

FIGURE 115.

The nucleus in human pyramidal cells.

This figure was published in Cajal, S. R. (1910) El núcleo de las células pyramidales del cerebro humano y de algunos mamíferos. *Trab. Lab. Invest. Biol. Univ. Madrid* 8, 27–62 (Figure 2). It has also been reproduced as Figure 47 in Cajal, S. R. (1933) ¿Neuronismo o reticularismo? Las pruebas objetivas de la unidad anatómica de las células nerviosas. *Arch. Neurobiol.* 13, 217–291, 579–646.

FIGURE LEGEND: Terminal nerve plexuses around the pyramidal cells. Cerebral cortex in an adult dog. *A*, Nucleolus of a giant pyramid; *B*, accessory body; *E*, basal neuroglial cell.

Original text: Plexos terminales situados en torno de las pirámides. Corteza cerebral del perro adulto: *A*, nucleolo de una pirámide gigante; *B*, cuerpo accesorio; *E*, corpúsculo neuróglico basal.

Note from the author (J. D.): The figure legend has been taken from" ¿Neuronismo o reticularismo?" In the legend of Cajal (1910), he writes: "Corte de la región motriz del hombre adulto; fijación en piridina al 50 por 100 y después en alcohol; método del nitrato de plata reducido. *A*, nucleolo con sus esférulas argentófilas; *B*, *D*, cuerpo accesorio; *C*, grano; *E*, célula de neuroglia." (Section of the motor cortex in an adult human. Fixation in 50% pyridine and then in alcohol. Reduced silver nitrate. *A*, Nucleolus with its argentophilic spherules; *B*, *D*, accessory body; *C*, small pyramid; *E*, neuroglial cell).

The nucleolar accessory bodies are now called *Cajal bodies* or *coiled bodies*.

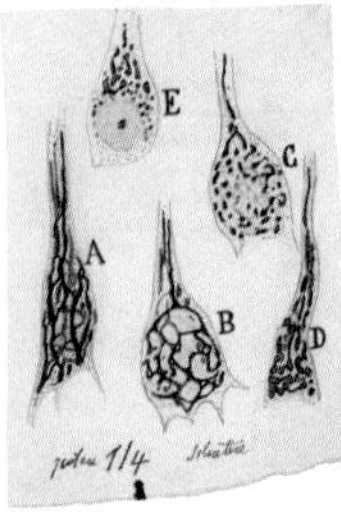

FIGURE 116.

Different types of large pyramidal cells of the cerebral cortex in a dog.

This figure was published in Cajal, S. R. (1914) Algunas variaciones fisiológicas y patológicas del aparato reticular de Golgi. *Trab. Lab. Invest. Biol. Univ. Madrid* 12, 127–227 (Figure 35).

FIGURE LEGEND: Different types of large pyramidal cells of the cerebral cortex in a one-month-old dog. *A*, *D*, Dark or retracted type; *B*, wide or light type; *E*, *G*, varieties of fragmented reticulum.

Original text: Diversos tipos de pirámides grandes tomados de la corteza del perro de un mes. *A*, *D*, tipos obscuros ó retraídos; *B*, tipo ancho ó claro; *E*, *G*, variedades de retículo fragmentado.

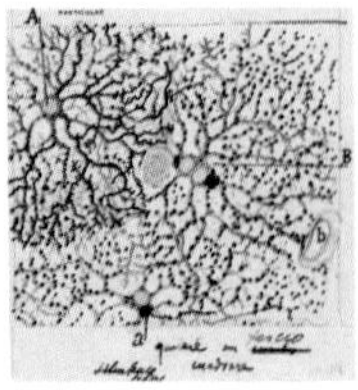

FIGURE 117.

Neuroglial plexus of the gray matter in the human brain.

This figure was published in Cajal, S. R. (1913) Contribución al conocimiento de la neuroglia del cerebro humano. *Trab. Lab. Invest. Biol. Univ. Madrid* 11, 255–315 (Figure 3).

FIGURE LEGEND: Neuroglial plexus of the gray matter impregnated by reduced silver nitrate (fixation for twenty-four hours in urano-formol). Brain tissue from a woman obtained from autopsy within two hours of postmortem. *A*, Heavily stained astrocyte; *B*, pair of astrocytes colored less strongly and in which gliosomes are observed; *a*, pigment in an astrocyte; *b*, blood vessel on which an end-foot is attached.

Original text: Plexo neuróglico de la substancia gris impregnado por el nitrato de plata reducido (fijación por veinticuatro horas en formol-urano). Cadáver de mujer, autopsiado á las dos horas. *A*, astrocito intensamente teñido; *B*, pareja de astrocitos coloreados menos vigorosamente y en los cuales se observan los gliosomas; *a*, pigmento en un astrocito; *b*, vaso sobre el cual se fija un apéndice chupador.

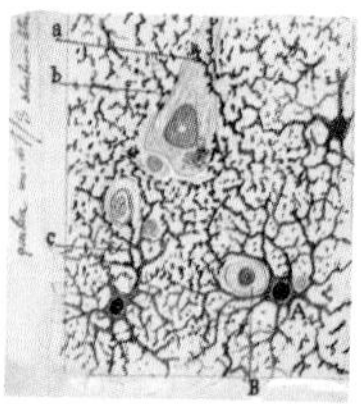

FIGURE 118.

Human cerebral cortex.

This figure was published in Cajal, S. R. (1913) Contribución al conocimiento de la neuroglia del cerebro humano. *Trab. Lab. Invest. Biol. Univ. Madrid* 11, 255–315 (Figure 7).

FIGURE LEGEND: Portion of a section of a normal adult human cerebral cortex. *A*, Protoplasmic astrocyte; *B*, neuron probably with a short axon; *a*, *b*, pericellular pedicles that continue as neuroglial appendages; *c*, fine perivascular pedicle. (Gold chloride staining.)

Original text: Trozo de un corte de la corteza cerebral del hombre adulto normal. *A*, astrocito protoplásmico; *B*, neurona probablemente de axon corto; *a*, *b*, pedículos pericelulares continuados con apéndices neuróglicos; *c*, fino pedículo perivascular. (Coloración por el cloruro de oro).

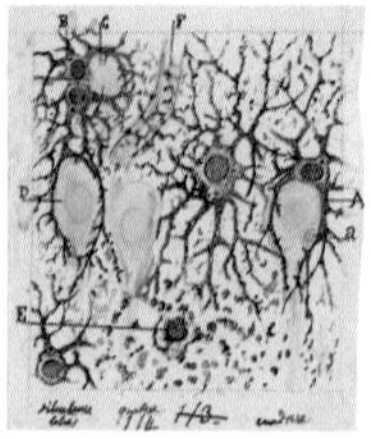

FIGURE 119.

Neuroglia of the stratum pyramidale and stratum radiatum of Ammon's horn.

This figure was published in Cajal, S. R. (1913) Contribución al conocimiento de la neuroglia del cerebro humano. *Trab. Lab. Invest. Biol. Univ. Madrid* 11, 255–315 (Figure 9).

FIGURE LEGEND: Neuroglia of the stratum pyramidale and stratum radiatum of Ammon's horn. Brain tissue from an adult man obtained from autopsy within 3 hours of postmortem. Gold chloride staining. *A*, Thick astrocyte embracing a pyramidal cell; *B*, twin astrocytes forming a nest around a cell (*C*). In addition, one of them sends two processes to another nest (*D*). *E*, Cell with signs of autolysis.

Original text: Neuroglia de la capa de las pirámides y estrato radiado del asta de Ammon. Hombre adulto autopsiado tres horas después de la muerte. Cloruro de oro. *A*, astrocito grueso abrazando una pirámide; *B*, astrocitos gemelos formando nido en torno de una célula (*C*), mientras uno de ellos envía dos brazos constitutivos de otro nido (*D*); *E*, célula con signos de autolisis.

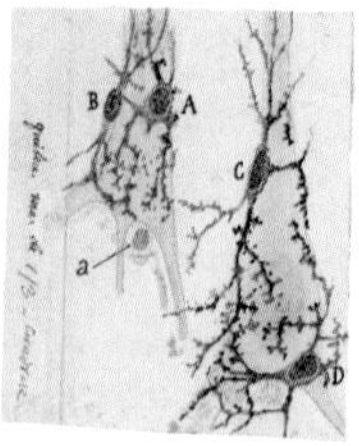

FIGURE 120.

Satellite neuroglial cells around large pyramids.

This figure was published in Cajal, S. R. (1913) Contribución al conocimiento de la neuroglia del cerebro humano. *Trab. Lab. Invest. Biol. Univ. Madrid* 11, 255–315 (Figure 10).

FIGURE LEGEND: Satellite neuroglial cells around large pyramids. Motor cortex in an adult cat. *A*, *B*, Lateral astrocytes; *C*, fusiform astrocyte located on the origin of the apical dendrite; *D*, basal astrocyte; *a*, *b*, satellite adendritic cells.

Original text: Células satélites neuróglicas en torno de gruesas pirámides. Cerebro motor del gato adulto. *A, B*, astrocitos laterales; *C*, astrocito fusiforme apoyado sobre el origen de la expansión radial; *D*, astrocito basal; *a, b*, corpúsculos satélites adendríticos.

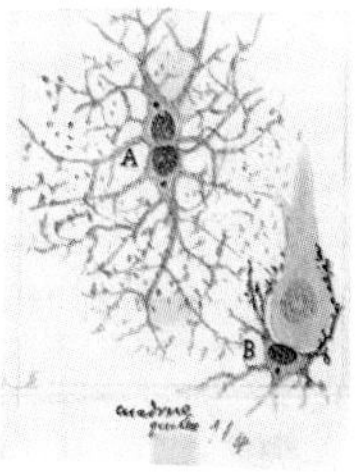

FIGURE 121.

Twin astrocytes in the cerebral cortex in an adult dog.

This figure was published in Cajal, S. R. (1913) Contribución al conocimiento de la neuroglia del cerebro humano. *Trab. Lab. Invest. Biol. Univ. Madrid* 11, 255–315 (Figure 13).

FIGURE LEGEND: *A*, Twin astrocytes in the cerebral cortex in an adult dog; *B*, gliomatous satellite cell showing the centrosome.

Original text: Astrocitos gemelos de la corteza cerebral del perro adulto (*A*); *B*, célula satélite gliomatosa mostrando el centrosoma.

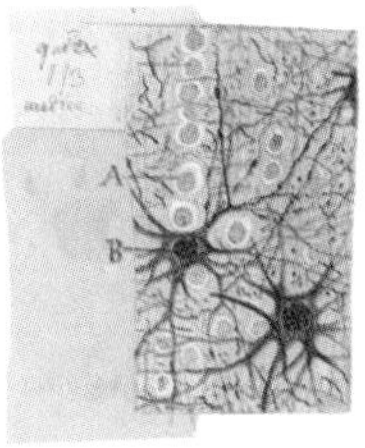

FIGURE 122.

White matter in an adult human brain.

This figure was published in Cajal, S. R. (1913) Contribución al conocimiento de la neuroglia del cerebro humano. *Trab. Lab. Invest. Biol. Univ. Madrid* 11, 255–315 (Figure 19).

FIGURE LEGEND: Portion of white matter in an adult human brain. *A*, "Stainable" astrocytes; *B*, small adendritic cells.

Original text: Trozo de la substancia blanca del hombre adulto. *A*, astrocitos coloreables; *B*, células pequeñas adendríticas.

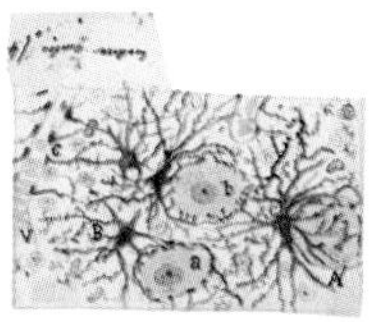

FIGURE 123.

Pericellular neuroglial cells of the gray matter of the spinal cord in a cat.

This figure was published in Cajal, S. R. (1920) Algunas consideraciones sobre la "mesoglia" de Robertson y Río-Hortega. *Trab. Lab. Invest. Biol. Univ. Madrid* 18, 109–127 (Figure 5).

FIGURE LEGEND: Pericellular neuroglial cells (*C, B*) of the gray matter of the spinal cord in a young cat. Formalin–uranyl nitrate method. *a, b*, Nerve cells focusing on the cell maximum diameter; *A*, pericellular neuroglial plexus focusing on the surface of the neuron; *c*, perivascular end-feet.

Original text: Células neuróglicas pericelulares (*C, B*) de la substancia gris de la médula espinal del gato joven. Método del urano-formol. *a, b*, células nerviosas vistas en enfoque ecuatorial; *A*, plexo neuróglico pericelular visto en enfoque superficial; *c*, pies de implantación perivascular.

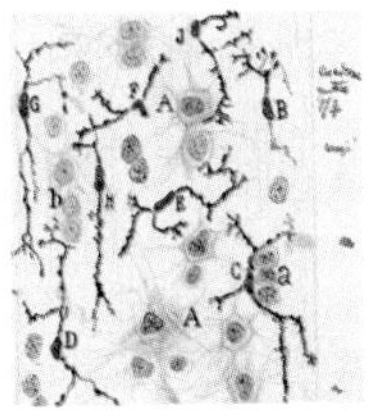

FIGURE 124.

Microglia of the white matter of the cerebellum in an adult cat.

This figure was published in Cajal, S. R. (1920) Algunas consideraciones sobre la "mesoglia" de Robertson y Río-Hortega. *Trab. Lab. Invest. Biol. Univ. Madrid* 18, 109–127 (Figure 7).

FIGURE LEGEND: Microglia of the white matter of the cerebellum in an adult cat. *A*, Common glial cell with long processes; *B, G, D, E*, common microglial cells; *H*, rod-shaped microglial cell; *C*, microglial cells surrounding a group of colorless cuboid cells (*a*); *b*, cuboid cells. (Modified Bielschowsky method.)

Original text: Microglía de la substancia blanca del cerebelo del gato adulto. *A*, corpúsculo glial ordinario de largas radiaciones; *B, G, D, E*, microglía común; *H*, microglía en bastoncito; *C*, microglía rodeando un grupo de células cuboides incoloreables (*a*); *b*, células cuboides. (Método de Bielschowsky modificado).

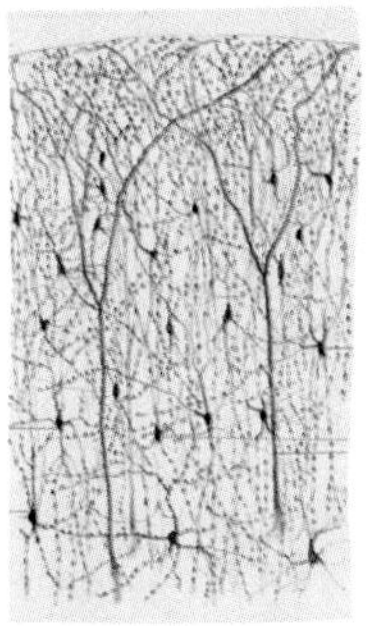

FIGURE 125.

Section of a cortical gyrus in an adult cat.

This figure was published in Cajal, S. R. (1899–1904) *Textura del sistema nervioso del hombre y de los vertebrados*. Madrid: Moya. (Figure 681).

FIGURE LEGEND: Section of a cortical gyrus in an adult cat (Ehrlich method). All the visible cells have short axons. *A*, Apical dendritic shaft of a large pyramidal cell; *B*, large bitufted cell; C, large cells with an arched short axon resolving itself into long branches; *D*, cells with ascending axon.

Original text: Corte de una circunvolución cerebral del gato adulto (método de Ehrlich). Todas las células que aparecen son de axon corto. *A*, tallo de pirámide grande; *B*, elemento bipenachado grueso; *C*, células grandes de axon corto arqueado y resuelto en largas ramas; *D*, células de axon ascendente.

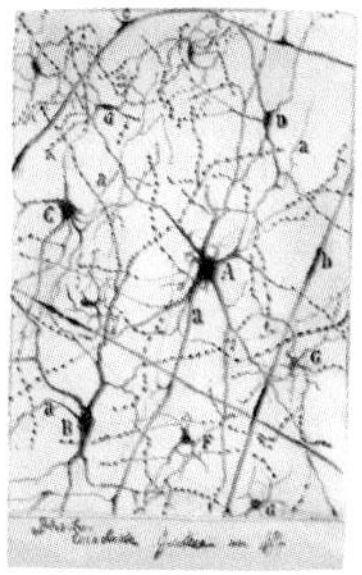

FIGURE 126.

Tangential section of the plexiform layer in an adult cat.

This figure was originally published in Cajal, S. R. (1897) Las células de cilindro-eje corto de la capa molecular del cerebro. *Rev. Trimest. Micrograf.* 2, 105–127 (Figure 2). It has also been reproduced as Figure 664 in Cajal, S. R. (1899–1904) *Textura del sistema nervioso del hombre y de los vertebrados*. Madrid: Moya.

FIGURE LEGEND: Tangential section of the plexiform layer in an adult cat. Ehrlich method. *A*, Horizontal or special cell of the cortex; *B, C, D*, voluminous short axon cells; *G, F*, cells with a short axon that arborizes near its origin; *a*, axon of a horizontal cell; *b*, other axons probably of the same nature; *c*, bifurcation of these fibers.

Original text: Corte horizontal de la capa plexiforme del gato adulto. Método de Ehrlich. *A*, célula horizontal ó especial de la corteza; *B, C, D*, elementos voluminosos de axon corto; *G, F*, células de axon corto ramificado á corta distancia; *a*, axon de un corpúsculo horizontal; *b*, otros axones probablemente de igual naturaleza; *c*, bifurcación de estas fibras.

Note from the author (J. D.): The legend of the figure in *Rev. Trimest. Micrograf.* is different from that in *Textura del sistema nervioso del hombre y de los vertebrados*. The legend in *Rev. Trimest. Micrograf* states: Superficie de una circunvolución cerebral del gato adulto. Método de Ehrilch. *A*, célula multipolar gigante con un axon robusto horizontal (*a*); *B*, célula de igual especie, pero menos voluminosa; *C, D*, corpúsculos de mediana talla; *F, G*, células más pequeñas; *a*, axones; *b*, estrangulaciones de tubos medulados robustos; *c*, colaterales. Translated as: Surface of a cerebral gyrus in an adult cat. Ehrlich method. *A*, Giant multipolar cell with a robust horizontal axon (*a*); *B*, cell of the same kind, but less voluminous; *C, D*, cells of medium size; *F, G*, smaller cells; *a*, axons; *b*, nodes of Ranvier of robust myelinated fibers; *c*, collaterals.

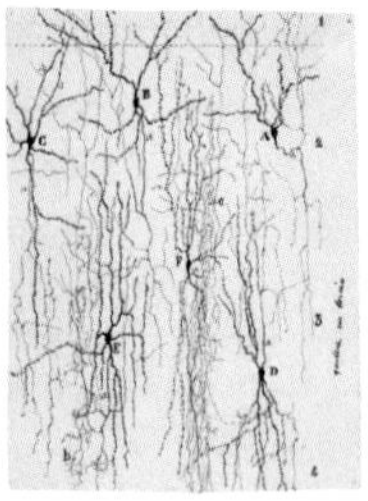

FIGURE 127.

Cells with a short axon in the second and third layers of the temporal cortex.

This figure was published in Cajal, S. R. (1900) Estudios sobre la corteza cerebral humana: III. Corteza acústica. *Rev. Trimest. Micrograf.* 5, 129–183 (Figure 5).

FIGURE LEGEND: Cells with a short axon observed in the second and third layers. 1, Plexiform layer; 2, small pyramids; 3, medium pyramids; *A, B, C*, large cells with an axon forming vertical small branches; *D, E, F*, several types of bitufted cells; *a*, axon.

Original text: Corpúsculos de axon corto observados en las zonas segunda y tercera. 1, zona plexiforme; 2, pequeñas pirámides; 3, medianas pirámides; *A, B, C*, células gruesas de axon descompuesto en ramillas verticales; *D, E, F*, diversos tipos de células bipenachadas; a, axon.

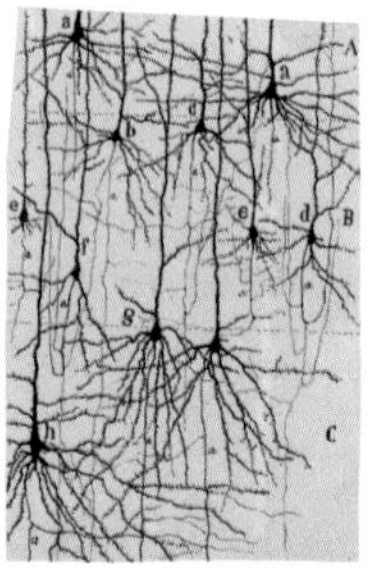

FIGURE 128.

Cells of fourth, fifth, and sixth layers of the superior temporal gyrus in a twenty-five-day-old infant.

This figure was originally published in Cajal, S. R. (1900) Estudios sobre la corteza cerebral humana: III. Corteza acústica. *Rev. Trimest. Micrograf.* 5, 129–183 (Figure 7). It has also been reproduced as Figure 711 in Cajal, S. R. (1899–1904) *Textura del sistema nervioso del hombre y de los vertebrados*. Madrid: Moya.

FIGURE LEGEND: Cells of the fourth (*A*), fifth (*B*), and sixth (*C*) layers of the superior temporal gyrus in a twenty-five-day-old infant. Golgi method. *a*, superficial large pyramids; *b, c*, small pyramids of the fifth layer; *e, d, f*, pyramidal cells with an axon dividing partially into arciform collaterals; *g, h*, large pyramids of the sixth layer.

Original text: Células de las zonas cuarta (*A*), quinta (*B*) y sexta (*C*) de la primera circunvolución esfenoidal del niño de veinticinco días. Método de Golgi. *a*, pirámides grandes superficiales; *b, c*, pirámides pequeñas de la capa quinta; *e, d, f*, pirámides de axon resuelto en parte en colaterales arciformes; *g, h*, pirámides grandes de la zona sexta.

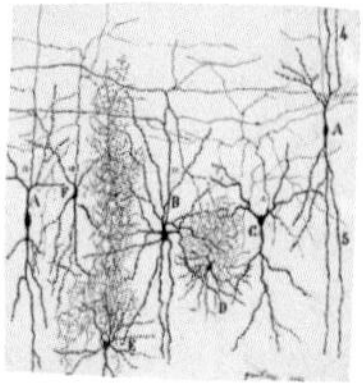

FIGURE 129.

Several types of cells with a short axon of the fifth layer in the human temporal cortex.

This figure was originally published in Cajal, S. R. (1900) Estudios sobre la corteza cerebral humana. III. Corteza acústica. *Rev. Trimest. Micrograf.* 5, 129–183 (Figure 8). It has also been reproduced as Figure 712 in Cajal, S. R. (1899–1904) *Textura del sistema nervioso del hombre y de los vertebrados*. Madrid: Moya.

FIGURE LEGEND: Several types of cells with a short axon of the fifth layer. Child of one month. *A*, fusiform cells with ascending axon; *B*, cell with axon resolving itself into very long horizontal branches; *C, F*, cells with less extensive axonal arborizations; *E*, neurogliaform cell with axon resolving itself into a very complicated plexus interspersed with nests; *D*, neurogliaform cell with a dense axonal arborization; *4*, layer of the superficial large pyramids; *5*, layer of granule cells.

Original text: Diversos tipos de células de axon corto de la zona quinta [de la primera circunvolución temporal]. Niño de un mes. Método de Golgi. *A*, células fusiformes de axón ascendente; *B*, célula de axon resuelto en larguísimas ramas horizontales; *C, F*, células de arborización nerviosa menos extensa; *E*, célula neurogliforme de axon resuelto en un plexo complicadísimo salpicado de nidos; *D*, célula neurogliforme de arborización nerviosa apretada; *4*, capa de las pirámides grandes superficiales; *5*, [capa de los] granos.

Note from the author (J. D.): In brackets is the text added in the French version of the *Textura*: Cajal, S. R. (1909–1911) *Histologie du système nerveux de l'homme et des vertébrés*, trans. L. Azoulay. Paris: Maloine.

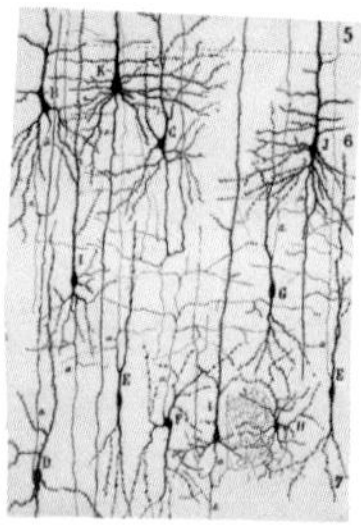

FIGURE 130.

Several cellular types of the sixth layer and beginning of the seventh in the human temporal cortex.

This figure was originally published in Cajal, S. R. (1900) Estudios sobre la corteza cerebral humana: III. Corteza acústica. *Rev. Trimest. Micrograf.* 5, 129–183 (Figure 11). It has also been reproduced as Figure 715 in Cajal, S. R. (1899–1904) *Textura del sistema nervioso del hombre y de los vertebrados*. Madrid: Moya.

FIGURE LEGEND: Several cellular types of the sixth layer and beginning of the seventh. Child one month old. Golgi method. *5*, Layer of the granule cells; *6*, layer of the deep medium pyramids; *D, B*, large cell with an ascending long axon; *J, K*, large pyramids with a long axon; *C*, large polygonal cell with a long axon that gives off three robust ascending collaterals; *E, G*, tiny cells with a long, ascending axon; *F*, cell with a short axon forming horizontal branches; *H*, neurogliaform type; *I*, small fusiform or pyramidal cells.

Original text: Diversos tipos celulares de la zona sexta y principio de la séptima [de la corteza temporal]. Niño de un mes. Método de Golgi. *5*, zona de los granos; *6*, zona de las medianas pirámides profundas; *D, B*, gruesas células de axon ascendente largo; *J, K*, gruesas pirámides de axon largo; *C*, célula gruesa poligonal de axon largo, cuyo cilindro-eje daba tres robustas colaterales ascendentes; *E, G*, menudas células de axon descendente largo; *F*, célula de axon corto resuelto en ramas horizontales; *H*, tipo neurogliforme; *I*, células fusiformes ó piramidales pequeñas.

Note from the author (J. D.): In brackets is the text added in the French version of the *Textura*: Cajal, S. R. (1909–1911) *Histologie du système nerveux de l'homme et des vertébrés*, trans. L. Azoulay. Paris: Maloine.

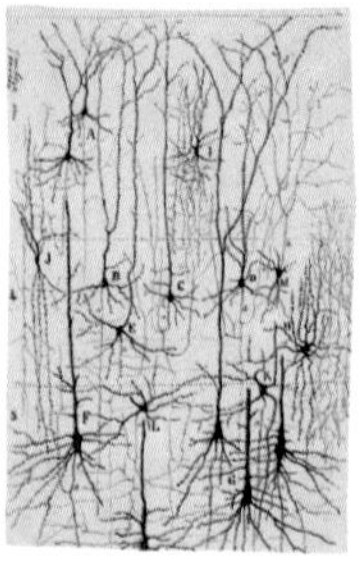

FIGURE 131.

Several cellular types of the temporal cortex in a cat.

This figure was originally published in Cajal, S. R. (1900) Estudios sobre la corteza cerebral humana: III. Corteza acústica. *Rev. Trimest. Micrograf.* 5, 129–183 (Figure 16). It has also been reproduced as Figure 718 in Cajal, S. R. (1899–1904) *Textura del sistema nervioso del hombre y de los vertebrados*. Madrid: Moya.

FIGURE LEGEND: Several cellular types of the temporal cortex in a cat of twenty-four days. Golgi method. *4*, Layer of the granule cells; *5*, layer of the giant pyramids; *A*, small and medium pyramids; *B*, medium common pyramid of the fourth layer; *C, D*, granule cells with ascending axon collaterals terminating in the second and third layers; E, stellate cell with radial dendritic shaft; *F*, G, giant pyramids; *H*, giant bitufted type with very dense axonal arborization; *J, I*, bitufted cell of medium size and with poorly branched axon; *K*, cell with a long descending axon; *L*, large stellate cell with a short axon dividing in long horizontal branches; M, cell with an ascending axon ramifying in the second and third layers.

Original text: Diversos tipos celulares de la corteza esfenoidal del gato de veinticuatro días. Método de Golgi. *4*, capa de los granos; *5*, capa de las pirámides gigantes; *A*, pirámides pequeñas y medianas; *B*, pirámide mediana común de la zona cuarta; *C, D*, granos con colaterales nerviosas ascendentes terminadas en las zonas segunda y tercera; *E*, célula estrellada con tallo radial; *F, G*, pirámides gigantes; *H*, tipo gigante bipenachado con tupida arborización nerviosa; *J, I*, bipenachada de mediana talla y axon poco arborizado; *K*, célula de axon largo descendente; *L*, célula estrellada grande de axon corto dividido en ramas largas horizontales; *M*, célula de axon ascendente ramificado en las zonas segunda y tercera.

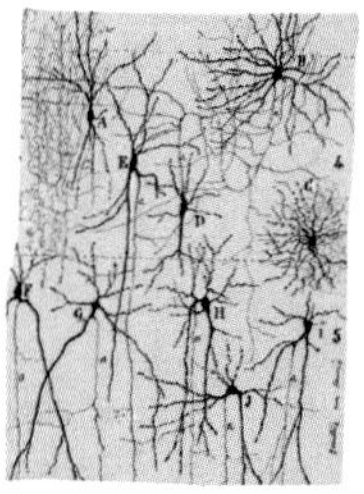

FIGURE 132.

Cells of the fourth and fifth layers in the temporal cortex in a cat.

This figure was originally published in Cajal, S. R. (1900) Estudios sobre la corteza cerebral humana: III. Corteza acústica. *Rev. Trimest. Micrograf.* 5, 129–183 (Figure 17). It has also been reproduced as Figure 719 in Cajal, S. R. (1899–1904) *Textura del sistema nervioso del hombre y de los vertebrados*. Madrid: Moya.

FIGURE LEGEND: Cells of the fourth and fifth layers in the cat temporal cortex. Golgi method. *4*, Layer of the granule cells; *5*, layer of the giant pyramids; *A*, type of bitufted cell; *C*, neurogliaform cell; *B*, stellate cell with a short axon; *D*, fusiform cell with a short axon divided in horizontal branches; *E, F, G, H, I, J*, morphological varieties of a cellular type devoid of an apical dendritic shaft and with a long descending axon.

Original text: Células de las capas cuarta y quinta del cerebro esfenoidal del gato. Método de Golgi. *4*, capa de los granos; *5*, capa de las pirámides gigantes; *A*, tipo de célula bipenachada; *C*, neurogliforme; *B*, célula estrellada de axon corto; *D*, célula fusiforme de axon corto dividido en ramas horizontales; *E, F, G, H, I, J*, variedades morfológicas de un tipo celular desprovisto de tallo radial y con axon largo descendente.

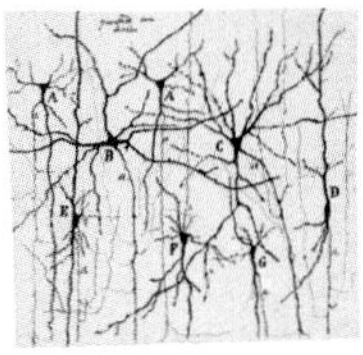

FIGURE 133.

Some cellular types of the seventh layer of the temporal cortex in a cat.

This figure was published in Cajal, S. R. (1900) Estudios sobre la corteza cerebral humana: III. Corteza acústica. *Rev. Trimest. Micrograf.* 5, 129–183 (Figure 18).

FIGURE LEGEND: Some cellular types of the seventh layer of the temporal cortex in a twenty-four-day-old cat. *A, G*, Cells devoid of radial dendritic shafts and with a long descending axon; *B, C*, giant stellate types with an axon incorporated into the white matter; *D, E*, fusiform types with a long axon and provided with a radial dendritic shaft; *F*, upside-down pyramidal cell or cell of Martinotti.

Original text: Algunos tipos celulares de la capa séptima de la corteza esfenoidal del gato de veinticuatro días. *A, G*, células desprovistas de tallo radial y con axon largo descendente; *B, C*, tipos estrellados gigantes de axon incorporado á la sustancia blanca; *D, E*, tipos fusiformes de axon largo provistos de tallo radial; *F*, célula piramidal al revés ó célula de Martinotti.

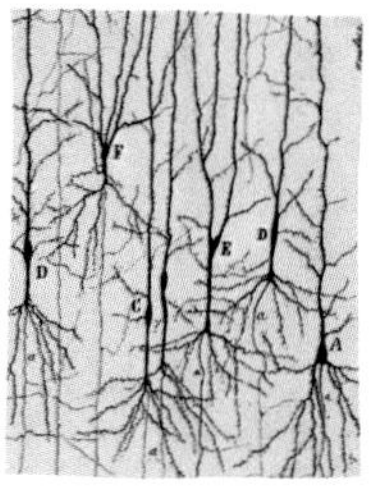

FIGURE 134.

Vertical section of the cortex of the insula in a child.

Part of this figure (see note) was originally published in Cajal, S. R. (1900) Estudios sobre la corteza cerebral humana: III. Corteza acústica. *Rev. Trimest. Micrograf.* 5, 129–183 (Figure 19). It has also been reproduced as Figure 720 in Cajal, S. R. (1899–1904) *Textura del sistema nervioso del hombre y de los vertebrados*. Madrid: Moya.

FIGURE LEGEND: Vertical section of the cortex of the insula in a child one month old. Fifth layer or layer of the pyramids and large fusiform cells. Golgi method. *A, B*, Ordinary, large pyramids; *D, C*, fusiform cells with a descending [dendritic] tuft; *E, F*, provided with two or more ascending [dendritic] shafts prolonged up to the first layer; *G*, stellate cell with two radial dendritic shafts; *H, I*, small cells with a long axon of the fourth layer; *a*, axon.

Original text: Corte vertical de la corteza de la ínsula del niño de un mes. Zona quinta ó de las pirámides y fusiformes grandes. Método de Golgi. *A, B*, pirámides grandes ordinarias; *D, C*, células fusiformes de penacho descendente; *E, F*, células provistas de dos ó más tallos ascendentes prolongados hasta la capa primera; *G*, célula estrellada con dos tallos radiales; *H, I*, células pequeñas de axon largo de la zona cuarta; *a*, axon.

Note from the author (J. D.): Cells labeled *B* and *G* do not appear in the original publication nor in the Textura (see Supplementary Figure S5).

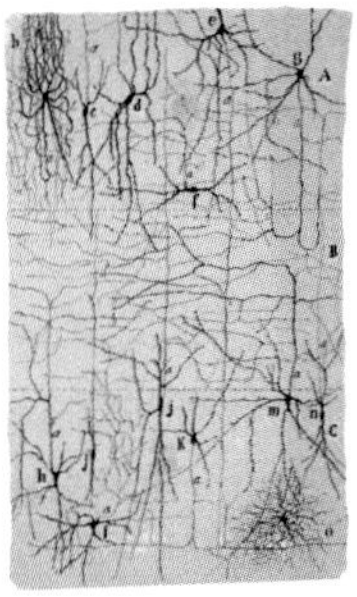

FIGURE 135.

Layers that contain small stellate cells of the precentral gyrus in a child.

This figure was published in Cajal, S. R. (1899) Estudios sobre la corteza cerebral humana: II. Estructura de la corteza motriz del hombre y mamíferos superiores. *Rev. Trimest. Micrograf.* 4, 117–200 (Figure 17).

FIGURE LEGEND: Layers that contain small stellate cells of the precentral gyrus in a child one month old. *A*, Superficial granular formation; *B*, layer of the superficial large pyramids; *C*, fifth layer or deep granular formation; *a*, axons; *b*, large bitufted cell; *c, d*, cells with an ascending axon of the superficial formation; *e*, small pyramid; *f*, cell with an axon resolving into horizontal branches; *g*, cell with a descending axon with arciform branches; *h, m*, cells with an axon ramified in the fourth layer; *j, n*, thin fusiform cells with a very long ascending axon.

Original text: Zonas que contienen pequeños elementos estrellados de la circunvolución frontal ascendente del niño de un mes. *A*, formación granular superficial; *B*, zona de las grandes pirámides superficiales; *C*, capa quinta ó formación granular profunda; *a*, axones; *b*, célula bipenachada gruesa; *c, d*, elementos de axon ascendente de la formación granular superficial; *e*, pirámide pequeña; *f*, célula de axon resuelto en ramas horizontales; *g*, célula de axon descendente con ramas arciformes; *h, m*, células cuyo axon se ramificaba en la zona cuarta; *j, n*, fusiformes finas de axon ascendente largísimo.

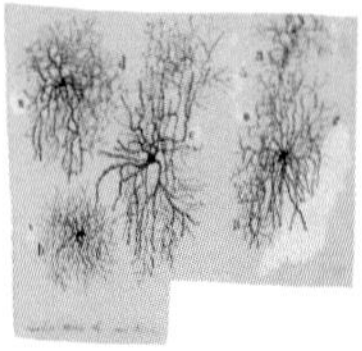

FIGURE 136.

Cells with a short axon from the region of the medium and large pyramids in a cat.

This figure was published in Cajal, S. R. (1899) Estudios sobre la corteza cerebral humana: II. Estructura de la corteza motriz del hombre y mamíferos superiores. *Rev. Trimest. Micrograf.* 4, 117–200 (Figure 22).

FIGURE LEGEND: Cells with a short axon from the region of medium and large pyramids in a twenty-five-day-old cat. *A, B*, Neurogliaform or small types; *C, D*, types of medium size; *a*, pericellular nerve plexuses; *c*, axon; *d*, axonal nests.

Original text: Células de axon corto tomadas de la region de las medianas y gruesas pirámides del gato de veiticinco días. *A, B*, tipos neurogliformes ó pequeños; *C, D*, tipos de mediano grosor; *a*, plexos nerviosos pericelulares; *c*, axon; *d*, nidos nerviosos.

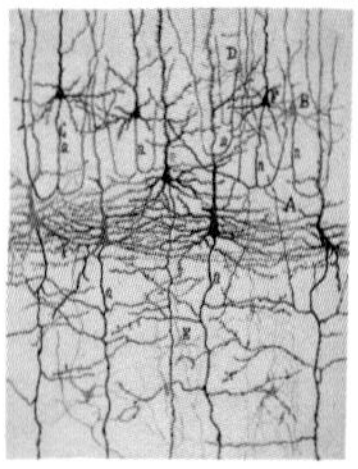

FIGURE 137.

Layers 5, 6, and 7 of the visual cortex in a cat.

This figure was published in Cajal, S. R. (1921) Textura de la corteza visual del gato. *Trab. Lab. Invest. Biol. Univ. Madrid* 19, 113–146 (Figure 8).

FIGURE LEGEND: Layers 5, 6, and 7 of the visual cortex in a cat of twenty five days old. Golgi method. *A*, Layer of the large solitary cells of Meynert; *B, C, D, F*, neurons with an arciform axon of the fifth layer (deep portion of the lamina granularis); *E*, neurons of the seventh layer; *a*, axons.

Original text: Zona 5, 6 y 7 de la corteza visual del gato de veinticinco días. Método de Golgi. *A*, zona de las neuronas grandes solitarias de Meynert; *B, C, D* y *F*, neuronas de axón arciforme de la capa 5.ª (porción inferior de la *lámina granularis*); *E*, neuronas de la capa 7.ª; *a*, axones.

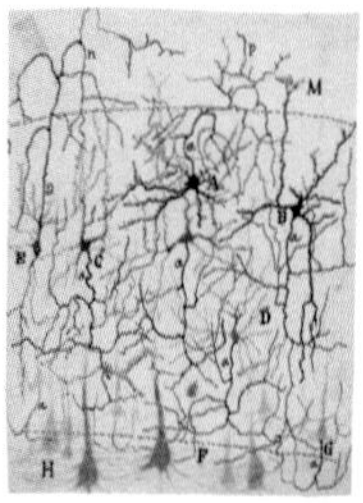

FIGURE 138.

Cells with a short axon of the layer of the stellate cells in the cat visual cortex.

This figure was published in Cajal, S. R. (1921) Textura de la corteza visual del gato. *Trab. Lab. Invest. Biol. Univ. Madrid* 19, 113–146 (Figure 9).

FIGURE LEGEND: Some cells with a short axon of the layer of the stellate cells (visual cortex in a twenty-day-old cat). *M*, Layer of superficial large pyramids; *F*, layer of solitary pyramidal cells of Meynert.

Original text: Algunas células de axón corto de la capa de las células estrelladas (corteza visual del gato de veinte días); *M*, zona de las grandes pirámides superficiales; *F*, zona de las pirámides solitarias de Meynert.

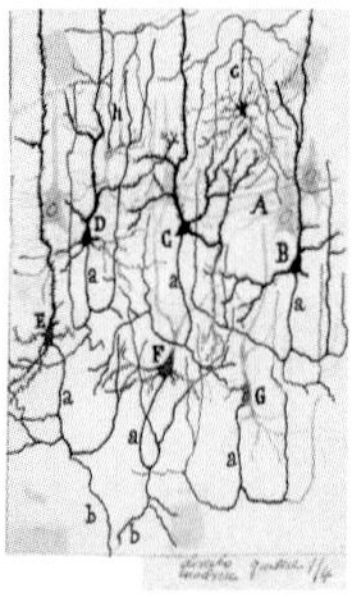

FIGURE 139.

Diverse neuronal types of layers 4, 5, and 6 of the visual cortex in a cat.

This figure was published in Cajal, S. R. (1921) Textura de la corteza visual del gato. *Trab. Lab. Invest. Biol. Univ. Madrid* 19, 113–146 (Figure 11).

FIGURE LEGEND: Diverse neuronal types of layers 4, 5, and 6. *A*, Layer of the solitary pyramids; *B, C, D, G*, pyramids with an arciform axon; *E, F*, pyramids with an arciform axon that give off a branch to the white matter; *c, h*, neurons with an ascending short axon of the fourth layer (deep sublayer).

Original text: Diversos tipos neuronales de las zonas 4, 5 y 6. *A*, capa de las pirámides solitarias; *Bi Ci D* y *G*, pirámides de axón arciforme; *E* y *F*, pirámides cuyo axón arciforme emitía una rama para la substancia blanca; *c* y *h* neuronas de axón corto ascendente de la capa 4ª (subzona profunda).

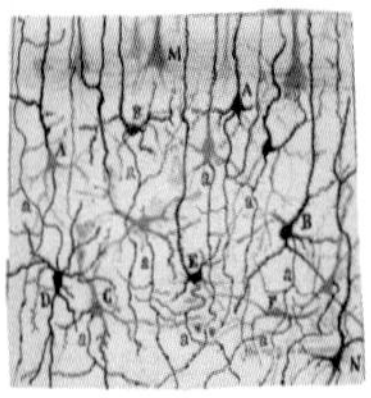

FIGURE 140.

Neurons of the layer of the polymorphic cells in the cat visual cortex.

This figure was published in Cajal, S. R. (1921) Textura de la corteza visual del gato. *Trab. Lab. Invest. Biol. Univ. Madrid* 19, 113–146 (Figure 12).

FIGURE LEGEND: Neurons of the layer of the polymorphic cells. *M*, Solitary pyramidal cells; *A, B*, pyramids with an axon directed to the white matter; *D*, cell with an ascending axon; *E, F, N*, triangular or stellate cells with a long axon.

Original text: Neuronas de la zona de los corpúsculos polimorfos. *M*, células piramidales solitarias; *A* y *B*, pirámides cuyos axones se dirigían a la substancia blanca; *D*, célula de axón ascendente; *E, F* y *N*, corpúsculos triangulares o estrellados de axón largo.

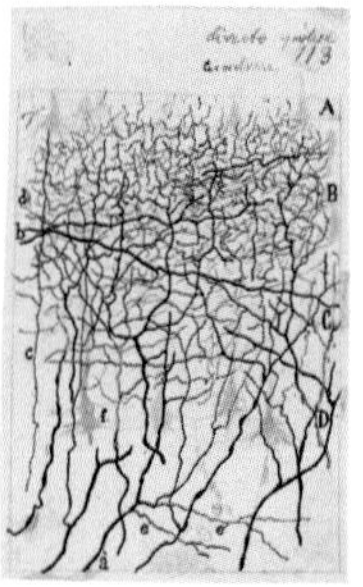

FIGURE 141.

Exogenous fibers of large caliber of the visual cortex in a cat.

This figure was published in Cajal, S. R. (1921) Textura de la corteza visual del gato. *Trab. Lab. Invest. Biol. Univ. Madrid* 19, 113–146 (Figure 14).

FIGURE LEGEND: Exogenous fibers of large caliber impregnated by the Golgi method (visual cortex in a cat twenty days old). *A*, Layer of the superficial large pyramidal cells; *B*, superficial portion of the plexus of Gennari; *a, D*, thick afferent fibers; *b*, horizontal arborizations.

Original text: Fibras exógenas de gran calibre impregnadas con el método de Golgi (corteza visual del gato de veinte días). *A*, zona de las células piramidales grandes superficiales; *B*, porción superficial del plexo de Gennari; *a* y *D*, fibras gruesas aferentes; *b*, arborizaciones horizontales.

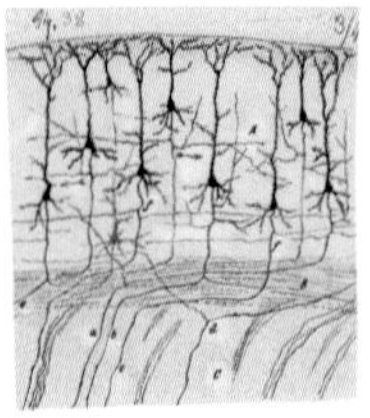

FIGURE 142.

Schematic representation of the enormous length of the cerebral axonal collaterals in a mouse.

This figure was published in Cajal, S. R. (1935) Die Neuronenlehre, trans. D. Miskolczy. *Handbuch der Neurologie*, vol. 1, ed. O. Bumke and O. Foerster, 887–994. Berlin: Springer.

FIGURE LEGEND: Schematic representation of the enormous length of the cerebral axonal collaterals in a fifteen-day-old mouse. *A*, Cerebral cortex; *B*, white matter; *C*, striatum; *f*, long axonal collaterals. Note that some long collaterals (*e*) in the white matter are converted into fibers of association.

Original text: Representación esquemática de la longitud enorme de las colaterales cerebrales en el ratón de quince días. *A*, corteza; *B*, substancia blanca; *C*, cuerpo estriado; *f*, largas colaterales nerviosas. Nótese que algunas colaterales largas (*e*) se convierten, llegadas a la substancia blanca, en fibras de asociación.

Note from the author (J. D.): This figure is an extended version of the figure that was originally published in Cajal, S. R. (1933) ¿Neuronismo o reticularismo? Las pruebas objetivas de la unidad anatómica de las células nerviosas. *Arch. Neurobiol.* 13, 1–144. (Figure 48 bis). The legend of the figure is from "¿Neuronismo o reticularismo?"

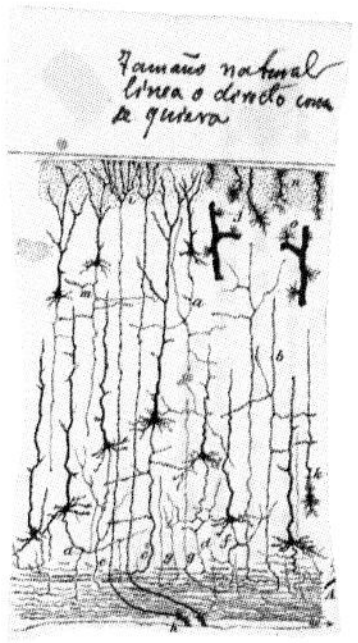

FIGURE 143.

Frontal section of the supraventricular region in the mouse cortex.

This figure was published in Cajal, S. R. (1891) Sur la structure de l´écorce cérébrale de quelques mammifères. *Cellule* 7, 1–54 (Figure 15).

FIGURE LEGEND: Frontal section of the supraventricular region of the cortex of a mouse age fifteen days. The layer of white matter shows the ensemble of callosal and projection fibers (transverse fascicle). The arrow indicates the direction of the corpus callosum or midline. *a*, Axon of a small pyramid; *b*, another continuous with an association fiber; *c*, axon of a giant pyramid, directed laterally and probably constituting an association fiber; *d*, globular cells of the fourth layer terminating in a T in the white matter, with the finer branch directed medially, similar to the fibers of the corpus callosum; *e*, association or callosal fiber (?) passing medially; *f*, another directed laterally; *g*, collaterals of the white matter; *h*, epithelial cells; *i*, external tuft of these cells; *j*, perivascular neuroglial cells; *k*, displaced epithelial cell; *n*, neuroglial cells of the molecular layer.

Original text: Coupe frontale de la région supra-ventriculaire de l'écorce de la souris àgée de 15 jours. La couche de substance blanche montre l'ensemble des fibres calleuses et des fibres d'association (faisceau transversal). La flèche indique la direction du corps calleux ou ligne moyenne; *a*, cylindre-axe d'une petite pyramide; *b*, un autre se continuant avec une fibre d'association; *c*, expansion nerveuse d'une pyramide géante, se dirigeant en dehors pour constituer problablement une fibre d'association; *d*, cellules globuleuses de la 4e couche se terminant en T dans la substance blanche; la branche plus fine se dirige en dedans, comme les fibrilles du corps calleux; *e*, fibre d'association ou calleuse (?) se portant en dedans; *f*, une autre se dirigeant en dehors; *g*, collatérales de la substance blanche; *h*, cellules épithéliales; *i*, panache externe de ces éléments; *j*, cellules de névroglie périvasculaires; *k*, cellule épithéliale déplacée; *n*, cellules névrogliques de la couche moléculaire.

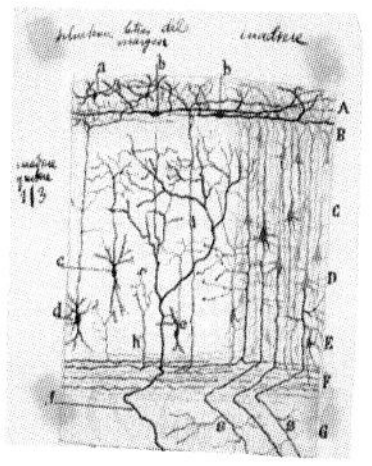

FIGURE 144.

Diagram of the cerebral cortex in a small mammal.

This figure was published in Cajal, S. R. (1917) *Recuerdos de mi vidai vol. 2: Historia de mi labor científica*. Madrid: Moya. (Figure 37).

FIGURE LEGEND: Diagram of a section of the cerebral cortex in a small mammal (rabbit, mouse, and so on). In this figure, some of my findings from 1890 and 1891 have been collected. *a*, Small stellate cells of the plexiform or superficial layer; *b*, horizontal fusiform cells; *c*, cell with an ascending axon ramifying in the layer of the medium pyramids; *d*, neuron located in the layer of polymorphic cells, with an axon that is ramifying in the molecular layer; *h*, collaterals of the white matter; *f*, terminal arborization of the sensory fibers; *g*, collateral of the axons of the pyramidal cells destined to the striatum; *A*, plexiform layer; *B*, layer of the small pyramidal cells; *C*, layer of the medium pyramidal cells; *D*, layer of the giant pyramidal cells; *E*, layer of the polymorphic cells; *F*, white matter; G, striatum.

Original text: Esquema de una sección de la corteza cerebral de un mamifero de pequeña talla (conejo, ratón, etc.). En esta figura se han reunido algunos de mis hallazgos de 1890 y 1891. *a*, células estrelladas pequeñas de la capa plexiforme ó superficial; *b*, corpúsculos fusiformes horizontales; *c*, elemento de axon ascendente arborizado en la zona de las medianas pirámides; *d*, neurona situada en la capa de corpúsculos polimorfos, cuyo axon se arboriza en la capa molecular; *h*, colaterales de la substancia blanca; *f*, ramificación terminal de las fibras sensitivas; *g*, colaterales de los axones de las pirámides destinadas al cuerpo estriado; *A*, zona plexiforme; *B*, de las pequeñas pirámides; *C*, de las medianas pirámides; *D*, de las pirámides gigantes; *E*, de los corpúsculos polimorfos; *F*, substancia blanca; G, cuerpo estriado.

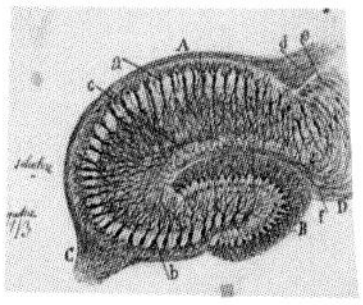

FIGURE 145.

Diagram of the architecture of Ammon's horn and fascia dentata.

This figure was published in Cajal, S. R. (1917) *Recuerdos de mi vidai vol. 2: Historia de mi labor científica*. Madrid: Moya. (Figure 41).

FIGURE LEGEND: Diagram of the architecture of Ammon's horn and fascia dentata as they appear in transverse sections. This figure shows the main types of neurons described by Golgi and Sala. *A*, Ammon's horn; *B*, fascia dentata; *D*, subiculum; *C*, fimbria; *a* pyramidal cells of the superior region; *b*, pyramidal cells of the inferior region.

Original text: Esquema de la arquitectura del asta de Ammon y *fascia dentata*, tal como aparece en los cortes transversales; en esta figura se han reproducido los principales tipos neuronales descritos por Golgi y Sala. *A*, Ammon's horn; *B*, cuerpo abollonado ó *fascia dentata; D*, subículo; *C*, fimbria; *a*, pirámide superior; *b*, pirámide de la región inferior.

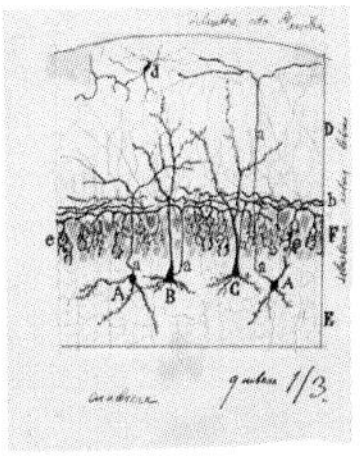

FIGURE 146.

Diagram of the fascia dentata.

This figure was published in Cajal, S. R. (1917) *Recuerdos de mi vidai vol. 2: Historia de mi labor científica*. Madrid: Moya. (Figure 43).

FIGURE LEGEND: Semischematic figure in which we reproduce our main findings of the fascia dentata. *A*, Cell with an ascending axon; *B, C*, pyramidal cells with an axon (*a*) terminated by nests or baskets (*e*), around the cell body of the granule cells; *D*, molecular layer; *F*, granular cell layer; *E*, plexiform layer; *e*, baskets terminations. NOTE: The region copied in the current figure corresponds to the small square plotted in Figure 145.

Original text: Figura semíesquemática donde reproducimos nuestros principales hallazgos en la *fascia dentata*. *A*, célula de axon ascendente. *B* y *C*, pirámides cuyo axon (*a*) se termina, mediante nidos ó cestas (*e*), que rodean el cuerpo de los granos; *D*, zona molecular; *F*, capa de los granos; *E*, zona plexiforme; *e*, cestas. NOTA: La región copiada en la presente figura corresponde al pequeño cuadrado trazado en la figura 145.

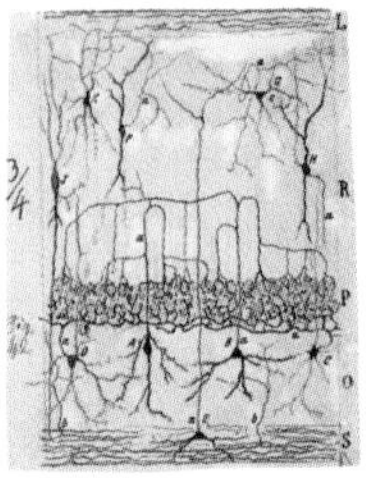

FIGURE 147.

Diagram of Ammon's horn.

This figure was published in Cajal, S. R. (1917) *Recuerdos de mi vida, vol. 2: Historia de mi labor científica*. Madrid: Moya. (Figure 44).

FIGURE LEGEND: My main findings on the horn of Ammon's horn (upper region), shown schematically. *A, B*, Neurons with an ascending axon that decomposes into arciform branches, forming nests around the deepest cell bodies of the pyramidal layer; *D, C*, neurons with a tangential axon forming nests destined to the cell bodies of the most superficial pyramidal neurons; *E*, cell with ascending axon (*a*); *F, K, G*, cells with a short axon distributed in the stratum radiatum; *J, H*, small, displaced pyramids. The current figure corresponds to the large square of the scheme in Figure 145.

Original text: Mis principales hallazgos en el asta de Ammon (región superior), mostrados esquemáticamente. *A, B*, neuronas cuyo axon ascendente se descompone en ramas arciformes, formadoras de nidos para los somas más profundo de la capa de las pirámides. *D, C*, neuronas de axon tangencial constructores de nidos destinados á los cuerpos de las neuronas piramidales más superficiales; *E*, célula de axon ascendente (*a*); *F, K, G*, células de axon corto distribuido por el *stratum radiatum; J, H*, pirámides dislocadas cortas. La figura actual corresponde al cuadrado grande del esquema de la figura 145.

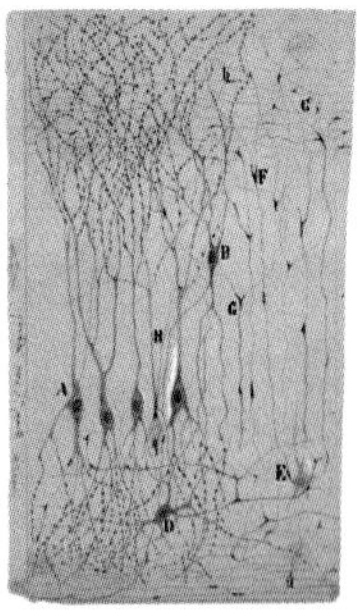

FIGURE 148.

Ammon's horn in a one-month-old rabbit.

This figure was published in Cajal, S. R. (1896) El azul de metileno en los centros nerviosos. *Rev. Trim. Micrograf. Madrid* 1, 151–203 (plate 2).

FIGURE LEGEND: Coronal section of Ammon' horn in a one-month-old rabbit. Upper region of Ammon's horn. Ehrlich-Bethe method. Objective 1.3 Zeiss. *A*, Typical pyramidal cells; *E*, stellate cell of the stratum radiatum; *C*, horizontal bundles of nerve fibers of the stratum lacunosum moleculare; *D*, cell with a horizontal axon branching at the level of the cell bodies of pyramidal cells; *E*, cell with an ascending axon to the molecular layer; *F*, bifurcation of one of these ascending axons; *G*, another similar bifurcation, but located below, in the stratum radiatum; *H*, small cell with an ascending axon, and with initial upper and lower parts of the cell body that are more intensely stained in blue; *a*, collateral of the white matter; *b*, collaterals of the nerve fibers of the stratum lacunosum moleculare.

Original text: Corte transversal del asta de Ammon del conejo de un mes. Región superior del órgano. Método de Ehrlich-Bethe. Objetivo 1'30 Zeiss. *A*, células piramidales típicas; *E*, célula estrellada del estrato radiado; *C*, fascículos horizontales de fibras nerviosas del estrato lacunoso; *D*, corpúsculo de cilindro- eje horizontal ramificado al nivel de los cuerpos de las pirámides; *E*, célula de cilindro-eje ascendente para la capa molecular; *F*, bifurcación de uno de estos cilindros-ejes ascendentes; *G*, otra bifurcación análoga, pero residente más abajo, en la zona radiada; *H*, célula pequeña de cilindro-eje ascendente, y en la cual el cuerpo presentaba polarizaciones de color azul; *a*, colateral de la substancia blanca; *b*, colaterales de las fibras nerviosas de la zona lacunosa.

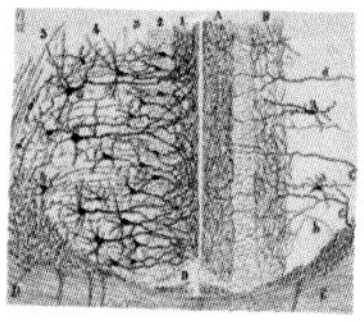

FIGURE 149.

Interhemispheric cortex in a mouse.

This figure was originally published in Cajal, S. R. (1901–1092) Estudios sobre la corteza cerebral humana: IV. Estructura de la corteza cerebral olfativa del hombre y mamíferos. *Trab. Lab. Invest. Biol. Univ. Madrid* 1, 1–140 (Figure 62). It has also been reproduced as Figure 832 in Cajal, S. R. (1899–1904) *Textura del sistema nervioso del hombre y de los vertebrados*. Madrid: Moya.

FIGURE LEGEND: Vertical transverse section of the interhemispheric cortex in a mouse eight days old. Golgi method. *A*, Superficial plexiform layer; *B*, deep plexiform layer; *D*, cingulum; *E*, corpus callosum; *a*, cells with an ascending axon; *b*, collaterals of the cingulum; *c, d*, terminal fibers of this; *g*, large pyramidal cell; *f, h*, cells with an ascending axon.

Original text: Corte transversal vertical de la corteza interhemisférica del ratón de ocho días. Método de Golgi. *A*, zona plexiforme superficial; *B*, zona plexiforme profunda; *D*, cíngulo; *E*, cuerpo calloso; *a*, célula de axon ascendente; *b*, colaterales del cíngulo; *c, d*, fibras terminales de éste; *g*, célula piramidal grande; *f, h*, células de axon ascendente.

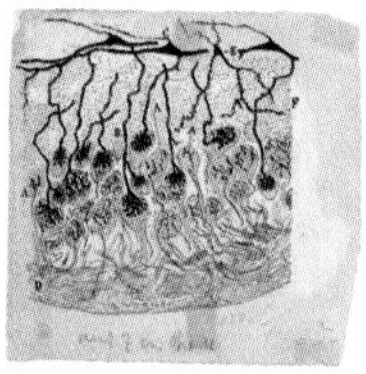

FIGURE 150.

Olfactory bulb in a duck.

This figure was published in Cajal, S. R. (1892) Nuevo concepto de la histología de los centros nerviosos. *Rev. Cienc. Méd. Barcelona* 18, 363–376, 457–476, 505–520, 529–540 (Figure 16).

FIGURE LEGEND: Sagittal section of the olfactory bulb in a duck. *A*, Arborization of the olfactory fibrils within the glomeruli; *B*, descending dendritic shafts of large, tufted cells, ending in grainy fringes in the glomeruli; *C*, large cells with dendritic tuft; *E*, inner granules.

Original text: Corte antero-posterior del bulbo olfatorio del pato: *A*, arborización de las fibrillas olfatorias dentro de los glomérulos; *B*, tallos descendentes de las grandes células empenachadas, terminados en fleco granuloso en los glomérulos; *C*, células grandes superiores con penacho; *E*, grano más inferior.

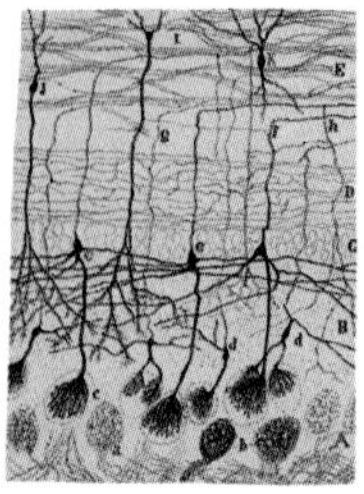

FIGURE 151.

Olfactory bulb in a kitten.

This figure was published in Cajal, S. R. (1901–1902) Estudios sobre la corteza cerebral humana: IV.

Estructura de la corteza cerebral olfativa del hombre y mamíferos. *Trab. Lab. Invest. Biol. Univ. Madrid* 1, 1–140 (Figure 2). It has also been reproduced as Figure 728 in Cajal, S. R. (1899–1904) *Textura del sistema nervioso del hombre y de los vertebrados*. Madrid: Moya.

FIGURE LEGEND: Section of the olfactory bulb in a kitten a few days old. Golgi method. *A*, Glomerular layer; *B*, outer plexiform layer; *C*, mitral cell layer; *D*, inner plexiform layer; E, granule cell layer and white matter; [*I*, *J*, inner granules]; *a*, terminal arborization of an olfactory fiber; *b*, glomeruli containing several [olfactory] endings; *c*, dendritic tuft of a mitral cell; *d*, tufted cells; [*h*, recurrent collateral of a mitral cell axon].

Original text: Corte del bulbo olfativo del gato de pocos días. Método de Golgi. *A*, capa de los glomérulos; *B*, capa plexiforme externa; *C*, capa de las células mitrales; *D*, capa plexiforme interna; *E*, capa de los granos y substancia blanca; [*I*, *J*, granos internos]; *a*, arborización terminal de una fibra olfativa; *b*, glomérulos con varias terminaciones [olfativas]; *c*, penacho de una mitral; *d*, células empenachadas; [*h*, colateral recurrente de un cilindro-eje de una célula mitral].

Note from the author (J. D.): In brackets is the text added in the French version of the *Textura*: Cajal, S. R. (1909–1911) *Histologie du système nerveux de l'homme et des vertébrés*, trans. L. Azoulay. Paris: Maloine.

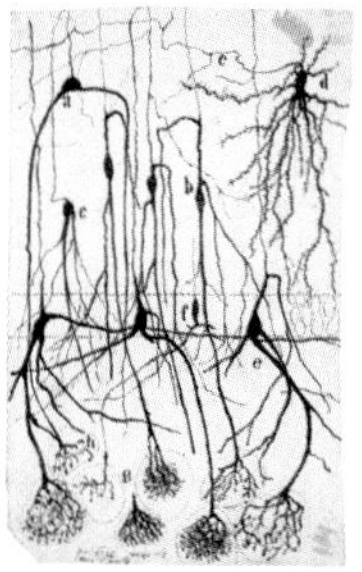

FIGURE 152.

Olfactory bulb in a cat.

This figure was originally published in Blanes, T. (1898) Sobre algunos puntos dudosos de la estructura del bulbo olfativo. *Rev. Trim. Micrograf. Madrid* 3, 99–127 (Figure 5). It has also been reproduced as Figure 733 in Cajal, S. R. (1899–1904) *Textura del sistema nervioso del hombre y de los vertebrados*. Madrid: Moya.

FIGURE LEGEND: Some cells of the olfactory bulb in a cat. [(Golgi method: after Blanes Viale.)] [*a*], *b*, Displaced mitral cells; *e*, mitral cell *with an axon that emanates from a dendrite*; [*f*, small mitral cell]; *h*, *g*, olfactory glomeruli; *d*, short axon cell *with numerous dendritic processes*; [*c*, inner granule cell].

Original text: Algunas células del bulbo olfativo del gato. [Método de Golgi. Según Blanes Viale]. [*a*], *b*, células mitrales dislocadas; *e*, células mitrales *cuyo axon emana de una dendrita*; [*f*, célula mitral pequeña]; *h*, *g*, glomérulos olfativos; *d*, célula de axon corto *con numerosas expansiones dendríticas*; [*c*, grano olfativo interno].

Note from the author (J. D.): In brackets is the text added in the French version of the *Textura*: Cajal, S. R. (1909–1911) *Histologie du système nerveux de l'homme et des vertébrés*, trans. L. Azoulay. Paris: Maloine. The text between asterisks appears in the original publication only.

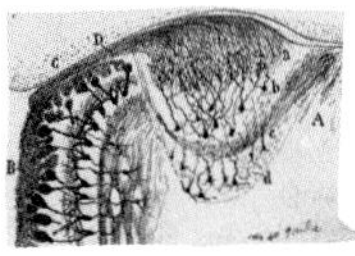

FIGURE 153.

Horizontal section of the olfactory bulb in a mouse.

This figure was originally published in Cajal, S. R. (1901b) Textura del lóbulo olfativo accesorio. *Trab. Lab. Invest. Biol. Univ. Madrid* 1, 1–140 (Figure 9). It has also been reproduced as Figure 744 in Cajal, S. R. (1899–1904) *Textura del sistema nervioso del hombre y de los vertebrados*. Madrid: Moya.

FIGURE LEGEND: Horizontal section of the olfactory bulb in a twenty-day-old mouse. Golgi method. *A*, Accessory olfactory lobe; *B*, typical olfactory cortex (inner aspect of the bulb); *C*, frontal pole of the cerebral cortex; *D*, nerve fiber bundle ending in the accessory olfactory lobe; *a*, glomerular layer; *b*, cells in contact with olfactory fibers; *c*, nerve fiber layer; *d*, granule cells of the accessory olfactory lobe.

Original text: Corte horizontal del bulbo olfativo del ratón de veinte días. Método de Golgi. *A*, lóbulo olfativo accesorio; *B*, corteza olfativa común (lado interno del bulbo); *C*, punta cerebral; *D*, nerviecito que se termina en el lóbulo accesorio; *a*, capa de los glomérulos; *b*, células relacionadas con las fibras olfativas; *c*, plano de fibras nerviosas; *d*, granos para dicho centro.

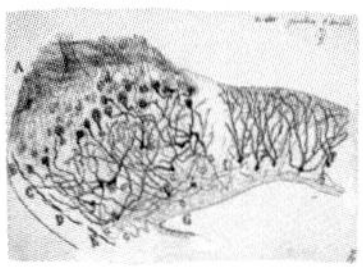

FIGURE 154.

Cerebral vesicle in an Iberian ribbed newt.

This figure was published in Cajal, S. R. (1899–1904) *Textura del sistema nervioso del hombre y de los vertebrados*. Madrid: Moya. (Figure 746).

FIGURE LEGEND: Horizontal rostrocaudal section of the cerebral vesicle in an Iberian ribbed newt. [(Urodele, *Pleurodeles Waltlii*, Mich.)] Golgi method, double impregnation. *A*, Fascicles of olfactory fibers; *B*, glomerular layer; *C*, molecular layer; *D*, layer of tufted cells; *E*, granule cell layer; *G*, ventricular cavity; *F*, cortical pyramidal cells; *a*, tufted cells; *b*, dendritic tuft of these cells; *c*, axons; *e*, granules; *d*, terminal arborizations of olfactory fibers; *f*, axons of tufted cells.

Original text: Corte horizontal y antero-posterior de la vesícula cerebral del gallipato. [Urodelo, *Pleurodeles Waltlii*, Mich.]. Método de Golgi-doble impregnación. *A*, fascículos de fibras olfatorias; *B*, capa de los glomérulos; *C*, capa molecular; *D*, capa de las células empenachadas; *E*, capa de los granos; *G*, cavidad ventricular; *F*, pirámides del cerebro; *a*, células empenachadas; *b*, penacho protoplásmico de éstas; c, cilindros-ejes; e, granos; *d*, arborizaciones terminales de fibras olfatorias; *f*, cilindros-ejes de células empenachadas

Note from the author (J. D.): In brackets is the text added in the French version of the *Textura*: Cajal, S. R. (1909–1911) *Histologie du système nerveux de l'homme et des vertébrés*, trans. L. Azoulay. Paris: Maloine.

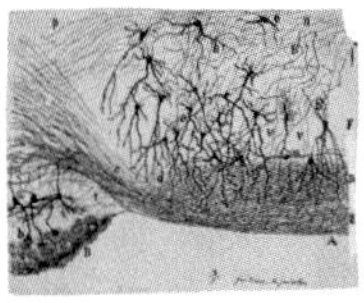

FIGURE 155.

Olfactory bulb and tract in a fifteen-day-old mouse.

This figure was originally published in Calleja, C. (1893) *La región olfatoria del cerebro*. Madrid: Moya. (Figure 10). It has also been reproduced as Figure 747 in Cajal, S. R. (1899–1904) *Textura del sistema nervioso del hombre y de los vertebrados*. Madrid: Moya.

FIGURE LEGEND: Rostrocaudal section of the olfactory bulb and tract in a fifteen-day-old mouse. Golgi method. *A*, Lateral olfactory tract; *B*, olfactory bulb; *C*, layer of polymorphic cells [of the gray matter deep to the lateral olfactory tract]; *D*, molecular layer [of this gray matter]; *E*, its fibrillar layer belonging to the lateral olfactory tract; *F*, pyramidal cell layer; *a*, mitral cells of the olfactory [bulb]; *b*, olfactory glomerulus; *c*, axons of tufted cells forming part of the lateral olfactory tract; *d*, collaterals of the [lateral] olfactory tract ramified in the molecular layer; *e*, *f*, pyramidal cells; *g*, large stellate cell; *h*, axon of a triangular cell; *o*, polymorphic cell; *m*, a horizontal fusiform cell; *n*, nerve fibers of the polymorphic cell layer; *s*, polymorphic cell; *r*, collaterals of the lateral olfactory tract for the olfactory bulb. (After C. Calleja.)

Original text: Corte antero-posterior del tractus y bulbo olfatorio del cerebro del ratón de quince días. Método de Golgi. *A*, raíz externa del nervio olfatorio; *B*, bulbo olfatorio; *C*, capa de las células polimorfas [de la substancia gris subyacente á la raíz]; *D*, capa molecular de [esta esta substancia gris]; *E*, su capa fibrilar perteneciente a la raíz externa; *F*, capa de las pirámides; *a*, células mitrales del bulbo [olfativo]; *b*, glomérulo olfativo; *c*, cilindros-ejes de células empenachadas constituyentes de la raíz externa; *d*, colaterales de la raíz [externa] distribuídas por la capa molecular; *e, f*, pirámides; *g*, gruesa célula estrellada; *h*, cilindro-eje de una célula triangular; *o*, célula polimorfa; *m*, una célula fusiforme horizontal; *n*, fibras nerviosas de la capa de las células polimorfas; *s*, célula polimorfa; *r*, colaterales de la raíz externa para el bulbo. (Tomado de C. Calleja).

Note from the author (J. D.): In brackets is the text added in the French version of the *Textura*: Cajal, S. R. (1909–1911) *Histologie du système nerveux de l'homme et des vertébrés*, trans. L. Azoulay. Paris: Maloine. The letter G should be in the upper part of the figure.

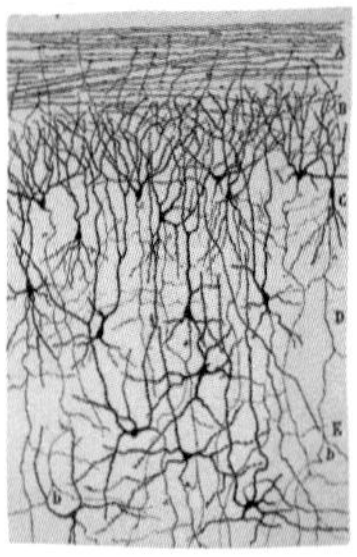

FIGURE 156.
Cortex of the frontal lobe covered by the lateral olfactory root.

This figure was originally published in Cajal, S. R. (1901–1902). Estudios sobre la corteza cerebral humana: IV. Estructura de la corteza cerebral olfativa del hombre y mamíferos. *Trab. Lab. Invest. Biol. Univ. Madrid* 1, 1–140 (Figure 10). It has also been reproduced as Figure 749 in Cajal, S. R. (1899–1904) *Textura del sistema nervioso del hombre y de los vertebrados*. Madrid: Moya.

FIGURE LEGEND: Cortex of the frontal lobe covered by the lateral olfactory root. Rabbit of twenty-five days. Golgi method. *A*, Layer of the olfactory fibers; *B*, plexiform layer; *C*, layer of the superficial polymorphic cells; *D*, layer of the pyramids; *E*, deep polymorphic cells; *b*, bifurcations of the axons.

Original text: Corteza de la región frontal cubierta por la raíz externa; [conejo de 25 días]. Método de Golgi. *A*, capa de las fibras olfativas; *B*, capa plexiforme; *C*, capa de las células polimorfas superficiales; *D*, capa de las pirámides; *E*, células polimorfas profundas; *b*, bifurcación de axones.

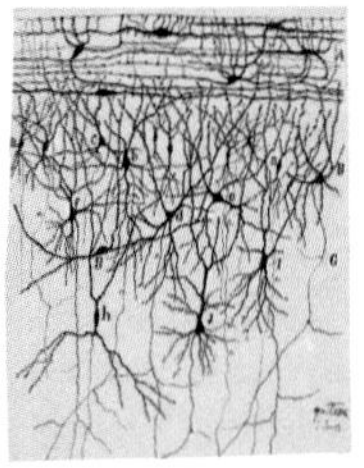

FIGURE 157.
Section of the first and second layers of the human entorhinal cortex.

This figure was published in Cajal, S. R. (1901–1902). Estudios sobre la corteza cerebral humana: IV. Estructura de la corteza cerebral olfativa del hombre y mamíferos. *Trab. Lab. Invest. Biol. Univ. Madrid* 1, 1–140 (Figure 17). It has also been reproduced as Figure 752 in Cajal, S. R. (1899–1904) *Textura del sistema nervioso del hombre y de los vertebrados*. Madrid: Moya.

FIGURE LEGEND: Section of the first and second layers of the entorhinal cortex in a 20-day-old child. Golgi method. *A*, Plexiform layer with horizontal neurons; *B*, layer of large polymorphic cells; *C*, beginning of the layer of small tasseled cells. (Region close to the presubiculum.)

Original text: Corte de las capas primera y segunda de la región olfativa de la circunvolución del hipocampo del niño de veinte días. Método de Golgi. *A*, zona plexiforme con sus células horizontales; *B*, zona de los corpúsculos polimorfos grandes; *C*, comienzo de la zona de las células borladas pequeñas. (Región poco alejada del presubículo).

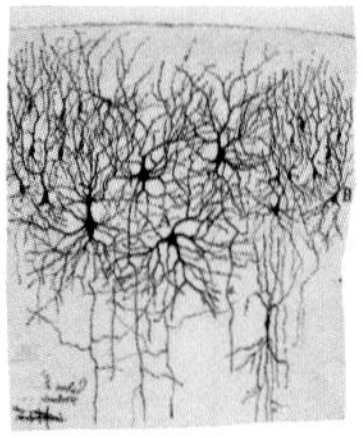

FIGURE 158.
Cells of the layer of the giant polymorphic cells of the human entorhinal cortex.

This figure was originally published in Cajal, S. R. (1901–1902). Estudios sobre la corteza cerebral humana: IV. Estructura de la corteza cerebral olfativa del hombre y mamíferos. *Trab. Lab. Invest. Biol. Univ. Madrid* 1, 1–140 (Figure 18). It has also been reproduced as Figure 753 in Cajal, S. R. (1899–1904) *Textura del sistema nervioso del hombre y de los vertebrados*. Madrid: Moya.

FIGURE LEGEND: Cells of the layer of the giant polymorphic cells of the entorhinal cortex in a one-month-old child. Golgi method. *A*, Island of giant polymorphic cells; *B*, island of small pyramidal cells.

Original text: Células de la capa de corpúsculos polimorfos gigantes de la región olfativa del hipocampo del niño de un mes. Método de Golgi. *A*, islotes de células [polimorfas] gigantes; *B*, islotes de pirámides pequeñas.

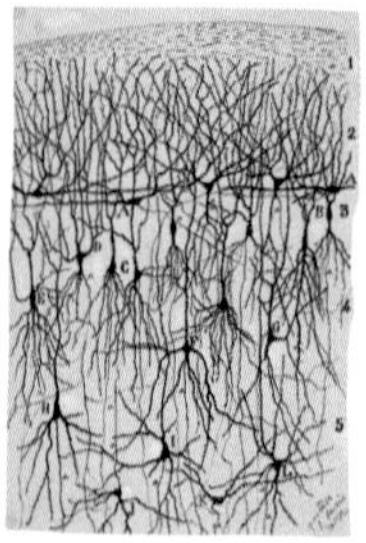

FIGURE 159.
Transverse section of the temporal lobe in a cat.

This figure was originally published in Cajal, S. R. (1901–1902). Estudios sobre la corteza cerebral humana: IV. Estructura de la corteza cerebral olfativa del hombre y mamíferos. *Trab. Lab. Invest. Biol. Univ. Madrid* 1, 1–140 (Figure 19). It has also been reproduced as Figure 754 in Cajal, S. R. (1899–1904) *Textura del sistema nervioso del hombre y de los vertebrados*. Madrid: Moya.

FIGURE LEGEND: Transverse section of the temporal lobe in a cat. Golgi method. *1*, Olfactory fibers; *2*, plexiform layer in the strict sense; *3*, layer of the large polymorphic cells; *4*, layer of the medium and small pyramids; *5*, layer of the triangular and fusiform cells; *A*, triangular and semilunar cells of the second layer; *B*, fusiform cells of the second layer; *C, D, E*, different types of tasseled cells.

Original text: Corte transversal del lóbulo esfenoidal del gato. Método de Golgi. *1*, fibras olfativas; *2*, zona plexiforme propiamente dicha; *3*, capa de los elementos polimorfos grandes; *4*, capa de las pirámides medianas y pequeñas; *5*, capa de las células triangulares y fusiformes; *A*, células triangulares y semilunares de la capa segunda; *B*, células fusiformes de la misma; *C, D, E*, diferentes tipos de células borladas.

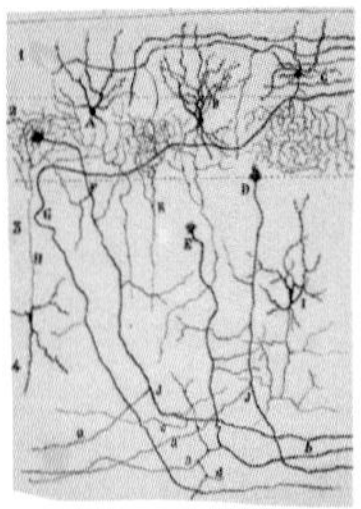

FIGURE 160.
Transverse section of the entorhinal cortex in a cat.

This figure was originally published in Cajal, S. R. (1901–1902). Estudios sobre la corteza cerebral humana: IV. Estructura de la corteza cerebral olfativa del hombre y mamíferos. *Trab. Lab. Invest. Biol. Univ. Madrid* 1, 1–140 (Figure 20). It has also been reproduced as Figure 756 in Cajal, S. R. (1899–1904) *Textura del sistema nervioso del hombre y de los vertebrados*. Madrid: Moya.

FIGURE LEGEND: Transverse section of the entorhinal cortex in a twenty-day-old cat. Golgi method. *A, B*, Cells with a long axon of the second layer; *C*, cell with an axon arborized in the second layer; *D, E, F, G*, axons of large cells located in the second and third layers; *H, K*, ascending fibers terminating in axonal nests in the second layer; *H*, cell with an ascending axon.

Original text: Corte transversal de la región esfenoidal olfativa del gato de veinte días. Método de Golgi. *A, B*, células de axon largo de la capa segunda; *C*, célula cuyo axon se arborizaba en la zona segunda; *D, E, F, G*, axones de células gruesas residentes en las zonas segunda y tercera; *H, K*, fibras ascendentes terminadas por nidos nerviosos en la segunda zona; *H*, célula de axon ascendente.

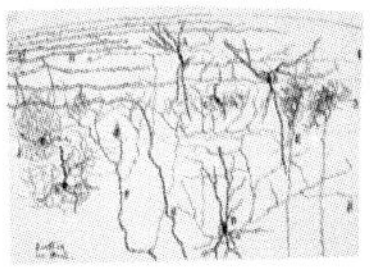

FIGURE 161.

Cells with a short axon in the cat entorhinal cortex.

This figure was originally published in Cajal, S. R. (1901–1902). Estudios sobre la corteza cerebral humana: IV. Estructura de la corteza cerebral olfativa del hombre y mamíferos. *Trab. Lab. Invest. Biol. Univ. Madrid* 1, 1–140 (Figure 21). It has also been reproduced as Figure 757 in Cajal, S. R. (1899–1904) *Textura del sistema nervioso del hombre y de los vertebrados*. Madrid: Moya.

FIGURE LEGEND: Cells with a short axon in the entorhinal cortex in a cat. Golgi method. *1*, Plexiform layer; *2*, layer of the large polymorphic cells; *3*, layer of the medium and large tasseled cells.

Original text: Células de axon corto de la corteza esfenoidal olfativa del gato. Método de Golgi. *1*, capa plexiforme; *2*, capa de las células polimorfas grandes; *3*, capa de las células borladas medianas y grandes.

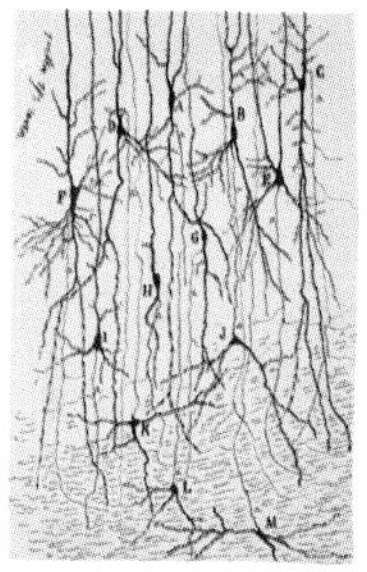

FIGURE 162.

Section of the deep layers in the human entorhinal cortex.

This figure was originally published in Cajal, S. R. (1901–1902). Estudios sobre la corteza cerebral humana: IV. Estructura de la corteza cerebral olfativa del hombre y mamíferos. *Trab. Lab. Invest. Biol. Univ. Madrid* 1, 1–140 (Figure 23). It has also been reproduced as Figure 759 in Cajal, S. R. (1899–1904) *Textura del sistema nervioso del hombre y de los vertebrados*. Madrid: Moya.

FIGURE LEGEND: Section of the deep layers of the entorhinal cortex in a one-month-old child. Golgi method. *A, B, C, D, E, F, G, H*, Several types of fusiform and triangular cells; *K, L, M*, cells of the white matter provided with an ascending axon.

Original text: Corte de las zonas profundas de la corteza esfenoidal olfativa del niño de un mes. Método de Golgi. *A, B, C, D, E, F, G, H*, diversos tipos de elementos fusiformes y triangulares; *K, L, M*, células de la substancia blanca provistas de axon ascendente.

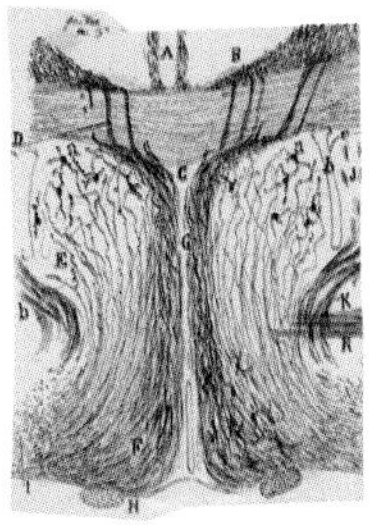

FIGURE 163.

Section of the septum in a newborn mouse.

This figure was published in Cajal, S. R. (1902). Estructura del septum lucidum. *Trab. Lab. Invest. Biol. Univ. Madrid* 1, 159–188 (Figure 19). It has also been reproduced as Figure 820 in Cajal, S. R. (1899–1904) *Textura del sistema nervioso del hombre y de los vertebrados*. Madrid: Moya.

FIGURE LEGEND: Coronal section of the septum in a newborn mouse. Golgi method. *A*, Interhemispheric fissure; *B*, cingulum; *C*, dorsal fornix merging with the radiation of Zuckerkandl (*G*); *D*, fibers of the dorsal fornix perforating the corpus callosum; *H*, optic nerve; *E*, lateral septal nucleus; *F*, medial arcuate fibers; *I*, site where arcuate fibers become sagittal; [*J*, corpus striatum; *K*, fascicles of the internal capsule;] *R*, anterior commissure; *a*, septal cells; *b*, centripetal fibers.

Original text: Corte frontal del septo del ratón recién nacido. Método de Golgi. *A*, cisura interhemisférica; *B*, cíngulo; *C, fornix longus* que se incorpora á la radiación de Zuckerkandl (*G*); *D*, fibras de éste que perforan el cuerpo calloso; *H*, nervio óptico; *E*, ganglio lateral del septo; *F*, fibras arciformes internas; *I*, punto en que las fibras arciformes se hacen sagitales; [*J*, cuerpo estriado; *K*, fascículos de la cápsula interna]; *R*, comisura anterior; *a*, células del septo; *b*, fibras centrípetas.

Note from the author (J. D.): In brackets is the text added in the French version of the *Textura*: Cajal, S. R. (1909–1911) *Histologie du système nerveux de l'homme et des vertébrés*, trans. L. Azoulay. Paris: Maloine.

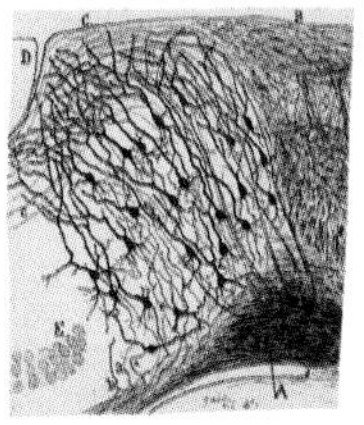

FIGURE 164.

Sagittal section of the subiculum in a mouse.

This figure was originally published in Cajal, S. R. (1901–1902). Estudios sobre la corteza cerebral humana: IV. Estructura de la corteza cerebral olfativa del hombre y mamíferos. *Trab. Lab. Invest. Biol. Univ. Madrid* 1, 1–140 (Figure 26). It has also been reproduced as Figure 762 in Cajal, S. R. (1899–1904) *Textura del sistema nervioso del hombre y de los vertebrados*. Madrid: Moya.

FIGURE LEGEND: Sagittal section of the subiculum in a fifteen-day-old mouse. Golgi method. *A*, Commissural bundle; *B*, presubiculum with its terminal plexuses; *C*, subiculum; *D*, dentate gyrus; *E*, beginning of the pyramids of Ammon's horn; *a, b*, subicular axons penetrating Ammon's horn.

Original text: Corte sagital del subículo del ratón de quince días. Método de Golgi. *A*, cordón comisural; *B*, presubículo con sus plexos terminales; *C*, subículo; *D*, fascia dentada; *E*, comienzo de las pirámides del asta de Ammon; *a, b*, axones subiculares penetrantes en el asta.

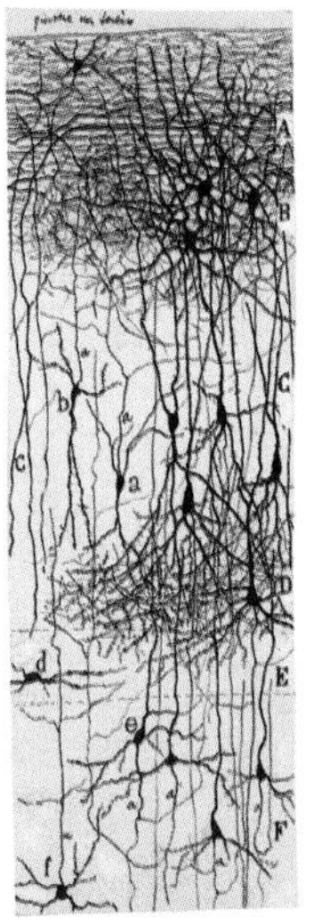

FIGURE 165.

Coronal section of the medial entorhinal cortex in a rabbit.

This figure was originally published in Cajal, S. R. (1902). Sobre un ganglio especial de la corteza esfeno-occipital. *Trab. Lab. Invest. Biol. Univ. Madrid* 1, 189–206 (Figure 6). It has also been reproduced as Figure 771 in Cajal, S. R. (1899–1904) *Textura del sistema nervioso del hombre y de los vertebrados*. Madrid: Moya.

FIGURE LEGEND: Coronal section of the medial entorhinal cortex in a six-day-old rabbit. Golgi method. *A*, Plexiform layer; *B*, layer of the stellate cells; *C*, medium pyramidal cells; *D*, deep plexiform layer; *E*, layer of the horizontal fusiform cells; *F*, granular layer.

Original text: Corte transversal del foco esfenoidal superior del conejo de seis días. Método de Golgi. *A*, capa plexiforme; *B*, capa de células estrelladas; *C*, pirámides medianas; *D*, capa plexiforme profunda; *E*, capa de las células fusiformes horizontales; *F*, granos.

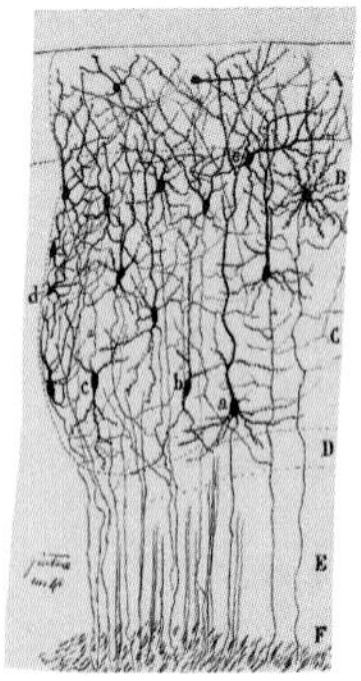

FIGURE 166.

Sagittal lateral section of the dorsal limit of the medial entorhinal cortex in a mouse.

This figure was originally published in Cajal, S. R. (1902). Sobre un ganglio especial de la corteza esfeno-occipital. *Trab. Lab. Invest. Biol. Univ. Madrid* 1, 189–206 (Figure 7). It has also been reproduced as Figure 772 in Cajal, S. R. (1899–1904) *Textura del sistema nervioso del hombre y de los vertebrados*. Madrid: Moya.

FIGURE LEGEND: Sagittal lateral section of the dorsal limit of the medial entorhinal cortex in a six-day-old mouse. Golgi method. *A*, Superficial plexiform layer; *B*, layer of stellate cells; *C*, layer of pyramidal cells; *D*, layer of horizontal cells; *E*, layer of the horizontal fusiform cells; *F*, granular layer; *a*, medium pyramidal cell; *b*, cell with an ascending axon; *c, d*, cells in the dorsal limit of the medial entorhinal cortex.

Original text: Corte sagital lateral de la extremidad superior de la corteza temporal superior del ratón de ocho días. Método de Golgi. *A*, capa plexíforme externa; *B*, células estrelladas; *C*, capa de las pirámides; *D*, capa de los elementos horizontales; *E*, zona de los granos; *a*, pirámide mediana; *b*, célula de axon ascendente; *c, d*, células del límite superior del foco esfenoidal caudal.

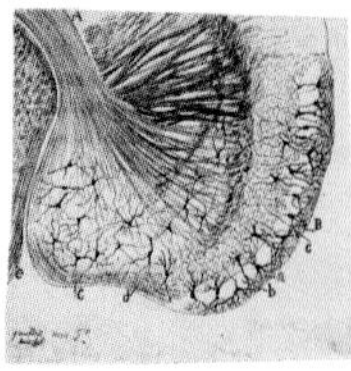

FIGURE 167.

Frontal section of the temporal cortex in a mouse.

This figure was published in Cajal, S. R. (1901–1902). Estudios sobre la corteza cerebral humana: IV. Estructura de la corteza cerebral olfativa del hombre y mamíferos. *Trab. Lab. Invest. Biol. Univ. Madrid* 1, 1–140 (Figure 36). It has also been reproduced as Figure 779 in Cajal, S. R. (1899–1904) *Textura del sistema nervioso del hombre y de los vertebrados*. Madrid: Moya.

FIGURE LEGEND: Frontal section of the temporal cortex in a fifteen-day-old mouse. Golgi method. *A*, Stria terminalis; *B*, olfactory cortex; *C*, amygdala; *a*, layer of olfactory fibers; *b*, layer of large polymorphic cells; *c*, plexus of the deep layers; *d*, tangential bundle of the amygdala; *e*, optic tract.

Original text: Corte frontal de la corteza esfenoidal del ratón de quince días. Método de Golgi. *A*, vía de proyección de la corteza esfenoidal; *B*, corteza olfativa; *C*, núcleo amigdalino; *a*, capa de las fibras olfativas; *b*, zona de las células polimorfas grandes; *c*, plexo de las capas profundas; *d*, haz tangencial de la amígdala; *e*, cinta óptica.

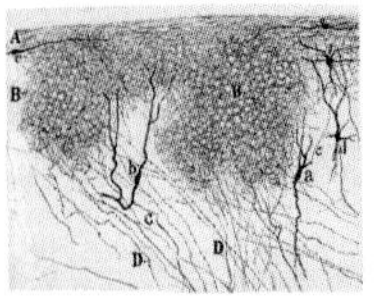

FIGURE 168.

Islands of pyramidal cells of the olfactory tubercle in a rabbit.

This figure was published in Calleja, C. (1893) *La región olfatoria del cerebro*. Madrid: Moya. (Figure 6). It has also been reproduced as Figure 784 in Cajal, S. R. (1899–1904) *Textura del sistema nervioso del hombre y de los vertebrados*. Madrid: Moya.

FIGURE LEGEND: Islands of pyramidal cells in a rabbit olfactory tubercle. Terminal axonal arborizations are impregnated with the Golgi method almost exlusively. [(After Calleja.)] *A*, Narrowed molecular layer; *B*, islands of pyramidal cells; *D*, nerve fibers ramified in the islands; *a*, fusiform cell with an ascending axon; *d*, typical pyramid cell; *b*, fusiform cell with a descending axon; *e*, fusiform cell of the molecular layer.

Original text: Islotes de pirámides del tubérculo olfativo del conejo. Se han teñido á favor del método de Golgi, casi exclusivamente, las arborizaciones nerviosas terminales. [(Según Calleja)]. *A*, capa molecular estrechada; *B*, islotes de pirámides; *D*, fibras nerviosas arborizadas en los islotes; *a*, célula fusiforme con cilindro-eje ascendente; *d*, una pirámide común; *b*, célula fusiforme de cilindro-eje descendente; *e*, fusiforme de la capa molecular.

Note from the author (J. D.): In brackets is the text added in the French version of the *Textura*: Cajal, S. R. (1909–1911) *Histologie du système nerveux de l'homme et des vertébrés*, trans. L. Azoulay. Paris: Maloine.

SECTION H

Degeneration and Regeneration of the Nervous System

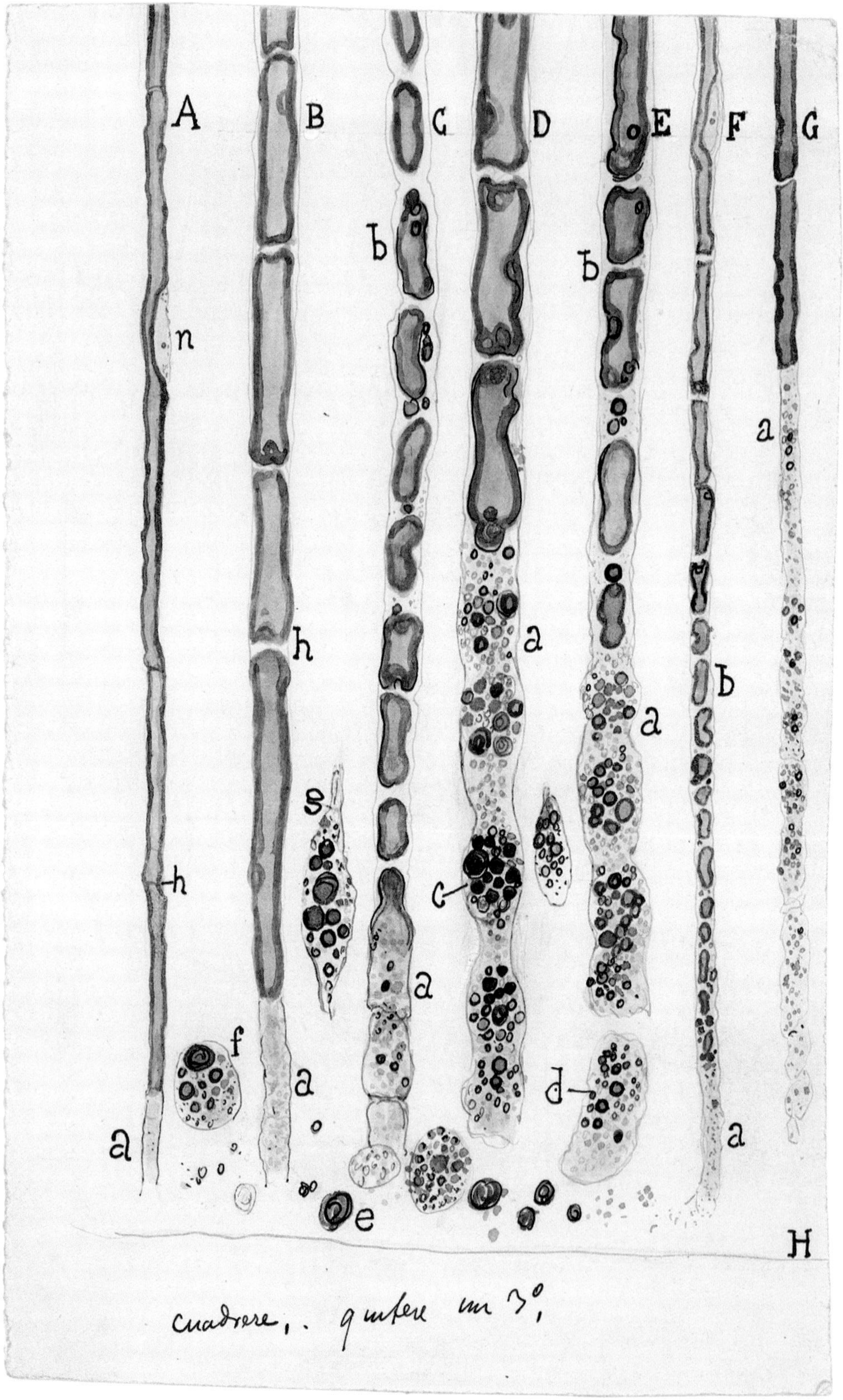

FIGURE 169. Myelinated fibers of the central stump.

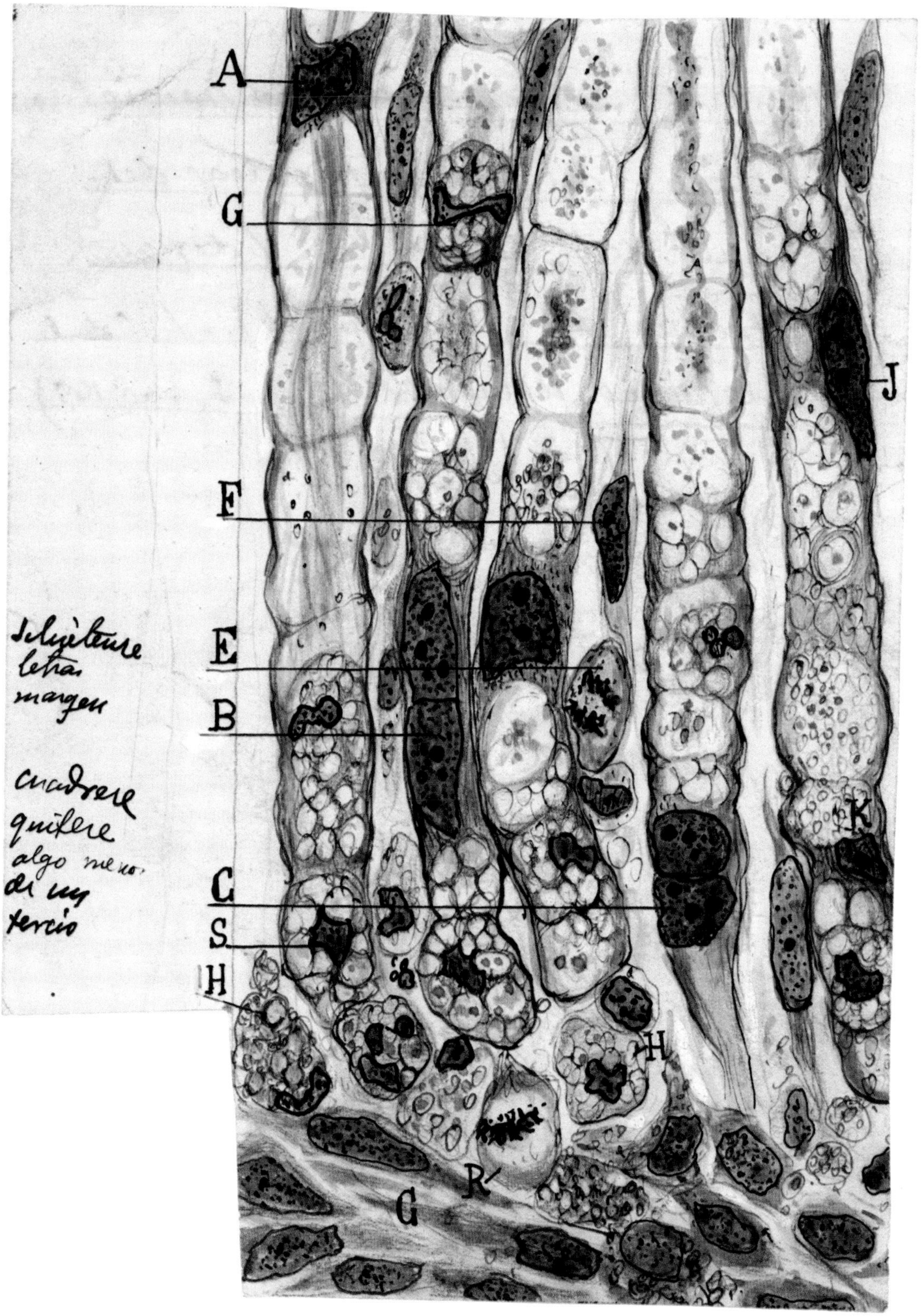

FIGURE 170. Central stump of the sciatic nerve in a cat three days after the operation.

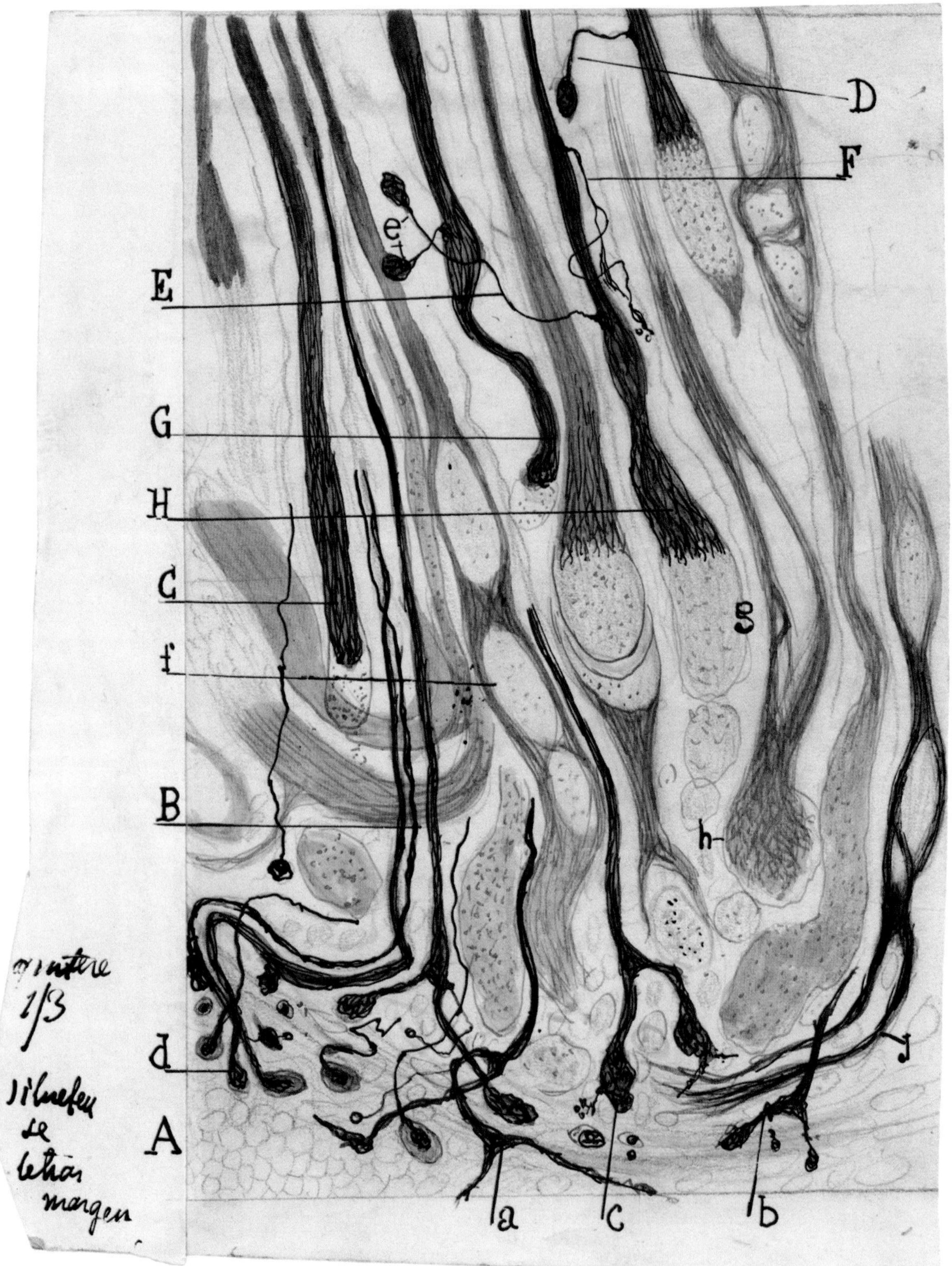

FIGURE 171. Central stump of the sciatic nerve in a rabbit six hours after the operation.

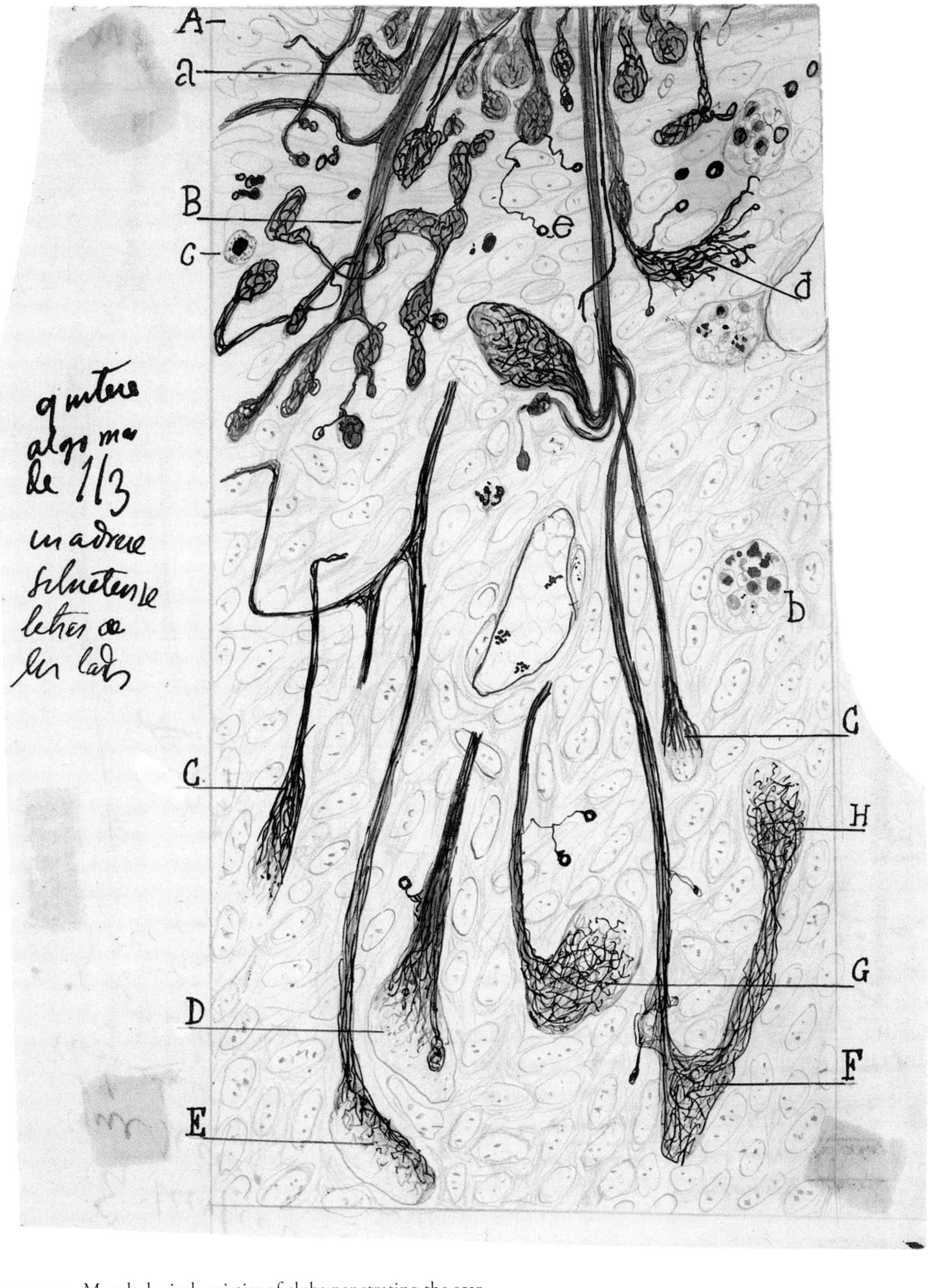

FIGURE 172. Morphological varieties of clubs penetrating the scar.

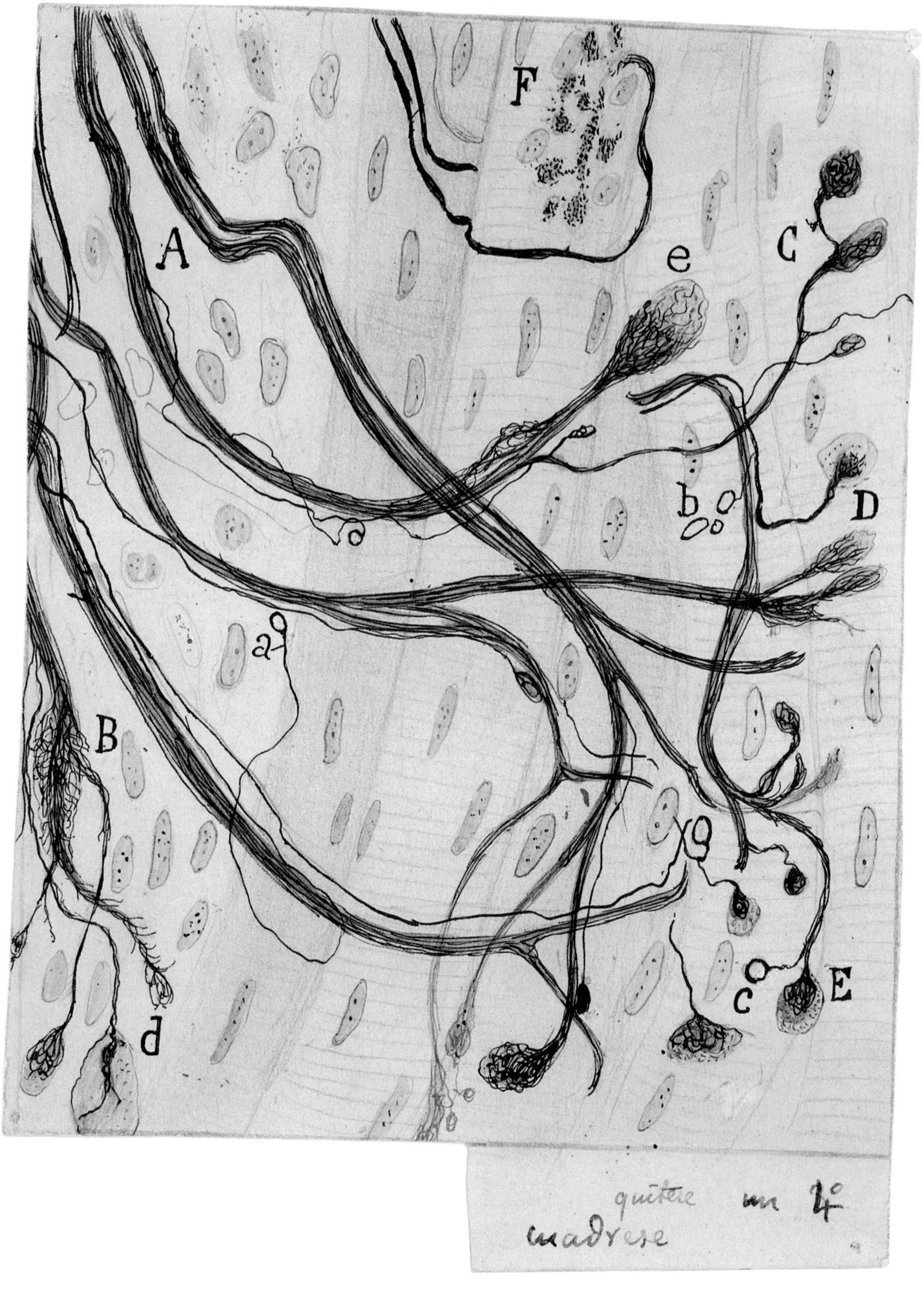

FIGURE 173. Nerve fibers lost in a muscle near to the central stump.

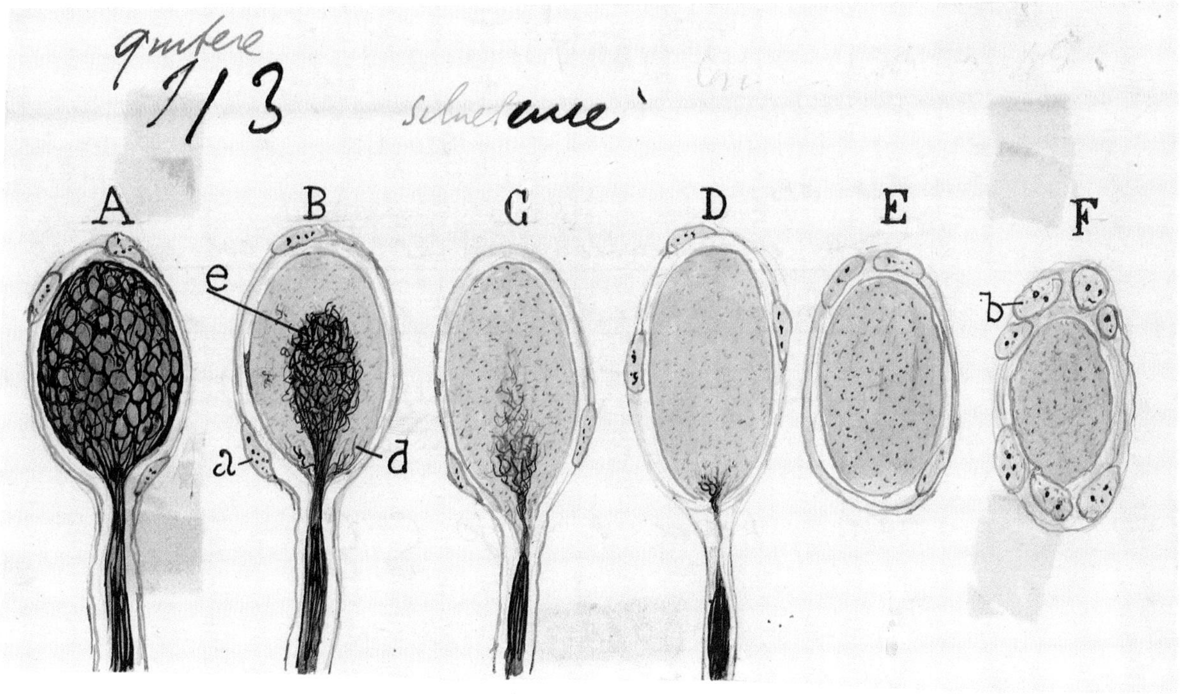

FIGURE 174. Degenerative phases of gigantic arrested balls.

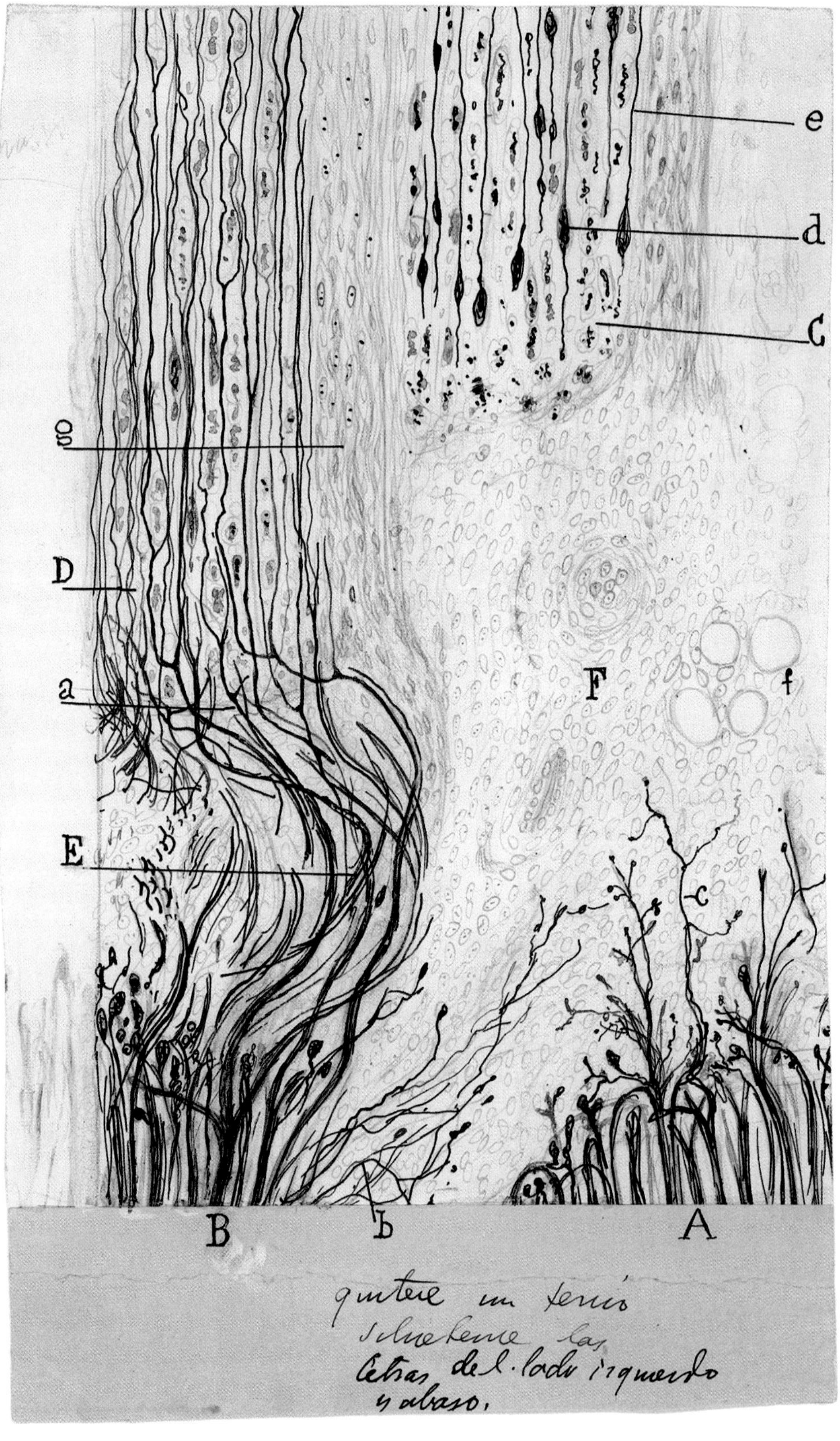

FIGURE 175. Rapid innervation of the peripheral stump.

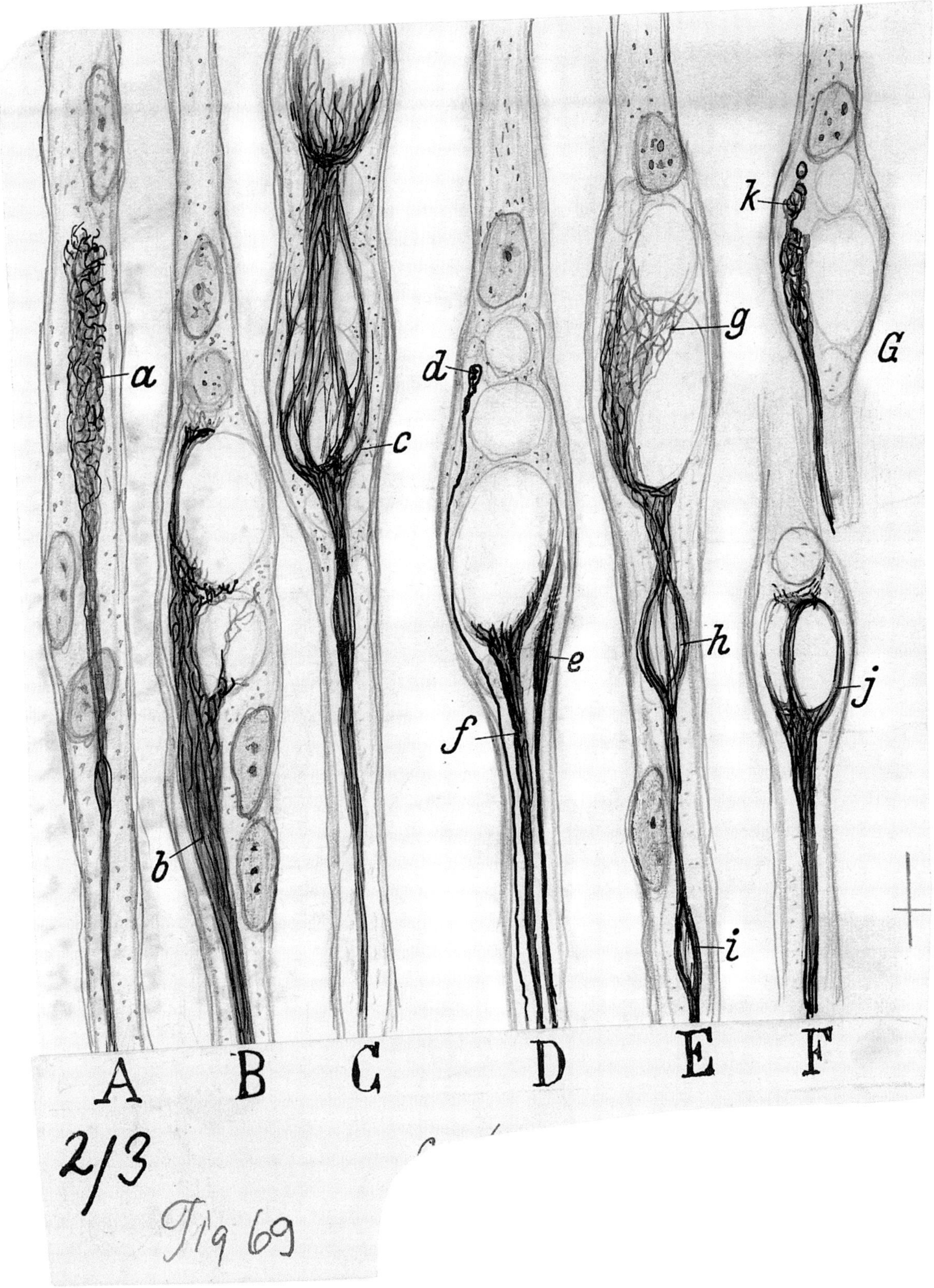

FIGURE 176. Growth cone of the sprouts that have penetrated into the old myelinated fibers of the peripheral stump.

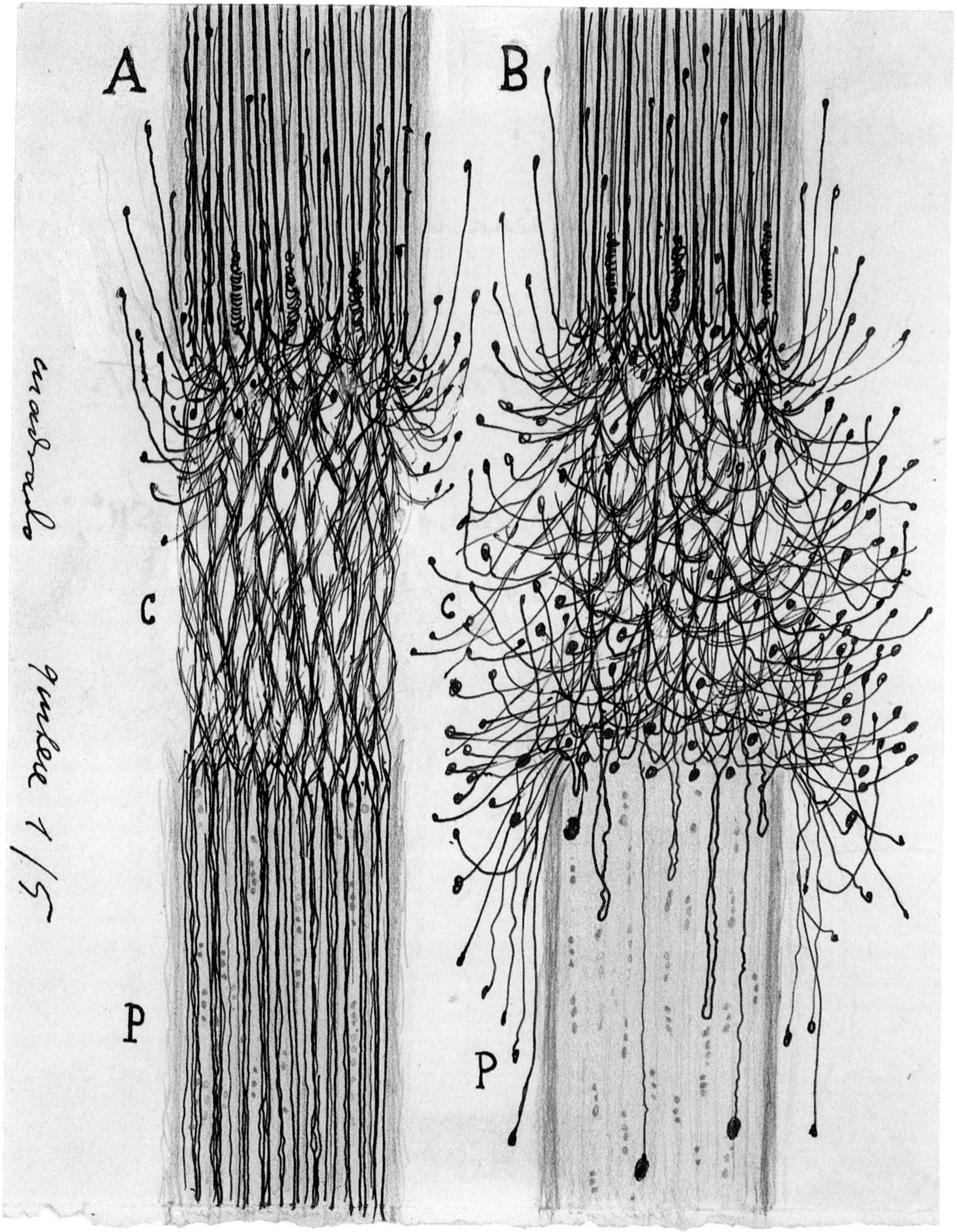

FIGURE 177. Path of the sprouts and mechanical factors.

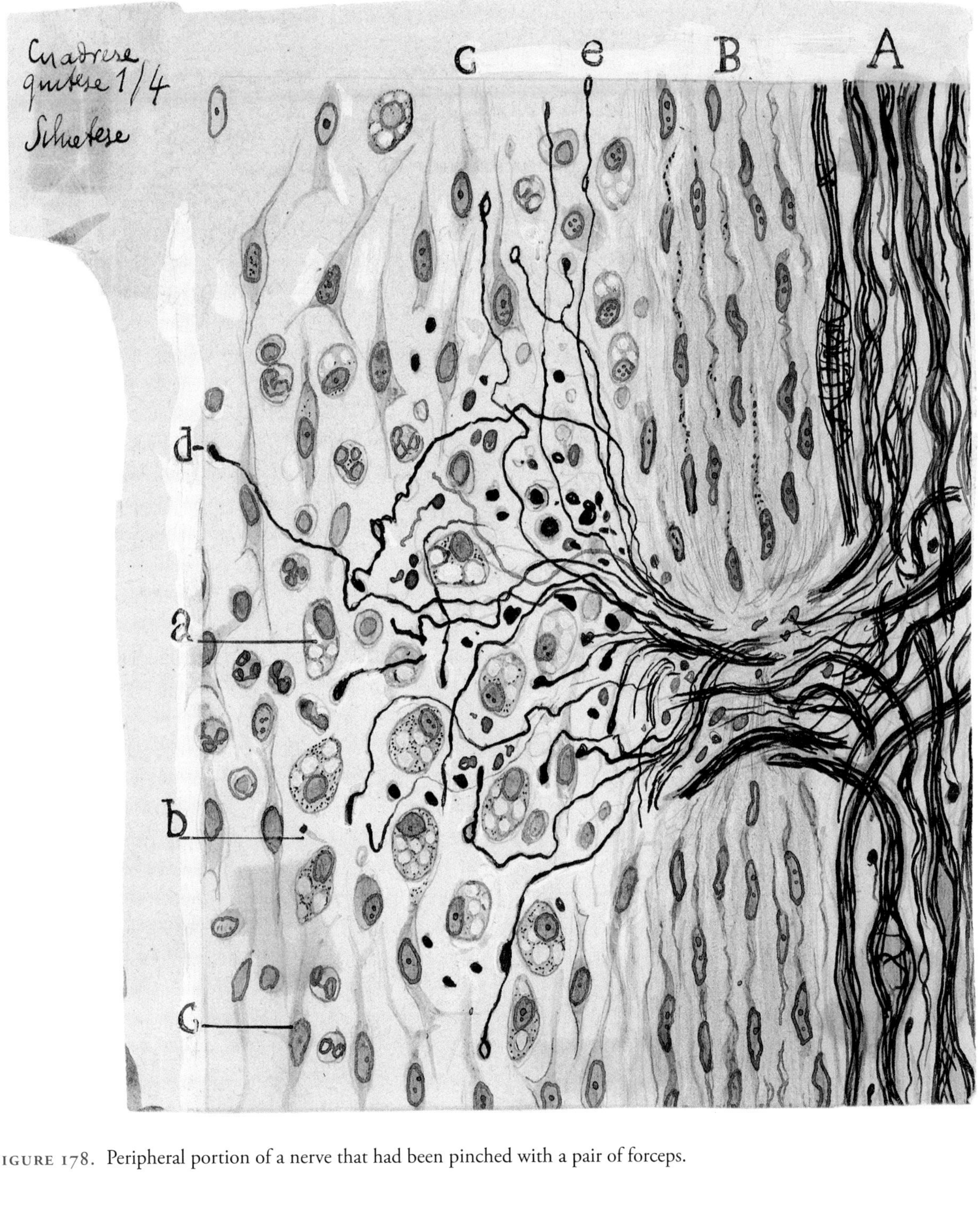

FIGURE 178. Peripheral portion of a nerve that had been pinched with a pair of forceps.

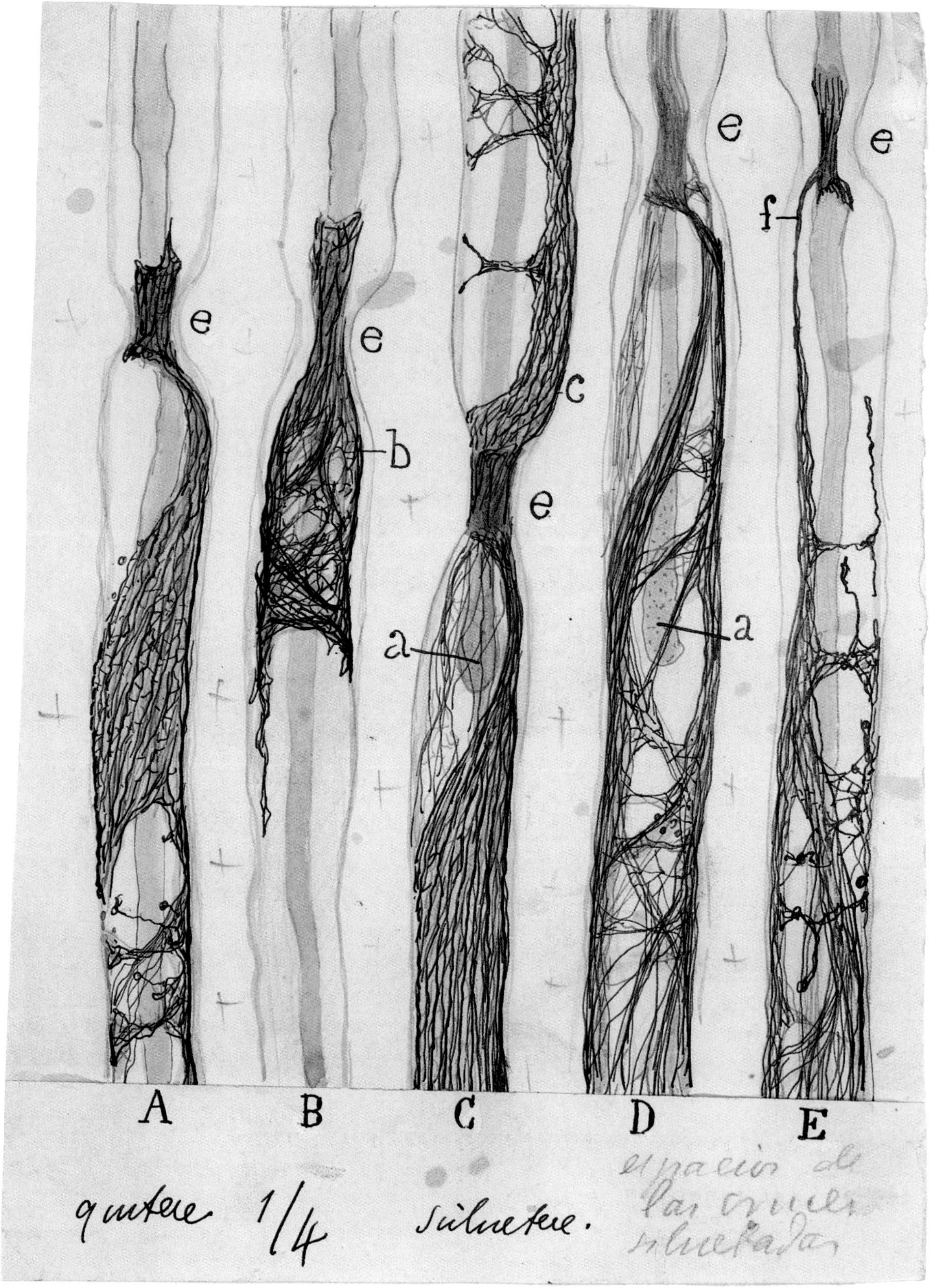

FIGURE 179. Central stump far from the ligature.

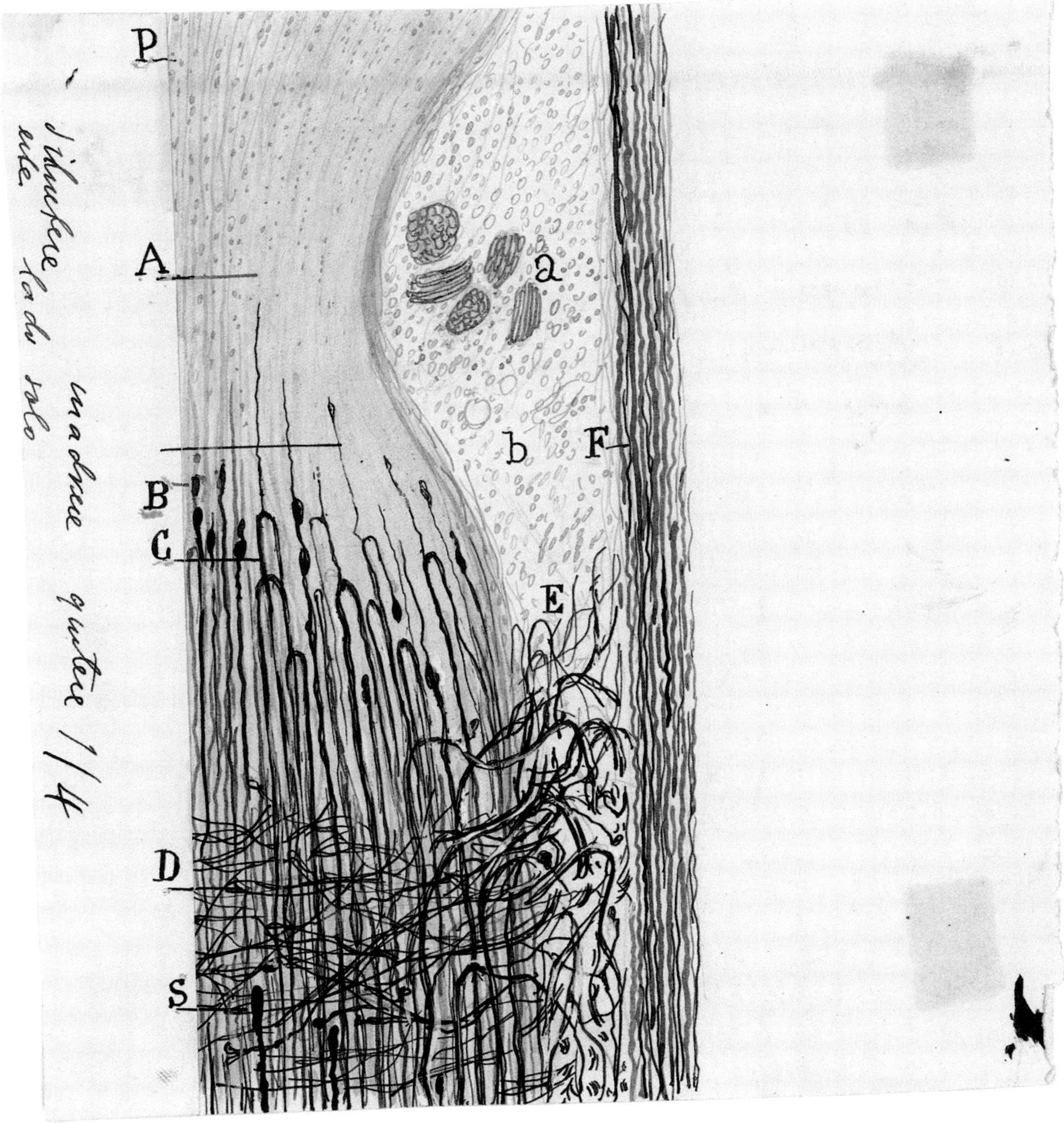

FIGURE 180. Sciatic nerve in a young rabbit.

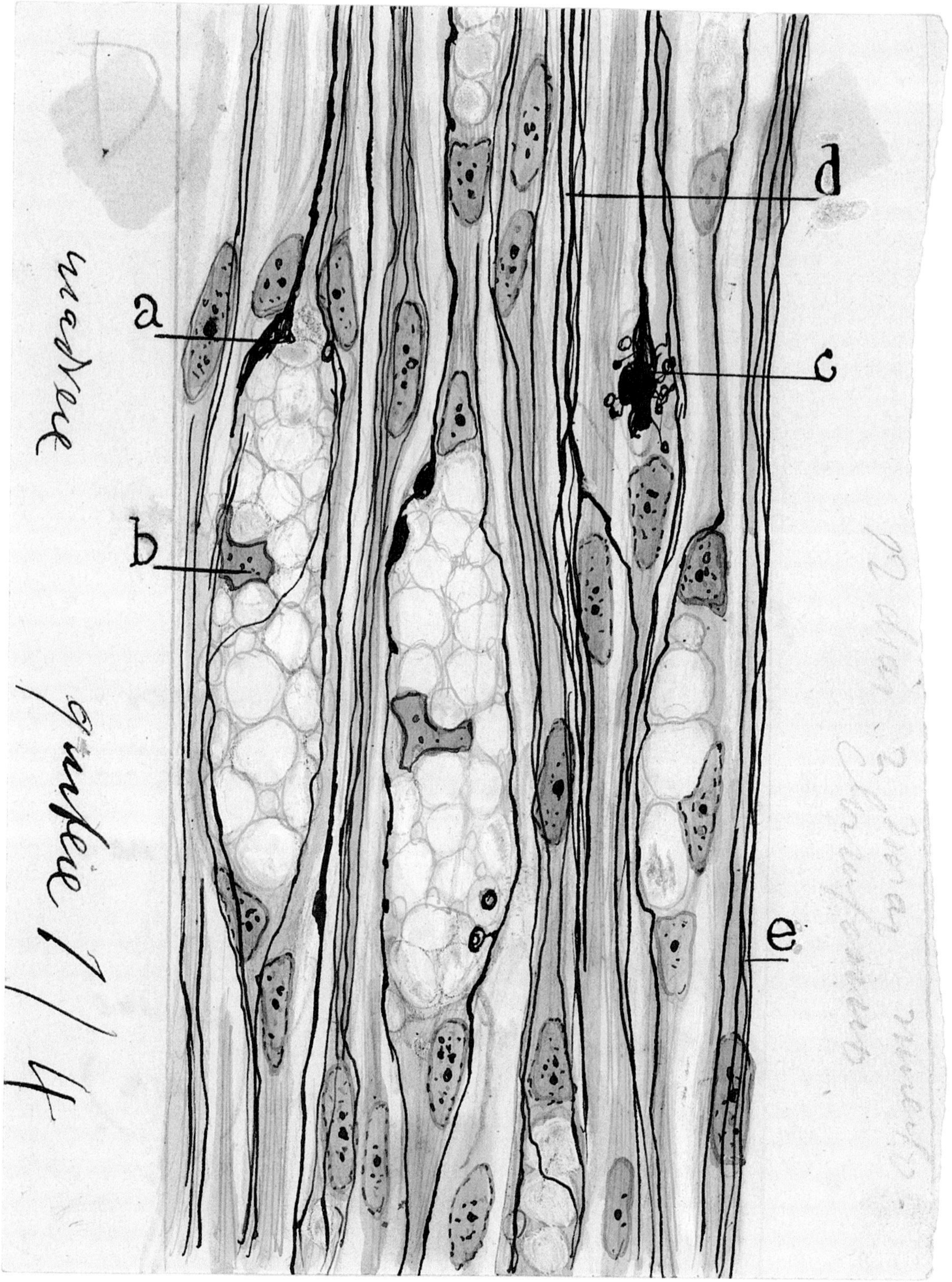

FIGURE 181. Details of the cortical region of a graft.

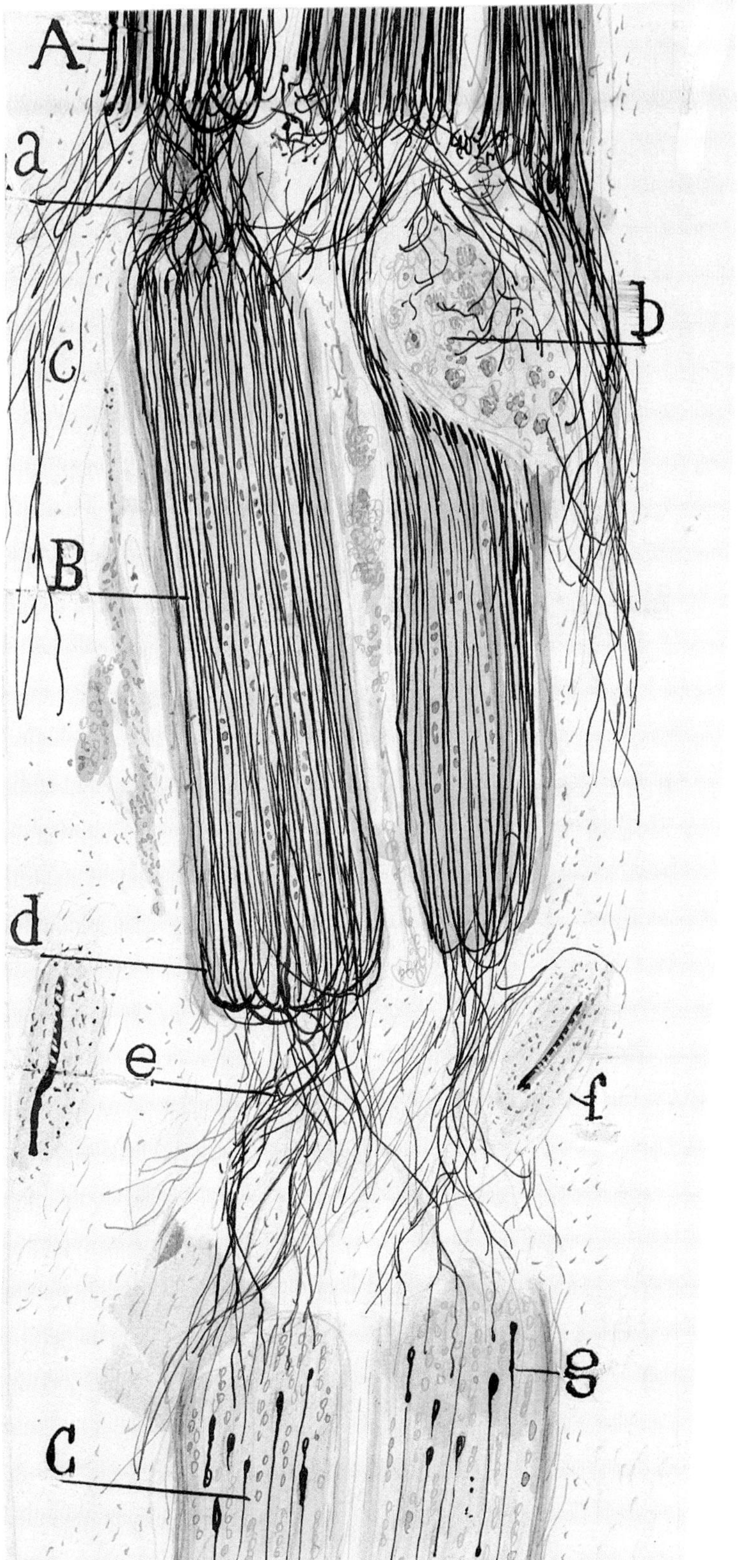

FIGURE 182. Graft of spinal roots on a wound of the sciatic.

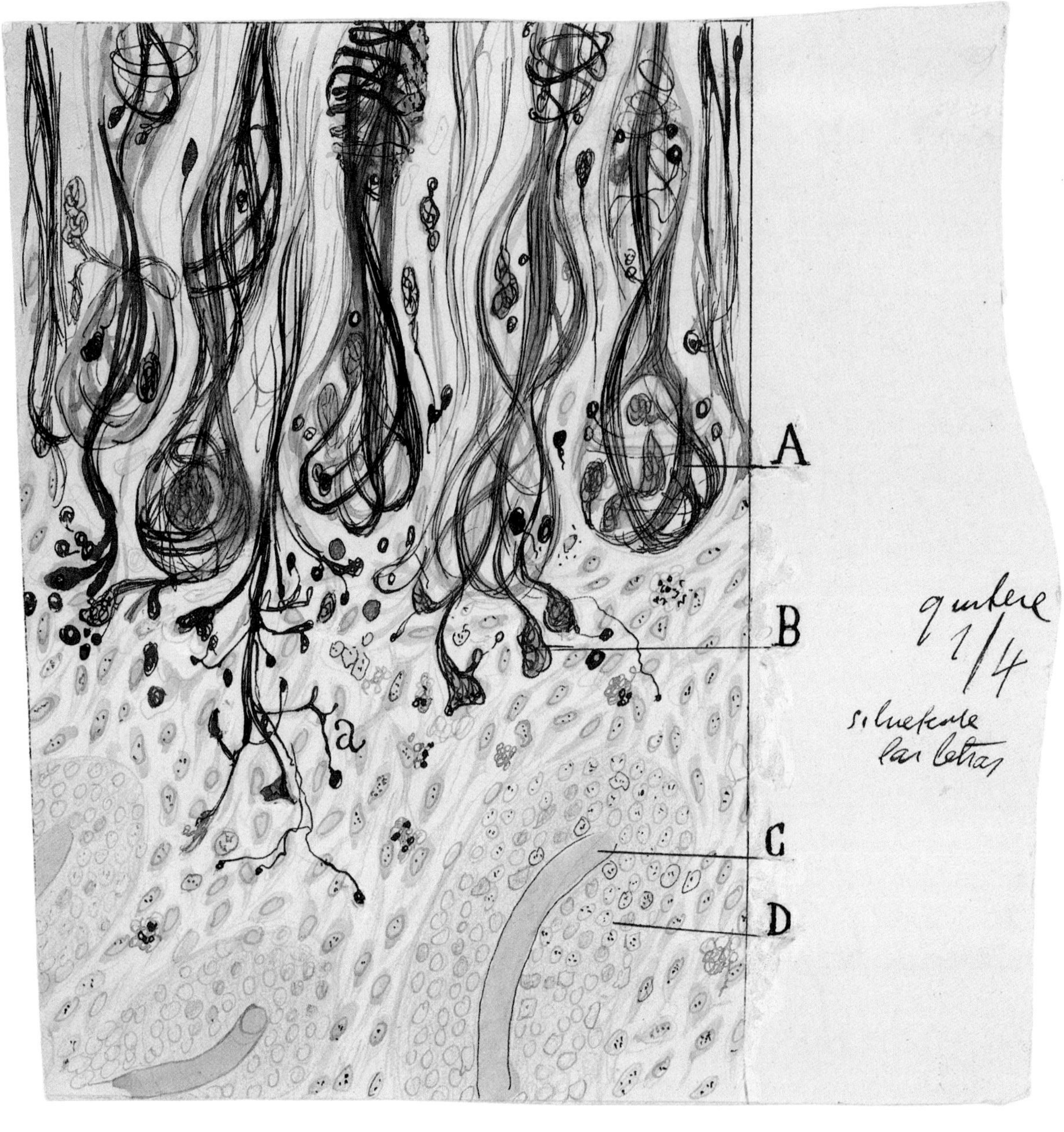

FIGURE 183. Piece of the central stump and scar in a near-adult rabbit.

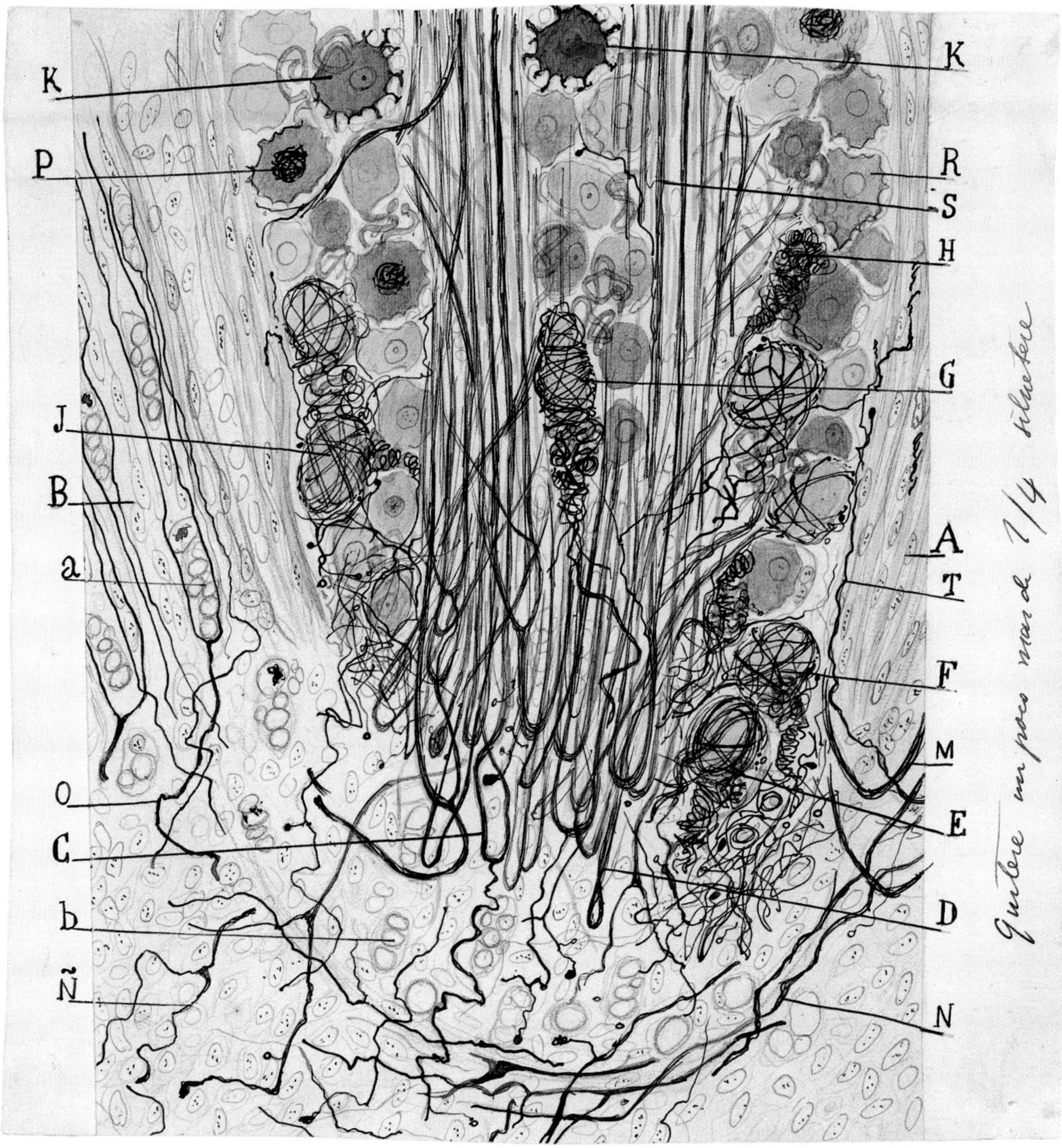

FIGURE 184. Axial section of a sensory ganglion of the sacral region.

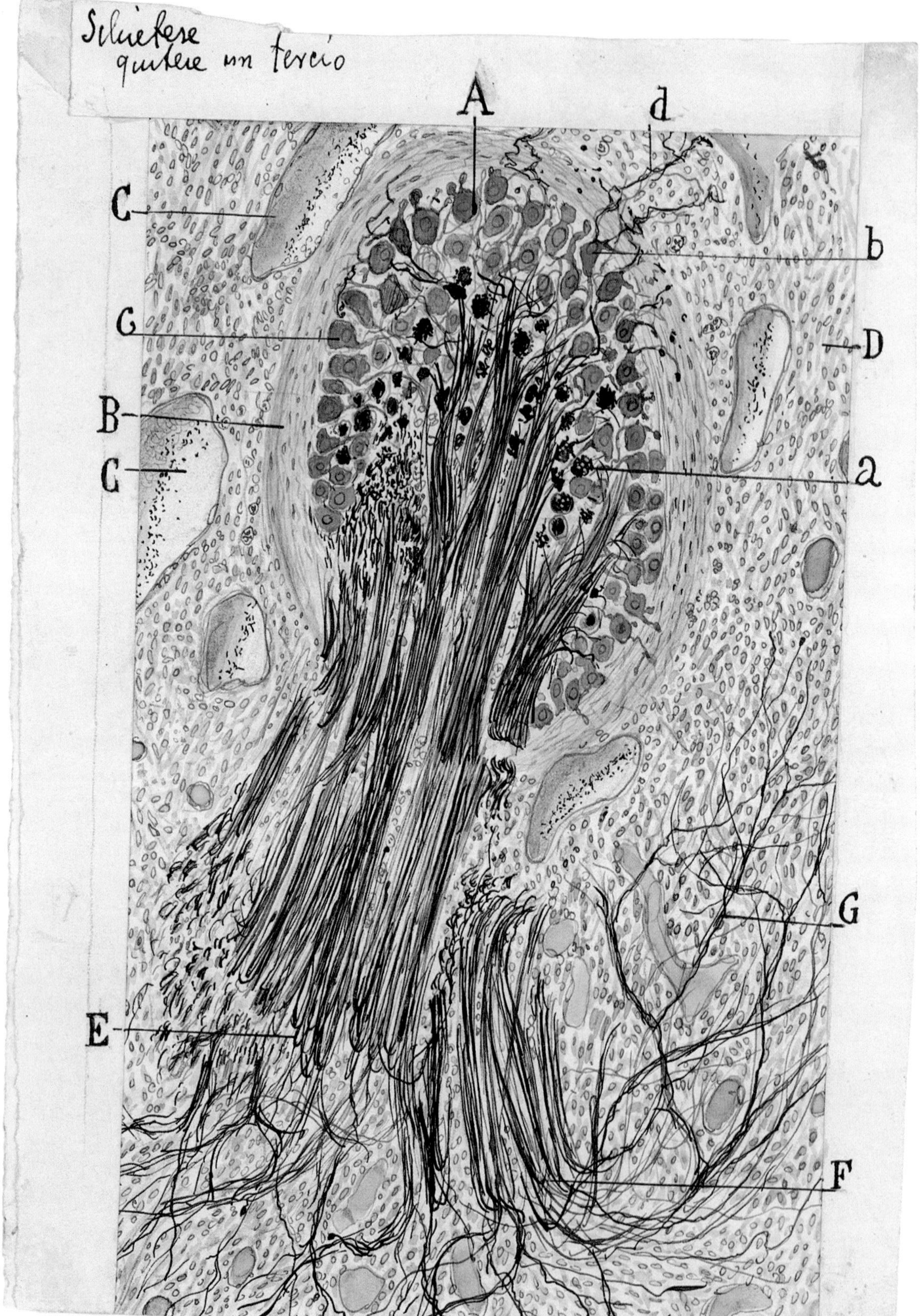

FIGURE 185. Small ganglion of the cauda equina in a cat a few days old.

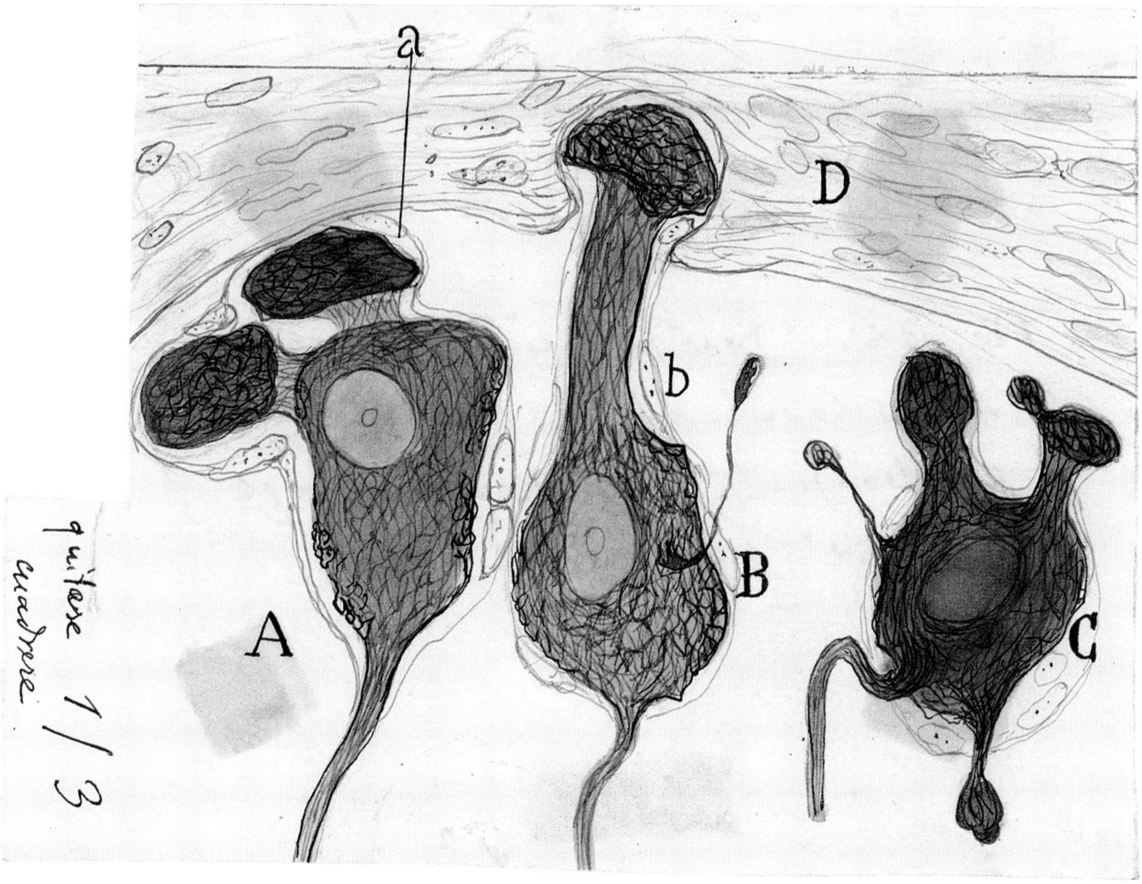

FIGURE 186. Small ganglion of the cauda equina in a cat a few days old, I.

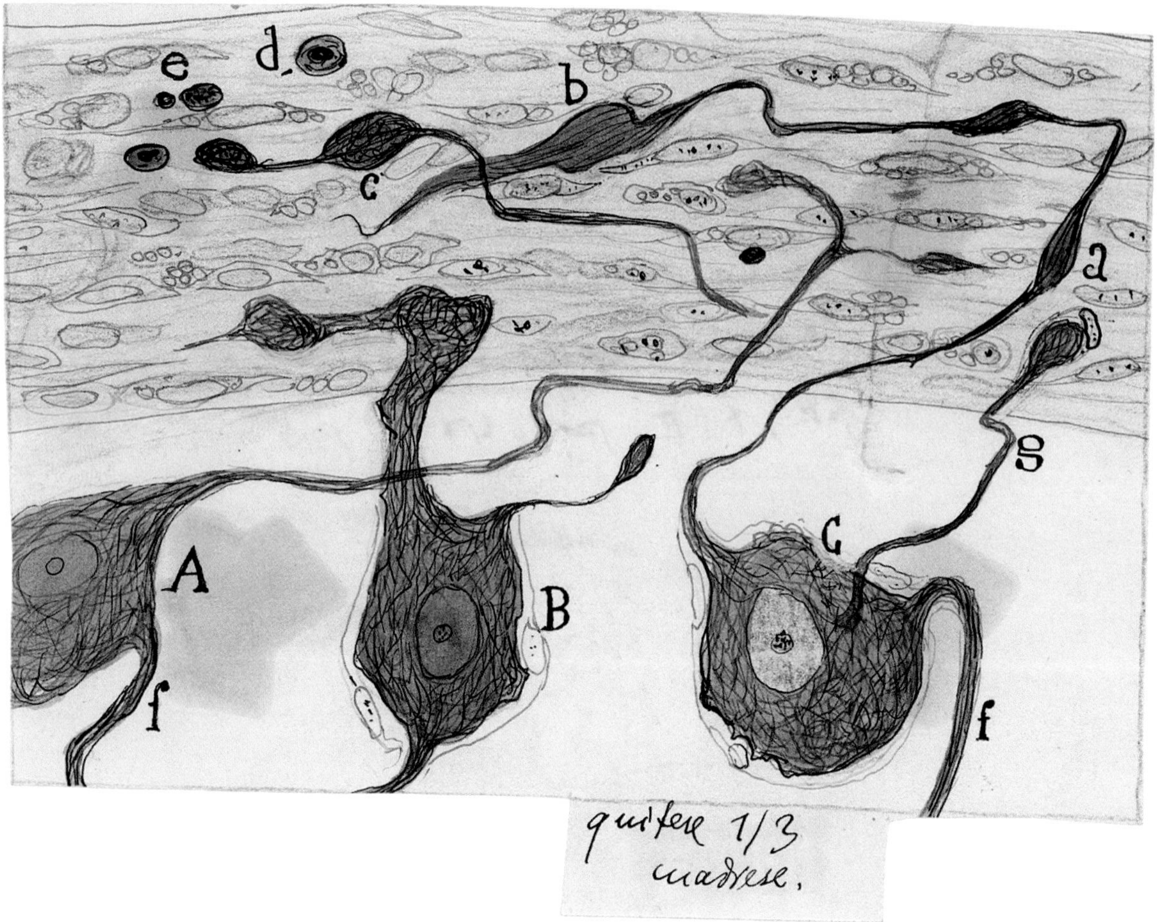

FIGURE 187. Small ganglion of the cauda equina in a cat a few days old, II.

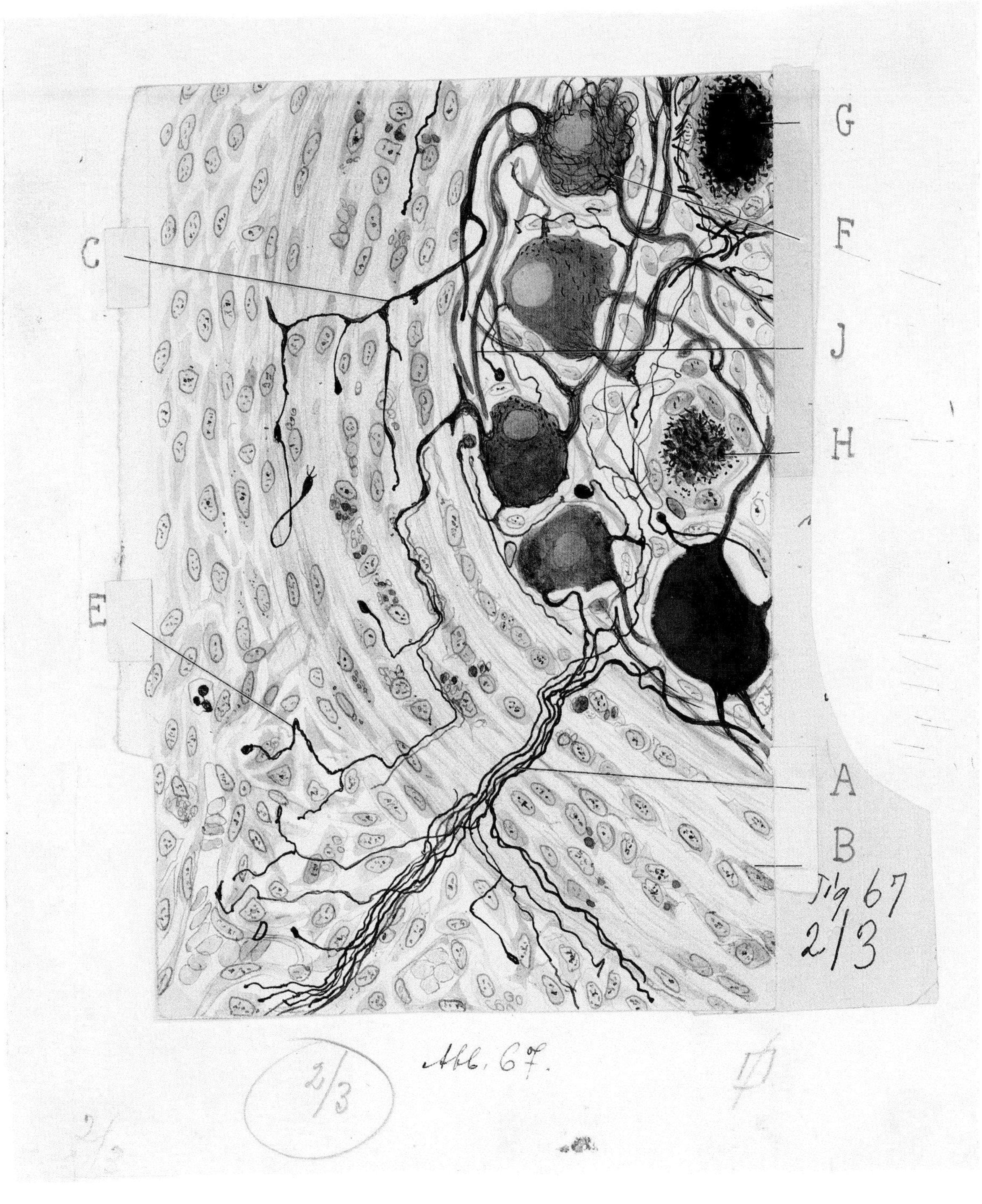

FIGURE 188. Graft of a ganglion in a dog a few days old.

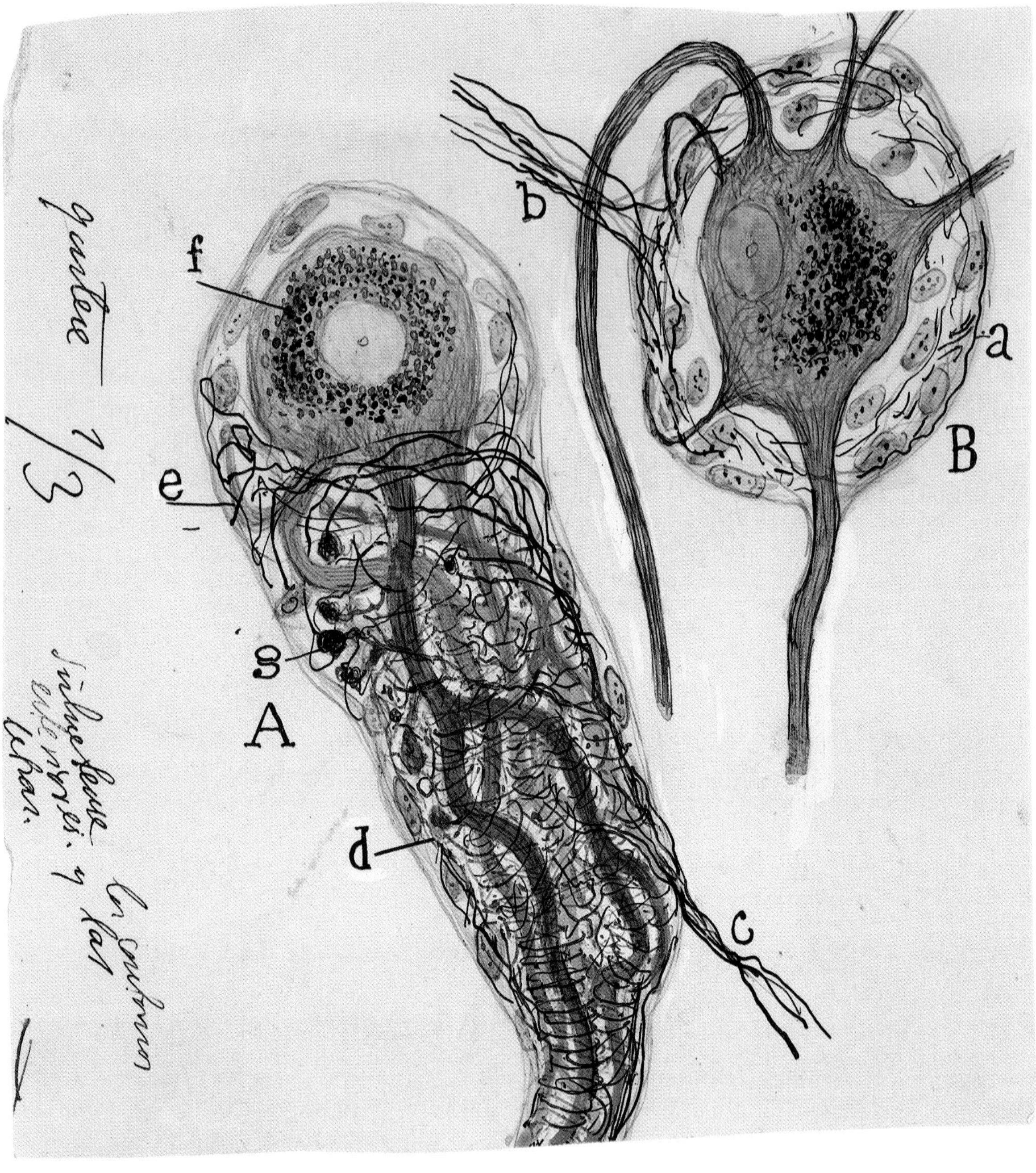

FIGURE 189. Atypical cells in an old horse.

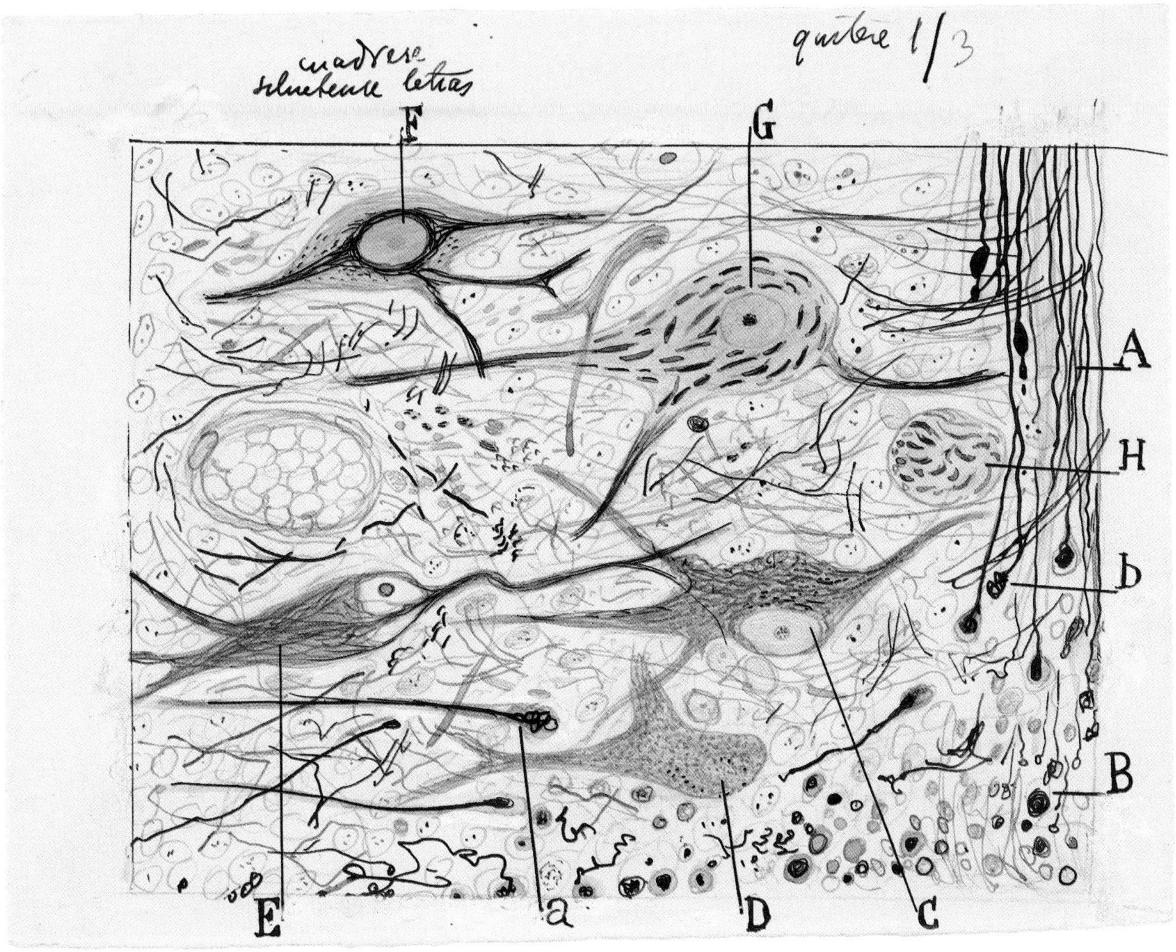

FIGURE 190. Nerve cells in the gray matter of the spinal cord in a young cat.

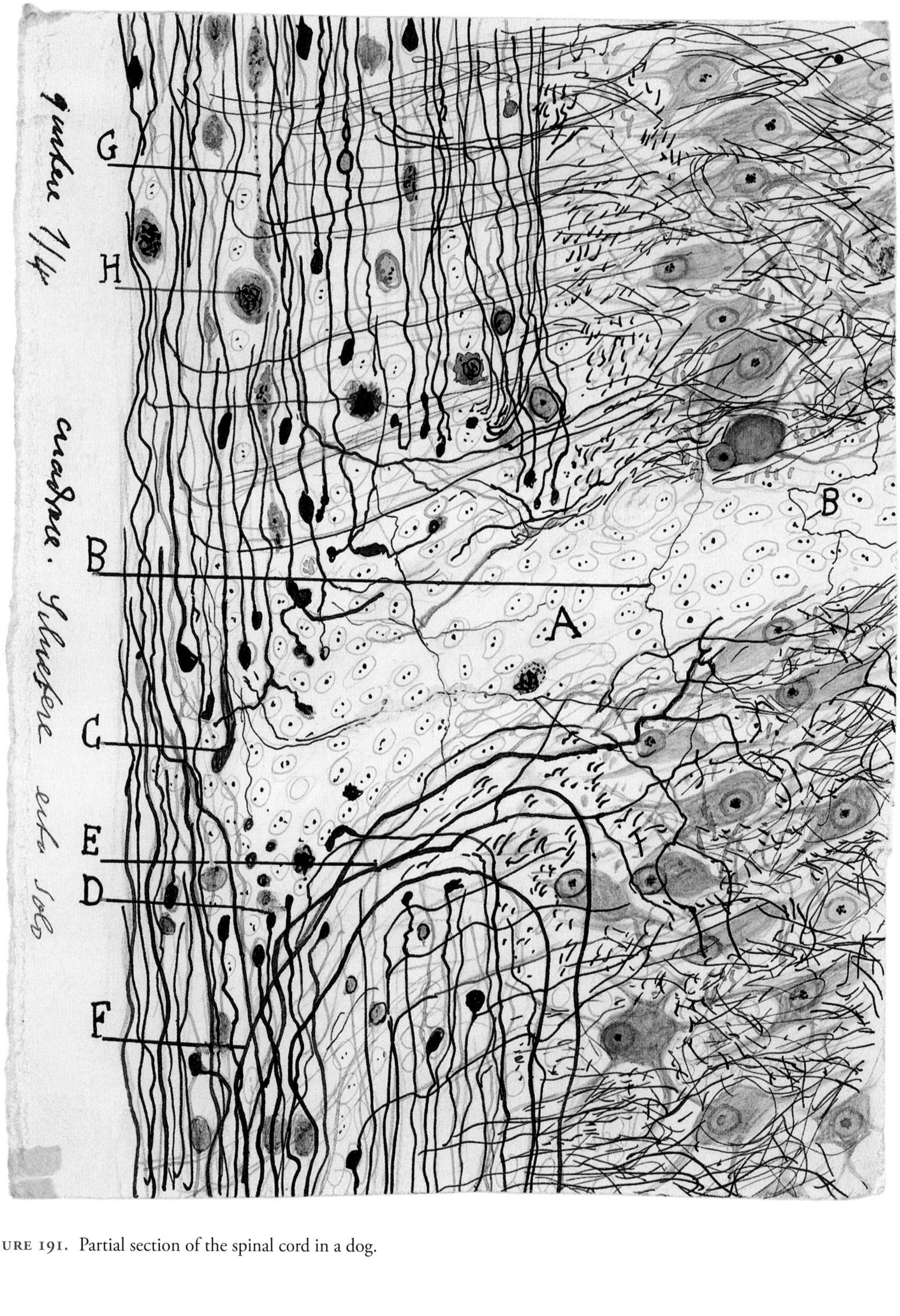

FIGURE 191. Partial section of the spinal cord in a dog.

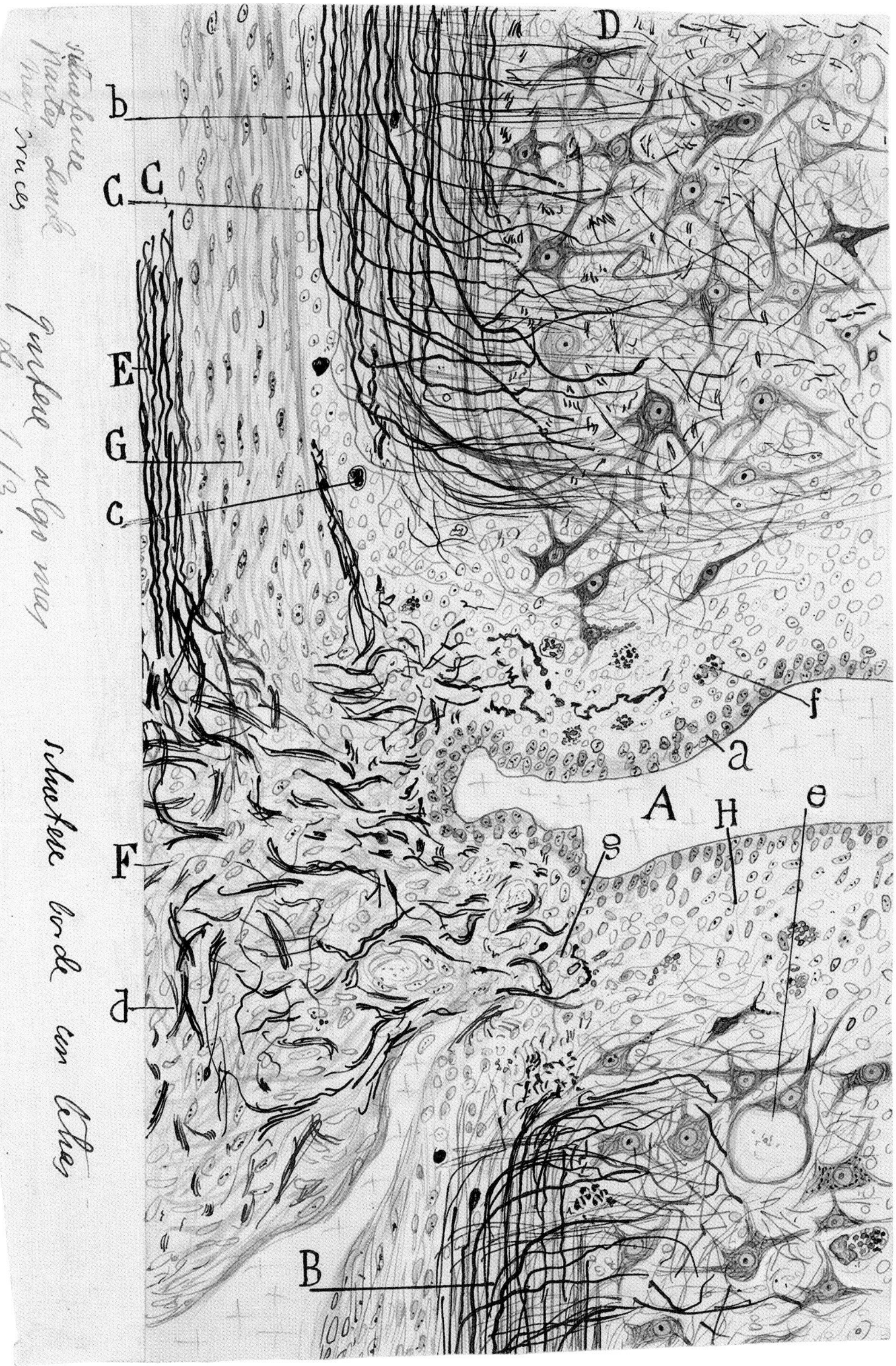

FIGURE 192. Complete section of the spinal cord in a rabbit.

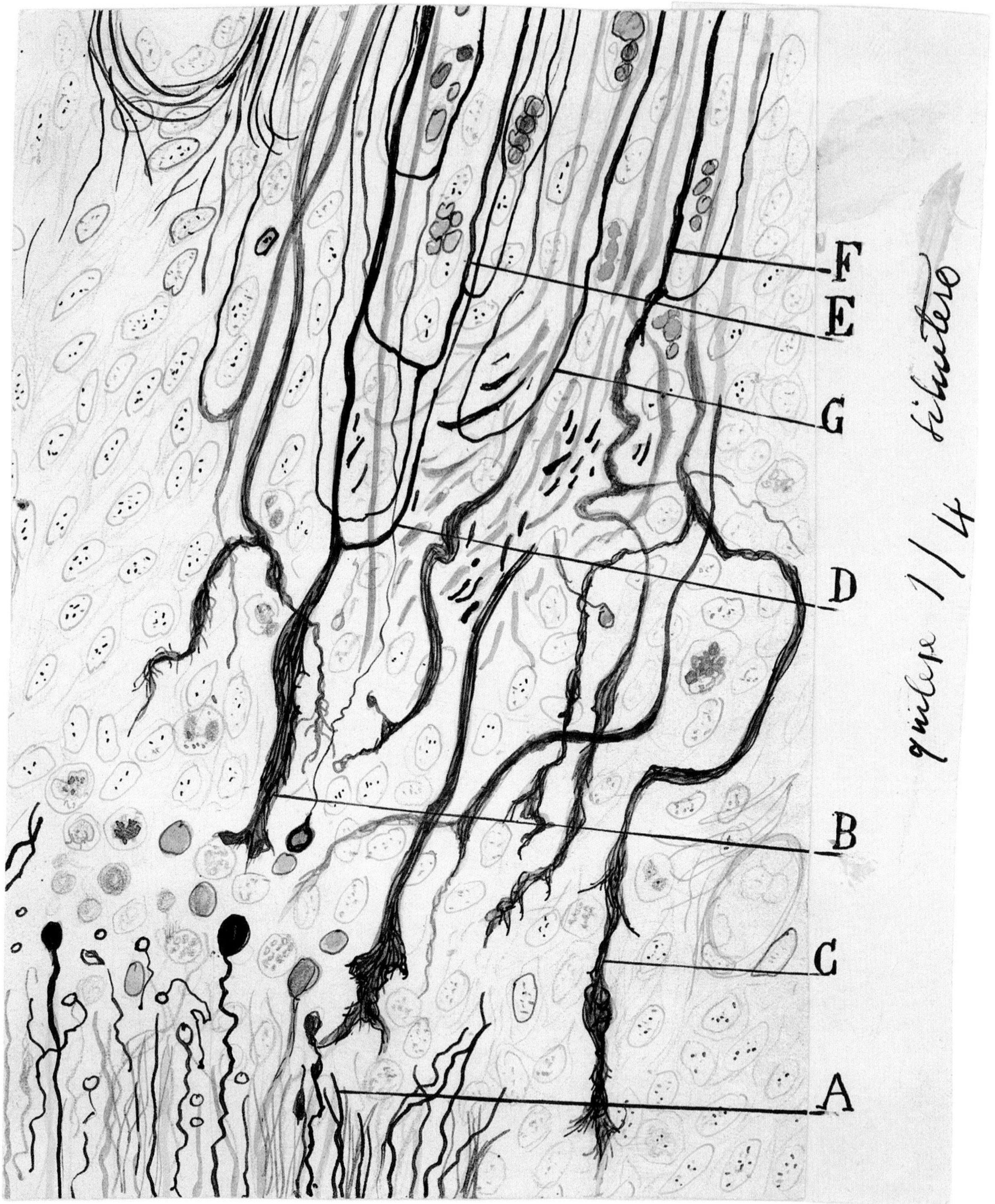

FIGURE 193. Juxtaspinal portion of a sensory root.

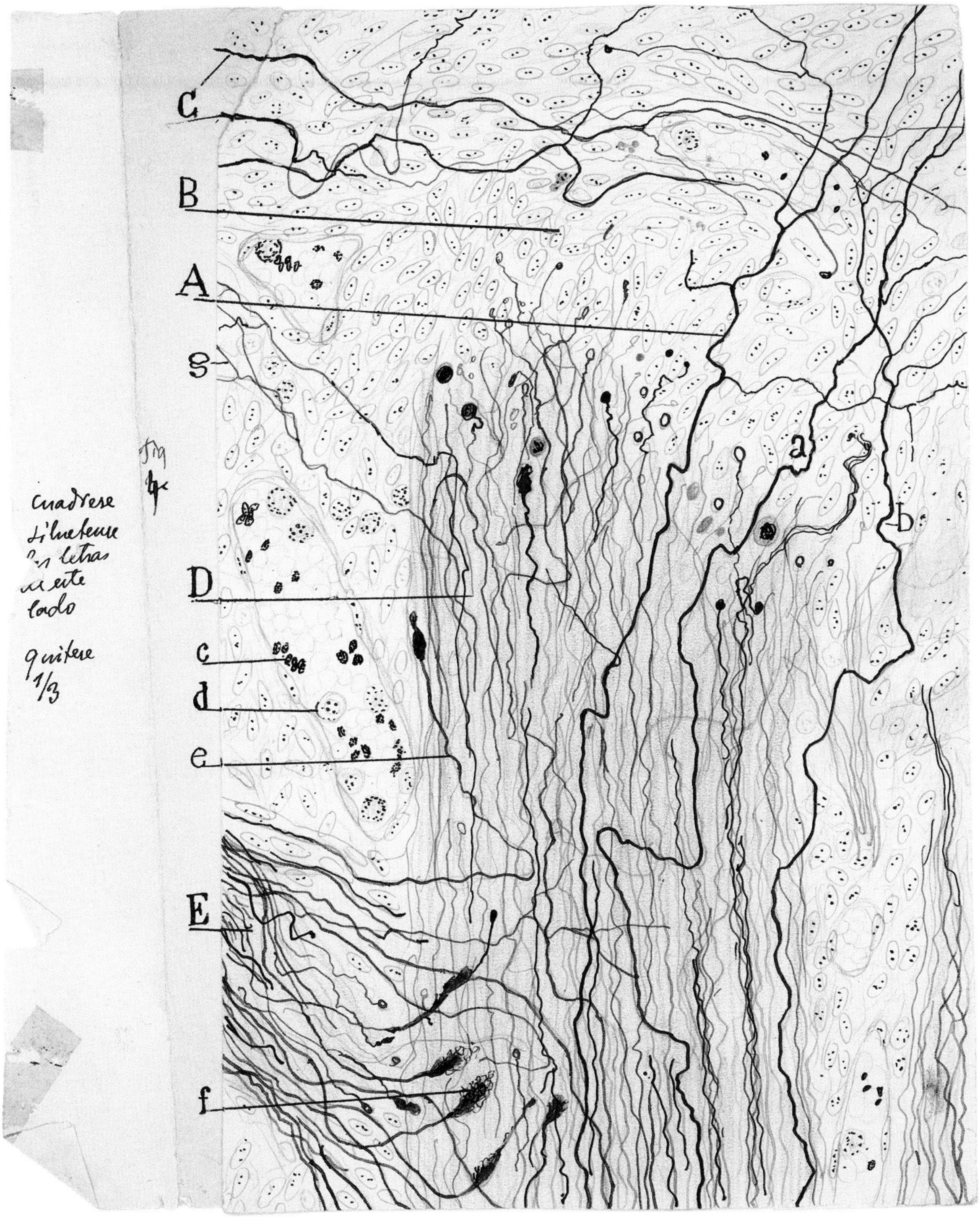

FIGURE 194. Longitudinal and tangential section of the posterior bundle in a dog.

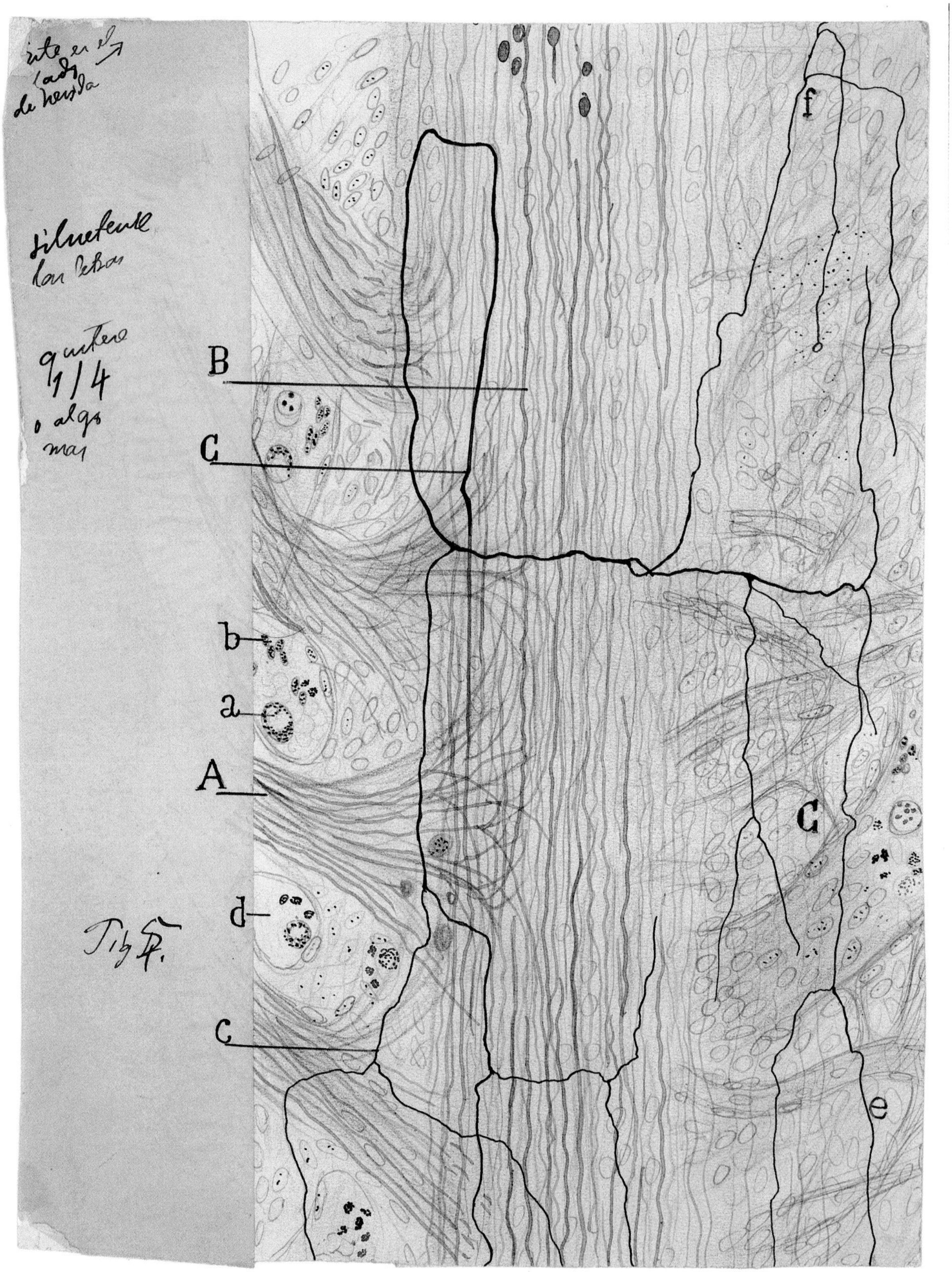

FIGURE 195. Tangential and longitudinal section of the posterior bundle near a spinal wound in a dog.

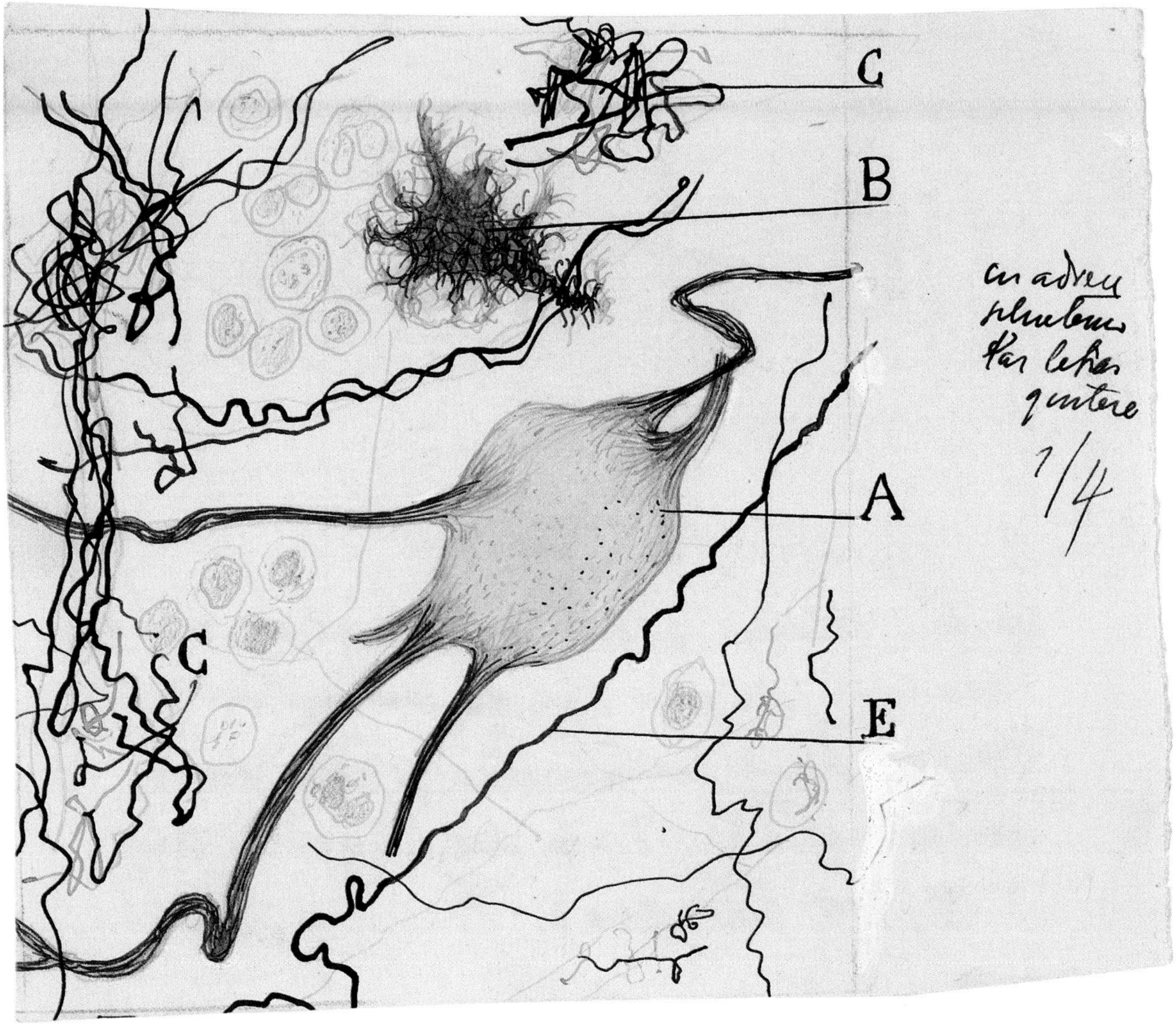

FIGURE 196. Cells and fibers floating in the exudate of a spinal cord wound.

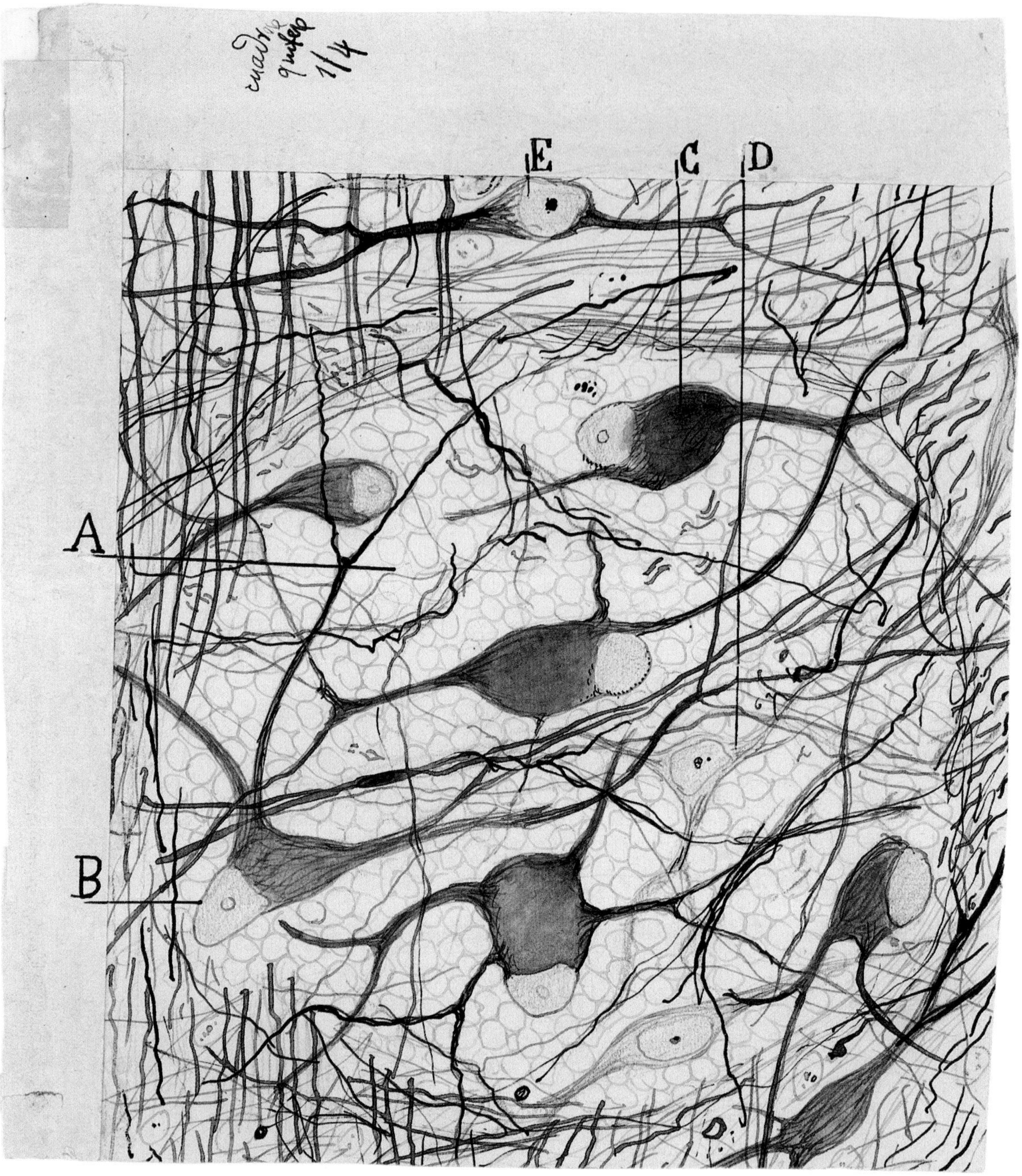

FIGURE 197. Cells lying in an interstitial hemorrhagic focus of the gray matter of the spinal cord.

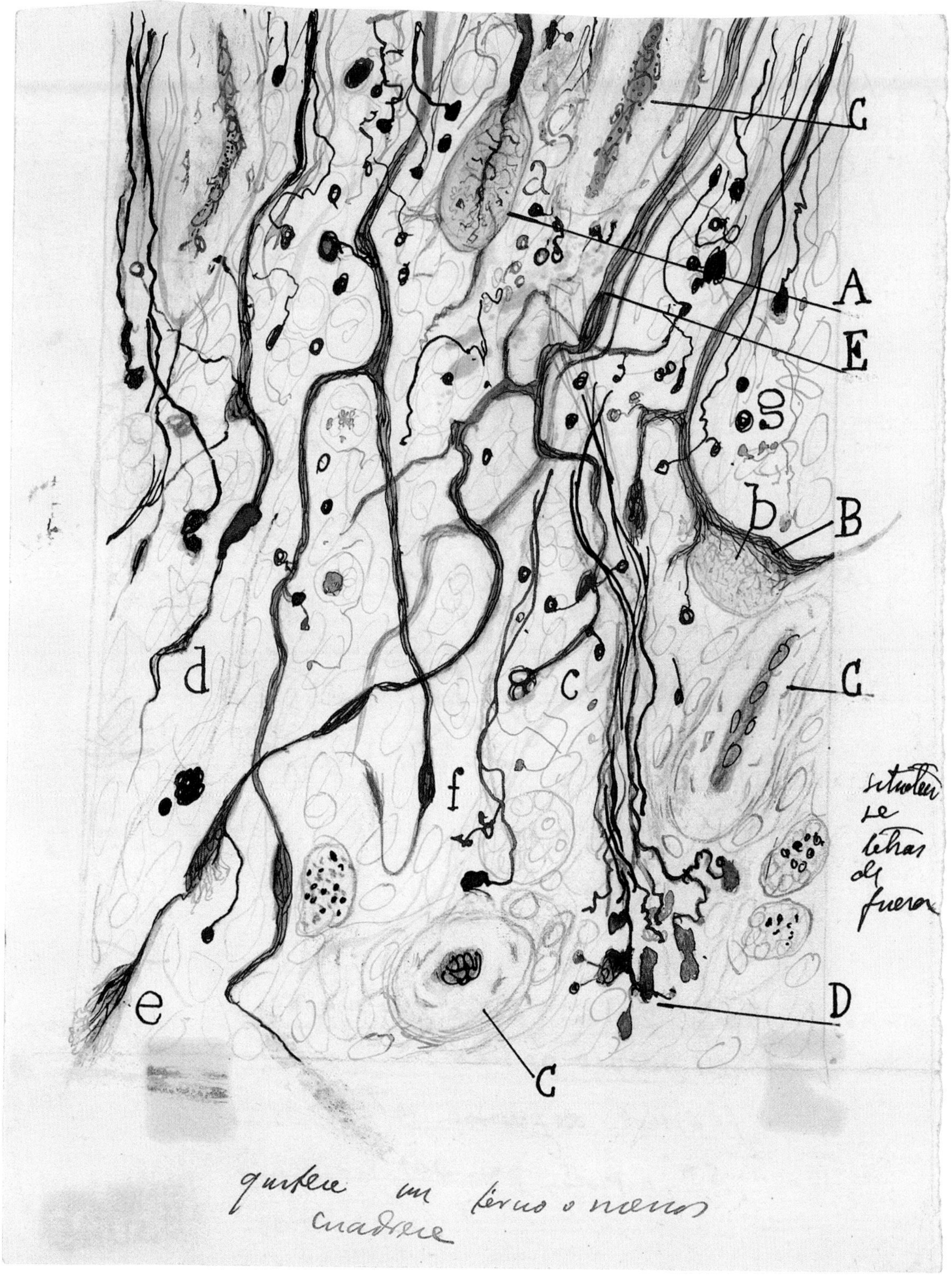

FIGURE 198. Retinal stump of the optic nerve in a rabbit.

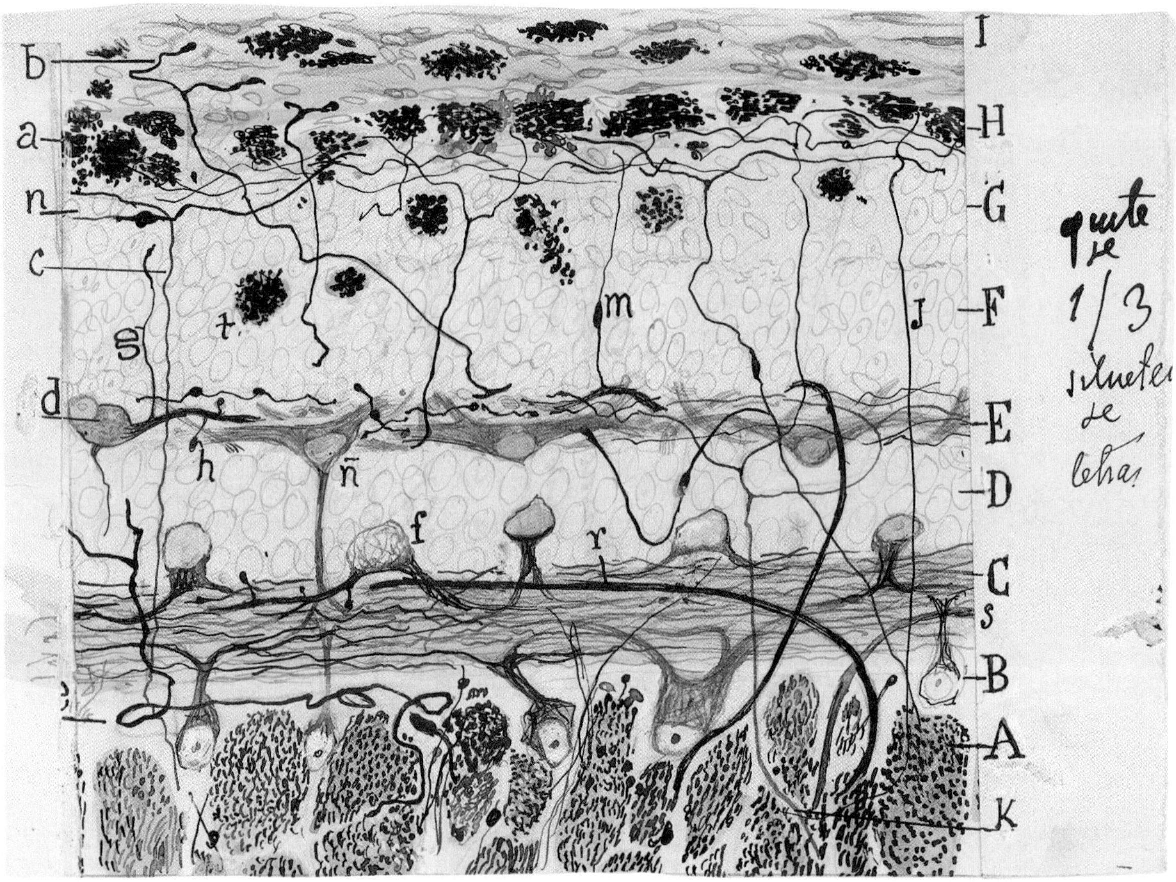

FIGURE 199. Phenomena of neoformation and dispersion of the optic fibers.

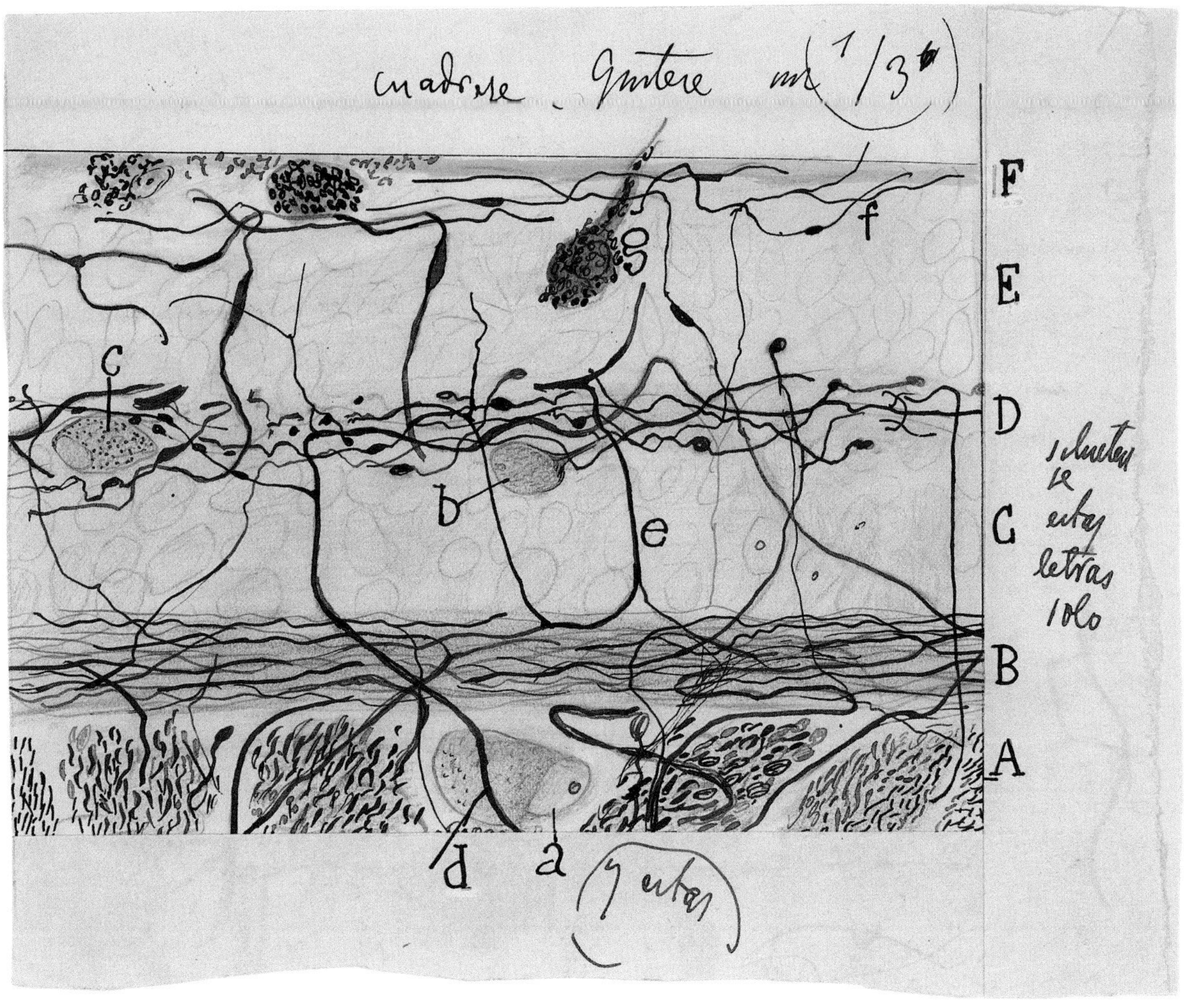

FIGURE 200. Regions in the retina from which nearly all the neurons had disappeared.

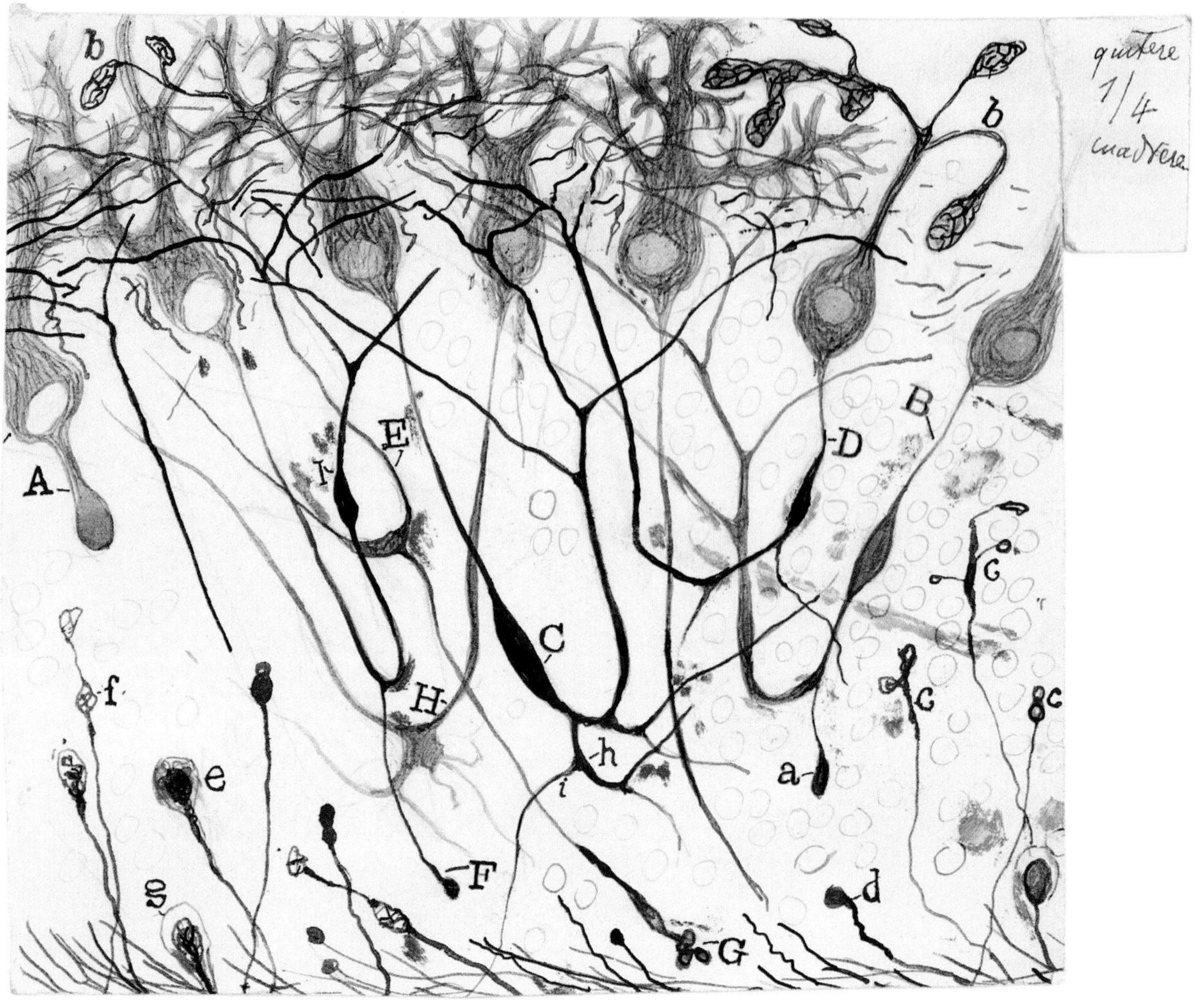

FIGURE 201. Disposition of Purkinje axons in the cerebellum in a cat.

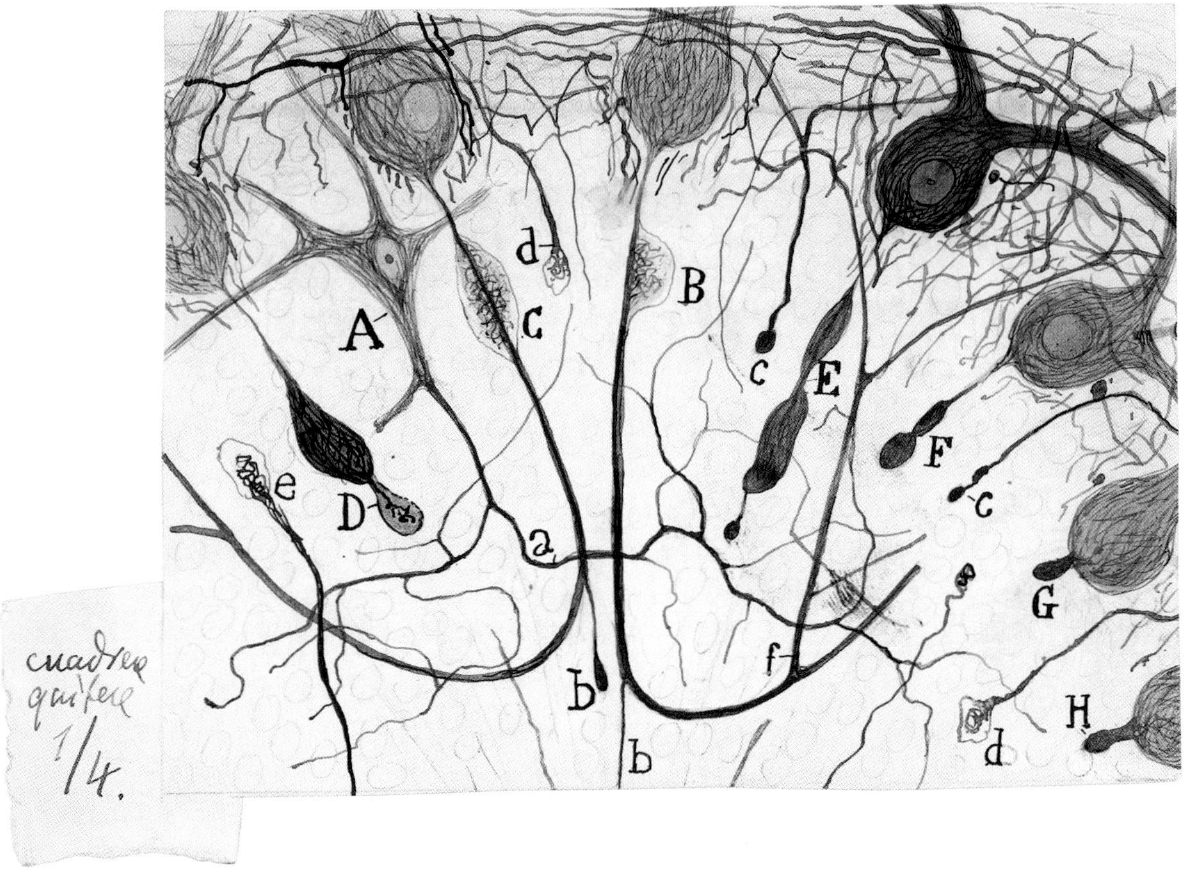

FIGURE 202. Section of a cerebellar folium.

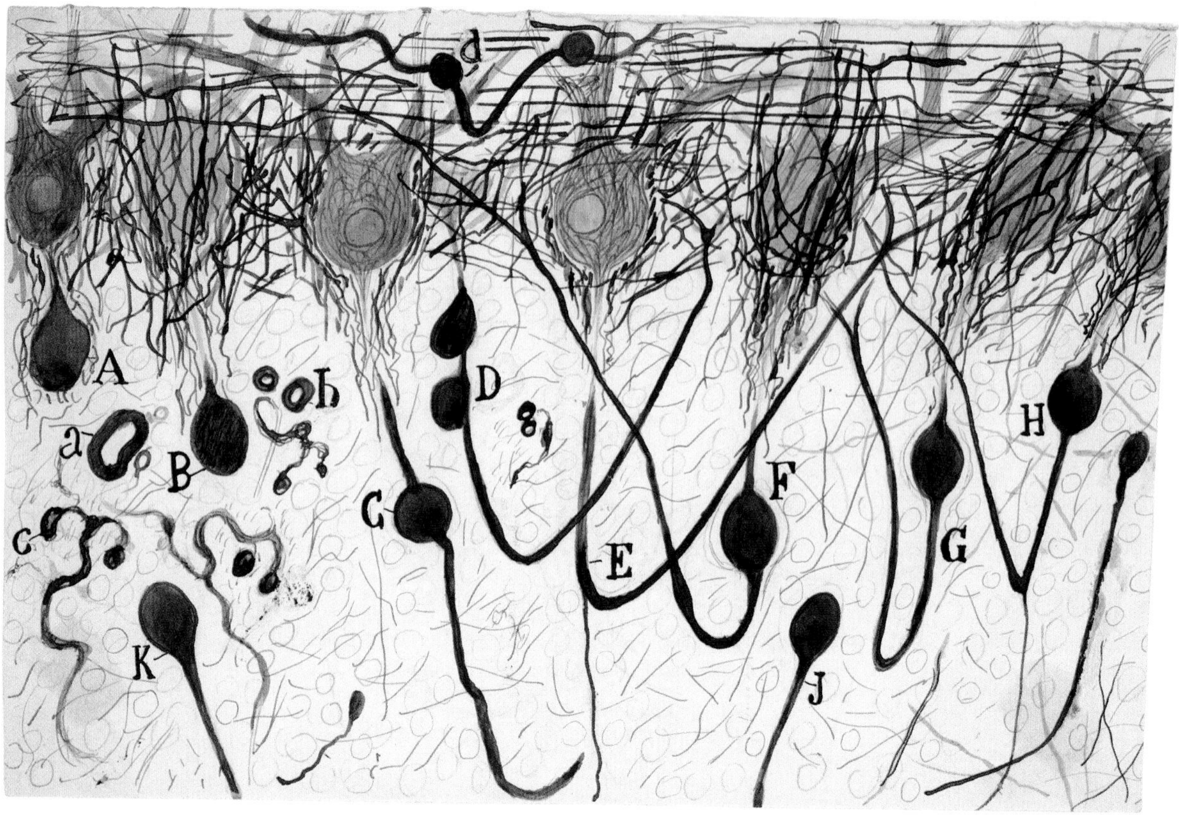

FIGURE 203. Lesions of the axon of Purkinje cells in the cerebellum in a human (drowned man).

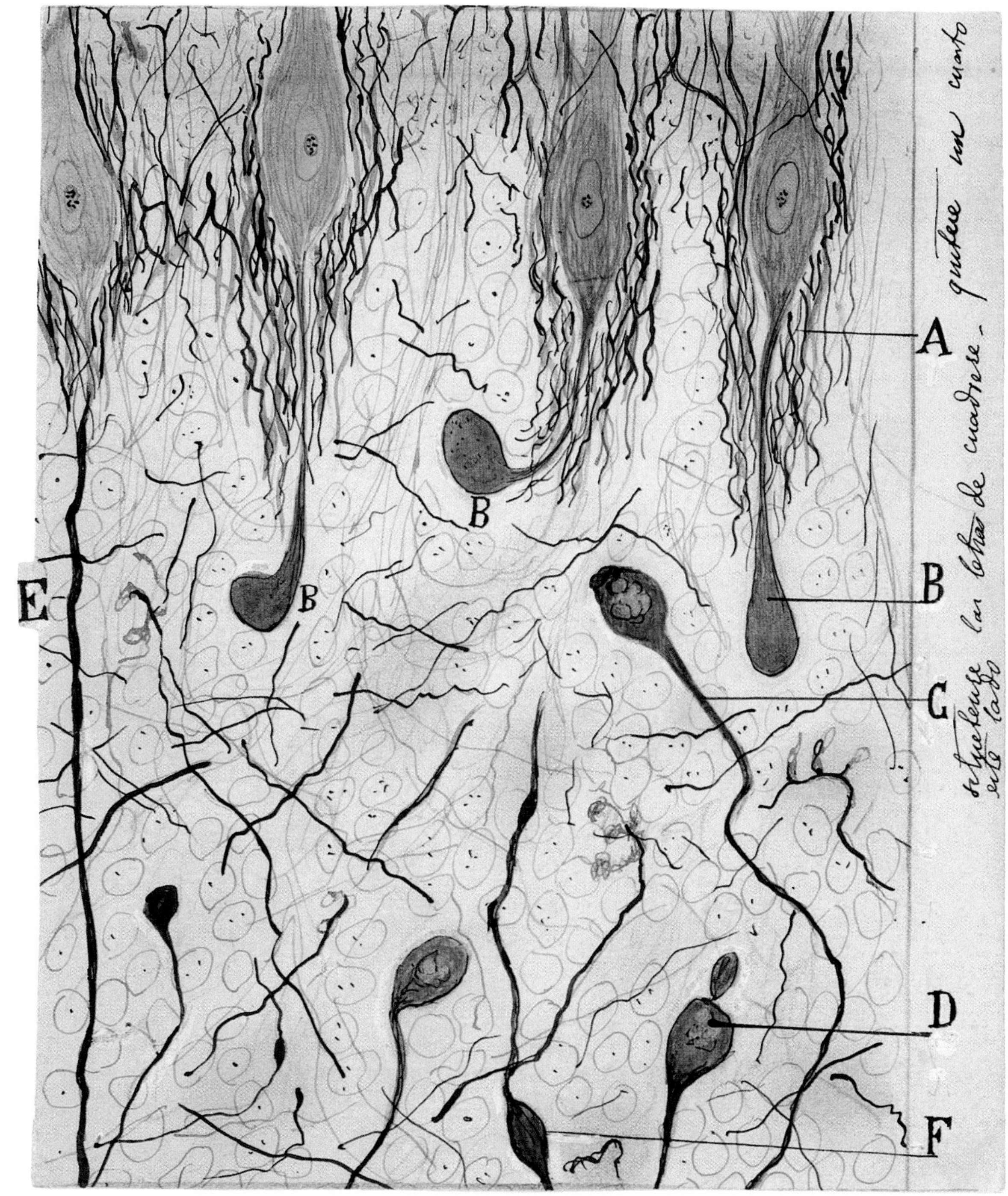

FIGURE 204. Section of a cerebellar folium in an adult rabbit.

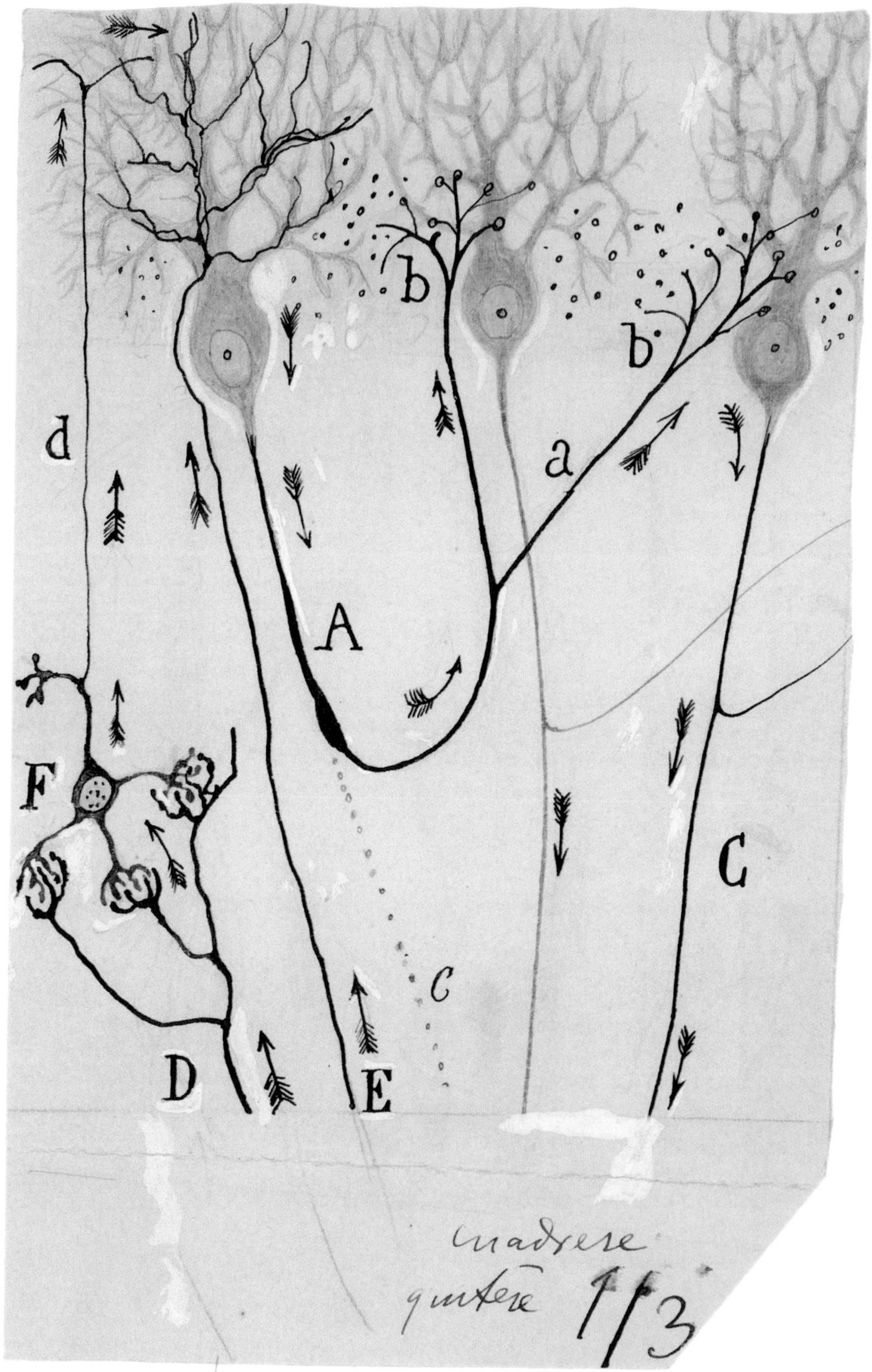

FIGURE 205. Path of the currents in the Purkinje cells that are deprived of the peripheral portion of the axon.

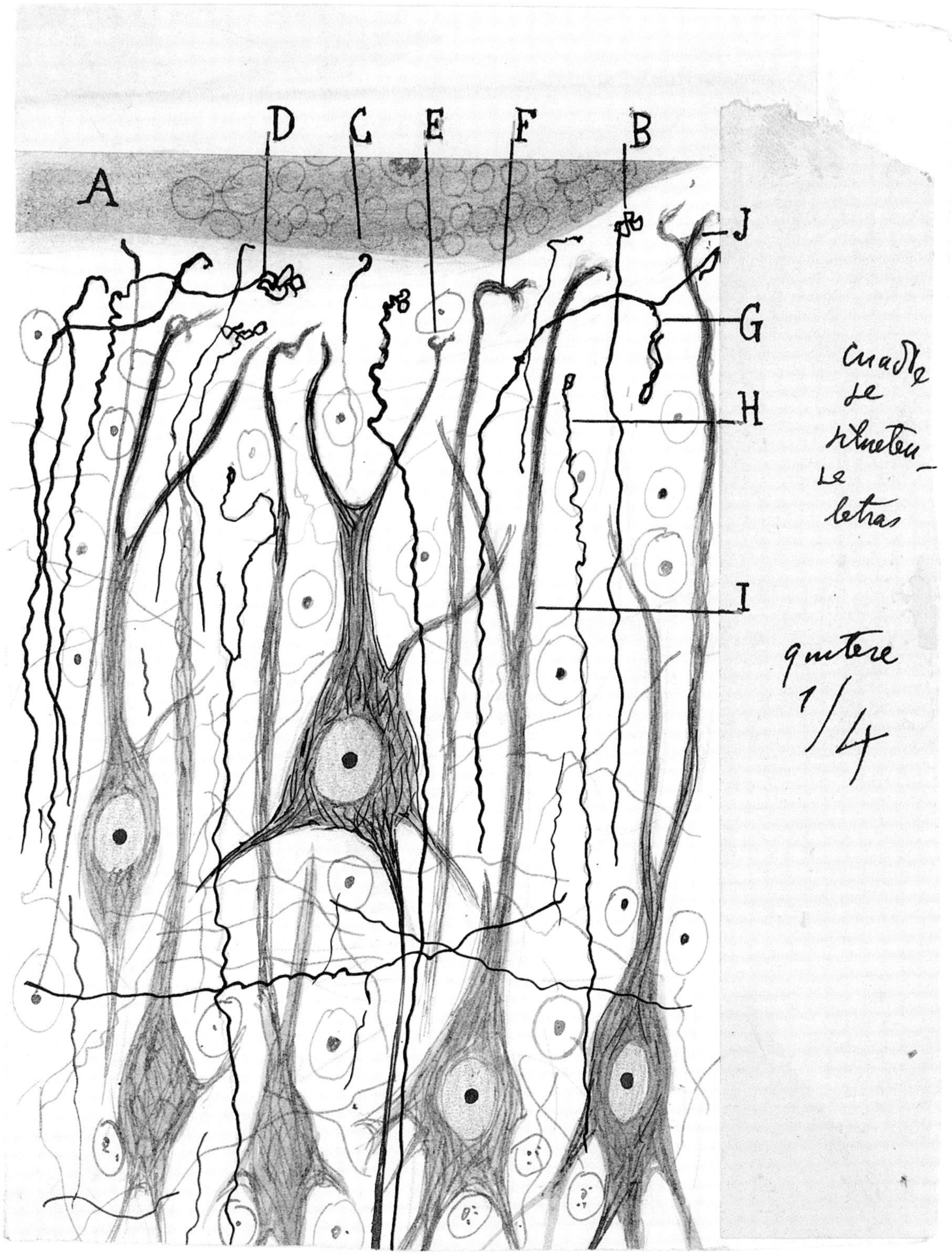

FIGURE 206. Pyramidal cells of the cerebral cortex in a cat in which a horizontal cut was made.

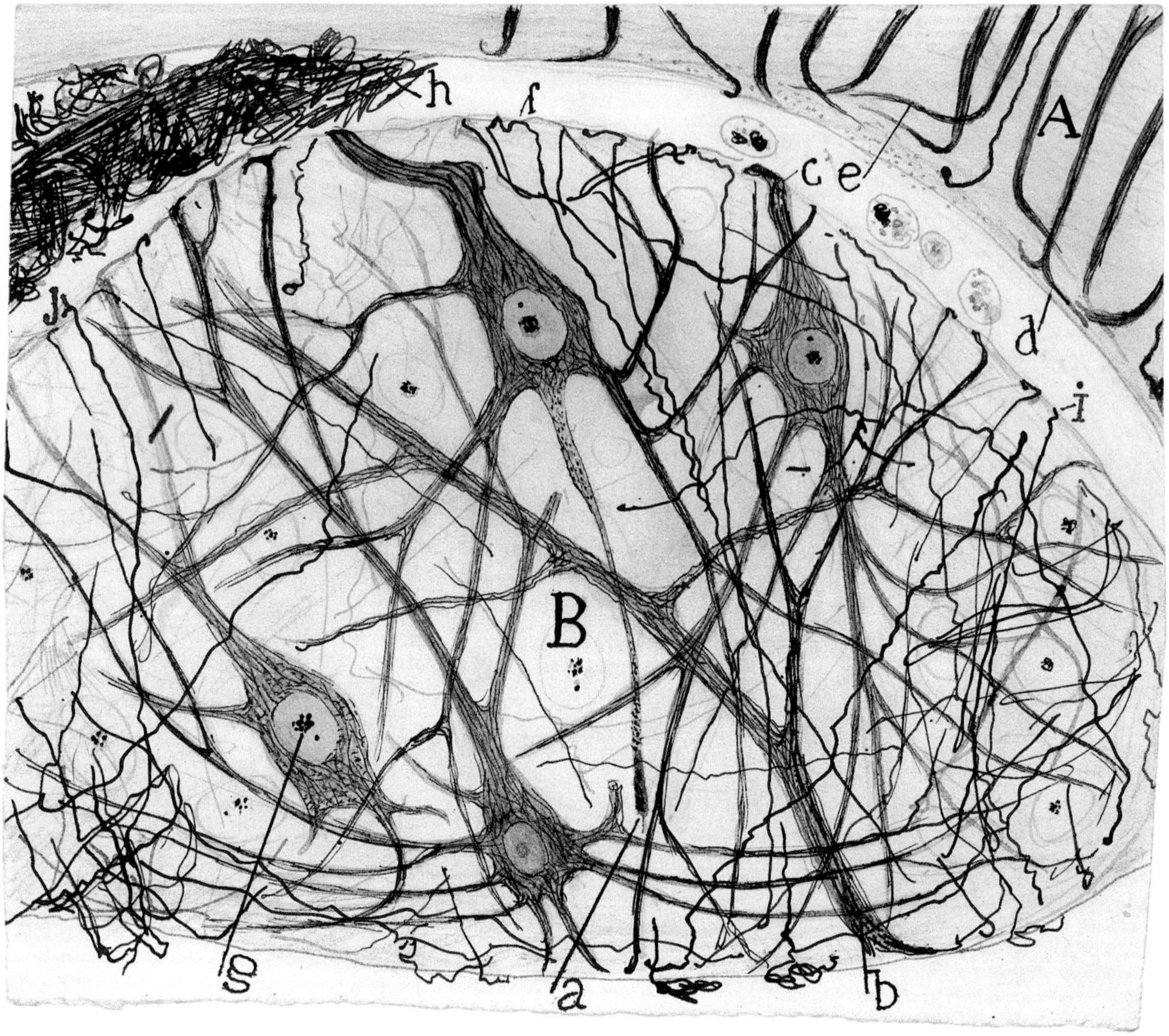

FIGURE 207. Cerebral sequestra in a cat.

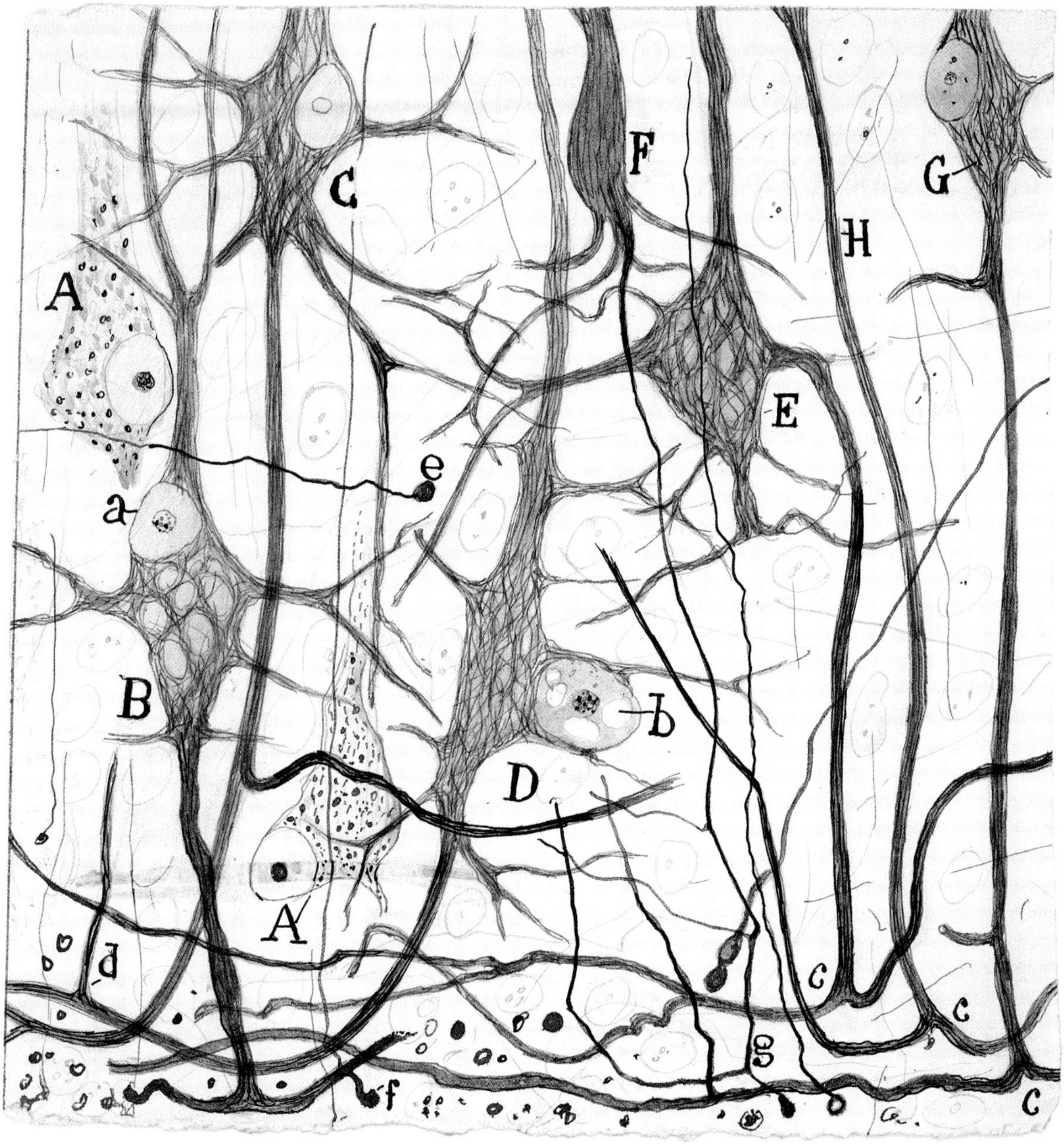

FIGURE 208. Section of the cerebral cortex in a dog two days old.

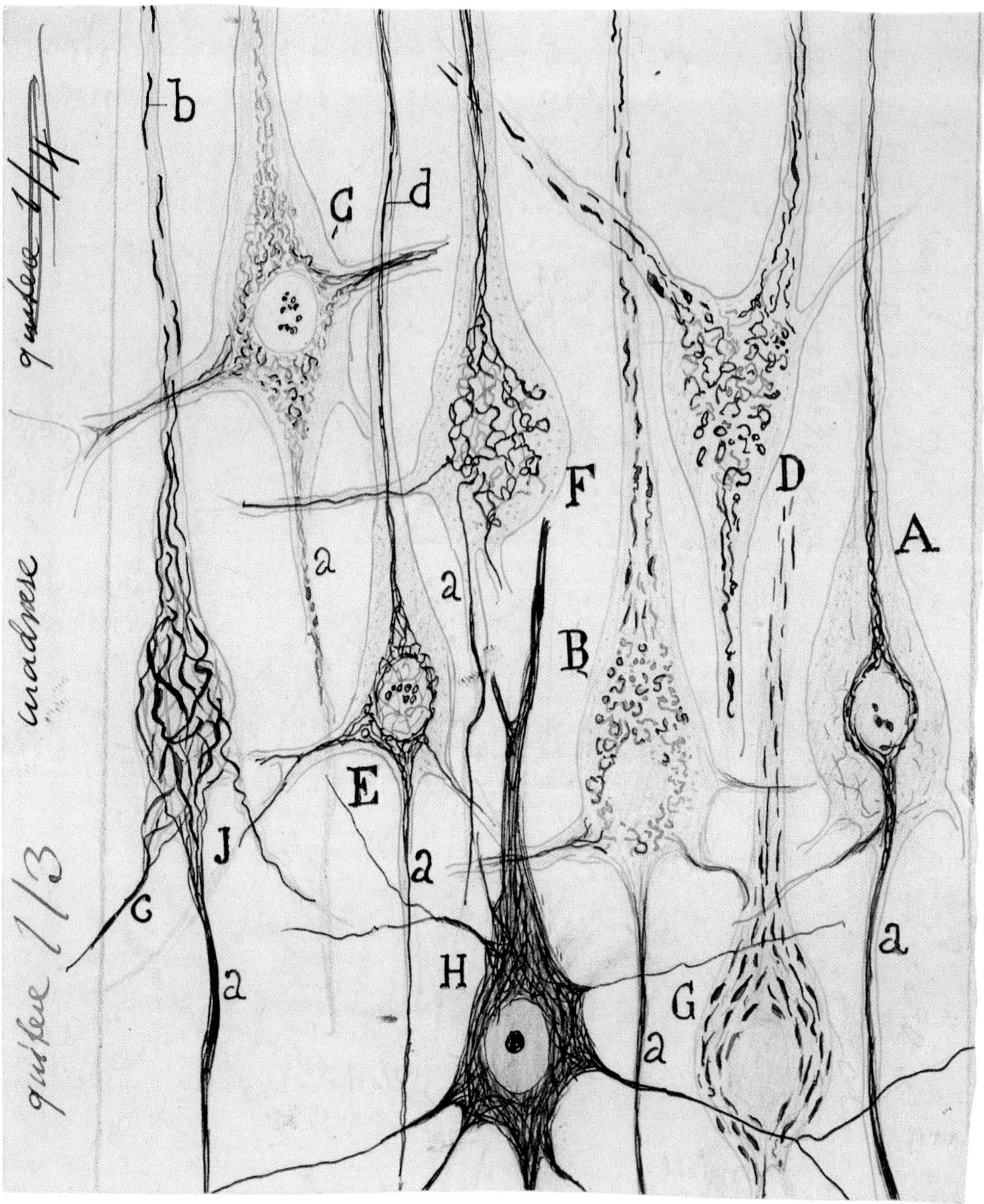

FIGURE 209. Edges of a contused cerebral wound in a cat.

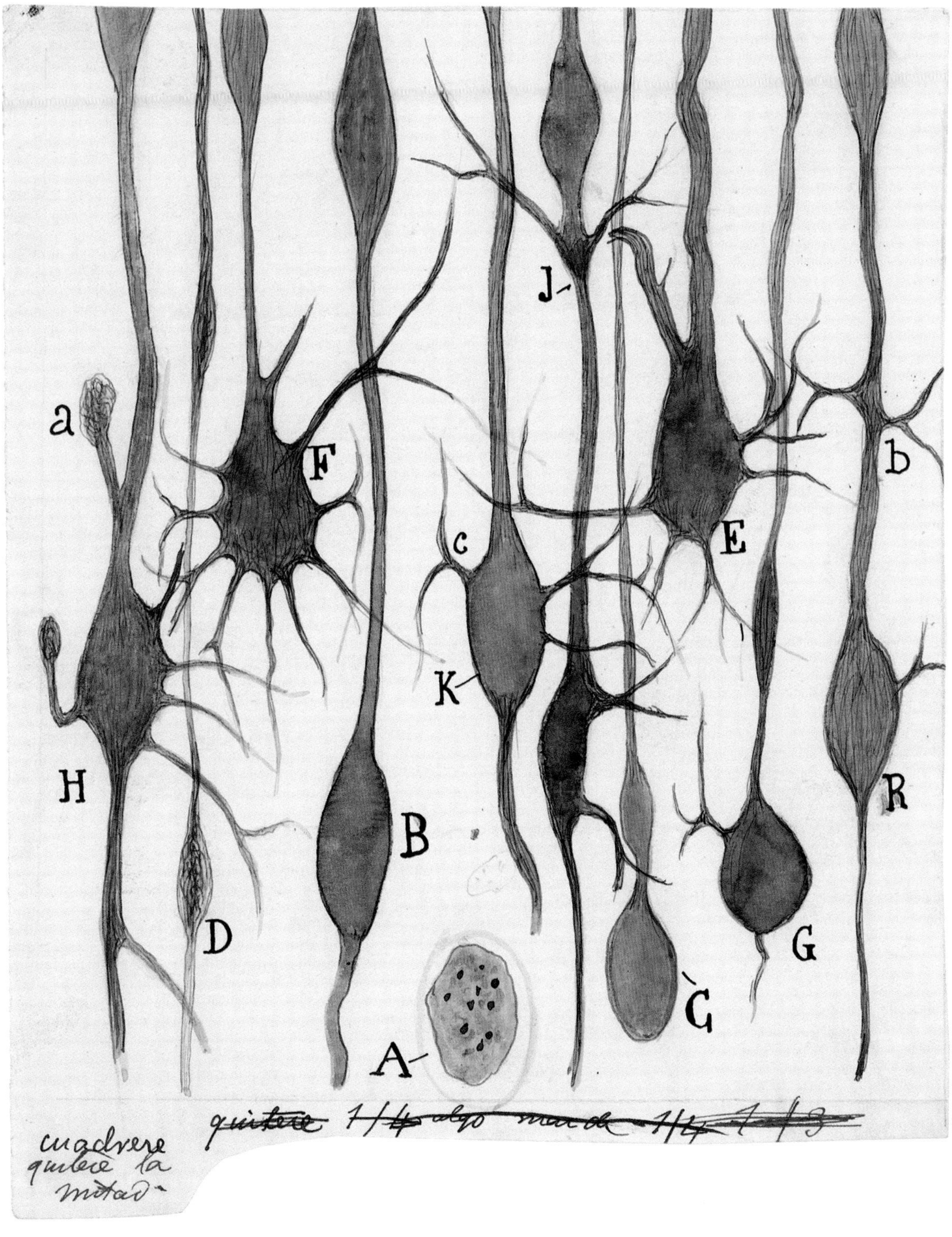

FIGURE 210. Various types of testudinoid structures as seen in a cerebral section in a dog.

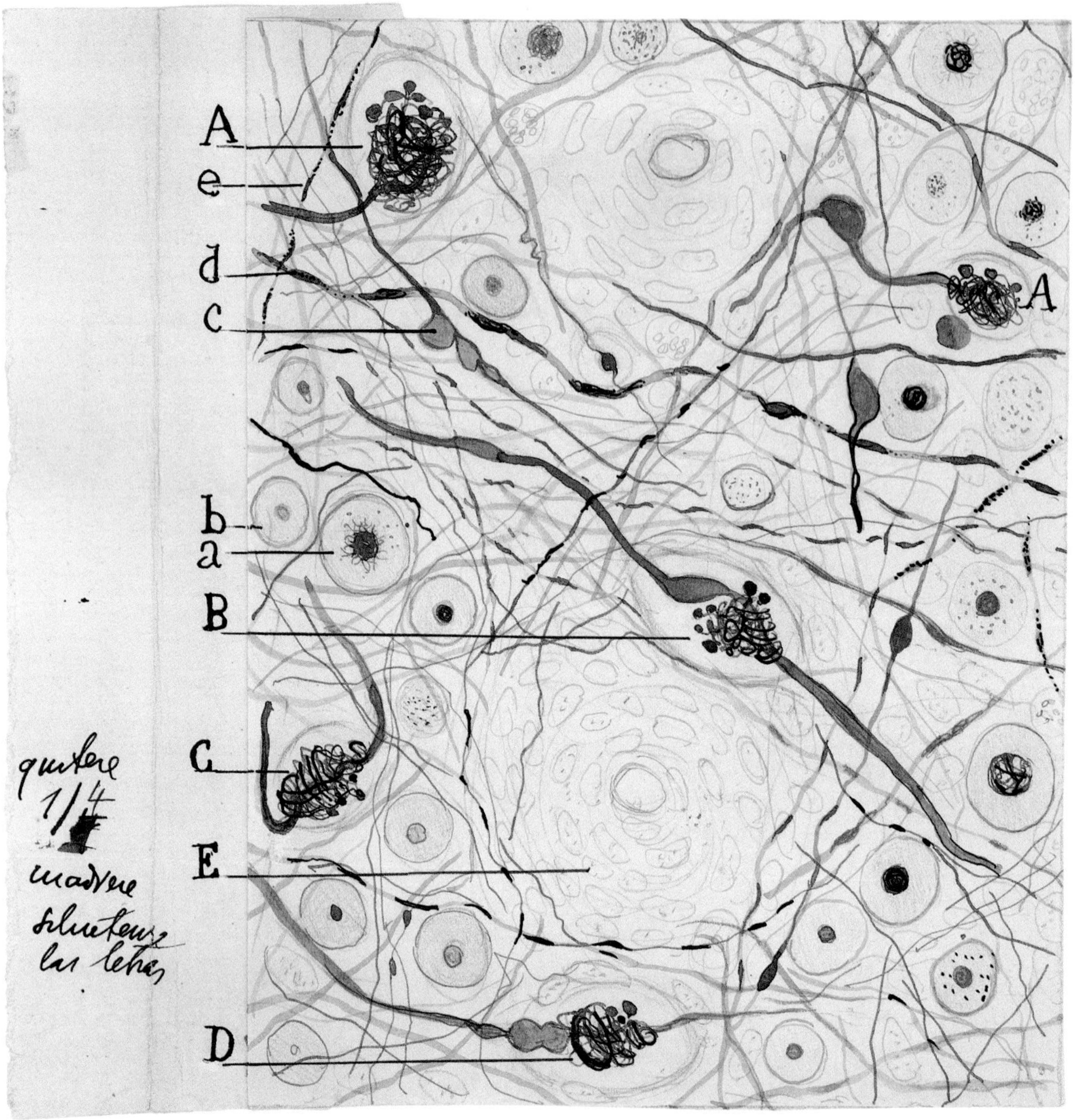

FIGURE 211. Central portion of a wound of the white matter in a dog.

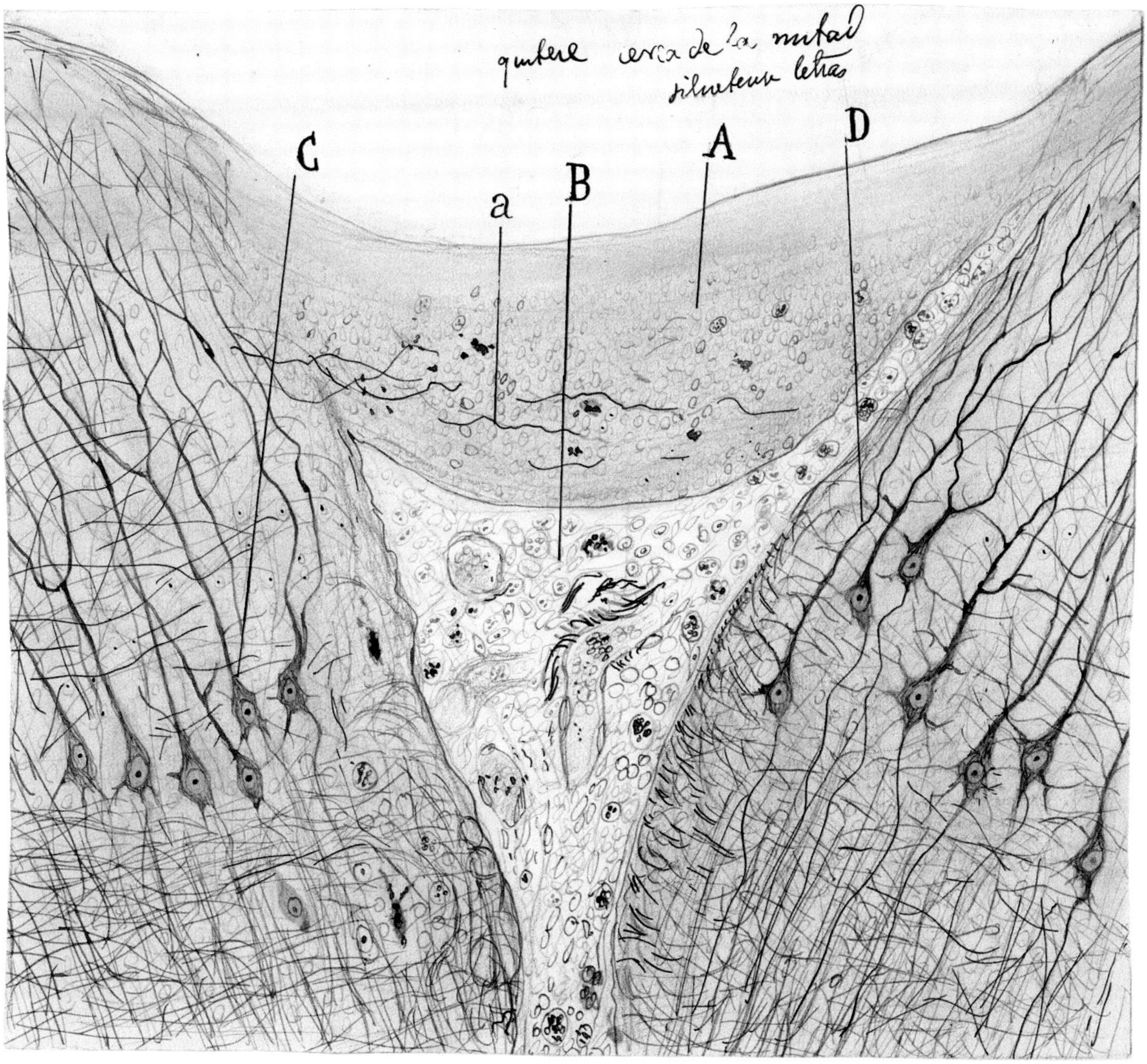

FIGURE 212. Transversal wound of the cerebrum in a young cat.

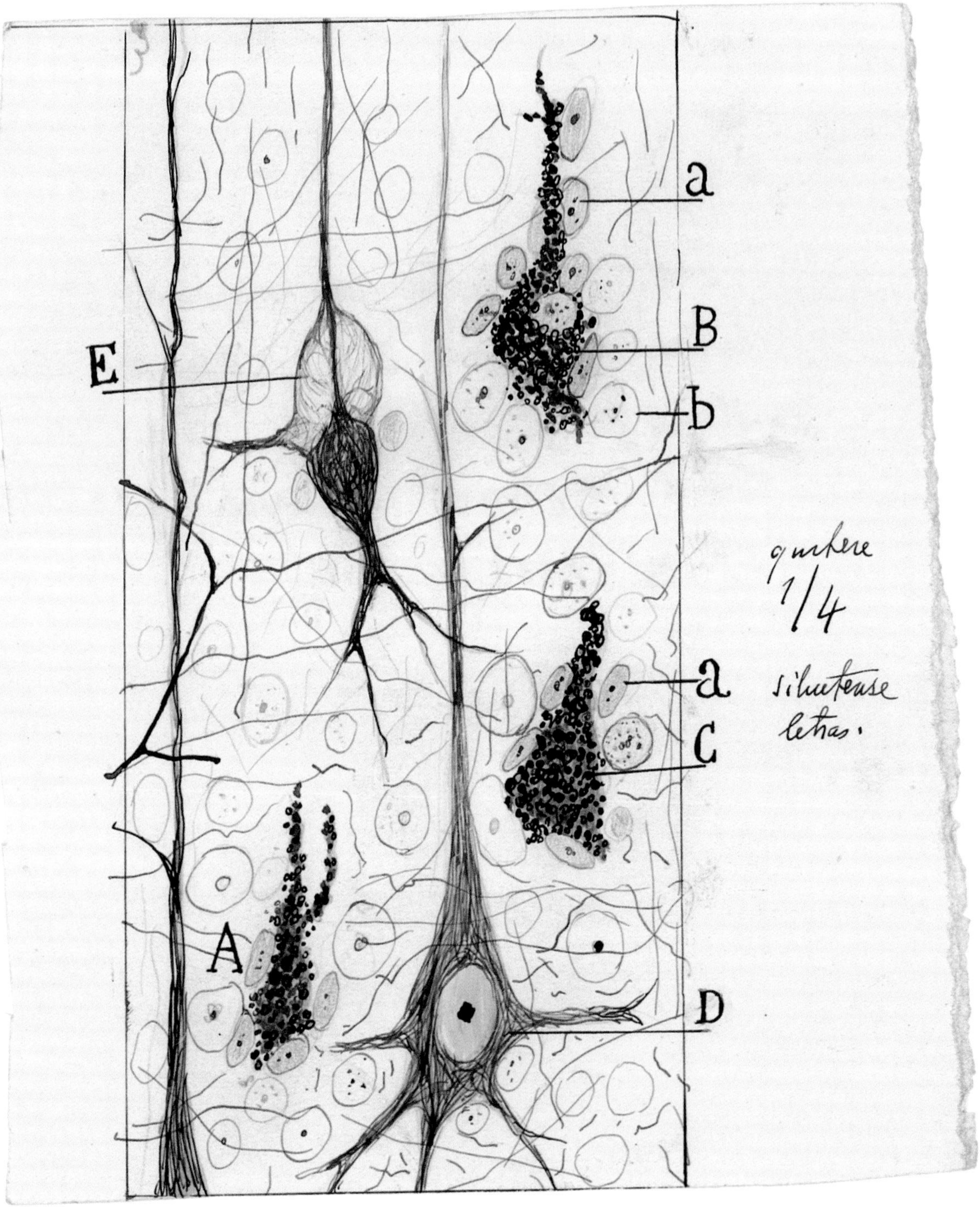

FIGURE 213. Necrosed pyramidal cells.

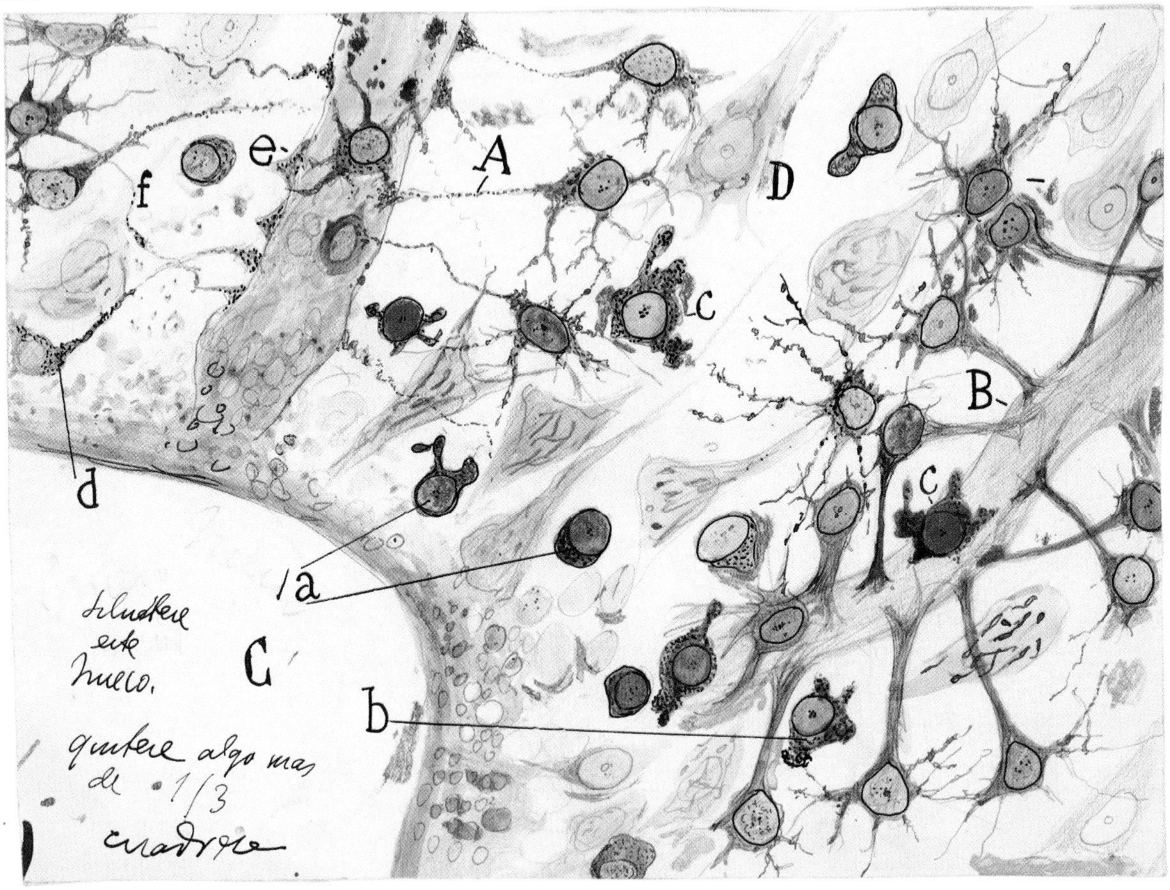

FIGURE 214. Edges of a cerebral transverse wound in a young cat.

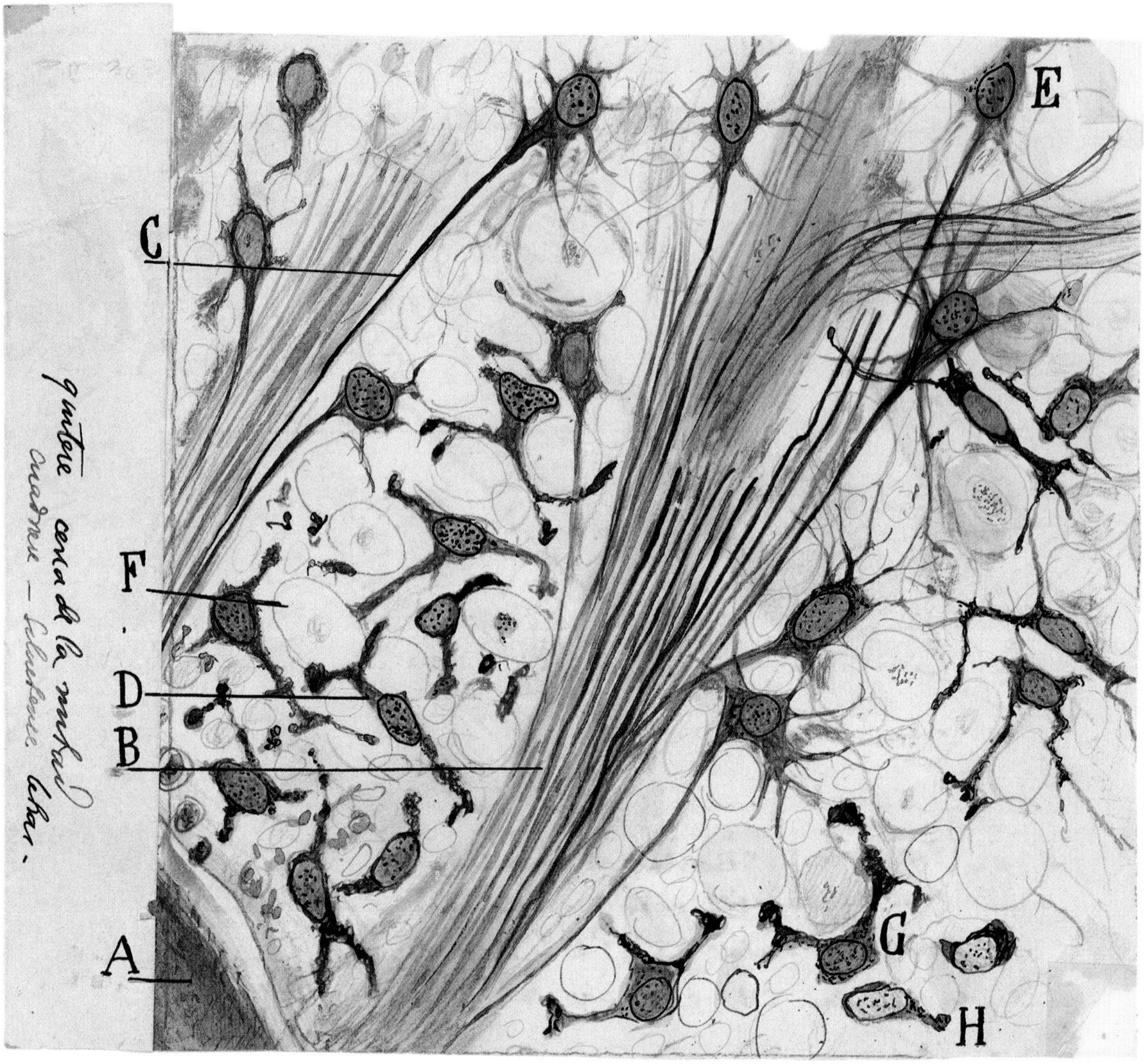

FIGURE 215. Edges of a transverse wound in a young cat.

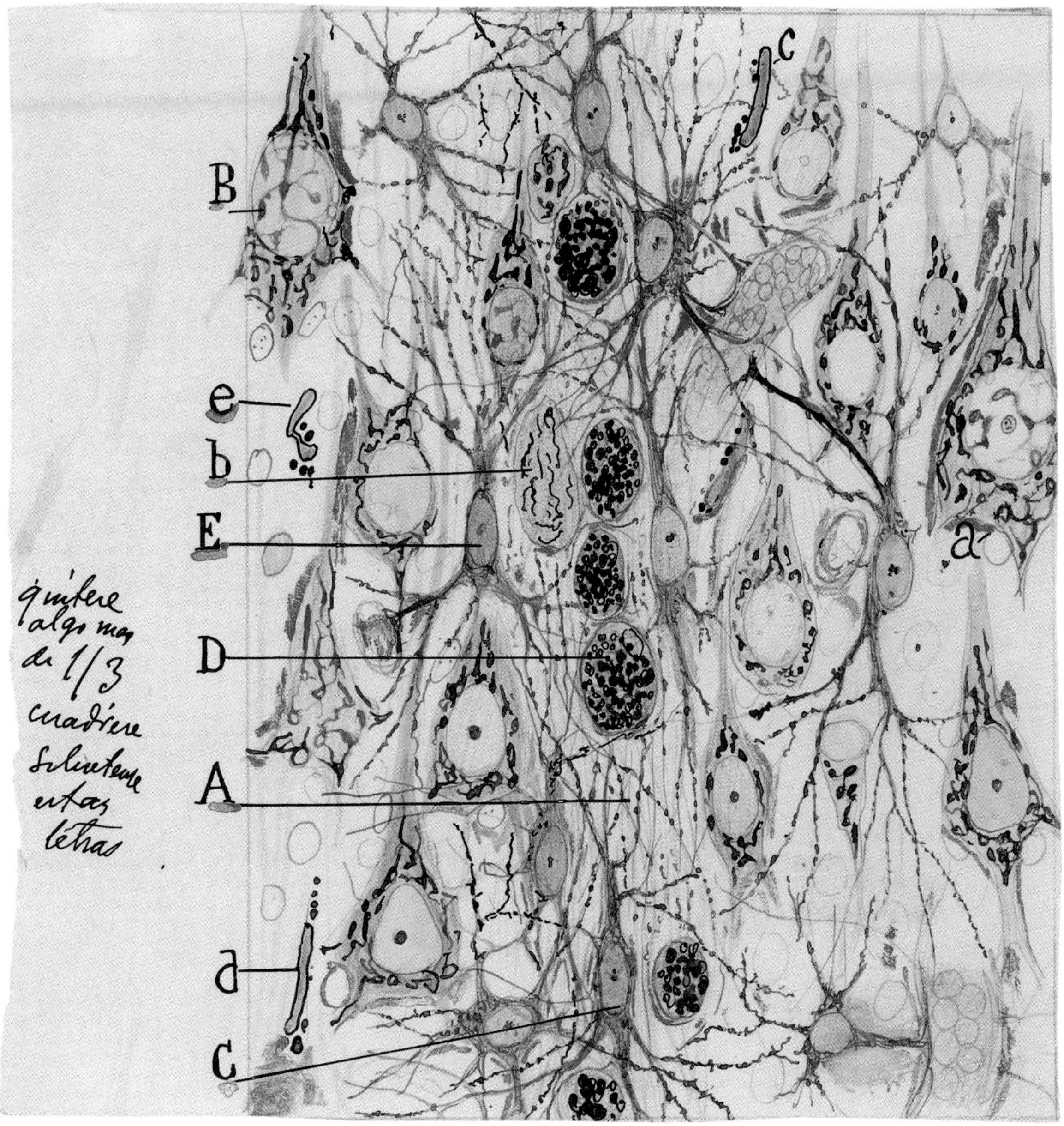

FIGURE 216. Linear scar of a radial wound in the cerebral cortex in a young cat.

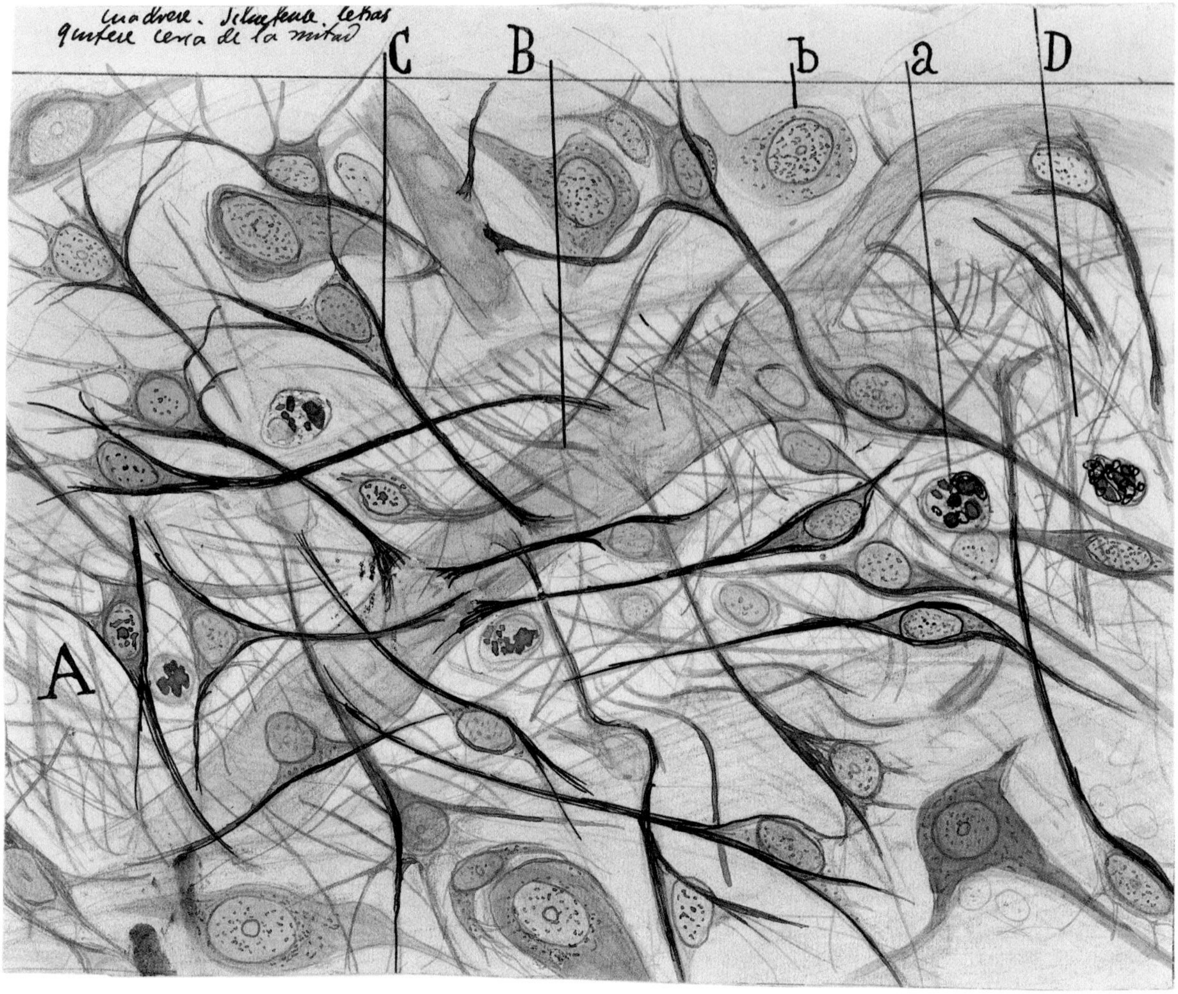

FIGURE 217. Linear and oblique scar of the cerebral cortex in a cat.

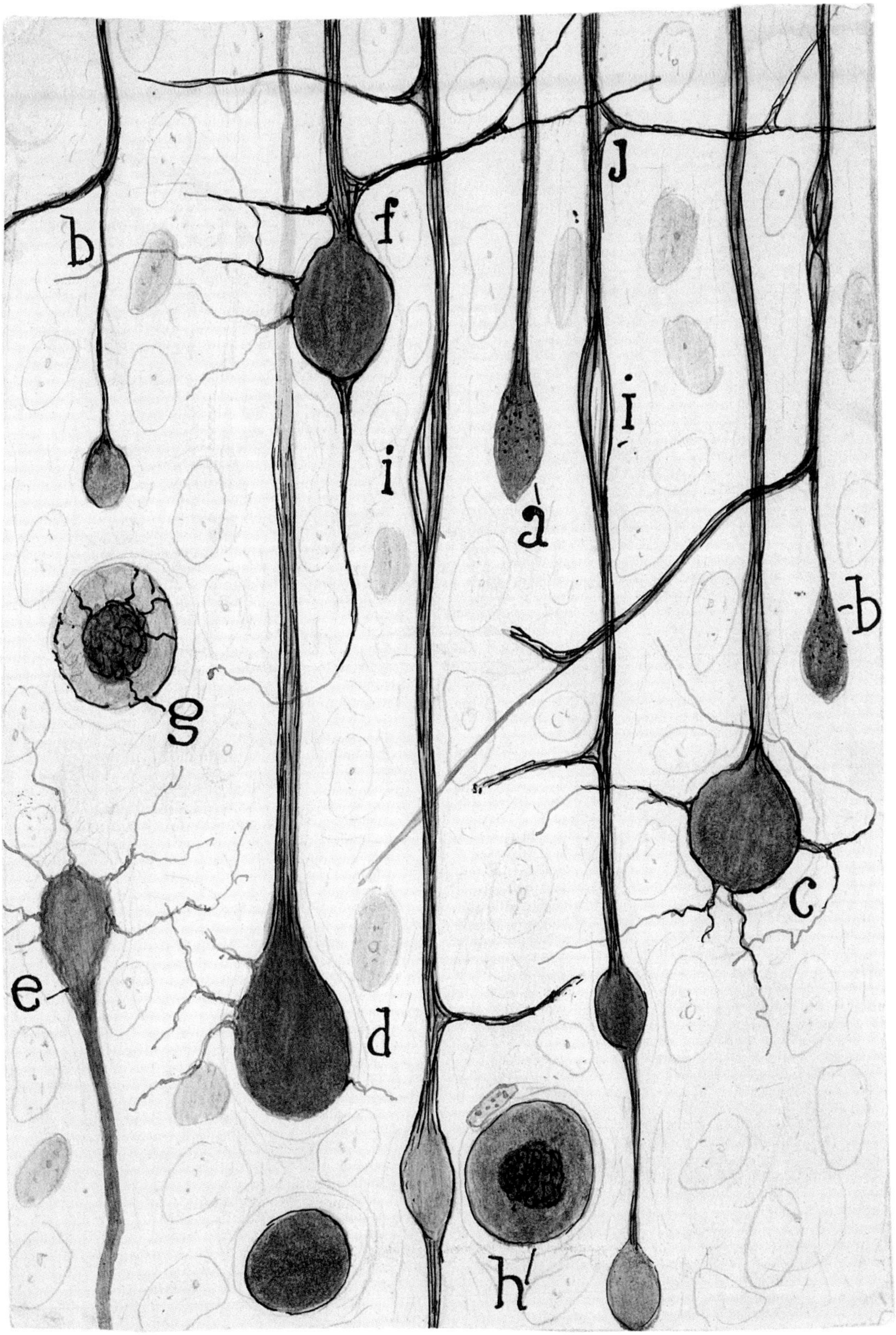

FIGURE 218. Degenerated region of the central stump of the axons of pyramidal cells.

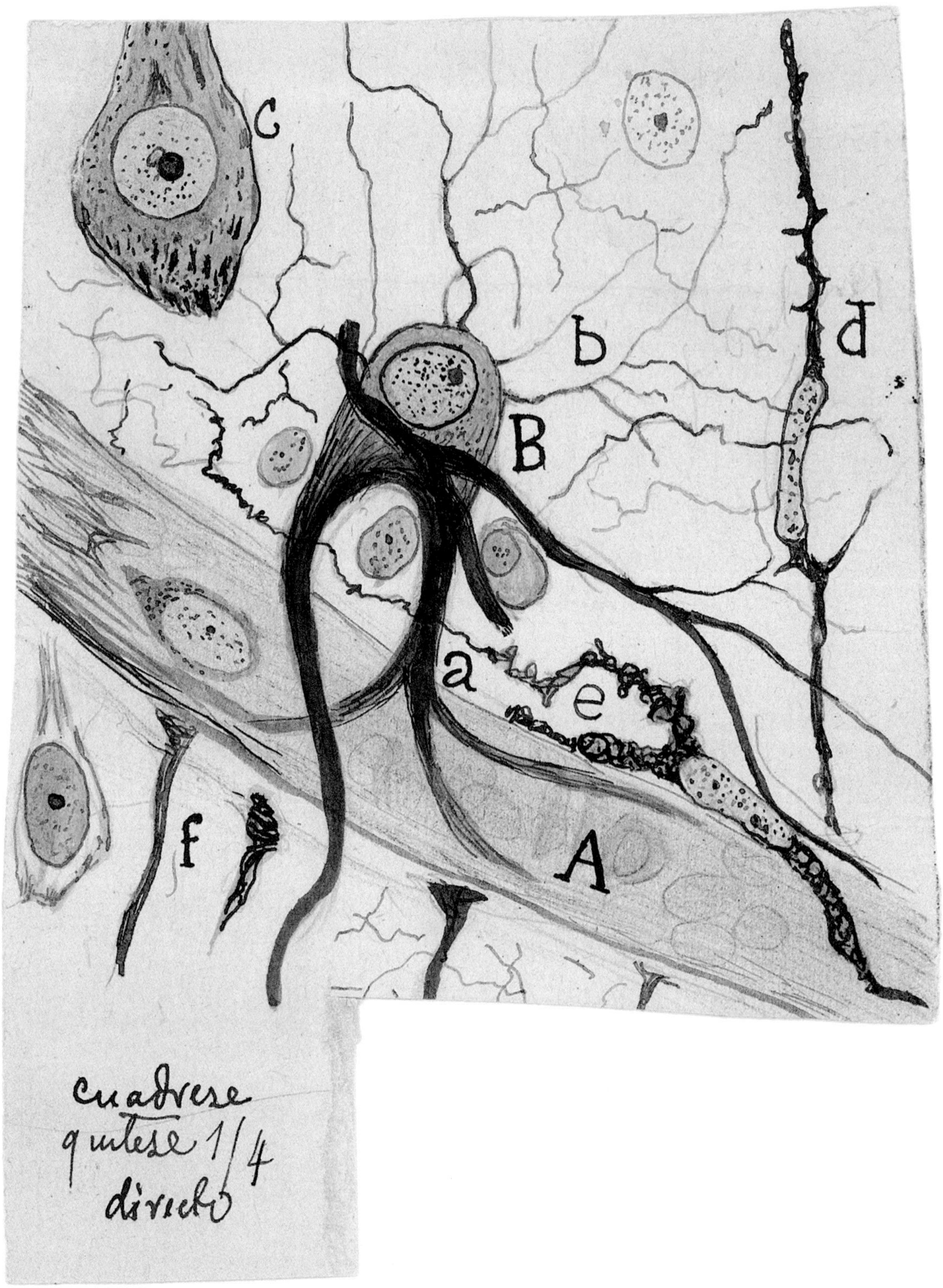

FIGURE 219. Giant neuroglial cell of the gray matter.

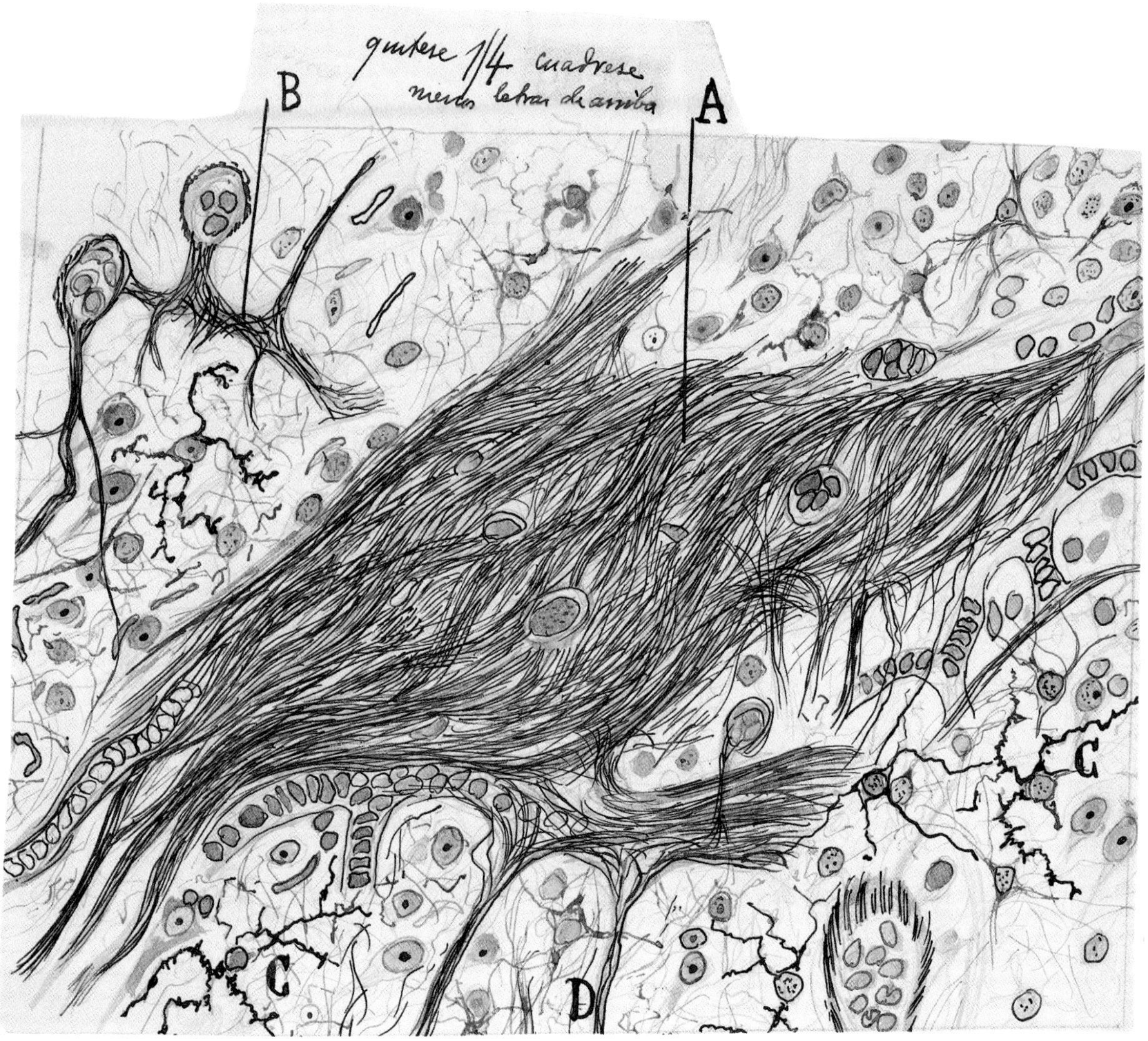

FIGURE 220. Large mass of Weigert fibers located in the gray matter.

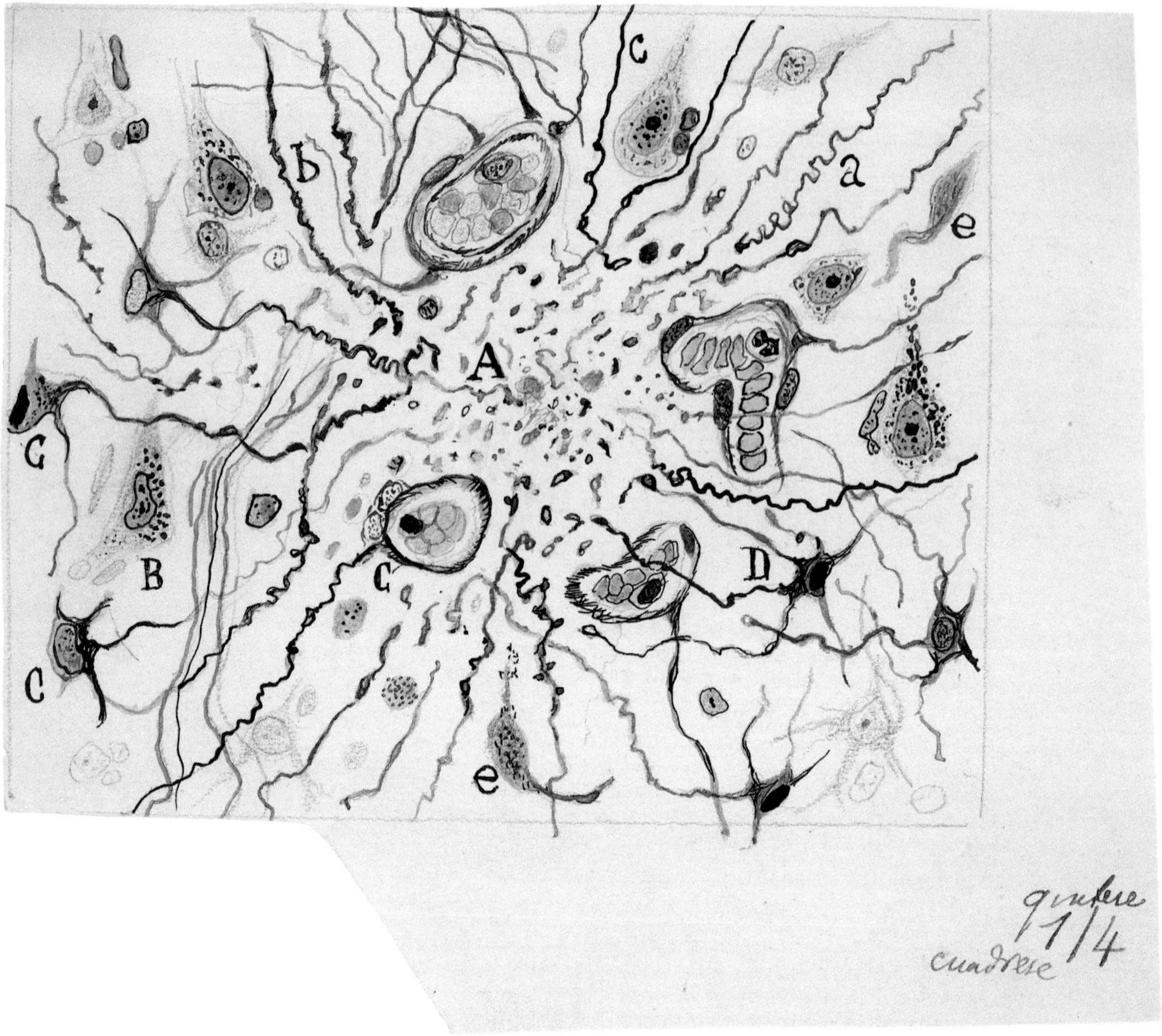

FIGURE 221. Perivascular end-feet uprooted around a focus of gray matter destruction

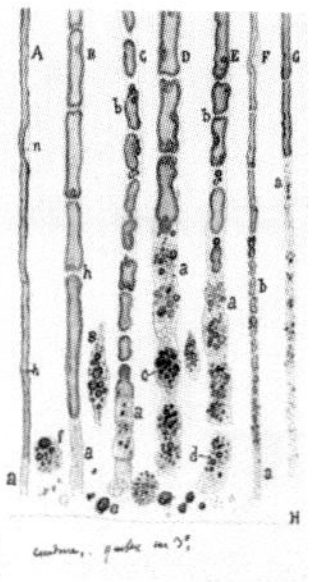

FIGURE 169.

Myelinated fibers of the central stump.

This figure was published in Cajal, S. R. (1920) Algunas observaciones contrarias a la hipótesis "syncytial" de la regeneración nerviosa y neurogénesis normal. *Trab. Lab. Invest. Biol. Univ. Madrid* 18, 275–302 (Figure 1). It has also been reproduced as Figure 46 in Cajal, S. R. (1913–1914) *Estudios sobre la degeneración y regeneración del sistema nervioso.* Madrid: Moya.

FIGURE LEGEND: Various conditions of the myelinated fibers of the central stump in a rabbit three days after section of the nerve (semischematic). Osmic acid. *H,* Level of the cut; *A, B,* fibers with a short necrotic segment (a); *D, E, F, G,* fibers with a long necrotic segment; *f, g,* free granular bodies; *c,* intratubal leukocytes with fatty droplets.

Original text: Diversos aspectos de las fibras meduladas del cabo central del conejo tres días después de la sección (semiesquema). Ácido ósmico. *H,* plano de la herida; *A, B,* fibras con segmento necrótico corto (a); *D, E, F, G,* tubos con segmento necrótico largo; *f, g,* corpúsculos granulosos libres; *c,* leucocitos intratubarios con gotas de grasa.

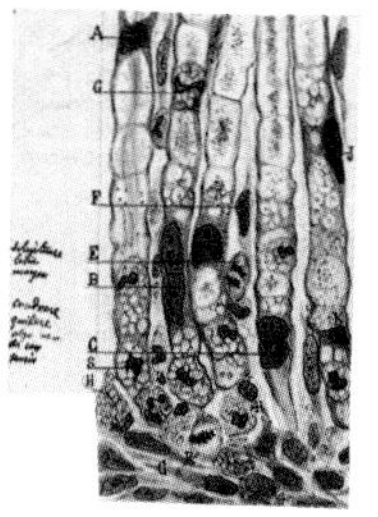

FIGURE 170.

Central stump of the sciatic nerve in a cat three days after the operation.

This figure was published in Cajal, S. R. (1913–1914) *Estudios sobre la degeneración y regeneración del sistema nervioso.* Madrid: Moya. (Figure 47).

FIGURE LEGEND: Central stump of the sciatic nerve in a cat three days after the section. *A, J,* Schwann cells in the degenerated portion; *B, C,* Schwann cells in the necrotic portion; *K,* Schwann cell that is contracted and probably necrotic because of its proximity to the wound; *G, S,* intratubal leukocytes; *H,* extratubal leukocytes that are full of fat; *E, R,* mitoses in connective tissue cells of the endoneurium; *F,* normal cell of the endoneurium.

Original text: Cabo central del nervio ciático del gato tres días después de la sección.- *A, J,* células de Schwann de la porción degenerada; *B, C,* células de Schwann de la porción necrótica; *K,* célula de igual clase encogida y probablemente necrótica por estar cerca de la herida; *G, S,* leucocitos intratubarios; *H,* leucocitos extratubarios llenos de grasa; *E, R,* mitosis en corpúsculos conectivos del endoneuro; *F,* célula normal de éste.

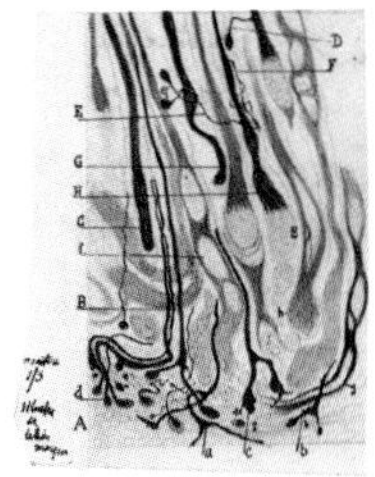

FIGURE 171.

Central stump of the sciatic nerve in a rabbit six hours after the operation.

This figure was published in Cajal, S. R. (1913–1914) *Estudios sobre la degeneración y regeneración del sistema nervioso.* Madrid: Moya. (Figure 48).

FIGURE LEGEND: Piece of the central stump of the sciatic nerve in a rabbit six hours after the operation. *A,* Wound and blood; *B,* nonmyelinated sprouting fibers; *f,* necrotic masses within axons; *g, h,* necrotic portion of large axons.

Original text: Trozo del cabo central del ciático del conejo seis horas después de la operación.- *A,* herida con hematíes; *B,* fibras de Remak en vías de retoñamiento; *f,* masas necróticas dentro de axones; *g, h,* porción necrótica de axones gruesos.

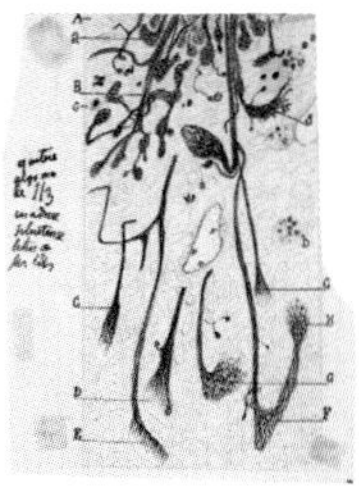

FIGURE 172.

Morphological varieties of clubs penetrating the scar.

This figure was published in Cajal, S. R. (1913–1914) *Estudios sobre la degeneración y regeneración del sistema nervioso.* Madrid: Moya. (Figure 71).

FIGURE LEGEND: Morphological varieties of clubs penetrating the scar. *A,* Border of the central stump; *B,* thick fiber terminating in a cluster of clubs; *C,* termination in the form of a brush; *D, E, H,* buds in which the neurofibrillar framework appears contracted and separated from the neuroplasm; *F,* folded clubs; *a,* kidney-shaped clubs; *d,* raveled club; *c,* segregated clubs; *e,* terminal rings.

Original text: Variedades morfológicas de las mazas penetrantes en la cicatriz.- *A,* frontera del cabo central; *B,* recia fibra terminada en un racimo de mazas; *C,* terminación en brocha ó pincel; *D, E, H,* botones en los cuales el esqueleto neurofibrillar aparece retraído y apartado del neuroplasma; *F,* mazas dobladas; *a,* mazas en forma de riñón; *d,* maza deshilachada; *c,* mazas segregadas; *e,* anillos terminales.

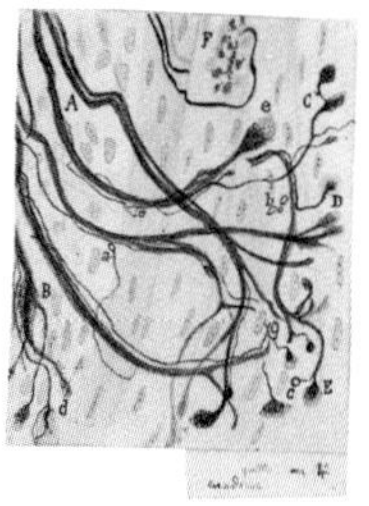

FIGURE 173.

Nerve fibers lost in a muscle near to the central stump.

This figure was published in Cajal, S. R. (1913–1914) *Estudios sobre la degeneración y regeneración del sistema nervioso.* Madrid: Moya. (Figure 79).

FIGURE LEGEND: Nerve fibers lost in a muscle near to the central stump. The animal was killed fifty hours after the operation.

Original text: Fibras nerviosas perdidas en un músculo próximo al cabo central. El animal fué sacrificado cincuenta horas después de la operación.

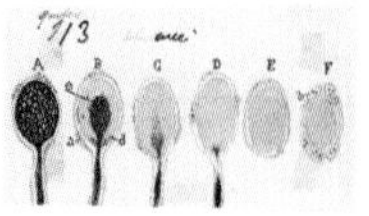

FIGURE 174.

Degenerative phases of gigantic arrested balls.

This figure was published in Cajal, S. R. (1913–1914) *Estudios sobre la degeneración y regeneración del sistema nervioso.* Madrid: Moya. (Figure 85).

FIGURE LEGEND: Degenerative phases of gigantic arrested balls. Note the progressive hyalinization. *a, b,* Nuclei of the capsule; *d,* hyaline zone of the ball; *e,* focus of persisting neurofibrils.

Original text: Fases degenerativas de las bolas colosales inmovilizadas. Nótese cómo la zona de hialinización va progresando. *a, b,* núcleos de la cápsula; *d,* zona hialina de la maza; *e,* foco de neurofibrillas persistentes.

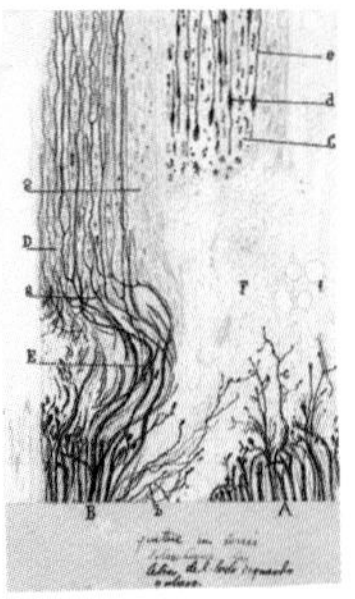

FIGURE 175.

Rapid innervation of the peripheral stump.

This figure was published in Cajal, S. R. (1913–1914) *Estudios sobre la degeneración y regeneración del sistema nervioso.* Madrid: Moya. (Figure 95).

FIGURE LEGEND: Rapid innervation of the peripheral stump. Section of the sciatic nerve in a twenty-day-old cat, killed five days after the operation. From the bundle on the right there was taken out a small piece of the peripheral stump, whereas the fascicle on the left remained relatively near the central stump. *A, B*, Central stumps; *D*, innervated peripheral stump; *C*, bundle of the resected peripheral stump; *F*, scar; *a*, bifurcations of the sprouts at the border of the peripheral stump; *b*, fibers of the central stump lost in the scar, having grown little because they did not receive trophic substances from the corresponding distal stump; *e, d*, agonal axons persisting in the peripheral stump; *c*, sprouts destined for the scar; *f*, adipose cells.

Original text: Inervación precoz del cabo periférico. Sección del ciático del gato de veinte días, sacrificado cinco después de la operación. En el haz de la derecha se resecó un pequeño trozo del cabo periférico, mientras que el fascículo de la izquierda permaneció relativamente cercano. *A* y *B*, cabos centrales; *D*, cabo periférico inervado; *C*, haz del cabo periférico resecado; F, cicatriz; *a*, dicotomas de los retoños en el híleo del cabo periférico; *b*, fibras del central perdidas en la cicatriz, y poco crecidas por no recibir substancias tróficas del cabo distal correspondiente; *e, d*, axones agónicos persistentes del cabo periféricos; *c*, retoños destinados á la cicatriz; *f*, células adiposas.

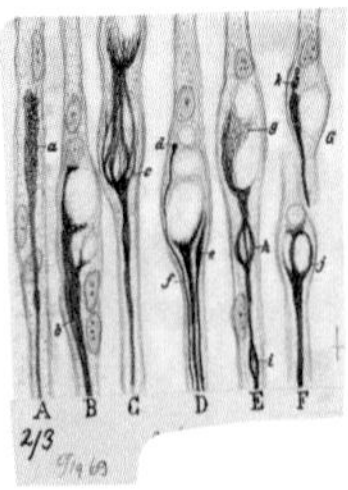

FIGURE 176.

Growth cone of the sprouts that penetrated the old myelinated fibers of the peripheral stump.

This figure was published in Cajal, S. R. (1913–1914) *Estudios sobre la degeneración y regeneración del sistema nervioso*. Madrid: Moya. (Figure 96).

FIGURE LEGEND: Details of the terminal or growth cone of the sprouts that have penetrated the old myelinated fibers of the peripheral stump during rapid nervous reunions. *a*, Cone in the shape of a boa (fur); *e, f*, lanceolate cones; *B*, fusiform ramified cones; *g, j*, cones in the shape of a chalice; *d*, terminal bud. Cat killed five days after the operation.

Original text: Detalles del cabo terminal ó cono de crecimiento de los retoños penetrados en los tubos viejos del cabo periférico durante las neurotizaciones rápidas. *a*, cono en forma de boa; *e, f*, conos lanceolados; *B*, conos fusiformes ramificados; *g, j*, conos en forma de cáliz; *d*, botón terminal. Gato sacrificado cinco días después de la operación.

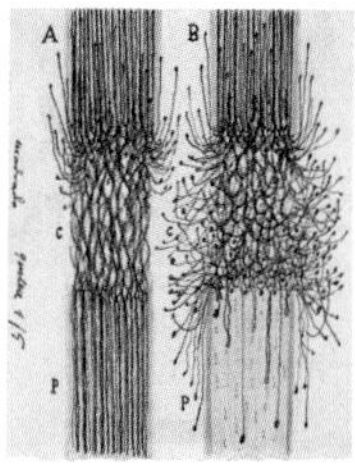

FIGURE 177.

Path of the sprouts and mechanical factors.

This figure was published in Cajal, S. R. (1913–1914) *Estudios sobre la degeneración y regeneración del sistema nervioso*. Madrid: Moya. (Figure 99).

FIGURE LEGEND: Figure to show what the path of the sprouts would be if only mechanical factors were involved. *B*, Central stump; *P*, peripheral stump. On the left (*A*) we show schematically the actual disposition.

Original text: Figura destinada á mostrar lo que sería la marcha de los retoños caso de que no actuaran sino factores mecánicos. *B*, cabo central; *P*, cabo periférico. A la izquierda (*A*) mostramos esquemáticamente la disposición real.

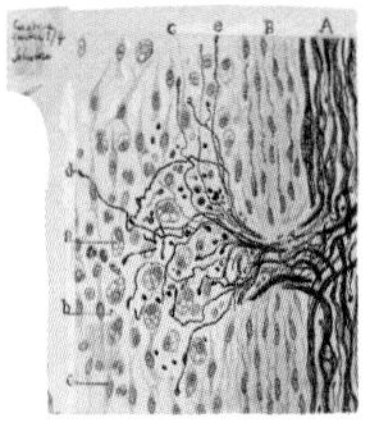

FIGURE 178.

Peripheral portion of a nerve that had been pinched with a pair of forceps.

This figure was published in Cajal, S. R. (1920) Algunas observaciones contrarias a la hipótesis "syncytial" de la regeneración nerviosa y neurogénesis normal. *Trab. Lab. Invest. Biol. Univ. Madrid* 18, 275–302 (Figure 1). It has also been reproduced as Figure 101A in DeFelipe, J., and Jones, E. G. (1991) *Cajal's degeneration and regeneration of the nervous system*. New York: Oxford University Press.

FIGURE LEGEND: Peripheral portion of a nerve that had been pinched with a pair of forceps. Young cat, killed two days after the operation. *A*, Tangential axons of the nerve in a productive phase; *B*, neurolemma; *C*, perinervous exudate through which grow many axonic sprouts; *a*, granular cell; *b*, neurite cut tangentially; *c*, fibroblast.

Original text: Porción periférica de un nervio apretado entre las pinzas. Gato joven sacrificado dos días después de la operación. *A*, axones tangenciales del nervio en fase productiva; *B*, neurilema; *C*, exudado perinervioso por el cual circulan numerosos retoños axónicos; *a*, célula granulosa; *b*, neurita vista de punta; *c*, fibroblasto.

Note from the author (J. D.): This figure is not included in Cajal, S. R. (1913–1914) *Estudios sobre la degeneración y regeneración del sistema nervioso*. Madrid: Moya.

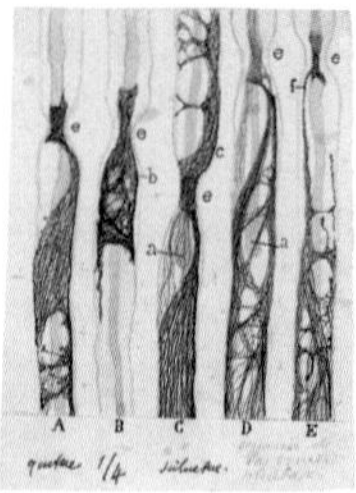

FIGURE 179.

Central stump far from the ligature.

This figure was published in Cajal, S. R. (1913–1914) *Estudios sobre la degeneración y regeneración del sistema nervioso*. Madrid: Moya. (Figure 114).

FIGURE LEGEND: Region of the central stump far from the ligature and in a state of divisive excitation. Adult rabbit killed two days after the lesion. Formation of germinative muffs near the nodes. *c*, Node; *b*, neoformation in the form of a membranous net; *a*, club of a preexisting axon.

Original text: Región del cabo central alejada de la ligadura y en vías de excitación divisoria. Conejo aduto sacrificado dos días después de la lesión. Formación de manguitos germinales cerca de las estrangulaciones. *c*, estrangulación; *b*, neoformación en forma de red submembranosa; *a*, maza de axon preexistente.

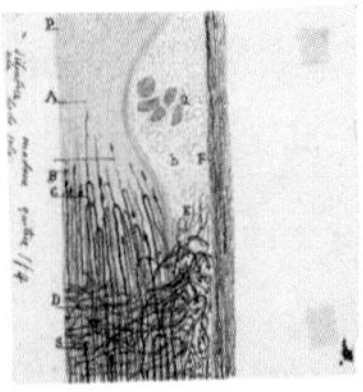

FIGURE 180.

Sciatic nerve in a young rabbit.

This figure was published in Cajal, S. R. (1913–1914) *Estudios sobre la degeneración y regeneración del sistema nervioso*. Madrid: Moya. (Figure 115).

FIGURE LEGEND: Sciatic nerve in a young rabbit. Partial ligature. The animal was killed thirteen days after the operation. *a*, Threads of the ligature; *A*, compressed region of the nerve; *D, E*, migrating fibers; *C*, retrograde fibers; *B*, arrested fibers; *P*, peripheral stump; *F*, nerve bundle that was not included in the ligature.

Original text: Nervio ciático de conejo joven. Ligadura parcial. El animal fue sacrificado trece días después de la operación. *a*, hilos de la ligadura; *A*, región apretada del nervio; *D, E*, fibras emigrantes; *C*, fibras retrógradas; *B*, fibras atascadas; *P*, cabo periférico; *F*, haz nervioso no comprendido en la ligadura.

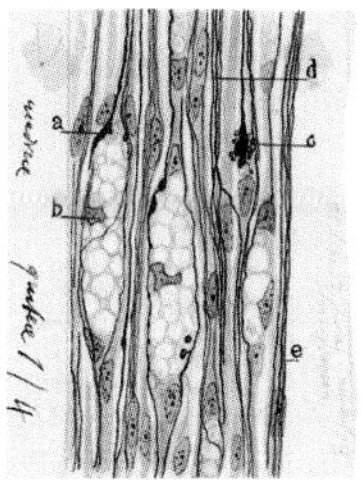

FIGURE 181.

Details of the cortical region of a graft.

This figure was published in Cajal, S. R. (1913) El neurotropismo y la transplantación de los nervios. *Trab. Lab. Invest. Biol. Univ. Madrid* 11, 81–102 (Figure 9). It has also been reproduced as Figure 141 in Cajal, S. R. (1913–1914). *Estudios sobre la degeneración y regeneración del sistema nervioso*. Madrid: Moya.

FIGURE LEGEND: Details of the cortical region of the same graft as in Figure 8. *a*, Intratubal cones of growth; *b*, nucleus of a phagocyte; *c*, free club with appendages ending in rings and excrescences; *e*, intratubal bundle; *d*, interstitial fibers. *Original text*: Detalles de la región cortical del mismo ingerto que en la figura 8. *a*, conos de crecimiento intratubarios; *b*, núcleo de fagocito; *c*, maza libre con apéndices acabados en anillo y excrecencias; *e*, haz intratubario; *d*, fibras intersticiales.

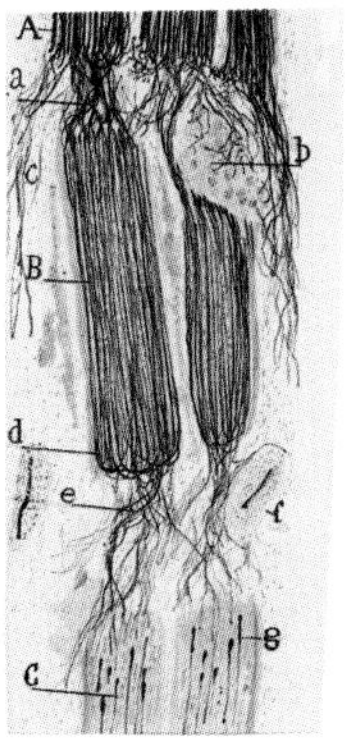

FIGURE 182.

Graft of spinal roots on a wound of the sciatic.

This figure was published in Cajal, S. R. (1913) El neurotropismo y la transplantación de los nervios. *Trab. Lab. Invest. Biol. Univ. Madrid* 11, 81–102 (Figure 12). It has also been reproduced as Figure 144 in Cajal, S. R. (1913–1914). *Estudios sobre la degeneración y regeneración del sistema nervioso*. Madrid: Moya.

FIGURE LEGEND: Graft of spinal roots on a wound of the sciatic. Young cat, killed fourteen days after the operation. *A*, Central stump, *B*, living roots; *C*, peripheral stump; *a*, bundles penetrating into the graft; *b*, remnants of a small ganglion, which is largely destroyed; *c*, nerve current that accompanies the graft at a distance; *d*, retrograde sprouts in the distal end of the graft; *e*, current that reaches the peripheral stump after passing through the graft; *f*, connective tissue surrounding a hair that is refractory to invasion by the sprouts. Semischematic figure.

Original text: Ingerto de raíces medulares sobre la herida del ciático. Gato joven sacrificado catorce días después de la operación. *A*, cabo central; *B*, raíces vivaces; *C*, cabo periférico; *a*, haces penetrantes en el ingerto; *b*, restos de un pequeño ganglio en gran parte destruido; *c*, corriente nerviosa que escolta á distancia el ingerto; *d*, retoños retrógrados en el cabo distal de éste; *e*, corriente que después de cruzar el ingerto aborda el cabo periférico; *f*, tejido conectivo envolvente de un pelo y refractario á la invasión de retoños. Figura semiesquemática.

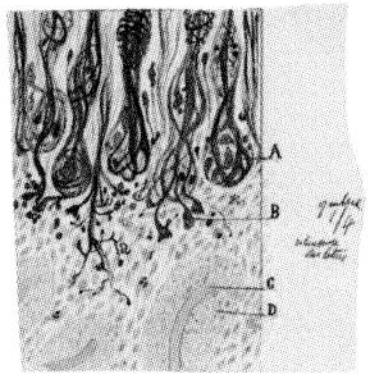

FIGURE 183.

Piece of the central stump and scar in a near-adult rabbit.

This figure was published in Cajal, S. R. (1913–1914) *Estudios sobre la degeneración y regeneración del sistema nervioso*. Madrid: Moya. (Figure 145).

FIGURE LEGEND: Piece of the central stump and scar in a near-adult rabbit in whose nerve wound had placed a piece of cotton saturated with concentrated methylene blue and then dried. The animal was killed ten days after the operation. Note the sparse growth of the sprouts and the swelling and enormous hypertrophy of the intratubal fibers. *A*, closed digestive chamber; *B*, emergent axons with large clubs; *D*, connective tissue closely pressed next to a cotton filament.

Original text: Trozo de cabo central y cicatriz del ciático de un conejo casi adulto, en cuya herida nerviosa se colocó un pedazo de algodón empapado en azul de metileno (algodón embebido en solución saturada y desecado después). El animal se sacrificó á los diez días de la operación. Nótese el escaso crecimiento de los retoños y la hinchazón é hipertrofia enorme de las fibras intratubarias. *A*, cámara digestiva cerrada; *B*, retoños emergentes con mazas gruesas; *D*, trama conectiva apretada en torno de un filamento de algodón.

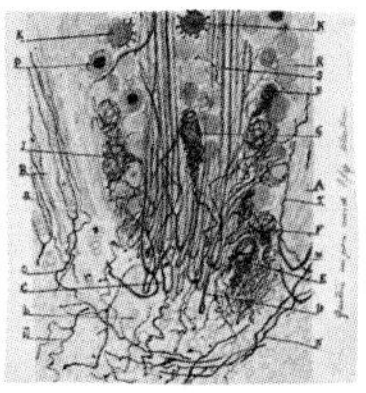

FIGURE 184.

Axial section of a sensory ganglion of the sacral region.

This figure was published in Cajal, S. R. (1910) Algunas observaciones favorables a la hipótesis neurotrópica. *Trab. Lab. Invest. Biol. Univ. Madrid* 8, 63–135 (Figure 5). It has also been reproduced as Figure 156 in Cajal, S. R. (1913–1914). *Estudios sobre la degeneración y regeneración del sistema nervioso*. Madrid: Moya.

FIGURE LEGEND: Axial section of a sensory ganglion of the sacral region, cut transversely. Young cat, killed six days after the operation. *A*, Connective tissue capsule of the ganglion; *B*, neighboring sensory root that was cut and is in full degeneration; *C, D*, curves described by pericellular nests on reaching the scar (frayed and growing axons); *E, F, G, J*, pericellular nests; *H*, periglomerular nest; *K*, frayed cells; *R*, angular cells; *P*, hirudiform cells; *M*, fibers coming from another neighboring root; *S*, axons with raveled collaterals; *N, Ñ*, sensory fibers ramified in the scar.

Original text: Corte axial de un ganglio sensitivo de la región sacra, cortado transversalmente (gato joven sacrificado seis días después de la operación). *A*, cápsula conjuntiva del ganglio; *B*, raíz sensitiva vecina seccionada y en plena degeneración; *C, D*, arcos trazados al llegar á la cicatriz, por manojos de hebras (axones deshilachados y en vías de crecimiento); *E, F, G, J*, nidos pericelulares; *H*, nido periglomerular; *K*, células desgarradas; *R*, células esquinadas; *P*, células hirudiformes; *M*, fibras llegadas de otra raíz vecina; *S*, axones en fase deshilachada; *N, Ñ*, fibras sensitivas ramificadas en la cicatriz.

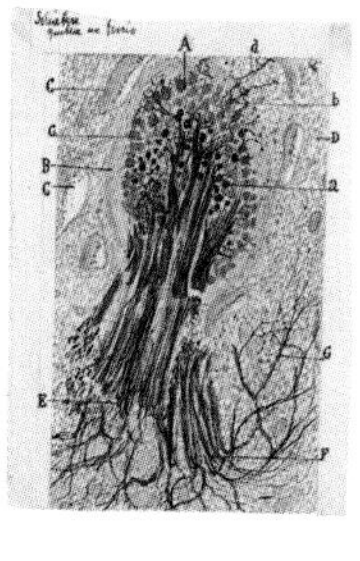

FIGURE 185.

Small ganglion of the cauda equina in a cat a few days old.

This figure was published in Cajal, S. R. (1913–1914) *Estudios sobre la degeneración y regeneración del sistema nervioso*. Madrid: Moya. (Figure 160).

FIGURE LEGEND: Small ganglion of the cauda equina in a cat a few days old that was grafted into an animal of the same age. This second animal was killed nine days after the operation. *A*, Ganglion; *B*, its fibrous capsule; *C*, periganglionic sanguineous cavities; *D*, embryonic connective tissue of the host; *E, F*, section of the peripheral branch of the ganglion, where numerous sprouts are seen innervating the newly formed connective tissue.

Original text: Pequeño ganglio de la cola del caballo del gato de pocos días, ingertado en un animal de la misma edad, que fue sacrificado nueve días después de la operación. *A*, ganglio; *B*, cápsula fibrosa de éste; *C*, senos sanguíneos periganglióncos; *D*, tejido conectivo embrionario del huésped; *E, F*, sección de la rama periférica del ganglio donde aparecen numerosos retoños inervadores de la trama conectiva neoformada.

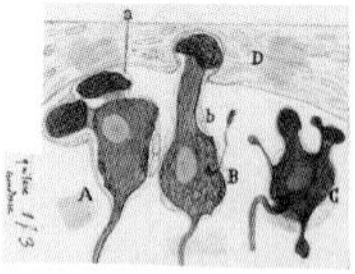

FIGURE 186.

Small ganglion of the cauda equina in a cat a few days old, I.

This figure was published in Cajal, S. R. (1913–1914) *Estudios sobre la degeneración y regeneración del sistema nervioso*. Madrid: Moya. (Figure 165).

FIGURE LEGEND: Various types of lobulated neurons. *D*, Capsule of the ganglion. Three-day-old graft in a young cat.

Original text: Diversos tipos de neuronas lobuladas. D, cápsula del ganglio. Ingerto del tercer día en el gato joven.

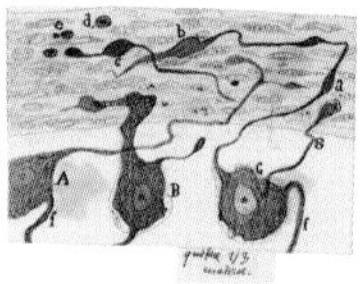

FIGURE 187.

Small ganglion of the cauda equina in a cat a few days old, II.

This figure was published in Cajal, S. R. (1913–1914) *Estudios sobre la degeneración y regeneración del sistema nervioso*. Madrid: Moya. (Figure 166).

FIGURE LEGEND: Cells with long appendages that penetrate the capsule of the ganglion, where they show varicosities as a result of arrests, and free spheres produced through autotomy. Nine-day-old graft in a young cat.

Original text: Células cuyos appendices largos penetran en la cápsula del ganglio, donde ofrecen varicosidades de detención y esferas sueltas (por autotomía). (Ingerto del noveno día en el gato joven).

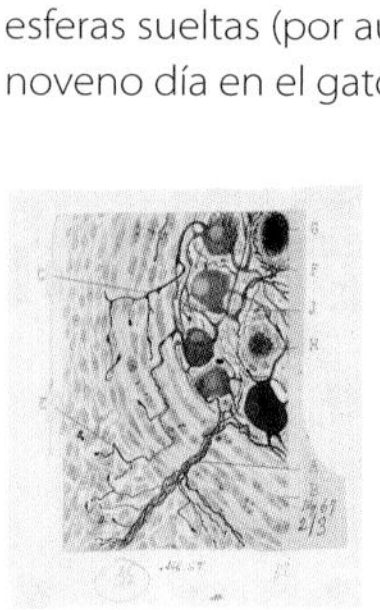

FIGURE 188.

Graft of a ganglion in a dog a few days old.

This figure was published in Cajal, S. R. (1913–1914) *Estudios sobre la degeneración y regeneración del sistema nervioso*. Madrid: Moya. (Figure 169).

FIGURE LEGEND: Graft of a ganglion in a dog a few days old, killed five days after the operation. *A*, Small nerve that crosses the ganglionic capsule; B, capsule infiltrated by embryonic connective cells; *C*, a perforating fiber that is ramified at the level of the connective interstices of the capsule; *E*, new fiber that is wandering through the connective tissue of the host; *F*, cell that has sent branches into the capsule; *G*, dead neuron surrounded by a nest; *H*, other dead neuron.

Original text: Ingerto de ganglio de perro de pocos días sacrificado al quinto de la operación. *A*, nerviecito que cruza la cápsula gangliónica; *B*, cápsula infiltrada de células conectivas embrionarias; *C*, una fibra perforante ramificada al nivel de los intersticios conectivos de la cápsula; *E*, fibra nueva errante por el tejido conectivo del huésped; *F*, célula que daba ramas á la cápsula; *G* neurona muerta rodeada de un nido; *H*, otra neurona muerta.

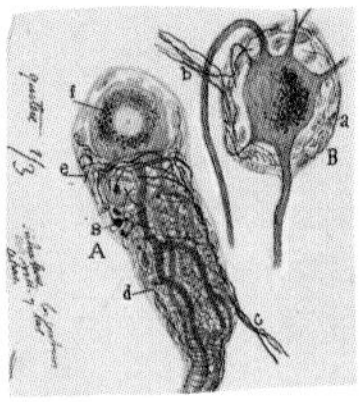

FIGURE 189.

Atypical cells in an old horse.

This figure was published in Cajal, S. R. (1913–1914) *Estudios sobre la degeneración y regeneración del sistema nervioso*. Madrid: Moya. (Figure 179).

FIGURE LEGEND: Atypical cells in an old horse. *A*, Comet-like type with nests: *B*, stellate type with pericellular nest; *c*, afferent fibers; *d*, capsule; *g*, bulbs and terminal clubs of certain fine dendritic appendages.

Original text: Corpúsculos atípicos de un caballo Viejo. *A*, tipo cometario cono nidos; *B*, tipo estrellado con nido pericelular; *c*, fibras aferentes; *d*, cápsula; *g*, bulbos y mazas terminales de ciertos apéndices dendríticos finos.

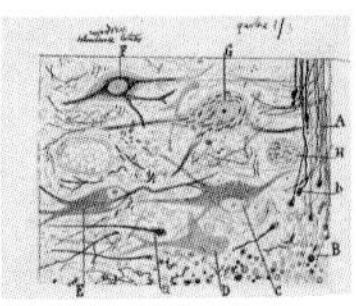

FIGURE 190.

Nerve cells in the gray matter of the spinal cord in a young cat.

This figure was published in Cajal, S. R. (1913–1914) *Estudios sobre la degeneración y regeneración del sistema nervioso*. Madrid: Moya. (Figure 202).

FIGURE LEGEND: Nerve cells in the gray matter of the spinal cord in a young cat killed twenty-four hours after the operation. *A*, White matter; *B*, edges of the wound; *C*, neuron with granular neurofibrils; *D*, necrotic cell; *E*, fish-like type of neuron; *F*, hirudiform type of neuron; *G*, neuron with fusiform neurofibrils; *a*, interrupted collateral.

Original text: Células nerviosas de la substancia gris de la médula espinal de un gato joven sacrificado veinticuatro horas después de la operación. *A*, substancia blanca; *B*, bordes de la herida; *D*, célula necrótica; *C*, neurona de neurofibrillas granulosas; *G*, neurona con neurofibrillas fusiformes; *F*, tipo hirudiforme; *E*, tipo pisciforme; *a*, colateral interrumpida.

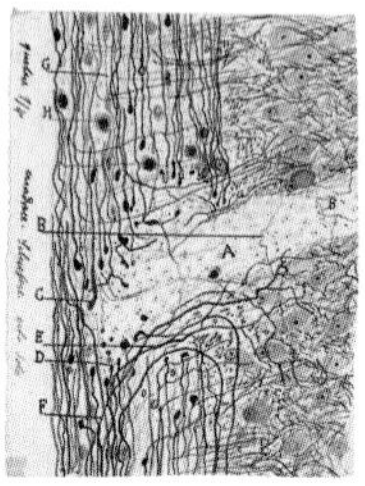

FIGURE 191.

Partial section of the spinal cord in a dog.

This figure was published in Cajal, S. R. (1910) Algunos hechos de regeneración parcial de la substancia gris de los centros nerviosos. *Trab. Lab. Invest. Biol. Univ. Madrid* 8, 197–236 (Figure 7). It has also been reproduced as Figure 206 in Cajal, S. R. (1913–1914). *Estudios sobre la degeneración y regeneración del sistema nervioso*. Madrid: Moya.

FIGURE LEGEND: Partial section of the spinal cord in a young dog that was killed six days after the lesion. *A*, Neuroglial scar; *B*, perforating fibers; *C, D*, balls at the end of the myelinated fibers of the interrupted white matter; *G*, beaded fibers; *F*, collaterals of motor roots.

Original text: Corte parcial de la médula espinal del perro joven sacrificado seis días después de la lesión. *A*, cicatriz neuróglica; *B*, fibras perforantes; *C, D*, bolas en el cabo final de tubos de la substancia blanca interrumpida; *G*, fibras arrosariadas; *F*, colaterales de radiculares motrices.

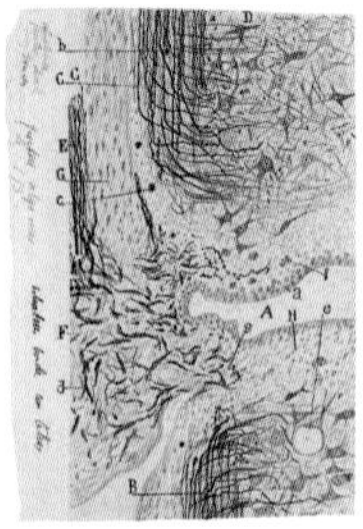

FIGURE 192.

Complete section of the spinal cord in a rabbit.

This figure was published in Cajal, S. R. (1913–1914) *Estudios sobre la degeneración y regeneración del sistema nervioso*. Madrid: Moya. (Figure 207).

FIGURE LEGEND: Complete section of the spinal cord in a rabbit one and a half months after the operation. *A*, Cyst coated by the ependyma; *B, C*, arciform fibers in both stumps of the white matter of the wound (anterior tract), *D*, cells of the gray matter; *E*, piece of an anterior root; *F*, connective scar invaded by sprouts arising from this anterior root; *c*, free balls; *f*, granular bodies.

Original text: Sección complete de la médula examinada en un conejo sacrificado mes y medio después de la operación. *A*, quiste revestido por el epéndimo; *B, C*, fibras arciformes en ambos cabos de la substancia blanca de la herida (cordón anterior); *D*, células de la substancia gris; *E*, trozo de una raíz anterior; *F*, cicatriz conjuntiva invadida por retoños nacidos de dicha raíz; *c*, bolas sueltas; *f*, cuerpos granulosos.

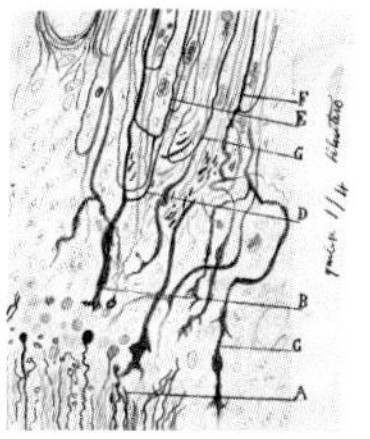

FIGURE 193.
Juxtaspinal portion of a sensory root.

This figure was published in Cajal, S. R. (1910) Algunas observaciones favorables a la hipótesis neurotrópica. *Trab. Lab. Invest. Biol. Univ. Madrid* 8, 63–135 (Figure 8). It has also been reproduced as Figure 216 in Cajal, S. R. (1913–1914). *Estudios sobre la degeneración y regeneración del sistema nervioso*. Madrid: Moya.

FIGURE LEGEND: Juxtaspinal portion of a sensory root that is intact but with an entrance into the posterior bundle that was intercepted by destruction of the white matter. *A*, Remnants of the posterior bundle; *B*, large roots ending in hirudiform stumps; *B, C*, other ramified axons; *E, F*, axons that give out retrograde fibers.

Original text: Porción yuxtamedular de una raíz sensitiva incólume, pero cuya entrada en el cordón posterior hallábase interceptada por destrucción de la substancia blanca. *A*, restos del cordón posterior; *B*, radiculares gruesas acabadas mediante cabos hirudiformes; *B, C*, otros axones ramificados; *E, F*, axones que suministraban fibras retrógradas.

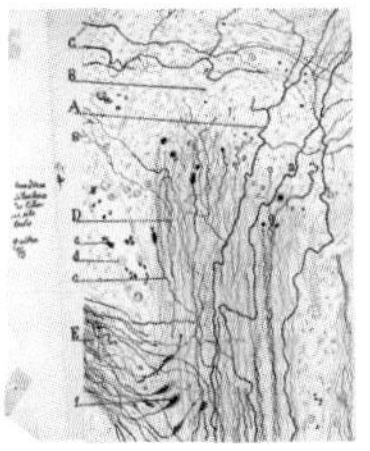

FIGURE 194.
Longitudinal and tangential section of the posterior bundle in a dog.

This figure was published in Cajal, S. R. (1910) Observaciones sobre la regeneración de la porción intramedular de las raíces sensitivas. *Trab. Lab. Invest. Biol. Univ. Madrid* 8, 177–196 (Figure 4). It has also been reproduced as Figure 217 in Cajal, S. R. (1913–1914). *Estudios sobre la degeneración y regeneración del sistema nervioso*. Madrid: Moya.

FIGURE LEGEND: Longitudinal and tangential section of the posterior bundle in a dog a few days old. *E*, Regenerated posterior root; *B*, wound of the posterior cordon filled by the scar; *D*, posterior bundle; *A*, Fibers of the posterior bundle in phase of excitatory division; *a, b*, other large fibers also ramified in the scar; *g*, fine fibers of the posterior bundle that have migrated; *f*, terminal clubs of regenerated root fibers; *c*, elements in a blood vessel; *C*, nerve fibers coming from a sensory radicular branch, which penetrate the scar.

Original text: Corte longitudinal y tangencial del cordón posterior del perro de pocos días. *E*, raíz posterior regenerada; *B*, herida del cordón posterior, suplida por la cicatriz: *D*, cordón posterior; *A*, fibras del cordón posterior en fase de excitación divisoria; *a, b*, otras fibras gruesas, también ramificadas en la cicatriz; *g*, fibras finas del cordón posterior emigradas; *f*, mazas terminales de radiculares regeneradas; *c*, plaquetas de un vaso sanguíneo; *C*, fibras nerviosas llegadas de una radicular sensitiva, penetrantes en la cicatriz.

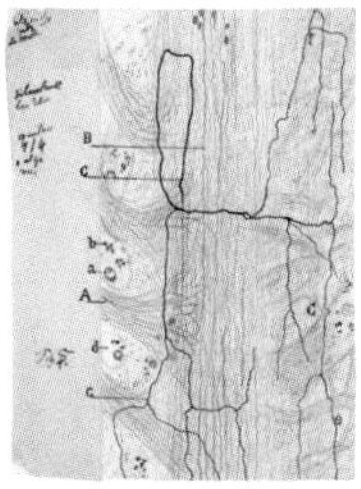

FIGURE 195.
Tangential and longitudinal section of the posterior bundle near a spinal wound in a dog.

This figure was published in Cajal, S. R. (1910) Observaciones sobre la regeneración de la porción intramedular de las raíces sensitivas. *Trab. Lab. Invest. Biol. Univ. Madrid* 8, 177–196 (Figure 5). It has also been reproduced as Figure 221 in Cajal, S. R. (1913–1914). *Estudios sobre la degeneración y regeneración del sistema nervioso*. Madrid: Moya.

FIGURE LEGEND: Tangential and longitudinal section of the posterior bundle near a spinal wound in a young dog. *A*, Almost-normal root fibers; *B*, posterior bundle; *C*, thick nerve fiber that, emerging from the posterior bundle, gives rise to an enormous terminal arborization; *c, e, f*, branches of this arborization; *a*, leukocytes; *b*, platelets in a blood vessel.

Original text: Corte tangencial y longitudinal del cordón posterior del perro joven en la proximidad de una herida medular. *A*, radiculares casi normales; *B*, cordón posterior; *C*, fibra nerviosa espesa que, saliendo del cordón posterior, genera enorme arborización terminal; *c, f, e*, ramas de esta arborización; *a*, leucocitos, y *b*, plaquetas de un vaso sanguíneo.

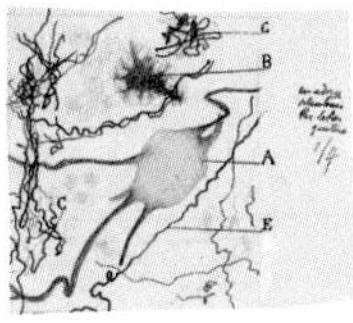

FIGURE 196.
Cells and fibers floating in the exudate of a spinal cord wound.

This figure was published in Cajal, S. R. (1911) Fibras nerviosas conservadas y fibras nerviosas degeneradas. *Trab. Lab. Invest. Biol. Univ. Madrid* 9, 181–215 (Figure 6).

FIGURE LEGEND: Cells and fibers floating in the exudate of a spinal cord wound of a month-old cat sacrificed five days after the operation. *A*, Free neuron; B, frayed or cotton-like cell; *C*, floating skeins of preserved axons.

Original text: Células y fibras flotantes en el exudado de una herida medular de un gato de un mes, sacrificado cinco días después de la operación. *A*, neurona suelta; *B*, célula desgarrada ó algodonosa; *C*, madejas flotantes de axones conservados.

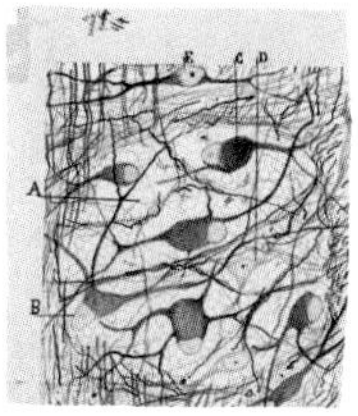

FIGURE 197.
Cells lying in an interstitial hemorrhagic focus of the gray matter of the spinal cord.

This figure was published in Cajal, S. R. (1911) Alteraciones de la substancia gris provocadas por conmoción y aplastamiento. *Trab. Lab. Invest. Biol. Univ. Madrid* 9, 217–253 (Figure 7). It has also been reproduced as Figure 227 in Cajal, S. R. (1913–1914). *Estudios sobre la degeneración y regeneración del sistema nervioso*. Madrid: Moya.

FIGURE LEGEND: Cells lying in an interstitial hemorrhagic center of the gray matter of the spinal cord in a twenty-day-old cat killed four days after the operation. *A*, Deposit of blood; *B, C*, cells with a marginal nucleus; *E*, fusiform cells of the margins of the hemorrhage.

Original text: Células yacentes en un foco intersticial hemorrágico de la substancia gris espinal de un gato de veinte días, sacrificado cuatro días después de la operación. *A*, depósito sanguíneo; *B, C*, células con núcleo marginal; *E*, células fusiformes de las márgenes del derrame sanguíneo.

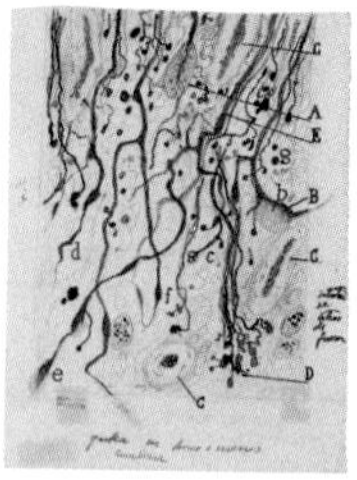

FIGURE 198.

Retinal stump of the optic nerve in a rabbit.

This figure was published in Cajal, S. R. (1913–1914) *Estudios sobre la degeneración y regeneración del sistema nervioso*. Madrid: Moya. (Figure 231).

FIGURE LEGEND: Retinal stump of the optic nerve in a rabbit, which was killed seven days after the operation. *A, B*, Terminal balls undergoing hyaline degeneration; *D*, bundle of fibers ending in balls and penetrating into the scar; *C*, blood vessels obstructed by anemia and consequent proliferation of the adventitial layer; *d*, growth cone; *E*, richly ramified fiber; *e*, terminal thickening in the form of a brush.

Original text: Cabo retiniano del nervio óptico del conejo sacrificado siete días después de la operación. *A, B*, bolas terminales en tránsito de degeneración hialina; D, manojo de fibras acabadas en bola y penetrantes en la cicatriz; *C*, vasos obstruidos por anemia y proliferación subsiguiente de la advertencia; *d*, cono de crecimiento; *E*, fibra ricamente arborizada; *e*, abultamiento final en forma de pincel.

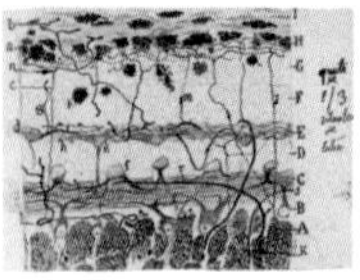

FIGURE 199.

Phenomena of neoformation and dispersion of the optic fibers.

This figure was published in Cajal, S. R. (1913–1914) *Estudios sobre la degeneración y regeneración del sistema nervioso*. Madrid: Moya. (Figure 235).

FIGURE LEGEND: Phenomena of neoformation and dispersion of the optic fibers after traumatic inflammation of the sclerotic and choroid coats. *A*, Layer of optic fibers full of sprouts; *B*, ganglion cells; *C*, internal plexiform layer; *D*, internal granular layer; *E*, external plexiform layer and horizontal cells; *F*, external granular layer; *G*, layer of rods and cones disorganized and invaded by pigment cells; *e, k, i, j, s*, dispersed nerve sprouts; *b*, axon with branches that penetrate the sclerotic coat; *d*, horizontal cell provided with an ascending sprout; *m*, another similar branch. (After Leoz and Arcaute.)

Original text: Fenornenos de neoformación y dispersión de las fibras ópticas consecutivas a la inflamacion traumática de la esclerótica y coroides. *A*, capa de fibras ópticas llena de retonos; *B*, celulas gangliónicas; *C*, plexiforme interna; *D*, granos internos; *E*, plexiforme externa y células horizontales; *F*, granos externos; *G*, capa de bastones y conos desorganizada e invadida por células pigmentarias; *e, k, s, j*, retoños nerviosos en dispersión; *b*, axon cuyas ramas penetran en la esclerótica; *d*, célula horizontal provista de retoño ascendente; *m*, otra rama semejante. (Según Leoz y Arcaute).

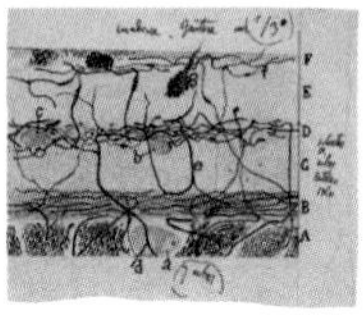

FIGURE 200.

Regions in the retina from which nearly all the neurons had disappeared.

This figure was published in Cajal, S. R. (1913–1914) *Estudios sobre la degeneración y regeneración del sistema nervioso*. Madrid: Moya. (Figure 236).

FIGURE LEGEND: Regions in the retina from which nearly all the neurons had disappeared, being replaced by layers of optic sprouts. *A*, Layer of optic fibers; *B*, internal plexiform layer; *C*, internal granular layer; *D*, external plexiform layer; *E*, external granular layer; *e, d*, optic fibers that are dispersed and ramified; *f*, horizontal plexus at the level of the pigmented layer; *b, c*, horizontal degenerated cells. (After Leoz and Arcaute.)

Original text: Regiones de la retina donde habían desaparecido casi del todo las neuronas, siendo sustituidas por capas de retoños ópticos. *A*, capa de fibras ópticas; *B*, plexiforme interna; *C*, granos internos; *D*, plexiforme externa; *E*, granos externos; *e, d*, fibras ópticas dispersas y ramificadas; *f*, plexo horizontal al nivel de la capa pigmentaria; *b, c*, células horizontales degeneradas. (Según Leoz y Arcaute).

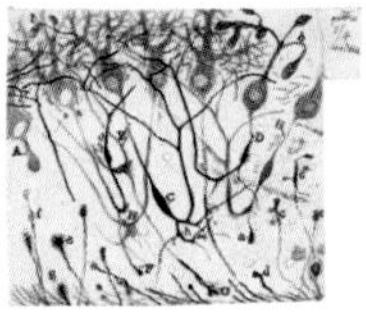

FIGURE 201.

Disposition of the Purkinje axons in the cerebellum in a cat.

This figure was published in Cajal, S. R. (1913–1914) *Estudios sobre la degeneración y regeneración del sistema nervioso*. Madrid: Moya. (Figure 239).

FIGURE LEGEND: Disposition of the Purkinje axons in the cerebellum in a twenty-day-old cat killed fifty-two hours after the operation. *A*, Short club; *B, I*, hypertrophic collaterals from which hangs the axon, terminating in a club; *C, H*, arciform thickenings from which many branches issue (*h*); *F*, terminal ball of a Purkinje axon; *a, G*, other balls of the same type; *b*, contracted dendrites (rosaliform type); *c*, altered mossy fibers; *d, e, g*, various type of clubs connected with fibers of the white matter; *f*, reticulated varicosities of fine fibers.

Original text: Disposición del axón de Purkinje del cerebelo del gato de veinte días, sacrificado cincuenta y dos horas después de la operación. *A*, maza corta; *B, I*, colaterales hipertróficas de que pendía el axón terminado en maza; *C, H*, espesamientos arciformes de que procedían numerosas ramas (*h*); *F*, bola terminal de un axón de Purkinje; *a, G*, otras bolas de igual especie; *b*, dendritas encogidas (tipo rosaliforme); *c*, musgosas alteradas; *d, e, g*, diversos tipos de mazas continuadas con fibras dela sustancia blanca; *f*, varicosidades reticuladas de fibras finas.

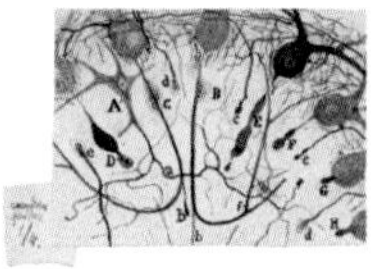

FIGURE 202.

Section of a cerebellar folium.

This figure was published in Cajal, S. R. (1913–1914) *Estudios sobre la degeneración y regeneración del sistema nervioso*. Madrid: Moya. (Figure 241).

FIGURE LEGEND: Section of a cerebellar folium in a twenty-five-day-old cat, one day after the section. *A*, Cell with a short axon; *B, C*, pale excrecences of the axon; *D, E, F*, varieties of double clubs; *G, H*, axon reduced to a digitiform appendage; *b*, continuation of the Purkinje axon, ending in a club; *c, d*, recurrent collaterals of the Purkinje axons with a retraction ball in their peripheral stump.

Original text: Corte de una laminilla cerebelosa. Gato de veinticinco días, uno después de la sección. *A*, corpúsculo de axon corto; *B, C*, excrecencias pálidas del axon; *D, E, F*, variedades de mazas dobles; *G, H*, axon reducido á apéndice digitiforme; *b*, continuación del axon de Purkinje acabado en maza, *c, d*, colaterales recurrentes de los axones de Purkinje con bola de retracción en su cabo periférico.

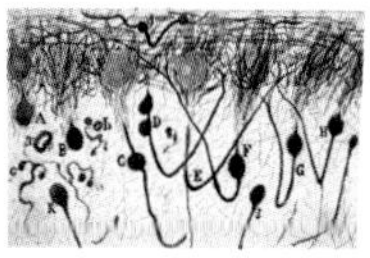

FIGURE 203.

Lesions of the axon of Purkinje cells in the cerebellum in a human (drowned man).

This figure was published in Cajal, S. R. (1911) Los fenómenos precoces de la degeneración neuronal en el cerebelo. *Trab. Lab. Invest. Biol. Univ. Madrid* 9, 1–38 (Figure 1). It has also been reproduced as Figure 244 in Cajal, S. R. (1913–1914). *Estudios sobre la degeneración y regeneración del sistema nervioso*. Madrid: Moya.

FIGURE LEGEND: Lesions of the axon of Purkinje cells in a human cerebellum (drowned man). In this figure have been drawn the principal lesions found in a single section. *A, B*, Terminal balls situated near the cell; *D*, arciform axon with a double ball; *C, G*, arciform axon with a ball that lies at some distance from the arc; *E, H*, arc formed by the recurrent collateral, in which the axon appears to be a collateral of the collateral; *J, K*, fibers ending in a club.

Original text: Lesiones del axon de las células de Purkinje del cerebelo humano (hombre ahogado). En esta figura se han copiado las principales lesiones halladas en un sólo corte. *A, B*, bolas finales situadas cerca de la célula; *D*, axon arciforme con doble bola; *C, G*, axon arciforme cuya bola yacía distante del arco; *E, H*, arco formado por la colateral recurrente y en que el axon parece colateral de la colateral; *J, K*, fibras acabadas en maza.

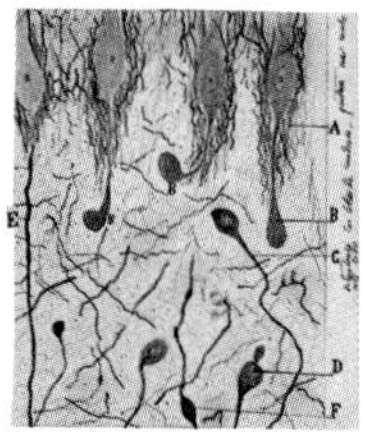

FIGURE 204.

Section of a cerebellar folium in an adult rabbit.

This figure was published in Cajal, S. R. (1907) Note sur la dégénérescence traumatique des fibres nerveuses du cervelet et du cerveau. *Trav. Lab. Recherches Biol. Univ. Madrid* 5, 105–116 (Figure 1).

FIGURE LEGEND: Section of a cerebellar folium in an adult rabbit. Examination eight days after the lesion. *A*, Baskets around Purkinje cells; *B*, retraction balls of the axon of Purkinje cells; *D*, balls with inner vacuoles; *E*, normal axon.

Original text: Coupe d'une lamelle cérébelleuse du lapin adulte. Examen 8 jours après la lésion. *A*, corbeilles de Purkinje; *B*, boules de retraction de l'axon des cellullales de Purkinje; *D*, boules avec vacuoles intérieures; *E*, axon sain.

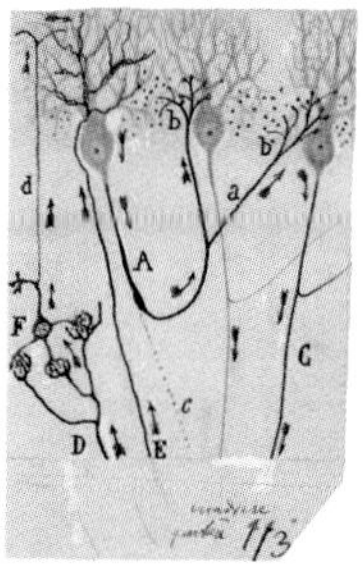

FIGURE 205.

Path of the currents in Purkinje cells deprived of the peripheral portion of the axon.

This figure was published in Cajal, S. R. (1913–1914) *Estudios sobre la degeneración y regeneración del sistema nervioso*. Madrid: Moya. (Figure 245).

FIGURE LEGEND: Schematic drawing designed to show the path of the currents in the Purkinje cells deprived of the peripheral portion of the axon. *A*, Arciform Purkinje cell; *D*, mossy fibers; *E*, climbing fiber; *F*, granule; *C*, normal Purkinje axons; *c*, position previously occupied by the axon that has disappeared.

Original text: Esquema destinado á mostrar la marcha de las corrientes en las células de Purkinje privadas de la porción periférica del axon. *A*, célula de Purkinje arciforme; *D*, fibras musgosas; *E*, fibra trepadora; *F*, grano; *C*, axones normales de Purkinje; *c*, lugar que ocupaba el axon desaparecido.

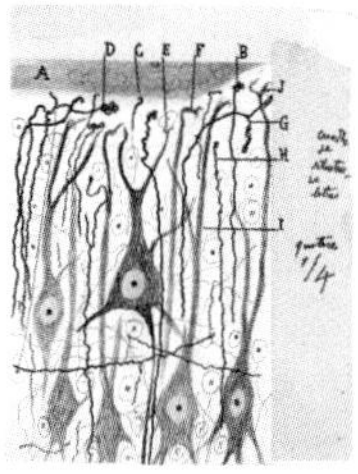

FIGURE 206.

Pyramidal cells of the cerebral cortex in a cat in which a horizontal cut was made.

This figure was published in Cajal, S. R. (1910) Algunos hechos de regeneración parcial de la substancia gris de los centros nerviosos. *Trab. Lab. Invest. Biol. Univ. Madrid* 8, 197–236 (Figure 4). It has also been reproduced as Figure 261 in Cajal, S. R. (1913–1914) *Estudios sobre la degeneración y regeneración del sistema nervioso*. Madrid: Moya.

FIGURE LEGEND: Pyramidal cells of the cerebral cortex in a two-month-old cat, in which a horizontal cut was made. *A*, Wound with remnants of the exudate; *B, C, D*, hooks and glomeruli because the ascending axons toward the molecular layer end in the wound; *E, F, J*, traumatized ends of the dendritic trunks.

Original text: Pirámides de la corteza cerebral del gato de dos meses, en la cual se hizo un corte horizontal. *A*, herida con restos de exudado; *B, C, D*, ganchos y glomérulos por qué terminan en la herida los axones ascendentes para la capa molecular; *E, F, J*, cabos traumatizados de los tallos dendríticos.

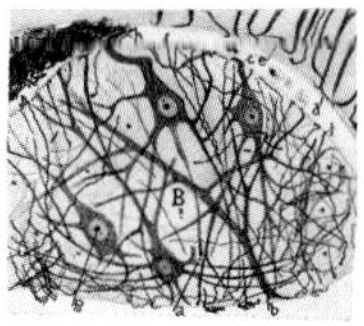

FIGURE 207.

Cerebral sequestra in a cat.

This figure was published in Cajal, S. R. (1910) Algunos hechos de regeneración parcial de la substancia gris de los centros nerviosos. *Trab. Lab. Invest. Biol. Univ. Madrid* 8, 197–236 (Figure 6). It has also been reproduced as Figure 263 in Cajal, S. R. (1913–1914) *Estudios sobre la degeneración y regeneración del sistema nervioso*. Madrid: Moya.

FIGURE LEGEND: Cerebral sequestrations in a one-month-old cat that was killed six days after the operation. *A*, Superficial portion in which the deep stumps of the dendritic trunks are being corroded; *B*, deep portion with an isolated cellular colony; *a*, degenerated axon; *b, c*, isolated trunks; *d*, bifurcated dendritic stump; *h*, block of dislocated nerve fibers; *g*, disintegrated nucleolus.

Original text: Secuestros cerebrales del gato de un mes sacrificado seis días después de la operación. *A*, secuestro superficial que muestra en corrosión los cabos profundos de los tallos dendriticos; *B*, secuestro profundo con una colonia celular aislada; *a*, axon degenerado; *b, c*, tallos aislados; *d*, cabo dendritico bifurcado; *h*, bloque de fibras nerviosas dislocadas; *g*, nucleolo desintegrado.

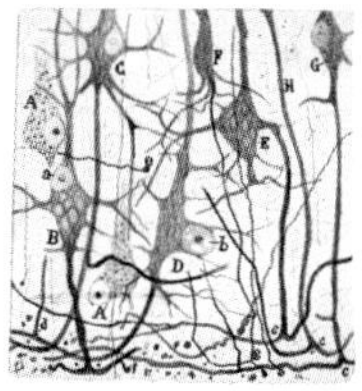

FIGURE 208.

Section of the cerebral cortex in a dog two days old.

This figure was published in Cajal, S. R. (1911) Los fenómenos precoces de la degeneración traumática de los cilindros-ejes del cerebro. *Trab. Lab. Invest. Biol. Univ. Madrid* 9, 39–96 (Figure 3). It has also been reproduced as Figure 282 in Cajal, S. R. (1913–1914) *Estudios sobre la degeneración y regeneración del sistema nervioso*. Madrid: Moya.

FIGURE LEGEND: Section of the cerebral cortex in a dog two days old (motor region); the animal was killed twenty-four hours after the operation. *A*, Gigantic necrosed pyramidal cell; B, pyramidal cell with an axon that appears to be bifurcated in the wound; *C, D*, pyramidal cells with axons that form an arc and are prolonged by horizontal or recurrent collaterals; *H, E, G*, cells with an axon that is prolonged by two hypertrophied ramified collaterals; *F*, small cell with a axon that ends in a ball below the point of origin of a hypertrophied arciform collateral; *a*, marginal nucleus; *b*, nucleus with vacuoles bulging between two appendages; *c*, bifurcation of the axon; *d*, secondary branches of nerve collaterals.

Original text: Corte de la corteza cerebral del perro de dos días (región motriz), sacrificado veinticuatro horas después de la operación. *A*, pirámide gigante necrosada; *B*, pirámide cuyo axon aparece bifurcado en la herida; *C, D*, pirámides cuyos axones se doblan en arco, continuándose con colaterales horizontales ó recurrentes; *H, E, G*, células de axon continuado con dos colaterales hipertróficas ramificadas; *F*, célula pequeña cuyo axon termina en bola por debajo del arranque de colateral arciforme hipertrófica; *a*, núcleo marginal; *b*, núcleo abultando entre dos apéndices y con vacuolas; *c*, bifurcación del axon; *d*, ramas secundarias de colaterales nerviosas.

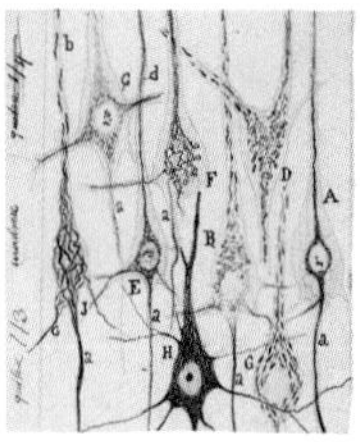

FIGURE 209.

Edges of a contused cerebral wound in a cat.

This figure was published in Cajal, S. R. (1911) Alteraciones de la substancia gris provocadas por conmoción y aplastamiento. *Trab. Lab. Invest. Biol. Univ. Madrid* 9, 217–253 (Figure 1). It has also been reproduced as Figure 289 in Cajal, S. R. (1913–1914) *Estudios sobre la degeneración y regeneración del sistema nervioso*. Madrid: Moya.

FIGURE LEGEND: Edges of a contused cerebral wound in a twenty-day-old cat that was killed twenty-one hours after the lesion. *A, E, F*, Hirudiform neurons; *B, C, D*, phases of granular formation of the hirudiform type; *G*, type with neurofibrillar spindles; *J*, type with hypertrophic neurofibrils; *a*, axon; *b*, neurofibrillary spindles.

Original text: Bordes de una herida cerebral contusa del gato de veinte días, sacrificado veintiuna horas después de la lesión. *A, E, F*, neuronas hirudiformes; *B, C, D*, fases de resolución granulosa del tipo hirudiforme; *G*, tipo con husos neurofibrillares; *J*, tipo con neurofibrillas hipertróficas; *a*, axon; *b*, husos neurofibrillares.

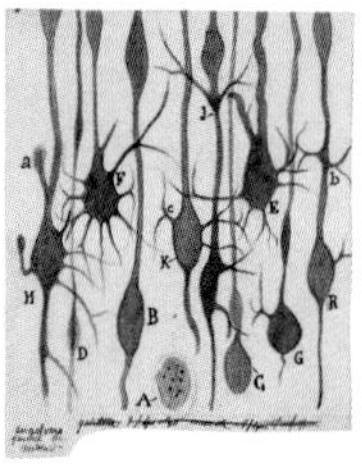

FIGURE 210.

Various types of testudinoid structures as seen in a cerebral section in a dog.

This figure was published in Cajal, S. R. (1911) Los fenómenos precoces de la degeneración traumática de los cilindros-ejes del cerebro. *Trab. Lab. Invest. Biol. Univ. Madrid* 9, 39–96 (Figure 11). It has also been reproduced as Figure 291 in Cajal, S. R. (1913–1914) *Estudios sobre la degeneración y regeneración del sistema nervioso*. Madrid: Moya.

FIGURE LEGEND: In this figure have been assembled various types of testudinoid structures as seen in a cerebral section in a two-month-old dog fifty-six hours after the operation. Region of the varicosities of the giant axons. *A*, Granular ball of axons that have been precociously destroyed; *B*, large varicose fiber; *D*, thin varicose fiber; *G, E, F*, terminal testudinoid structures; *H, K, J, R*, collateral testudinoid structures; *a*, appendage ending in a reticulated ball; *c*, appendages ending a pale point.

Original text: En esta figura se han reunido diversos tipos de aparatos testudoides hallados en un corte cerebral de perro de dos meses, sacrificado cincuenta y seis horas después de la operación. Región de las varicosidades de los axones gigantes. *A*, bola granulosa de axones precozmente destruídos; *B*, fibra varicosa gruesa; *D*, fibra varicosa delgada; *G, E, F*, aparatos testudoides terminales; *H, K, J, R*, aparatos testudoides colaterales; *a*, apéndice terminado en bola reticulada; c, apéndices acabados en punta pálida.

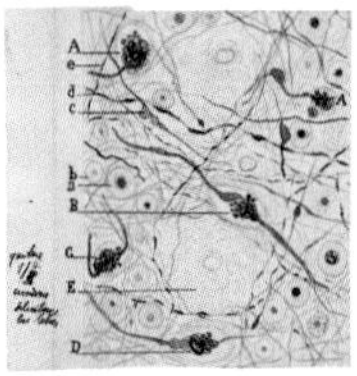

FIGURE 211.

Central portion of a wound of the white matter in a dog.

This figure was published in Cajal, S. R. (1911) Los fenómenos precoces de la degeneración traumática de los cilindros-ejes del cerebro. *Trab. Lab. Invest. Biol. Univ. Madrid* 9, 39–96 (Figure 14). It has also been reproduced as Figure 295 in Cajal, S. R. (1913–1914) *Estudios sobre la degeneración y regeneración del sistema nervioso*. Madrid: Moya.

FIGURE LEGEND: Central portion, very largely degenerated, of a wound of the white matter in a dog, twenty-five to thirty days old, killed one week after the operation. *A*, Terminal tangles; *B, C, D*, tangles along the fibers; *E*, embryonic nodules situated around blood vessels; *a*, free balls with a central portion still stained with colloidal silver; *b*, other ball with a center that appears granular; *c*, varicosities along the fibers; *d, e*, degenerated axons.

Original text: Porción central, degenerada en grande extensión, de una herida de la substancia blanca del perro de veinticinco á treinta días, sacrificado una semana después de la operación. *A*, ovillos terminales; *B, C, D*, ovillos de trayecto; *E*, nódulos embrionarios situados en torno de vasos sanguíneos; *a*, bolas sueltas con porción central todavía coloreable por la plata coloidal; *b*, otra bola cuyo centro aparece granuloso; *c*, varicosidades de trayecto; *d, e*, axones degenerados.

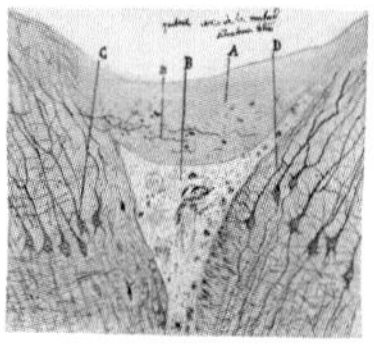

FIGURE 212.

Transverse wound of the cerebrum in a young cat.

This figure was published in Cajal, S. R. (1913–1914) *Estudios sobre la degeneración y regeneración del sistema nervioso*. Madrid: Moya. (Figure 296).

FIGURE LEGEND: Transverse wound of the cerebrum in a young cat killed fourteen days after the operation. *A*, Superficial portion of the gray matter, which is atrophied and sunk in relation to the general plane of the neighboring circumvolutions; *B*, wound in process of cicatrization; *C, D*, neighboring cortical portions that have retained their nerve cells; *a*, persistence of a few exogenous fibers in the atrophied cortex.

Original text: Herida transversal del cerebro del gato joven sacrificado catorce días después de la operación. *A*, porción superficial de la substancia gris atrofiada y hundida con relación al plano general de las circunvoluciones vecinas; *B*, herida en vías de cicatrización; *C, D*, porciones corticales vecinas que han conservado sus células nerviosas; *a*, persistencia de algunas fibras exógenas en la corteza atrofiada.

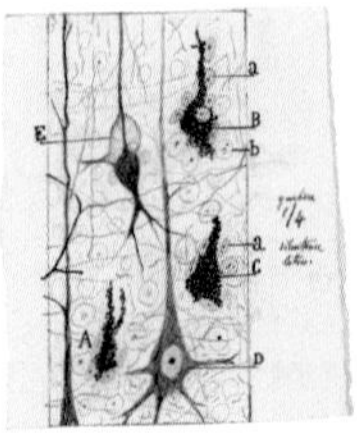

FIGURE 213.

Necrosed pyramidal cells.

This figure was published in Cajal, S. R. (1913–1914) *Estudios sobre la degeneración y regeneración del sistema nervioso.* Madrid: Moya. (Figure 299).

FIGURE LEGEND: Details of a few cells of sector B from Figure 297 [in Cajal (1913–1914)]. *A, B, C,* Necrosed pyramidal cells reduced to disintegrated granules; *a*, proliferated satellite cells; *D*, normal neuron; *E*, neuron vacuolated in its apical portion.

Original text: Detalles de algunas células del sector B de la figura 297 [en Cajal (1913–1914)]. *A, B, C,* pirámides necrosadas y reducidas á granulos disgregados; *a*, corpúsculos satélites proliferados; *D*, neurona normal; *E*, otra vacuola en la porción apical.

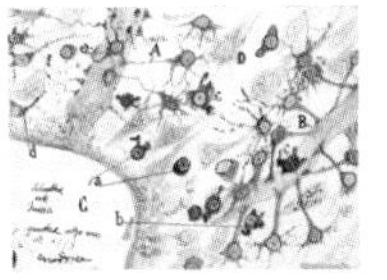

FIGURE 214.

Edges of a cerebral transverse wound in a young cat.

This figure was published in Cajal, S. R. (1913–1914) *Estudios sobre la degeneración y regeneración del sistema nervioso.* Madrid: Moya. (Figure 304).

FIGURE LEGEND: Edges of a cerebral transverse wound in a young cat killed three days after the operation. Uranium nitrate method. *a*, adendritic small cells; *b, c,* small amoeboid cells; *B*, normal capillary surrounded by neuroglial pedicles; *C*, obstructed capillary with gliomatous appendages that have become striated and atrophied; *D*, neuron.

Original text: Bordes de una herida cerebral transversal de un gato joven, sacrificado tres días después de la operación. Método del nitrato de urano. *a*, células adendríticas pequeñas; *b, c,* células amiboides menudas; *B*, capilar normal rodeado de pedículos neuróglicos; *C*, capilar obstruido, cuyos pedículos gliomatosos se estiran y caen en atrofia; *D*, neurona.

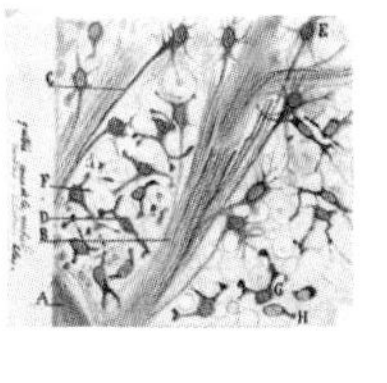

FIGURE 215.

Edges of a transverse wound in a young cat.

This figure was published in Cajal, S. R. (1913–1914) *Estudios sobre la degeneración y regeneración del sistema nervioso.* Madrid: Moya. (Figure 305).

FIGURE LEGEND: Edges of a transverse wound in a young cat killed three days after the operation. *A*, Blood clot in the wound; *B*, vessel surrounded by neuroglial appendages that are notably elongated and with cells of origin that seem to withdraw from the wound; *C*, one of these appendages; *G, H,* free glia cells in the course of alteration. Sublimate–gold method.

Original text: Bordes de una herida transversal del gato joven, sacrificado tres días después de la operación. *A*, coágulo sanguíneo situado en la herida, *B*, vaso rodeado de apéndices neuróglicos notablemente estirados y cuyas células de origen parecen huir de la herida; *C*, uno de estos apéndices; *G, H,* astrocitos emancipados en vías de alteración. Método del sublimado-oro.

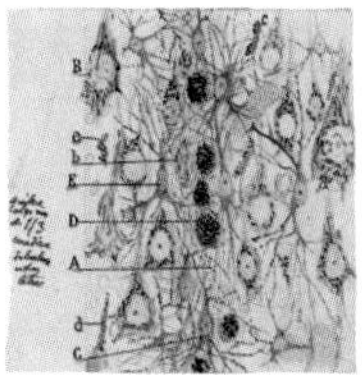

FIGURE 216.

Linear scar of a radial wound in the cerebral cortex in a young cat.

This figure was published in Cajal, S. R. (1913–1914) *Estudios sobre la degeneración y regeneración del sistema nervioso.* Madrid: Moya. (Figure 307).

FIGURE LEGEND: Linear scar of a radial wound in the cortex of the young cat killed eighteen days after the operation. Uranium nitrate method. *A*, Scar; *B*, normal pyramidal cells; *C, E,* neuroglial cells of the scar; *D*, granular cell with carbon granules; *c, d, e,* rod-like cells with inclusions in their protoplasm.

Original text: Cicatriz lineal de una herida radial de la corteza del gato joven sacrificado dieciocho días después de la operación. Método del nitrato de urano. *A*, cicatriz; *B*, pirámides normales; *C, E,* células neuróglicas de la cicatriz; *D*, célula granulosa con granos de carbón; *c, d, e,* células en bastoncito con inclusiones en su protoplasma.

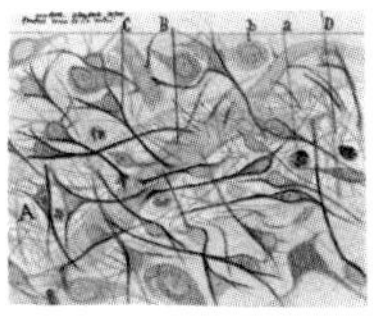

FIGURE 217.

Linear and oblique scar of the cerebral cortex in a cat.

This figure was published in Cajal, S. R. (1913–1914) *Estudios sobre la degeneración y regeneración del sistema nervioso.* Madrid: Moya. (Figure 308).

FIGURE LEGEND: Linear and oblique scar of the cerebral cortex in a cat that was killed one month after the operation. Sublimate–gold method. *A*, Region of the scar; *B*, newly formed vessel in the scar to which converge numerous pedicles or feet of neuroglial cells; *C*, newly formed glia in which fibrils have differentiated; *D*, neuroglial plexus; *a*, granular cell; *b*, cerebral pyramidal cell.

Original text: Cicatriz lineal y oblicua de la corteza cerebral del gato, sacrificado un mes después de la operación. Método del sublimado-oro. *A*, región de la cicatriz; *B*, vaso neoformado en la cicatriz, al cual convergen numerosos pedículos ó aparatos chupadores de células neuróglicas; *C*, glía de nueva formación, donde se han diferenciado fibrillas; *D*, plexo neróglico; *a*, célula granulosa; *b*, pirámide cerebral.

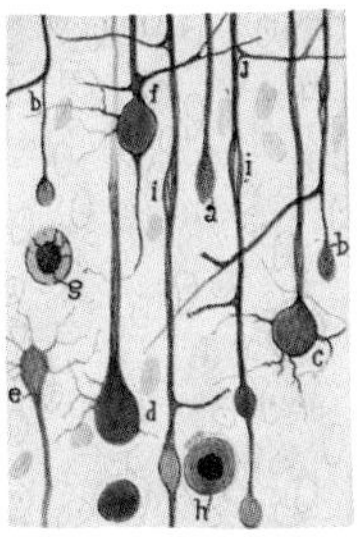

FIGURE 218.

Degenerated region of the central stump of the axons of pyramidal cells.

This figure was published in Cajal, S. R. (1913–1914) *Estudios sobre la degeneración y regeneración del sistema nervioso.* Madrid: Moya. (Figure 316).

FIGURE LEGEND: Details of the degenerated region of the central stump of the axons of pyramidal cells in a young dog killed eight days after the operation. *a, b,* Retraction buds; *d, e, f,* retraction balls provided with sprouts; *b*, axons with a collateral that appears hypertrophied a short distance from the retraction ball; *i*, unraveling of certain hypertrophied axons; *h, g,* free spheres (nervous autotomy). Figure taken from our communication of 1907 [(Cajal, 1907)].

Original text: Detalles de la región degenerada del cabo central de los axones de las pirámides cerebrales. Perro joven sacrificado ocho días después de la operación. *a, b,* botones de retracción; *d, e, f,* bolas de retracción provistas de retoños; *b*, axones cuya colateral aparece hipertrofiada á corta distancia de la bola de retracción; *i*, deshilachamiento de ciertos axones hipertrofiados; *h, g,* esferas sueltas (autonomía nerviosa). Figura tomada de nuestra comunicación de 1907 [(Cajal, 1907)].

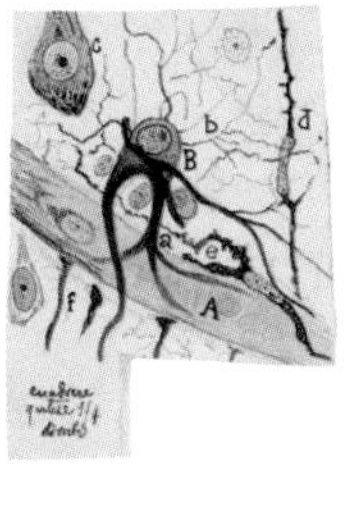

FIGURE 219.

Giant neuroglial cell of the gray matter.

This figure was published in Cajal, S. R. (1925) Contribution à la connaissance de la néuroglie cérébrale et cérébélleuse dans la paralysie générale progressive. *Trav. Lab. Recherches Biol. Univ. Madrid* 23, 157–216 (Figure 1).

FIGURE LEGEND: Giant neuroglial cell of the gray matter: *A*, A vessel on which a robust, branched end-foot is attached (*a*); *b*, thin processes emanating from the opposite vascular pole; *e, d*, microglia; *c*, neuron.

Original text: Corpuscule névroglique géant de la substance grise: *A*, vaisseau sur lequel s'étend un robuste pied ramifié (*a*); *b*, fines expansions émanées du pôle contre-vasculaire; *e, d*, microglie; *c*, neurone.

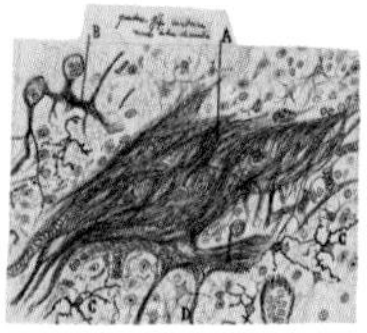

FIGURE 220.

Large mass of Weigert fibers located in the gray matter.

This figure was published in Cajal, S. R. (1925) Contribution à la connaissance de la néuroglie cérébrale et cérébélleuse dans la paralysie générale progressive. *Trav. Lab. Recherches Biol. Univ. Madrid* 23, 157–216 (Figure 5).

FIGURE LEGEND: Large mass of Weigert fibers (*A*) located in the thickness of the gray matter; *B, D*, bundles of perivascular fibers converging in the sclerotic nodule; *C*, scarcely altered macroglial cells.

Original text: Grand massif de fibres de Weigert (*A*) situé dans l'épaisseur de la substance grise; *B, D*, faisceaux de fibres périvasculaires qui convergent dans le nodule sclérotique; *C*, corpuscules de macroglie peu altérés.

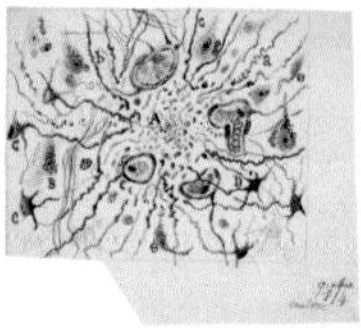

FIGURE 221.

Perivascular end-feet uprooted around a focus of gray matter destruction.

This figure was published in Cajal, S. R. (1925) Contribution à la connaissance de la néuroglie cérébrale et cérébélleuse dans la paralysie générale progressive. *Trav. Lab. Recherches Biol. Univ. Madrid* 23, 157–216 (Figure 8).

FIGURE LEGEND: Convergent orientation of perivascular end-feet uprooted around a focus of gray matter destruction (*A*). Note the varicosity of the fibers, their spiroidal trajectories, and their termination in thorns or pale clubs. In the center, remnants of fragmented end-feet are visible. *B*, Neurons; *c*, atrophied macroglia.

Original text: Orientation convergente des pieds périvasculaires déracinés autour d'un foyer de destruction de la substance grise (*A*). Remarquer la varicosité des fibres leurs trajets spiroïdaux et leur terminaison en pointes ou en massues pâles. On aperçoit au centre des restes de pieds fragmentés; *B*, neurones; *c*, macroglie atrophiée.

SECTION I

Retina and Optic Centers of Cephalopods

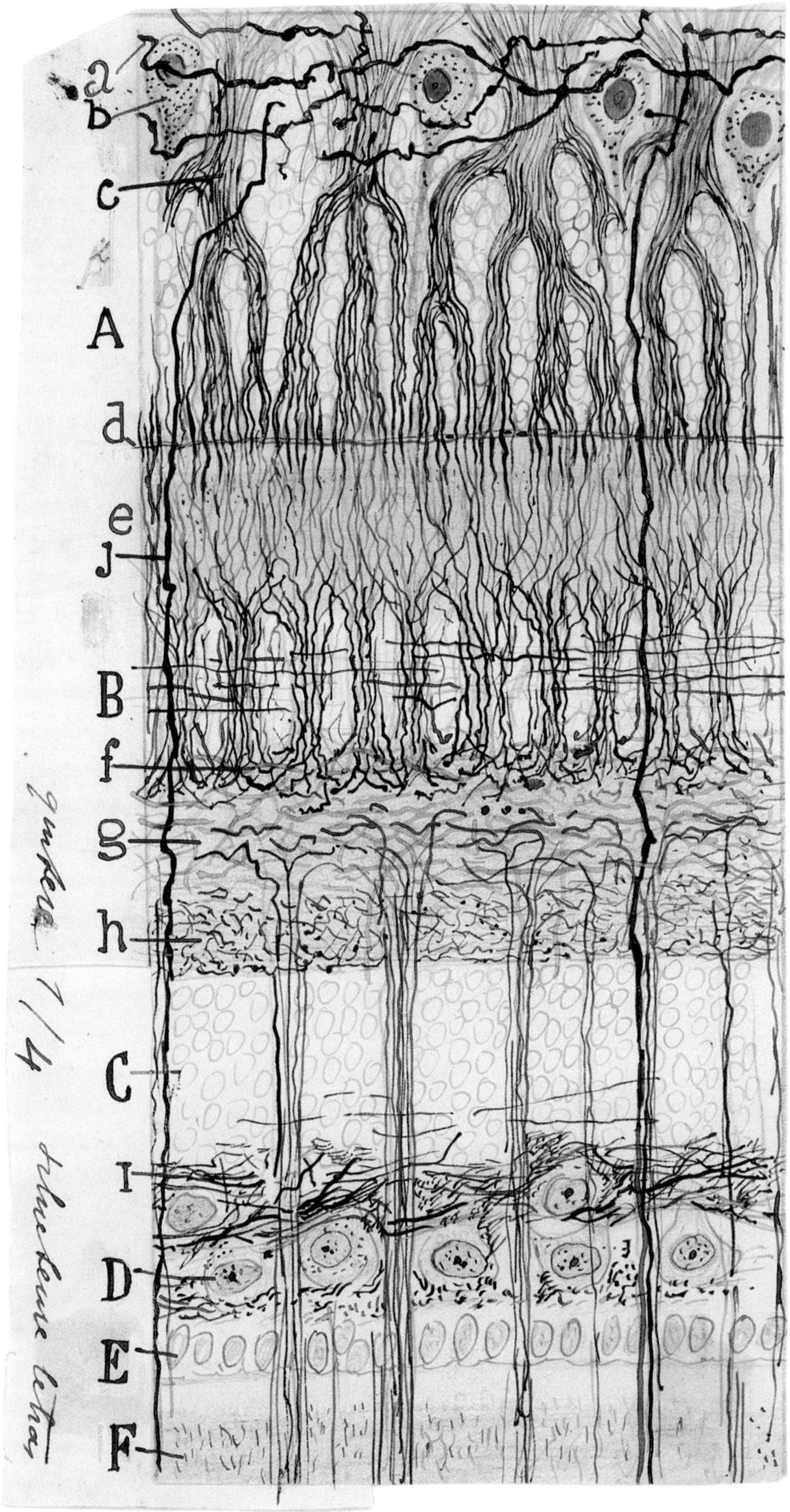

FIGURE 222. Perpendicular section of the deep retina in an adult sepia.

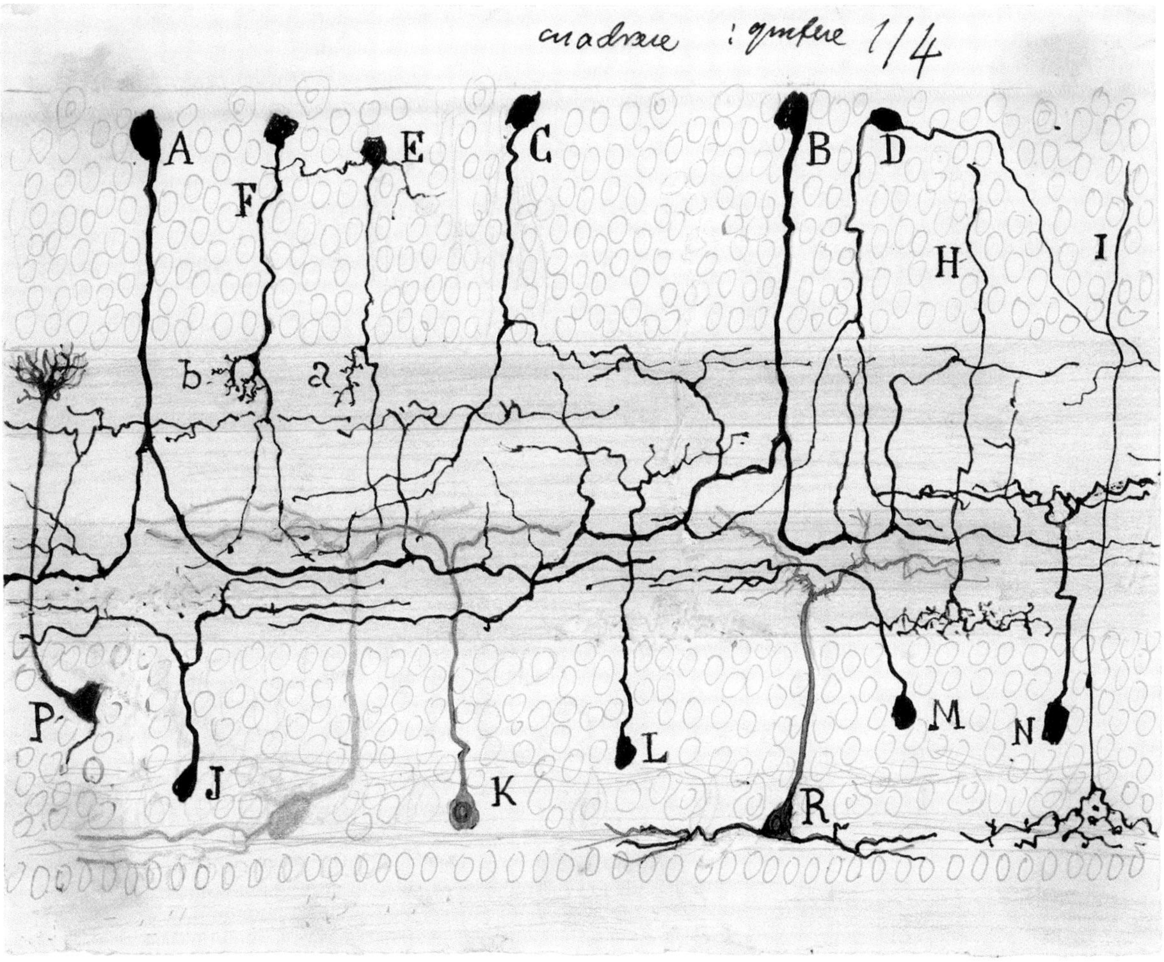

FIGURE 223. Deep retina in a sepia.

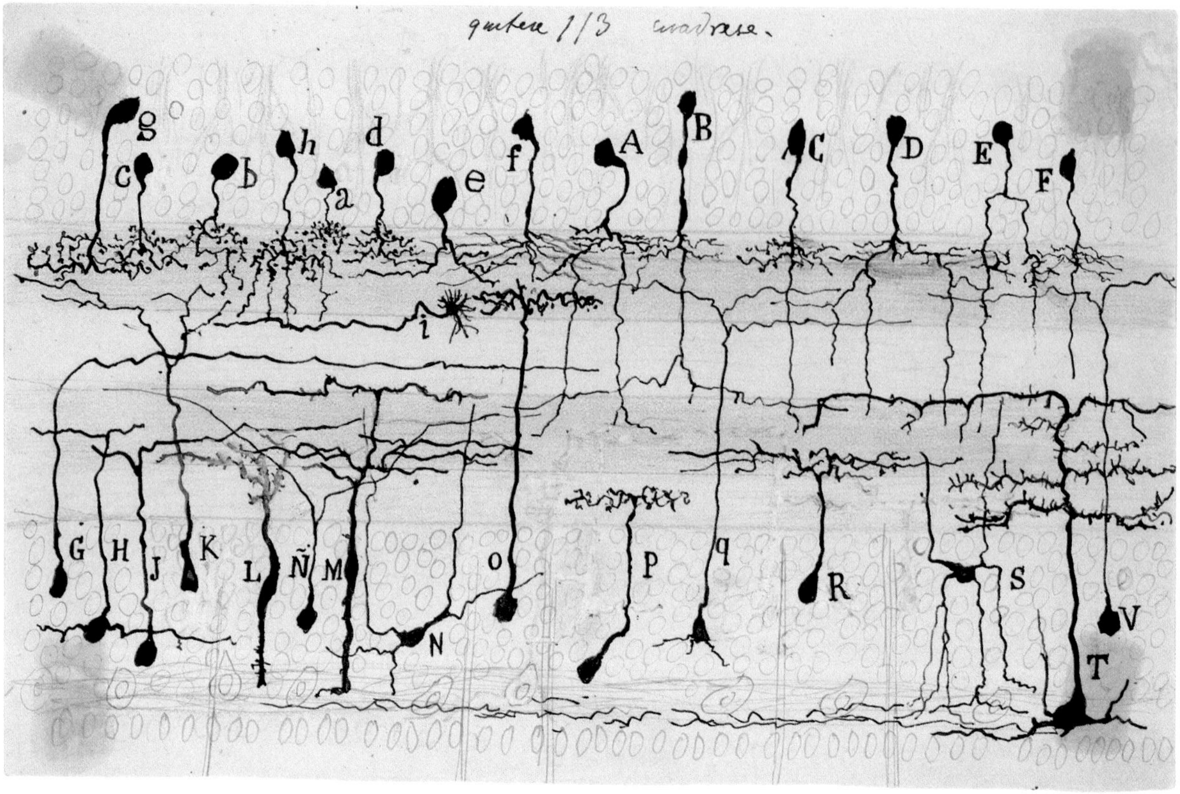

FIGURE 224. Intermediate retina in a sepia.

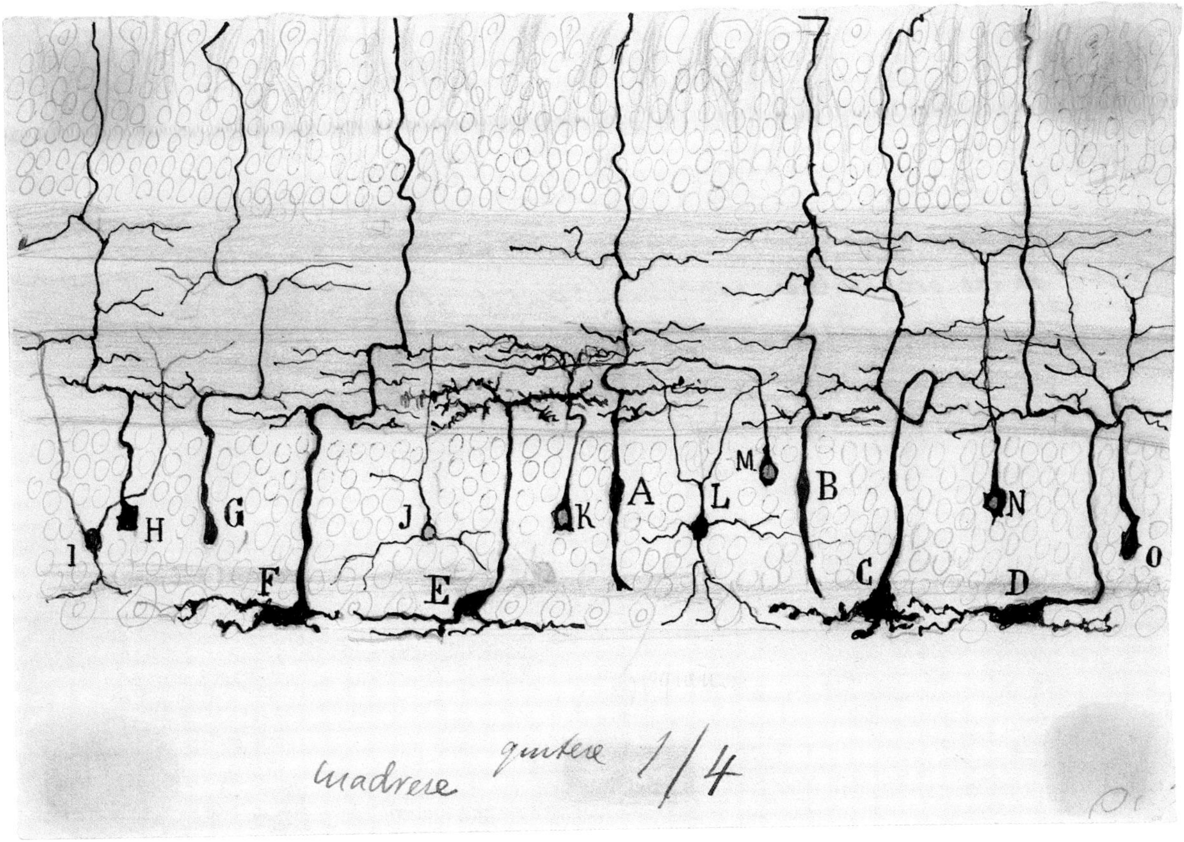

FIGURE 225. Amacrine and granule cells.

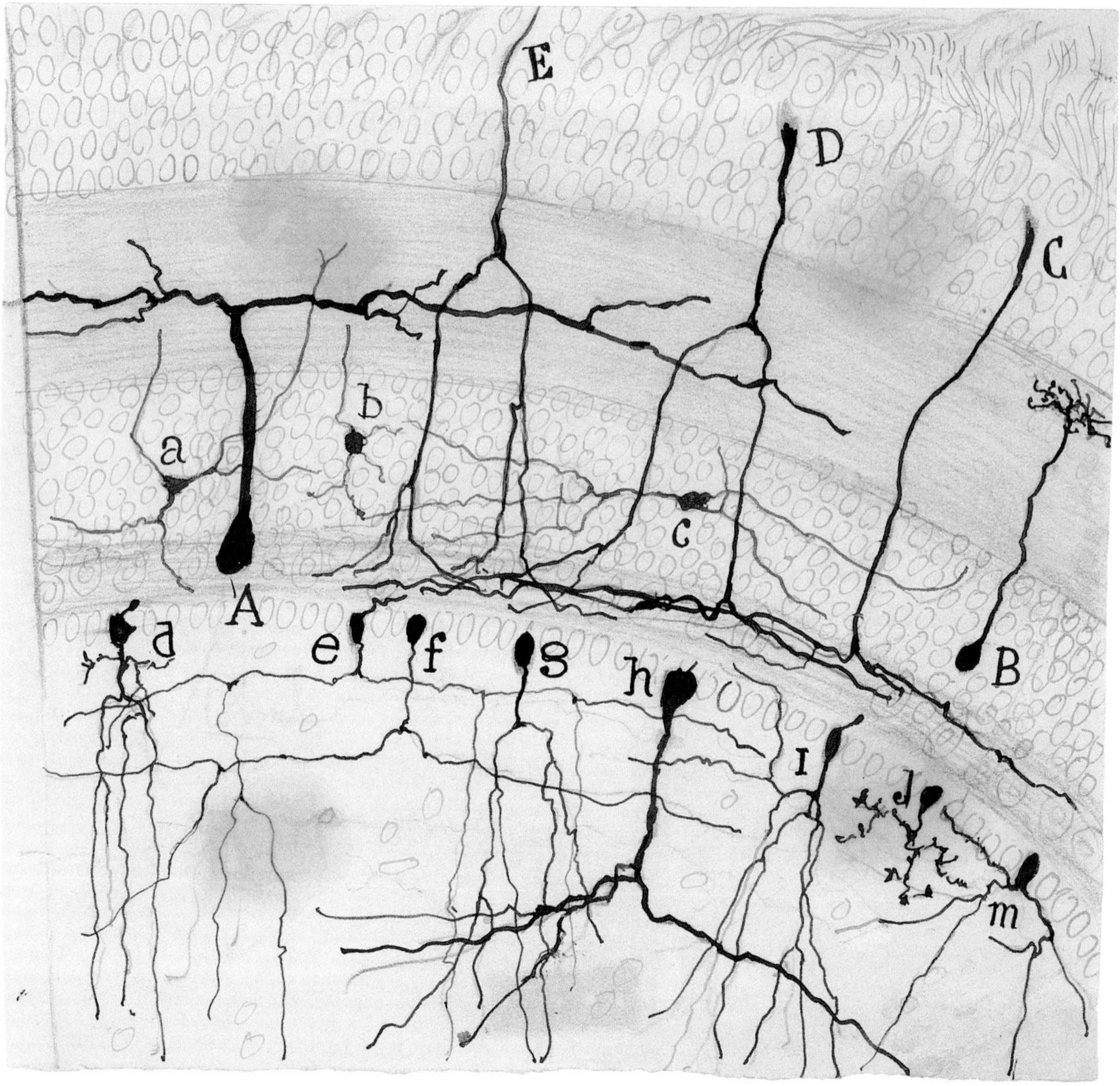

FIGURE 226. Deep retina in the near-adult squid.

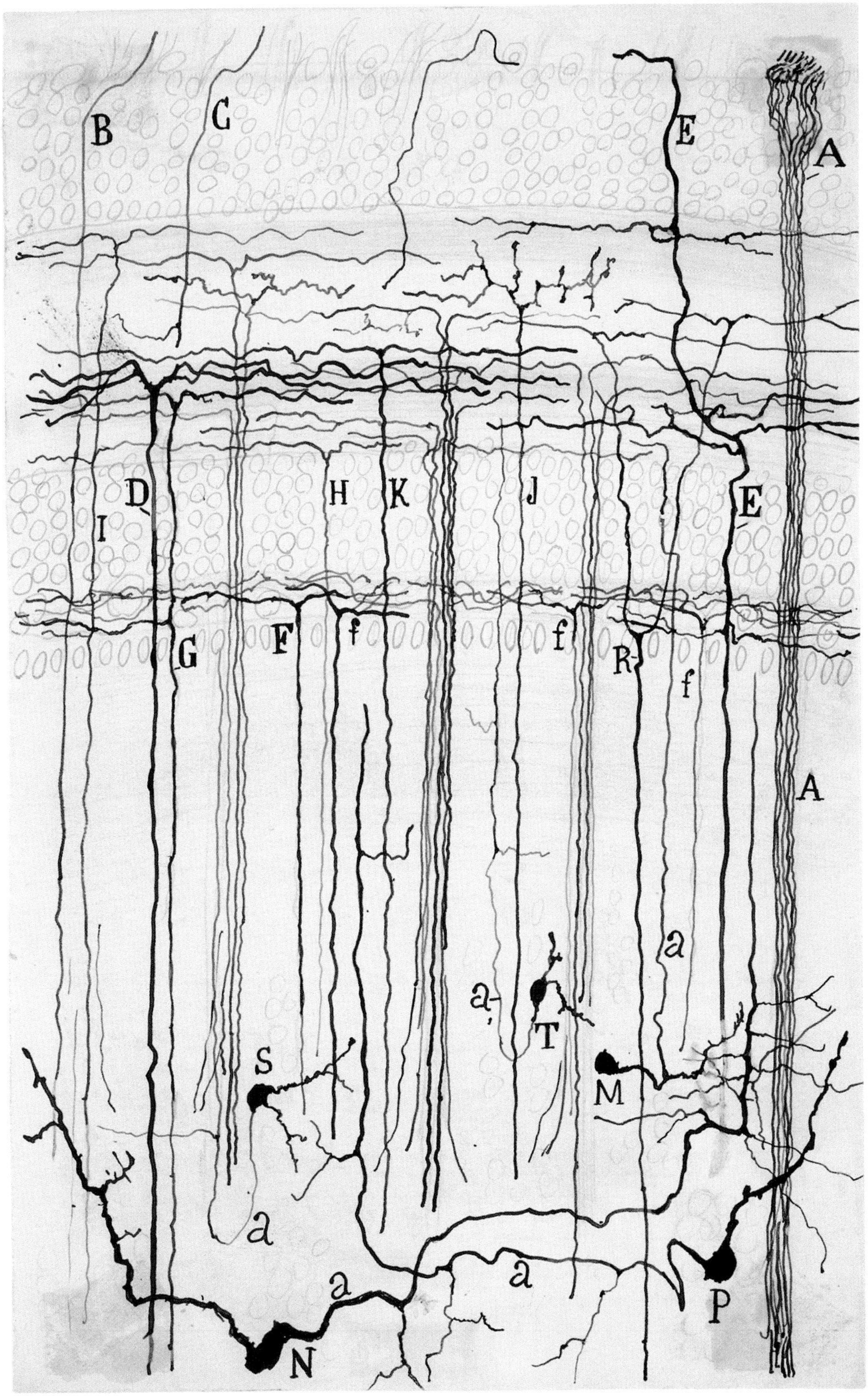

FIGURE 227. Assembly of centrifugal fibers branching onto the intermediate retina.

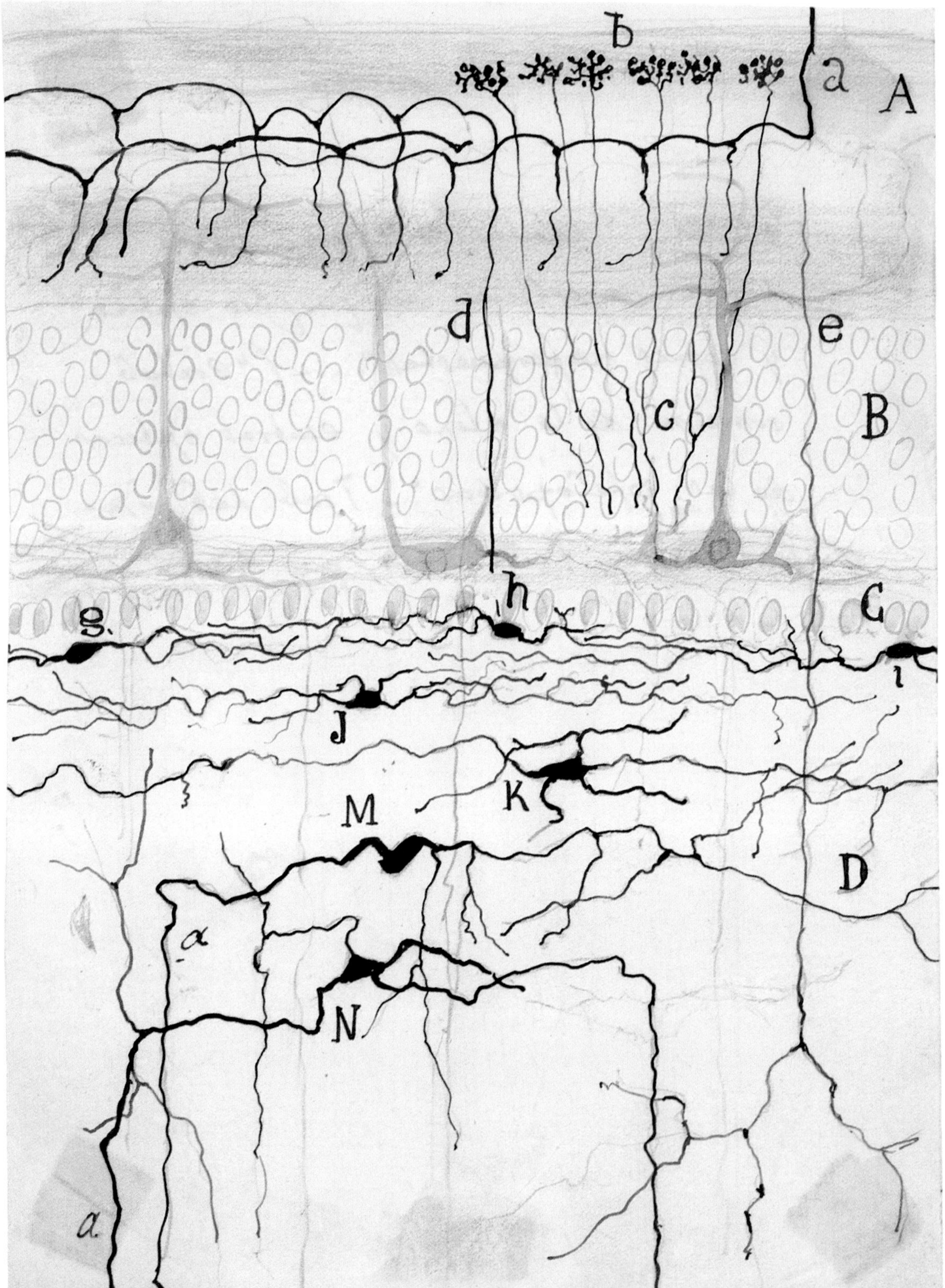

FIGURE 228. Cells of the superficial plexiform layer of the optic ganglion and superimposed layers.

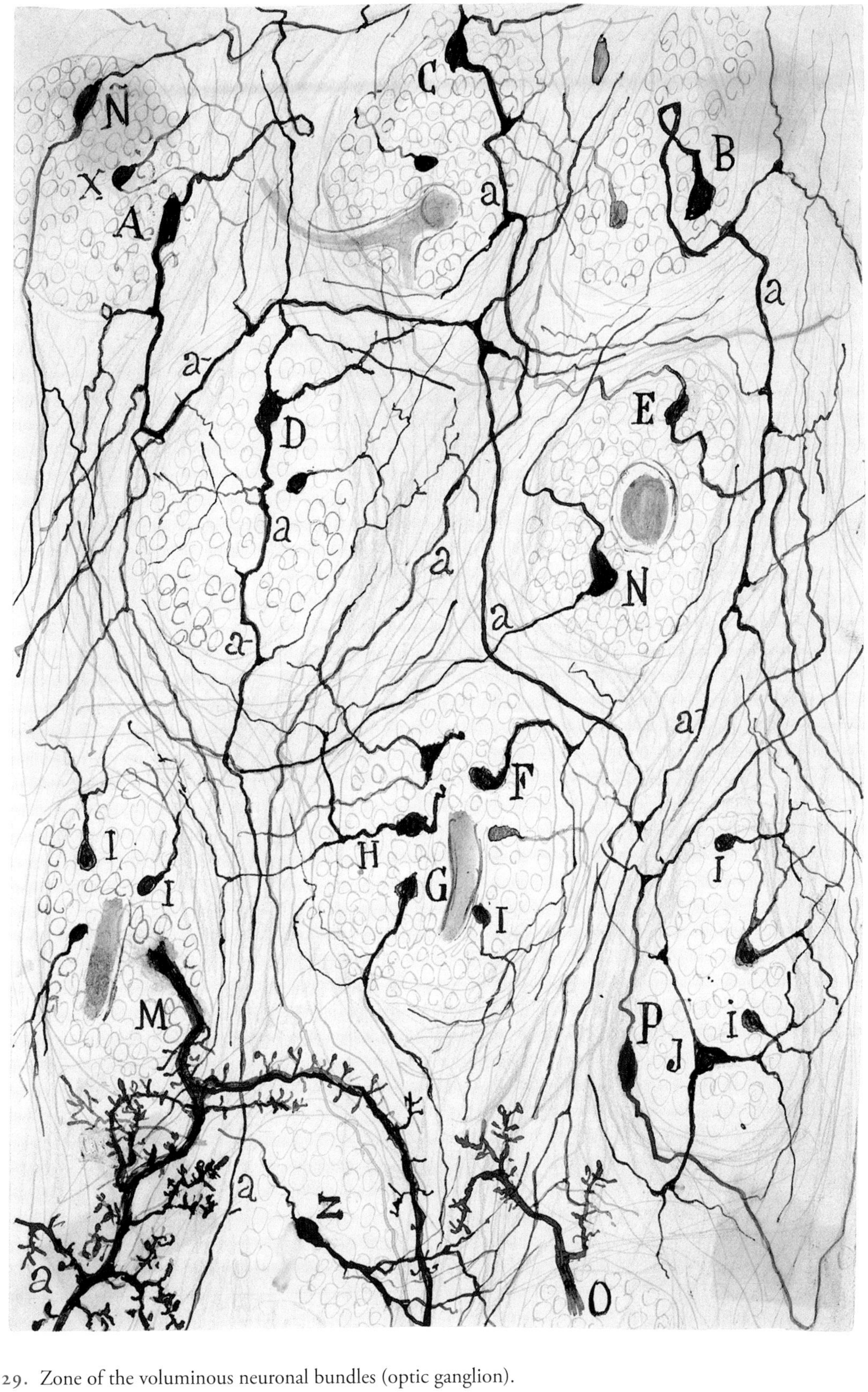

FIGURE 229. Zone of the voluminous neuronal bundles (optic ganglion).

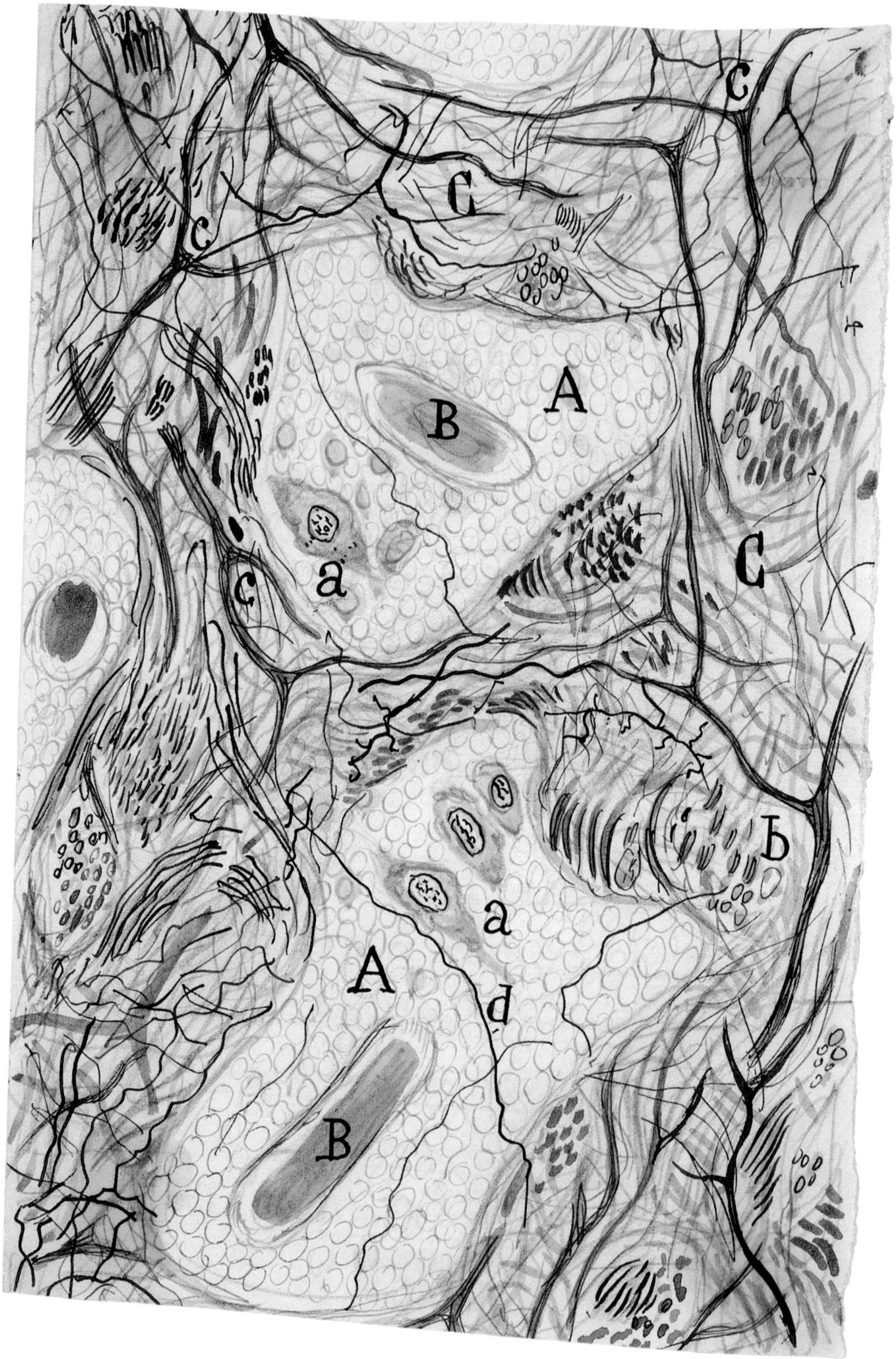

FIGURE 230. Zone of the deep plexiform bundles.

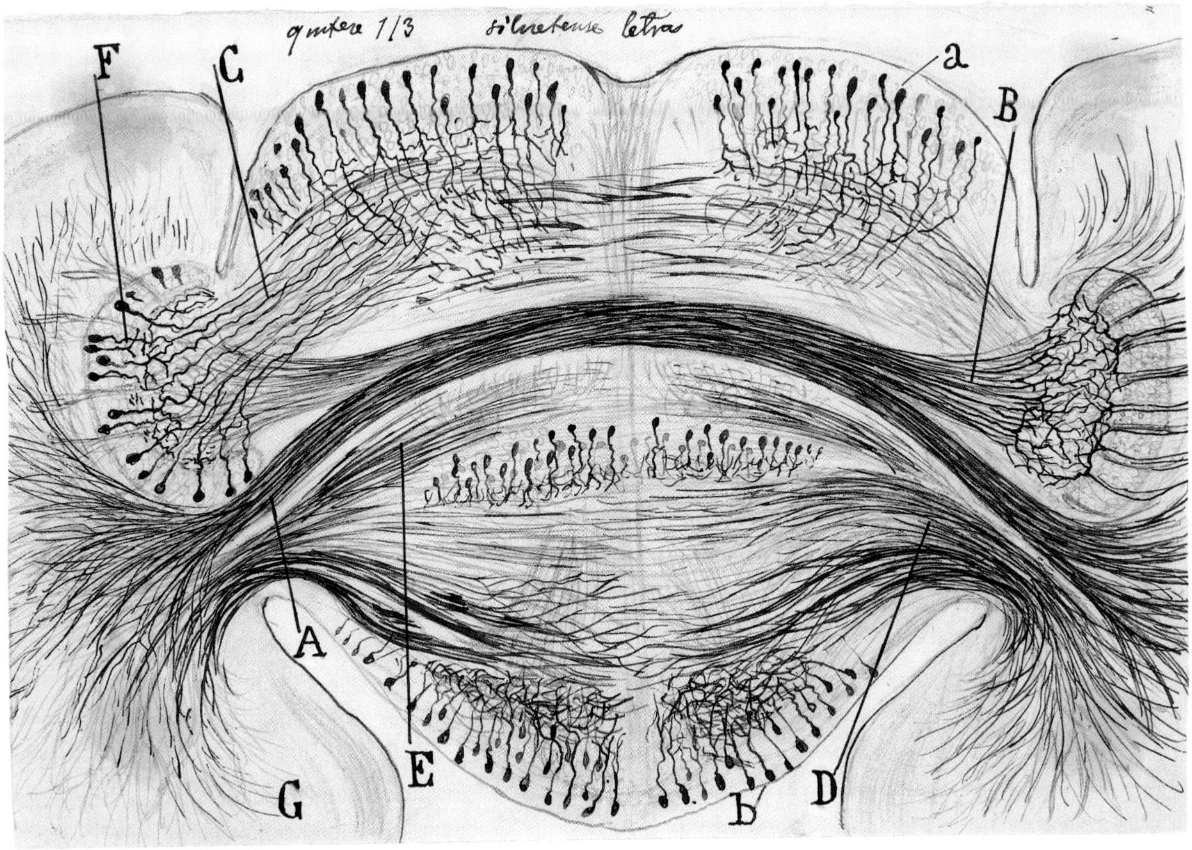

FIGURE 231. Horizontal section of the cerebral ganglion in a sepia.

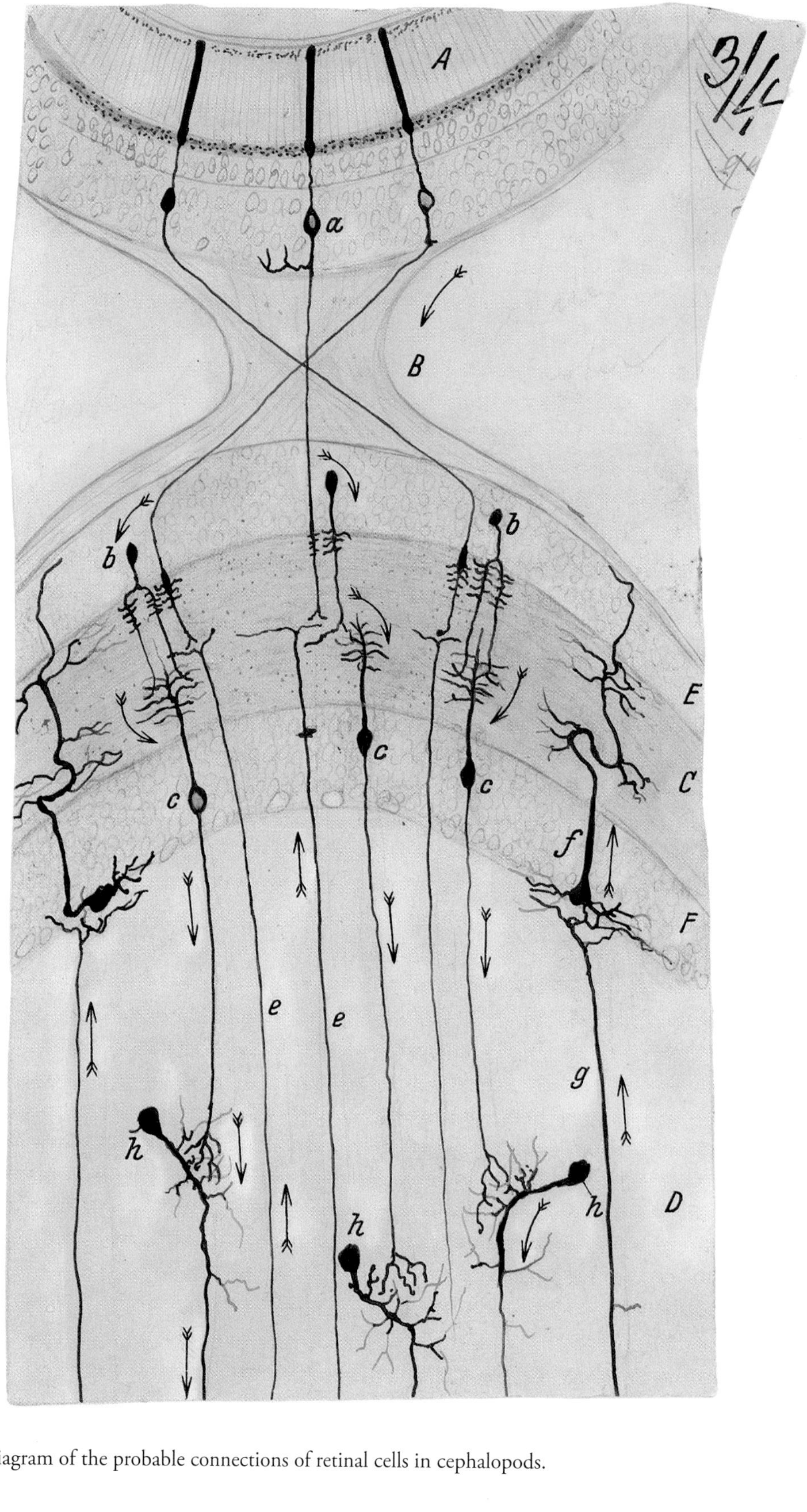

FIGURE 232. Diagram of the probable connections of retinal cells in cephalopods.

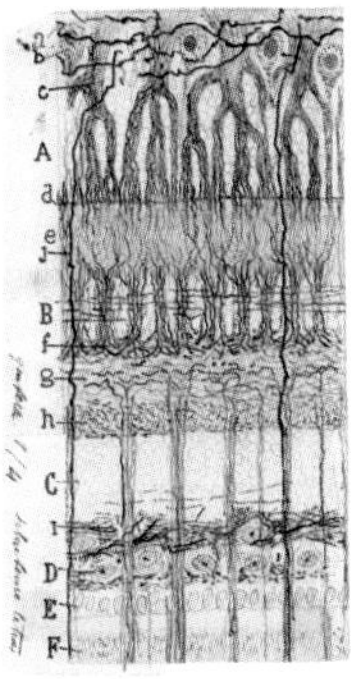

FIGURE 222.

Perpendicular section of the deep retina in an adult sepia.

This figure was published in Cajal, S. R. (1917) Contribución al conocimiento de la retina y centros ópticos de los cefalópodos. *Trab. Lab. Invest. Biol. Univ. Madrid* 15, 1–82 (Figure 15).

FIGURE LEGEND: Perpendicular section of the deep retina in an adult sepia. Reduced silver nitrate method. *A*, Outer layer of amacrine cells; *B*, plexiform layer; *C*, inner layer of amacrine cells; *D*, layer of the lower giant cells; *E*, cellular palisade; *F*, bundles of optical fibers crossing the granule cell layer; *g*, bundles of terminal processes of visual fibers.

Original text: Sección perpendicular de la retina profunda de la sepia adulta. Impregnación con el proceder del nitrato de plata reducido. *A*, capa de las amacrinas externas; *B*, zona plexiforme; *C*, zona de las amacrinas internas; *D*, capa de las células gigantes inferiores; *E*, empalizada celular; *F*, manojos de fibras ópticas cruzando la capa de los granos; *g*, haces de expansiones terminales de fibras visuales.

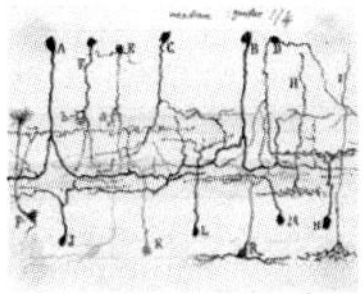

FIGURE 223.

Deep retina in a sepia.

This figure was published in Cajal, S. R. (1917) Contribución al conocimiento de la retina y centros ópticos de los cefalópodos. *Trab. Lab. Invest. Biol. Univ. Madrid* 15, 1–82 (Figure 17).

FIGURE LEGEND: Section of the deep retina in a sepia. Golgi method. In this figure, cells scattered in various preparations have been collected. *A, B, C, D*, and so on, various types of giant amacrine cells; *P, J, K, L*, and so forth, lower or descending amacrine cells; *H, I*, thin descending Kopsch fibers.

Original text: Corte de la retina profunda de la sepia. Método de Golgi. En este dibujo se han reunido células tomadas de varios cortes. *A, B, C, D*, etc., diversas modalidades de amacrinas gigantes; *P, J, K, L*, etc., amacrinas inferiores o descendentes; *H, I*, fibras finas descendentes de Kopsch.

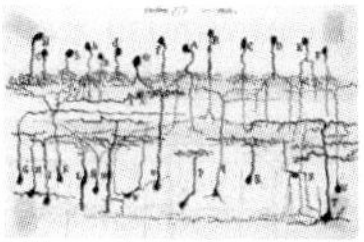

FIGURE 224.

Intermediate retina in a sepia.

This figure was published in Cajal, S. R. (1917) Contribución al conocimiento de la retina y centros ópticos de los cefalópodos. *Trab. Lab. Invest. Biol. Univ. Madrid* 15, 1–82 (Figure 18).

FIGURE LEGEND: Section of the intermediate retina in a sepia. *A, B, C, E, F*, Cells of Lenhossék; *G, H, J, K*, lower amacrine cells; *S*, multipolar amacrine cell; *F*, bistratified lower amacrine cell.

Original text: Corte de la retina intermediaria de la sepia. *A, B, C, E, F*, células de Lenhossék; *G, H, J, K*, amacrinas inferiores; *S*, amacrina multipolar; *F*, amacrina inferior biestratificada.

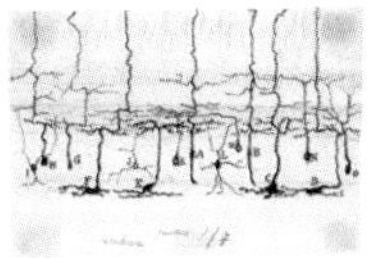

FIGURE 225.

Amacrine and granule cells.

This figure was published in Cajal, S. R. (1917) Contribución al conocimiento de la retina y centros ópticos de los cefalópodos. *Trab. Lab. Invest. Biol. Univ. Madrid* 15, 1–82 (Figure 21).

FIGURE LEGEND: Lower amacrine cells and cells of the inner granule cell layer. *A, B*, Bipolar centrifugal cells; *K, L, H, O*, lower amacrine cells; *F, C, D*, centrifugal collosal cells.

Original text: Células amacrinas inferiores y corpúsculos de la formación de los granos internos. *A* y *B*, células centrífugas bipolares; *K, L, H, O*, amacrinas inferiores; *F, C, D*, células colosales centrífugas.

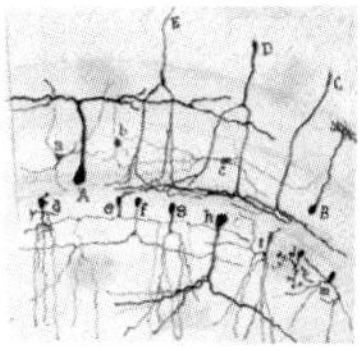

FIGURE 226.

Deep retina in the near-adult squid.

This figure was published in Cajal, S. R. (1917) Contribución al conocimiento de la retina y centros ópticos de los cefalópodos. *Trab. Lab. Invest. Biol. Univ. Madrid* 15, 1–82 (Figure 23).

FIGURE LEGEND: Section of the deep retina in the near-adult squid. *A*, Giant lower amacrine cell; *B*, amacrine cell with a short tuft; *C, D, E*, amacrine cells (?) destined to the fibrillar stria; *b, c*, multipolar cells of the inner granule cell layer; *d, e, f, g, h, i, j, m*, cells of the palisade of Kopsch.

Original text: Corte de la retina profunda del calamar casi adulto. *A*, amacrina inferior gigante; *B*, amacrína de penacho recogido; *C, D, E*, amacrinas (?) destinadas a la estría fibrilar; *b, c*, celulas multipolares de la capa de los granos internos; *d, e, f, g, h, i, j, m*, corpúsculos de la empalizada de Kopsch.

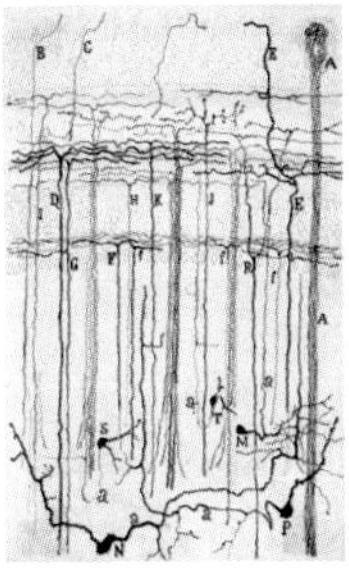

FIGURE 227.

Assembly of centrifugal fibers branching onto the intermediate retina.

This figure was published in Cajal, S. R. (1917) Contribución al conocimiento de la retina y centros ópticos de los cefalópodos. *Trab. Lab. Invest. Biol. Univ. Madrid* 15, 1–82 (Figure 24).

FIGURE LEGEND: Assembly of centrifugal fibers branching onto the intermediate retina. Adult sepia. Golgi method. In this figure, fibers observed in various preparations have been collected.

Original text: Conjunto de las fibras centrífugas arborizadas por la retina intermediaria. Sepia adulta. Método de Golgi. En esta figura se han reunido fibras recogidas en varios cortes.

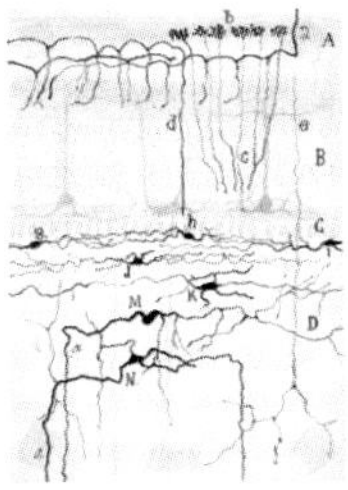

FIGURE 228.

Cells of the superficial plexiform layer of the optic ganglion and superimposed layers.

This figure was published in Cajal, S. R. (1917) Contribución al conocimiento de la retina y centros ópticos de los cefalópodos. *Trab. Lab. Invest. Biol. Univ. Madrid* 15, 1–82 (Figure 26).

FIGURE LEGEND: Cells of the superficial plexiform layer of the optic ganglion and superimposed layers. Near-adult sepia. *g, h, i, j*, Small horizontal cells; *M, N*, cells with an apparently long axon that represents modifications of the mitral type; *J, A*, plexiform layer of the deep retina; *B*, inner layer of amacrine cells; *d*, arciform fibers. The letter *a* indicates the probable axon.

Original text: Células de la zona plexiforme superficial del ganglio óptico y capas superpuestas. Sepia casi adulta. *g, h, i, j*, pequeños elementos horizontales; *M, N*, corpúsculos al parecer de axon largo, variantes del tipo mitral; *J, A*, zona, plexiforme de la retina profunda; *B*, zona de las amacrinas internas; *d*, fibras arciformes; la letra *a* marca el axon probable.

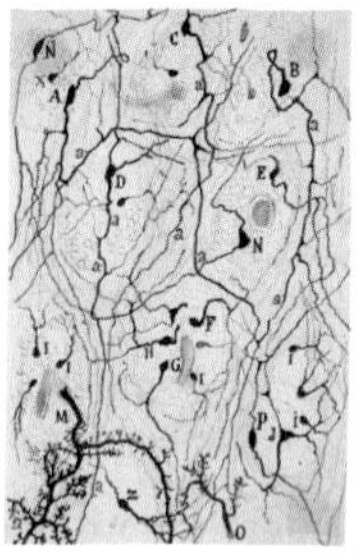

FIGURE 229.

Zone of the voluminous neuronal bundles (optic ganglion).

This figure was published in Cajal, S. R. (1917) Contribución al conocimiento de la retina y centros ópticos de los cefalópodos. *Trab. Lab. Invest. Biol. Univ. Madrid* 15, 1–82 (Figure 31).

FIGURE LEGEND: Zone of the voluminous neuronal bundles (optic ganglion). *I*, Minute cells of the cellular nests; *F, G, H*, cells in T; *E, N*, bipolar cells; *A, D, B, C*, cells with descending axon; *M*, cells with downy shafts.

Original text: Zona de los cordones neuronales voluminosos (ganglio óptico). *I*, corpúsculos diminutos de los nidos celulares; *F, G, H*, células en T; *E, N*, corpúsculos bipolares; *A, D, B, C*, células de axon descendente; *M*, corpúsculos de tallos vellosos.

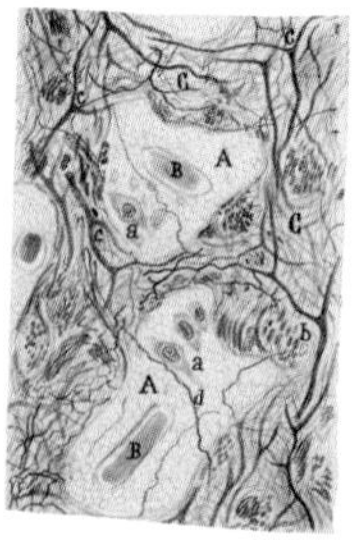

FIGURE 230.

Zone of the deep plexiform bundles.

This figure was published in Cajal, S. R. (1917) Contribución al conocimiento de la retina y centros ópticos de los cefalópodos. *Trab. Lab. Invest. Biol. Univ. Madrid* 15, 1–82 (Figure 33).

FIGURE LEGEND: Zone of the deep plexiform bundles as seen in preparations stained with reduced silver nitrate. *A*, Cell nests; *B*, blood vessels; *e*, plexiform bundles; *a*, giant neurons; *b*, bifurcations of nerve fibers; *d*, fibrils that cross the nests.

Original text: Aspecto de la zona de los cordones plexiformes profundos en los preparados del nitrato de plata reducido. *A*, nidos celulares; *B*, vasos sanguíneos; *e*, cordones plexiformes; *a*, neuronas gigantes; *b*, bifurcaciones de fibras nerviosas; *d*, fibrillas que cruzan los nidos.

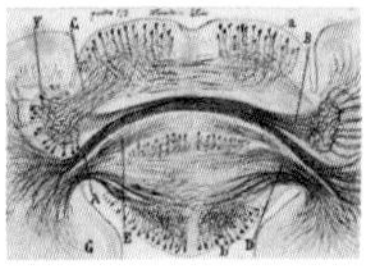

FIGURE 231.

Horizontal section of the cerebral ganglion in a sepia.

This figure was published in Cajal, S. R. (1917) Contribución al conocimiento de la retina y centros ópticos de los cefalópodos. *Trab. Lab. Invest. Biol. Univ. Madrid* 15, 1–82 (Figure 38).

FIGURE LEGEND: Horizontal section of the cerebral ganglion in a sepia a few weeks old. Semischematic figure. *A*, Crossed optical bundle; *B*, termination of this bundle in the opposite peduncular nucleus; *C*, reflex optic pathway originating in the peduncular nucleus; *D*, bundle of the optic corona radiata destined to the anterior lobe of the cerebral nucleus; *E*, bundle destined to the middle lobe; *F*, cortex of the peduncular nucleus.

Original text: Corte horizontal del centro cerebroide de la sepia de algunas semanas. Figura semiesquemática. *A*, cordón óptico cruzado; *B*, terminación de este cordón en el foco peduncular contrapuesto; *C*, vía óptica refleja nacida en el núcleo peduncular; *D*, manojo de la corona óptica radiante destinada al lóbulo anterior del foco cerebroide; *E*, cordón destinado al lóbulo medio; *F*, corteza del núcleo peduncular.

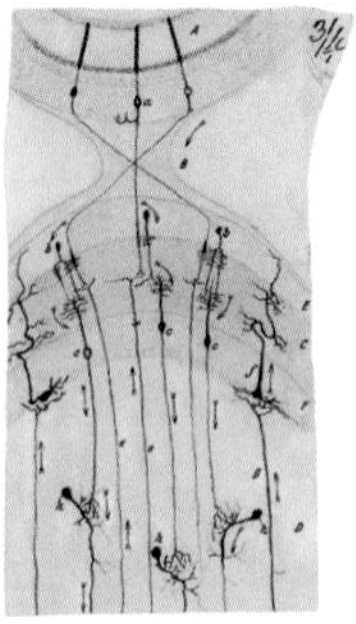

FIGURE 232.

Diagram of the probable connections of retinal cells in cephalopods.

This figure was published in Cajal, S. R. (1917) Contribución al conocimiento de la retina y centros ópticos de los cefalópodos. *Trab. Lab. Invest. Biol. Univ. Madrid* 15, 1–82 (Figure 42).

FIGURE LEGEND: Diagram of the probable connections of retinal cells in cephalopods. *A*, Retina with the rods; *B*, chiasmatic bundle; *C*, deep retina; *D*, optic ganglion; *E*, outer granule cells; *F*, inner granule cells; *a*, rod or first visual neuron; *b*, bipolar cell or second visual neuron; *c*, ganglion cell or third visual neuron; *h*, cell of the optic ganglion (fourth visual neuron); *e*, centrifugal fiber with an arborization that ends at the foot of the rods and tuft of amacrine cells; *g*, centrifugal fiber to the colossal cells with ascending axon (*f*).

Original text: Esquema de las conexiones probables de las células de la retina de los cefalópodos. *A*, retina con los bastones; *B*, cordón kiasmático; *C*, retina profunda; *D*, ganglio óptico; *E*, granos externos; *F*, granos internos; *a*, bastón o primera neurona visual; *b*, céula bipolar o segunda neurona visual; *c*, célula gangliónica o tercera neurona visual; *h*, corpúsculo del ganglio óptico (cuarta neurona visual); *e*, fibra centrífuga cuya arborización concurre en el pie de los bastones y penacho de las amacrinas; *g*, centrífuga para los elementos colosales de axon ascendente (*f*).

SECTION J

Insect Brain: Visual System

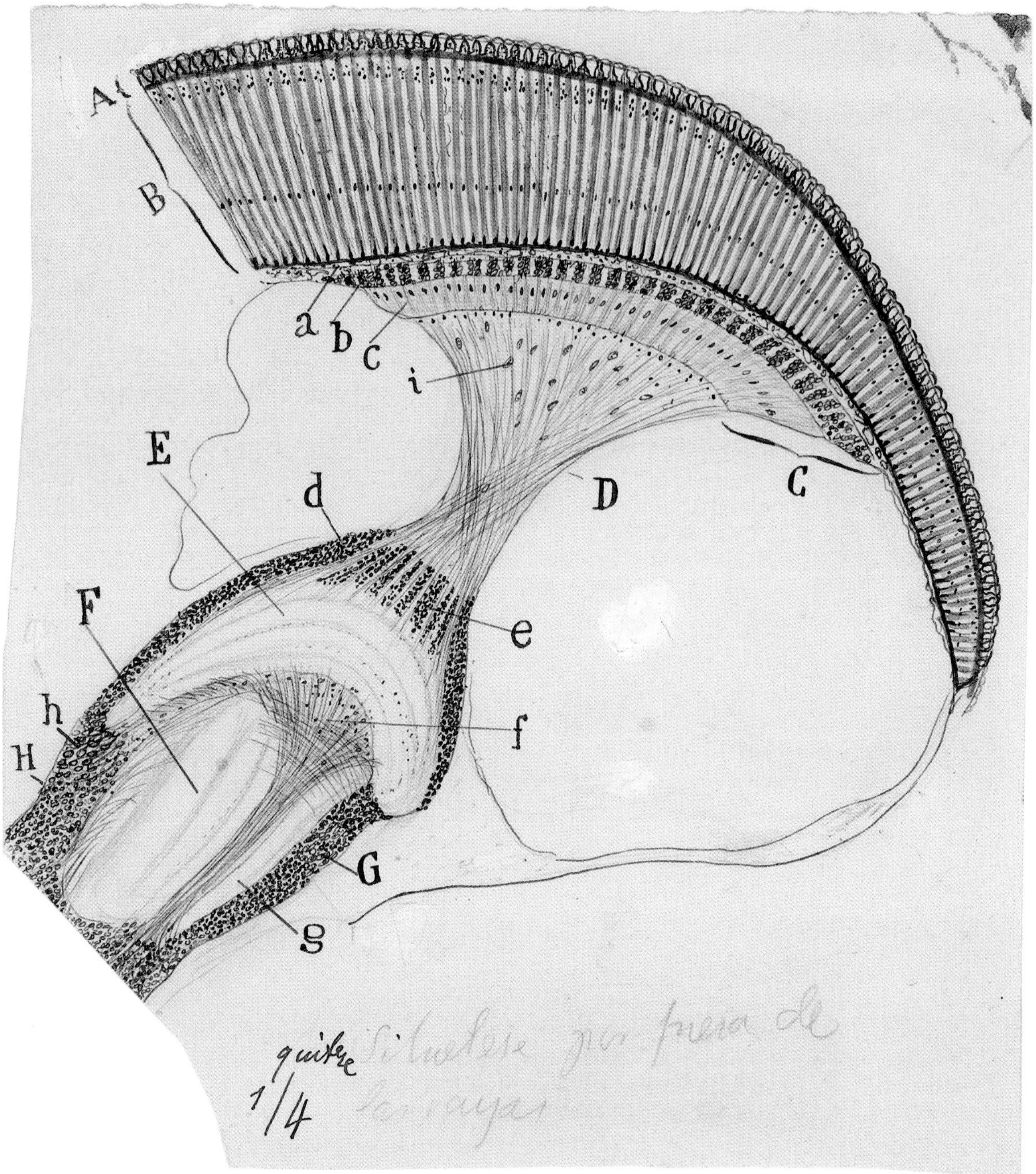

FIGURE 233. Frontal section of the eye and optic lobe in *Musca vomitoria*.

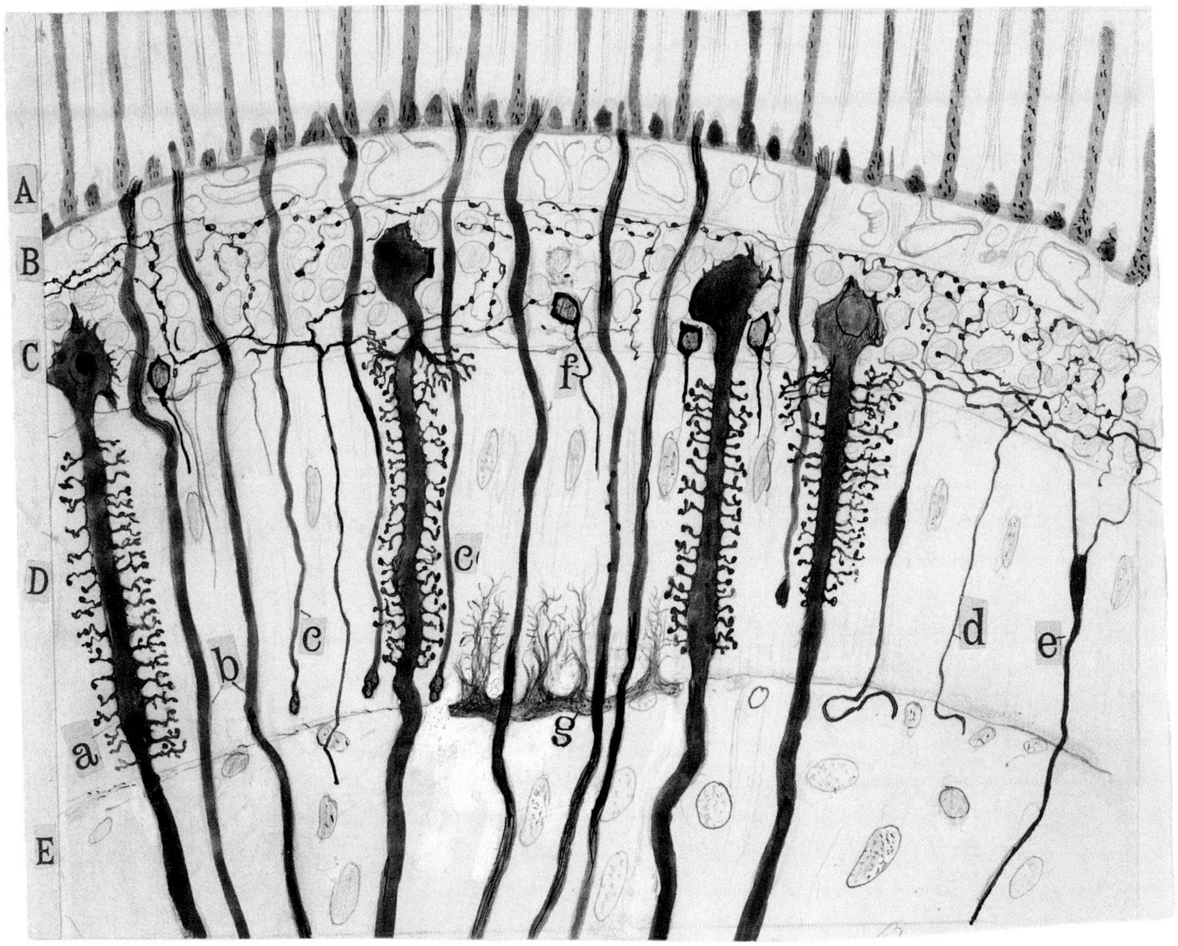

FIGURE 234. Detail from a perioptic frontal section in *Musca vomitoria.*

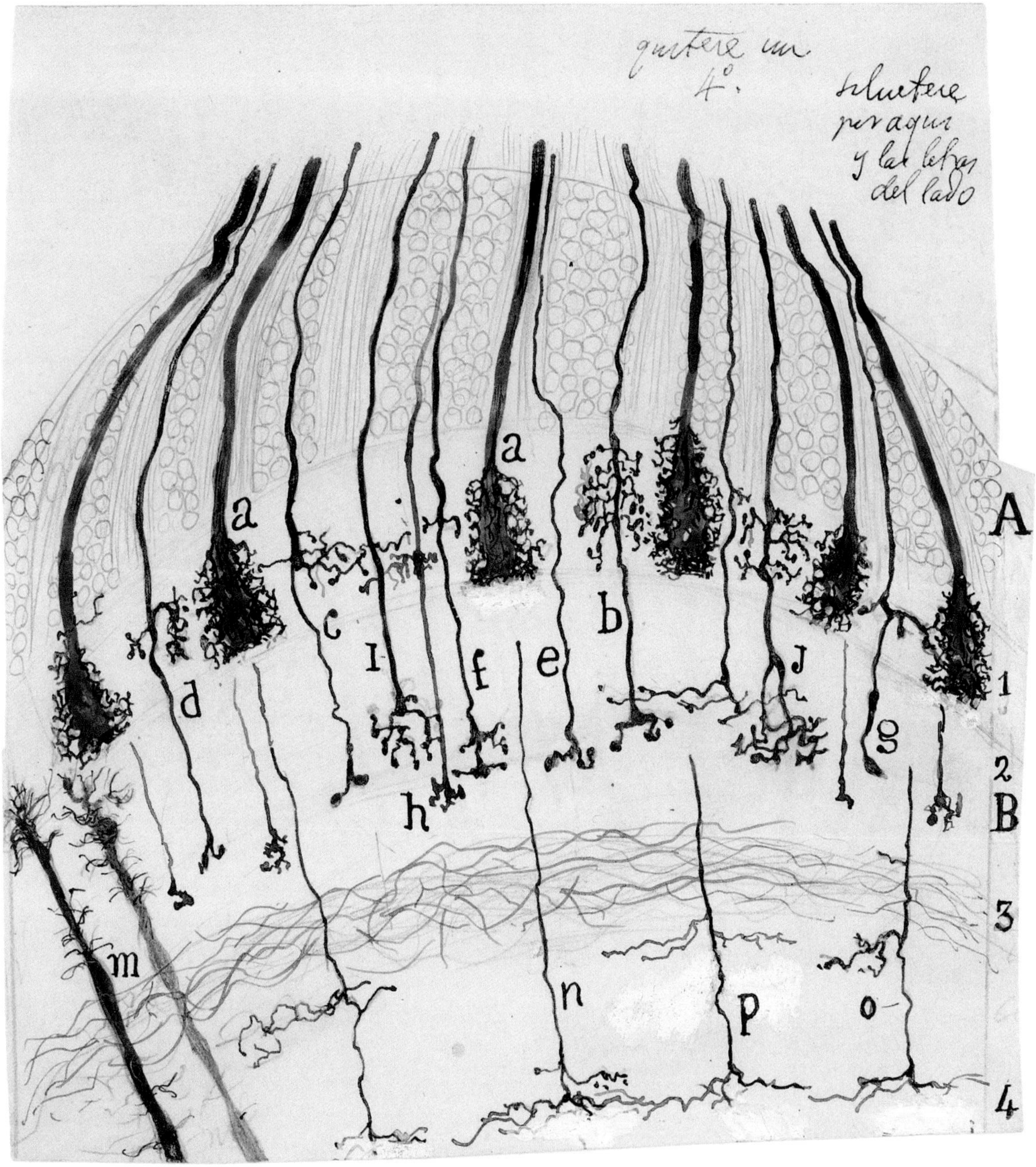

FIGURE 235. Detail of a frontal section from the optic lobe in *Musca vomitoria*.

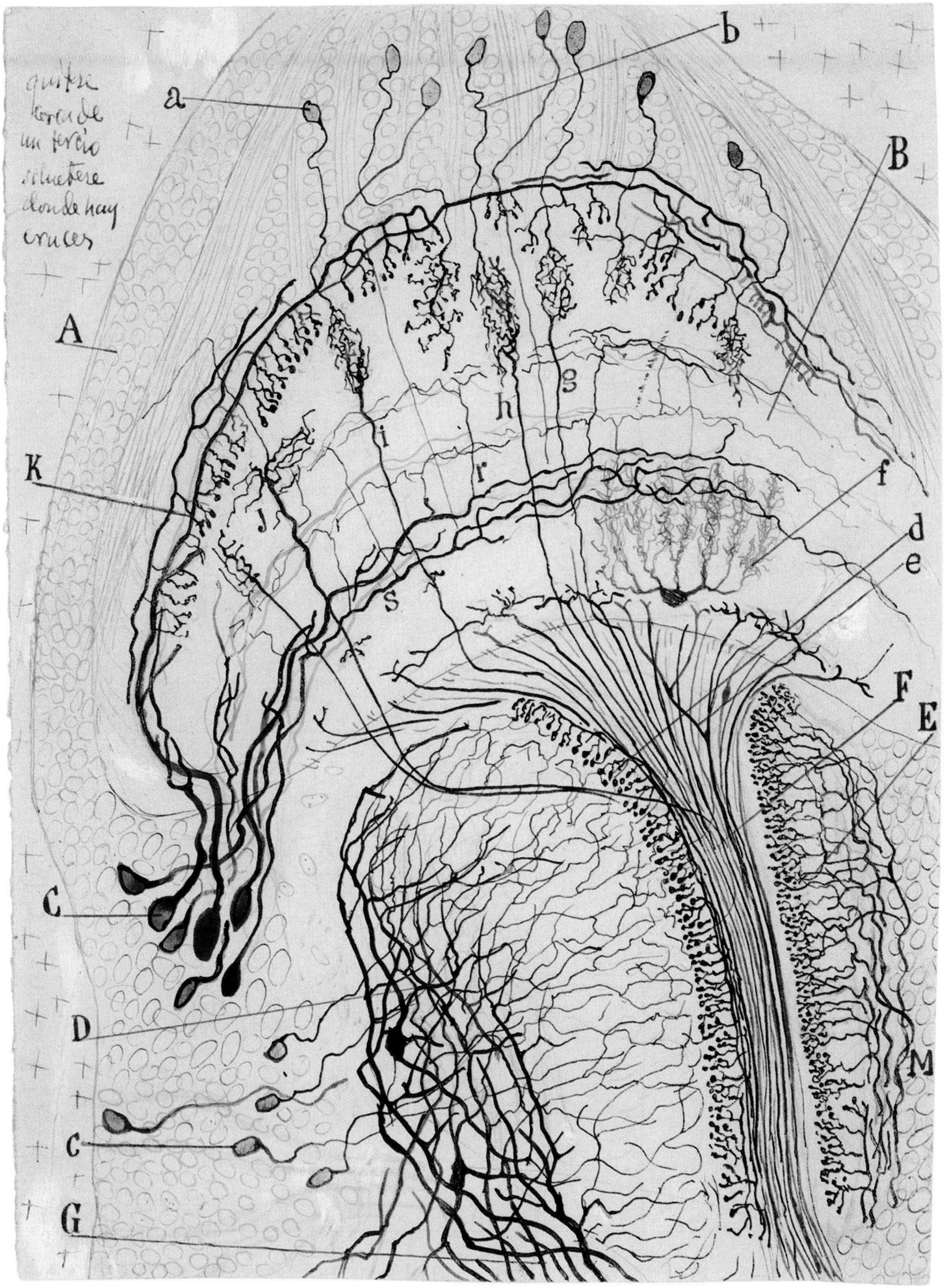

FIGURE 236. Optic lobe (epioptic) and internal medullary mass of a muscid.

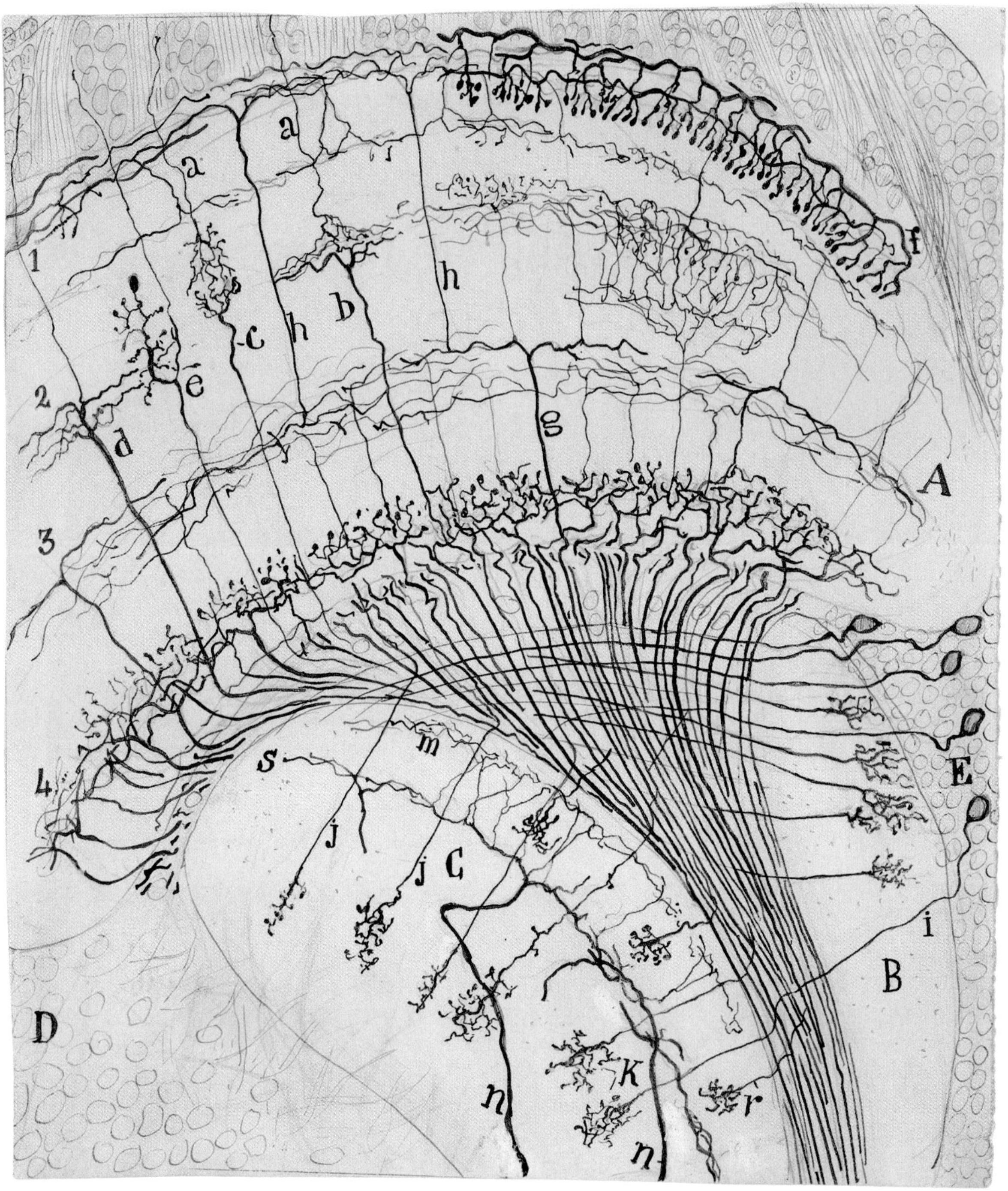

FIGURE 237. Frontal section of the epioptic and internal medullary mass of a muscid.

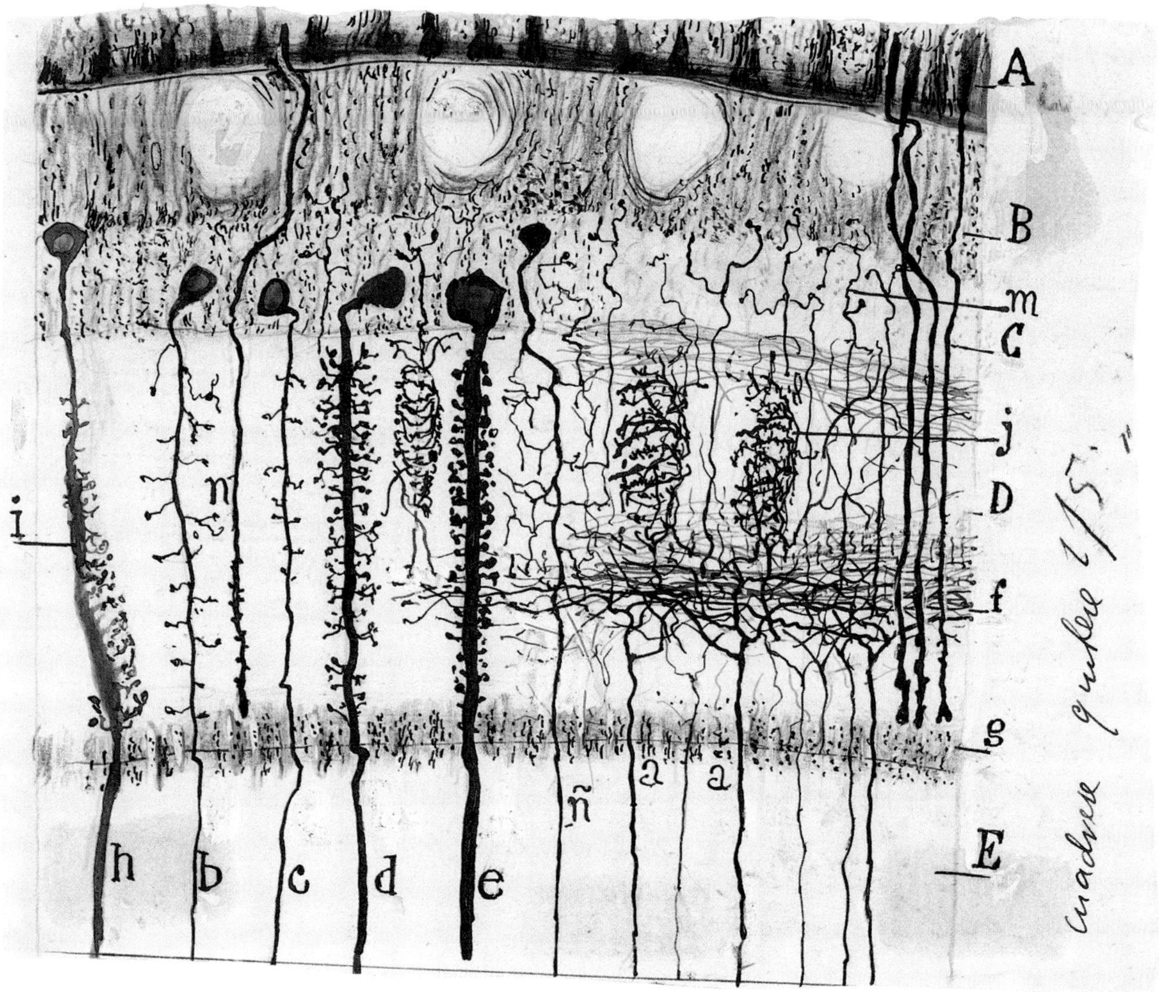

FIGURE 238. Intermediate retina in *Libellula*.

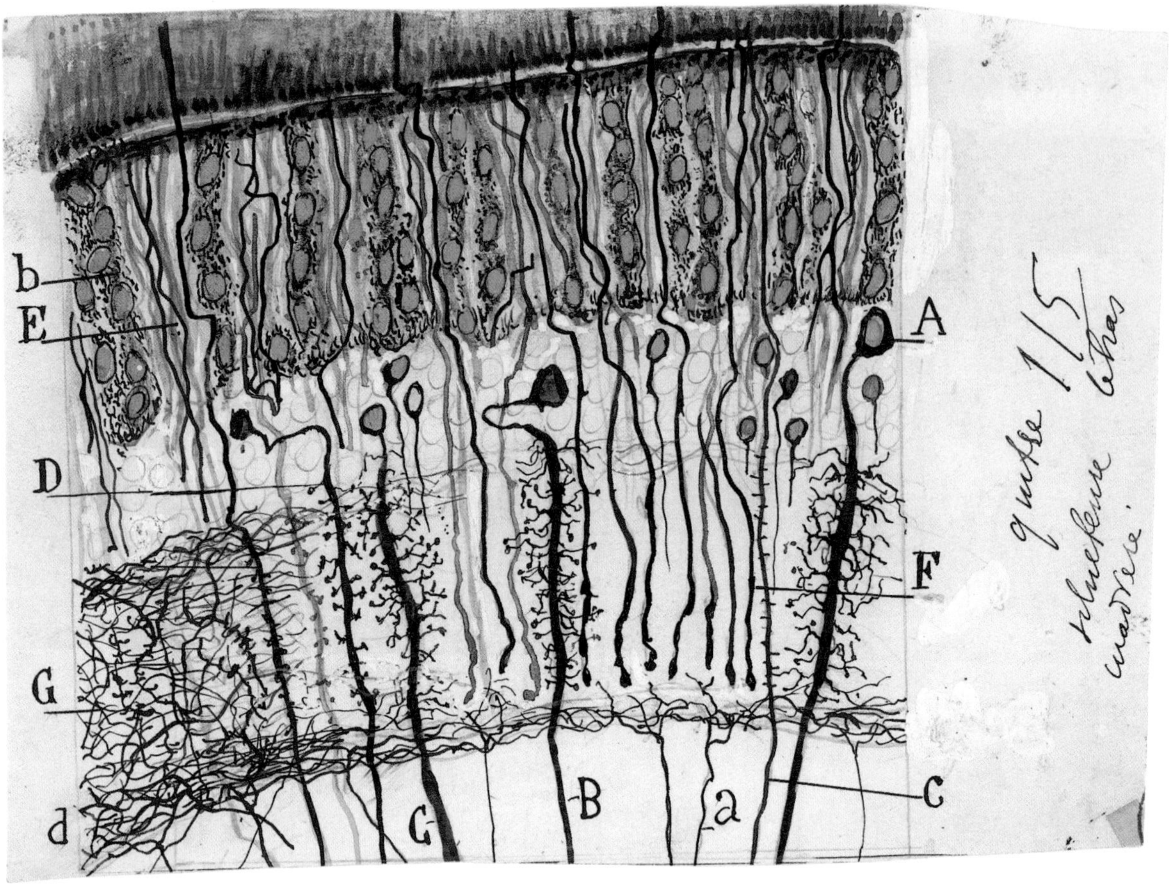

FIGURE 239. Intermediate retina in a lepidopteran.

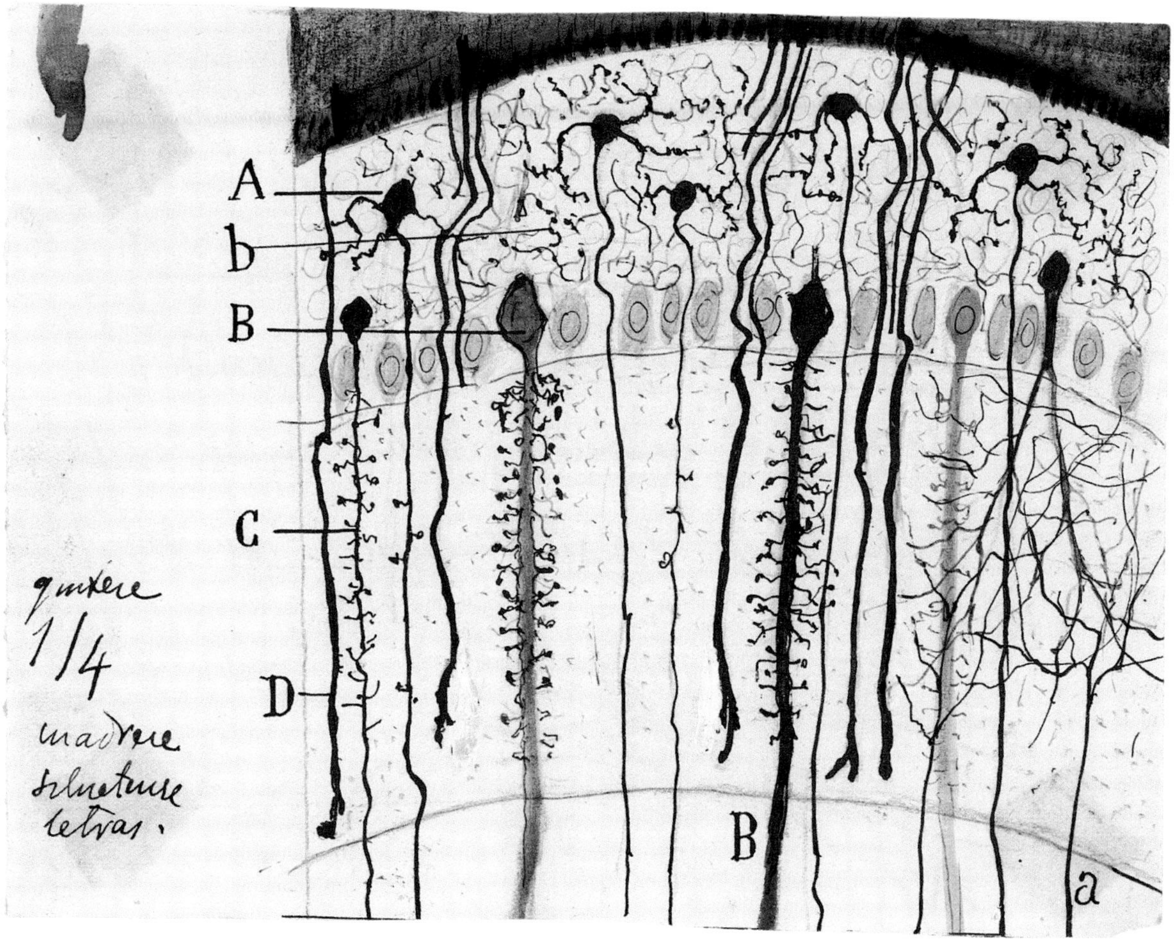

FIGURE 240. Intermediate retina in *Agrion.*

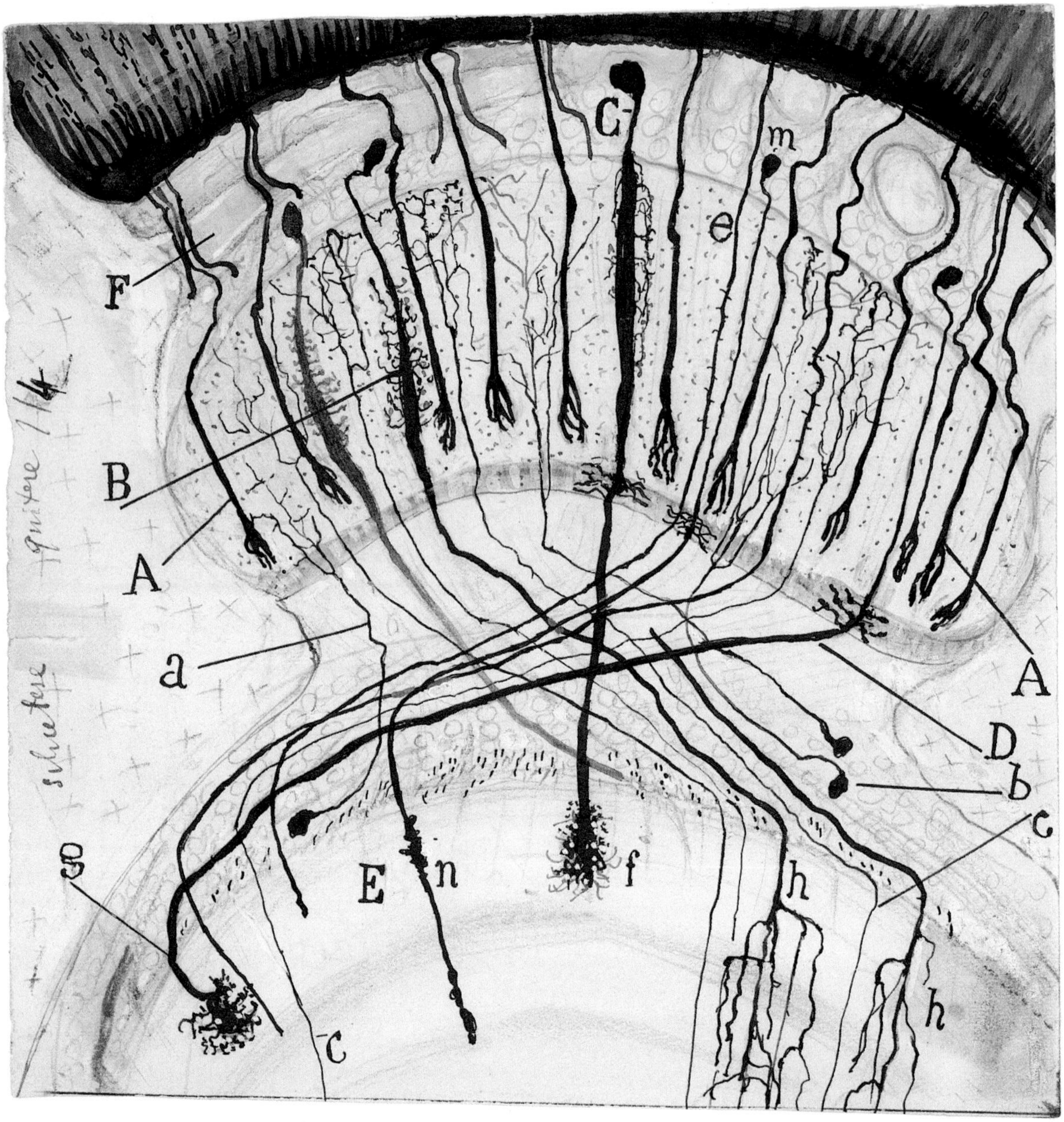

FIGURE 241. Horizontal section of the retina in a bee.

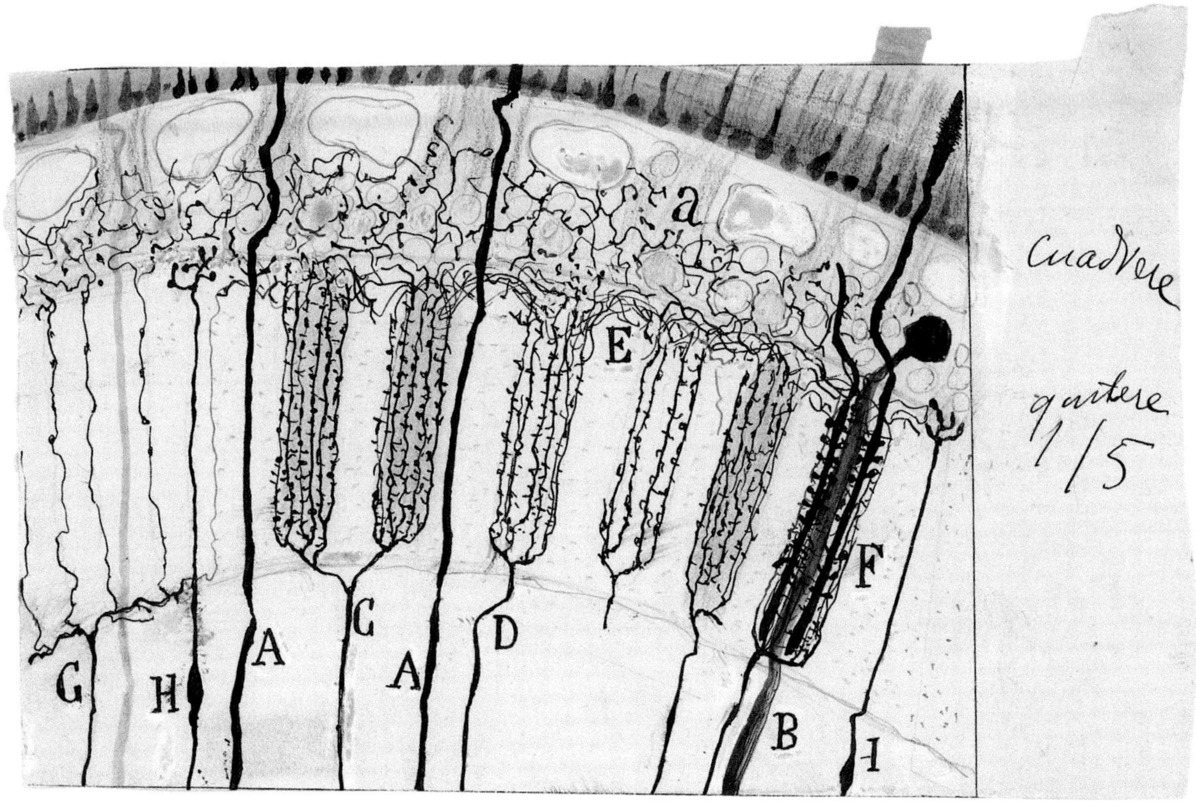

FIGURE 242. Nervous plexi of the intermediate retina in a blowfly.

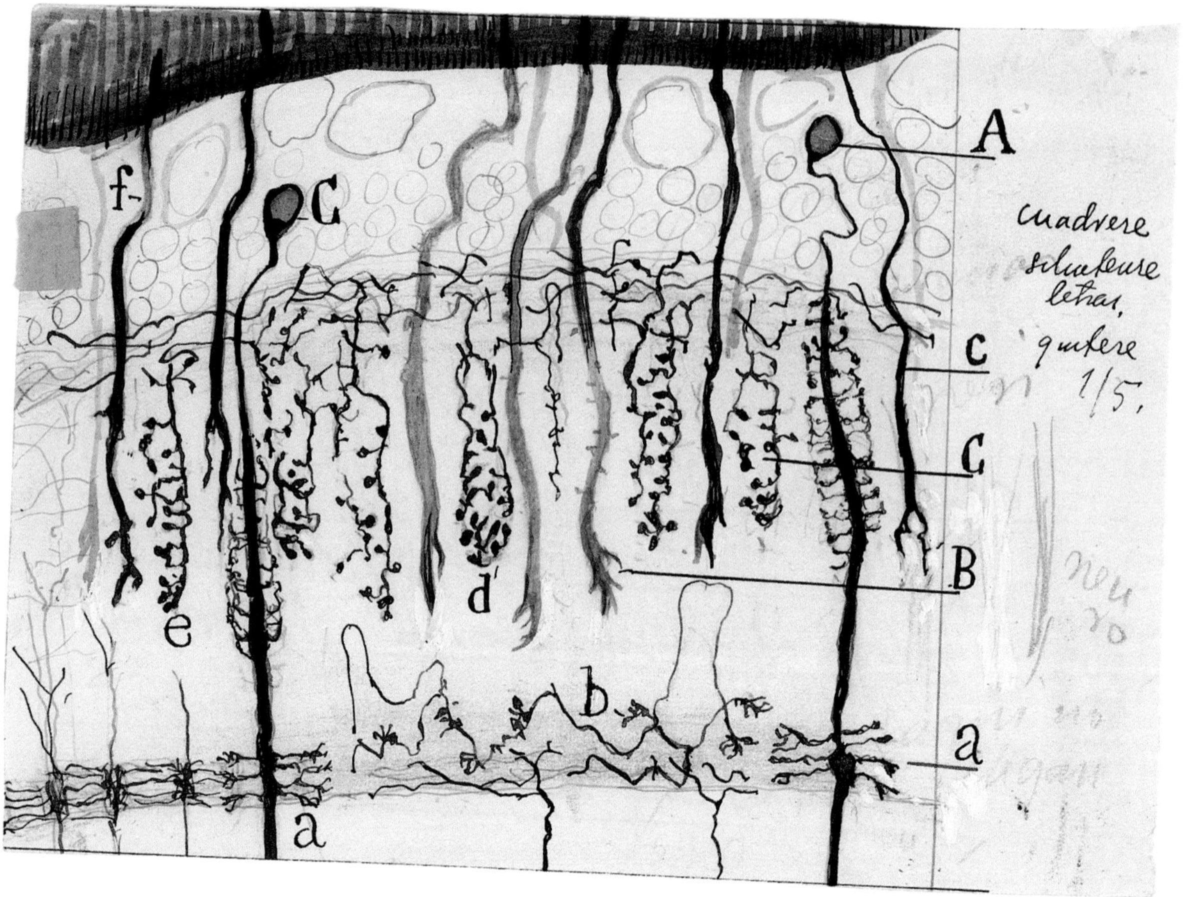

FIGURE 243. Nervous prominences from intermediate retina in a honeybee.

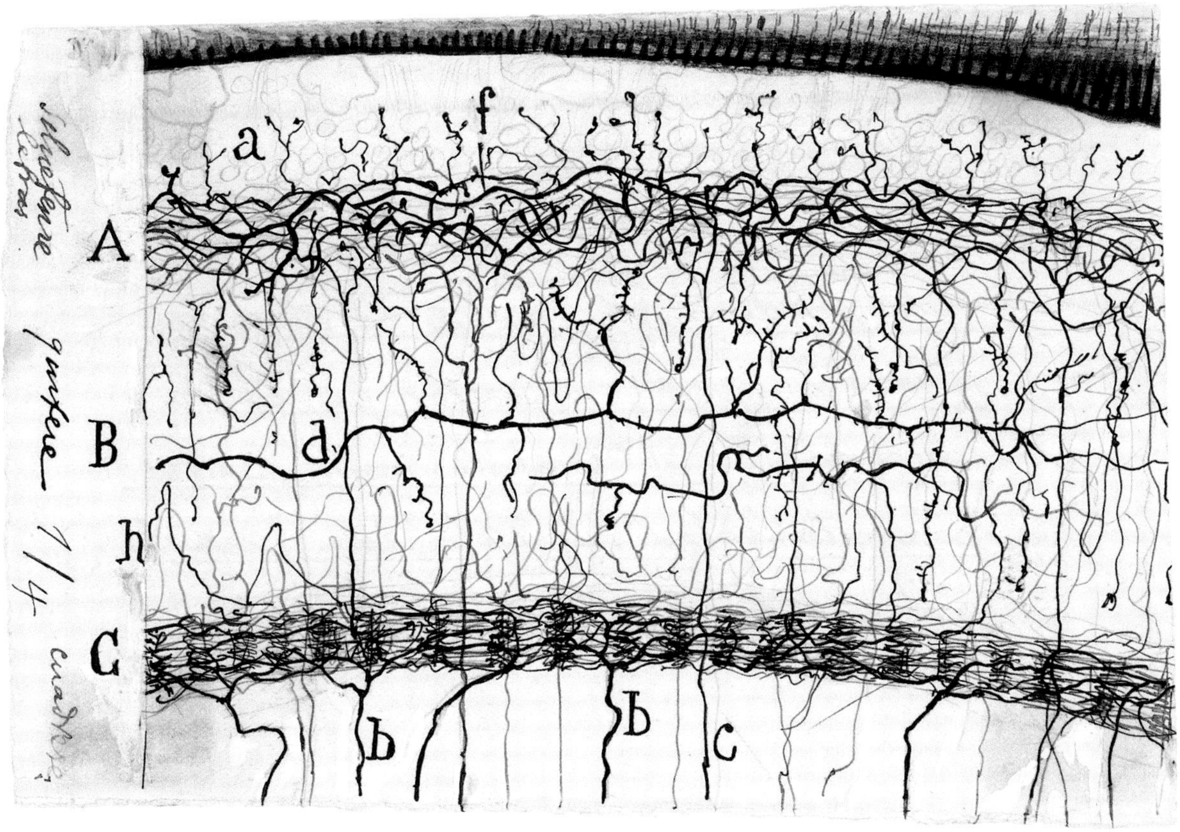

FIGURE 244. Frontal section of the intermediate retina in a honeybee.

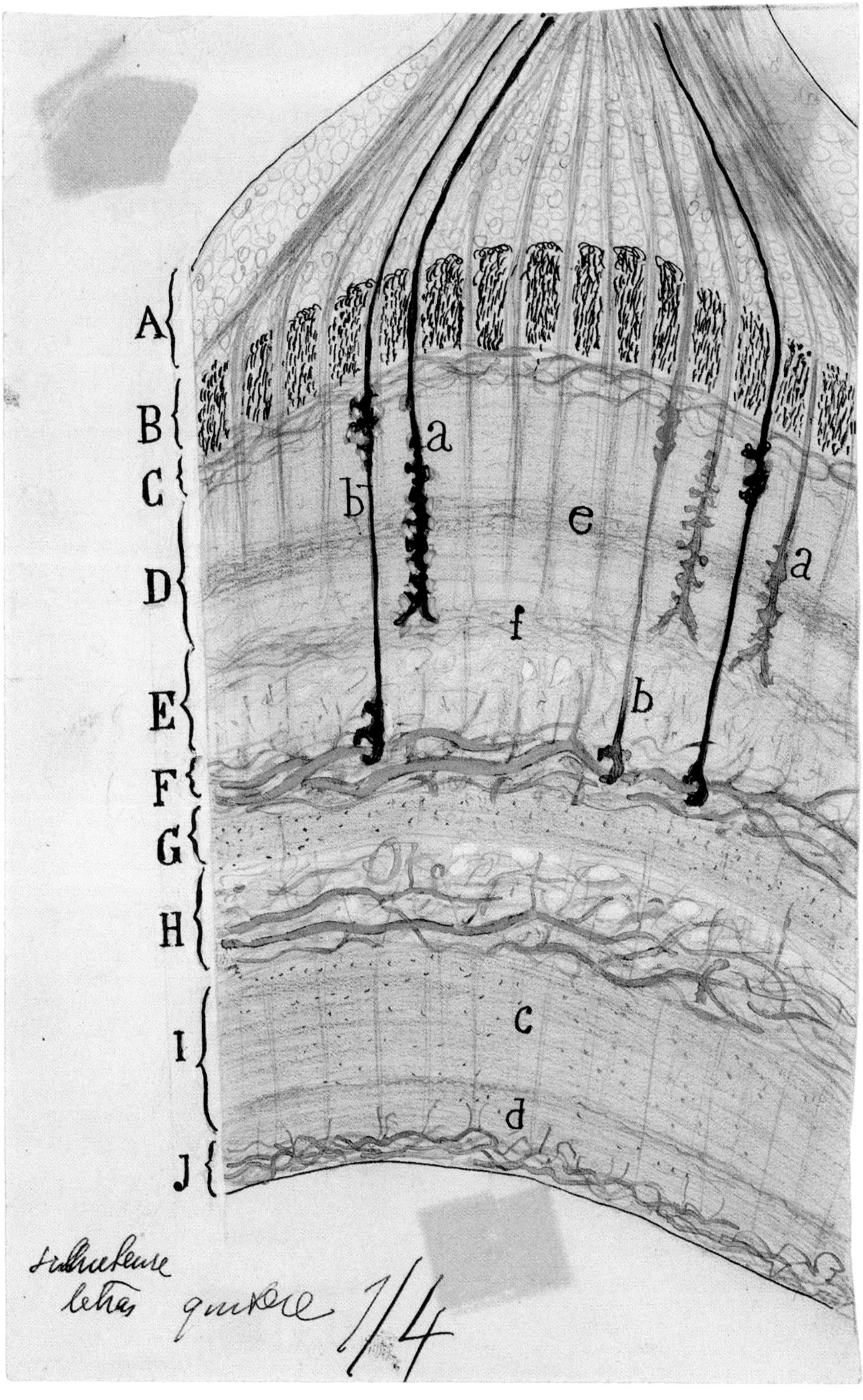

FIGURE 245. Layers of connections from the plexiform formation in the deep retina in a gadfly.

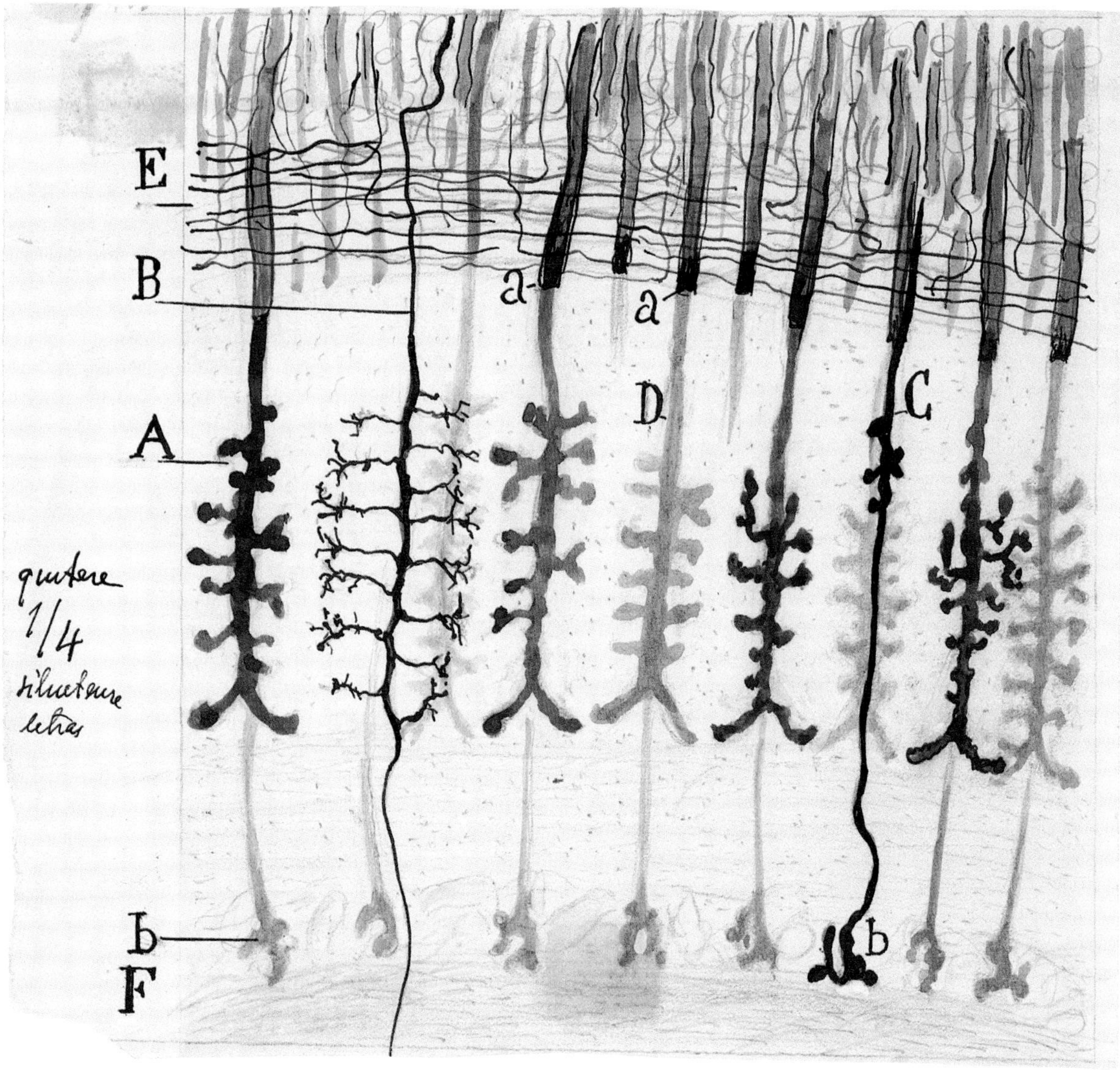

FIGURE 246. Frontal section from the deep retina in a gadfly.

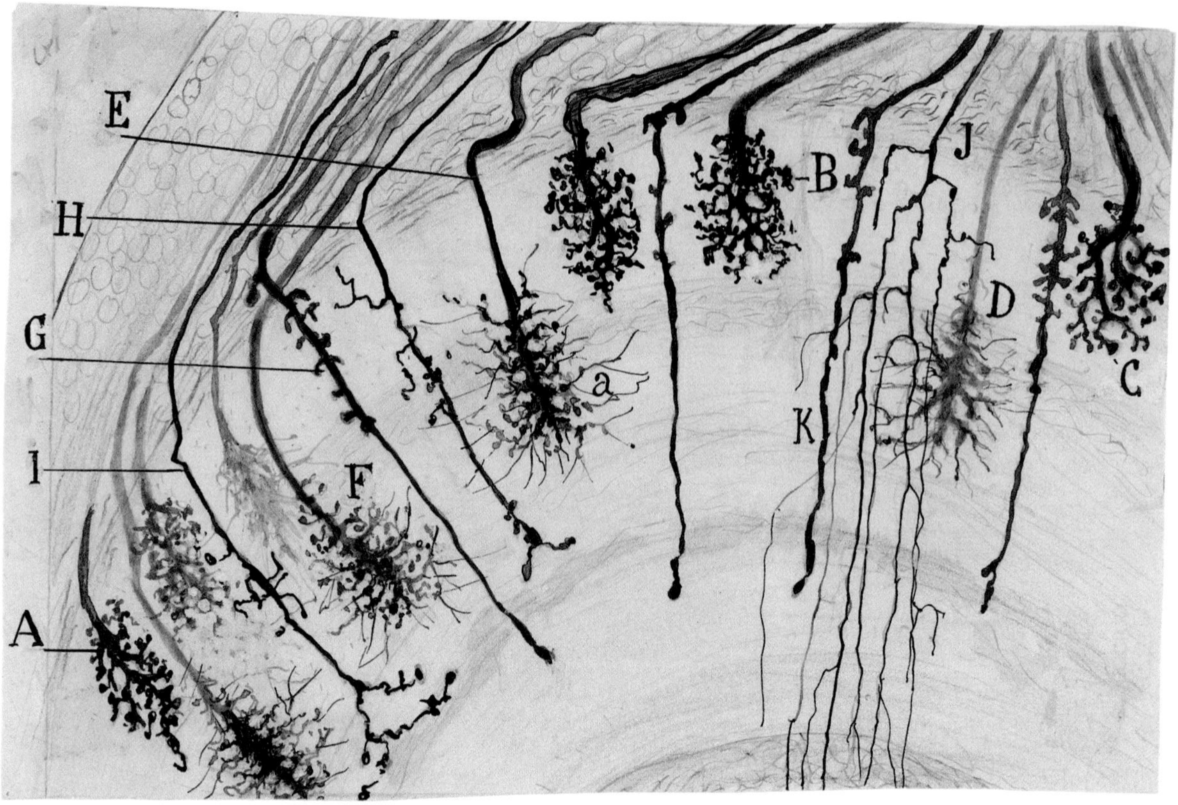

FIGURE 247. Slightly oblique section from the deep retina in a bee.

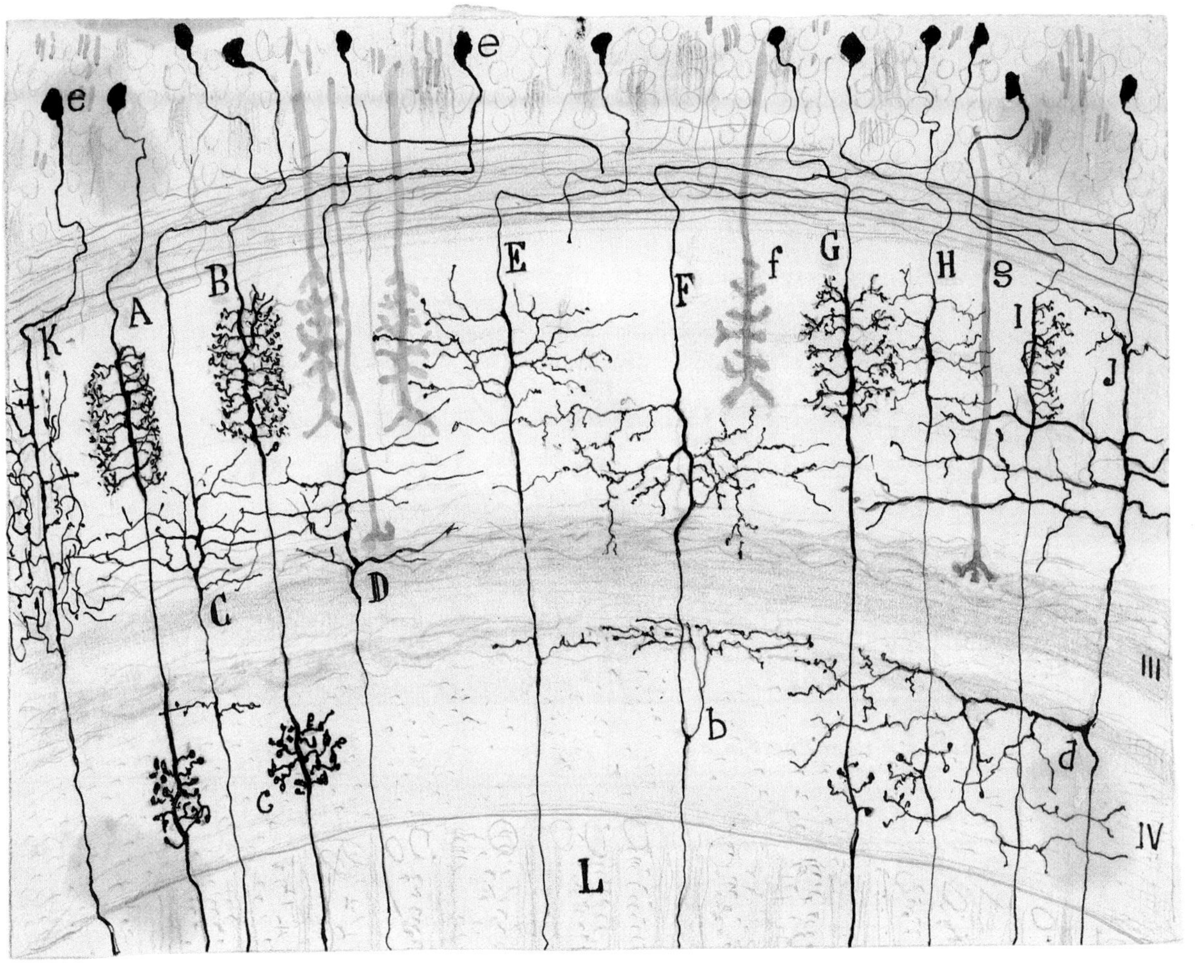

FIGURE 248. Frontal section of the deep retina in a gadfly.

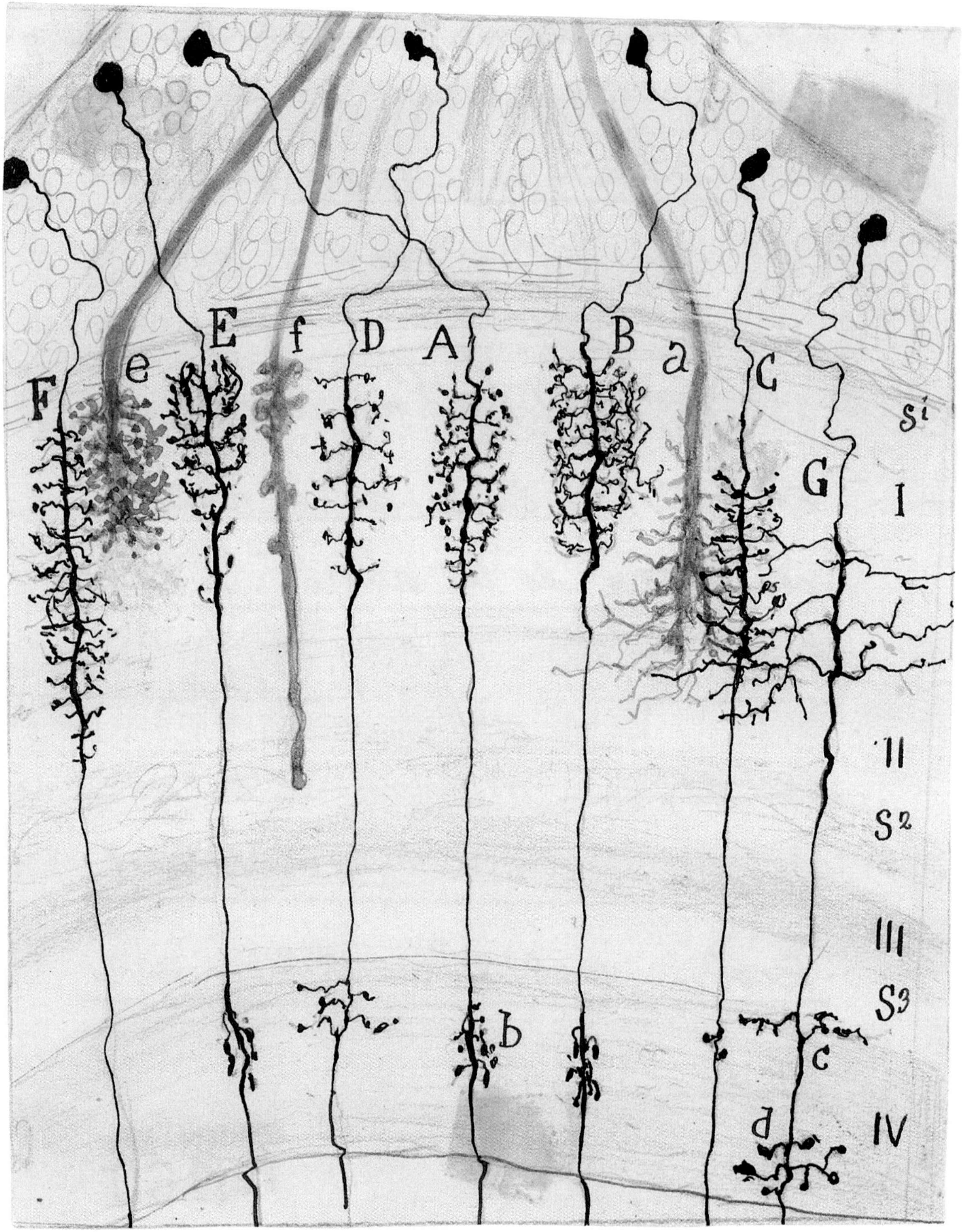

FIGURE 249. Section from the deep retina in a bee.

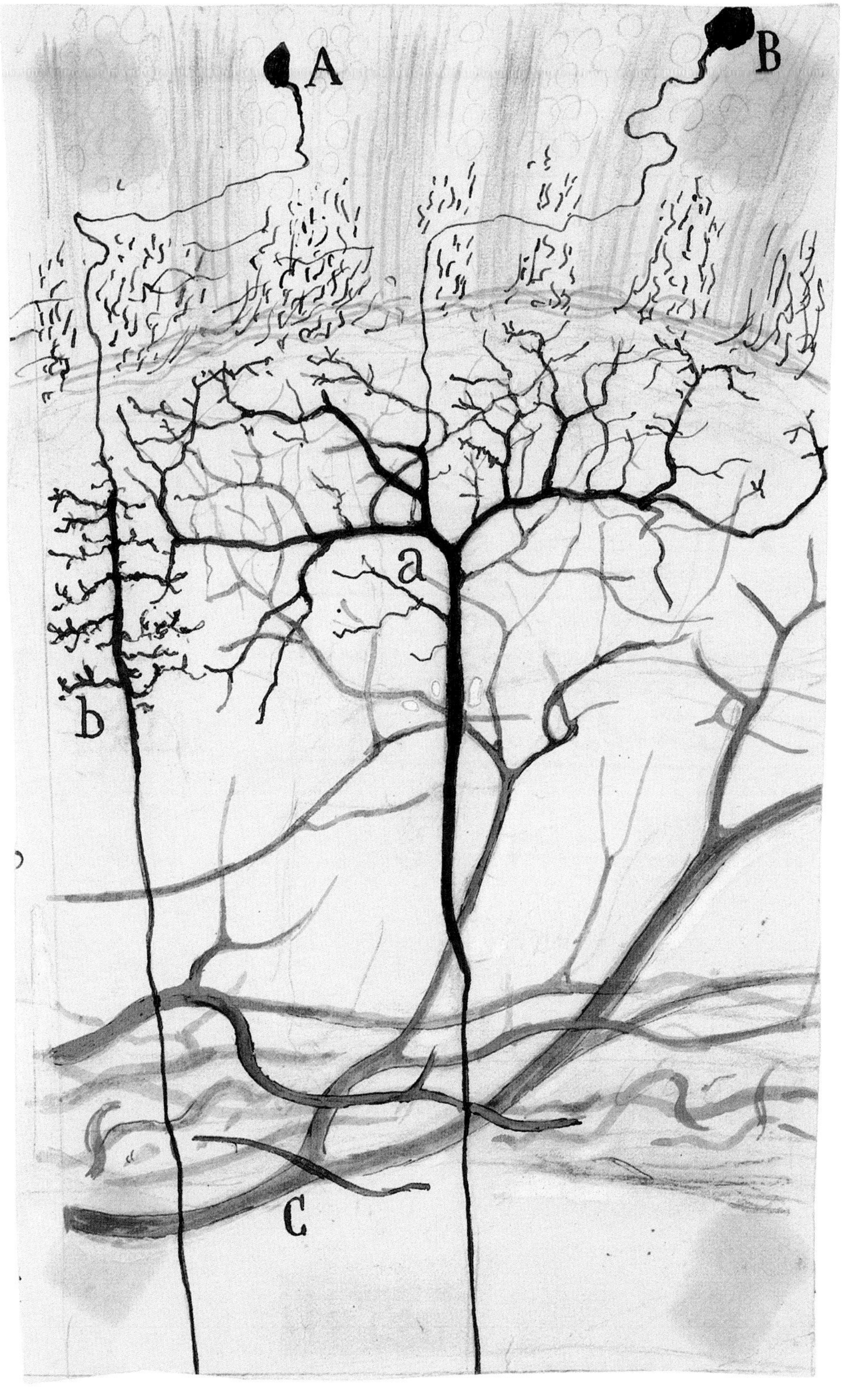

FIGURE 250. Giant ganglion cell from the epioptic in a gadfly.

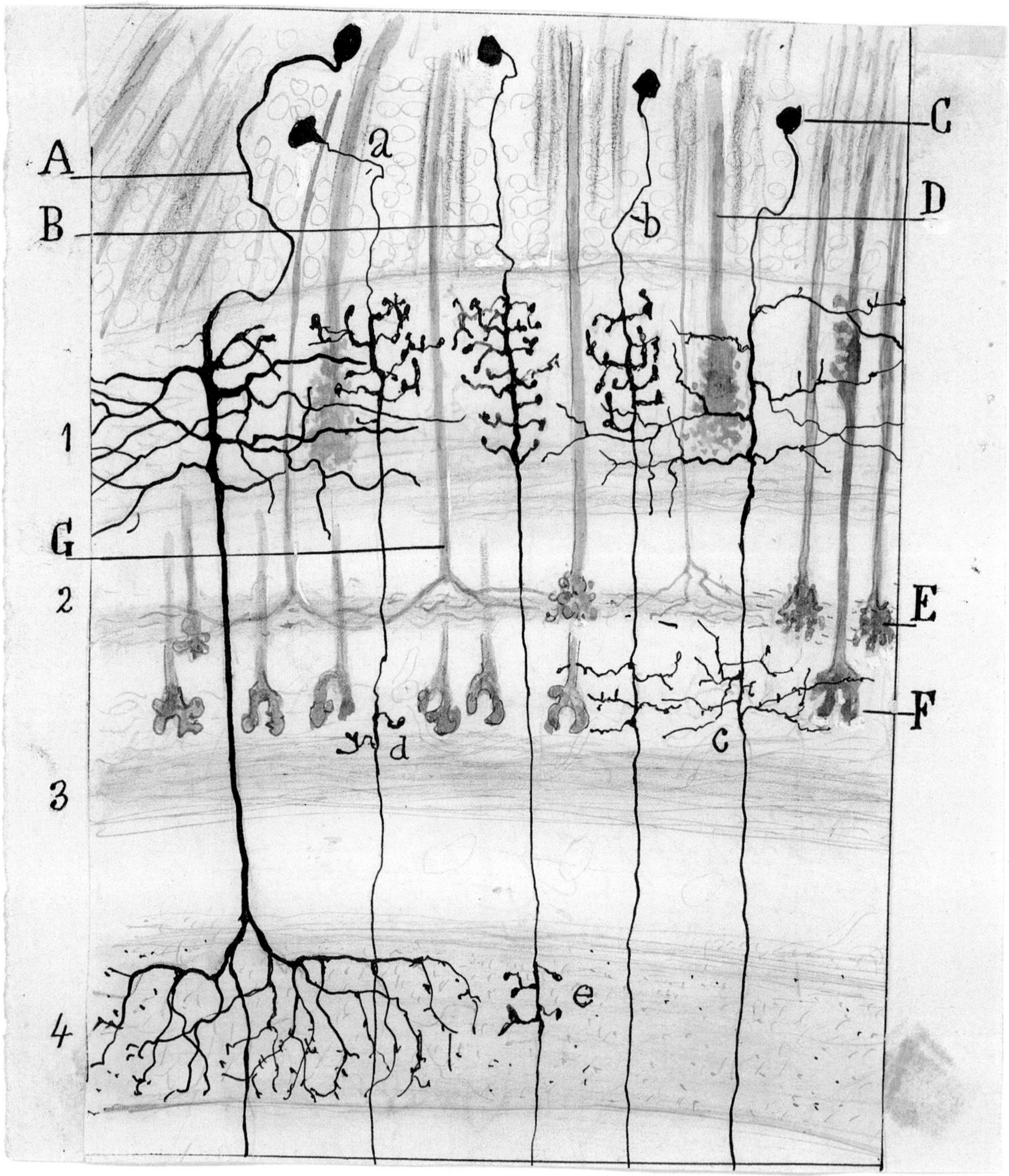

FIGURE 251. Section from the deep retina in a fly.

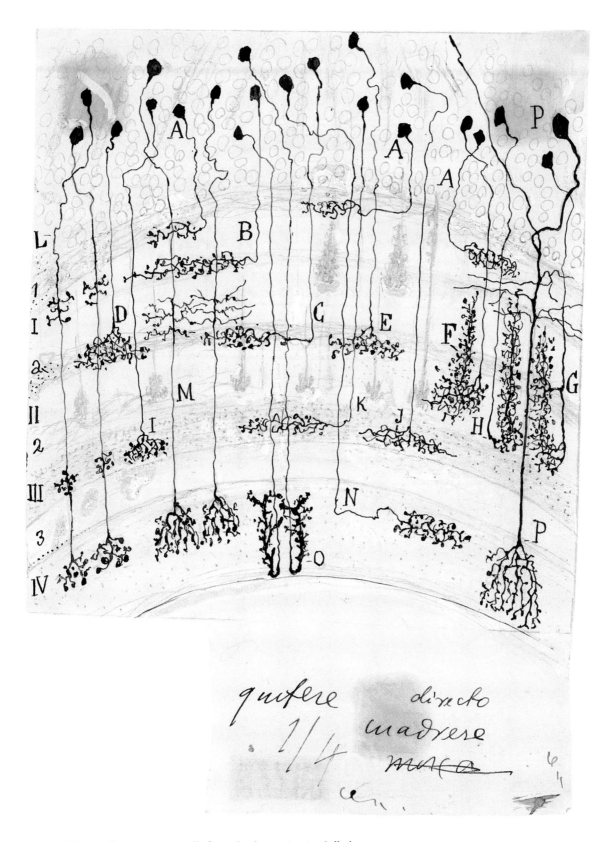

FIGURE 252. Type I cells or amacrine cells from the deep retina in *Calliphora.*

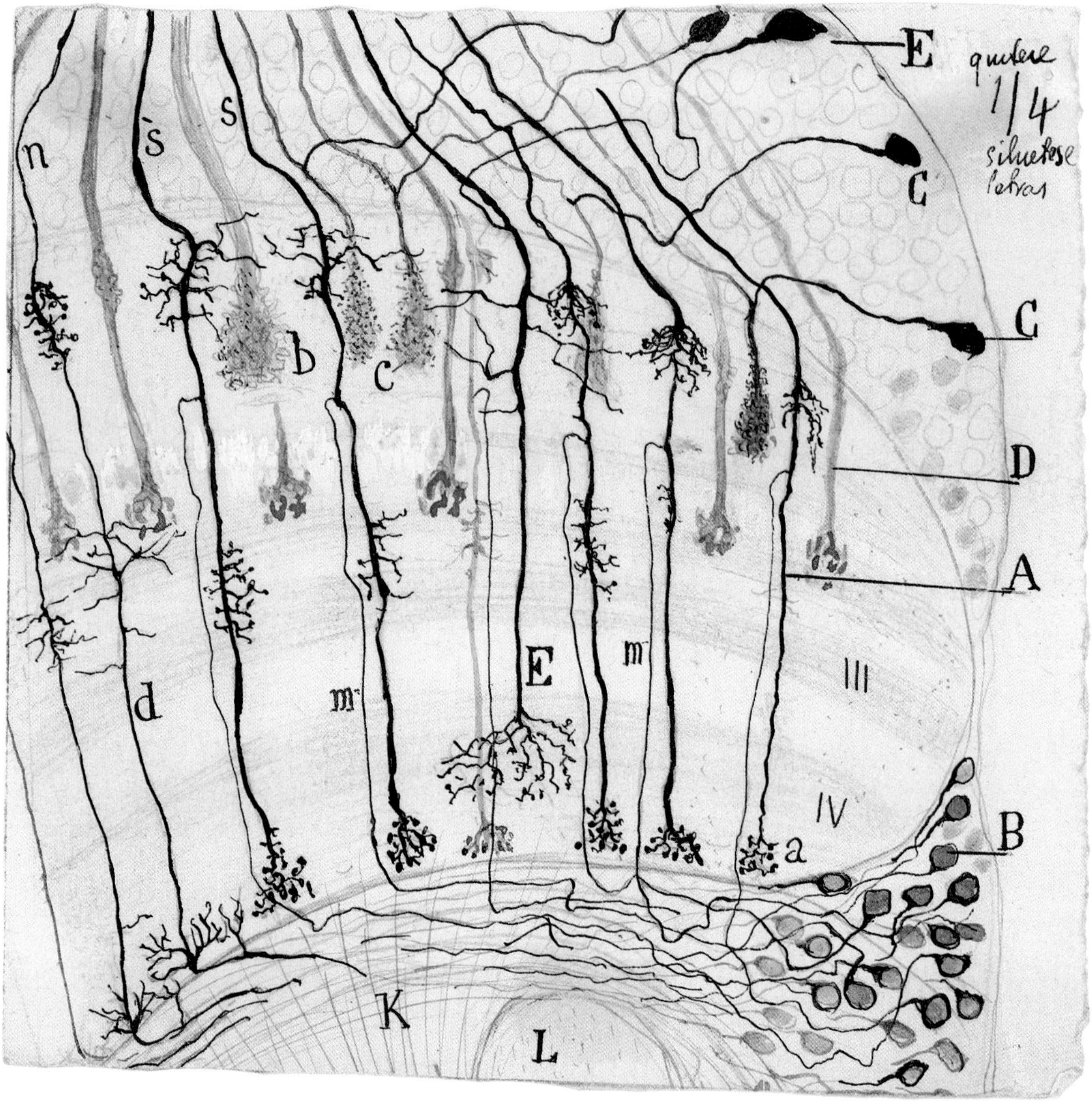

FIGURE 253. Horizontal section from the deep retina in *Calliphora.*

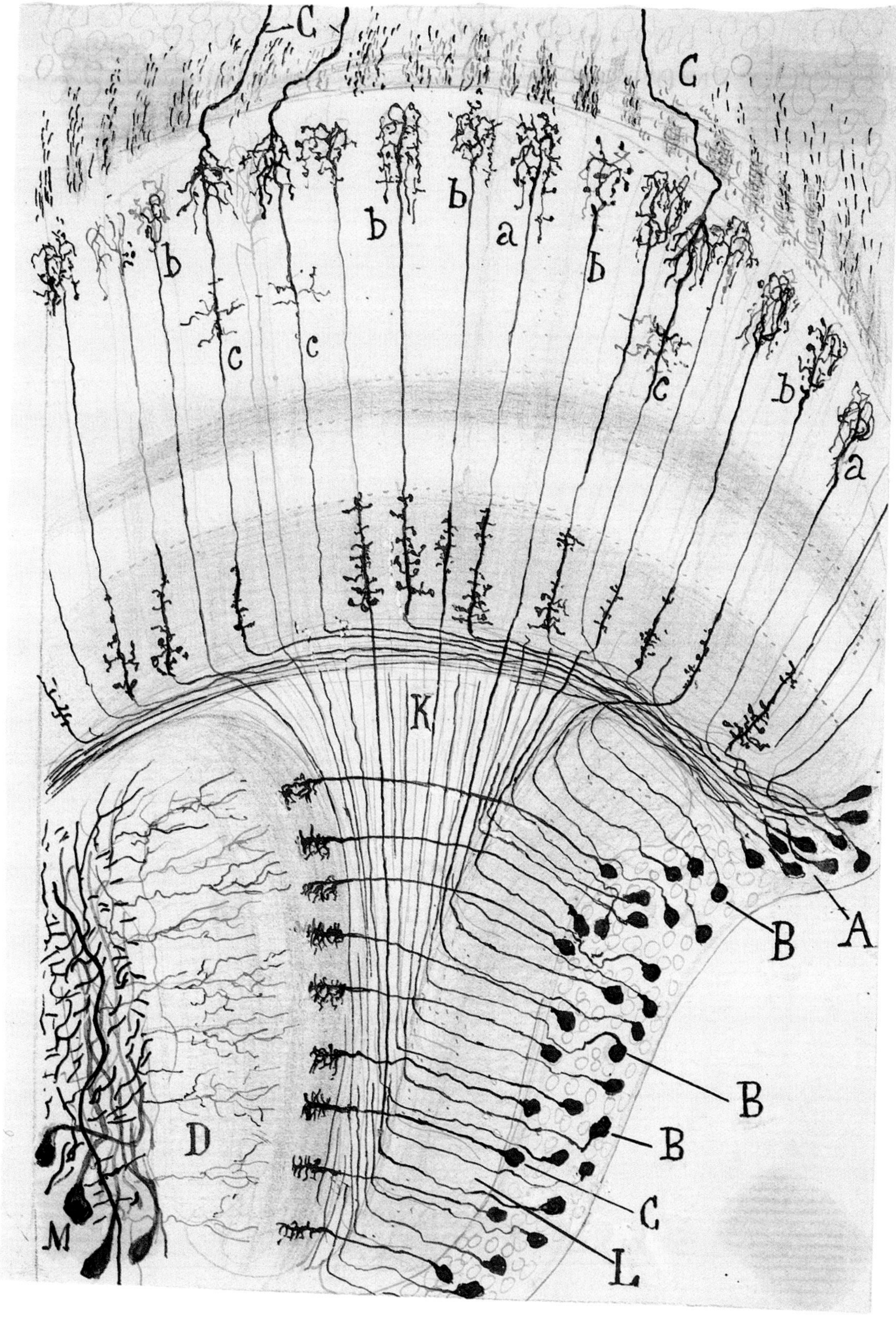

FIGURE 254. Horizontal section from the deep retina and optic lobe in a gadfly.

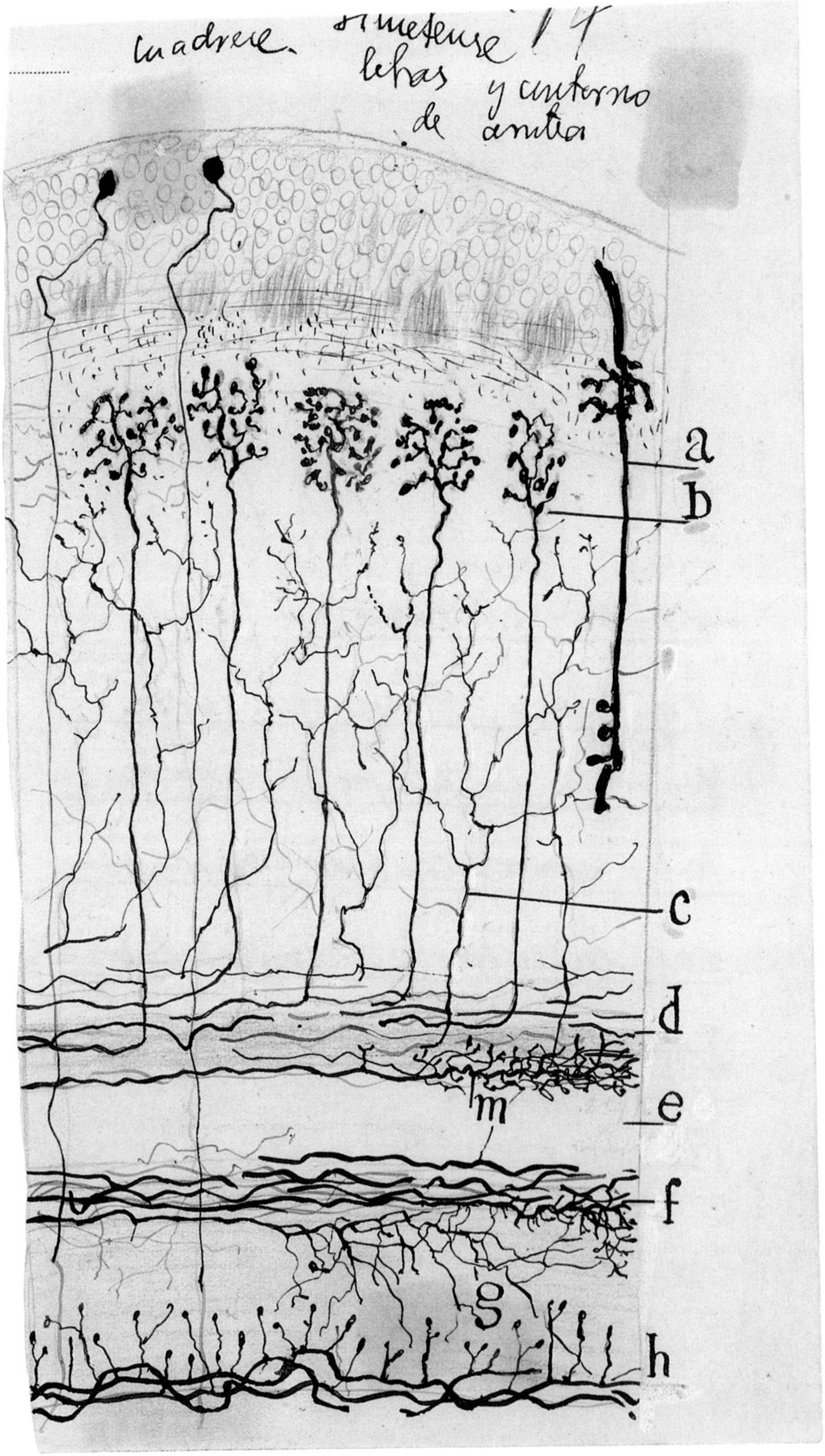

FIGURE 255. Section from the epioptic in a honeybee.

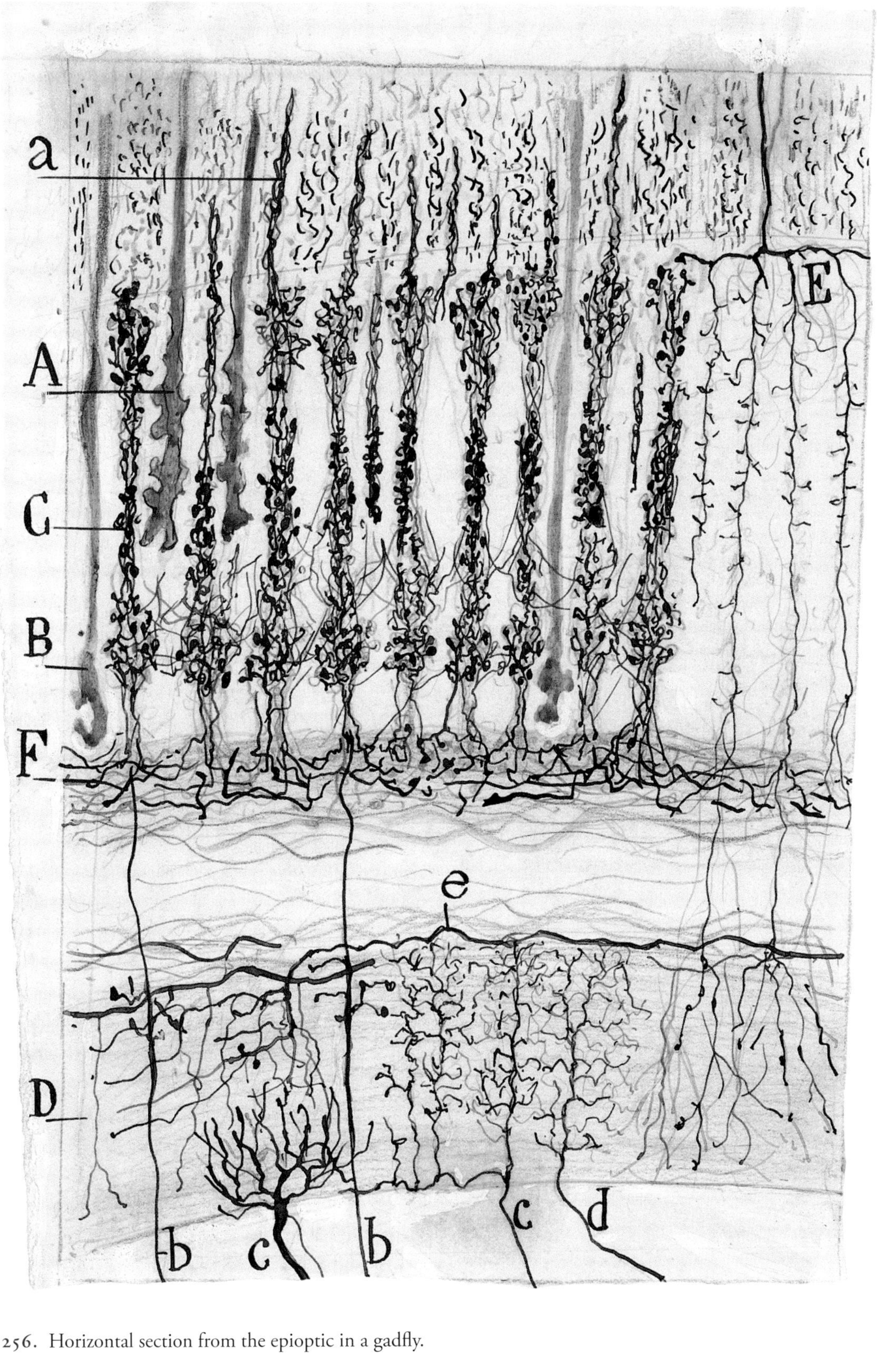

FIGURE 256. Horizontal section from the epioptic in a gadfly.

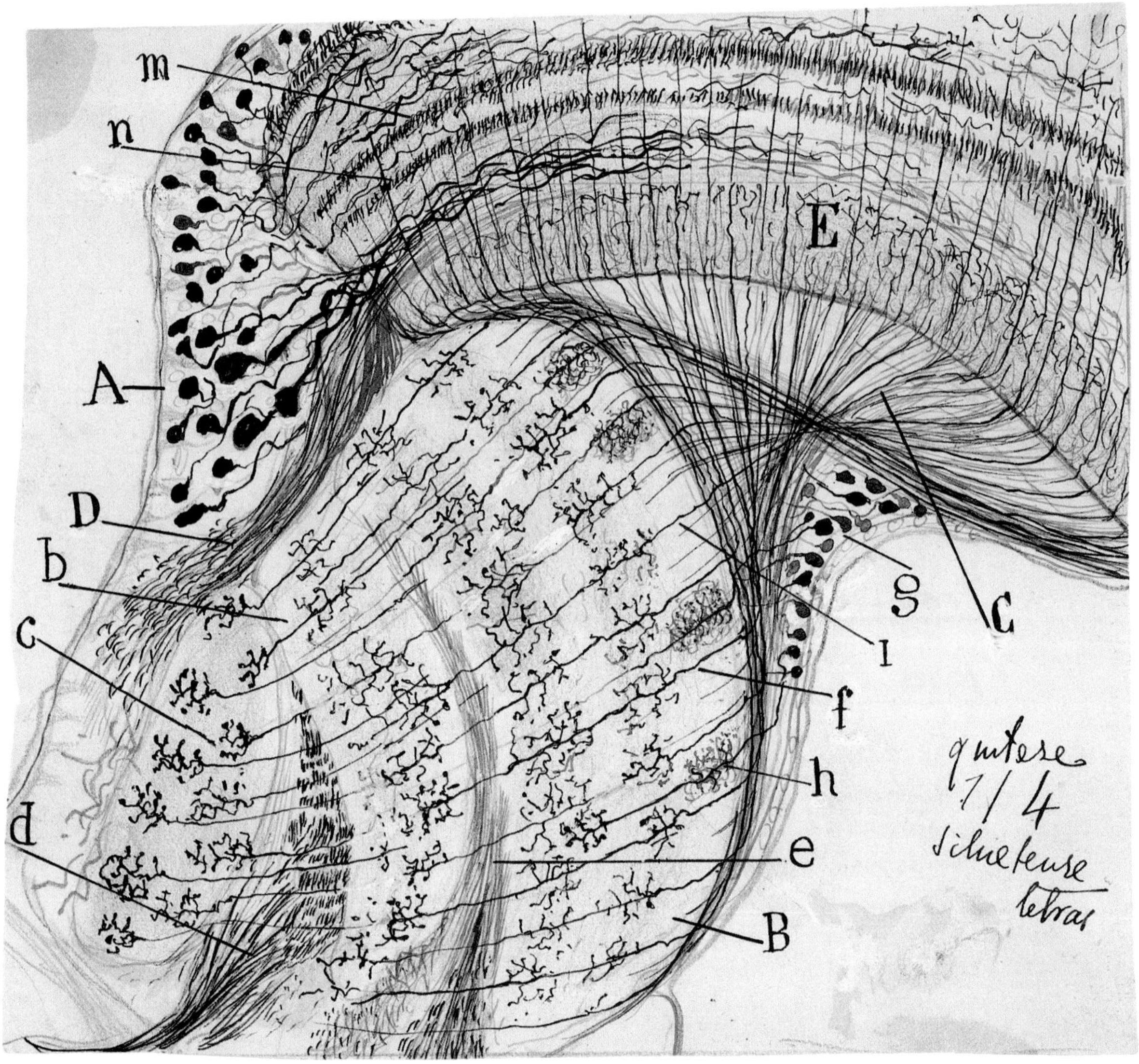

FIGURE 257. Optic lobe and internal chiasm in *Libellula*.

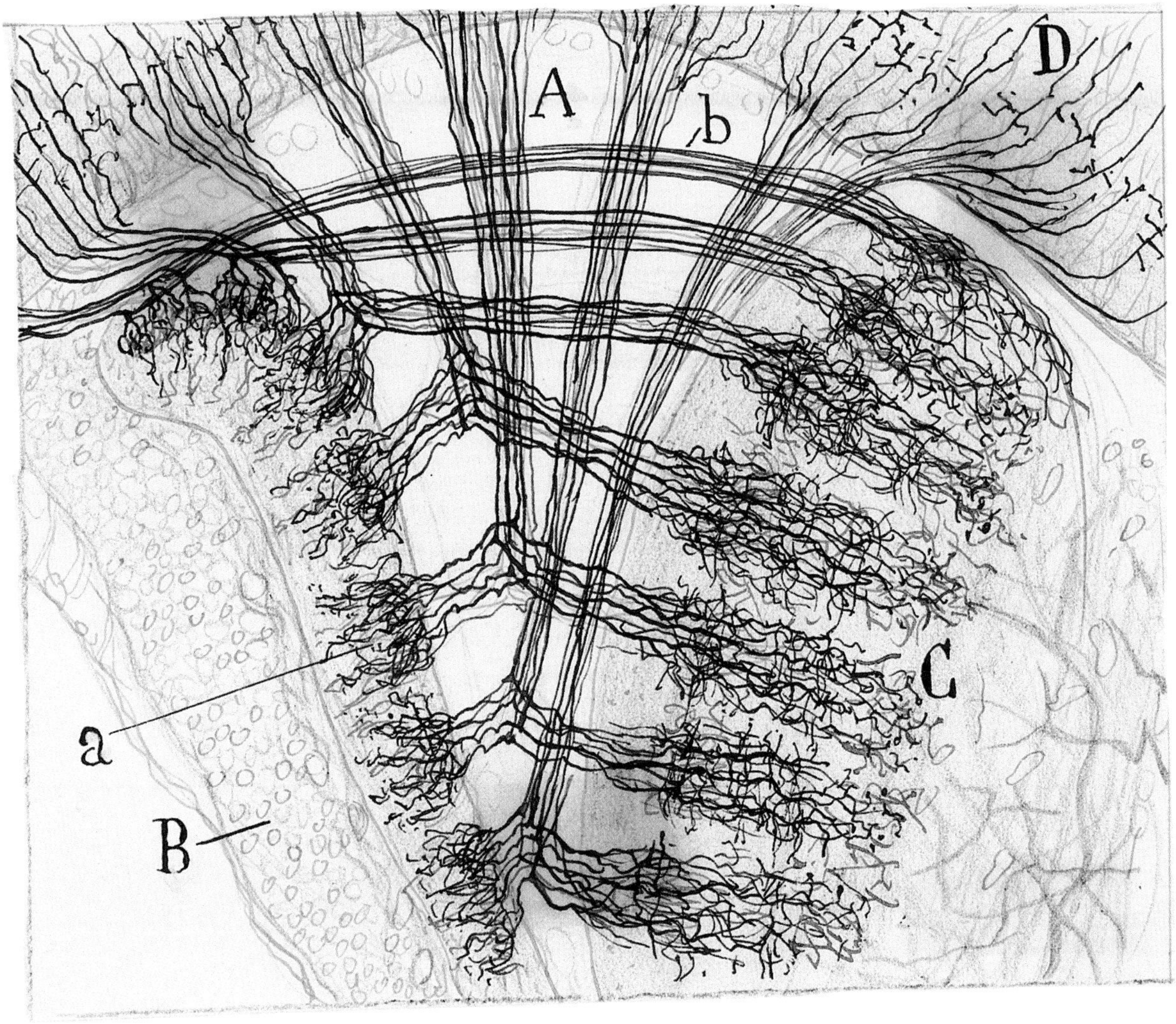

FIGURE 258. Horizontal section from the internal chiasm region and optic lobe in a gadfly.

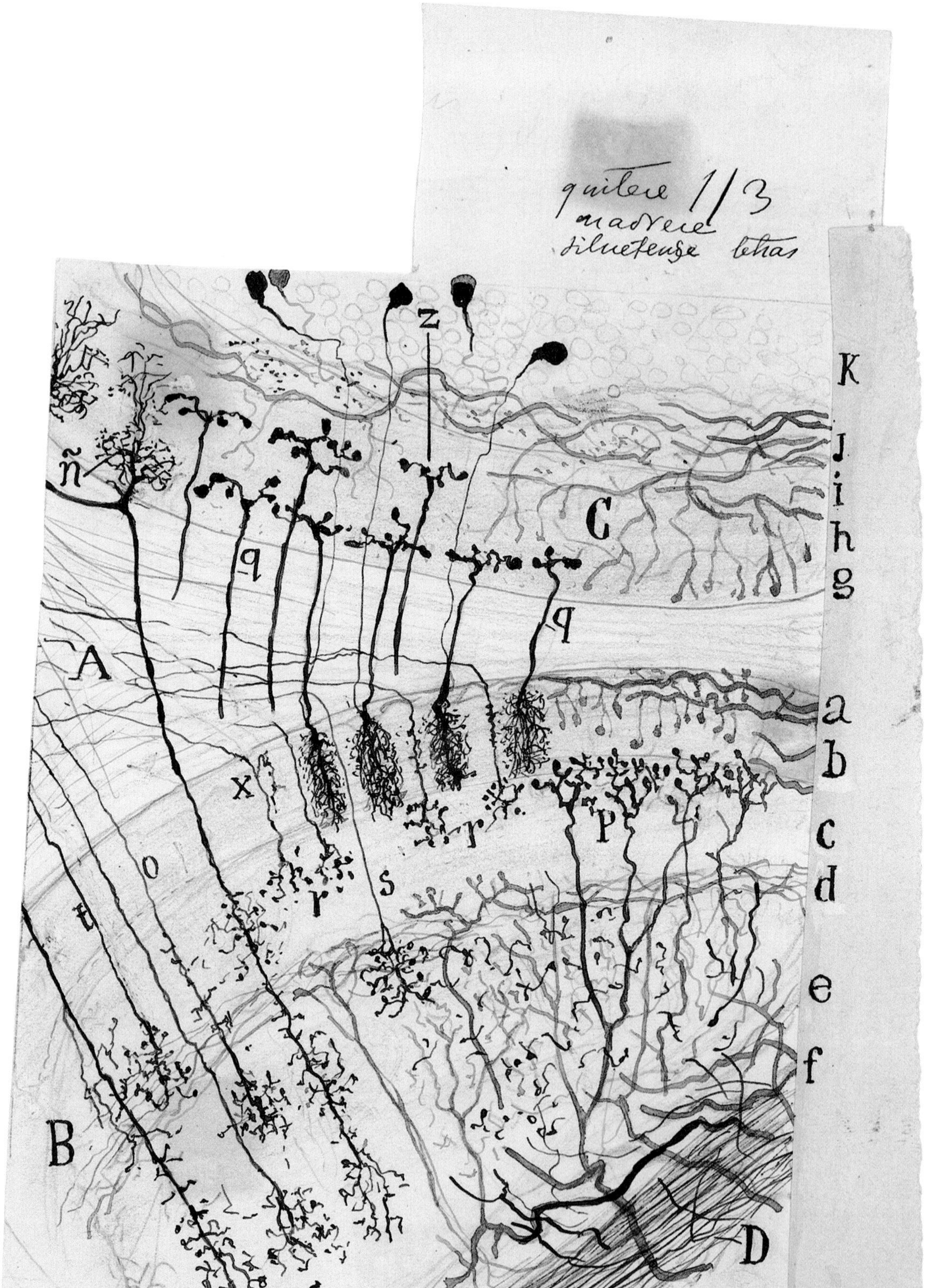

FIGURE 259. Section of the two segments of the optic lobe in a gadfly retina.

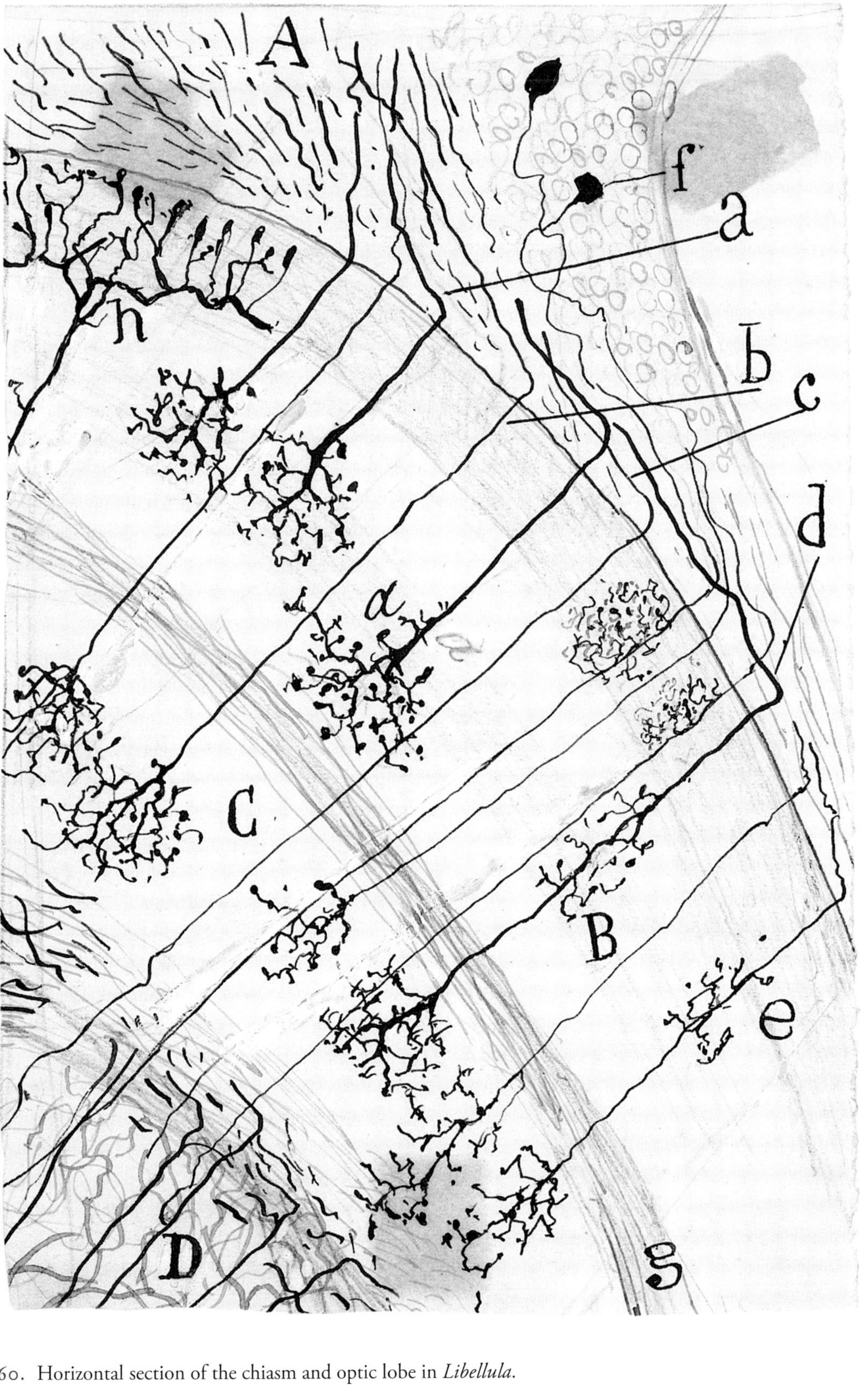

FIGURE 260. Horizontal section of the chiasm and optic lobe in *Libellula*.

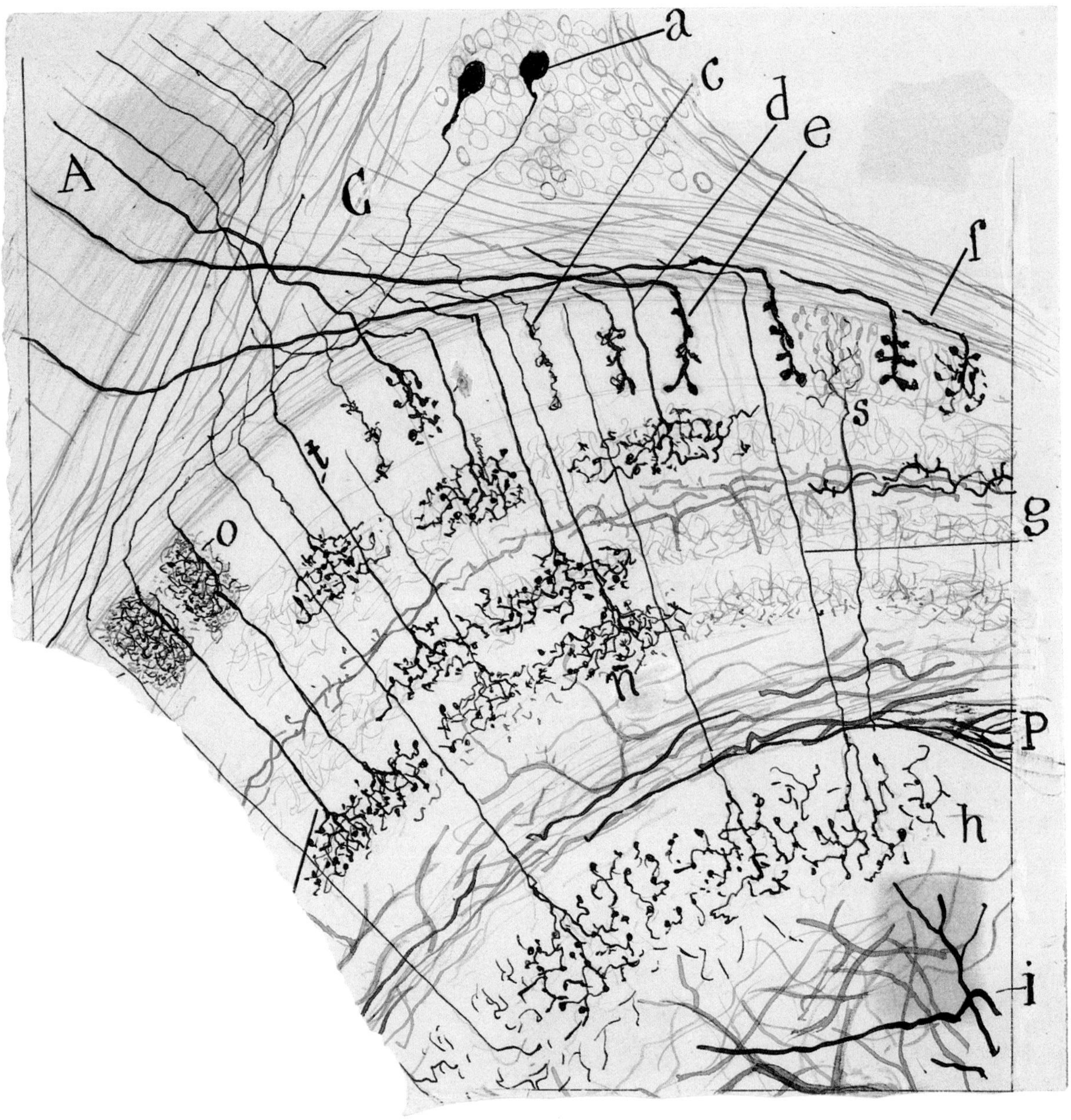

FIGURE 261. Horizontal section from the optic lobe in a bee.

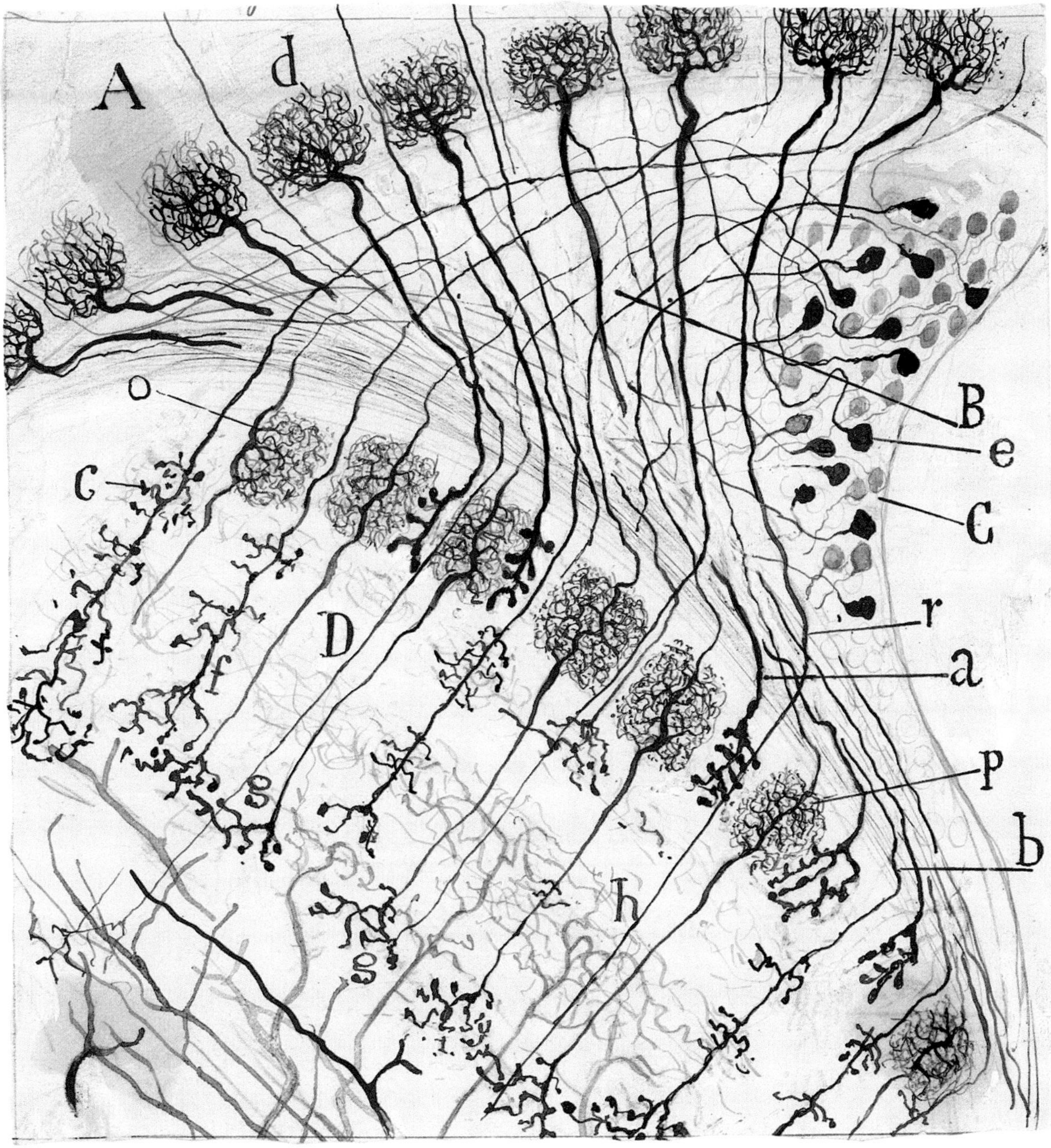

FIGURE 262. Region of the chiasm and optic lobe in a bee.

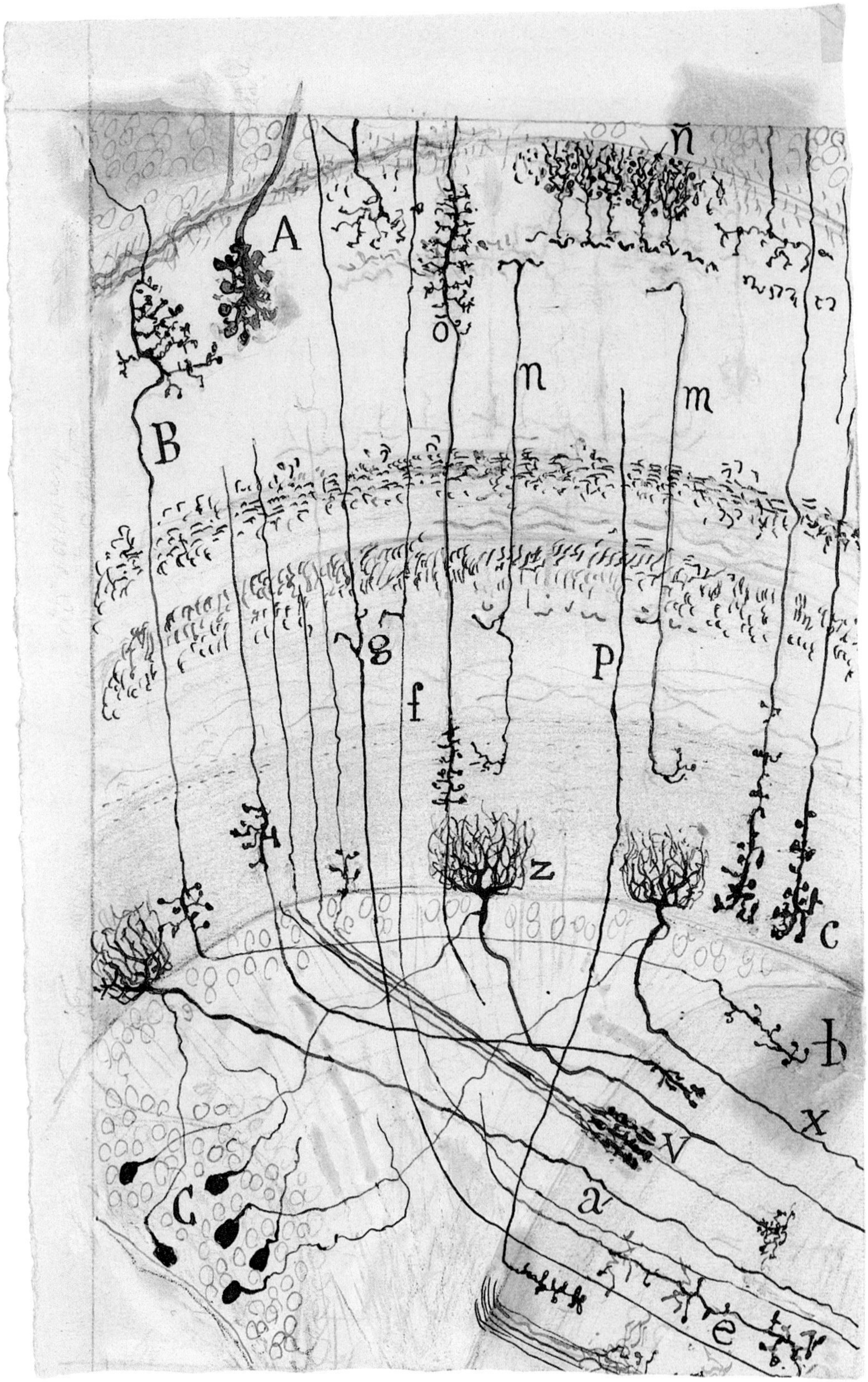

FIGURE 263. Epioptic, internal chiasm, and optic lobe in a bee.

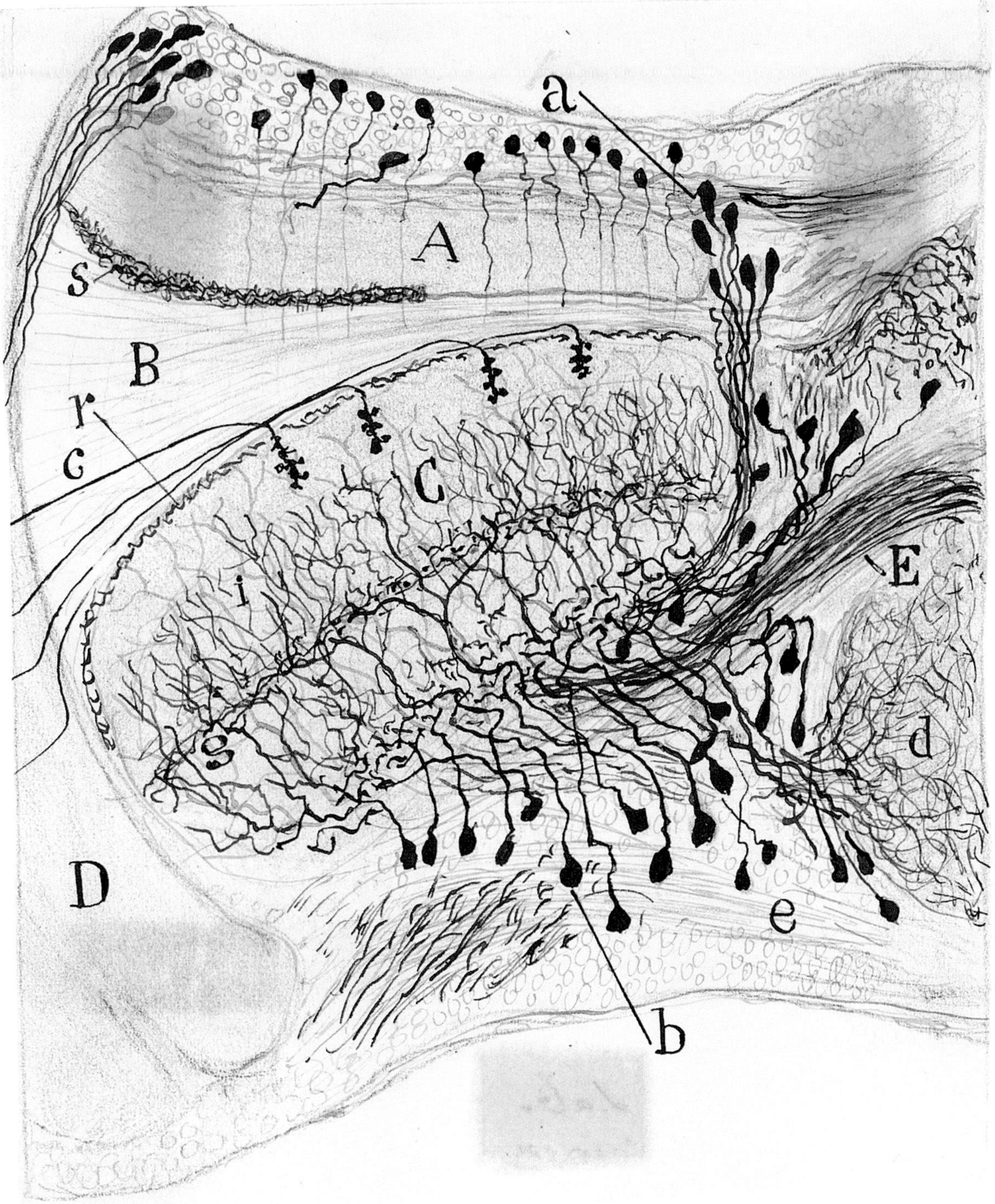

FIGURE 264. Optic lobe in a blowfly.

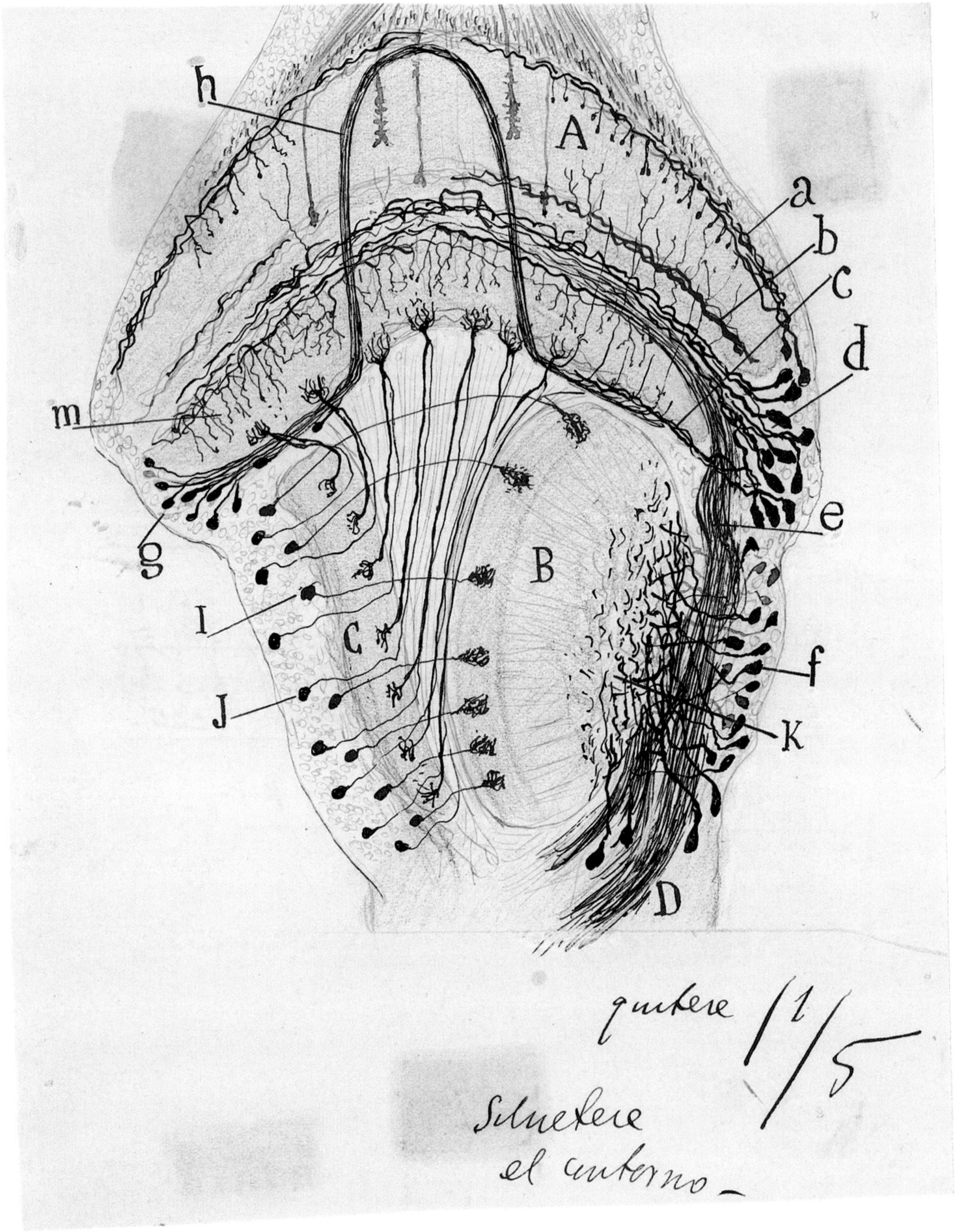

FIGURE 265. Retina and optic lobe in a gadfly.

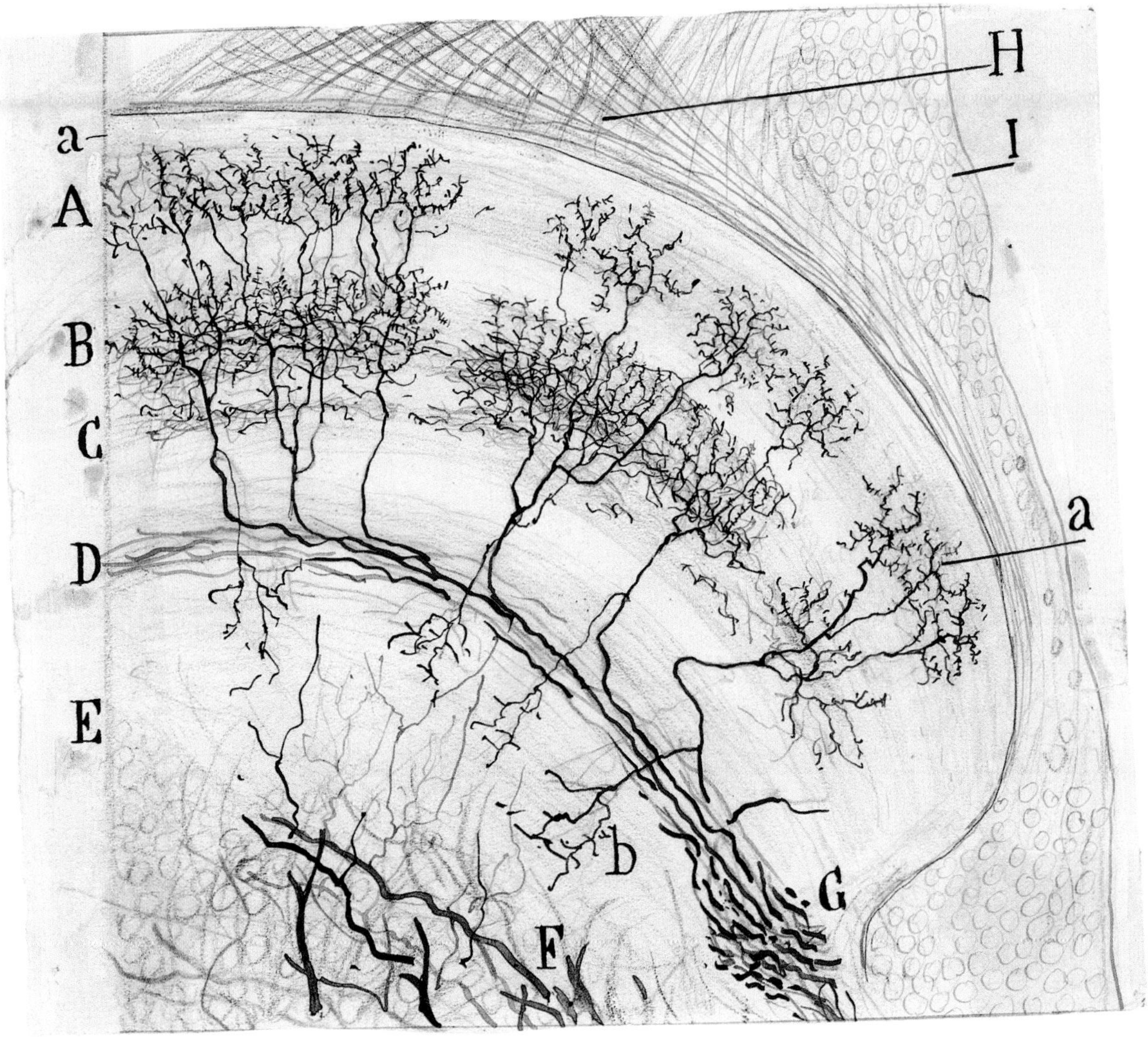

FIGURE 266. Optic lobe in a bee.

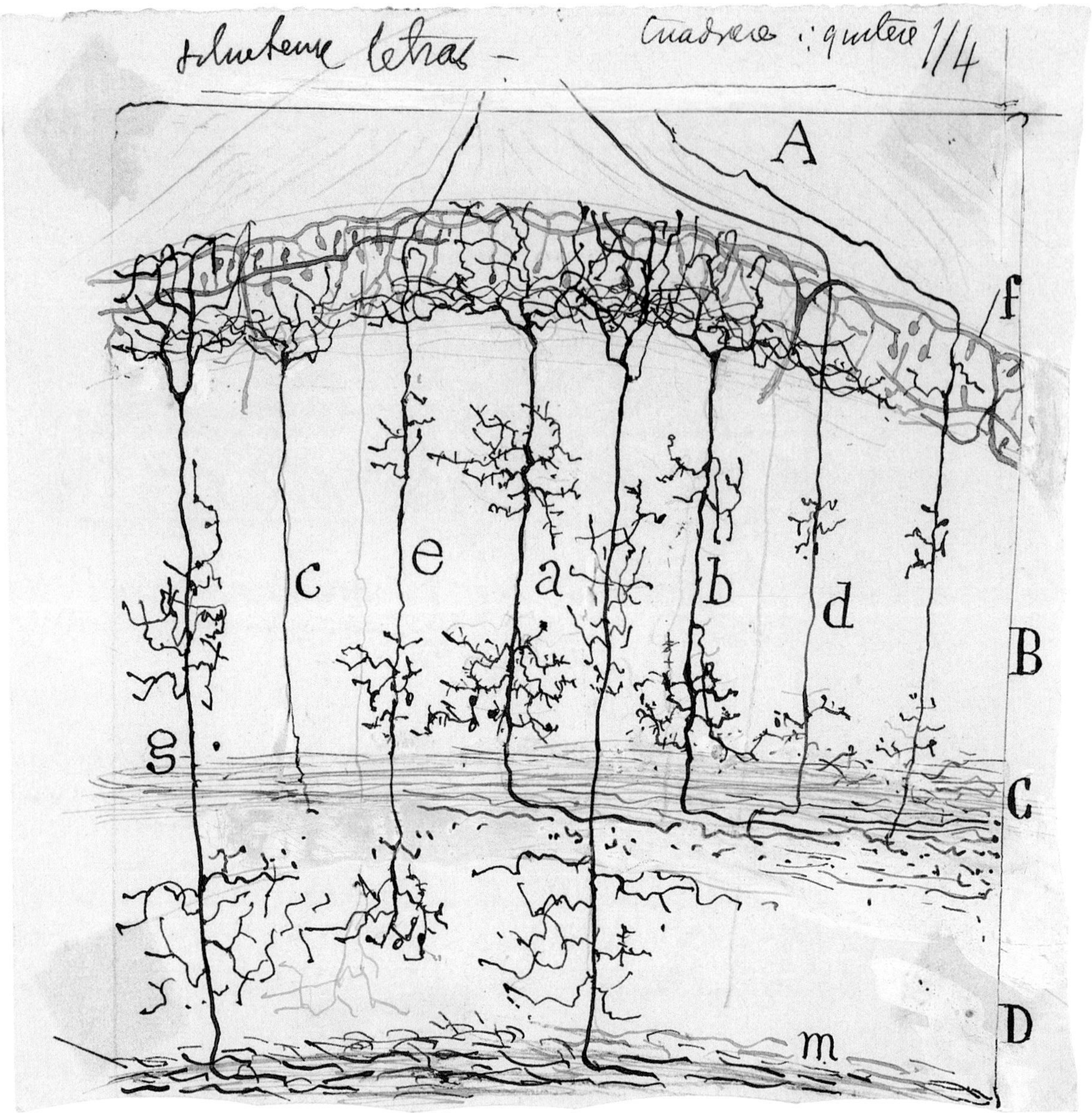

FIGURE 267. First and second segments of the optic lobe in *Libellula*.

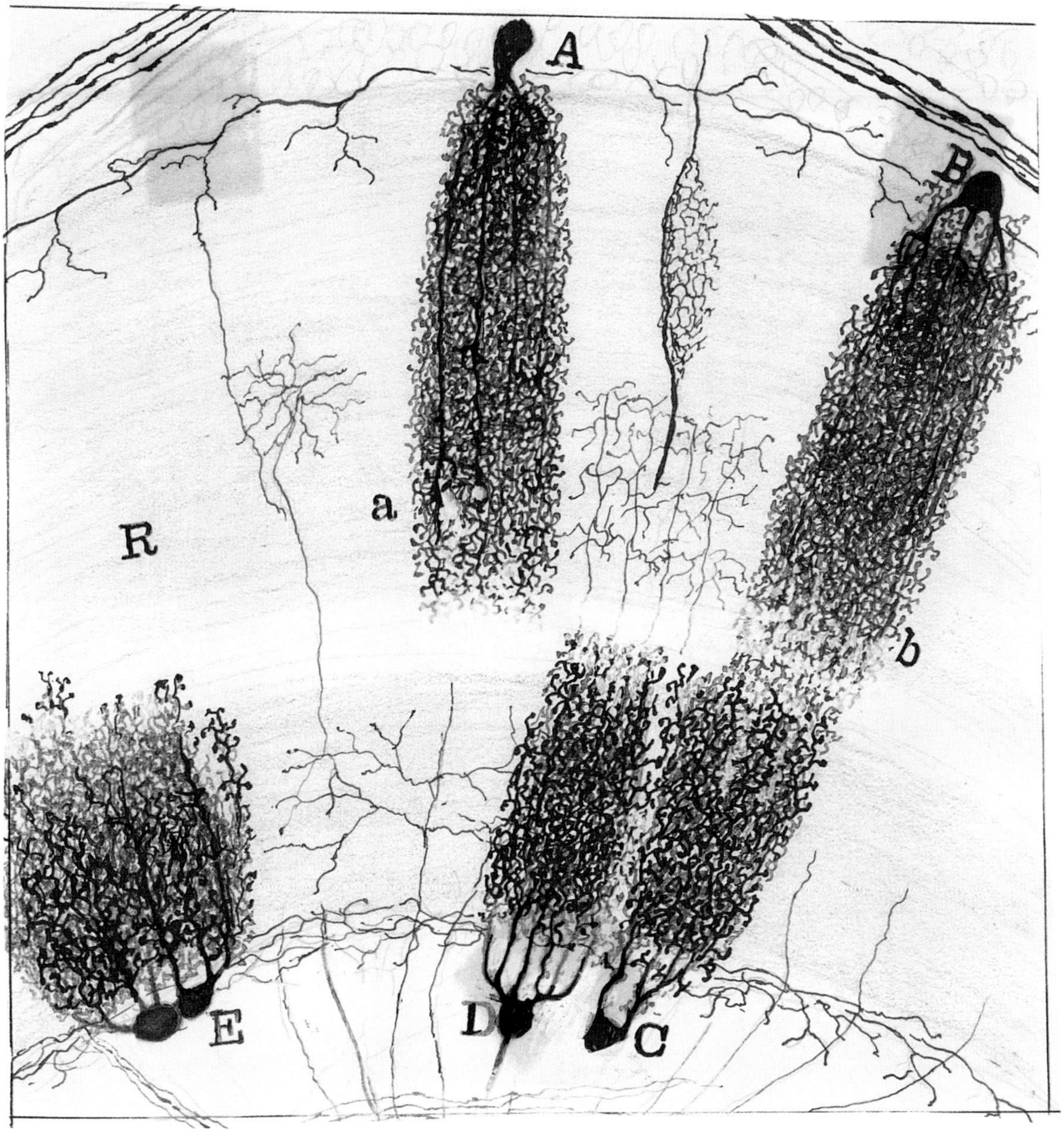

FIGURE 268. Neuroglia from the deep retina in a gadfly.

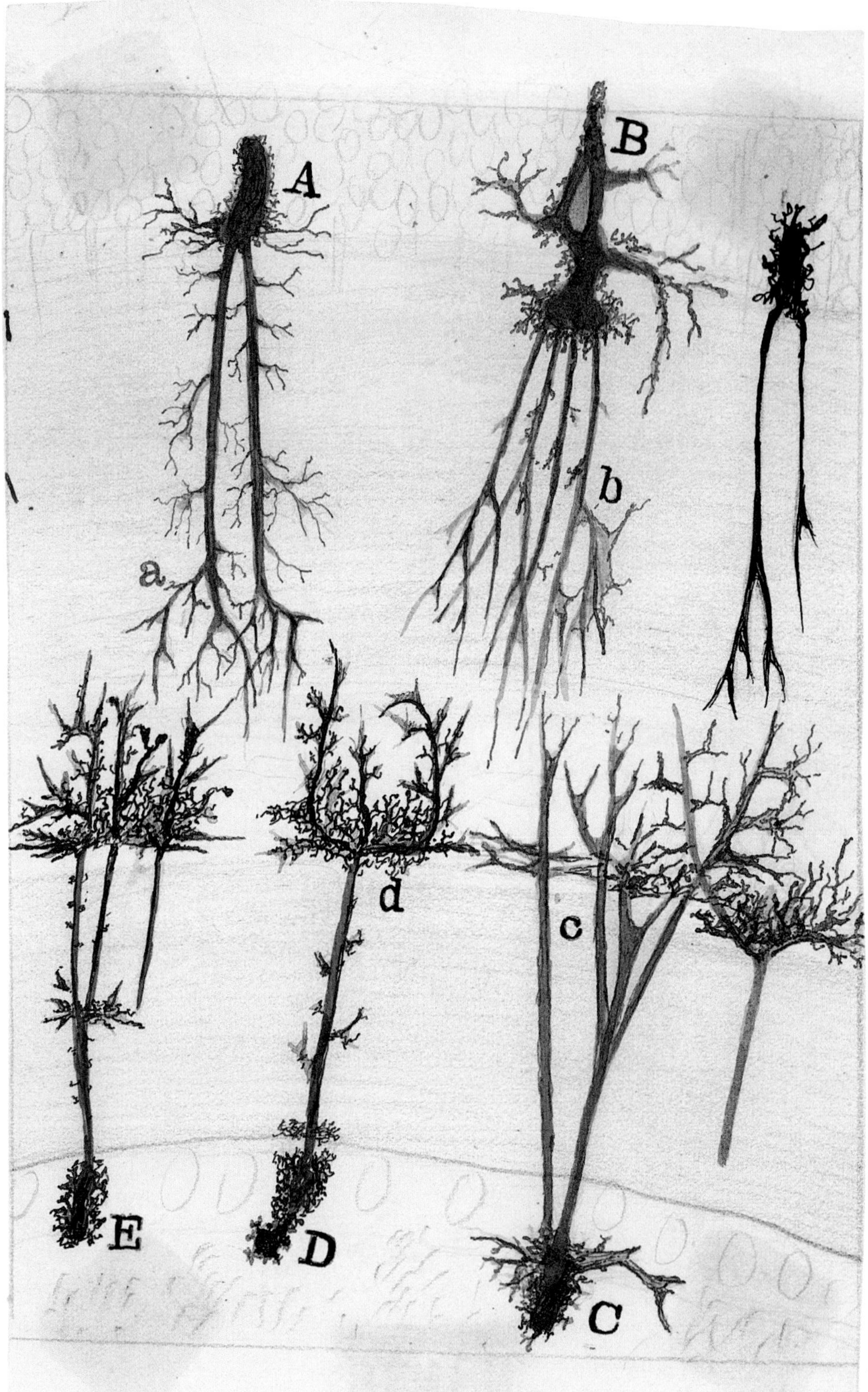

FIGURE 269. Neuroglia devoid of cotton-like filaments.

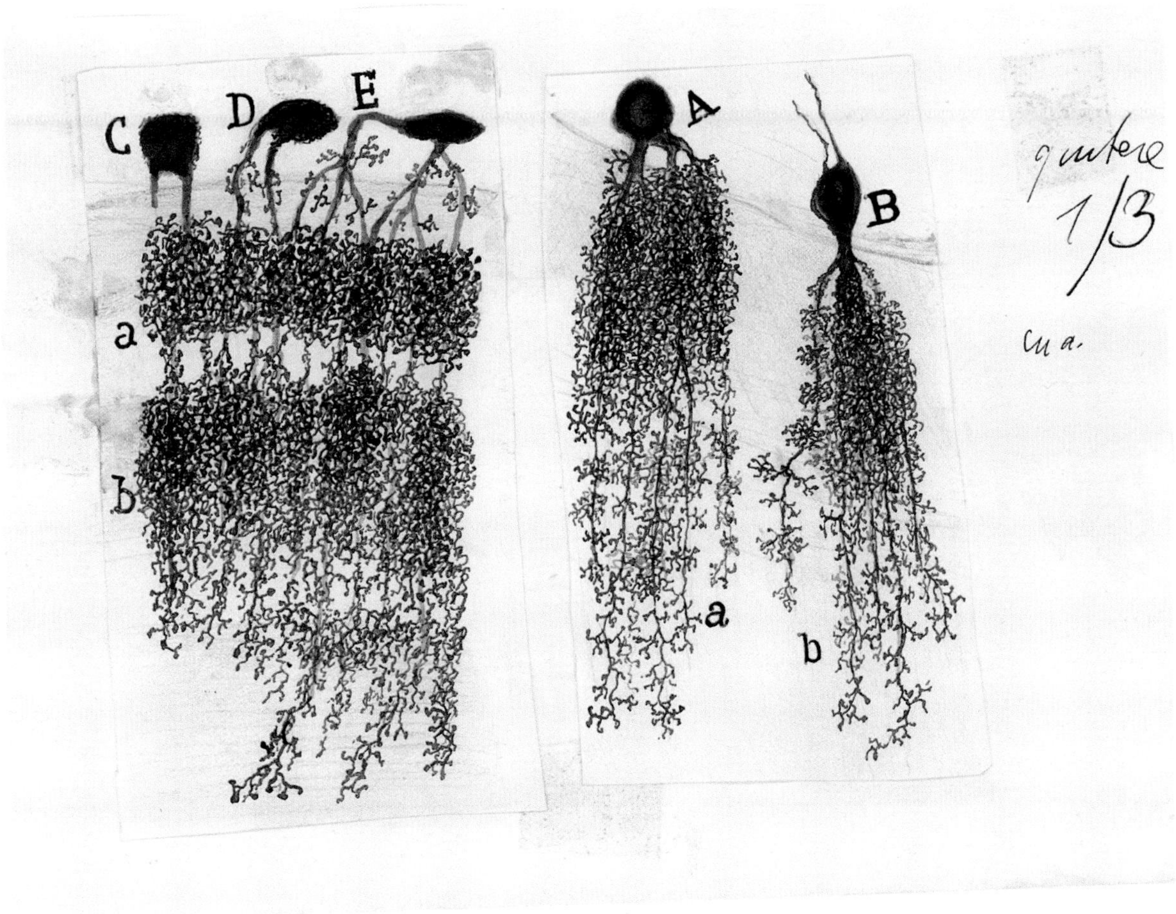

FIGURE 270. Some neuroglial cells in a bee.

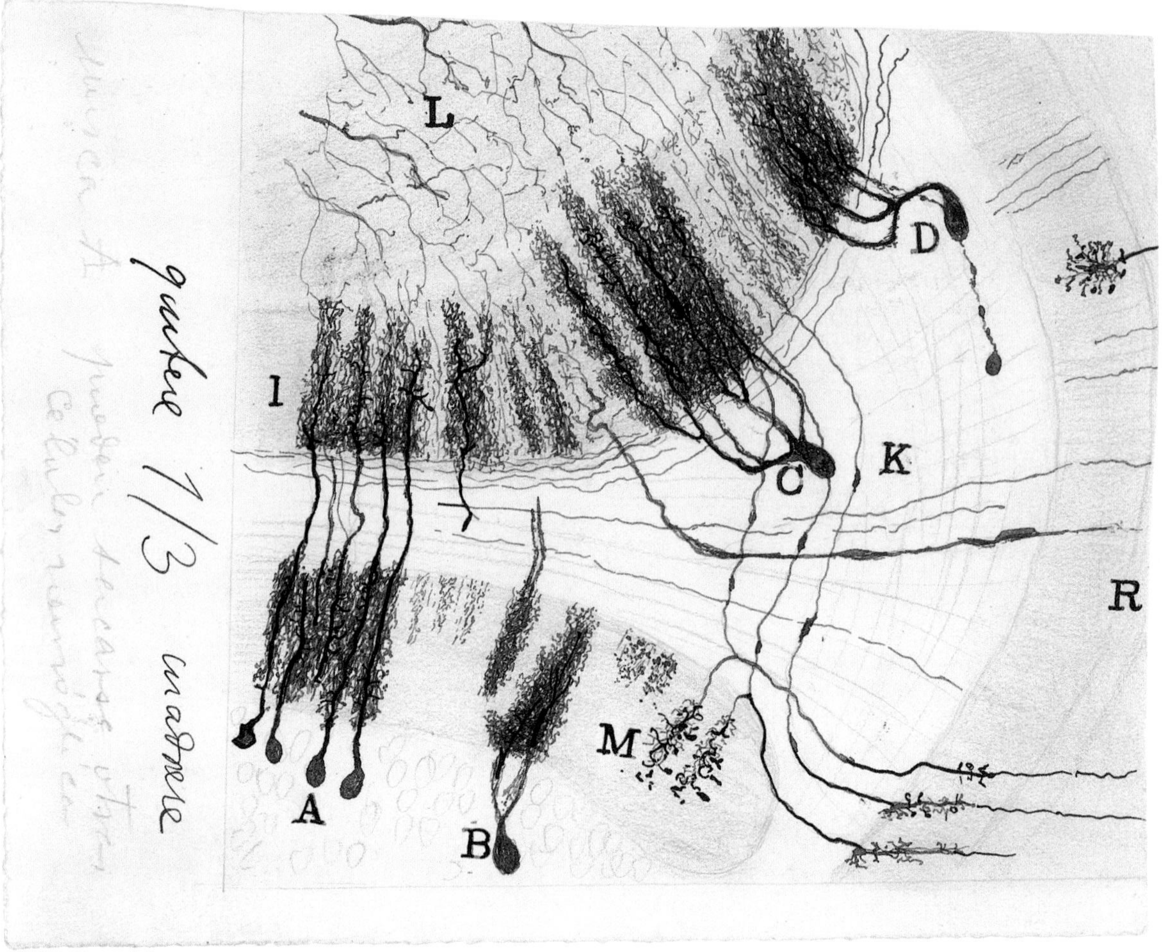

FIGURE 271. Neuroglial cells from the optic lobe in a blowfly.

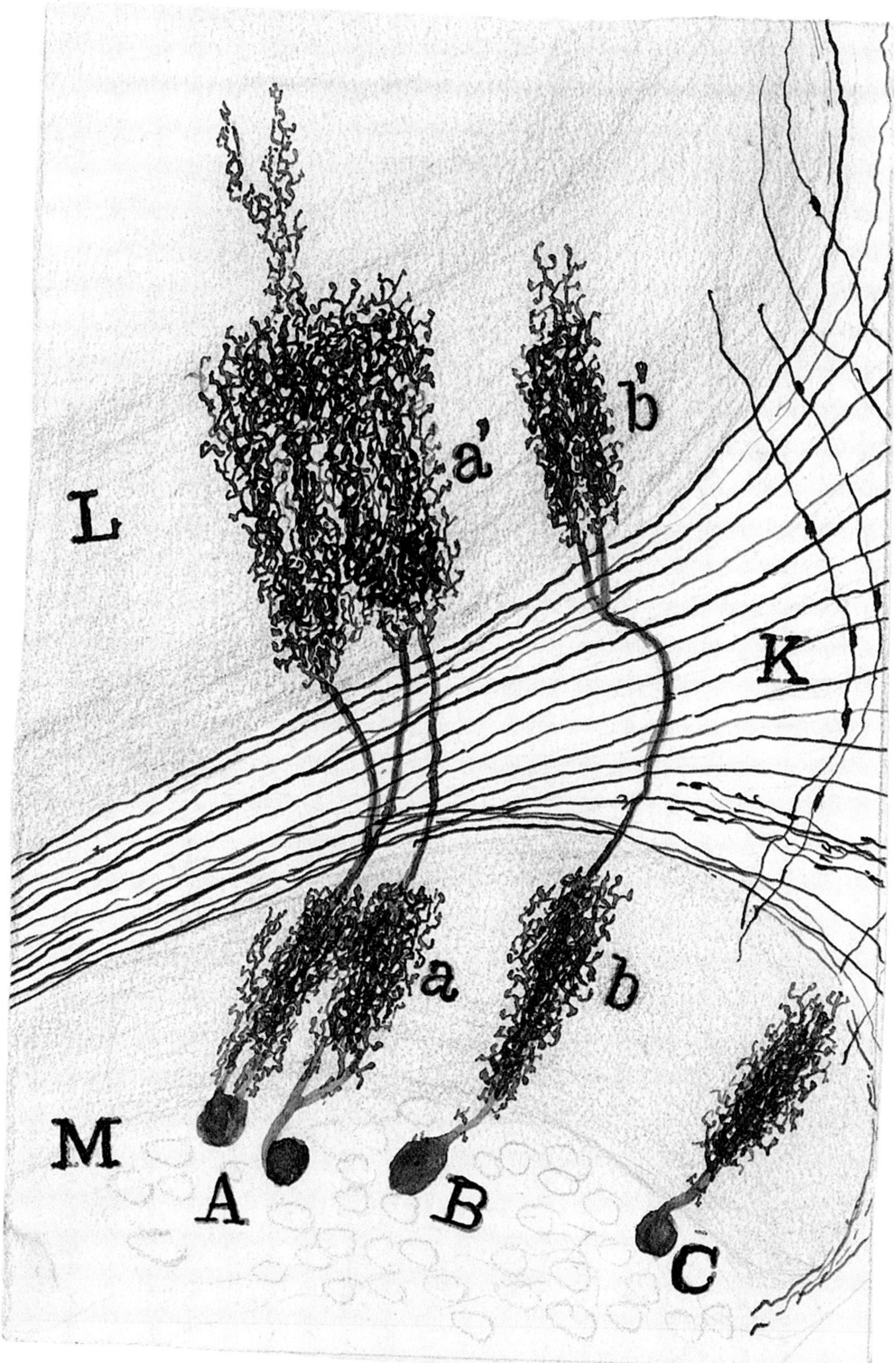

FIGURE 272. Bitufted neuroglial elements from the optic lobe in a gadfly.

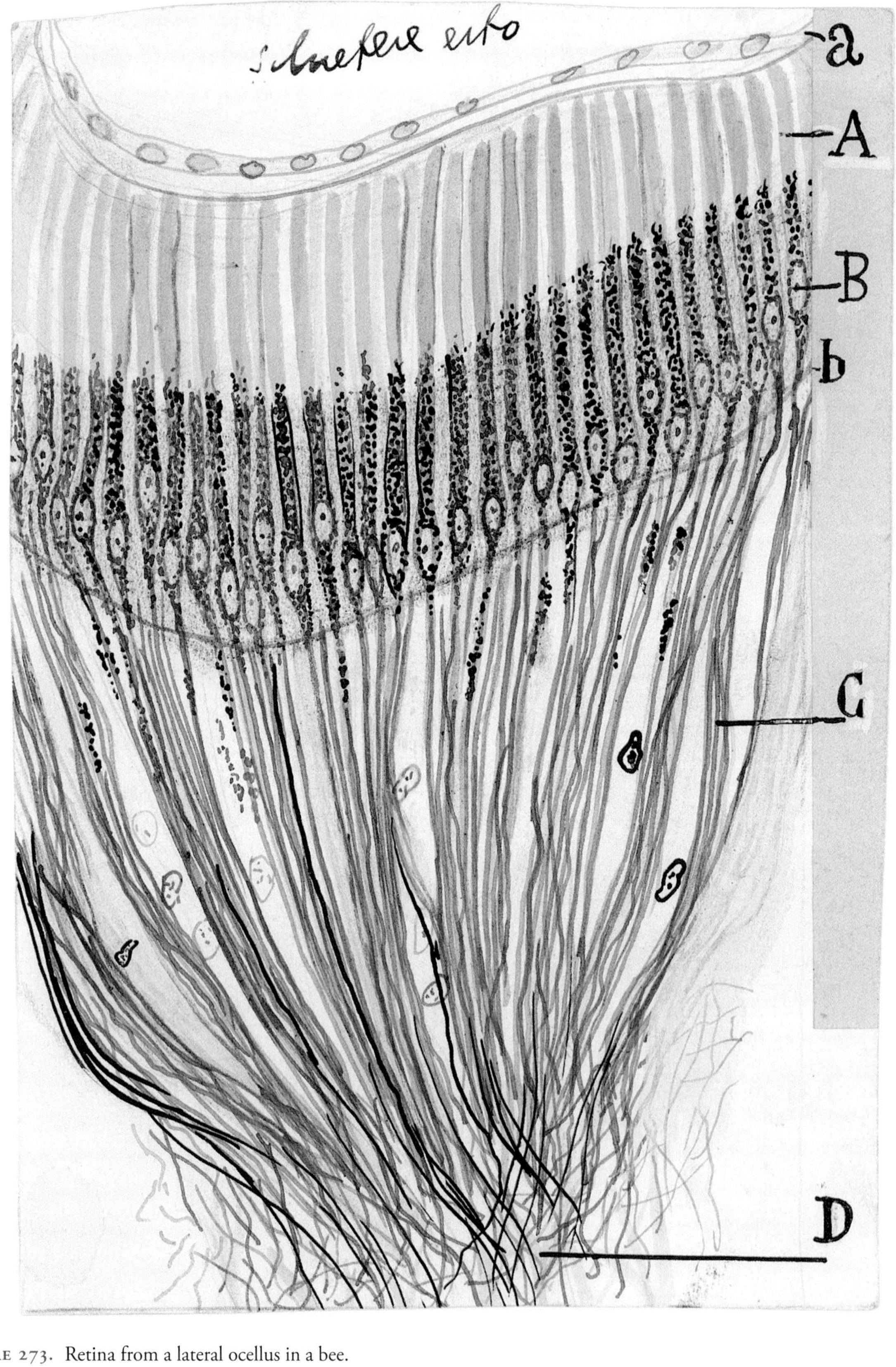

FIGURE 273. Retina from a lateral ocellus in a bee.

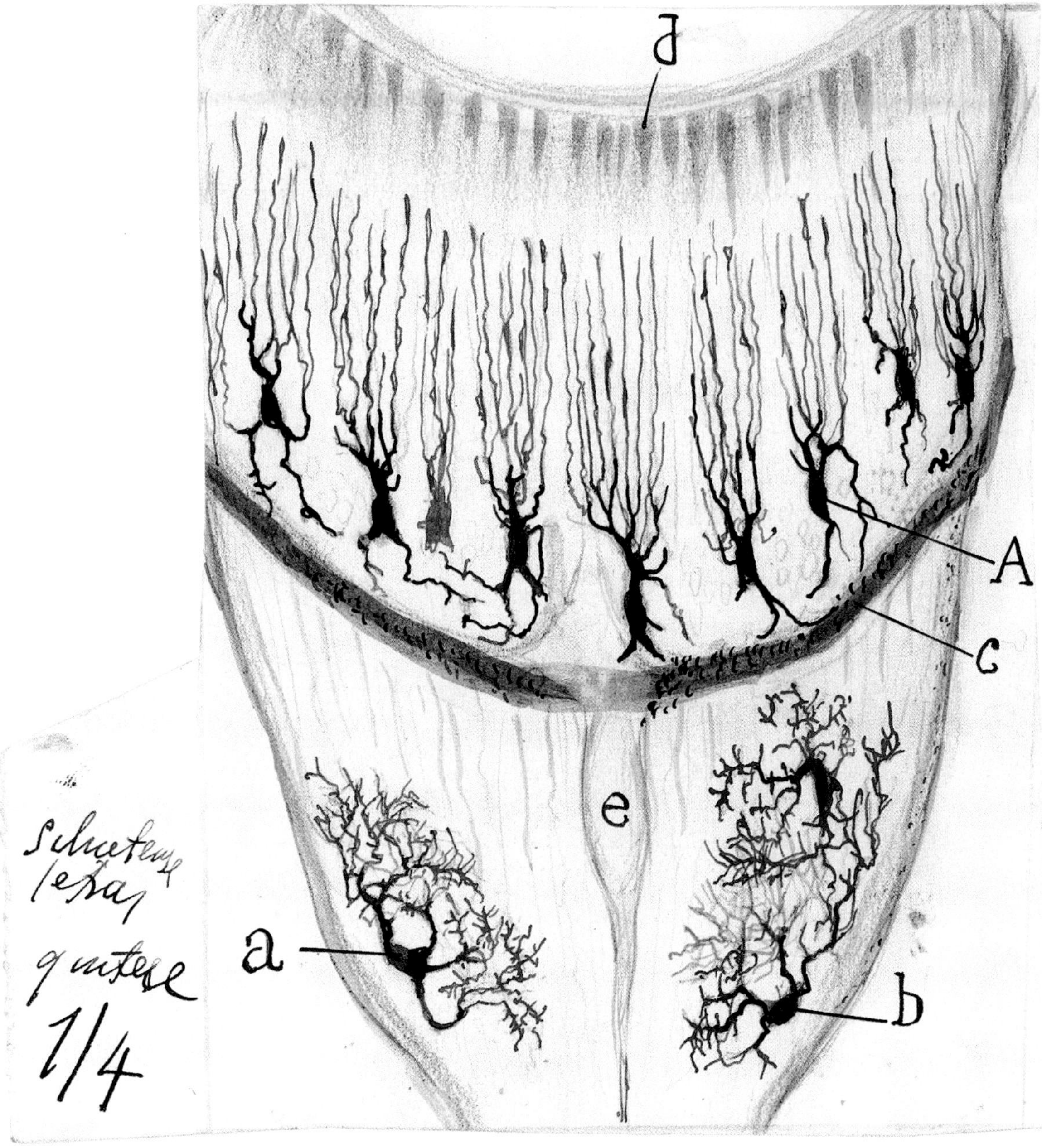

FIGURE 274. Neuroglia of the retina and retinal region from the middle ocellus in *Libellula*.

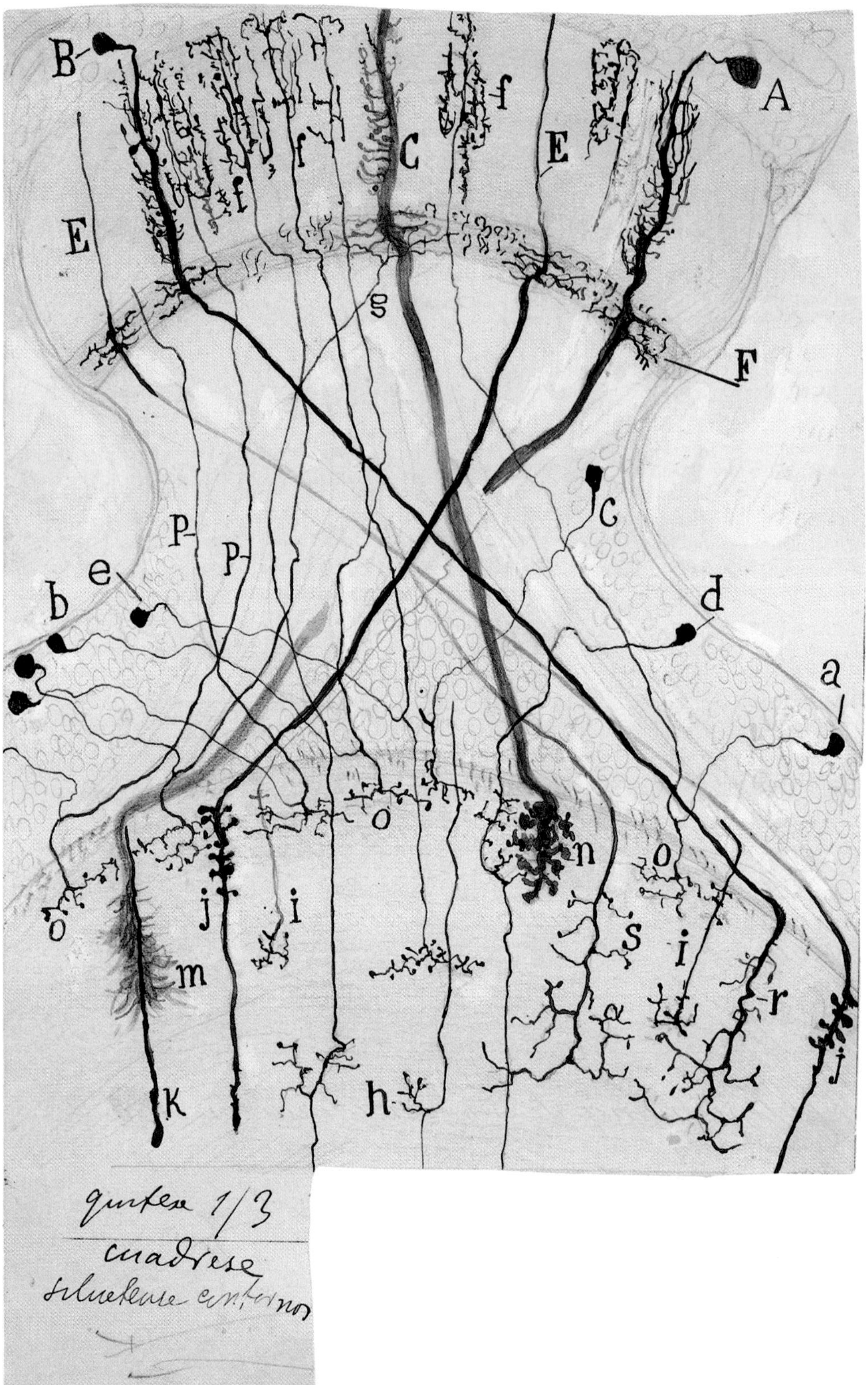

FIGURE 275. Some elements in a bee retina.

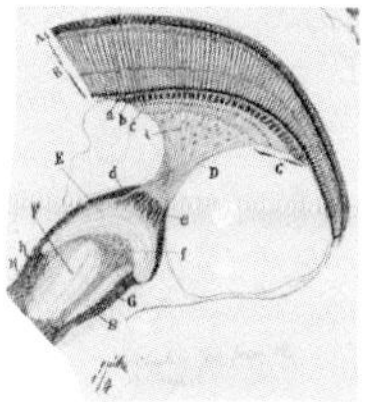

FIGURE 233.

Frontal section of the eye and optic lobe of *Musca vomitoria*.

This figure was published in Cajal, S. R. (1909) Nota sobre la estructura de la retina de la mosca (*M. vomitoria L.*). *Trab. Lab. Invest. Biol. Univ. Madrid* 7, 217–257 (Figure 1).

FIGURE LEGEND: Frontal section of the eye and optic lobe of *M. vomitoria*. *A*, Corneal and pseudocone layer; *B*, rods and rhabdomeric layer; *C*, perioptic or external ganglion sheet, formed by three subzones, *a, b, c*, named, respectively, fenestrated, granular, and plexiform membranes; *D*, optic nerve; E, optic lobe (epioptic or external medullary mass); *F*, internal medullary mass; *d, e*, amacrine cells area of the optic lobe; *G*, posterior ganglion mass; *H*, anterior ganglionic mass; *g*, laminar ganglion or superficial plexiform layer of the internal medullary mass; *f*, internal chiasm region.

Original text: Corte frontal de un ojo y lóbulo óptico de la *Musca vomitoria*. *A*, Capa de las corneolas y pseudoconos; *B*, Capa de los bastones y rabdomas; *C*, Perióptico o lámina ganglionar externa, con sus tres subzonas *a, b, c*, llamadas respectivamente, fenestrada, de los granos y plexiforme; *D*, Nervio óptico; E, Lóbulo óptico (epióptico ó masa medular externa; *F*, Masa medular interna; *d, e*, Subzona de células amacrinas del lóbulo óptico; *G*, Masa ganglionar posterior; *H*, Masa ganglionar anterior; *g*, ganglio laminar ó capa plexiforme superficial de la masa medular interna; *f*, Región del llamado kiasma interno.

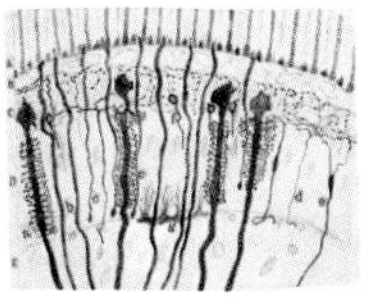

FIGURE 234.

Detail from a perioptic frontal section of *Musca vomitoria*.

This figure was published in Cajal, S. R. (1909) Nota sobre la estructura de la retina de la mosca (*M. vomitoria L.*). *Trab. Lab. Invest. Biol. Univ. Madrid* 7, 217–257 (Figure 4).

FIGURE LEGEND: Detail from a perioptic (external medullary sheet) frontal section of *M. vomitoria*. Golgi method. *A*, Rod layer; *B*, fenestrated subzone; *C*, granulated subzone; *D*, plexiform subzone; *E*, optic nerve; *a*, spiny shaft of perioptic large neurons; *b*, long optical fibers; *c*, short optical fibers; *d, e*, centrifugal fibers; *f*, small monopolar elements; *g*, neuroglial cells.

Original text: Trozo de un corte frontal del perióptico o lámina medular externa de la *Musca vomitoria*. Método de Golgi. *A*, Capa de los bastones; *B*, Subzona fenestrada; *C*, Subzona de los granos; *D*, Subzona plexiforme; *E*, Nervio óptico; *a*, Tallo espinoso de las neuronas gruesas del perióptico; *b*, Fibras ópticas largas; *c*, Fibras ópticas cortas; *d, e*, Fibras centrífugas; *f*, Pequeños elementos monopolares; *g*, Corpúsculos neuróglicos.

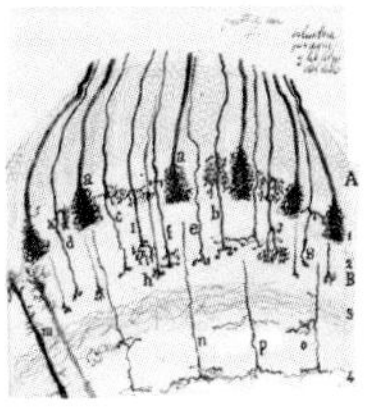

FIGURE 235.

Detail of a frontal section from the optic lobe of *Musca vomitoria*.

This figure was published in Cajal, S. R. (1909) Nota sobre la estructura de la retina de la mosca (*M. vomitoria L.*). *Trab. Lab. Invest. Biol. Univ. Madrid* 7, 217–257 (Figure 8).

FIGURE LEGEND: Detail of a frontal section from the optic lobe of *M. vomitoria*. Golgi method. In this figure, fibers found in various sections have been collected. *A*, Epioptic granular layer; *B*, epioptic plexiform area; *a*, terminal cones of perioptic (external ganglion sheet) large neurons; *b, d, e*, terminal feet from thin afferent fibers, probably in continuity with long optical fibers; *j, i, f*, thin afferent fibers showing an elaborate terminal tuft; *o, p, n*, thin descending fibers branching on lower levels of the plexiform layer; *m*, epithelial cells. (Consecutive numbers indicate stratified strata of the plexiform layer.)

Original text: Trozo de un corte frontal del lóbulo óptico de la *Musca vomitoria*. Método de Golgi. En esta figura se han reunido fibras encontradas en varios cortes. *A*, Capa granular del epióptico; *B*, Zona plexiforme de éste; *a*, Cono terminal de las gruesas neuronas del perióptico o lámina ganglionar externa; *b, d, e*, Pies terminales de fibras aferentes delgadas, probalemente continuadas con fibras ópticas largas; *j, i, f*, Fibras de igual especie, pero provistas de un penacho terminal más complicado; *o, p, n*, Fibras descendentes delgadas arborizadas en los pisos profundos de la capa plexiforme; *m*, Células epiteliales. (Los números de orden señalan pisos de estratificación de la zona plexiforme.

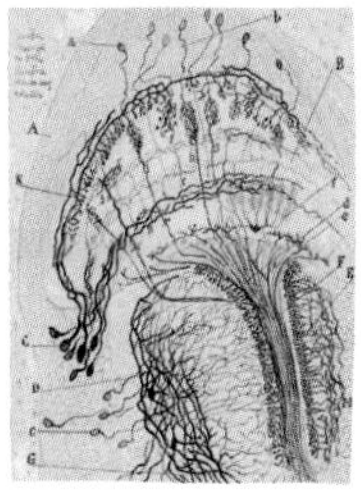

FIGURE 236.

Optic lobe (epioptic) and internal medullary mass of a muscid.

This figure was published in Cajal, S. R. (1909) Nota sobre la estructura de la retina de la mosca (*M. vomitoria L.*). *Trab. Lab. Invest. Biol. Univ. Madrid* 7, 217–257 (Figure 10).

FIGURE LEGEND: Frontal section of the optic lobe (epioptic) and internal medullary mass of Muscidae. Golgi method. *A*, Granular layer; *B*, plexiform layer; *C*, thick cells from the anterior ganglionic mass; *D*, internal medullary mass or ovoid body; *E*, superficial plexiform layer of the internal medullary mass; *F*, fibrillar layer of the internal medullary mass; *G*, central nervous tract ending in the ovoid body; *K, S*, dendritic plexi of the epioptic; *M*, posterior ganglionic mass; *a, b*, granule cells; *g, h, i*, centrifugal fibers; *c*, granule cells of the anterior ganglionic mass; *f*, neuroglial cell.

Original text: Corte frontal del lóbulo óptico (epióptico) y masa medular interna de un muscido. Método de Golgi. *A*, Corona granular; *B*, Capa plexiforme; *C*, Células gruesas de la masa gangliónica anterior; *D*, Masa medular interna ó cuerpo ovoideo; *E*, Capa plexiforme superficial de la masa medular interna; *F*, Capa fibrilar de este foco; *G*, Vía nerviosa central terminada en el cuerpo ovoideo; *K, S*, Plexos dendríticos del epióptico; *M*, Masa gangliónica posterior; *a, b*, Granos; *g, h, i*, Fibras centrífugas; *c*, Granos de la masa gangliónica anterior; *f*, Célula neuróglica.

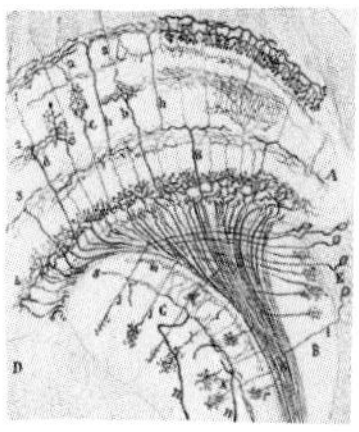

FIGURE 237.

Frontal section of the epioptic and internal medullary mass of a muscid.

This figure was published in Cajal, S. R. (1909) Nota sobre la estructura de la retina de la mosca (*M. vomitoria L.*). *Trab. Lab. Invest. Biol. Univ. Madrid* 7, 217–257 (Figure 11).

FIGURE LEGEND: Detail of a frontal section of the epioptic and internal medullary mass of a muscid (*Musca carnaria*). *A*, Epioptic plexiform layer; *B*, superficial plexiform layer of the internal medullary mass; *C*, deep plexiform layer of the internal medullary mass (Cucatti ovoid nucleus); *D*, anterior ganglionic mass; *E*, posterior ganglionic mass; *a*, deep expansions of the granule cells; *b, c*, discrete centrifugal fibers; *d, e*, peripheral filament from centrifugal fibers; *g, h*, collateral branches from plexi formed by diffuse centrifugal fibers; *j*, afferent fibers ending in the internal medullary mass, and so on. Numbers indicate branching layers of the epioptic plexiform layer.

Original text: Trozo de un corte frontal del epióptico y masa medular interna de un muscido (*M. carnaria*). *A*, Capa plexiforme del epióptico con sus pisos de arborización; *B*, Capa plexiforme superficial de la masa medular interna; *C*, Porción plexiforme profunda de este mismo foco o núcleo ovoideo de Cucatti; *D*, Masa gangliónica anterior; *E*, Masa ganglionica posterior; *a*, Expansiones profundas de los granos; *b, c*, Fibras centrífugas discretas; *d, e*, Fibras centrífugas, de cuya arborización nace un filamento periférico; *g, h*, Ramas colaterales de los plexos formados por fibras centrífugas difusas; *j*, Fibras aferentes acabadas en la masa medular interna, etc. Los números de orden señalan pisos de arborización de la capa plexiforme del epióptico.

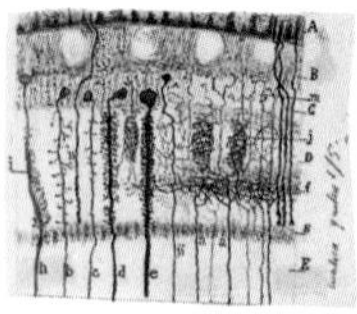

FIGURE 238.

Intermediate retina of *Libellula*.

This figure was published in Cajal, S. R., and Sánchez, D. (1915) Contribución al conocimiento de los centros nerviosos de los insectos. *Trab. Lab. Invest. Biol. Univ. Madrid* 13, 1–164 (Figure 8).

FIGURE LEGEND: Intermediate retina of *Libellula*. *A*, Peripherical retina; *B*, fenestrated layer scattered with pigment cells; *C*, layer of monopolar cells; *D*, external plexiform layer; *E*, chiasm region; *a*, centrifugal fibers from the intermediate nervous plexus; *j*, basket terminals; *e, d, h*, large monopolar cells; *b, c, ñ*, small monopolar cells; *g*, limiting layer of pigmentary elements.

Original text: Retina intermediaria de la *Libelula*. *A*, retina periférica; *B*, zona fenestrada salpicada de células de pigmento; *C*, zona de los corpúsculos monopolares; *D*, capa plexiforme externa; *E*, región del kiasma; *a*, fibras centrífugas para el plexo nervioso intermediario; *j*, cestas nerviosas; *e, d, h*, diversos tipos de monopolares grandes; *b, c, ñ*, monopolares pequeñas; *g*, capa limitante de elementos pigmentarios.

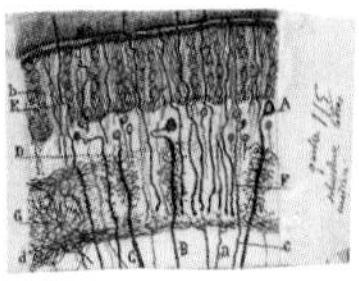

FIGURE 239.

Intermediate retina in a lepidopteran.

This figure was published in Cajal, S. R., and Sánchez, D. (1915) Contribución al conocimiento de los centros nerviosos de los insectos. *Trab. Lab. Invest. Biol. Univ. Madrid* 13, 1–164 (Figure 11).

FIGURE LEGEND: Intermediate retina in a lepidopteran (*Sphinx*). *A, B, C*, Several types of large monopolar cells; *D*, small monopolar cells; *E*, rods; *G*, nervous plexus of the external plexiform layer; *b*, pigmentary cells; *d*, inferior nervous plexus; *c*, rod or long visual fiber.

Original text: Retina intermediaria de un lepidóptero (*Sphinx*). *A, B, C*, tipos de células monopolares grandes; *D*, monopolar pequeña; *E*, paquete de bastones; *G*, plexo nervioso de la zona plexiforme externa; *b*, células pigmentarias; *d*, plexo nervioso limitante inferior; *c*, bastón o fibra visual larga.

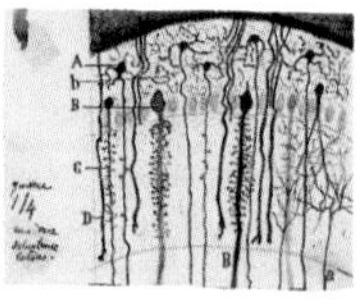

FIGURE 240.

Intermediate retina in *Agrion*.

This figure was published in Cajal, S. R., and Sánchez, D. (1915) Contribución al conocimiento de los centros nerviosos de los insectos. *Trab. Lab. Invest. Biol. Univ. Madrid* 13, 1–164 (Figure 12).

FIGURE LEGEND: Section of the intermediate retina in *Agrion*. *A*, Singular multipolar elements of the layer of granule cells; *B*, monopolar collosal cells; *C*, small monopolar cells; *D*, short rods; *a*, centrifugal fiber; *b*, interstitial plexus of the layer of the granule cells or monopolar neurons. (In this figure cells scattered in various consecutive sections have been collected).

Original text: Corte de la retina intermediaria del *Agrion*. *A*, singulares elementos multipolares de la zona de los granos; *B*, monopolares colosales; *C*, monopolares pequeñas; *D*, bastones cortos; *a*, fibra centrífuga; *b*, plexo intersticial de la zona de los granos ó neuronas monopolares. (Figura compuesta con las células de varios cortes sucesivos).

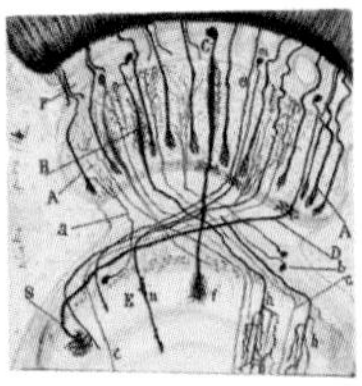

FIGURE 241.

Horizontal section of the retina in a bee.

This figure was published in Cajal, S. R., and Sánchez, D. (1915) Contribución al conocimiento de los centros nerviosos de los insectos. *Trab. Lab. Invest. Biol. Univ. Madrid* 13, 1–164 (Figure 15).

FIGURE LEGEND: Horizontal section of the retina in a bee. *A*, Short rods ending in brush-shape appendages; *B, C*, large monopolar cells; *E*, deep retina; *a*, long visual fibers; *b*, cells generating ascending centrifugal fibers. (In this figure cells scattered in various consecutive sections have been collected.)

Original text: Corte horizontal de la retina de la abeja. *A*, bastones cortos acabados por un pincel de apéndices; *B, C*, monopolares grandes; *E*, retina profunda; *a*, fibras visuales largas; *b*, corpúsculos generadores de fibras centrífugas ascendentes. (Figura compuesta con células halladas en cortes sucesivos.

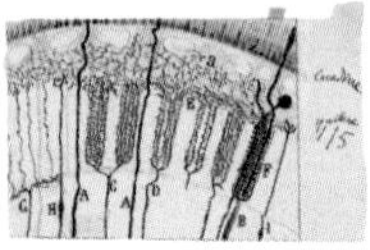

FIGURE 242.

Nervous plexi of the intermediate retina in a blowfly.

This figure was published in Cajal, S. R., and Sánchez, D. (1915) Contribución al conocimiento de los centros nerviosos de los insectos. *Trab. Lab. Invest. Biol. Univ. Madrid* 13, 1–164 (Figure 17).

FIGURE LEGEND: Nervous plexi of the intermediate retina in a blowfly. *A*, Long visual fibers; *B*, shaft of a monopolar collosal cell; *C, D*, centrifugal fibers ending in nervous prominences; *E*, external fibrillar connections between adjacent nervous prominences; *H, I*, a kind of centrifugal fiber ramifying moderately on the external border of the plexiform layer; *G*, other type of centrifugal fiber; *a*, nervous plexus located between the somas of the monopolar cells; *F*, optical cartridge.

Original text: Plexos nerviosos de la retina intermediaria de la mosca azul. *A*, fibras visuales largas; *B*, tallo de monopolar colosal; *C, D*, fibras centrífugas acabadas en bolsas nerviosas; *E*, comunicaciones fibrilares externas entre bolsas contiguas; *H, I*, otro tipo de fibra centrífuga sobriamente ramificado en la frontera externa de la zona plexiforme; *G*, otra variedad de centrífuga; *a*, plexo nervioso situado entre los somas de las monopolares; *F*, cartucho óptico.

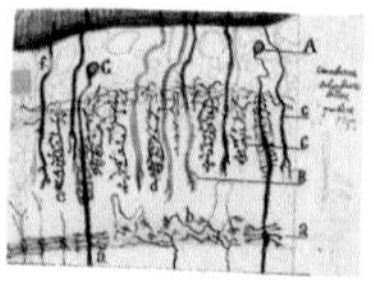

FIGURE 243.

Nervous prominences from intermediate retina in a honeybee.

This figure was published in Cajal, S. R., and Sánchez, D. (1915) Contribución al conocimiento de los centros nerviosos de los insectos. *Trab. Lab. Invest. Biol. Univ. Madrid* 13, 1–164 (Figure 19).

FIGURE LEGEND: Nervous prominences from intermediate retina in a honeybee. *A, C*, Monopolar cells; *B, c, f*, rods ending in the middle third of the plexiform layer; *e, d*, nervous prominences; *a*, group of appendages of a monopolar cell in contact with centrifugal cells of the inferior limiting plexus; *b*, varicosities and rosette structures of some plexus fibers.

Original text: Bolsas nerviosas en la retina intermediaria de la abeja. *A, C*, células monopolares; *B, c, f*, bastones terminados en el tercio medio de la zona plexiforme; *e, d*, bolsas nerviosas; *a*, penacho de apéndices de una monopolar en contacto con las centrífugas del plexo limitante inferior; *b*, varicosidades y rosáceas de algunas fibras de este plexo.

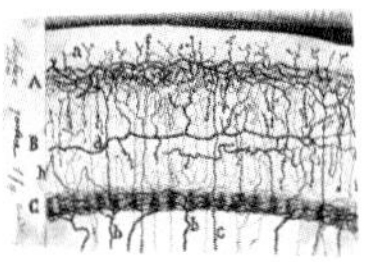

FIGURE 244.

Frontal section of the intermediate retina in a honeybee.

This figure was published in Cajal, S. R., and Sánchez, D. (1915) Contribución al conocimiento de los centros nerviosos de los insectos. *Trab. Lab. Invest. Biol. Univ. Madrid* 13, 1–164 (Figure 20).

FIGURE LEGEND: Frontal section in a bee intermediate retina showing the nervous plexi. *A*, External limiting plexus; *B*, intermediate plexus; *C*, internal limiting plexus; *a*, neuronal branches ending in a layer of monopolar cells; *b*, centrifugal fibers at the inferior plexus; *c*, centrifugal fibers at the external plexus.

Original text: Corte frontal de la retina intermediaria de la abeja destinada a mostrar los plexos nerviosos. *A*, plexo limitante externo; *B*, plexo intermediario; *C*, plexo limitante interno; *a*, ramas acabadas en la capa de los corpúsculos monopolares; *b*, centrífugas para el plexo inferior; *c*, centrífugas para el plexo externo.

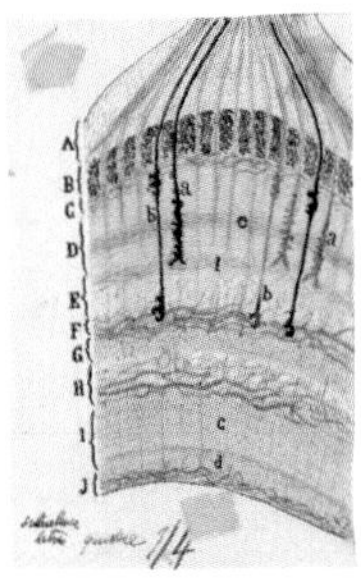

FIGURE 245.

Layers of connections from the plexiform formation in the deep retina in a gadfly.

This figure was published in Cajal, S. R., and Sánchez, D. (1915) Contribución al conocimiento de los centros nerviosos de los insectos. *Trab. Lab. Invest. Biol. Univ. Madrid* 13, 1–164 (Figure 21).

FIGURE LEGEND: Layers of connections from the plexiform formation in the deep retina in a gadfly. Illustration showing a combination of morphological features obtained from reduced silver nitrate preparations and from sections stained with the Golgi method. *A*, Granular formation; *B*, layer of fine tangential fibers; *C*, first layer of winding fibers; *D*, first diffuse nervous plexus; *E*, second diffuse nervous plexus; *F*, second or central layer of winding fibers; *H*, third layer of winding fibers; *G*, third diffuse plexus; *I*, fourth diffuse plexus; *J*, fourth layer of winding fibers; *a*, foot of a monopolar collosal cell; *b*, foot of a long visual fiber.

Original text: Pisos de conexión de la formación plexiforme de la retina profunda del tábano. Esquema en que se han combinado aspectos de las preparaciones del nitrato de plata reducido y algunas revelaciones del método de Golgi. *A*, formación granular; *B*, capa de las fibras tangenciales finas; *C*, primera lámina de fibras serpenteantes; *D*, primer plexo nervioso difuso; *E*, segundo plexo nervioso difuso; *F*, segunda lámina de fibras serpenteantes ó central; *H*, tercera lámina de fibras serpenteantes; *G*, Tercer plexo difuso; *I*, cuarto plexo difuso; *J*, cuarta lámina de fibras serpenteantes; *a*, pie de una monopolar colosal; *b*, pie de una fibra visual larga.

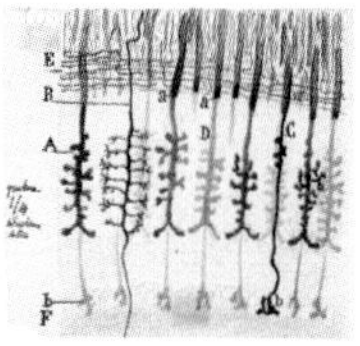

FIGURE 246.

Frontal section from the deep retina in a gadfly.

This figure was published in Cajal, S. R., and Sánchez, D. (1915) Contribución al conocimiento de los centros nerviosos de los insectos. *Trab. Lab. Invest. Biol. Univ. Madrid* 13, 1–164 (Figure 22).

FIGURE LEGEND: Frontal section from the deep retina in a gadfly. *A*, Branching of a monopolar collosal cell as seen in a frontal view; *B*, shaft of a ganglion cell; *D*, a single branch stained gray from osmic acid; *C*, long visual fiber; *E*, layer of fine tangential fibers; *F*, third diffuse plexiform layer; *a*, end of the sheath surrounding visual fibers; *b*, layer of long visual fibers.

Original text: Corte frontal de la retina profunda del tábano. *A*, arborización, vista de plano, de una monopolar colosal; *B*, Tallo de un corpúsculo ganglionar; *D*, una arborización teñida solamente en gris por el ácido ósmico; *C*, fibra visual larga; *E*, zona de las fibras finas tangenciales; *F*, tercer piso plexiforme difuso; *a*, terminación de la vaina que acompaña á las fibras visuales; *b*, piso de las fibras visuales largas.

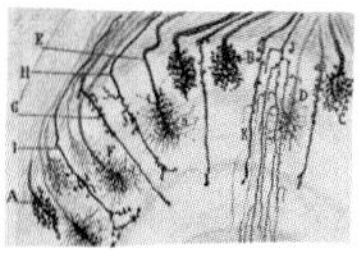

FIGURE 247.

Slightly oblique section from the deep retina in a bee.

This figure was published in Cajal, S. R., and Sánchez, D. (1915) Contribución al conocimiento de los centros nerviosos de los insectos. *Trab. Lab. Invest. Biol. Univ. Madrid* 13, 1–164 (Figure 23).

FIGURE LEGEND: Slightly oblique section from the deep retina in a bee. Different types of fibers arriving from the intermediate retina (perioptic). *A, B, C*, Thick branches of the first layer; *D, E, F*, branching of the second layer; *H, G, K, I*, long visual fibers; *J*, a descending brush-shape branch.

Original text: Corte algo oblicuo de la retina profunda de la abeja. Diversas especies de fibras llegadas de la retina intermediaria ó perióptico. *A, B, C*, arborizaciones groseras del primer piso; *D, E, F*, arborizaciones del segundo piso; *H, G, K, I*, fibras visuales largas; *J*, arborización descendente en forma de pincel.

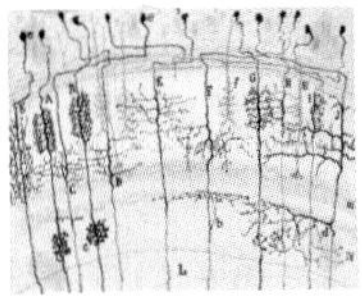

FIGURE 248.

Frontal section of the deep retina in a gadfly.

This figure was published in Cajal, S. R., and Sánchez, D. (1915) Contribución al conocimiento de los centros nerviosos de los insectos. *Trab. Lab. Invest. Biol. Univ. Madrid* 13, 1–164 (Figure 26).

FIGURE LEGEND: Frontal section of the deep retina in a gadfly showing several types of ganglion cells. *A, B, G*, Types of proximal, short-ending dendrites; *H, E*, modalities of diffuse initial branching; *J*, giant modality; *C, D, F*, ganglionic cells with their dendrites distributed in the second nervous plexus; *e*, somas; *c*, basal branching; *f*, foot of a short visual fiber; *g*, long visual fiber.

Original text: Corte frontal de la retina profunda del tábano, donde se observan diversos tipos de células gangliónicas. *A, B, G*, tipos de dendritas próximas y prontamente terminadas; *H, E*, modalidades de arborización inicial difusa; *J*, modalidad gigante; *C, D, F*, ganglionares cuyas dendritas se distribuyen por el segundo plexo nervioso; *e*, somas; *c*, arborización basal; *f*, pie de una visual corta; *g*, visual larga.

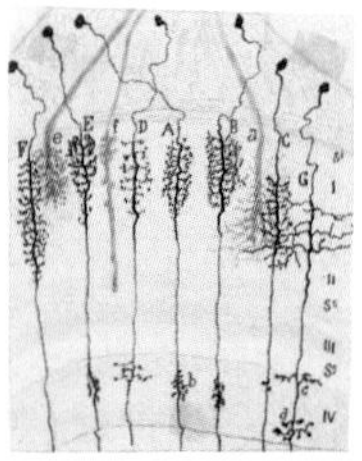

FIGURE 249.

Section from the deep retina in a bee.

This figure was published in Cajal, S. R., and Sánchez, D. (1915) Contribución al conocimiento de los centros nerviosos de los insectos. *Trab. Lab. Invest. Biol. Univ. Madrid* 13, 1–164 (Figure 27).

FIGURE LEGEND: Section from the deep retina in a bee. Different types of ganglion cells. *A, B*, Types of patchy terminations; *G*, variety of diffuse ramification; *e*, foot of a monopolar collosal cell; *f*, long visual fiber; *b, c, d*, basal branches. Roman numerals indicate diffuse nervous plexi; S^1, first winding layer; S^2, second winding layer, and so on.

Original text: Corte de la retina profunda de la abeja. Diversos tipos de células ganglionares. *A, B*, tipos de arborización concreta; *G*, variedad de ramificación difusa; *e*, pie de una monopolar colosal; *f*, fibra visual larga; *b, c, d*, arborizaciones basales. Los números romanos señalan los plexos nerviosos difusos; S^1, lámina serpenteante primera; S^2, serpenteante segunda, etc.

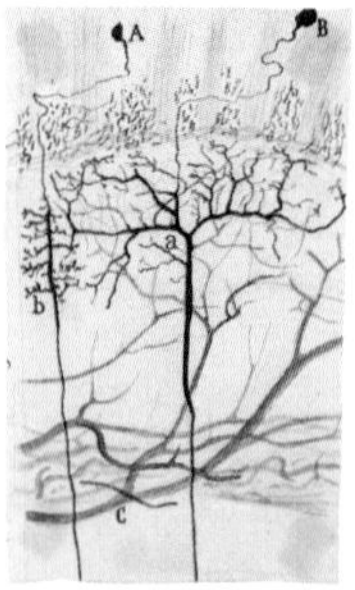

FIGURE 250.

Giant ganglion cell from the epioptic in a gadfly.

This figure was published in Cajal, S. R., and Sánchez, D. (1915) Contribución al conocimiento de los centros nerviosos de los insectos. *Trab. Lab. Invest. Biol. Univ. Madrid* 13, 1–164 (Figure 28).

FIGURE LEGEND: *B*, Giant ganglion cell from the epioptic in a gadfly; *A*, common ganglion cell; *a*, thick dendrites of a giant ganglion cell; *C*, robust branches arriving from winding horizontal fibers of the third layer.

Original text: B, ganglionar gigante del epióptico del tábano; *A*, gangliónica común; *a*, gruesas dendritas de la ganglionar gigante; *C*, robustas ramas llegadas de la tercera lámina de conductores horizontales serpenteantes.

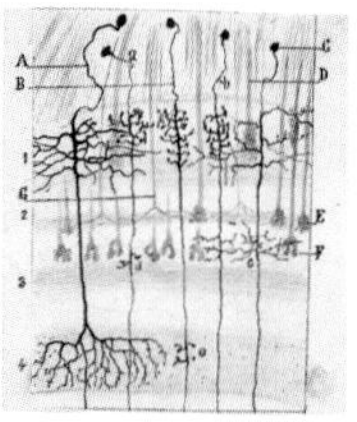

FIGURE 251.

Section from the deep retina in a fly.

This figure was published in Cajal, S. R., and Sánchez, D. (1915) Contribución al conocimiento de los centros nerviosos de los insectos. *Trab. Lab. Invest. Biol. Univ. Madrid* 13, 1–164 (Figure 30).

FIGURE LEGEND: Section from the deep retina in a fly. *A*, Giant ganglion cell; *B*, a type of patchy branching; *C*, type of diffuse branching; *D*, foot of a monopolar collosal cell; *E, F*, feet of long visual fibers; *G*, robust branching fibers in a special nervous plexus located in the thickness of the second diffuse plexus.

Original text: Corte de la retina profunda de la mosca. *A*, gangliónica gigante; *B*, tipo de arborización concreta; *C*, tipo de arborización difusa; *D*, pie de una monopolar colosal; *E, F*, pies de fibras visuales largas; *G*, recias fibras arborizadas en un plexo nervioso especial situado en el espesor del plexo difuso segundo.

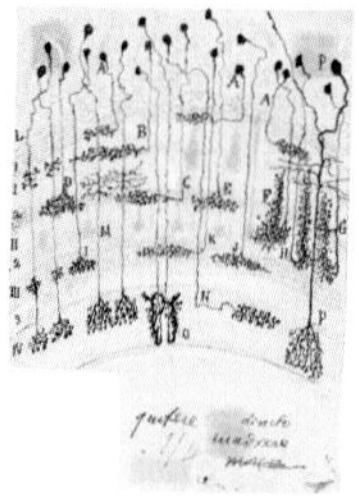

FIGURE 252.

Type I cells or amacrine cells from the deep retina in *Calliphora.*

This figure was published in Cajal, S. R., and Sánchez, D. (1915) Contribución al conocimiento de los centros nerviosos de los insectos. *Trab. Lab. Invest. Biol. Univ. Madrid* 13, 1–164 (Figure 31).

FIGURE LEGEND: Type I or amacrine cells from the deep retina in *Calliphora*. In this figure, elements from several sections have been put together. *A*, Cells with their tuft extending through the first winding layer; *B*, cells with their tufts located in the thickness of the first diffuse plexus; *C, D, E*, others cells with their tufts located in a secondary striation that divides the second diffuse plexus into two subzones; *J, K, I*, amacrine cells located on the third diffuse plexus; *N*, folded amacrine cell in the fourth diffuse plexus; *L, M*, bistratified and tristratified amacrines; *F, G, O*, retrograde amacrines.

Original text: Células del I tipo ó amacrinas de la retina profunda de la *Calliphora*; en esta figura se han reunido los elementos encontrados en varios cortes. *A*, células cuyo penacho se extiende por la primera lámina serpenteante; *B*, células cuyo penacho se distribuye en el espesor del plexo difuso primero; *C, D, E*, otras para una estría secundaria que divide el plexo difuso segundo en dos subzonas; *J, K, I*, amacrinas para el plexo difuso tercero; *N*, amacrina doblada para el plexo difuso cuarto; *L, M*, amacrinas bi y triestratificadas; *F, G, O*, amacrinas retrógradas.

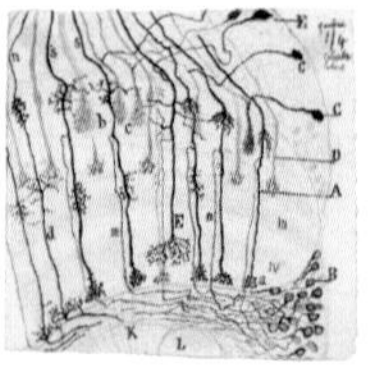

FIGURE 253.

Horizontal section from the deep retina in *Calliphora.*

This figure was published in Cajal, S. R., and Sánchez, D. (1915) Contribución al conocimiento de los centros nerviosos de los insectos. *Trab. Lab. Invest. Biol. Univ. Madrid* 13, 1–164 (Figure 37).

FIGURE LEGEND: Horizontal section from the deep retina in *Calliphora. A*, Deep centrifugal arcuate peduncular cells; *B*, deep ganglion where the soma of these cells is located; *C*, cell divided in T; *D*, long visual fiber; *b*, visual collosal club; *E*, element divided in T, with a robust ascending centrifugal process to the intermediate retina; *K*, deep chiasm; *L*, optic lobe (laminar nucleus); *m*, arcuate peduncle.

Original text: Corte horizontal de la retina profunda de la *Calliphora. A*, centrífugas profundas de mango arciforme; *B*, ganglio profundo donde reside el soma de esas células; *C*, célula en T; *D*, fibra visual larga; *b*, maza colosal visual; *E*, elemento dividido en T, con robusta expansión centrífuga ascendente para la retina intermediaria; *K*, kiasma profundo; *L*, lóbulo óptico (foco laminar); *m*, mango arciforme.

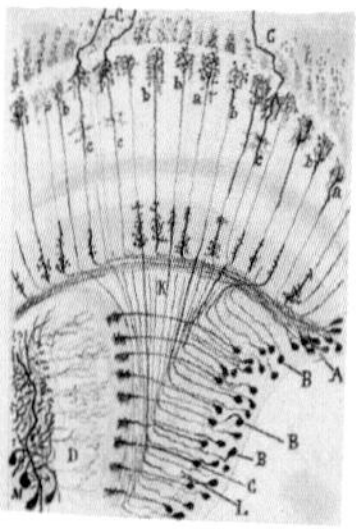

FIGURE 254.

Horizontal section from the deep retina and optic lobe in a gadfly.

This figure was published in Cajal, S. R., and Sánchez, D. (1915) Contribución al conocimiento de los centros nerviosos de los insectos. *Trab. Lab. Invest. Biol. Univ. Madrid* 13, 1–164 (Figure 40).

FIGURE LEGEND: Horizontal section of the deep retina and optic lobe in a gadfly. *A*, Group of neurons with branching centrifugal fibers in the epioptic (*a, c*); *B*, granular cortex of the optic lobe where are located the somas of cells with centrifugal fibers ending in the first diffuse plexus of the plexiform internal layer (*b*); *C*, long or perforating centrifugal cells for the intermediate retina, with their somas located in the angular ganglion *A; D*, ovoid ganglion of the optic lobe; *L*, laminar nucleus; *K*, deep chiasm.

Original text: Sección horizontal de la retina profunda y lóbulo óptico del tábano. *A*, acúmulo de neuronas generadoras de fibras centrífugas arborizadas en el epióptico (*a, c*); *B*, corteza granular del lóbulo óptico donde residen los somas de centrífugas acabadas en el plexo primero difuso de la zona plexiforme interna (*b*); *C*, centrifugas largas ó perforantes para la retina intermediaria y cuyo soma reside en el ganglio angular *A; D*, ganglio ovoideo del lóbulo óptico; *L*, foco laminar; *K*, kiasma profundo.

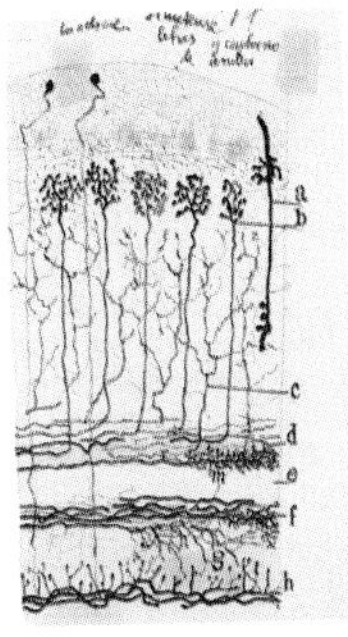

FIGURE 255.

Section from the epioptic in a honeybee.

This figure was published in Cajal, S. R., and Sánchez, D. (1915) Contribución al conocimiento de los centros nerviosos de los insectos. *Trab. Lab. Invest. Biol. Univ. Madrid* 13, 1–164 (Figure 44).

FIGURE LEGEND: Section from the epioptic in a honeybee. *a*, Long visual fiber; *b*, terminal branching of fibers from the third diffuse plexus; *h*, winding layer IV; *f*, winding layer III; *m*, terminal branching of a thin horizontal fiber; *g*, terminal ramification of a fiber of the winding layer III.

Original text: Corte del epióptico de la abeja. *a*, fibra visual larga; *b*, arborización terminal de fibras venidas del plexo difuso tercero; *h*, lámina serpenteante IV; *f*, lámina serpenteante III; *m*, ramificación terminal de una fibra fina horizontal; *g*, arborización terminal de un conductor de la lámina serpenteante III.

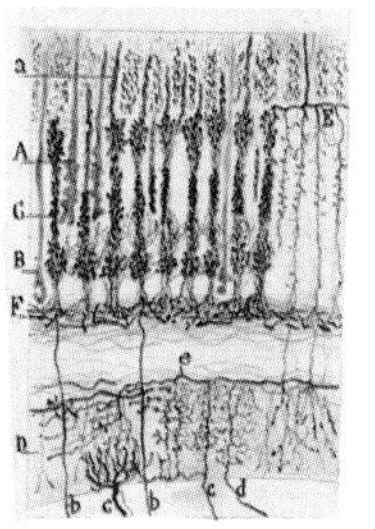

FIGURE 256.

Horizontal section from the epioptic in a gadfly.

This figure was published in Cajal, S. R., and Sánchez, D. (1915) Contribución al conocimiento de los centros nerviosos de los insectos. *Trab. Lab. Invest. Biol. Univ. Madrid* 13, 1–164 (Figure 45).

FIGURE LEGEND: Horizontal section from the epioptic in a gadfly. *A*, Foot of the large monopolar cells arriving from the intermediate retina; *B*, long visual fibers; *C*, climbing plexi apparently located around the shafts of ganglion neurons (*b*); *D*, diffuse plexus IV; *F*, diffuse plexus III.

Original text: Corte horizontal del epióptico del tábano. *A*, pie de las monopolares grandes llegadas de la retina intermediaria; *B*, fibras visuales largas; *C*, plexos trepadores situados al parecer en torno de los tallos de las neuronas ganglionares (*b*); *D*, plexo difuso IV; *F*, plexo difuso III.

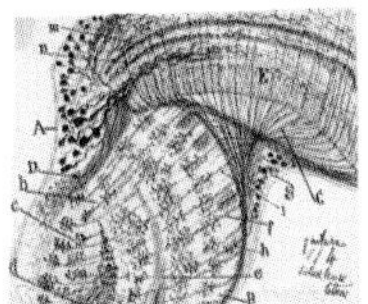

FIGURE 257.

Optic lobe and internal chiasm in *Libellula.*

This figure was published in Cajal, S. R., and Sánchez, D. (1915) Contribución al conocimiento de los centros nerviosos de los insectos. *Trab. Lab. Invest. Biol. Univ. Madrid* 13, 1–164 (Figure 49).

FIGURE LEGEND: Semischematic horizontal section of the optic lobe and internal chiasm in *Libellula*. *A*, Area of the frontal granule cells and angular nucleus; *B*, optic lobe (first segment); *C*, internal chiasm; *E*, deep diffuse plexus of the epioptic; *f, i*, multistratified visual fibers; *h*, cotton-like tufts of the amacrine cells destined to the optic lobe; *g*, dorsal granular accumulation.

Original text: Corte horizontal semiesquemático del lóbulo óptico y kiasma interno de la *libelula*. *A*, zona de los granos frontales y foco angular; *B*, lóbulo óptico (primer segmento); *C*, kiasma interno; *E*, plexo difuso profundo del epióptico; *f, i*, fibras visuales multiestratificadas; *h*, penachos algodonosos de las amacrinas destinados al lóbulo óptico; *g*, acúmulo granular dorsal.

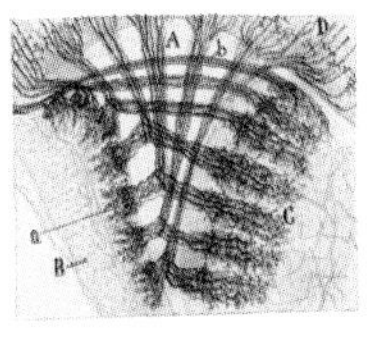

FIGURE 258.

Horizontal section from the internal chiasm region and optic lobe in a gadfly.

This figure was published in Cajal, S. R., and Sánchez, D. (1915) Contribución al conocimiento de los centros nerviosos de los insectos. *Trab. Lab. Invest. Biol. Univ. Madrid* 13, 1–164 (Figure 53).

FIGURE LEGEND: Horizontal section from the internal chiasm region and optic lobe in a gadfly. *A*, Bundles of optic fibers (shafts); *b*, fascicles of branches destined to the ovoid nucleus; *a*, arborizations destined to the laminar nucleus; *D*, epioptic; *B*, granule cells of the laminar nucleus; *C*, ovoid nucleus.

Original text: Corte horizontal de la región del kiasma interno y lóbulo óptico del tábano. *A*, haces de fibras ópticas (tallos); *b*, fascículos de ramas para el foco ovoideo; *a*, arborizaciones destinadas al foco laminar; *D*, epióptico; *B*, granos del foco laminar; *C*, foco ovoideo.

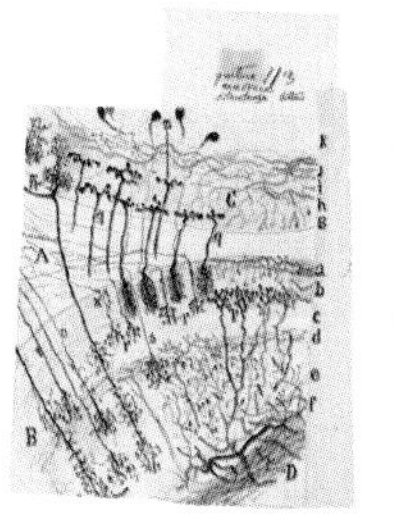

FIGURE 259.

Section of the two segments of the optic lobe in a gadfly retina.

This figure was published in Cajal, S. R., and Sánchez, D. (1915) Contribución al conocimiento de los centros nerviosos de los insectos. *Trab. Lab. Invest. Biol. Univ. Madrid* 13, 1–164 (Figure 54).

FIGURE LEGEND: Horizontal section of the two segments of the optic lobe in a gadfly retina. *A*, Internal chiasm; *B*, ovoid nucleus; *C*, laminar nucleus; *x, t, o, s, r*, different types of monostratified visual fibers; *ñ*, forked visual fiber with the tuft directed to the laminar nucleus; *q*, bitufted amacrines or with arcuate peduncle.

Original text: Corte horizontal de los dos segmentos del lóbulo óptico de la retina del tábano. *A*, kiasma interno; *B*, foco ovoideo; *C*, foco laminar; *x, t, o, s, r*, diversos tipos de fibras visuales monoestratificadas; *ñ*, fibra visual bifurcada con el penacho destinada al foco laminar; *q*, amacrinas bipenachadas ó de mango retrógrado.

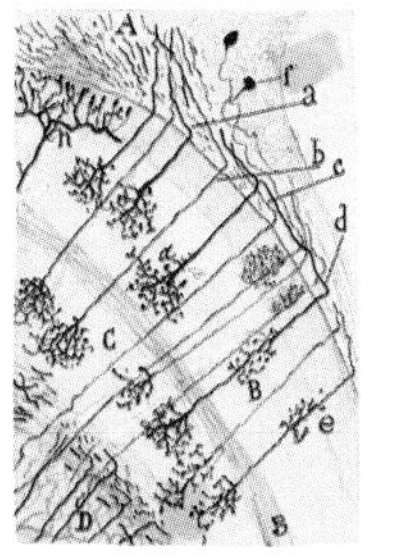

FIGURE 260.

Horizontal section of the chiasm and optic lobe in *Libellula.*

This figure was published in Cajal, S. R., and Sánchez, D. (1915) Contribución al conocimiento de los centros nerviosos de los insectos. *Trab. Lab. Invest. Biol. Univ. Madrid* 13, 1–164 (Figure 57).

FIGURE LEGEND: Detail of the horizontal section of the chiasm and optic lobe in *Libellula*. *a*, Branched optic fibers in the second diffuse plexus; *e*, branched optical fibers in the second segment of the lobe; *g*, bundle of concentric nervous fibers; *A*, chiasm; *B*, first segment of the optic lobe; *C*, second segment; *D*, third segment.

Original text: Trozo de un corte horizontal del kiasma y lóbulo óptico de la libelula. *a*, fibras ópticas ramificadas en el segundo plexo difuso; *e*, fibras ópticas arborizadas en el segundo segmento del lóbulo; *g*, faja de fibras nerviosas concéntricas; *A*, kiasma; *B*, primer segmento del lóbulo óptico; *C*, segundo segmento; *D*, tercer segmento.

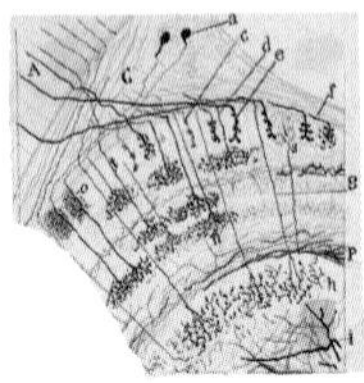

FIGURE 261.

Horizontal section from the optic lobe in a bee.

This figure was published in Cajal, S. R., and Sánchez, D. (1915) Contribución al conocimiento de los centros nerviosos de los insectos. *Trab. Lab. Invest. Biol. Univ. Madrid* 13, 1–164 (Figure 58).

FIGURE LEGEND: Horizontal section from the optic lobe in a bee. *A*, Deep retina; *B*, optic lobe; *a, b*, bistratified amacrine cells; *c*, fine optic fibers destined to the first plexus; *e, f*, thick optic fibers destined to the first plexus; *d*, optic fiber destined to the second plexus; *t, ñ, h*, other arborizations in deep plexi.

Original text: Corte horizontal del lóbulo óptico de la abeja. *A*, retina profunda; *B*, lóbulo óptico; *a, b*, amacrinas biestratificadas; *c*, fibras ópticas finas para el primer plexo; *e, f*, fibras ópticas gruesas para el mismo; *d*, fibra óptica destinada al segundo plexo; *t, ñ, h*, otras arborizadas en plexos profundos.

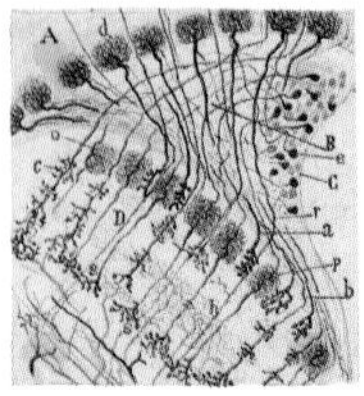

FIGURE 262.

Region of the chiasm and optic lobe in a bee.

This figure was published in Cajal, S. R., and Sánchez, D. (1915) Contribución al conocimiento de los centros nerviosos de los insectos. *Trab. Lab. Invest. Biol. Univ. Madrid* 13, 1–164 (Figure 59).

FIGURE LEGEND: Horizontal section of the region of the chiasm and optic lobe in a bee. *A*, Epioptic; *B*, chiasm; *C*, neuronal agglomeration of the optic lobe; *D*, plexiform portion of the optic lobe; *a*, thick optic fibers destined to the first diffuse plexus; *b, c, f*, polystratified visual fibers; *d*, external tuft of arcuate peduncle neurons; *e*, soma of these same cells; *r*, processes in the optic lobe of the same neurons; *o, p*, superficial cotton-like arborizations of the amacrine cells of the optic lobe; g, deep tuft of amacrine cells.

Original text: Sección horizontal de la región del kiasma y lóbulo óptico de la abeja. *A*, epióptico; *B*, kiasma; *C*, aglomeración neuronal del lóbulo óptico; *D*, porción plexiforme del lóbulo óptico; *a*, fibras ópticas gruesas destinadas al primer plexo difuso; *b, c, f*, fibras visuales poliestratificadas; *d*, penacho externo de las neuronas de mango retrógrado; *e*, soma de estas células; *r*, expansión para el lóbulo óptico de estos mismos elementos; *o, p*, arborizaciones superficiales algodonosas de las amacrinas del lóbulo óptico; g, penacho profundo de estos elementos.

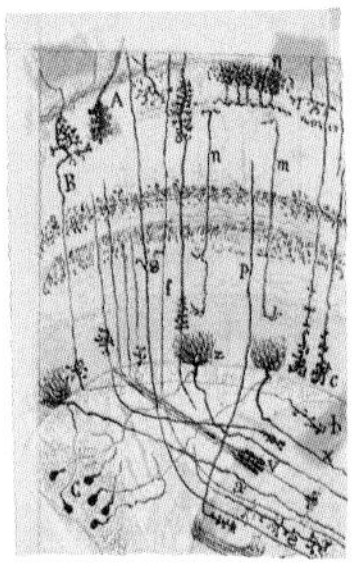

FIGURE 263.

Epioptic, internal chiasm, and optic lobe in a bee.

This figure was published in Cajal, S. R., and Sánchez, D. (1915) Contribución al conocimiento de los centros nerviosos de los insectos. *Trab. Lab. Invest. Biol. Univ. Madrid* 13, 1–164 (Figure 60).

FIGURE LEGEND: Horizontal section of the epioptic, internal chiasm, and optic lobe in a bee. Semischematic figure. *A*, Foot of monopolar collosal cells of the intermediate retina; *B*, fiber from a ganglion cell that gives rise to a visual branch in the first diffuse plexus of the optic lobe (*b*); *C*, neuronal mass of the optic lobe; *z*, external tuft of arcuate peduncle neurons; *f*, longer perforating fiber; *m, n*, singular fibers forming a loop; *f, g*, perforating fibers showing a vertical branch to the cellular regions of the epioptic; *e*, polystratified visual fiber; *c*, amacrine cells to the epioptic(?); *P*, thick visual fiber to the first diffuse plexus of the optic lobe; *ñ* [in the top of the figure], rose-shape branches from vertical fibers in the first zone of the epioptic.

Original text: Sección horizontal del epióptico, kiasma interno y lóbulo óptico de la abeja. Figura semiesquemática. *A*, pie de las monopolares colosales de la retina intermediaria; *B*, célula gangliónica continuada con una arborización visual para el primer plexo difuso del lóbulo óptico (*b*); *C*, macizo neuronal del lóbulo óptico; *z*, penacho externo de las neuronas de mango retrógrado; *f*, fibra perforante larguísima; *m, n*, singulares fibras en asa; *f, g*, fibras perforantes que emiten una rama vertical para las regiones celulares del epióptico; *e*, fibra visual poliestratificada; *c*, amacrinas para el epióptico? *P*, fibra visual gruesa para el primer plexo difuso del lóbulo óptico; *ñ*, arborizaciones rosaliformes para la primera zona del epióptico, originadas de fibras verticales.

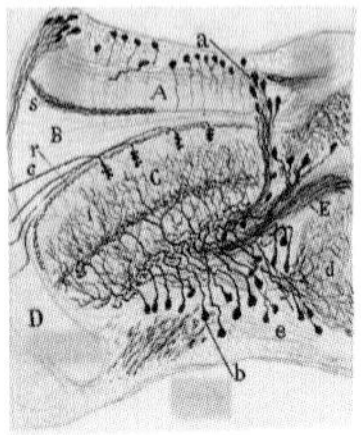

FIGURE 264.

Optic lobe in a blowfly.

This figure was published in Cajal, S. R., and Sánchez, D. (1915) Contribución al conocimiento de los centros nerviosos de los insectos. *Trab. Lab. Invest. Biol. Univ. Madrid* 13, 1–164 (Figure 61).

FIGURE LEGEND: Horizontal section from the optic lobe in a blowfly. *A*, Laminar nucleus; *B*, chiasm; *C*, ovoid nucleus; *D*, deep retina; *a*, dorsal cells with processes that penetrate the ovoid nucleus; *b*, frontal or anterior cells with processes to the oval ganglion plexi; *s*, tangential plexus of the laminar nucleus; *r*, tangential plexus of the ovoid nucleus.

Original text: Sección horizontal del lóbulo óptico de la mosca azul. *A*, foco laminar; *B*, kiasma; *C*, foco ovoideo; *D*, retina profunda; *a*, corpúsculos dorsales cuya expansión penetra en el foco ovoideo; *b*, células frontales ó anteriores destinadas á los plexos del ganglio oval; *s*, plexo tangencial del foco laminar; *r*, plexo tangencial del foco ovoideo.

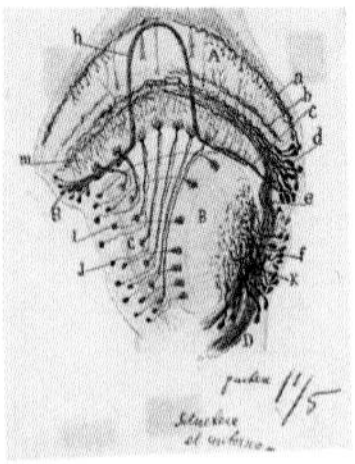

FIGURE 265.

Retina and optic lobe in a gadfly.

This figure was published in Cajal, S. R., and Sánchez, D. (1915) Contribución al conocimiento de los centros nerviosos de los insectos. *Trab. Lab. Invest. Biol. Univ. Madrid* 13, 1–164 (Figure 62).

FIGURE LEGEND: Horizontal section of the retina and optic lobe in a gadfly (lower magnification than previous figures). This illustration shows schematically some elements found in several successive sections. *A*, Internal plexiform layer of the deep retina; *B*, main or ovoid nucleus of the optic lobe; *C*, accessory or laminar nucleus; *D*, central pathway from the protocerebrum; *a, b, c*, laminar or winding plexi; *d*, anterior angular nucleus; *g*, posterior angular nucleus; *h*, arcuate funiculus of centrifugal fibers; *J*, soma of retrograde peduncle centrifugal cells; *I*, amacrine cells of the optic lobe.

Original text: Corte horizontal de la retina y lóbulo óptico del tábano. Aumento menor que en las figuras anteriores. En este grabado se han dibujado algo esquemáticamente elementos encontrados en varios cortes sucesivos. *A*, capa plexiforme interna de la retina profunda; *B*, foco principal ú ovoideo del lóbulo óptico; *C*, foco accesorio ó laminar; *D*, vía central llegada del protocerebrón; *a, b, c*, plexos laminares ó serpenteantes; *d*, foco angular anterior; *g*, foco angular posterior; *h*, cordón arciforme de fibras centrífugas; *J*, soma de las centrífugas de mango retrógrado; *I*, amacrinas del lóbulo óptico.

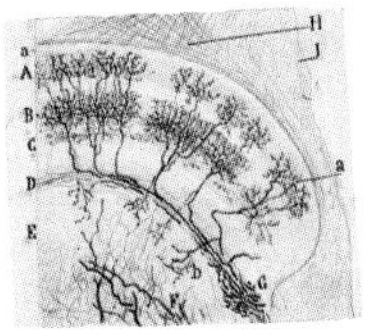

FIGURE 266.

Optic lobe in a bee.

This figure was published in Cajal, S. R., and Sánchez, D. (1915) Contribución al conocimiento de los centros nerviosos de los insectos. *Trab. Lab. Invest. Biol. Univ. Madrid* 13, 1–164 (Figure 65).

FIGURE LEGEND: Horizontal section from the optic lobe in a bee. Terminal arborization of centrifugal fibers. *A*, Arborizations located in the first diffuse plexus; *B*, arborizations located in the second and third plexi; *D*, layer of horizontal fibers; *b*, recurrent collaterals; *H*, chiasm; *I*, posterior granular mass of the optic lobe.

Original text: Corte horizontal del lóbulo óptico de la abeja. Arborización terminal de fibras centrífugas. *A*, arborizaciones para el plexo difuso primero; *B*, arborizaciones para el plexo segundo y tercero; *D*, capa de fibras horizontales; *b*, colaterales recurrentes; *H*, kiasma; *I*, macizo granular posterior del lóbulo óptico.

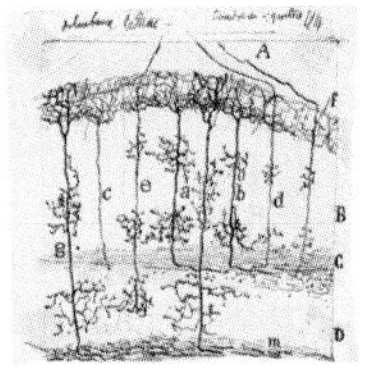

FIGURE 267.

First and second segments of the optic lobe in *Libellula*.

This figure was published in Cajal, S. R., and Sánchez, D. (1915) Contribución al conocimiento de los centros nerviosos de los insectos. *Trab. Lab. Invest. Biol. Univ. Madrid* 13, 1–164 (Figure 66).

FIGURE LEGEND: Horizontal section of the first and second segments from the optic lobe in *Libellula*. *A*, Region of the internal chiasm; *B, D*, first and second segments of the optic lobe; *a, b*, centrifugal fibers arriving from the first fibrillary layer; *g*, centrifugal fibers arriving from the second fibrillary layer; *e*, stratified visual fiber; *d*, centrifugal fibers ascending towards the epioptic.

Original text: Sección horizontal de los segmentos primero y segundo del lóbulo óptico de la libélula. *A*, región del kiasma interno; *B* y *D*, segmentos primero y segundo del citado lóbulo; *a, b*, fibras centrífugas llegadas de la primera capa fibrilar; *g*, centrífugas desprendidas de la segunda lámina fibrilar; *e*, fibra visual estratificada; *d*, centrífugas que ascienden hasta el epióptico.

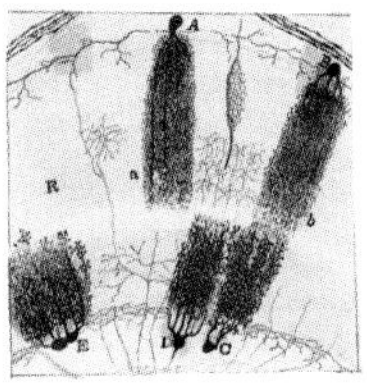

FIGURE 268.

Neuroglia from the deep retina in a gadfly.

This figure was published in Cajal, S. R., and Sánchez, D. (1915) Contribución al conocimiento de los centros nerviosos de los insectos. *Trab. Lab. Invest. Biol. Univ. Madrid* 13, 1–164 (Figure 74).

FIGURE LEGEND: Neuroglia from the deep retina in a gadfly. *A, B*, External radiated cells; *C, D, E*, internal radiated cells; *a, b*, small terminal branches.

Original text: Neuroglia de la retina profunda del tábano. *A, B*, células radiadas externas; *C, D, E*, células radiadas internas; *a, b*, ramitas terminales.

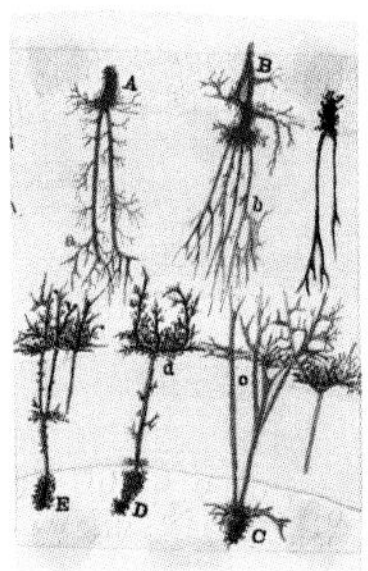

FIGURE 269.

Neuroglia devoid of cotton-like filaments.

This figure was published in Cajal, S. R., and Sánchez, D. (1915) Contribución al conocimiento de los centros nerviosos de los insectos. *Trab. Lab. Invest. Biol. Univ. Madrid* 13, 1–164 (Figure 75).

FIGURE LEGEND: Dislocated epithelial cells or neuroglia showing no cotton-like filaments. Epioptic in a gadfly.

Original text: Células epiteliales dislocadas ó neuroglia desprovista de filamentos algodonosos. Epióptico del tábano.

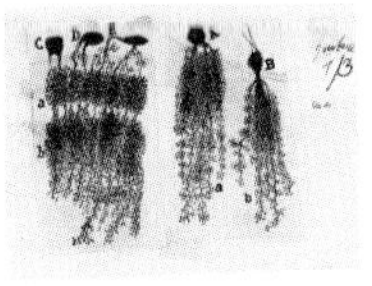

FIGURE 270.

Some neuroglial cells in a bee.

This figure was published in Cajal, S. R., and Sánchez, D. (1915) Contribución al conocimiento de los centros nerviosos de los insectos. *Trab. Lab. Invest. Biol. Univ. Madrid* 13, 1–164 (Figure 76).

FIGURE LEGEND: Some neuroglial cells in a bee. *A, B*, Internal radiated cells of the epioptic; *C, D, E*, posterior cells of the optic lobe.

Original text: Algunas células neuróglicas de la abeja. *A, B*, corpúsculos radiados internos del epióptico; *C, D, E*, corpúsculos posteriores del lóbulo óptico.

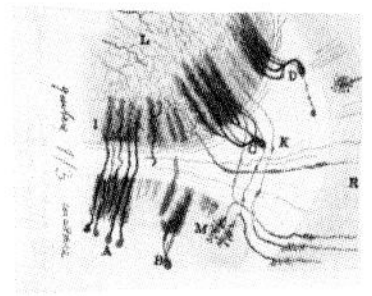

FIGURE 271.

Neuroglial cells from the optic lobe in a blowfly.

This figure was published in Cajal, S. R., and Sánchez, D. (1915) Contribución al conocimiento de los centros nerviosos de los insectos. *Trab. Lab. Invest. Biol. Univ. Madrid* 13, 1–164 (Figure 79).

FIGURE LEGEND: Neuroglial cells from the optic lobe in a blowfly. *A*, Cells destined to the two nuclei of this lobe; *C, D*, dorsal neuroglial elements ramifying exclusively in the ovoid nucleus; *K*, chiasm; *R*, epioptic; *L*, ovoid ganglion; *M*, laminar nucleus.

Original text: Células neuróglicas del lóbulo óptico de la mosca azul. *A*, células destinadas á los dos focos de este lóbulo; *C, D*, elementos neuróglicos dorsales ramificados exclusivamente en el foco ovoideo; *K*, kiasma; *R*, epióptico; *L*, ganglio ovoideo; *M*, foco laminar.

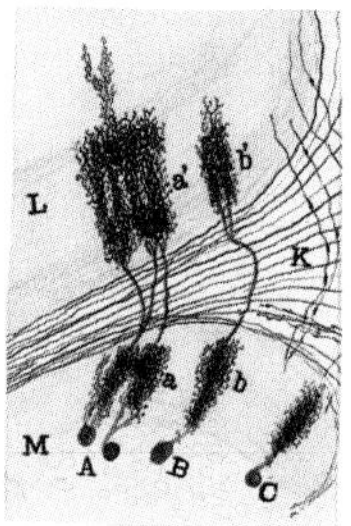

FIGURE 272.

Bitufted neuroglial elements from the optic lobe in a gadfly.

This figure was published in Cajal, S. R., and Sánchez, D. (1915) Contribución al conocimiento de los centros nerviosos de los insectos. *Trab. Lab. Invest. Biol. Univ. Madrid* 13, 1–164 (Figure 80).

FIGURE LEGEND: Some dorsal bitufted neuroglial elements from the optic lobe in a gadfly. *K*, Internal chiasm; *L*, internal lobe.

Original text: Algunos elementos neuróglicos dorsales bipenachados del lóbulo óptico del tábano. *K*, kiasma interno; *L*, lóbulo interno.

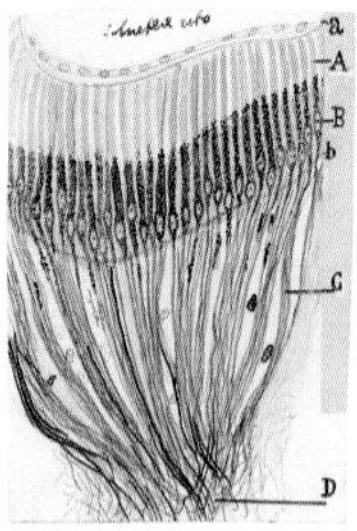

FIGURE 273.

Retina from a lateral ocellus in a bee.

This figure was published in Cajal, S. R. (1918) Observaciones sobre la estructura de los ocelos y vías nerviosas ocelares de algunos insectos. *Trab. Lab. Invest. Biol. Univ. Madrid* 16, 109–139 (Figure 2).

FIGURE LEGEND: Semischematic section from retina of a bee lateral ocellus. Impregnation of the rods with reduced silver nitrate. *a*, Corneogenous layer; *A*, outer segment of small rods; *B*, inner segment with nucleus and pigment; *b*, basal; *C*, fascicles formed by deep prolongations of the small rods; *D*, terminal plexus of the subretina.

Original text: Corte semiesquemático de la retina de un ocelo lateral de la abeja. Impregnación de los bastones por el nitrato de plata reducido. *a*, capa corneógena; *A*, artículo externo de los bastoncitos; *B*, artículo interno donde reside el núcleo y el pigmento; *b*, basal; *C*, paquetes formados por las prolongaciones profundas de los bastoncitos; *D*, plexo terminal subretiniano.

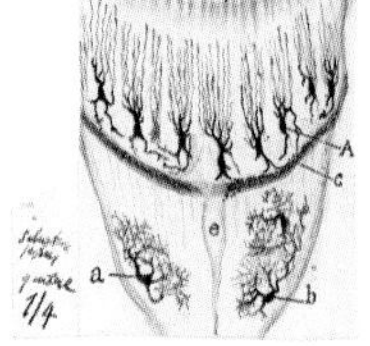

FIGURE 274.

Neuroglia of the retina and retinal region from the middle ocellus in *Libellula*.

This figure was published in Cajal, S. R. (1918) Observaciones sobre la estructura de los ocelos y vías nerviosas ocelares de algunos insectos. *Trab. Lab. Invest. Biol. Univ. Madrid* 16, 109–139 (Figure 5).

FIGURE LEGEND: Neuroglia of the retina and retinal region from the middle ocellus in *Libellula*. *A*, Neuroglial cells from the layer of rods; *a*, *b*, neuroglia of the subretinal region; *c*, choroid; *d*, superficial ends of the rods; *e*, central septum dividing the optic nerve in two halves (Golgi method).

Original text: Neuroglia de la retina y región retiniana del ocelo medio de la libélula. *A*, corpúsculos neuróglicos de la zona de los bastones. *a* y *b*, neuroglia de la región subretiniana; *c*, coroides; *d*, cabos superficiales de los bastones; *e*, tabique medio que divide el nervio óptico en dos mitades (método de Golgi).

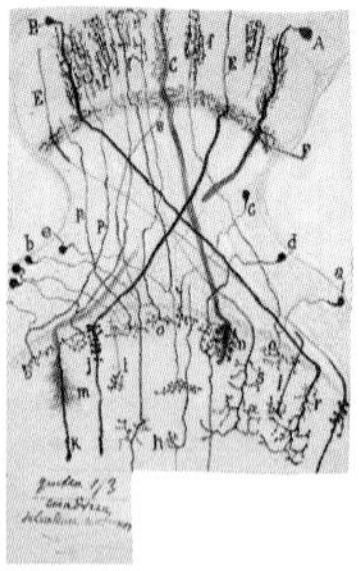

FIGURE 275.

Some elements in a bee retina.

This figure was published in Cajal, S. R., and Sánchez, D. (1915) Contribución al conocimiento de los centros nerviosos de los insectos. *Trab. Lab. Invest. Biol. Univ. Madrid* 13, 1–164 (Figure 85).

FIGURE LEGEND: Some elements in a bee retina. Horizontal section. *A*, *C*, Monopolar collosal cells ending in a serrated, coarse foot (*n*); *B*, monopolar cells ending in a diffuse arborization; *E*, monopolar cells showing descending fibers (*K*, *J*); *a*, *b*, T cells; *e*, T cell showing a descending tuft ending on a deeper plane; *h*, long centrifugal fibers ending in the intermediate retina.

Original text: Algunos elementos de la retina de la abeja. Sección horizontal. *A*, *C*, monopolares colosales terminadas mediante pie dentellado y grosero (*n*); *B*, monopolares acabadas á favor de ramaje difuso; *E*, monopolares continuadas con fibras descendentes (*K*, *J*); *a*, *b*, células en T; *e*, célula en T, cuyo penacho descendente acaba en plano más profundo que los elementos congéneres; *h*, fibras centrífugas largas terminadas en la retina intermediaria.

SECTION K

Supplementary Figures

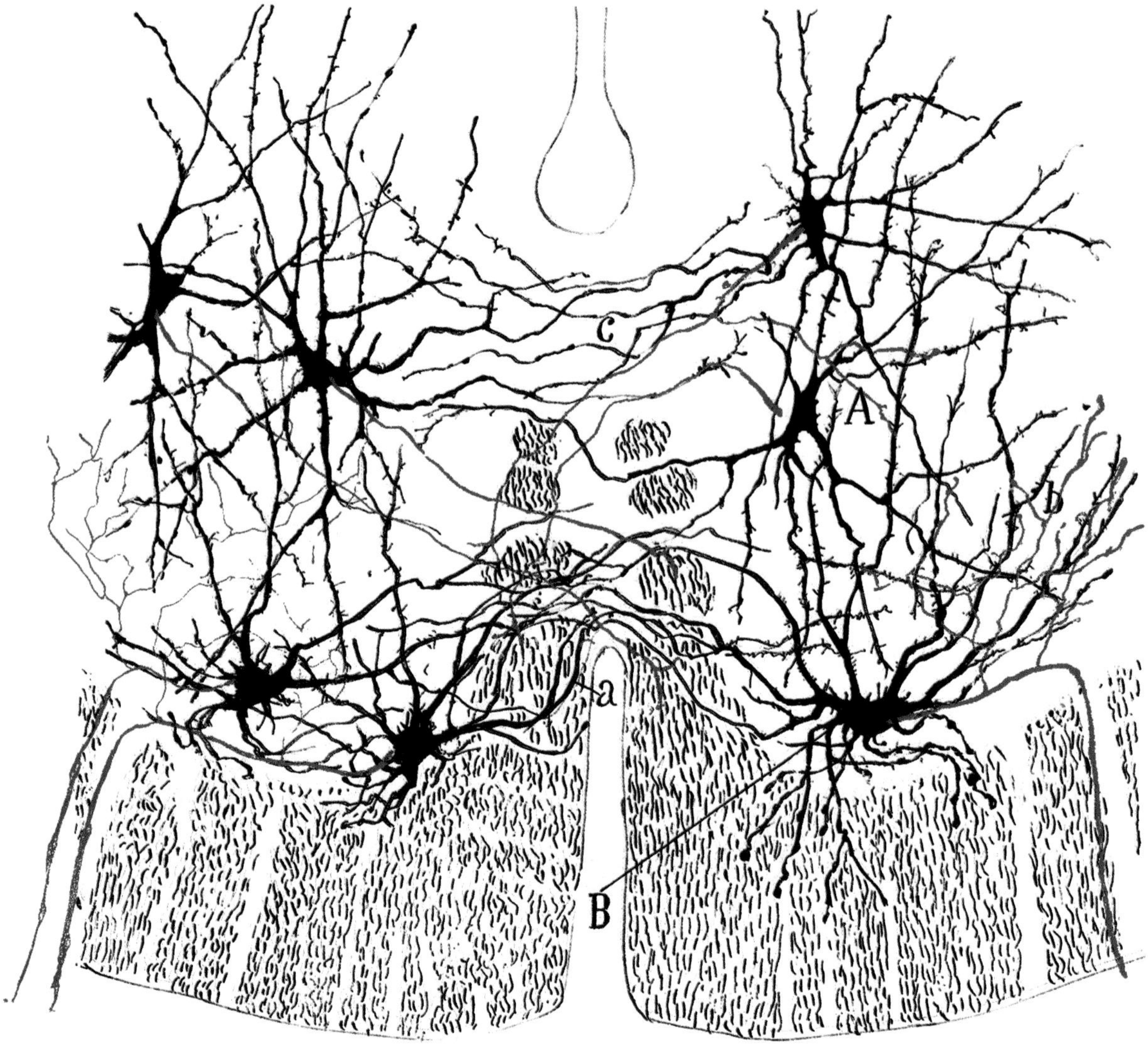

SUPPLEMENTARY FIGURE S1. Radicular and commissural cells of the thoracic spinal cord in a cat fetus. See Figure 10 (Part II, page 156) for the figure legend and further details.

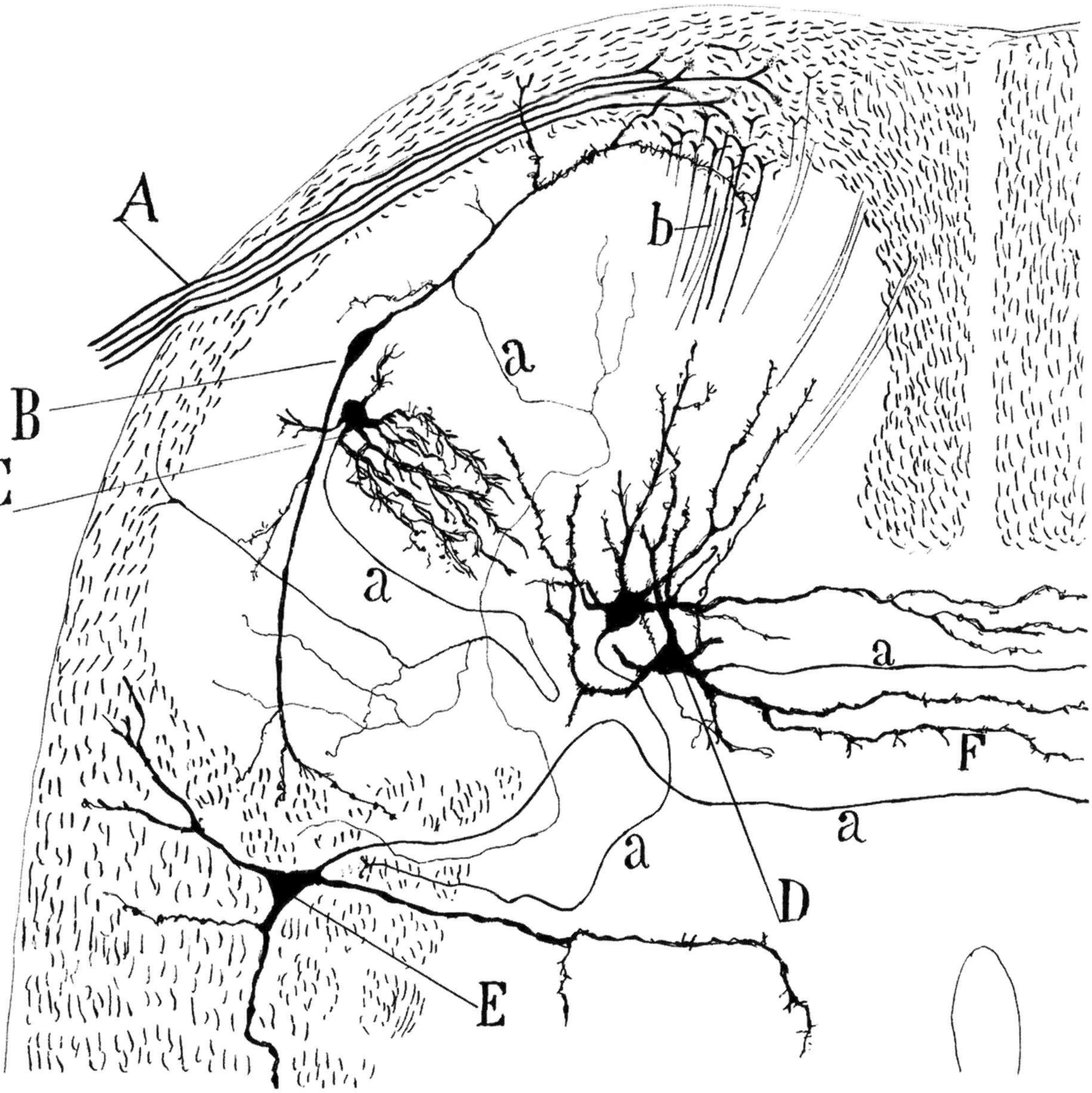

SUPPLEMENTARY FIGURE S2. Cells of the dorsal horn in a chick embryo on day 15 of incubation. See Figure 11 (Part II, page 156) for the figure legend and further details.

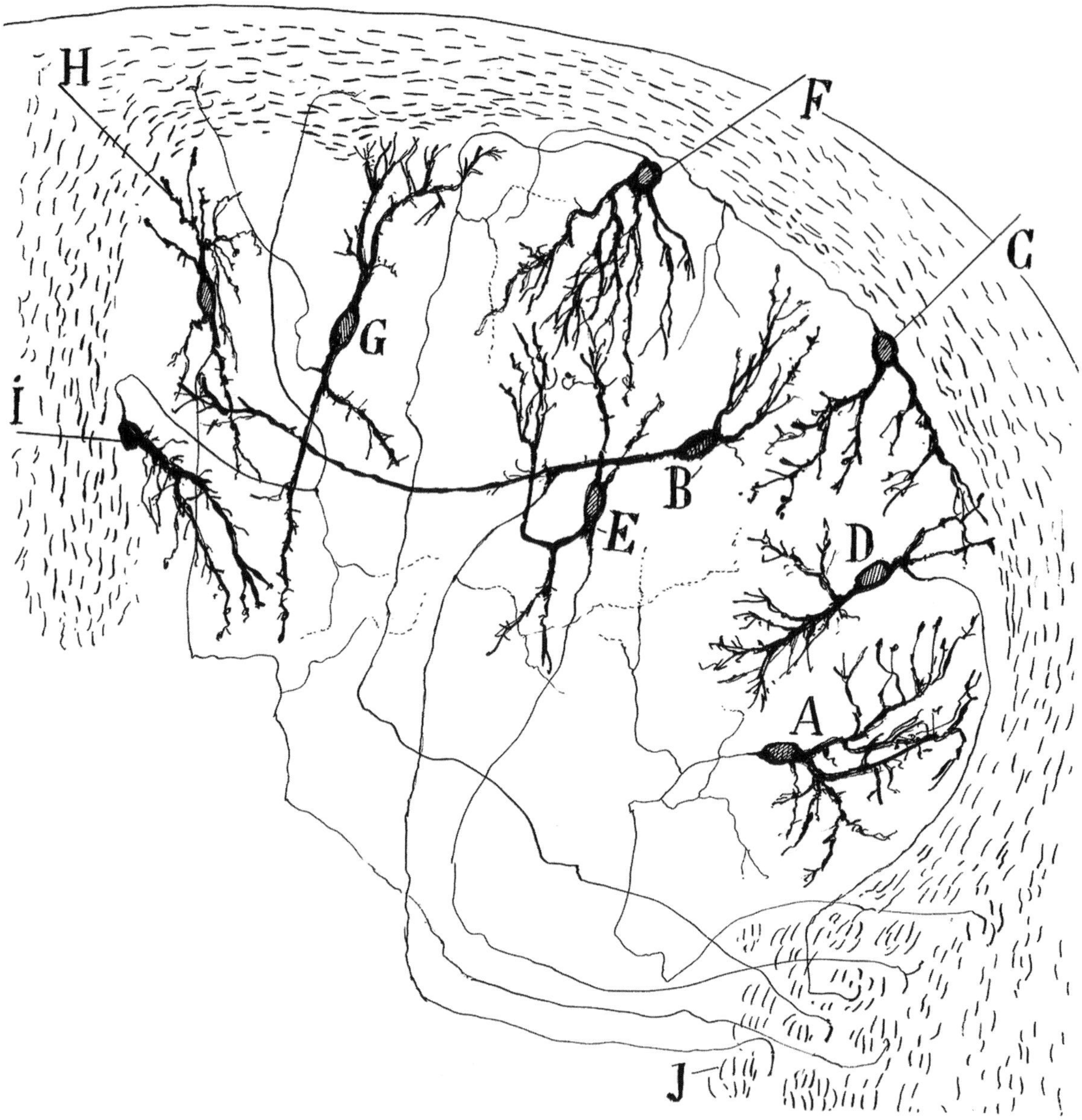

SUPPLEMENTARY FIGURE S3. Cells of the substantia gelatinosa in a chick embryo on day 19 of incubation. See Figure 12 (Part II, page 156) for the figure legend and further details.

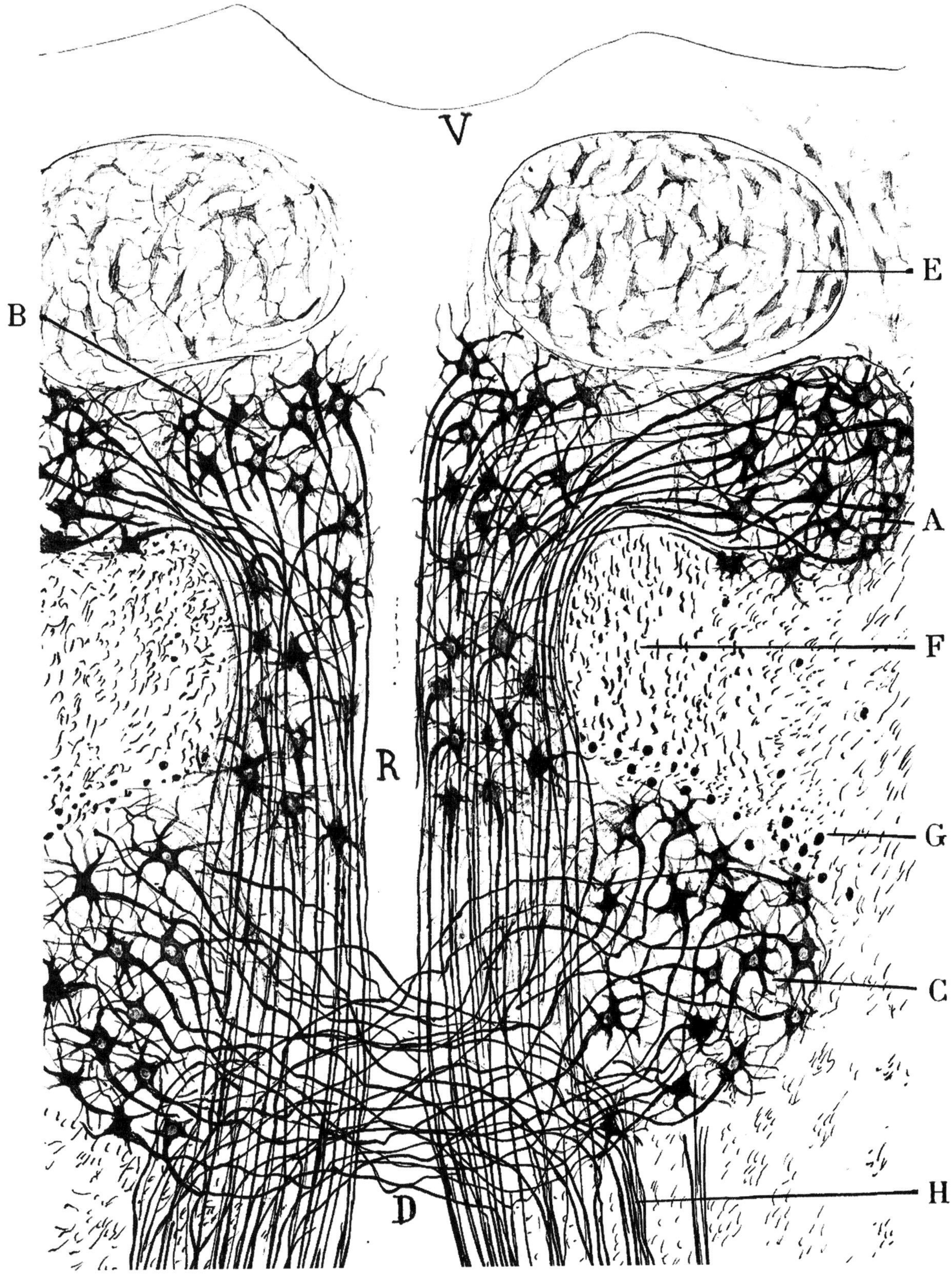

SUPPLEMENTARY FIGURE S4. Section through cell groups forming the oculomotor nucleus in a kite. See Figure 34 (Part II, page 199) for the figure legend and further details.

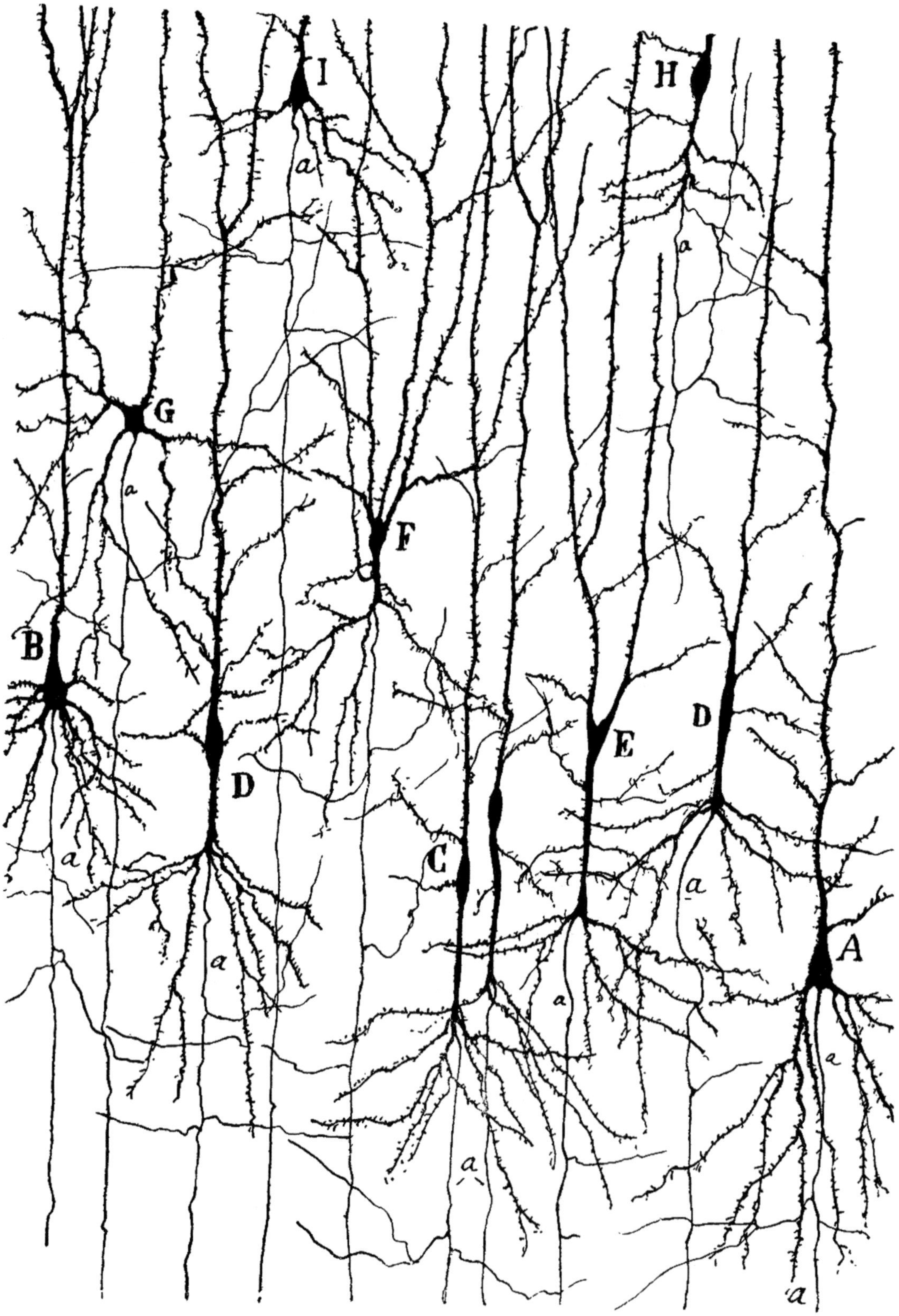

SUPPLEMENTARY FIGURE S5. Vertical section of the cortex of the insula in a child. See Figure 134 (Part II, page 339) for the figure legend and further details.

INDEX